Sports and Exercise Nutrition

Third Edition

Sports and Exercise Nutrition

Third Edition

WILLIAM D. McARDLE

Professor Emeritus
Department of Family, Nutrition, and Exercise Science
Queens College of the City University of New York
Flushing, New York

FRANK I. KATCH

International Research Scholar
Faculty of Public Health, Sport, and Nutrition
Agder University College
Kristiansand, Norway

Instructor and Board Member
Certificate Program in Fitness Instruction
University of California at Los Angeles (UCLA) Extension
Los Angeles, California

Former Professor and Chair of Exercise Science
University of Massachusetts, Amherst
Amherst, Massachusetts

VICTOR L. KATCH

Professor, Department of Movement Science
Division of Kinesiology
Associate Professor, Pediatrics
School of Medicine
University of Michigan
Ann Arbor, Michigan

Wolters Kluwer | Lippincott Williams & Wilkins
Health

Philadelphia · Baltimore · New York · London
Buenos Aires · Hong Kong · Sydney · Tokyo

Acquisitions Editor: Emily Lupash
Managing Editor: Karen Ruppert
Marketing Manager: Christen Murphy
Production Editor: John Larkin
Creative Director: Doug Smock
Compositor: Maryland Composition

Third Edition

Copyright © 1999, 2005, 2009 Lippincott Williams & Wilkins, a Wolters Kluwer business.

351 West Camden Street
Baltimore, MD 21201

530 Walnut Street
Philadelphia, PA 19106

Printed in China

9 8 7 6 5 4 3

Library of Congress Cataloging-in-Publication Data

McArdle, William D.
  Sports and exercise nutrition / William D. McArdle, Frank I. Katch, Victor L. Katch. — 3rd ed.
    p. ; cm.
  Includes bibliographical references and index.
  ISBN 978-0-7817-7037-8 (alk. paper)
  1. Athletes—Nutrition. 2. Physical fitness—Nutritional aspects. 3. Exercise—Physiological aspects. I. Katch, Frank I. II. Katch, Victor L. III. Title.
  [DNLM: 1. Sports. 2. Energy Metabolism—physiology. 3. Exercise—physiology. 4. Nutrition Physiology. QT 260 M478s 2007]
  TX361.A8M38 2007
  613.2'024796—dc22

2007041529

DISCLAIMER

Care has been taken to confirm the accuracy of the information present and to describe generally accepted practices. However, the authors, editors, and publisher are not responsible for errors or omissions or for any consequences from application of the information in this book and make no warranty, expressed or implied, with respect to the currency, completeness, or accuracy of the contents of the publication. Application of this information in a particular situation remains the professional responsibility of the practitioner; the clinical treatments described and recommended may not be considered absolute and universal recommendations.

The authors, editors, and publisher have exerted every effort to ensure that drug selection and dosage set forth in this text are in accordance with the current recommendations and practice at the time of publication. However, in view of ongoing research, changes in government regulations, and the constant flow of information relating to drug therapy and drug reactions, the reader is urged to check the package insert for each drug for any change in indications and dosage and for added warnings and precautions. This is particularly important when the recommended agent is a new or infrequently employed drug.

Some drugs and medical devices presented in this publication have Food and Drug Administration (FDA) clearance for limited use in restricted research settings. It is the responsibility of the health care provider to ascertain the FDA status of each drug or device planned for use in their clinical practice

To purchase additional copies of this book, call our customer service department at **(800) 638-3030** or fax orders to **(301) 223-2320**. International customers should call **(301) 223-2300**.

Visit Lippincott Williams & Wilkins on the Internet: http://www.lww.com. Lippincott Williams & Wilkins customer service representatives are available from 8:30 am to 6:00 pm, EST.

Dedication

To all those who have provided stimulation, instruction, encouragement, and creativity. We also gratefully acknowledge our former professors, mentors, and many undergraduate and graduate students.

Preface

In the first and second editions of *Sports and Exercise Nutrition*, we were hopeful that the emergence of "sports nutrition" courses of study would meld with the established field that incorporates the exercise sciences to create a new field that we originally titled Exercise and Sports Nutrition. We are pleased this has begun to evolve as undergraduate and graduate programs embrace courses that now have a mainstream component that includes the science of human exercise nutrition. At full maturity, exercise nutrition (or some variant of this title) will take its deserved place as a respectable academic field of study. The evolution is far from complete, but exercise physiology and nutrition continue to become more integrated, owing to an ever-expanding knowledge base. Interwoven within this fabric are the clear relationships that emerge from this research, particularly regarding sound nutritional practices, regular, moderate-intensity physical activity, and optimal health for individuals of all ages. Students of exercise science and nutrition science now demand coursework related to the specifics of exercise nutrition, and we hope our text contributes to this goal.

Organization

As with the second edition, we have designed the text for a one-semester course with what we feel provides logical sequencing of material. For example, one cannot reasonably understand carbohydrate's use during exercise without first reviewing the rudiments of human digestion and then the composition and effect of carbohydrate on the body. Similarly, ergogenic aids, fluid replacement, and achieving an "optimal weight" (all critical topics to sports and exercise nutrition) can best be evaluated by understanding basic bioenergetics, nutrient and exercise metabolism, energy balance, and temperature regulation.

Section I integrates information about digestion, absorption, and nutrient assimilation. Section II explains how the body extracts energy from ingested nutrients. We stress nutrition's role in energy metabolism: how nutrients metabolize, and how exercise training affects nutrient metabolism. This section ends with the measurement and quantification of the energy content of foods, and the energy requirements of diverse physical activities. Section III focuses on aspects of nutrition to optimize exercise performance and training responsiveness. We also discuss how to make prudent decisions in the nutrition–fitness marketplace. Section IV describes fundamental mechanisms and adaptations for thermal regulation during heat stress, including strategies for optimizing fluid replacement. Section V consists of two chapters on pharmacologic, chemical, and nutritional ergogenic aids. We integrate the latest findings related to their effectiveness and implications for health and safety. The three chapters in Section VI explain body composition assessment (laboratory and field methods), sport-specific guidelines about body composition and its assessment, energy balance, and weight control (losing and gaining weight), and the increasing prevalence of eating disorders among diverse groups of athletes and other physically active people.

New to the Third Edition

Components of the entire text have been upgraded to reflect current research findings, including updated recommendations about nutrition and physical activity.

Significant Additions and Modifications to the Text Include:

- Inclusion of the latest Dietary Reference Intakes including MyPyramid, radically new and more comprehensive approaches to nutritional recommendations that include a physical activity component in planning and assessing diets for healthy people.
- Presentation of the USDA-designed Healthy Eating Index to monitor changes in diet quality over time. This 100-point analytic tool evaluates how well a person's diet conforms to such recommendations as MyPyramid and *Dietary Guidelines for Americans* based on dietary balance, moderation, and variety.
- Updated discussion of potential ergogenic effects of different nutritional supplements.
- Expanded information on characteristic features and warning signs of anorexia nervosa and bulimia nervosa to help coaches and trainers identify athletes with eating disorders.
- Inclusion of current standards for overweight and obesity in the United States and worldwide.
- Latest information about the health risks and trends about overweight and obesity and their economic impact on individuals, societies, and countries.
- Discussion of functional muscular strength exercise and training related to bone density and bone health.
- New information regarding exercise and GI disorders, including information about exercise and digestion, and the effects of exercise on digestive processes and functions.
- Updated information about direct and indirect (performance) tests of human energy-generating capacities.

- Latest information on the topics related to nutrient timing to optimize the training response.
- New section on food's meaning from a social and physiologic perspective, and on the various factors that affect food choices.
- Current information about fast foods and food labeling and dietary supplement labeling.
- Discussion of the growing trend toward organic farming and how it relates to nutritional quality.
- A new section on comparisons of what people eat who live in different world regions.
- Updated information about the nutrient composition of different beverages.
- Internet links within the text to relevant governmental and non-governmental web sites.
- Updated information about the nutritional composition of foods from the most popular fast food restaurants.

Pedagogic Features

Each chapter contains numerous pedagogic features to engage the student and promote comprehension.

TEST YOUR KNOWLEDGE. Each chapter begins with 10 True–False statements about relevant chapter material. Tackling these questions before reading the chapter allows students to assess changes in their comprehension after completing the chapter. This approach also provides students the opportunity to evaluate the completeness of their answers with the answer key and the rationale for each answer provided at the end of the chapter.

CASE STUDY/PERSONAL HEALTH AND EXERCISE NUTRITION. Each chapter also contains at least one case study or topic related to personal health and exercise nutrition. This unique aspect more actively engages the student in specific areas of nutritional assessment and health appraisal, application of dietary guidelines, weight control, body composition assessment, overuse syndrome, and physical activity recommendations.

EQUATIONS AND DATA. Important equations, data, and reference to websites are highlighted throughout the text for easy reference.

KEY TERMS. Key terms are bolded within the chapter.

REFERENCES. A current reference list is included at the end of every chapter.

WEB SITES. Where applicable, we have included relevant web sites related to nutrition, exercise, and health.

Art Program

The full-color art program continues to be a stellar feature of the textbook. More than 250 figures are included to illustrate important concepts in the text. Fifty new figures have been added, redrawn, or enhanced to complement the new and updated content.

Student Resources

To enhance the student learning experience outside of the classroom, a companion web site is available with purchase of the third edition of *Sports and Exercise Nutrition*, and includes the appendices from the text and a student quiz. Refer to the inside cover of this book for information on how to access the site.

Instructor Resources

We understand the demand on instructor's time, so to help make your job easier, you will have access to Instructor Resources available on a companion web site upon adoption of the third edition of *Sports and Exercise Nutrition*. These resources include a test generator from Brownstone; PowerPoint slides for every chapter; an image bank that contains figures from the textbook; and a WebCT/Blackboard-ready cartridge. Refer to the inside cover of this book for information on how to access the site.

The student quizzes, test generator questions, and PowerPoint presentations were revised and updated by Melissa Langone.

How to Use this Book

T his User's Guide explains all of the key features found in the third edition of *Sports and Exercise Nutrition.* Become familiar with them so you can get the most out of each chapter and gain a strong foundation in the science of exercise nutrition and bioenergetics and gain insight to how the principles work in the real world of human physical activity and sports medicine.

Introductory Section

Outlines the historical precedent for exercise nutrition, helping you strengthen and ground your knowledge of the field.

Vivid Full-Color Illustrations and Photographs

Enhance learning of important topics and add visual impact.

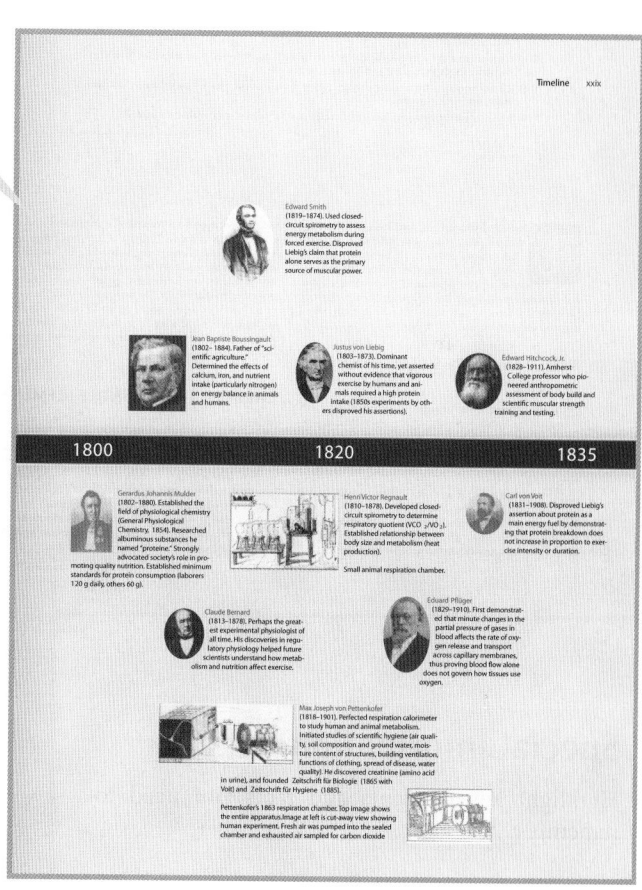

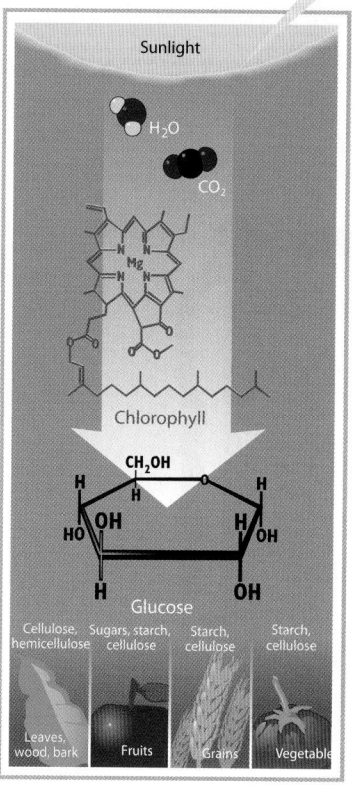

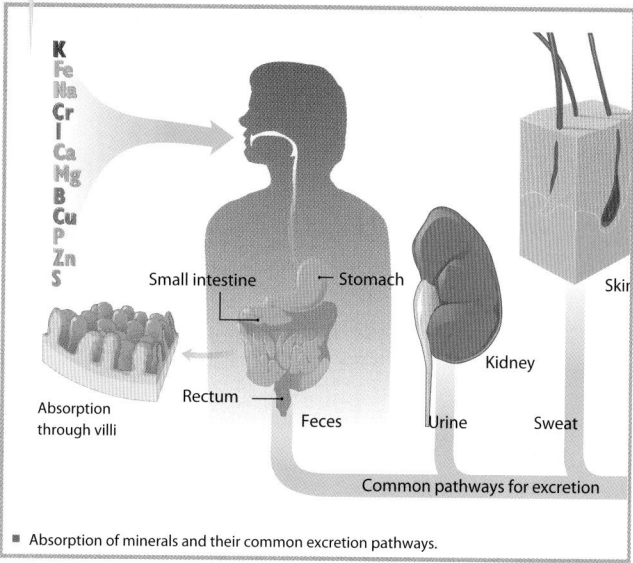

■ Absorption of minerals and their common excretion pathways.

Test Your Knowledge

Answer these 10 statements about carbohydrates, lipids, and proteins. Use the scoring key at the end of the chapter to check your results. Repeat this test after you have read the chapter and compare your results.

1. **T F** Carbohydrates consist of atoms of carbon, oxygen, nitrogen, and hydrogen.
2. **T F** Glucose can be synthesized from amino acids in the body.
3. **T F** Dietary fiber's main function is to provide energy for biologic work.
4. **T F** Carbohydrate intake for most physically active individuals should make up about 45% of the total caloric intake.
5. **T F** Individuals who consume simple carbohydrates run little risk of gaining weight.
6. **T F** A given quantity of sugar, lipid, and protein contains about the same amount of energy.
7. **T F** Although cholesterol is found predominantly in the animal kingdom, certain plant forms also contain cholesterol.
8. **T F** Vegans are at greater risk for nutrient and energy malnutrition than are individuals who consume foods from plant and animal sources.
9. **T F** Consuming an extra amount of high-quality protein above recommended levels facilitates increases in muscle mass.
10. **T F** The protein requirement (per kg of body mass) for men is greater than for women.

The carbohydrate, lipid, and protein nutrients ultimately provide energy to maintain body functions during rest and all forms of physical activity. In addition to their role as biologic fuels, these large nutrients called **macronutrients** also maintain the organism's structural and functional integrity. This chapter focuses on each macronutrient's structure, function, and source in the diet.

ATOMS: NATURE'S BUILDING BLOCKS

Of the 103 different atoms or elements identified in nature, the mass of the human organism contains about 3% nitrogen, 10% hydrogen, 18% carbon, and 65% oxygen. These atoms play the major role in chemical composition of nutrients and make up structural units for the body's biologically active substances.

The union of two or more atoms forms a molecule whose particular properties depend on its specific atoms and their arrangement. Glucose is glucose because of the arrangement of three different kinds of 24 atoms within its molecule. Chemical bonding involves a common sharing of electrons between atoms, as occurs when hydrogen and oxygen atoms join to form a water molecule. The force of attraction between positive and negative charges serves as bonding, or "chemical cement," to keep the atoms within a molecule together. A larger aggregate of matter (a substance) forms when two or more molecules bind chemically. The substance can take the form of a gas, liquid, or solid, depending on forces of interaction among molecules. Altering forces by removing, transferring, or exchanging electrons releases energy, some of which powers cellular functions.

CARBON: THE VERSATILE ELEMENT

All nutrients contain carbon except water and minerals. Almost all substances within the body consist of carbon-containing (**organic**) compounds. Carbon atoms share chemical bonds with other carbon atoms and with atoms of other elements to form large carbon-chain molecules. Specific linkages of carbon, hydrogen, and oxygen atoms form lipids and carbohydrates, while addition of nitrogen and certain minerals creates a protein molecule. Carbon atoms linked with hydrogen, oxygen, and nitrogen also serve as atomic building blocks for the body's exquisitely formed structures.

Test Your Knowledge Boxes

Offer True-False statements at the beginning of each chapter to quiz and challenge your current knowledge, allowing you to assess your comprehension after completing the chapter.

Special Information Boxes

Highlight key concepts and facts you need to remember.

Caffeinism

Refers to caffeine intoxication characterized by restlessness, tremulousness, nervousness, excitement, insomnia, flushed face, dieresis, gastrointestinal complaints, rambling flow of thought and speech, tachycardia or cardiac arrhythmia, periods of inexhaustibility, and/or psychomotor agitation.

FIGURE 11.8 shows that subjects exercised for 90.2 minutes with 330 mg of pre-exercise caffeine compared with 75.5 minutes without it. Despite similar heart rate and oxygen uptake values during the two trials, the caffeine made the work "feel easier." Consuming caffeine 60 minutes before exercise in-

creased exercise fat catabolism and reduced carbohydrate oxidation as assessed by plasma glycerol and free fatty acids levels and the respiratory quotient. The ergogenic effect of caffeine on endurance performance also applies to similar exercise performed at high ambient temperatures.[48]

Caffeine provides an ergogenic benefit during maximal swimming for durations less than 25 minutes. In a double-blind, crossover research design, competent male and female distance swimmers (<25 min for 1500-m swims) consumed caffeine (6 mg · kg body mass^{-1}) 2.5 hours before swimming 1500 m. FIGURE 11.9 illustrates that split times improved with caffeine for each 500-m of the swim. Total swim time averaged 1.9% faster with caffeine than without it (20:58.6 vs 21:21.8). Enhanced performance associated with lower plasma potassium concentration before exercise and higher blood glucose levels at the end of the trial. These responses

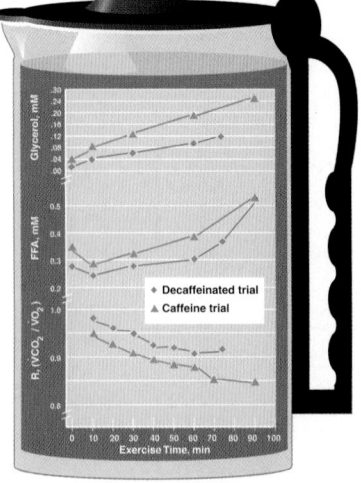

FIGURE 11.8 ■ Average values for plasma glycerol, free fatty acids *(FFA)*, and the respiratory exchange ratio *(R)* during endurance exercise trials after ingesting caffeine and decaffeinated liquids. (From Costill DL, et al. Effects of caffeine ingestion on metabolism and exercise performance. *Med Sci Sports* 1978;10:155.)

Case Studies and Personal Health and Exercise Nutrition Activities

Engage readers in specific areas of nutritional assessment and health appraisal, application of dietary guidelines, weight control, body composition, overuse syndrome, and physical activity recommendations.

Case Study

Personal Health And Exercise Nutrition 1–2

Adult Hyperlipidemia

The following data were obtained on a 58-year-old executive who has not had an annual physical examination in 5 years. He has gained weight and is now concerned about his health status.

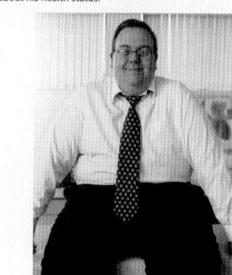

Medical History

No history of chronic diseases or major hospitalization. He does not take medications or dietary supplements and has no known food allergies.

Family History

Father died from a heart attack at age 61; his younger brother has had triple bypass surgery, and his uncle has type 2 diabetes. His mother, physically inactive for most of her adult life, classifies as obese with high serum cholesterol and triacylglycerol levels.

Social History

Overweight since high school. He has gained 15 lb during the last year, which he attributes to his job and changes in eating habits (eats out more frequently). J.M. wants to improve his diet but does not know what to do. He typically eats only two meals daily, with at least one meal consumed at a restaurant and several snacks interspersed. He drinks three to five cups of coffee throughout the day and two to three alcoholic drinks every evening. He also smokes one pack of cigarettes daily and reports high stress in his job and at home (two teenage children). Patient states he has little opportunity for exercise or leisure time activities given his present schedule.

Physical Examination/Anthropometric/Laboratory Data

- Blood pressure: 135/90 mm Hg
- Height: 6 feet (182.9 cm)
- Body weight: 215 lb (97.1 kg)
- BMI: 29.0
- Abdominal girth: 40.9 inches (104 cm)
- Laboratory data
  - Nonfasting total cholesterol: 267 mg $\cdot dL^{-1}$
  - HDL-C: 34 mg $\cdot dL^{-1}$
  - LDL-C: 141 mg $\cdot dL^{-1}$
  - Blood glucose: 124 mg $\cdot dL^{-1}$
- Dietary intake from 24-hour food recall
  - Calories: 3001 kCal
  - Protein: 110 g (14.7% of total kCal)
  - Lipid: 121 g (36.3% of total kCal)
  - Carbohydrate: 368 g (49% of total kCal)
  - Saturated fatty acids: 18% of total kCal
  - Monounsaturated fatty acids (MUFA): 7% of total kCal
  - Cholesterol: 390 mg $\cdot dL^{-1}$
  - Fiber: 10 g
  - Folic acid: 200 μg
- General impressions: overly fat male with possible metabolic syndrome

Case Questions

1. Provide an overall assessment of patient's health status.
2. What other laboratory tests could be performed?
3. Interpret the blood lipid profile based on his history, physical examination, and laboratory data.
4. Give recommendations for improving the adequacy of patient's diet.
5. Create the best dietary approach for the patient.
6. What course of action should the patient consider to improve his blood lipid profile?

Answers

1. Based on available data it appears that the patient is hypercholesterolemic (elevated cholesterol, low HDL-C, elevated LDL-C) and perhaps prediabetic (elevated blood glucose) with a high risk for coronary

---

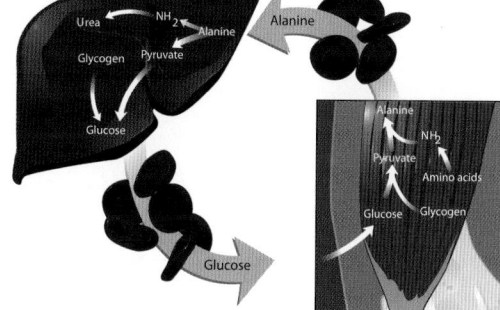

FIGURE 1.19 ■ The alanine–glucose cycle. Alanine, synthesized in muscle from glucose-derived pyruvate via transamination, is released into the blood and converts to glucose and urea in the liver. Glucose release into the blood coincides with its subsequent delivery to the muscle for energy. During exercise, increased production and output of alanine from muscle helps to maintain blood glucose for nervous system and active muscle needs. Exercise training augments processes of hepatic gluconeogenesis. (From Felig P, Wahren J. Amino acid metabolism in exercising man. J Clin Invest 1971;50:2703.)

Summary

1. Proteins differ chemically from lipids and carbohydrates because they contain nitrogen in addition to sulfur, phosphorus, and iron.
2. Proteins form from subunits called amino acids. The body requires 20 different amino acids, each containing an amino radical (NH_2) and an organic acid radical called a carboxyl group (COOH). Amino acids contain a side-chain that defines the amino acid's particular chemical characteristics.
3. An almost infinite number of possible protein structures can form because of the diverse combinations possible for the 20 different amino acids.
4. The body cannot synthesize 8 of the 20 amino acids. These are the essential amino acids that must be consumed in the diet.
5. Animal and plant cells contain protein. Proteins with all the essential amino acids are called complete (higher quality) proteins; the others are called incomplete (lower quality) proteins. Examples of higher quality, complete proteins include animal proteins in eggs, milk, cheese, meat, fish, and poultry.
6. The diets of many physically active persons and competitive athletes consist predominantly of nutrients from plant sources. Consuming a variety of plant foods provides all of the essential amino acids because each food source contains a different quality and quantity of them.
7. Proteins provide the building blocks for synthesizing cellular material during anabolic processes. Amino acids also contribute their "carbon skeletons" for energy metabolism.
8. The RDA, the recommended quantity for nutrient intake, represents a liberal yet safe level of excess to meet the nutritional needs of practically all healthy persons. For adults, the protein RDA equals 0.83 g per kg of body mass.

Section Summaries

Help readers reinforce and review key concepts and material.

Listings of Relevant Web Sites

Direct you to reliable online exercise nutrition resources.

Not Without Risk

The indiscriminate use of alleged ergogenic substances increases the likelihood of adverse side effects ranging from relatively benign physical discomfort to life-threatening episodes.[8] Many of these compounds fail to conform to labeling requirements to correctly identify the strength of the product's ingredients.[96,128] Results from a study at the Institute of Biochemistry at the German Sports University of Cologne (www.dopinginfo.de) and supported by the Medical Commission of the International Olympic Committee (IOC) indicate that up to 20% of the nutritional supplements sam-

General References

Boyle M. Personal Nutrition. 4th ed. Belmont, CA: Wadsworth Publishing, 2001.

Brody T. Nutritional Biochemistry. 2nd ed. New York: Academic Press, 1999.

Brown J. Nutrition Now. 5th ed. Belmont, CA: Wadsworth Publishing, 2007.

Campbell MK, Farrell SO. Biochemistry. 5th ed. Philadelphia: WB Saunders, 2005.

Emken EA. Metabolism of dietary stearic acid relative to other fatty acids in human subjects. *Am J Clin Nutr* 1994;60(suppl):1023S.

Fox SI. Human Physiology. 10th ed. New York: McGraw-Hill, 2007.

Groff JL, Gropper SS. Advanced Nutrition and Human Metabolism. 4th ed. Belmont, CA: Thomson Learning, 2004.

Guyton AC, et al. Textbook of Medical Physiology. 11th ed. Philadelphia: WB Saunders, 2005.

Kraut J. How do enzymes work? Science 1988;242:533.

Mahan LK, Escott-Stump S. Krause's Food, Nutrition, & Diet Therapy. Philadelphia: WB Saunders, 2004.

Marieb EN. Essentials of Human Anatomy and Physiology. 8th ed. Menlo Park, CA: Pearson Education: Benjamin Cummings, 2005.

References

At the end of each chapter list additional classic and up-to-date resources.

Additional Learning and Teaching Resources

This textbook features a companion web site: http://thepoint.lww.com/McArdleNutrition3e, which includes components listed below.

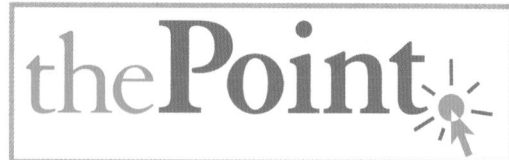

Student Resource Center

- Appendices from the book
- Student Quiz Bank

Instructor's Resource Center

- Test generator
- Image collection
- PowerPoint presentations

Acknowledgments

We gratefully acknowledge the following individuals at Lippincott Williams & Wilkins for their dedication and expertise with this project: Emily Lupash, Executive Editor, and John Larkin, Production Editor, for helpful editing and quality suggestions; to Christen D. Murphy, Marketing Manager, for creatively promoting our text and interpreting its unique aspects to the appropriate markets; and a very special thanks to Karen Ruppert and Laura Horowitz, Managing Editors, for tolerating our unique idiosyncrasies, for gently keeping us focused and "on track," and for making what often becomes a difficult task a relatively enjoyable experience. We are also grateful to the numerous undergraduate and graduate students at our respective universities for keeping our "motors" going during our work on various projects related to this text.

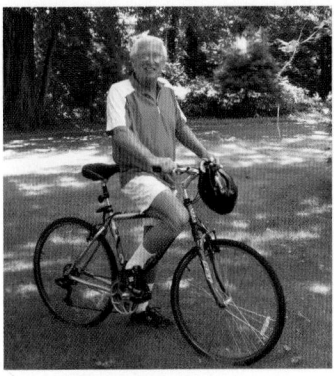

WILLIAM McARDLE
Sound Beach, NY

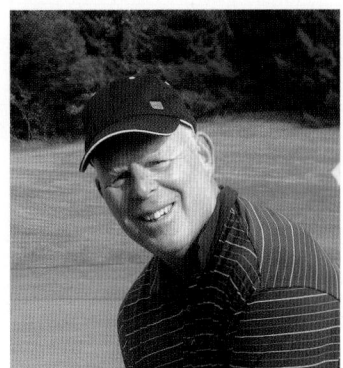

FRANK KATCH
Santa Barbara, CA

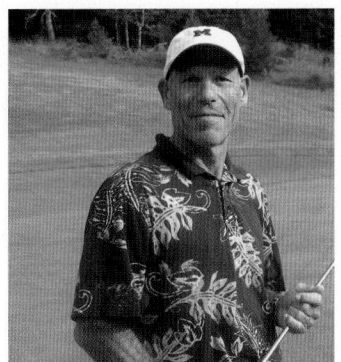

VICTOR KATCH
Ann Arbor, MI

Contents

Introduction

Food provides the source of essential elements and building blocks for preserving lean body mass, synthesizing new tissue, optimizing skeletal structure, repairing existing cells, maximizing oxygen transport and use, maintaining optimal fluid and electrolyte balance, and regulating all metabolic processes. "Good nutrition" encompasses more than preventing nutrient deficiencies related to disease, including overt endemic diseases ranging from beriberi (vitamin deficiency disease from inadequate thiamine [vitamin B_1]; damages heart and nervous system) to xerophthalmia (caused by vitamin A deficiency and general malnutrition leading to night blindness, corneal ulceration, and blindness). It also encompasses the recognition of individual differences in need for and tolerance of specific nutrients and the role of genetic heritage on such factors. Borderline nutrient deficiencies (i.e., less than required to cause clinical manifestations of disease) negatively impact bodily structure and function and thus the capacity for exercise.

Proper nutrition also forms the foundation for physical performance; it provides the fuel for biologic work and the chemicals for extracting and using food's potential energy. Not surprisingly then, from the time of the ancient Olympics to the present, almost every conceivable dietary practice has been used to enhance exercise performance. Writings from the first Olympic games in 776 BC to today's computerized era provide a glimpse at what athletes consume. Poets, philosophers, writers, and the physicians of ancient Greece and Rome tell of diverse strategies athletes undertook to prepare for competitions. They consumed various animal meats (oxen, goat, bull, deer), moist cheeses and wheat, dried figs, and special "concoctions" and liquors. For the next two thousand years, however, little reliable information existed about the food preferences of top athletes (except for rowers and pedestrian walkers during the nineteenth century). The 1936 Berlin Olympics offered a preliminary assessment of the food consumed by world-class athletes. From the paper by Schenk,[1]

> . . . the Olympic athletes competing at Berlin frequently focused upon meat, that athletes regularly dined on two steaks per meal, sometimes poultry, and averaged nearly half a kilogram of meat daily . . . pre-event meals regularly consisted of one to three steaks and eggs, supplemented with "meat-juice" extract. . . . Other athletes stressed the importance of carbohydrate. . . . Olympic athletes from England, Finland and Holland regularly consumed porridge, the Americans ate shredded wheat or corn flakes in milk, and the Chileans and Italians feasted on pasta . . . members of the Japanese team consumed a pound of rice daily.

During the 2004 Olympic Games in Athens, about 12,000 athletes from 197 countries consumed an inordinate amount of food. During this Olympiad, some countries applied specific dietary regimens, while athletes from less industrialized countries had free choice of what they ate, often combining ritual with novelty foods. The majority of athletes probably consumed dietary supplements including vitamins and minerals; a smaller percentage most likely ingested stimulants, narcotics, anabolic agents, diuretics, peptides, glycoprotein hormones and analogs, alcohol, marijuana, local anesthetics, corticosteroids, beta blockers, beta-2 agonists, and used blood doping, all prohibited by the International Olympic Committee. In the war against illegal drug use, the Beijing 2008 Olympic Games will perform about 4500 drug tests. This is a major increase compared to 2800 tests at the 2000 Sydney Games and 3700 tests at the 2004 Athens Games.

Feeding Olympic Athletes

At the Olympic Village, meals were prepared for approximately 22,000 customers on a 24-hour basis. Approximately 50,000 meals were served daily from 1500 international recipes requiring about 100 tons of food and creating 55 tons of waste! The following supplies were used to prepare 6000 meals each hour in the Village: 15,000 liters of milk, 2500 dozen eggs, 300 tons of fruits and vegetables, 120 tons of meats, 85 tons of seafood, 25,000 loafs of bread, 2 million liters of potable water, and 3 million refreshments.

Even today's technologically savvy world is inundated with trendy theories, misinformation, and outright quackery about links between nutrition and physical performance. Accomplishments during the last 100 years of Olympic competition have undeniably improved (FIG. I.1), but no one has yet established universal ties between food and these remarkable physical achievements. Athletes have every reason to desire any substance that might confer a competitive advantage because winning ensures glory and multimillion dollar endorsement contracts. Their eagerness to shave milliseconds from a run or add centimeters to a jump convinces them to experiment with nutrition and polypharmacy supplementation, including illegal drugs.

The search for the Holy Grail to enhance physical performance has not been limited to the last few decades. Athletes and trainers in ancient civilization also sought to improve athletic prowess. Although lacking objective proof, they routinely experimented with nutritional substances and rituals, trusting that the natural and supernatural would provide an advantage. Over the past 25 centuries, the scientific method has gradually replaced dogma and ritual as the most effective approach to healthful living and optimal physical

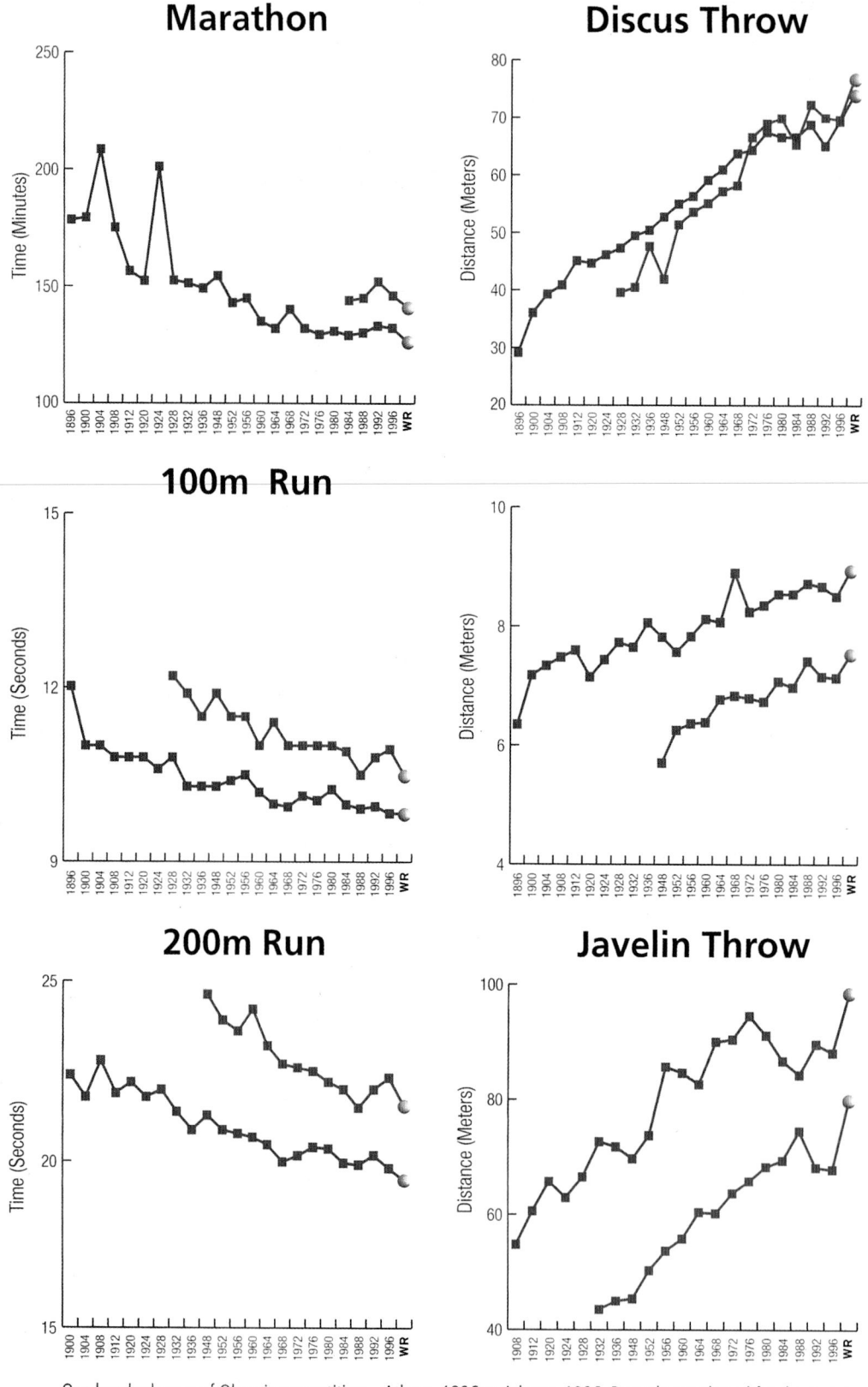

One hundred years of Olympic competition—Athens, 1896 to Atlanta, 1996. Records are plotted for the men in **blue** and women in **red**. The last point of each graph marks the world record (WR).

(World records as of November 9, 1997)

FIGURE I.1 ■ One hundred years of Olympic competition—Athens, 1896 to Atlanta, 1996—in selected events for men in blue and women in red.

Nutritional Enhancement • Optimal nutrition vs. optimal nutrition for exercise • Environmental stressors • Military • Spaceflight dynamics	**Health and Longevity** • Eating patterns • Exercise patterns • Nutrition–physical activity interactions • Reproduction • Mortality and morbidity • Epidemiology
Energy Balance and Body Composition • Metabolism • Exercise dynamics • Assessment • Weight control/overfatness • Body size, shape, and proportion	**Peak Physiologic Function** • Protein, carbohydrate, and lipid requirement • Oxidative stress • Fatigue and staleness • Tissue repair and growth • Micronutrient needs • Gender related effects
Optimal Growth • Normal and abnormal • Bone, muscle, other tissues • Life span • Effects on cognitive behaviors • Effects of chronic exercise • Sport-specific interactions	**Safety** • Disordered eating • Ergogenic/ergolytic substances • Thermal stress and fluid replacement • Nutrient abuse

FIGURE I.2 ■ Six core areas for research and study in the field of Exercise Nutrition.

performance. The emerging field of exercise nutrition uses the ideas of pioneers in medicine, anatomy, physics, chemistry, hygiene, nutrition, and physical culture to establish a robust body of knowledge.

A sound understanding of exercise nutrition enables one to appreciate the importance of adequate nutrition, and to critically evaluate the validity of claims concerning nutrient supplements and special dietary modifications to enhance physique, physical performance, and exercise training responses. Knowledge of the nutrition–metabolism interaction forms the basis for the preparation, performance, and recuperation phases of intense exercise and/or training. Not surprisingly, many physically active individuals, including some of the world's best athletes, obtain nutritional information in the locker room, and from magazine and newspaper articles, advertisements, video "infomercials," training partners, health-food shops, and testimonials from successful athletes, rather than from well-informed and well-educated coaches, trainers, physicians, and physical fitness and exercise nutrition professionals. Far too many devote considerable time and energy striving for optimum performance and

training, only to fall short from inadequate, counterproductive, and sometimes harmful nutritional practices.

We hope the third edition of *Sports and Exercise Nutrition* continues to provide "cutting edge" scientific information for all people involved in regular physical activity and exercise training, not just the competitive athlete.

Exercise Nutrition for the Future: A Fresh Look

And if we are ignorant of our past, if we are indifferent to our story and those people who did so much for us, we're not just being stupid, we're being rude. (From 146th Beloit College Commencement. May 12, 1996. Pulitzer Prize-winner David McCollough)

The accompanying timeline presents an historical overview of selected individuals, from the Renaissance to the 21st century, whose work and scientific experiments demonstrated the intimate interconnections among medicine, physiology, exercise, and nutrition. Their important accomplishments provide a powerful rationale for developing an integrated subject field of study that we call exercise nutrition.

Some consider an exercise nutrition curriculum (at a college or university) as a subset of nutrition, but we believe this designation requires updating. First we recommend a change in name from "sports nutrition" to "exercise nutrition." The term exercise encompasses more than the word sports, and more fully reflects the many active men and women who are not necessarily "sportspeople." An academic program would have as its core academic content applicable to the ever-increasing number of physically active individuals. Such a curriculum would neither be housed in a Department of Nutrition nor a Department of Exercise Science or Kinesiology. Rather, the curriculum deserves a unique identity. FIGURE I.2 presents six core areas for research and study that constitute exercise nutrition, with specific topics listed within each area.

The focus of exercise nutrition becomes cross-disciplinary. It synthesizes knowledge from the separate but related fields of nutrition and kinesiology. A number of existing fields take a cross-disciplinary approach. Biochemists do not receive in-depth training as chemists or biologists. Instead, their training as biochemists makes them more competent biochemists than more narrowly focused chemists or biologists. The same inclusivity characterizes a biophysicist, a radio astronomer, a molecular biologist, and a geophysicist.

Historical precedents exist for linking two fields: those involving nutrition and those involving exercise. The chemist Lavoisier, for example, employed exercise to study respiration, probably not thinking that his discoveries would impact fields other than chemistry. A.V. Hill, a competent mathematician and physiologist, won a Nobel Prize in Physiology or Medicine, not for his studies of mathematics or physiology per se, but for his integrative work with muscle that helped to unravel secrets about the biochemistry of muscular contraction.

In the cross-discipline of exercise nutrition, students specialize neither in exercise nor nutrition. Instead, they are trained in aspects of *both* fields. Our concept of an academic discipline agrees with Professor Franklin Henry's ideas promoted in the late 1960s.[2] It is an organized body of information collectively embraced in a formal course of instruction worthy of pursuit on its own merits.

Exercise nutrition synthesizes data from physiology, chemistry, exercise physiology, biochemistry, medicine, and nutrition. Students of exercise nutrition may not be full-fledged chemists, exercise physiologists, or nutritionists; however, their cross-disciplinary training gives them a broader and more appropriate perspective to advance their discipline. The renal physiologist studies the kidney as an isolated organ to determine its functions, often utilizing exercise as the stressor. The exercise scientist measures the effects of exercise on kidney function. Here the researcher emphasizes exercise physiology more than renal physiology. By contrast, the exercise nutritionist might investigate how combining diet and exercise impact kidney function in general and in specific circumstances like physical activity under heat stress.

We urge the establishment of a separate discipline to unite previously disparate fields. We hope others share our vision.

REFERENCES

1. Grivetti LE, Applegate EA. From Olympia to Atlanta: a cultural-historical perspective on diet and athletic training. *J Nutr* 1997;127:860S–868S.
2. Henry FM. Physical education: An academic discipline. Proceedings of the 67th Annual Meeting of the National College Physical Education Association for Men, AAHPERD, Washington DC, 1964.

TIMELINE: Exercise Nutrition Through the Ages

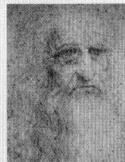

Leonardo da Vinci
(1452–1519). Master anatomist produced exquisite drawings of the heart and circulation which showed that air reached pulmonary arteries via bronchi, not directly through the heart as taught by Galenic medicine.

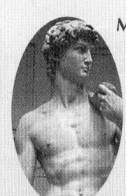

Michelangelo Buonarroti
(1475–1564). Realistic sculpture of "David" combined scientific anatomy with ideal body proportions.

"David"

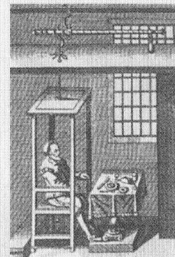

Santorio (1561–1636). Accurately recorded changes in body weight over a 30-year period to understand metabolism. Published *De Medicina Statica Aphorismi* (Medical Aphorisms), 1614.

Santorio's scale used to assess his weight.

1450   1500   1600

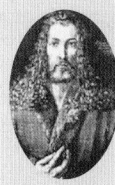

Albrecht Dürer
(1471–1528). "Quadrate Man" illustrated age-related differences in body segment ratios.

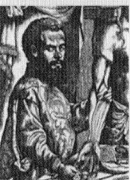

Andreas Vesalius
(1514–1564). Incomparable De Humani Corporis Fabrica (On the Composition of the Human Body) and De Fabrica (1543) based on his own dissections demolished traditional Galenic pronouncements about human anatomy.

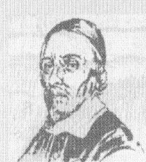

William Harvey
(1578–1657). Proved the heart pumped blood one way through a closed circulatory system.

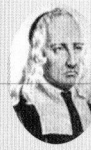

Giovanni Alfonso Borelli
(1608–1679). Used
mathematical models to explain
locomotion (*De Motu Animaliu*,
1680, 1681). Showed that the
lungs filled with air because the
chest volume increased when
diaphragm moved downward. Disproved the
Galenic claim that air cooled the heart by
showing how respiration, not circulation,
required diffusion of air in the alveoli.

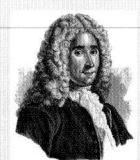

**René-Antoine Fercault de
Réaumur**
(1683–1757). Proved by
regurgitation experiments
that gastric secretions digest
foods (*Digestion in Birds*,
1752).

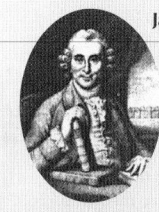

James Lind
(1716–1794).
Eradicated scurvy by
adding citrus fruits to
sailors' diets.

1620   1700   1735

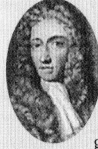

Robert Boyle
(1627–1691). Proved that combustion and respiration required
air. Boyle's Law of Gases states
that at constant temperature, the
pressure (P) of a given mass of
gas varies inversely proportional to
its volume (V): $P_1V_1 = P_2V_2$.

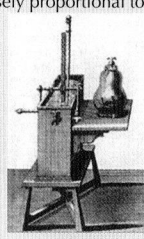

Boyle's "Pneumatical
Engine" apparatus

Joseph Priestley
(1733-1804). Discovered
oxygen by heating red oxide
of mercury in a closed vessel
(*Observations on Different
Kinds of Air*, 1773).

Priestley's
laboratory

Stephen Hales
(1677–1761). *Vegetable Statics* (1727) described how chemical changes occurred in solids and liquids upon calcination (oxidation during combustion), and how the nervous system governed muscular contraction.

Hale's combustion apparatus.

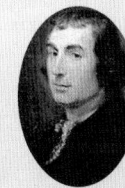

Joseph Black
(1728–1799). Isolated carbon dioxide gas in air produced by fermentation (*Experiments Upon Magnesia Alba, Quicklime, And Some Other Alcaline Substances*, 1756).

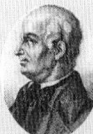

Lazzaro Spallanzani
(1729–1799). Proved that tissues of the heart, stomach, and liver consume oxygen and liberate carbon dioxide, even in creatures without lungs.

1620   **1700**   **1735**

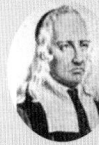

Giovanni Alfonso Borelli
(1608–1679). Used mathematical models to explain locomotion (De Motu Animaliu, 1680, 1681). Showed that the lungs filled with air because the chest volume increased when diaphragm moved downward. Disproved the Galenic claim that air cooled the heart by showing how respiration, not circulation, required diffusion of air in the alveoli.

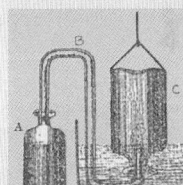

Henry Cavendish
(1731–1810). Identified hydrogen produced when acids combined with metals (*On Factitious Air*, 1766). Proved that water formed when "inflammable air" (hydrogen) combined with "deflogisticated air" (oxygen) (*Experiments in Air*, 1784).

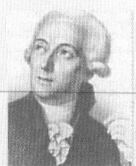

Antoine Laurent Lavoisier
(1743–1794). Quantified
effects of muscular work on
metabolism by measuring
increases in oxygen uptake,
pulse rate, and respiration
rate. Proved that atmospheric air provides oxygen for
animal respiration and that the "caloric" (heat)
liberated during respiration is itself the source
of the combustion.

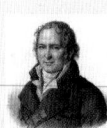

A.F. Fourcroy
(1755–1809). Demonstrated
that the same proportions of
nitrogen occur in animals
and plants.

1740   **1755**   **1775**

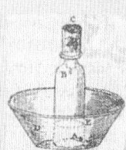

Carl Wilhelm Scheele
(1742–1786). Described
oxygen ("fire air") independently of Priestley, and "foul
air" (phlogisticated air—later
called nitrogen) in a famous
experiment with bees
(*Chemical Treatise on Air and Fire,* 1777).
Scheele's bees living in "fire air" in a closed
vessel submerged in limewater.

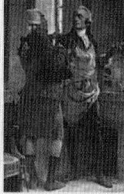

Claude Louis Berthollet
(1748–1822). Proved that
animal tissues do not contain ammonia but that
hydrogen united with nitrogen during fermentation to
produce ammonia. He dis-
agreed with Lavoisier's concept of heat production: "the
quantity of heat liberated in
the incomplete oxidation of a substance is
equal to the difference between the total
caloric value of the substance and that of the
products formed."

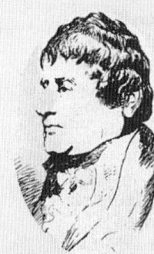

Joseph Louis Proust
(1755–1826). Formulated
"Law of Definite
Proportions" (chemical
constancy of substances
permits future analysis
of major nutrients,
including metabolic
assessment by oxygen
consumption).

Nineteenth Century Metabolism and Physiology

The untimely death of Lavoisier (1794) did not terminate fruitful research in nutrition and medicine. During the next half century, scientists discovered the chemical composition of carbohydrates, lipids, and proteins, and further clarified the energy balance equation.

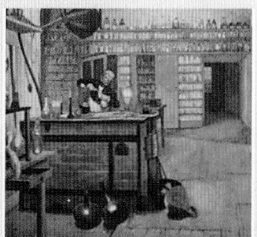

Davey's chemistry laboratory where he isolated 47 elements

François Magendie

(1783–1855). Established experimental physiology as a science and founded its first journal (*Journal de Physiologie Expérimentale*). Proved that anterior spinal nerve roots control motor activities, while posterior roots control sensory functions. Categorized foods as nitrogenous or non-nitrogenous (*Précis élémentaire de Physiologie*, 1816), arguing that foods, not air, provided nitrogen to tissues.

1778   1800   1735

Humphrey Davey

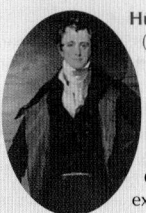

(1778–1829). Consolidated all of the contemporary chemical data related to nutrition, including 47 elements he isolated (*Elements of Agricultural Chemistry*, 1813). Tried to explain how heat and light affect the blood's ability to contain oxygen.

Joseph-Louis Gay-Lussac

(1778–1850). Proved that 20 animal and vegetable substances differed depending on the proportion of H to O atoms. Named one class of compounds ("saccharine") later identified as carbohydrates. Proved the equivalency of oxygen percentage in air at altitude and sea level.

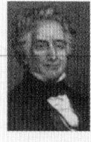

Michel Eugène Chevreul
(1786–1889). Explained that fats consist of fatty acids and glycerol (*Chemical Investigations of Fat*, 1823). Coined the term margarine, and showed that lard consists of two main fats he called "stearine and elaine." With Gay-Lussac, patented the manufacture of the stearic acid candle (still used today).

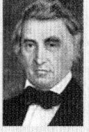

William Beaumont
(1785–1853). Explained in vivo and in vitro human digestion.

1778

1800

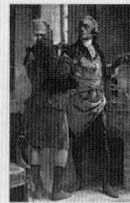

Claude Louis Berthollet
(1748–1822). Proved that animal tissues do not contain ammonia but that hydrogen united with nitrogen during fermentation to produce ammonia. He disagreed with Lavoisier's concept of heat production: "the quantity of heat liberated in the incomplete oxidation of a substance is equal to the difference between the total caloric value of the substance and that of the products formed."

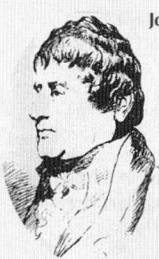

Joseph Louis Proust
(1755–1826). Formulated "Law of Definite Proportions" (chemical constancy of substances permits future analysis of major nutrients, including metabolic assessment by oxygen consumption).

William Prout
(1785–1850). First to separate foodstuffs into the modern classification of carbohydrates, fats, and proteins. Measured the carbon dioxide exhaled by men exercising to fatigue (*Annals of Philosophy*, 2: 328, 1813). Showed that walking raised carbon dioxide production to a plateau (ushering in the modern concept of steady-state gas exchange). Proved that free HCl appeared in the stomach's gastric juice. First prepared pure urea. Extolled milk as the perfect food in *Treatise on Chemistry, Meteorology, and the Function of Digestion* (1834).

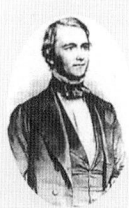

Edward Smith
(1819–1874). Used closed-circuit spirometry to assess energy metabolism during forced exercise. Disproved Liebig's claim that protein alone serves as the primary source of muscular power.

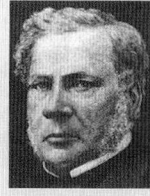

Jean Baptiste Boussingault
(1802– 1884). Father of "scientific agriculture." Determined the effects of calcium, iron, and nutrient intake (particularly nitrogen) on energy balance in animals and humans.

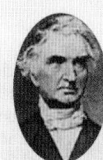

Justus von Liebig
(1803–1873). Dominant chemist of his time, yet asserted without evidence that vigorous exercise by humans and animals required a high protein intake (1850s experiments by others disproved his assertions).

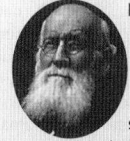

Edward Hitchcock, Jr.
(1828–1911). Amherst College professor who pioneered anthropometric assessment of body build and scientific muscular strength training and testing.

1800   1820   1835

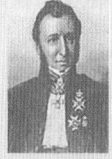

Gerardus Johannis Mulder
(1802–1880). Established the field of physiological chemistry (*General Physiological Chemistry*, 1854). Researched albuminous substances he named "proteine." Strongly advocated society's role in promoting quality nutrition. Established minimum standards for protein consumption (laborers 120 g daily, others 60 g).

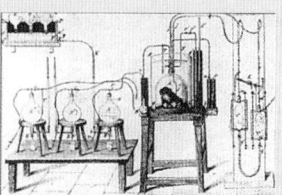

Henri Victor Regnault
(1810–1878). Developed closed-circuit spirometry to determine respiratory quotient ($\dot{V}CO_2/\dot{V}O_2$). Established relationship between body size and metabolism (heat production). Small animal respiration chamber.

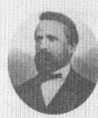

Carl von Voit
(1831–1908). Disproved Liebig's assertion about protein as a main energy fuel by demonstrating that protein breakdown does not increase in proportion to exercise intensity or duration.

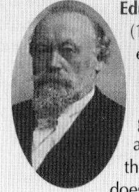

Claude Bernard
(1813–1878). Perhaps the greatest experimental physiologist of all time. His discoveries in regulatory physiology helped future scientists understand how metabolism and nutrition affect exercise.

Eduard Pflüger
(1829–1910). First demonstrated that minute changes in the partial pressure of gases in blood affects the rate of oxygen release and transport across capillary membranes, thus proving blood flow alone does not govern how tissues use oxygen.

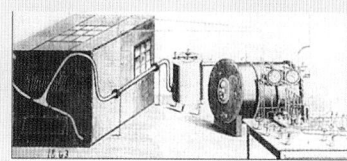

Max Joseph von Pettenkofer
(1818–1901). Perfected respiration calorimeter to study human and animal metabolism. Initiated studies of scientific hygiene (air quality, soil composition and ground water, moisture content of structures, building ventilation, functions of clothing, spread of disease, water quality). He discovered creatinine (amino acid in urine), and founded *Zeitschrift für Biologie* (1865 with Voit) and *Zeitschrift für Hygiene* (1885).

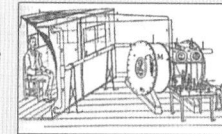

Pettenkofer's 1863 respiration chamber. Top image shows the entire apparatus. Image at right is cut-away view showing human experiment. Fresh air was pumped into the sealed chamber and exhausted air sampled for carbon dioxide

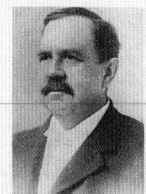

Wilbur Olin Atwater
(1844–1907). Published the chemical composition of 2600 American foods (1896) still used in modern databases of food consumption; performed human calorimetric studies. Confirmed that the Law of Conservation of Energy governs transformation of matter in the human body and inanimate world.

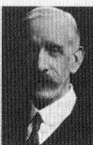

Frederick Gowland Hopkins
(1861–1947). Isolated and identified the structure of the amino acid tryptophan (1929 Nobel Prize in Medicine or Physiology).

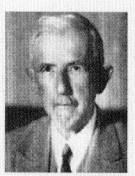

Russel Henry Chittenden
(1856–1943). Refocused scientific attention on man's minimal protein requirement while resting or exercising (no debilitation occurred from protein intake less than 1 g · kg^{-1} body mass in either normal and athletic young men (*Physiological Economy In Nutrition, With Special Reference To The Minimal Proteid Requirement Of The Healthy Man. An Experimental Study,* 1897).

1835   **1850**   **1860**

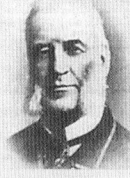

Austin Flint, Jr.
(1836–1915). Prolific author and physiology researcher who chronicled topics of importance to the emerging science of exercise physiology and future science of exercise nutrition. His 987-page compendium of five prior textbooks (*The Physiology of Man; Designed to Represent the Existing State of Physiological Science as Applied to the Functions of the Human Body,* 1877) summarized knowledge about exercise, circulation, respiration, and nutrition from French, German, English, and American literature.

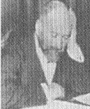

Nathan Zuntz
(1847–1920). Devised first portable metabolic apparatus to assess respiratory exchange in animals and humans at different altitudes. Proved that carbohydrates are precursors of lipid synthesis, and that lipids and carbohydrates should not be consumed equally. Zuntz produced 430 articles concerning blood and blood gases, circulation, mechanics and chemistry of respiration, general metabolism and metabolism of specific foods, energy metabolism and heat production, and digestion.

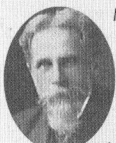

Max Rubner
(1854–1932). Discovered the Isodynamic Law and the calorific heat values of foods (4.1 kCal · g^{-1} for protein and carbohydrates, 9.3 kCal · g^{-1} for lipids). Rubner's Surface Area Law states that resting heat production is proportional to body surface area, and that consuming food increases heat production (SDA effect).

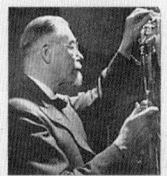

August Krogh (1874–1949). 1920 Nobel Prize in Physiology or Medicine for discovering the mechanism that controls capillary blood flow in resting and active muscle (in frogs). Krogh's 300 published scientific articles link exercise physiology with nutrition and metabolism.

1870   1900

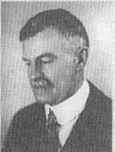

Francis Gano Benedict (1870–1957). Conducted exhaustive studies of energy metabolism in newborn infants, growing children and adolescents, starving people, athletes, and vegetarians. Devised "metabolic standard tables" on sex, age, height, and weight to compare energy metabolism in normals and patients.

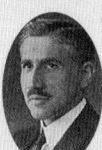

Otto Fritz Meyerhof (1884–1951). 1923 Nobel Prize in Physiology or Medicine with A.V. Hill for elucidating the cyclic characteristics of intermediary cellular energy transformation.

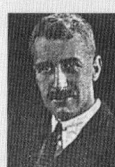

Archibald Vivian (A.V.) Hill (1886– 1977). 1922 Nobel Prize in Physiology or Medicine with Meyerhof for discoveries about the chemical and mechanical events in muscle contraction.

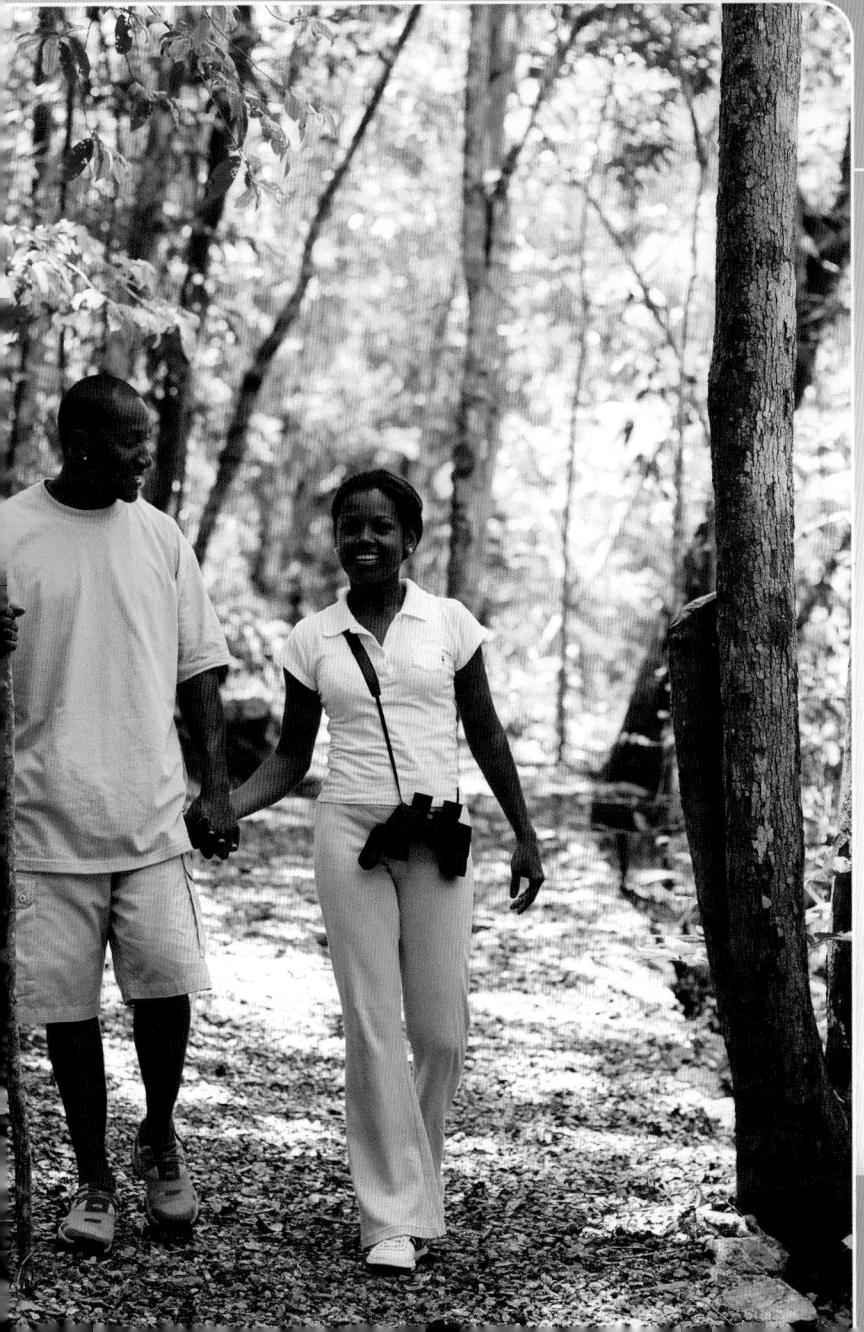

Chapter 1

The Macronutrients

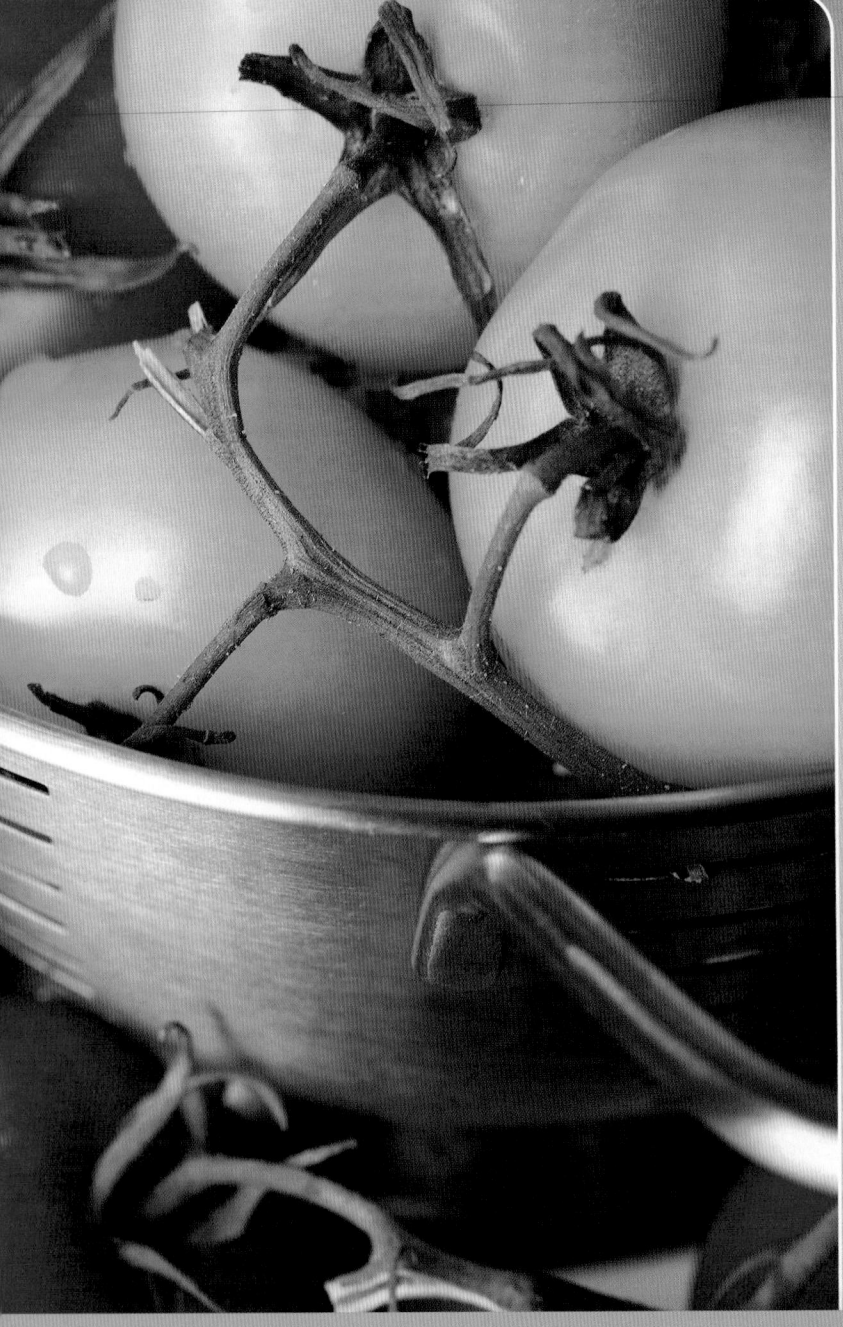

Outline

- Atoms: Nature's Building Blocks
- Carbon: The Versatile Element

Carbohydrates

- Nature of Carbohydrates
- Kinds and Sources of Carbohydrates
- Recommended Dietary Carbohydrate Intake
- Role of Carbohydrate in the Body

Lipids

- Nature of Lipids
- Kinds and Sources of Lipids
- Recommended Dietary Lipid Intake
- Role of Lipid in the Body

Proteins

- Nature of Proteins
- Kinds of Proteins
- Recommended Dietary Protein Intake
- Role of Protein in the Body
- Dynamics of Protein Metabolism

Test Your Knowledge

Answer these 10 statements about carbohydrates, lipids, and proteins. Use the scoring key at the end of the chapter to check your results. Repeat this test after you have read the chapter and compare your results.

1. **T F** Carbohydrates consist of atoms of carbon, oxygen, nitrogen, and hydrogen.
2. **T F** Glucose can be synthesized from amino acids in the body.
3. **T F** Dietary fiber's main function is to provide energy for biologic work.
4. **T F** Carbohydrate intake for most physically active individuals should make up about 45% of the total caloric intake.
5. **T F** Individuals who consume simple carbohydrates run little risk of gaining weight.
6. **T F** A given quantity of sugar, lipid, and protein contains about the same amount of energy.
7. **T F** Although cholesterol is found predominantly in the animal kingdom, certain plant forms also contain cholesterol.
8. **T F** Vegans are at greater risk for nutrient and energy malnutrition than are individuals who consume foods from plant and animal sources.
9. **T F** Consuming an extra amount of high-quality protein above recommended levels facilitates increases in muscle mass.
10. **T F** The protein requirement (per kg of body mass) for men is greater than for women.

The carbohydrate, lipid, and protein nutrients ultimately provide energy to maintain body functions during rest and all forms of physical activity. In addition to their role as biologic fuels, these large nutrients called **macronutrients** also maintain the organism's structural and functional integrity. This chapter focuses on each macronutrient's structure, function, and source in the diet.

ATOMS: NATURE'S BUILDING BLOCKS

Of the 103 different atoms or elements identified in nature, the mass of the human organism contains about 3% nitrogen, 10% hydrogen, 18% carbon, and 65% oxygen. These atoms play the major role in chemical composition of nutrients and make up structural units for the body's biologically active substances.

The union of two or more atoms forms a molecule whose particular properties depend on its specific atoms and their arrangement. Glucose is glucose because of the arrangement of three different kinds of 24 atoms within its molecule. Chemical bonding involves a common sharing of electrons between atoms, as occurs when hydrogen and oxygen atoms join to form a water molecule. The force of attraction between positive and negative charges serves as bonding, or "chemical cement," to keep the atoms within a molecule together. A larger aggregate of matter (a substance) forms when two or more molecules bind chemically. The substance can take the form of a gas, liquid, or solid, depending on forces of interaction among molecules. Altering forces by removing, transferring, or exchanging electrons releases energy, some of which powers cellular functions.

CARBON: THE VERSATILE ELEMENT

All nutrients contain carbon except water and minerals. Almost all substances within the body consist of carbon-containing (**organic**) compounds. Carbon atoms share chemical bonds with other carbon atoms and with atoms of other elements to form large carbon-chain molecules. Specific linkages of carbon, hydrogen, and oxygen atoms form lipids and carbohydrates, while addition of nitrogen and certain minerals creates a protein molecule. Carbon atoms linked with hydrogen, oxygen, and nitrogen also serve as atomic building blocks for the body's exquisitely formed structures.

Carbohydrates

NATURE OF CARBOHYDRATES

All living cells contain carbohydrates, a class of organic molecules that includes monosaccharides, disaccharides, and polysaccharides. Except for lactose and a small amount of glycogen from animals, plants provide the major source of carbohydrate in the human diet. As the name suggests, carbohydrates contain carbon and water. Combining atoms of carbon, hydrogen, and oxygen forms a carbohydrate (sugar) molecule with the general formula $(CH_2O)n$, where n equals 3 to 7 carbon atoms, with single bonds attaching to hydrogen and oxygen. Carbohydrates with 5 and 6 atoms interest nutritionists the most.

FIGURE 1.1 displays the chemical structure of **glucose,** the most typical sugar, along with other carbohydrates synthesized by plants during photosynthesis. Glucose contains 6 carbon, 12 hydrogen, and 6 oxygen atoms, having the chemical formula $C_6H_{12}O_6$. Each carbon atom has four bonding sites that link to other atoms, including carbons. Carbon bonds not linked to other carbon atoms remain "free" to accept hydrogen (with only one bond site), oxygen (with two bond sites), or an oxygen–hydrogen combination (OH), termed a hydroxyl. **Fructose** and **galactose,** two other simple sugars, have the same chemical formula as glucose, but with a slightly different carbon-to-hydrogen-to-oxygen linkage. This makes fructose, galactose, and glucose uniquely different in function, each with its own distinctive biochemical characteristics.

KINDS AND SOURCES OF CARBOHYDRATES

Four categories of carbohydrates include **monosaccharides, disaccharides, oligosaccharides,** and **polysaccharides.** The number of simple sugars linked within the molecule distinguishes each carbohydrate type.

Monosaccharides

The monosaccharide molecule represents the basic unit of carbohydrates. More than 200 monosaccharides exist in nature. The number of carbon atoms in their ringed structure determines the category. The Greek word for this number, ending with "ose," indicates they represent sugars. For example, 3-carbon monosaccharides are trioses, 4-carbon sugars are tetroses, 5-carbon are pentoses, 6-carbon are hexoses, and 7-carbon sugars are heptoses. The hexose sugars glucose, fructose, and galactose make up the nutritionally important monosaccharides. Glucose, also called dextrose or blood sugar, occurs naturally in food. The digestion of more complex carbohydrates also produces glucose. Furthermore, animals produce glucose by **gluconeogenesis,** synthesizing it (primarily in the liver) from carbon skeletons of specific amino acids and from

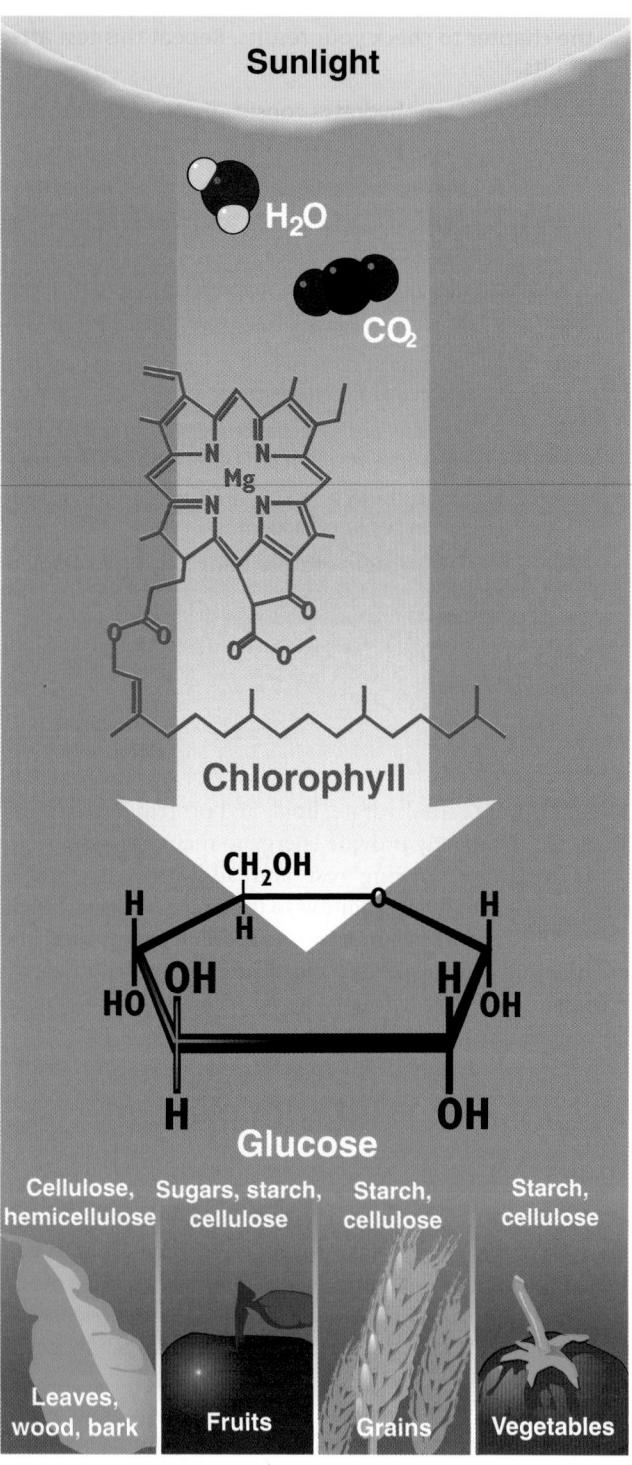

FIGURE 1.1 ■ Three-dimensional ring structure of the simple sugar molecule glucose, formed during photosynthesis when the energy from sunlight interacts with water, carbon dioxide, and the green pigment chlorophyll. The molecule resembles a hexagonal plate to which H and O atoms attach. About 75% of the plant's dry matter consists of carbohydrate.

glycerol, pyruvate, and lactate. The small intestine absorbs glucose, where it then can be (1) used directly by cells for energy, (2) stored as glycogen in muscles and liver for later use, or (3) converted to fat and stored for energy.

Fructose (also called levulose or fruit sugar), the sweetest of the simple sugars, occurs in large amounts in fruits and honey. It accounts for about 9% of the average energy intake in the United States. The small intestine absorbs some fructose directly into the blood, and the liver slowly converts it to glucose. Galactose does not occur freely in nature; rather, it forms milk sugar (lactose) in the mammary glands of lactating animals. In the body, galactose converts to glucose for energy metabolism.

Disaccharides and Oligosaccharides

Combining two monosaccharide molecules forms a disaccharide or double sugar. The monosaccharides and disaccharides are collectively called sugars or **simple sugars.**

Each disaccharide includes glucose as a principle component. The three disaccharides of nutritional significance include:

1. **Sucrose:** The most common dietary disaccharide, consists of glucose plus fructose; it constitutes up to 25% of the total caloric intake in the Unites States. Sucrose occurs naturally in most foods that contain carbohydrates, particularly in beet and cane sugar, brown sugar, sorghum, maple syrup, and honey. Honey, sweeter than table sugar because of its greater fructose content, offers no advantage nutritionally or as an energy source.
2. **Lactose:** Found in natural form only in milk (called milk sugar), consists of glucose plus galactose. The least sweet of the disaccharides, lactose can be artificially processed and is often present in carbohydrate-rich, high-calorie liquid meals. A substantial segment of the world's population is lactose intolerant; these individuals lack adequate quantities of the enzyme lactase that splits lactose into glucose and galactose during digestion.
3. **Maltose:** Composed of two glucose molecules, occurs in beer, cereals, and germinating seeds. Also called malt sugar, maltose makes only a small contribution to the carbohydrate content of a person's diet.

Oligosaccharides (*oligo* in Greek, meaning a few) form from combining three to nine monosaccharide residues. The main dietary sources for the oligosaccharides are vegetables, particularly seed legumes.

Sugar by Any Other Name

Many different terms refer to monosaccharides and disaccharides or to products containing these simple sugars. TABLE 1.1 gives names for sugars present either naturally in food products or added during their manufacture. Food labels (see Chapter 9) place all these simple carbohydrates into one category, "sugars."

Sugars Give Flavor and Sweetness to Foods

Receptors in the tip of the tongue recognize diverse sugars and even some noncarbohydrate substances. Sugars vary in

TABLE 1.1 Terms That Denote Sugar
Sugar
Sucrose
Brown sugar
Confectioner's sugar (powdered sugar)
Turbinado sugar
Invert sugar
Glucose
Sorbitol
Levulose
Polydextrose
Lactose
Mannitol
Honey
Corn syrup
Natural sweeteners
High-fructose corn syrup
Date sugar
Molasses
Maple sugar
Dextrin
Dextrose
Fructose
Maltose
Caramel
Fruit sugar

sweetness on a per gram basis. For example, fructose is almost twice as sweet as sucrose under either acid or cold conditions; sucrose is 30% sweeter than glucose, and lactose is less than half as sweet as sucrose. Because of sweetness variations, some sugars improve the palatability of many foods and thus enhance the eating experience. TABLE 1.2 lists the sweetness of selected sugars and alternative sweeteners and their typical dietary sources.

Polysaccharides

The term *polysaccharide* refers to the linkage of 10 to thousands of monosaccharide residues by **glycosidic bonds.** Polysaccharides classify into plant and animal categories. Cells that store carbohydrate for energy link simple sugar molecules into the more complex polysaccharide form. This reduces the osmotic effect within the cell that would result from storage of an equal energy value of a larger number of simple sugar molecules.

TABLE 1.2	Relative Sweetness of Simple Sugars and Alternative Sweeteners	
Type of Sweetener	Relative Sweetness (sucrose = 1.0)	Dietary Sources
Sugars		
Lactose	0.2	Dairy products
Maltose	0.4	Sprouted seeds
Glucose	0.7	Corn syrup
Sucrose	1.0	Table sugar
Invert sugar	1.3	Candies, honey
Fructose	1.2–1.8	Fruit, honey, some soft drinks
Sugar alcohols		
Sorbitol	0.6	Dietetic candies
Mannitol	0.6	Dietetic candies
Xylitol	0.75	Sugarless gum
Alternative sweeteners		
Cyclamate	30	Not currently in use in U.S.
Aspartame	200	Diet soft drinks, diet fruit drinks,
Acesulfame-K	200	sugarless gum,
Saccharin	500	powdered diet sweetener, diet drink mixes, puddings, gelatin desserts
Sucralose	600	None

Plant Polysaccharides

Starch and **fiber** represent the two common forms of plant polysaccharides.

STARCH. Starch serves as the storage form of carbohydrate in plants and represents the most familiar form of plant polysaccharide. Starch appears as large granules in the cell's cytoplasm and is plentiful in seeds, corn, and various grains that make bread, cereal, spaghetti, and pastries. Large amounts also exist in peas, beans, potatoes, and roots, where starch serves as an energy store for the plant's future use. Plant starch remains an important source of carbohydrate in the American diet, accounting for approximately 50% of the total carbohydrate intake. Daily starch intake, however, has decreased about 30% since the turn of the 20th century, whereas simple sugar consumption correspondingly has increased from 30 to about 50% of total carbohydrate intake. The term **complex carbohydrate** commonly refers to dietary starch.

The Form Makes a Difference. Starch exists in two forms: **amylose,** a long, straight chain of glucose units twisted into a helical coil, and **amylopectin,** a highly branched monosaccharide linkage (FIG. 1.2). The relative proportion of each starch form determines the specific characteristics of the starch in a particular plant species. For example, the predominance of one form or the other determines the "digestibility" of a food containing starch. The branching of the amylopectin polymer exposes greater surface area to digestive enzymes than starches whose glucose units link in a straight

chain. Chapters 7 and 8 cover more about the importance of the different carbohydrate forms in feedings before, during, and after strenuous exercise.

Differing Structure Affects Digestion Rate

Starches with a relatively large amount of amylopectin digest and absorb rapidly, whereas starches with high amylose content have a slower rate of chemical breakdown **(hydrolysis).**

FIBER: The Unheralded "Nutrient." Fiber, classified as a non-starch, structural polysaccharide, includes cellulose, the most abundant organic molecule on earth. Fibrous materials resist hydrolysis by human digestive enzymes, although a portion ferments by action of intestinal bacteria and ultimately participates in metabolic reactions following intestinal absorption. *Fibers exist exclusively in plants; they make up the structure of leaves, stems, roots, seeds, and fruit coverings.* Fibers differ widely in physical and chemical characteristics and physiologic action. They are located mostly within the cell wall as cellulose, gums (substances dissolved or dispersed in water that give a gelling or thickening effect), hemicellulose (sugar units containing 5 or 6 carbons; insoluble in water but soluble in alkali), pectin (forms gels with sugar and acid and imparts a crispy texture to freshly picked apples), and the noncarbohydrate lignins that give rigidity to plant cell walls (increase in content with plant maturity).

Health Implications. Dietary fiber has received considerable attention by researchers and the lay press, largely from epidemiologic studies linking high fiber intake (particularly whole grains[66,78,99]) with lower occurrence of obesity, insulin resistance, systemic inflammation, the metablic syndrome, type 2 diabetes, hyperlipidemia, hypertension, intestinal disorders, and heart disease.[4,29,47,71,72,81,92,94] The Western diet, high in fiber-free animal foods and low in natural plant fiber lost through processing (refining), contributes to more intestinal disorders in industrialized countries compared to countries that consume a more primitive-type diet high in unrefined, complex carbohydrates. For example, the typical American diet contains a daily fiber intake of about 12 to 15 g. In contrast, the fiber content of diets from Africa and India range between 40 and 150 g per day.

Fiber retains considerable water and thus gives "bulk" to the food residues in the large intestine, often increasing stool weight and volume by 40 to 100%. Dietary fiber may aid gastrointestinal functions by (1) exerting a scraping action on the cells of the gut wall, (2) binding or diluting harmful chemicals or inhibiting their activity, and (3) shortening the transit time for food residues (and possibly carcinogenic materials) to pass through the digestive tract. The potential protective effect of fiber on rates and risks of colon cancer remains an inconclusive, hotly debated topic.[38] However, two recent studies—one by American scientists and one by a British team—showed that fibrous foods, particularly grains, cereals, and fruits, provide significant protection.[9,88]

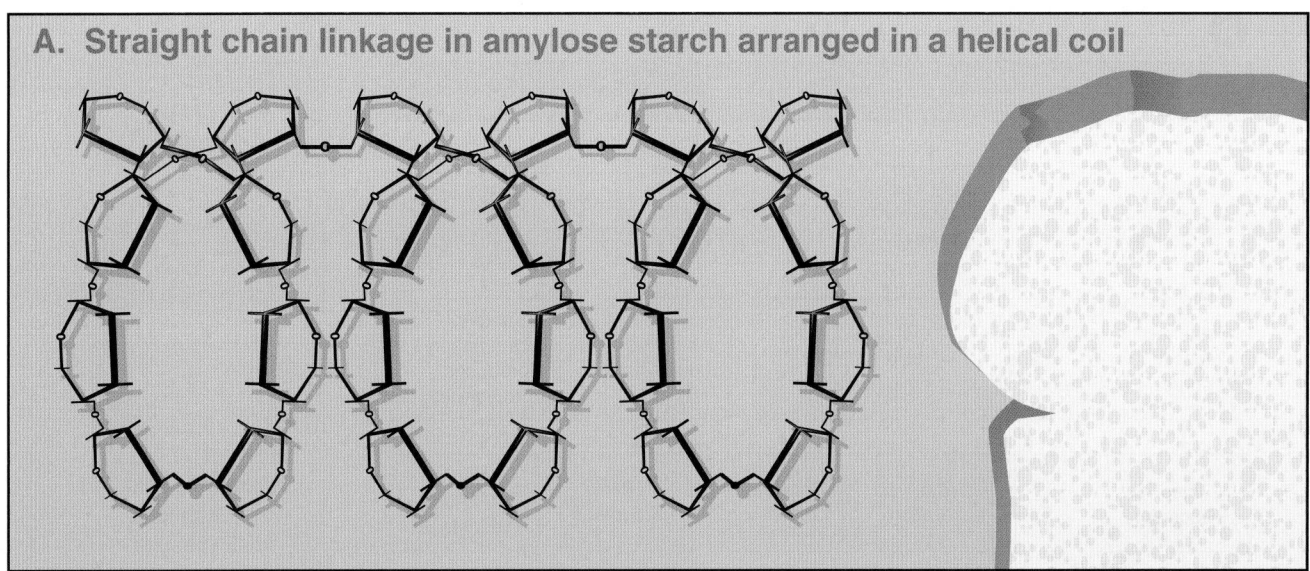

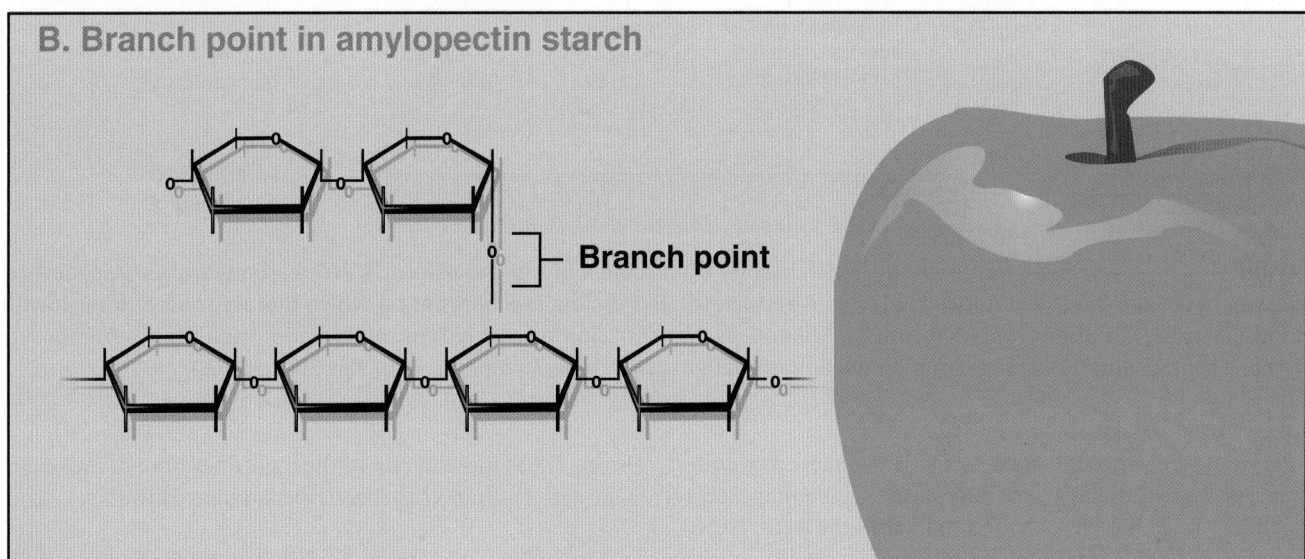

FIGURE 1.2 ■ The two forms of plant starch. **A.** Straight-chain linkage with unbranched bonding of glucose residues (glycosidic linkages) in amylose starch. **B.** Branch point in the highly branched amylopectin starch molecule. The amylopectin structure appears linear, but in reality it exists as a helical coil.

Increased fiber intake modestly reduces serum cholesterol, particularly the **water-soluble** mucilaginous fibers such as pectin and guar gum in oats (rolled oats, oat bran, oat flour), legumes, barley, brown rice, peas, carrots, psyllium, and a variety of fruits (all rich in diverse phytochemicals and antioxidants).[4,30,52] In patients with type 2 diabetes, a daily dietary fiber intake (50 g; 25 g soluble and 25 g insoluble) above that recommended by the American Diabetes Association (24 g; 8 g soluble and 16 g insoluble) improved glycemic control, decreased hyperinsulinemia, and lowered plasma lipid concentrations.[16] A high-fiber oat cereal favorably altered low-density lipoprotein (LDL) cholesterol particle size and number in middle-aged and older men, without adversely changing blood triacylglycerol or high-density lipoprotein (HDL) cholesterol concentrations.[23] Increasing daily intake of guar gum fiber reduced cholesterol by lowering the harmful LDL component of the cholesterol profile.[10,30] In contrast, the **water-insoluble** fibers of cellulose, hemicellulose, lignin, and cellulose-rich wheat bran failed to lower cholesterol.[11] Manufacturers of oatmeal and other oat-based cereals can now claim that their products may reduce heart disease risk, provided the health claim advises one to also eat "diet(s) low in saturated fat and cholesterol."

How dietary fibers favorably affect serum cholesterol remains unknown, although multiple mechanisms likely operate (FIG. 1.3A). Perhaps individuals who consume the most dietary fiber also lead more healthy overall lifestyles that include engaging in more physical activity, smoking fewer cigarettes, and eating a more nutritious diet.[123] Adding fiber to the diet also replaces cholesterol- and saturated fat-laden food choices. In addition, water-soluble fibers may hinder cholesterol absorption or reduce cholesterol metabolism in the gut. These ac-

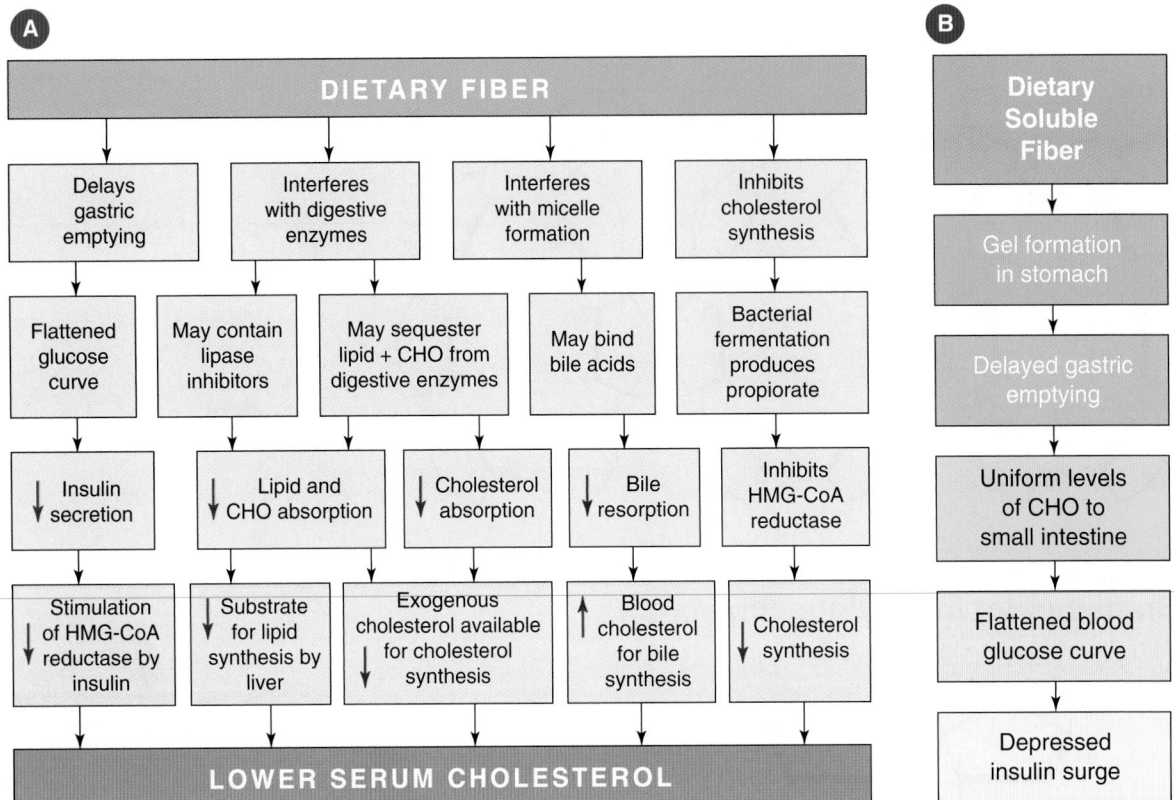

FIGURE 1.3 ■ **A.** Possible mechanism by which dietary fiber lowers blood cholesterol. (*CHO,* carbohydrate; *HMG-CoA reductase,* hydroxy-3-methylglutaryl–coenzyme A reductase). **B.** Possible mechanisms by which dietary soluble fiber lowers blood glucose. (Modified from McIntosh M, Miller C. A diet containing food rich in soluble and insoluble fiber improves glycemic control and reduces hyperlipidemia among patients with type 2 diabetes. *Nutr Rev* 2001;59:52.)

tions would limit hepatic lipogenesis (less glucose as a substrate and less insulin as an activator) while facilitating excretion of existing cholesterol bound to fiber in the feces. Heart disease and obesity protection may relate to dietary fiber's regulatory role in favorably reducing insulin secretion by slowing nutrient absorption by the small intestine following a meal (Fig. 1.3B).[68] For nearly 69,000 middle-aged nurses, each 5-g daily increase in cereal fiber (¹/₂ cup of bran flake cereal contains 4 g of fiber) translated into a 37% decrease in coronary risk.[121] Dietary fiber also contains micronutrients, particularly magnesium, which reduce risk for type 2 diabetes.[96] Magnesium possibly increases the body's sensitivity to insulin, thus reducing the required level of insulin production per unit rise in blood sugar.

The overall health benefits of a high-fiber diet may also come from other components in the food sources. One should obtain the diverse fibers from food in the daily diet, not from fiber supplements. Obtaining fiber in food rather than from over-the-counter supplements ensures intake of other important nutrients. Chapter 9 points out that the nutrition labeling law requires packaged food to list fiber content. Examples of high-fiber common foods include ²/₃ cup brown rice (3 g), ¹/₂ cup cooked carrots (3 g), 1 cup Wheaties (3 g), oatmeal (4 g), shredded wheat (5 g), 1 whole wheat pita (5 g), ¹/₂ grapefruit (6 g), 1 cup Cracklin' Oat Bran (6 g), lentils (7 g), and Raisin

Bran (7 g). One-half cup of the high-fiber bran cereals Fiber One and All-Bran With Extra Fiber contain 14 to 15 g.

The Latest Recommendations

Present nutritional wisdom advocates consuming 38 g of fiber per day (ratio of 3:1 for water-insoluble to soluble fiber) for men and 25 g for women up to age 50 and 30 g for men and 21 g for women older than age 50. Obtain this fiber by following the recommendations of the MyPyramid from the United States Department of Agriculture (see Chapter 7).

TABLE 1.3 lists recommended daily fiber intake by age and gender and the total fiber content of common grains and grain products, nuts and seeds, vegetables and legumes, fruits, and baked goods. Individuals who experience frequent constipation (infrequent or nonexistent bowel movements) should increase daily fiber intake. Seed coats of grains and legumes, and the skins and peels of fruits and vegetables, contain a relatively high fiber content. Adding the pulpy residues from the juices of fruits and vegetables increases the fiber content of biscuits, breads, and other homemade dishes.

TABLE 1.3 Recommended Daily Fiber Intake by Age and Gender and Sources of Total Fiber (g)[a] in Common Grains and Grain Products, Nuts and Seeds, Vegetables and Legumes, Fruits, and Baked Goods

Recommended Daily Fiber Intake (g)	
Children 1–3 years	19
Children 4–8 years	25
Boys 9–13 years	31
Boys 14–18 years	38
Girls 9–18 years	26
Men 19–50 years	38
Men 51 years and older	30
Women 19–50 years	25
Women 51 years and older	21

Food	Serving	Fiber/Serving	Food	Serving	Fiber/Serving
Grains			Broccoli, raw	1 cup	2.9
Oat bran	1 cup	16.4	Black beans	1 oz	2.5
Refined white flour, bleached	1 cup	3.4	Green beans, raw, cooked	1 cup	2.5
Spaghetti, whole wheat	1 cup	5.0	Artichoke, raw	1 oz	2.3
Penne, whole wheat	1 cup	10.0	Carrot	1	2.3
Bran muffin	1	4.0	Baked potato	1	2.3
Whole wheat flour	1 cup	15.1	Tomato, raw	1	1.8
Wheat germ, toasted	1 cup	15.6	Onions, sliced, raw	1 cup	1.8
Couscous	1 cup	8.7	Lentils, stir fry	1 oz	1.1
Popcorn, air-popped	1 cup	1.3	Chili w/beans	1 oz	0.9
Rice bran	1 oz	21.7	**Fruits**		
Millet	1 cup	17.0	Avocado	1	22.9
Corn grits	1 cup	4.5	Loganberries, fresh	1 cup	9.3
Barley, cooked, whole	1 cup	4.6	Pear, Bartlett	1	4.6
Bulgur wheat	1 cup	25.6	Figs	2	4.1
Rye flour-dark	1 cup	17.7	Blueberries	1 cup	3.9
Wild rice	1 cup	4.0	Strawberries, fresh	1 cup	3.9
All-Bran cereal	1/2 cup	8.5	Apple, raw	1	3.5
Barley	1 cup	31.8	Orange, navel	1	3.4
Oatmeal, cooked	1 cup	4.1	Grapefruit, sections, fresh	1	3.0
Grape Nuts	1 cup	10.0	Banana	1	2.3
Macaroni, cooked enriched	1 cup	2.2	Pineapple, chunks	1 cup	2.3
Rice, white	1 oz	1.5	Grapes, Thompson, seedless	1 cup	1.9
Almonds, dried	1 oz	3.5	Peach, fresh	1	1.5
Peanut butter	1 Tbsp	1.0	Plum, small	1	0.6
Macadamia nuts, dried	1 oz	1.5	**Baked goods**		
Low-fat granola	1 cup	4.5	Whole wheat toast	Slice	2.3
Cherrios	1 cup	5.0	Waffle, homemade	1	1.1
Nuts and seeds			Pumpkin pie	Slice	5.4
Pumpkin seeds, roasted, unsalted	1 oz	10.2	Oatmeal bread	Slice	1.0
Chestnuts, roasted	1 oz	3.7	French bread	Slice	0.7
Peanuts, dried, unsalted	1 oz	3.5	Danish pastry, plain	1	0.7
Sunflower seeds, dry	1 oz	2.0	Fig bar cookie	1	0.6
Walnuts, chopped, black	1 oz	1.6	Chocolate chip cookie, homemade	1	0.2
Vegetables and legumes			White bread	Slice	0.6
Pinto beans, dry, cooked	1 cup	19.5	Pumpernickel bread	Slice	1.7
Lima beans, fresh, cooked	1 cup	16.0	Rye bread	Slice	1.9
Black eyed peas, cooked from raw	1 cup	12.2	Seven-grain bread	Slice	1.7
Mixed vegetables (corn, carrots, beans)	1 cup	7.2			
Corn on cob	1	3.2			

Data from the United States Department of Agriculture.
[a] The crude fiber content of foods reported in food composition tables (including the foods in the above table) refers to the organic portion of the dry, acid, and alkali-extracted residue from the ashing of the food after it is ground up, dried to a constant weight in a low-temperature oven, and had the fat removed with solvents. The fat-free food sample is then boiled in hot sulfuric acid, rinsed in hot water, and then boiled again in dilute sodium hydroxide to yield the food's crude fiber content.

FIGURE 1.4 shows a sample daily 2200-kCal menu that includes 31 g of fiber (21 g of insoluble fiber). In this meal plan, lipid calories account for 30% (saturated fat, 10%), protein 16%, and carbohydrate 54% of total caloric intake. Each 10-g increase in a subpar diet's fiber content reduces coronary risk by about 20%. Five daily servings of fruits and vegetables combined with 6 to 11 servings of grains (particularly whole grains) ensures dietary fiber intake at recommended levels.

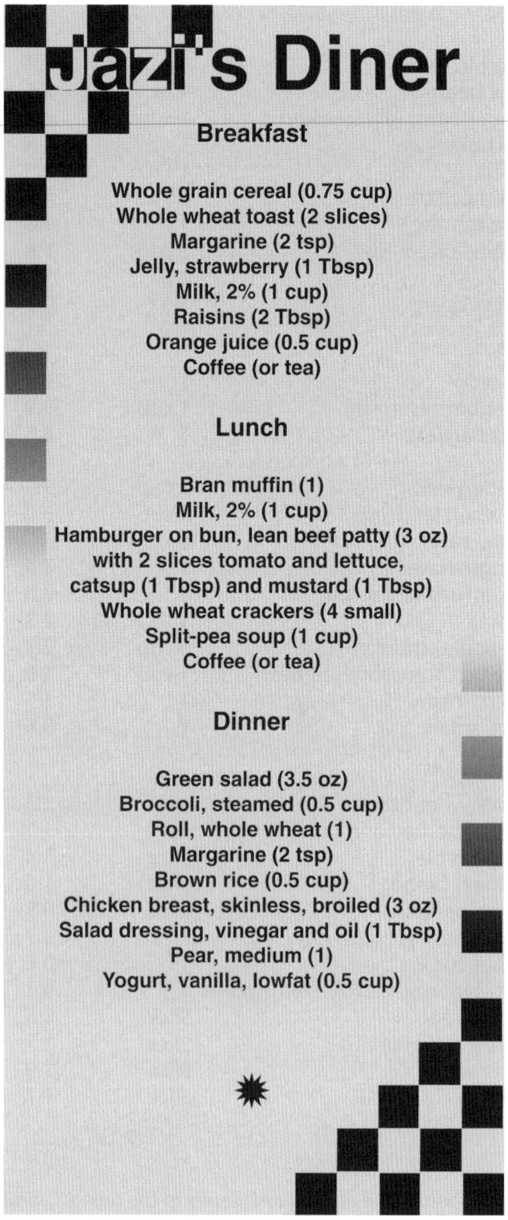

Jazi's Diner

Breakfast

Whole grain cereal (0.75 cup)
Whole wheat toast (2 slices)
Margarine (2 tsp)
Jelly, strawberry (1 Tbsp)
Milk, 2% (1 cup)
Raisins (2 Tbsp)
Orange juice (0.5 cup)
Coffee (or tea)

Lunch

Bran muffin (1)
Milk, 2% (1 cup)
Hamburger on bun, lean beef patty (3 oz)
with 2 slices tomato and lettuce,
catsup (1 Tbsp) and mustard (1 Tbsp)
Whole wheat crackers (4 small)
Split-pea soup (1 cup)
Coffee (or tea)

Dinner

Green salad (3.5 oz)
Broccoli, steamed (0.5 cup)
Roll, whole wheat (1)
Margarine (2 tsp)
Brown rice (0.5 cup)
Chicken breast, skinless, broiled (3 oz)
Salad dressing, vinegar and oil (1 Tbsp)
Pear, medium (1)
Yogurt, vanilla, lowfat (0.5 cup)

FIGURE 1.4 ■ Sample menu for breakfast, lunch, and dinner (2200 kCal) containing 31 g of dietary fiber. The diet's total cholesterol content is less than 200 mg, and total calcium equals 1242 mg.

(See Chapter 7 concerning actual serving size, which is smaller than the typical portion size eaten by Americans.) Whole grains provide a nutritional advantage over refined grains because they contain more fiber, vitamins, minerals, and diverse phytochemicals, all of which favorably affect health status.[73] Excessive fiber intake (particularly high-fiber foods with seed coats and thus large amounts of phytates) are ill advised for individuals with marginal levels of nutrition; these compounds generally blunt intestinal absorption of the major minerals calcium and phosphorus and some trace minerals, including iron.

Animal Polysaccharides

Glycogen, the storage polysaccharide found in mammalian muscle and liver, consists of an irregularly shaped, branched polysaccharide polymer similar to amylopectin in plant starch. This macromolecule, synthesized from glucose during **glucogenesis,** ranges from a few hundred to thousands of glucose molecules linked together like a chain of sausages, with some branch points for additional glucose linkage. FIGURE 1.5 shows that glycogen synthesis occurs by adding individual glucose units to an already existing glycogen polymer.

FIGURE 1.6 *illustrates that a well-nourished 80-kg person stores approximately 500 g of carbohydrate.* Of this, the largest reserve (approximately 400 g) exists as muscle glycogen, 90 to 110 g as liver glycogen (highest concentration that represents 3 to 7% of the liver's weight), and only about 2 to 3 g as blood glucose. Because each gram of either glycogen or glucose contains about 4 kCal of energy, the typical person stores between 1500 and 2000 kCal of carbohydrate energy—enough total energy to power a high-intensity 20-mile run.

GLYCOGEN DYNAMICS. Several factors determine the rate and quantity of glycogen breakdown and subsequent synthesis. Muscle glycogen serves as the *major source* of carbohydrate energy for active muscles during exercise. In contrast to muscle glycogen, liver glycogen reconverts to glucose (controlled by a specific **phosphatase enzyme**) for transport in the blood to the working muscles. **Glycogenolysis** describes this reconversion process; it provides a rapid extramuscular glucose supply. Depleting liver and muscle glycogen through either (1) dietary restriction or (2) high-intensity exercise stimulates glucose synthesis from the structural components of other nutrients, principally amino acids, through gluconeogenic metabolic pathways.

Hormones control the level of circulating blood glucose and play an important role in regulating liver and muscle glycogen stores. Elevated blood glucose levels cause the beta cells of the pancreas to secrete additional **insulin,** forcing peripheral tissues to take up the excess glucose. This feedback mechanism inhibits further insulin secretion, which maintains blood glucose at an appropriate physiologic concentration. In contrast, when blood glucose falls below the normal range, the pancreas' alpha cells immediately secrete insulin's opposing hormone, **glucagon,** to normalize blood glucose levels. This "insulin antagonist" hormone stimulates liver

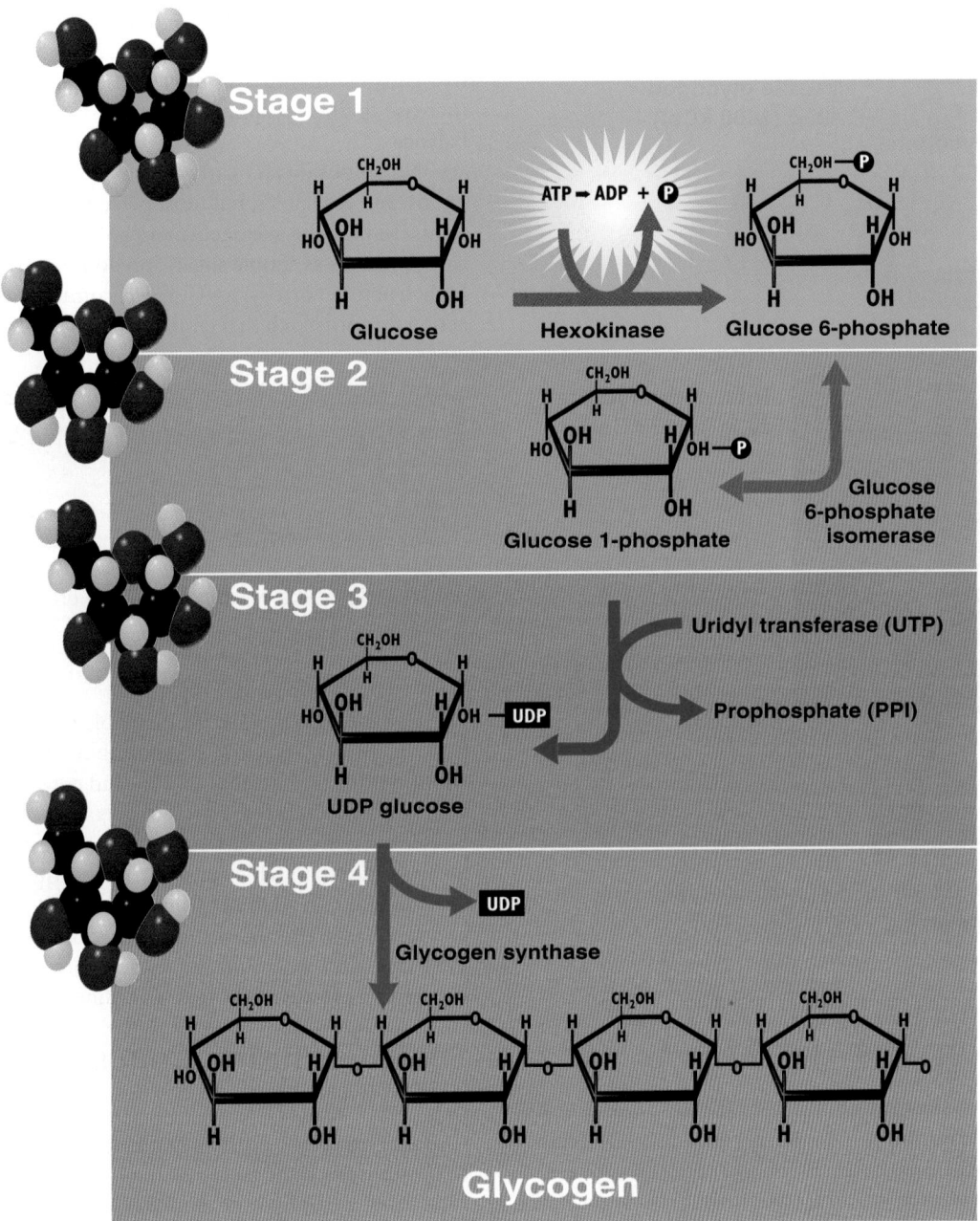

FIGURE 1.5 ■ Glycogen synthesis is a four-step process. *Stage 1,* ATP donates a phosphate to glucose to form glucose 6-phosphate. This reaction involves the enzyme hexokinase. *Stage 2,* Glucose 6-phosphate isomerizes to glucose 1-phosphate by the enzyme glucose 6-phosphate isomerase. *Stage 3,* The enzyme uridyl transferase reacts uridyl triphosphate (UTP) with glucose 1-phosphate to form UDP-glucose (a phosphate is released as UTP → UDP). *Stage 4,* UDP-glucose attaches to one end of an existing glycogen polymer chain. This forms a new bond (known as a glycoside bond) between the adjacent glucose units, with the concomitant release of UDP. For each glucose unit added, 2 moles of ATP converts to ADP and phosphate.

glycogenolysis and gluconeogenesis to raise the blood glucose concentration.

The body stores comparatively little glycogen, so one's diet profoundly affects the amount available. For example, a 24-hour fast or a low-carbohydrate, normal-calorie (isocaloric) diet greatly reduces glycogen reserves. In contrast, maintaining a carbohydrate-rich isocaloric diet for several days enhances the body's carbohydrate stores to a level almost twice that of a normal, well-balanced diet.

Limited Stores of an Important Compound for Exercise

The body's upper limit for glycogen storage averages about 15 g per kilogram (kg) of body mass, equivalent to 1050 g for an average-sized, 70-kg man and 840 g for a typical 56-kg woman.

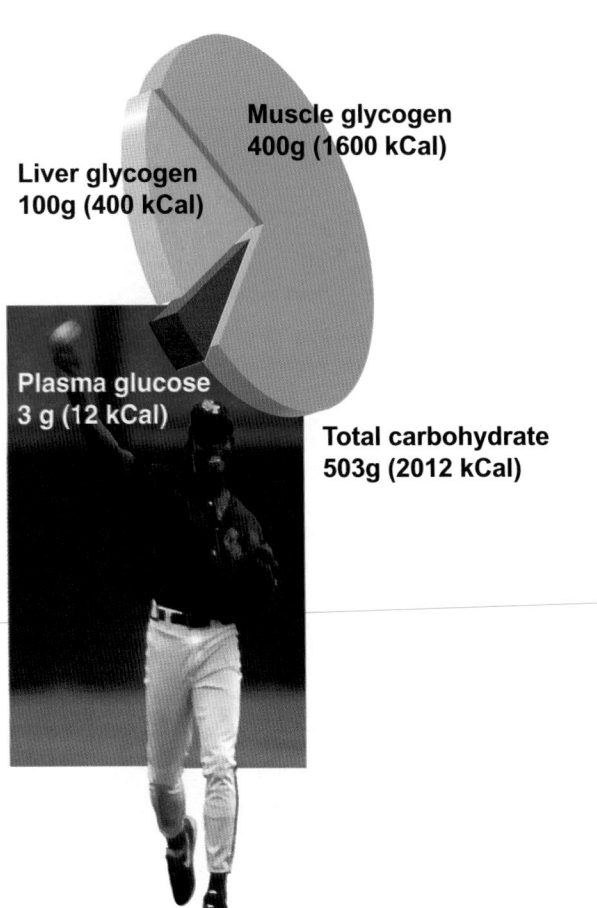

Muscle glycogen
400g (1600 kCal)

Liver glycogen
100g (400 kCal)

Plasma glucose
3 g (12 kCal)

Total carbohydrate
503g (2012 kCal)

FIGURE 1.6 ■ Distribution of carbohydrate energy for an average 80-kg man.

RECOMMENDED DIETARY CARBOHYDRATE INTAKE

FIGURE 1.7 (TOP) illustrates the carbohydrate content of selected foods. Rich carbohydrate sources include cereals, cookies, candies, breads, and cakes. Fruits and vegetables appear to be less valuable sources because carbohydrate percentage derives from the food's total weight, including water content. The dried portions of these foods, however, exist as almost pure carbohydrate. This makes them an ideal lightweight, "dehydrated" food source during hiking or long treks when one must transport the food supply during the activity. The bottom of the figure lists the amount of carbohydrate in various food categories.

On a worldwide basis, carbohydrates represent the most prevalent source of calories. In Africa, for example, nearly 80% of total caloric intake comes from carbohydrates, while in Caribbean countries the value reaches 65%. *Carbohydrates account for between 40 and 50% of the total calories in the typical American diet.* For a sedentary 70-kg person, this translates to a daily carbohydrate intake of about 300 g. For individuals who engage in regular physical activity, carbohydrates should supply about 60% (400–600 g) of total daily calories, predominantly as unrefined, fiber-rich fruits, grains, and vegetables.

This quantity replenishes, in a nutrient-rich package, the carbohydrate used to power the increased level of physical activity. During intense training, carbohydrate intake should increase to 70% of total calories consumed when in energy balance.

Nutritious dietary carbohydrate sources consist of fruits, grains, and vegetables, but most persons do not consume these foods. In fact, the average American consumes about 50% of carbohydrates as simple sugars, predominantly as sucrose and high-fructose corn syrup (formed commercially by enzyme action on cornstarch that emphasizes fructose formation).

Too Much Carbohydrate in Simple Form

Simple sugar intake represents more than the yearly equivalent of 70 lb of table sugar (18 teaspoons of sucrose a day) and 50 lb of corn syrup. About 100 years ago, the yearly intake of simple sugars averaged only 4 lb per person!

Consuming excessive fermentable carbohydrate (principally sucrose) *causes* tooth decay, but dietary sugar's contributing role to diabetes, obesity, and coronary heart disease still remains an area of controversy (see next section). Substituting fructose for sucrose, a monosaccharide nearly 80% sweeter than table sugar, provides equal sweetness with fewer calories. In addition, fructose does not stimulate pancreatic insulin secretion. Consuming fructose thus helps to stabilize blood glucose and insulin levels. More is said in Chapter 8 concerning pre-exercise fructose feedings.

Some Confusion Concerning Dietary Carbohydrates

Concern exists about the negative effects of the typical diet that imposes a high **glycemic load**—an index that incorporates both carbohydrate quantity and glycemic index (see Chapter 8)—on risk for obesity, type 2 diabetes, abnormal blood lipids, and coronary heart disease, particularly among sedentary individuals.[21,64,65,77,87,102,109,111,120] Frequent and excessive consumption of more rapidly absorbed forms of carbohydrate (i.e., those with high glycemic index) may alter the metabolic profile and increase disease risk, particularly for individuals with excess body fat. For example, eating a high-carbohydrate, low-fat meal reduces fat breakdown and increases fat synthesis more in overweight men than in lean men.[70] Dietary patterns of women followed over 6 years showed that those who consumed a high-glycemic starchy diet (potatoes and low-fiber, processed white rice, pasta, and white bread, along with nondiet soft drinks) suffered 2.5 times the rate of diabetes of women who consumed less of those foods and more fiber-containing whole-grain cereals, fruits, and vegetables.[96] Participants who became diabetic developed type 2 diabetes, the most common form of the dis-

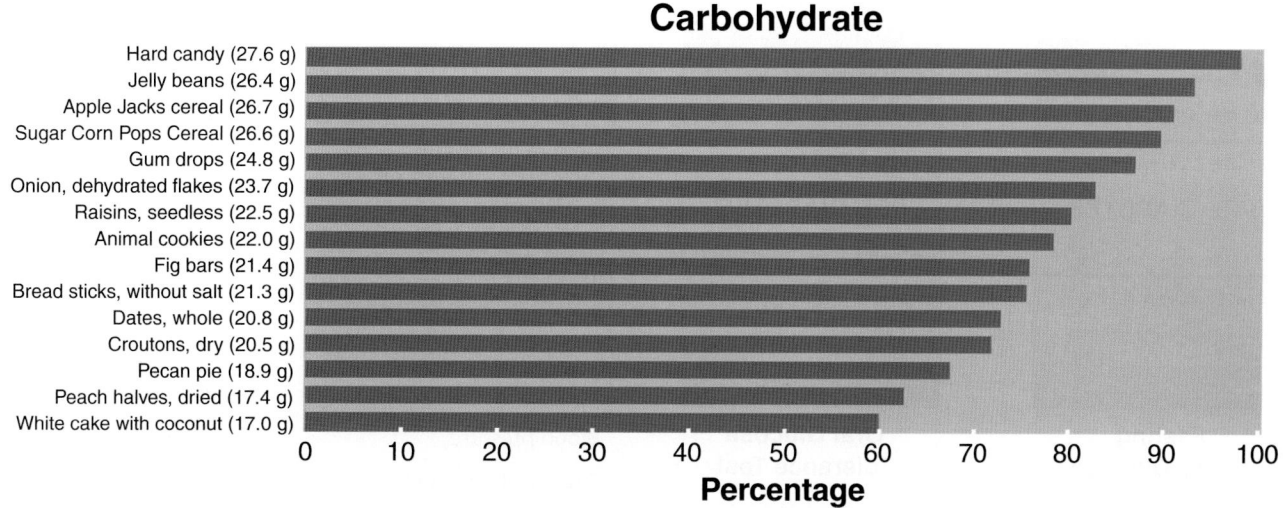

FIGURE 1.7 ■ *Top.* Percentage of carbohydrate in selected foods arranged by food type. The number in parentheses indicates the number of grams of carbohydrate per ounce (28.4 g) of the food. *Bottom.* The amount of carbohydrate in various foods grouped by category.

ease that afflicts more than 18 million people in the United States. High blood glucose levels in type 2 diabetes can result from (1) decreased effect of insulin on peripheral tissue (**insulin resistance**), (2) inadequate insulin production by the pancreas to control blood sugar (**relative insulin deficiency**), or (3) the combined effect of both factors. FIGURE 1.8 illus-

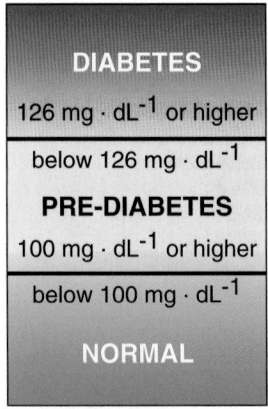

DIABETES	DIABETES
126 mg · dL^{-1} or higher	200 mg · dL^{-1} or higher
below 126 mg · dL^{-1}	below 200 mg · dL^{-1}
PRE-DIABETES	**PRE-DIABETES**
100 mg · dL^{-1} or higher	140 mg · dL^{-1} or higher
below 100 mg · dL^{-1}	below 140 mg · dL^{-1}
NORMAL	NORMAL
Fasting Blood Glucose	**Oral Glucose Tolerance Test**

FIGURE 1.8 ■ Classification for normal, prediabetes, and type 2 diabetes based on blood glucose levels in a fasting blood glucose test or an oral glucose tolerance test.

TABLE 1.4	Clinical Identification of the Metabolic Syndrome
Risk Factor	**Defining Level**
Abdominal obesity[a] (waist circumference)[b]	
Men	>102 cm (>40 in)
Women	>88 cm (>35 in)
Triacylglycerols	≥150 mg/dL
High-density lipoprotein cholesterol	
Men	<40 mg/dL
Women	<50 mg/dL
Blood pressure	≥130/≥85 mm Hg
Fasting blood glucose	≥110 mg/dL

[a]*Overweight and obesity associate with insulin resistance and the metabolic syndrome. The presence of abdominal obesity highly correlates more with the metabolic risk factors than an elevated body mass index (BMI). The simple measure of waist circumference is recommended to identify the body weight component of the metabolic syndrome.*

[b]*Some male patients can develop multiple metabolic risk factors when the waist circumference is marginally increased, e.g., 94 to 102 cm (37 to 40 in). Such patients may have strong genetic contribution to insulin resistance and they should benefit from changes in life habits, similarly to men with categorical increases in waist circumference.*

trates blood glucose levels for classification as normal, prediabetic, and type 2 diabetic. Insulin, produced by the pancreas, facilitates the transfer of glucose from the blood into the cells of the body. Type 1 diabetes exists when no insulin is produced. If the pancreas produces insulin but your cells are inefficient in removing glucose, you are insulin resistant or demonstrate poor insulin sensitivity. If blood sugar rises only slightly, you have prediabetes. If blood sugar goes even higher, you have type 2 diabetes. The blood sugar cutoffs depend on whether your blood is tested after a 12-hour fast (fasting blood sugar) or 2 hours after consuming a glucose-laden drink (oral glucose tolerance test).

Diet-induced insulin resistance/hyperinsulinemia often precedes manifestations of the **metabolic syndrome**—defined as having three or more of the criteria indicated in TABLE 1.4.[6,83,101] In essence, the syndrome reflects a concurrence of four factors:

1. Disturbed glucose and insulin metabolism
2. Overweight and abdominal fat distribution
3. Mild dyslipidemia
4. Hypertension

These individuals exhibit a high risk for cardiovascular disease, diabetes, and all-cause mortality.[58] Estimates place the age-adjusted prevalence of the metabolic syndrome in the United States at 25%, or about 47 million men and women.[35] The percentage increases with age and poor levels of cardiovascular fitness[31] and is particularly high among Mexican Americans and African Americans.[20] The syndrome also has emerged among obese children and adolescents.[116]

Not All Carbohydrates Are Physiologically Equal

Digestion rates of different carbohydrate sources possibly explain the carbohydrate intake–diabetes link. Low-fiber processed starches (and simple sugars) digest quickly and enter the blood at a relatively rapid rate (high glycemic index),

whereas slow-release forms of high-fiber, unrefined complex carbohydrates minimize surges in blood glucose. The rapid rise in blood glucose with refined, processed starch intake increases insulin demand, stimulates overproduction of insulin by the pancreas to accentuate hyperinsulinemia, increases plasma triacylglycerol concentrations, and stimulates fat synthesis. Consuming such foods for prolonged periods may eventually reduce the body's sensitivity to insulin (more insulin resistant), thus requiring progressively greater insulin output to control blood sugar levels. *Type 2 diabetes results when the pancreas cannot produce sufficient insulin to regulate blood glucose.* In contrast, diets with fiber-rich, low-glycemic carbohydrates tend to lower blood glucose and insulin response after eating, improve the blood lipid profile, and increase insulin sensitivity.[39,76,79,90,113]

Regularly consuming high-glycemic foods can increase cardiovascular risk because elevated blood glucose precipitates oxidative damage and inflammation that elevates blood pressure, stimulates clot formation, and reduces blood flow. For individuals with type 1 diabetes who require exogenous insulin, consumption of low–glycemic index foods causes more favorable physiologic adaptations for glycemic control, HDL cholesterol concentrations, serum leptin levels, resting energy expenditure, voluntary food intake, and nitrogen balance.[1,12]

A Role in Obesity?

About 25% of the population produce excessive insulin from consuming rapidly absorbed carbohydrates. These insulin-resistant individuals increase their risk for obesity if they consistently consume such a diet. Weight gain occurs because abnormal quantities of insulin (1) promote glucose entry into cells and (2) facilitate the liver's conversion of glucose to triacylglycerol, which then becomes stored as body fat in adipose tissue.[37]

The insulin surge in response to a sharp rise in blood glucose following ingestion of high-glycemic carbohydrates often abnormally decreases blood glucose. This **rebound hypoglycemia** sets off hunger signals that cause the person to overeat. This repetitive scenario of high blood sugar followed by low blood sugar exerts the most profound effect on the sedentary obese individual who shows the greatest insulin resistance and consequently the greatest insulin surge to a blood glucose challenge. For physically active people, regular low-to-moderate physical activity produces the following three beneficial effects:

1. Exerts a potent influence for weight control
2. Stimulates plasma-derived fatty acid oxidation, which decreases fatty acid availability to the liver and blunts any increase in plasma very low-density-lipoprotein cholesterol–triacylglycerol concentrations
3. Improves insulin sensitivity, thus reducing the insulin requirement for a given glucose uptake

To reduce the risks for type 2 diabetes and obesity, consuming more slowly absorbed, unrefined complex carbohydrate foods provides a form of "slow-release" carbohydrate without producing rapid fluctuations in blood sugar. If rice, pasta, and bread remain the carbohydrate sources of choice, they should be consumed in unrefined form as brown rice and whole-grain pastas and breads. The same dietary modification would benefit individuals involved in intense physical training and endurance competition. Their daily dietary carbohydrate intake should approach 800 g (8–10 g per kg of body mass; see Chapter 7).

ROLE OF CARBOHYDRATES IN THE BODY

Carbohydrates serve four important functions related to energy metabolism and exercise performance.

Energy Source

Carbohydrates primarily serve as an energy fuel, particularly during high-intensity exercise. Energy derived from blood-borne glucose and liver and muscle glycogen breakdown ultimately powers the contractile elements of muscle and other forms of more "silent" biologic work.

Carbohydrates exhibit the most dramatic use and depletion in intense exercise and heavy training, compared with fat and protein. For physically active people, adequate daily carbohydrate intake maintains the body's relatively limited glycogen stores. In contrast, exceeding the cells' capacity to store glycogen triggers conversion and storage of excess dietary carbohydrate calories as fat.

Affects Metabolic Mixture and Spares Protein

Carbohydrate availability affects the metabolic mixture catabolized for energy. TABLE 1.5 shows the effect of reduced energy intake during a 40-hour fast and 7 days of total food deprivation on plasma glucose and fat breakdown components. After almost 2 days of fasting, blood glucose decreases 35% but does not decrease to a lower level during further prolonged food abstinence. Concurrently, circulating fatty acid and ketone levels (acetoacetate and β-hydroxybutyrate by-products of incomplete fat breakdown) increase rapidly, with plasma ketones rising dramatically after 7 days of starvation.

Adequate carbohydrate intake preserves tissue proteins. Normally, protein serves a vital role in tissue maintenance, repair, and growth and, to a lesser degree, as a nutrient energy source. Glycogen reserves readily deplete during (1) starvation, (2) reduced energy intake and low-carbohydrate diets, and (3) prolonged strenuous exercise. Reduced glycogen reserves and plasma glucose levels trigger glucose synthesis from both protein (amino acids) and the glycerol portion of the fat (triacylglycerol) molecule. This gluconeogenic conversion provides a metabolic option to augment carbohydrate availability (and to maintain plasma glucose levels) with depleted glycogen stores. The price paid, however, strains the body's protein components, particularly muscle protein. In the extreme, gluconeogenesis reduces lean tissue mass and produces an accompanying solute load on the kidneys, which must excrete the nitrogen-containing by-products of protein breakdown.

Metabolic Primer/Prevents Ketosis

Components of carbohydrate catabolism serve as "primer" substrate for fat catabolism. Insufficient carbohydrate metabolism—either through limitations in glucose transport into the cell (as in diabetes from too little insulin production or insulin insensitivity) or glycogen depletion through inadequate diet, particularly low-carbohydrate diets, or prolonged exercise—causes more fat mobilization than oxidation. This produces incomplete fat breakdown and the accumulation of acetone-like by-products (chiefly acetoacetate and hydroxybutyrate) called **ketone bodies.** Excessive ketone formation increases body fluid acidity, a harmful condition called acido-

TABLE 1.5	Changes in the Plasma Concentrations of Glucose, Fatty Acids, and Ketones following 40 Hours of Fasting and Subsequent 7 Days of Starvation		
Nutrient (mmol · L^{-1})	Normal	40 Hours Fasting	7 Days Starvation
Glucose	5.5	3.6	3.5
Fatty acids	0.3	1.15	1.19
Ketones	0.01	2.9	4.5

Adapted from Bender DA. Introduction to Nutrition and Metabolism. London: UCL Press, 1993.

sis, or with regard to fat breakdown, **ketosis.** Chapter 5 continues the discussion of carbohydrate as a primer for fat catabolism.

Fuel for the Central Nervous System

The central nervous system requires carbohydrate to function properly. Under normal conditions, the brain relies on blood glucose almost exclusively as its fuel. In poorly regulated diabetes, during starvation, or with a chronic low carbohydrate intake, the brain adapts after about 8 days by metabolizing relatively large amounts of fat (in the form of ketones) for alternative fuel. Adaptations also occur in skeletal muscle to chronic low-carbohydrate, high-fat diets by increasing fat use during exercise, which spares muscle glycogen.[60]

Liver glycogenolysis primarily maintains normal blood glucose levels at rest and during exercise, usually at 100 mg · dL^{-1} (5.5 mM). In prolonged, intense exercise, blood glucose eventually falls below normal levels because liver glycogen

A Tightly Regulated Macronutrient

Blood sugar usually remains regulated within narrow limits for two main reasons: the important role of glucose (1) in nerve tissue metabolism and (2) as the energy fuel for red blood cells.

depletes and active muscles continue to use the available blood glucose. Symptoms of an abnormally reduced blood glucose or **hypoglycemia** include weakness, hunger, and dizziness. Reduced blood glucose ultimately impairs exercise performance and partially explains "central" fatigue associated with prolonged exercise. Sustained and profound hypoglycemia (e.g., induced by an overdose of exogenous insulin) can trigger loss of consciousness and produce irreversible brain damage.

Case Study

Personal Health and Exercise Nutrition 1–1

Diabetes 2007 Facts

Each year, at least 1.5 million people in the United States will be added to the number of people diagnosed with diabetes, predominantly of the type 2 variety. This segment on personal health and exercise nutrition is of a general nature in that it applies to the population rather than to a single individual. It reflects the latest statistics about how diabetes—the body's inability to produce sufficient insulin (insulin insufficiency) or use it effectively (insulin resistance) to metabolize sugar—affects this country's 20.8 million adults and children (7% of the population). Slightly more men (10.9 million) than women (9.7 million) have diabetes. About 21% of people older than age 60 (10.3 million) have diabetes. The NIH (National Institutes of Health: www.nih.gov) estimates that 850,000 to 1.7 million Americans have type 1 diabetes. This translates to about 1 in every 400 to 600 children and adolescents. The remainder have type 2 diabetes, and millions more are not yet diagnosed. A chronic elevation in blood glucose level can lead to the following medical complications:

1. *Heart disease:* This is the leading cause of diabetes-related deaths. Adults with diabetes have heart disease death rates two to four times higher than those of adults without diabetes.

2. *Stroke:* Individuals with diabetes exhibit a two to four times higher stroke risk than do those without diabetics.

3. *High blood pressure:* About 73% of adults with diabetes have elevated blood pressure of 140/90 mm Hg or higher or use prescription medications to control their hypertension.

4. *Blindness:* Diabetes is the leading cause of new cases of blindness among adults 20 to 74 years old. Diabetic retinopathy causes 12,000 to 24,000 new cases of blindness yearly.

5. *Kidney disease:* Diabetes is the leading cause of treated, end-stage renal disease, accounting for 43% of new cases. In 2000, 41,046 people with diabetes began treatment for end-stage renal disease, and 129,183 diabetics underwent dialysis or kidney transplantation.

6. *Nervous system disease:* About 60 to 70% of persons with diabetes have mild-to-severe nervous system damage. This impairs sensation or pain in the feet or hands, slows digestion of food, and produces carpal tunnel syndrome and other nerve pathologies.

7. *Amputations:* More than 60% of nontraumatic lower limb amputations in the United States occur among

patients with diabetes. In 2002, about 82,000 of these amputations were performed.

8. *Dental disease:* Periodontal or gum diseases are more common among individuals with diabetes than among those who do not have diabetes. Young adults with diabetes experience twice the risk for these disorders. Almost one third of people with diabetes have severe periodontal diseases with loss of attachment of the gums to the teeth measuring 5 mm or more.

9. *Complications of pregnancy:* Poorly controlled diabetes before conception and during the first trimester causes major birth defects in 5 to 10% of pregnancies and spontaneous abortions in 15 to 20% of pregnancies. Poorly controlled diabetes during the second and third trimesters often results in excessively large babies, posing a risk to the mother and child.

10. *Other complications:* Uncontrolled diabetes often leads to biochemical imbalances and acute life-threatening diabetic ketoacidosis and hyperosmolar (nonketotic) coma.

Statistics About Diabetes

- Diabetes is the sixth leading cause of death in the United States.
- An estimated 14.6 million Americans have been diagnosed with diabetes, and about 6 million additional Americans have the disease but remain undiagnosed.
- Diabetes is the leading cause of blindness among adults between 20 and 74 years of age.
- Of American Indians and Alaska Natives who are at least 20 years old and receive care from the Indian Health Service, 14.9% have diabetes. On average, American Indians and Alaska Natives are 2.3 times as likely to have diabetes as non-Hispanic whites of similar age.
- Of non-Hispanic blacks aged 20 years or older, 1.4% have diabetes. On average, non-Hispanic blacks are 1.6 times as likely to have diabetes as non-Hispanic whites of a similar age.
- Of non-Hispanic whites aged 20 years or older, 8.4% have diabetes.
- Of Hispanics aged 20 years or older, 8.2% have diabetes. On average, Hispanic Americans are 1.5 times more likely to have diabetes as non-Hispanic whites of similar age.
- Native Hawaiians and Japanese and Filipino residents of Hawaii aged 20 years or older are twice as likely to have diabetes as white residents of Hawaii.
- Direct medical and indirect expenditures attributable to diabetes in 2002 were estimated at $132 billion, with direct medical expenditures alone totaling $91.8 billion.
- Individuals can reduce the risk of diabetes by 50 to 70% by reducing their body weight by 5 to 7% and exercising at a moderate intensity for about 150 minutes weekly.

Summary

1. Atoms provide the basic building blocks of all matter and play the major role in the composition of food nutrients and biologically active substances.

2. Carbon, hydrogen, oxygen, and nitrogen serve as the primary structural units for most of the body's biologically active substances. Specific combinations of carbon with oxygen and hydrogen form carbohydrates and lipids. Proteins consist of combinations of carbon, oxygen, and hydrogen, with nitrogen and minerals.

3. Simple sugars consist of chains of 3 to 7 carbon atoms, with hydrogen and oxygen in the ratio of 2:1. Glucose, the most common simple sugar, contains a 6-carbon chain: $C_6H_{12}O_6$.

4. There are three kinds of carbohydrates: monosaccharides (sugars such as glucose and fructose), disaccharides (combinations of two monosaccharides as in sucrose, lactose, and maltose), and oligosaccharides (3 to 9 glucose residues). Polysaccharides that contain 10 or more simple sugars form starch and fiber in plants and glycogen, the large glucose polymer in animals.

5. Glycogenolysis reconverts glycogen to glucose, whereas gluconeogenesis synthesizes glucose predominantly from the carbon skeletons of amino acids.

6. The two basic starch configurations are (1) amylose, consisting of a long, straight chain of glucose units; and (2) amylopectin, constructed from a highly branched mono-

Summary *continued*

saccharide linkage. The "digestibility" of a starch-containing food depends on the predominance of one starch form or the other.

7. Fiber, a nonstarch structural plant polysaccharide, resists human digestive enzymes. Technically not a nutrient, water-soluble and water-insoluble dietary fibers confer health benefits for gastrointestinal functioning and reduce cardiovascular disease risks.

8. Heart disease and obesity protection may relate to dietary fiber's regulatory role in favorably reducing insulin secretion by slowing nutrient absorption in the small intestine following a meal.

9. Americans typically consume 40 to 50% of total calories as carbohydrates. Greater sugar intake in the form of sweets (simple sugars) occurs commonly in the population with possibly harmful effects for glucose-insulin regulation, cardiovascular disease, and obesity.

10. Physically active men and women should consume about 60% of daily calories as carbohydrates (400–600 g), pre-

dominantly in unrefined complex form. During intense training and prolonged physical activities, carbohydrate intake should increase to 70% of total calories or 8 to 10 g per kg of body weight.

11. Frequent and excessive consumption of carbohydrates with a high glycemic index may alter the metabolic profile and increase risk for the metabolic syndrome of obesity, insulin resistance, glucose intolerance, dyslipidemia, and hypertension.

12. Carbohydrates stored in limited quantity in liver and muscles (1) serve as a major source of energy, (2) spare protein breakdown for energy, (3) function as a metabolic primer for fat metabolism, and (4) provide fuel for the central nervous system.

13. A carbohydrate-deficient diet rapidly depletes muscle and liver glycogen This profoundly affects high-intensity anaerobic and long-duration aerobic exercise capacity.

Lipids

NATURE OF LIPIDS

Lipid (from the Greek *lipos,* meaning fat), the general term for a heterogeneous group of compounds, includes oils, fats, and waxes and related compounds. Oils become liquid at room temperature, whereas fats remain solid. A lipid molecule contains the same structural elements as carbohydrate except that it differs markedly in its linkage of atoms. Specifically, the lipid's ratio of hydrogen to oxygen considerably exceeds that of carbohydrate. For example, the formula $C_{57}H_{110}O_6$ describes the common lipid stearin, with an H to O ratio of 18.3:1; for carbohydrate, the ratio is 2:1. Approximately 98% of dietary lipids exist as triacylglycerols, while about 90% of the body's total fat resides in the adipose tissue depots of the subcutaneous tissues.

KINDS AND SOURCES OF LIPIDS

Plants and animals contain lipids in long hydrocarbon chains. Lipids are generally greasy to touch and remain insoluble in water but soluble in organic solvents such as ether, chloroform, and benzene. According to common classification, lipids belong to one of three main groups: **simple lipids, compound lipids,** and **derived lipids.** TABLE 1.6 lists the general classification for lipids, with specific examples of each form.

Simple Lipids

The simple lipids, or "neutral fats," consist primarily of **tri-acylglycerols,** the most plentiful fats in the body. They constitute the major storage form of fat in adipose (fat) cells. This

TABLE 1.6	General Classification of Lipids
Type of Lipid	**Example**
I. Simple lipids	
Neutral fats	Triglycerides (triacylglycerols)
Waxes	Beeswax
II. Compound lipids	
Phospholipids	Lecithins, cephalins, lipositols
Glycolipids	Cerebrosides, gangliosides
Lipoproteins	Chylomicrons, very low-density lipoproteins (VLDLs), low-density lipoproteins (LDLs), high-density lipoproteins (HDLs)
III. Derived lipids	
Fatty acids	Palmitic acid, oleic acid, stearic acid, linoleic acid
Steroids	Cholesterol, ergosterol, cortisol, bile acids, vitamin D, estrogens, progesterone, androgens
Hydrocarbons	Terpenes

molecule consists of two different clusters of atoms. One cluster, **glycerol,** consists of a 3-carbon alcohol molecule that by itself does not qualify as a lipid because of its high solubility in water. Three clusters of carbon-chained atoms, usually in even number, termed **fatty acids,** attach to the glycerol molecule. Fatty acids consist of straight hydrocarbon chains with as few as 4 carbon atoms or more than 20 in their chain, although chain lengths of 16 and 18 carbons prevail.

Three molecules of water form when glycerol and fatty acids join in the synthesis (**condensation**) of the triacylglycerol molecule. Conversely, during hydrolysis, when the fat molecule cleaves into its constituents by the action of **lipase enzymes,** three molecules of water attach at the point where the molecule splits. FIGURE 1.9 illustrates the basic structure of **saturated fatty acid** and **unsaturated fatty acid** molecules. All lipid-containing foods consist of a mixture of different proportions of saturated and unsaturated fatty acids. Fatty acids get their name because the organic acid (COOH) molecule forms part of their chemical structure.

Saturated Fatty Acids

A saturated fatty acid contains only single covalent bonds between carbon atoms; all of the remaining bonds attach to hydrogen. The fatty acid molecule is referred to as saturated because it holds as many hydrogen atoms as chemically possible.

Saturated fatty acids occur primarily in animal products such as beef (52% saturated fatty acids), lamb, pork, chicken, and egg yolk and in dairy fats of cream, milk, butter (62% saturated fatty acids), and cheese. Saturated fatty acids from the plant kingdom include coconut and palm oil (liquid at room temperature because they have short fatty acid chains), veg-

etable shortening, and hydrogenated margarine; commercially prepared cakes, pies, and cookies also contain plentiful amounts of these fatty acids.

Unsaturated Fatty Acids

Unsaturated fatty acids contain one or more double bonds along the main carbon chain. Each double bond reduces the number of potential hydrogen-binding sites; therefore, the molecule remains unsaturated relative to hydrogen. A **monounsaturated fatty acid** contains one double bond along the main carbon chain. Examples include canola oil, olive oil (77% monounsaturated fatty acids), peanut oil, and the oil in almonds, pecans, and avocados. A **polyunsaturated fatty acid** contains two or more double bonds along the main carbon chain; safflower, sunflower, soybean, and corn oil serve as examples.

Fatty acids from plant sources are generally unsaturated and tend to liquefy at room temperature. Lipids with longer (more carbons in the chain) and more saturated fatty acids remain solid at room temperature, whereas those with shorter and more unsaturated fatty acids stay soft. Oils exist as liquid and contain unsaturated fatty acids. **Hydrogenation** changes oils to semisolid compounds. This chemical process bubbles liquid hydrogen into vegetable oil, which reduces double bonds in the unsaturated fatty acid to single bonds to capture more hydrogen atoms along the carbon chain. This creates firmer fat because adding hydrogen to the carbons increases the lipid's melting temperature. Hydrogenated oil thus behaves as a saturated fat. The most common hydrogenated fats include lard substitutes and margarine.

Triacylglycerol Formation

FIGURE 1.10 outlines the sequence of reactions in triacylglycerol synthesis, a process termed **esterification.** Initially, a fatty acid substrate attached to coenzyme A forms fatty acyl-CoA that transfers to glycerol (as glycerol 3-phosphate). In subsequent reactions, two additional fatty acyl-CoAs link to a single glycerol backbone as the composite triacylglycerol molecule forms. Triacylglycerol synthesis increases following a meal for the following two reasons: (1) increased blood levels of fatty acids and glucose from food absorption and (2) a relatively high level of circulating insulin, which facilitates triaclyglycerol synthesis.

Butter Versus Margarine: A Health Risk in *Trans* Fatty Acids

One cannot distinguish butter and margarine by caloric content but rather by their fatty acid composition. Butter contains about 62% saturated fatty acids (which dramatically raise LDL cholesterol) compared with 20% in margarine. During manufacturing, margarine and other vegetable shortenings such as unsaturated corn, soybean, or sunflower oil become partially hydrogenated. This process rearranges the chemical structure of the original polyunsaturated oil. The lipid remains hardened (saturated), but not as hard as butter. A ***trans*** **unsaturated fatty acid** forms in margarine when one of the hydrogen atoms along the restructured carbon chain moves from its naturally occurring *cis* position to the oppo-

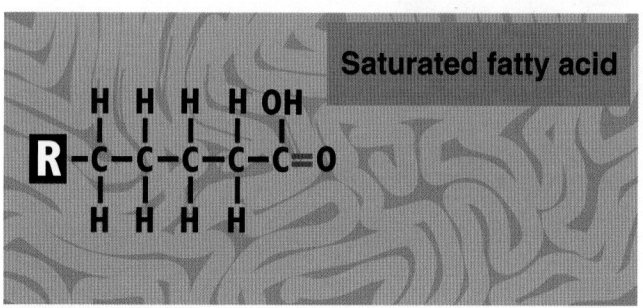

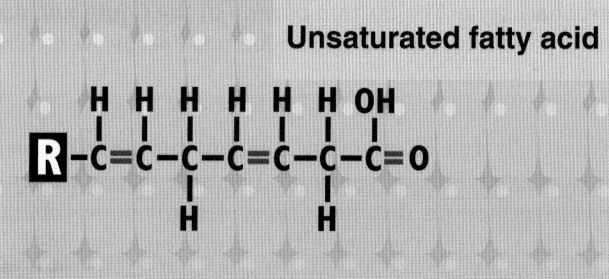

FIGURE 1.9 ■ The presence or absence of double bonds between the carbon atoms constitutes the major structural difference between saturated and unsaturated fatty acids. **R** represents the glycerol portion of the triacylglycerol molecule.

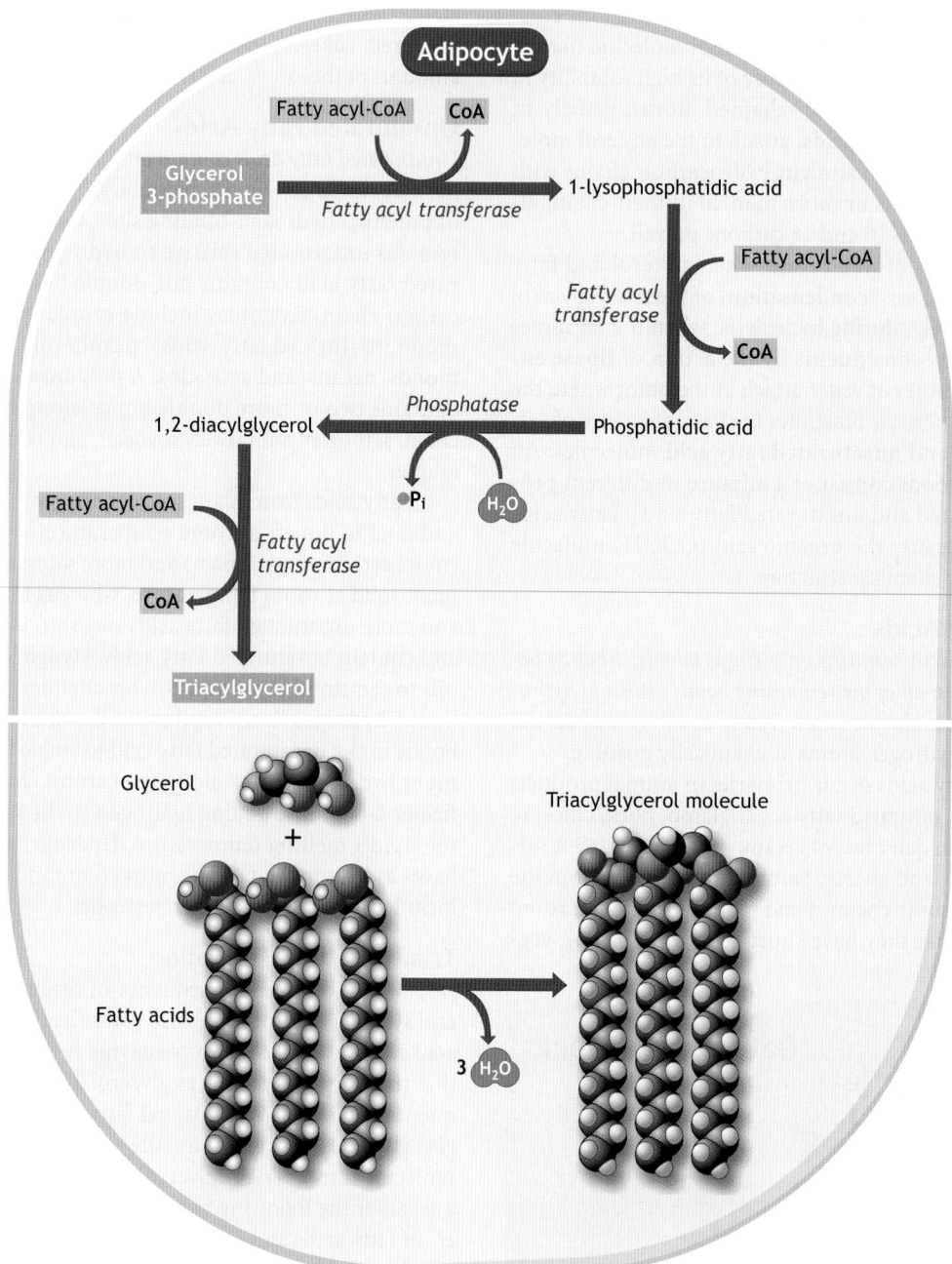

FIGURE 1.10 ■ *Top,* Triacylglycerol formation in adiopocytes (and muscle) tissue involves a series of reactions (dehydration synthesis) that link three fatty acid molecules to a single glycerol backbone. The *bottom portion* of the figure summarizes this linkage. (Reprinted with permission from McArdle W, Katch F, and Katch V. *Exercise Physiology Energy, Nutrition, and Human Performance.* 6th ed. Baltimore: Lippincott Williams & Wilkins, 2007:22.)

site side of the double bond that separates two carbon atoms (*trans* position). Although *trans* fatty acids are close in structure to most unsaturated fatty acids, the opposing hydrogens on its carbon chain make the physical properties similar to those of saturated fatty acids. Seventeen to twenty-five percent of margarine's fatty acids exist as *trans* unsaturated fatty acids, compared with only 7% in butterfat. Many popular fast foods contain considerably high levels of *trans* fats.[105] A serving of French fries can contain up to 3.6 g of *trans* fat, and doughnuts and pound cake can have 4.3 g. (Liquid vegetable oils normally have no *trans* fatty acids, but they are sometimes added to extend the oil's shelf life.) Because margarine consists of vegetable oil, it contains no cholesterol; butter, on the other hand, originates from a dairy source and contains between 11 and 15 mg of cholesterol per teaspoon. *Trans* fatty acids represent about 5 to 10% of the fat in the typical American diet.

A diet high in margarine and commercial baked goods and deep-fried foods prepared with hydrogenated (hardened) vegetable oils increases LDL cholesterol concentrations by about the same amount as a diet high in saturated fatty acids. Unlike saturated fats, hydrogenated oils decrease the beneficial HDL cholesterol concentration and adversely affect markers of inflammation and endothelial dysfunction.[48,67,74,80,82] *Trans* fatty acids also elevate plasma levels of triacylglycerols and may impair arterial wall flexibility and function.

Dietary *trans* fatty acids account for 30,000 deaths annually from heart disease.[117] In addition, a prospective study of more than 84,204 healthy middle-aged women demonstrated that diets high in *trans* fatty acids promote resistance to insulin, increasing the risk for type 2 diabetes.[97] Women with high tissue levels of *trans* fatty acids are also 40% more likely than those with the lowest levels to develop breast cancer.

Trans Fat on the Label: When Zero does not Mean Zero

Food labels must now contain the quantity of *trans* fatty acids a food contains. Be aware, however, that if the label indicates zero it does not necessarily indicate the absence of *trans* fat because the government allows 0.5 g to still be considered zero.

Lipids in the Diet

FIGURE 1.11 shows the approximate percentage contribution of some common food groups to the total lipid content of the typical American diet. Plants generally contribute about 34% to the daily lipid intake; the remaining 66% comes from animal sources.

The average person in the United States consumes about 15% of total calories (over 50 lb yearly) as saturated fats. The relationship between saturated fatty acid intake and coronary

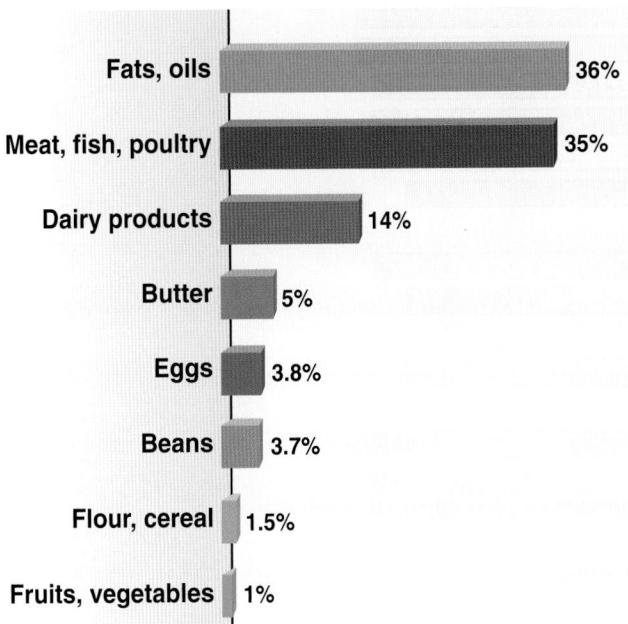

FIGURE 1.11 ■ The major food source's contribution to the lipid content of the typical American diet.

heart disease risk has prompted nutritionists and medical personnel to recommend replacing at least a portion of the saturated fatty acids and nearly all *trans* fatty acids in the diet with nonhydrogenated monounsaturated and polyunsaturated fatty acids.[13,85] Consuming both forms of unsaturated fatty acids lowers coronary risk even below normal levels. From a public health perspective, individuals are advised to consume no more than 10% of total energy intake as saturated fatty acids (about 250 kCal or 25 to 30 g per day for the average young adult male) and all lipid intake to less than 30% of total calories.

FISH OILS (AND FISH) ARE HEALTHFUL. Studies of the health profiles of Greenland Eskimos, who consume large quantities of lipid from fish, seal, and whale yet have a low incidence of coronary heart disease, indicated the potential for two essential long-chain polyunsaturated fatty acids to confer diverse health benefits. These oils, eicosapentaenoic acid (EPA) and docosahexaenoic acid (DHA), belong to an **omega-3** family of fatty acids (also termed n-3, characterized by the presence of a double bond 3 carbons from the n end of the molecule) found primarily in the oils of shellfish and cold-water herring, salmon, sardines, bluefish, and mackerel and sea mammals. Plant sources for α-linolenic acid, another omega-3 oil and precursor of EPA and DHA, include dark green leafy vegetables and flax, hemp, canola, soy, and walnut oils.

Regular fish intake (two meals a week) and fish oil exert multiple physiologic effects that protect against coronary artery disease.[28,54] It may benefit one's lipid profile (particularly plasma triacylglycerol),[57,98,103] overall heart disease risk (particularly risk of ventricular fibrillation and sudden death),[24,49,50,62,122] inflammatory disease risk,[12,19] and (for smokers) risk of contracting chronic obstructive pulmonary disease.[100] A long-term study of employees of the Western Electric Company in Chicago noted a reduction of 42% in heart attacks among men who ate 7 oz or more of fish a week compared with men who rarely ate fish.[22] This benefit from regular yet moderate fish intake remained even when considering numerous other factors known to affect heart disease risk. Omega-3 fish oils, particularly DHA, may also prove beneficial in treating diverse psychological disorders and Alzheimer's disease. The intake of fish and marine fatty acids probably does not reduce cancer risk.[69,108]

Several mechanisms explain how eating fish—with its additional cardioprotective nutrients of selenium, various natural antioxidants, and protein not present in fish oil—protects against death from heart disease. Fish oil may act as an antithrombogenic agent to prevent blood clot formation on arterial walls. It also may inhibit the growth of atherosclerotic plaques, reduce pulse pressure and total vascular resistance (increase arterial compliance), and stimulate endothelial-derived nitric oxide to facilitate myocardial perfusion.[19,84] The oil's lowering effect on triacylglycerol also confers protection because plasma triacylglycerol level strongly predicts coronary heart disease risk.[27] On the negative side, elevation in atherogenic LDL cholesterol may accompany the triacylglycerol-lowering effect of fish oil supplements.[41] For men with moderate hypercholesterolemia, daily supplements of 12 g of fish oil in capsule form for 12 weeks decreased triacylglycerols by 37.3%, reduced total cholesterol by 11.5%, but increased harmful LDL cholesterol by 8.5%.

Perhaps the most powerful cardioprotective benefit of fish oils relates to their antiarrhythmic effect on myocardial tissue.[2,18] This protection against ventricular arrhythmias occurs from the unique effects of dietary n-3 fatty acids on the respective n-3 fatty acid content of the myocardial cell membranes. In the event of severe physiologic stress (e.g., ischemic attack from reduced myocardial blood flow), the n-3 fatty acids in the cell membrane are released and locally protect the myocardium from the development and propagation of a rapid heart rate (tachycardia), which often causes cardiac arrest and sudden death.

ALL LIPID INTAKE IN MODERATION. In the quest for good health and optimal exercise performance, prudent practice entails cooking with and consuming lipids derived primarily from vegetable sources. This approach may be too simplistic, however, because total saturated *and* unsaturated fatty acid intake may constitute a risk for diabetes and heart disease. If so, then one should reduce the intake of all lipids, particularly lipids high in saturated fatty acids and *trans* fatty acids. Concerns also exist over the association of high-fat diets with ovarian, colon, endometrial, and other cancers.

FIGURE 1.12 lists the saturated, monounsaturated, and polyunsaturated fatty acid content of various sources of dietary lipid. All fats contain a mix of each fatty acid type, although different fatty acids predominate in certain lipid sources. In foods, α-linolenic acid is the major omega-3 fatty acid; linoleic acid is the major omega-6 fatty acid; and oleic acid is the major omega-9 fatty acid. These fatty acids provide components for vital body structures, perform important roles in immune function and vision, help form and maintain the integrity of plasma membranes, and produce hormone-like compounds called eicosanoids.

One can obtain omega-3 and omega-6 polyunsaturated fatty acids (abundant in most vegetable oils except tropical ones) only through the diet. Because of their role as precursors of other fatty acids that the body cannot synthesize, they have been termed **essential fatty acids.** About 1 to 2% of the total energy intake should come from linoleic acid. For a 2500-kCal intake, this corresponds to about 1 tablespoon of plant oil per day. Mayonnaise, cooking oils, and salad dressings, whole grains, vegetables, and other foods readily provide this amount. Fatty fish (salmon, tuna, or sardines) or canola, soybean, safflower, sunflower, sesame, and flax oils provide the best sources for α-linolenic acid or its related omega-3 fatty acids, EPA and DHA.

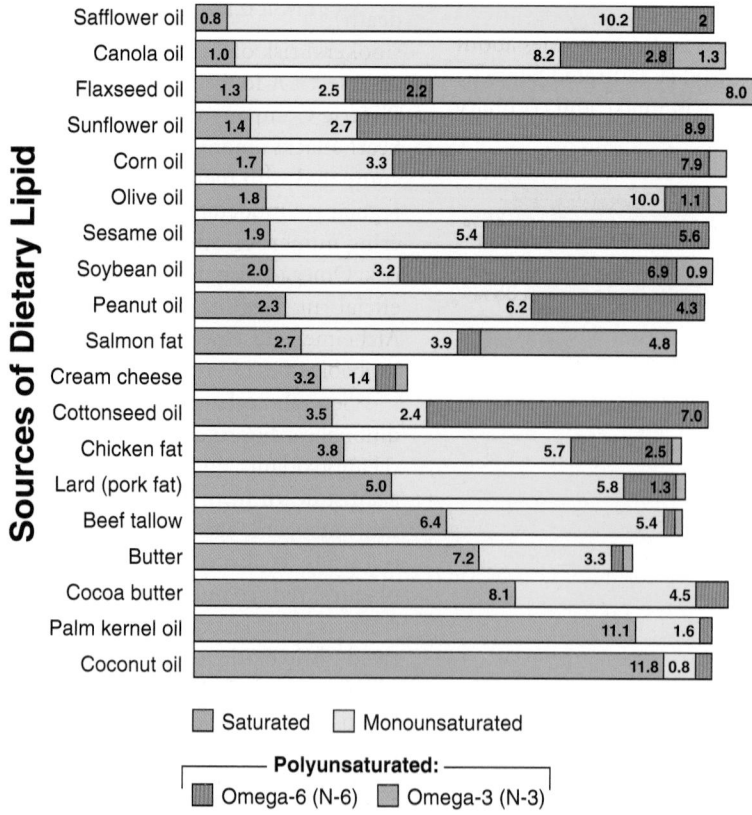

**Fatty Acid Content
(grams per tablespoon)**

FIGURE 1.12 ■ Saturated, monounsaturated, and polyunsaturated fatty acid content of various sources of dietary lipid.

Lipids: The Good, the Bad, and the Ugly

Subjective terms describe the impact of the various forms of fatty acids in the diet. Unsaturated fatty acids, which contain one (monounsaturated) or more (polyunsaturated) double bonds along their main carbon chain, classify as desirable in that they lower blood cholesterol, particularly the harmful LDL cholesterol. In contrast, consumption of saturated fatty acids, which contain only single bonds between carbon atoms, stimulates the liver's production of LDL cholesterol. Even more disturbing, the consumption of partially hydrogenated unsaturated vegetable oils to produce *trans* fatty acids not only increases LDL concentrations but also lowers the beneficial HDL cholesterol.

Compound Lipids

Compound lipids consist of a triacylglycerol molecule combined with other chemicals and represent about 10% of the body's total fat. One group of modified triacylglycerols, the **phospholipids,** contains one or more fatty acid molecules combined with a phosphorus-containing group and a nitrogenous base. These lipids form in all cells, although the liver synthesizes most of them. The phosphorus part of the phospholipids within the plasma membrane bilayer attracts water (hydrophilic), whereas the lipid portion repels water (hydrophobic). Thus, phospholipids interact with water and lipid to modulate fluid movement across cell membranes. Phospholipids also maintain the structural integrity of the cell, play an important role in blood clotting, and provide structural integrity to the insulating sheath around nerve fibers. **Lecithin,** the most widely distributed phospholipid in food sources (liver, egg yolk, wheat germ, nuts, soybeans), functions in fatty acid and cholesterol transport and use. Lecithin does not qualify as an essential nutrient because the body manufactures the required amount.

Other compound lipids include **glycolipids** (fatty acids bound with carbohydrate and nitrogen) and water-soluble **lipoproteins** (formed primarily in the liver when protein joins with either triacylglycerols or phospholipids). *Lipoproteins provide the major avenue for lipid transport in the blood.* If blood lipids did not bind to protein, they literally would float to the top like cream in nonhomogenized fresh milk.

High- and Low-Density-Lipoprotein Cholesterol

FIGURE 1.13 illustrates the general dynamics of dietary cholesterol and the lipoproteins, including their transport among the small intestine, liver, and peripheral tissues. Four types of lipoproteins exist according to gravitational density. **Chylomicrons** form when emulsified lipid droplets (including long-chain triacylglycerols, phospholipids, and free fatty acids) leave the intestine and enter the lymphatic vasculature. Under normal conditions, the liver metabolizes chylomicrons and sends them for storage in adipose tissue. Chylomicrons also transport the fat-soluble vitamins A, D, E, and K.

Lipoproteins: Particle Size Matters

Cholesterol is transported on a family of lipid-carrying proteins termed *lipoproteins.* The lipoprotein's protein component determines its behavior—whether it stimulates plaque development, extracts cholesterol from plaque, or passes to the liver for disposal.

LDL: LDL is made up of various-sized particles that differ in their potential to cause heart disease. The size difference in LDL particles is crucial in predicting heart disease risk, with small particles (high number) being the most destructive. Thus, heart attack can occur when the LDL particle number (number of LDL particles in 1 mL of blood) is high despite a relatively low LDL level. LDL is generally measured indirectly as apoprotein B, the major protein particle of LDL. Because a single apoprotein B links to an LDL particle, apoprotein B level indicates LDL particle number. Small LDL particles wreak maximum arterial damage because they effectively penetrate arterial walls. When oxidized, they promote release of inflammatory and adhesive proteins to enhance the atherogenic process. Estimates indicate that a large number of small LDL particles triple heart disease risk.

HDL: A family of HDL particles make up total HDL, with the beneficial HDL being the larger HDL_{2b} component responsible for reverse cholesterol transport, which extracts cholesterol from plaque.

The liver and small intestine produce **HDL.** HDL contains the greatest percentage of protein (about 50%) and the least total lipid (about 20%) and cholesterol (about 20%) compared with the other lipoproteins. Degradation of a **very low-density lipoprotein (VLDL)** produces an **LDL.** VLDL, formed in the liver from fats, carbohydrates, alcohol, and cholesterol, contains the greatest percentage of lipid (95%), of which about 60% consists of triacylglycerol. VLDL transports triacylglycerols to muscle and adipose tissue. Action of the enzyme **lipoprotein lipase** produces a denser LDL molecule because now it contains less lipid. LDL and VLDL have the most lipid and least protein components.

"BAD" CHOLESTEROL. Among the lipoproteins, LDL, which normally carries between 60 and 80% of the total serum cholesterol, has the greatest affinity for cells of the arterial wall. LDL delivers cholesterol to arterial tissue, where LDL oxidizes and participates in the proliferation of smooth muscle cells and other unfavorable changes that damage and narrow arteries. Regular aerobic exercise, visceral fat accumulation, and the diet's macronutrient composition all affect serum LDL concentrations.

"GOOD" CHOLESTEROL. Unlike LDL, HDL protects against heart disease. HDL acts as a scavenger in the **reverse transport of cholesterol** by removing cholesterol from the arterial wall. It then delivers it to the liver for incorporation into bile and subsequent excretion via the intestinal tract.

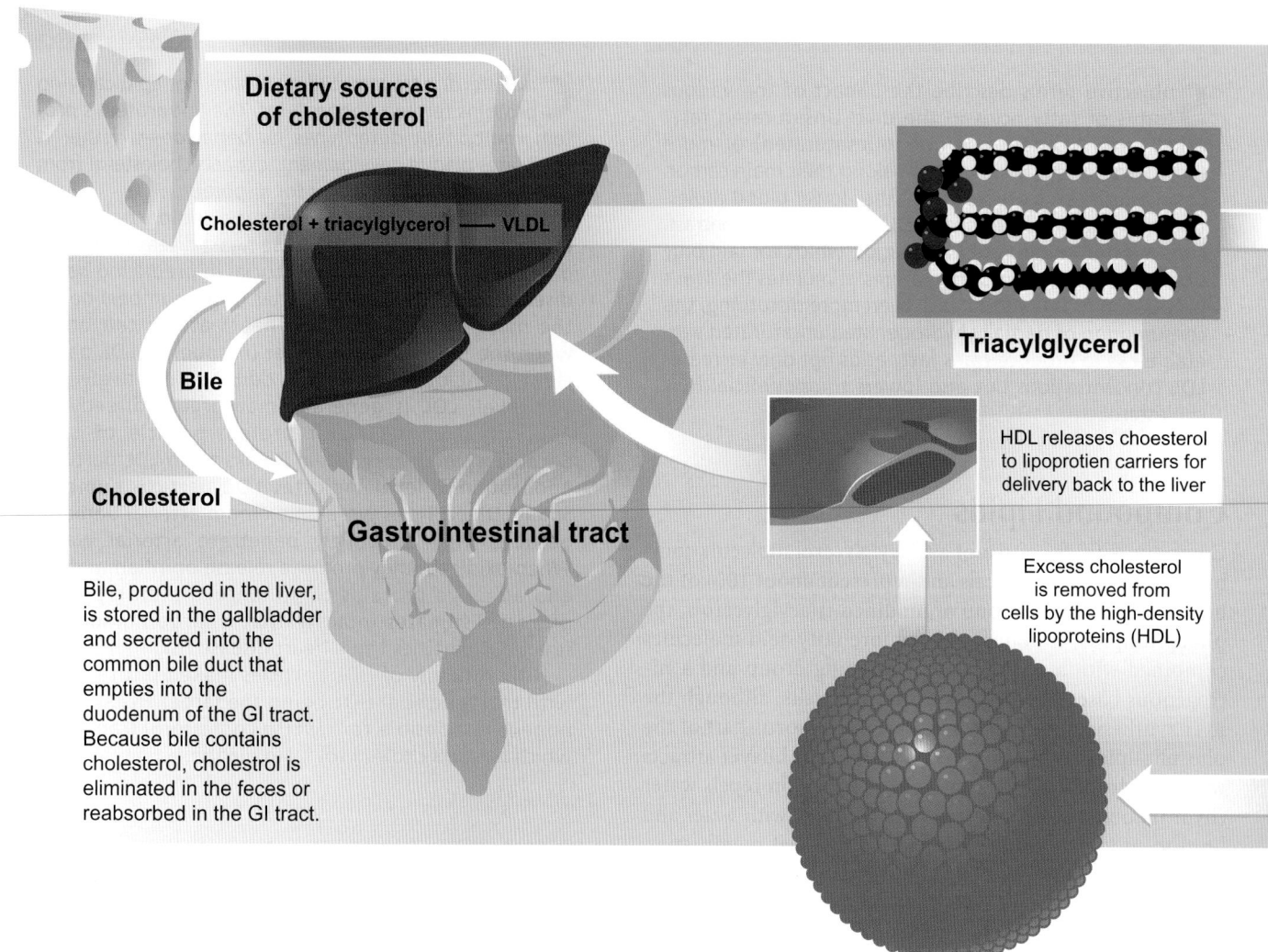

Dietary sources of cholesterol

Cholesterol + triacylglycerol ——— VLDL

Bile

Cholesterol

Gastrointestinal tract

Triacylglycerol

HDL releases choesterol to lipoprotien carriers for delivery back to the liver

Excess cholesterol is removed from cells by the high-density lipoproteins (HDL)

Bile, produced in the liver, is stored in the gallbladder and secreted into the common bile duct that empties into the duodenum of the GI tract. Because bile contains cholesterol, cholestrol is eliminated in the feces or reabsorbed in the GI tract.

FIGURE 1.13 ■ General interaction between dietary cholesterol and the lipoproteins and their transport among the small intestine, liver, and peripheral tissues.

The amount of LDL and HDL cholesterol and their specific ratios (e.g., HDL ÷ total cholesterol) and subfractions provide more meaningful indicators of coronary artery disease risk than does total cholesterol alone. Regular aerobic exercise and abstinence from cigarette smoking increase HDL, lower LDL, and favorably alter the LDL ÷ HDL ratio.[56,63,104,119]

Check It Out

An online computer program calculates the risk and the appropriate cholesterol levels for adults (www.nhlbi.nih.gov/guidelines/cholesterol/index.htm).

Derived Lipids

Derived lipids form from simple and compound lipids. Unlike the neutral fats and phospholipids with hydrocarbon chains, derived lipids contain hydrocarbon rings. *Cholesterol, the most widely known derived lipid, exists only in animal tissue.* The chemical structure of cholesterol provides the backbone for synthesizing all of the body's steroid compounds (e.g., bile salts, vitamin D, sex hormones, and adrenocortical hormones). Cholesterol does not contain fatty acids but shares some of the physical and chemical characteristics of lipids. Thus, from a dietary viewpoint, cholesterol is considered a lipid.

Cholesterol, widespread in the plasma membrane of all cells, is obtained either through the diet (**exogenous cholesterol**) or through cellular synthesis (**endogenous cholesterol**).

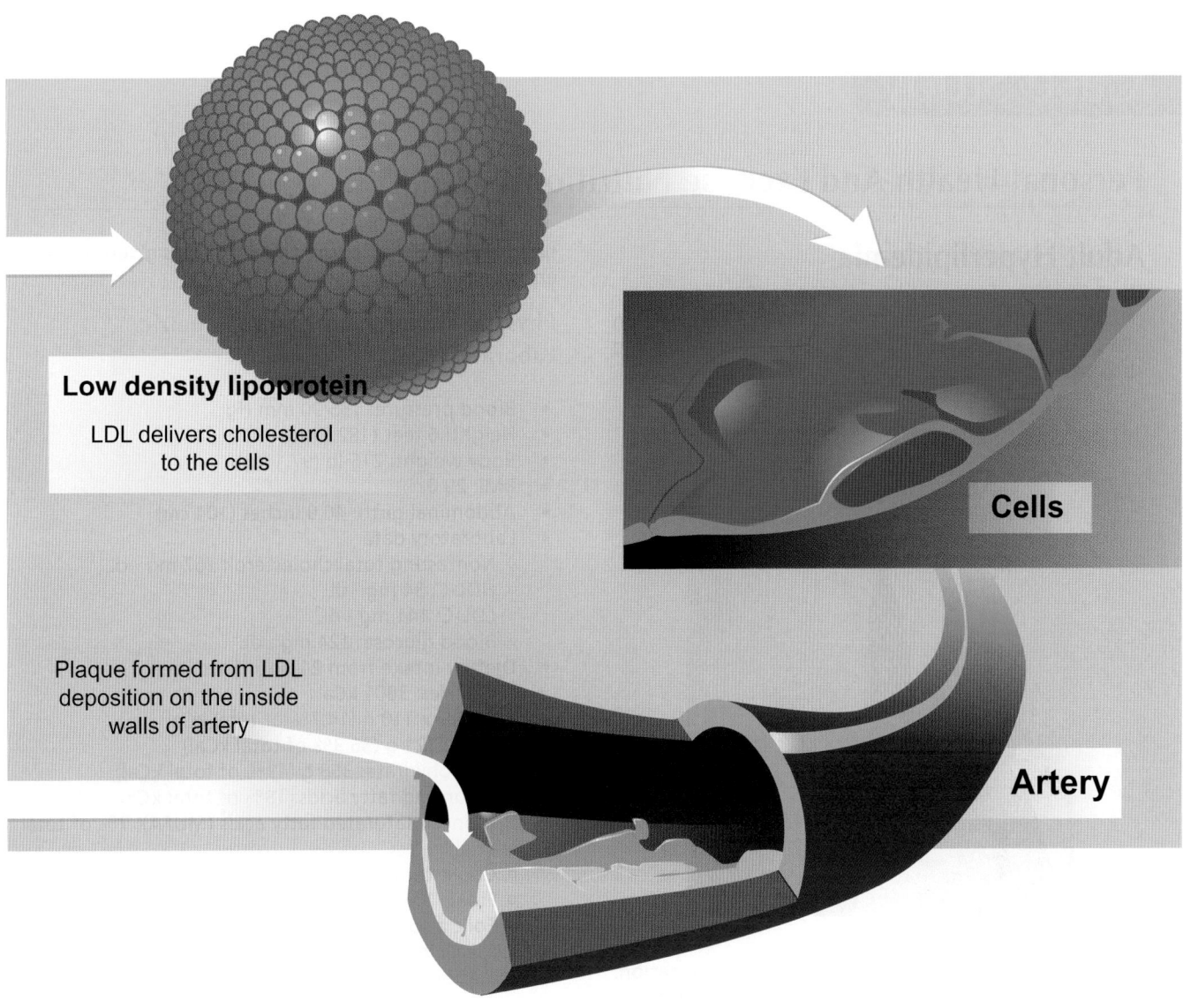

Low density lipoprotein

LDL delivers cholesterol
to the cells

Cells

Plaque formed from LDL
deposition on the inside
walls of artery

Artery

FIGURE 1.13 ■ *continued*

Even if an individual maintains a "cholesterol-free" diet, endogenous cholesterol synthesis varies between 0.5 and 2.0 g per day. More endogenous cholesterol forms with a diet high in saturated fatty acids, which facilitate cholesterol synthesis by the liver.[25,26] Although the liver synthesizes about 70% of the body's cholesterol, other tissues—including the walls of the arteries and intestines—also synthesize it. The rate of endogenous synthesis usually meets the body's needs; hence, severely reducing cholesterol intake, except in pregnant women and infants, probably causes little harm.

Functions of Cholesterol

Cholesterol participates in many complex bodily functions, including building plasma membranes and as a precursor in synthesizing vitamin D and adrenal gland hormones, as well as the sex hormones estrogen, androgen, and progesterone. Cholesterol provides a crucial component for the synthesis of bile, which emulsifies lipids during digestion and plays an important role in forming tissues, organs, and body structures during fetal development.

TABLE 1.7 presents the cholesterol content per serving of common foods from meat and dairy sources. Egg yolk contributes a rich source of cholesterol, as do red meats and organ meats (liver, kidney, and brains). Shellfish, particularly shrimp, and dairy products (ice cream, cream cheese, butter, and whole milk) contain relatively large amounts of cholesterol. Foods of plant origin contain *no* cholesterol.

Cholesterol and Heart Disease

Powerful predictors of coronary artery disease include high levels of total serum cholesterol and the cholesterol-rich LDL molecule. The risk becomes particularly apparent when combined with other risk factors such as cigarette smoking, physical inactivity, obesity, and untreated hypertension. A continuous and graded relationship exists between serum cholesterol and death from coronary artery disease; thus, low-

Case Study

Personal Health And Exercise Nutrition 1–2

Adult Hyperlipidemia

The following data were obtained on a 58-year-old executive who has not had an annual physical examination in 5 years. He has gained weight and is now concerned about his health status.

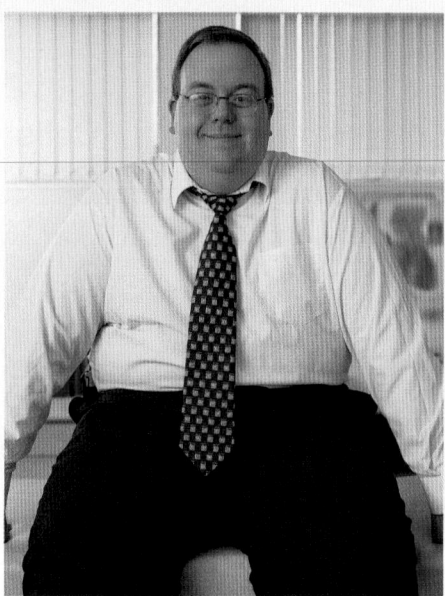

Medical History
No history of chronic diseases or major hospitalization. He does not take medications or dietary supplements and has no known food allergies.

Family History
Father died from a heart attack at age 61; his younger brother has had triple bypass surgery, and his uncle has type 2 diabetes. His mother, physically inactive for most of her adult life, classifies as obese with high serum cholesterol and triacylglycerol levels.

Social History
Overweight since high school. He has gained 15 lb during the last year, which he attributes to his job and changes in eating habits (eats out more frequently). J.M. wants to improve his diet but does not know what to do. He typically eats only two meals daily, with at least one meal consumed at a restaurant and several snacks interspersed. He drinks three to five cups of coffee throughout the day and two to three alcoholic drinks every evening. He also smokes one pack of cigarettes daily and reports high stress in his job and at home (two teenage children). Patient states he has little opportu-

nity for exercise or leisure time activities given his present schedule.

Physical Examination/Anthropometric/Laboratory Data

- Blood pressure: 135/90 mm Hg
- Height: 6 feet (182.9 cm)
- Body weight: 215 lb (97.1 kg)
- BMI: 29.0
- Abdominal girth: 40.9 inches (104 cm)
- Laboratory data
  - Nonfasting total cholesterol: 267 mg · dL^{-1}
  - HDL-C: 34 mg · dL^{-1}
  - LDL-C: 141 mg · dL^{-1}
  - Blood glucose: 124 mg · dL^{-1}
- Dietary intake from 24-hour food recall
  - Calories: 3001 kCal
  - Protein: 110 g (14.7% of total kCal)
  - Lipid: 121 g (36.3% of total kCal)
  - Carbohydrate: 368 g (49% of total kCal)
  - Saturated fatty acids: 18% of total kCal
  - Monounsaturated fatty acids (MUFA): 7% of total kCal
  - Cholesterol: 390 mg · dL^{-1}
  - Fiber: 10 g
  - Folic acid: 200 µg
- General impressions: overly fat male with possible metabolic syndrome

Case Questions

1. Provide an overall assessment of patient's health status.
2. What other laboratory tests could be performed?
3. Interpret the blood lipid profile based on his history, physical examination, and laboratory data.
4. Give recommendations for improving the adequacy of patient's diet.
5. Create the best dietary approach for the patient.
6. What course of action should the patient consider to improve his blood lipid profile?

Answers

1. Based on available data it appears that the patient is hypercholesterolemic (elevated cholesterol, low HDL-C, elevated LDL-C) and perhaps prediabetic (elevated blood glucose) with a high risk for coronary

heart disease (elevated cholesterol; elevated glucose; elevated diastolic blood pressure; high BMI; family history of chronic disease and larger than normal abdominal girth). According to the National Cholesterol Education Program (NCEP; www.nhlbi.nih. gov/guidelines/cholesterol/index.htm), all adults age 20 and older should have cholesterol and HDL cholesterol measured at least every 5 years. Perform a fasting blood lipid profile when cholesterol exceeds 240 mg · dL^{-1}.

2. A fasting lipid profile is warranted on the basis of his cholesterol level and number of risk factors. The fasting blood sample should include total triacylglycerol level. Additionally, plasma homocysteine and lipoprotein (a) levels should be measured based on the family history of heart disease. Perform a fasting blood glucose determination to rule out glucose intolerance or type 2 diabetes.

   The following 12-hour fasting blood profile indicates:
   a. Total cholesterol: 266 mg · dL^{-1} (desirable <200 mg · dL^{-1})
   b. HDL-C: 31 mg · dL^{-1} (desirable >40 mg · dL^{-1})
   c. LDL-C: 150 mg · dL^{-1} (desirable <130 mg · dL^{-1})
   d. Triacylglycerol: 341 mg · dL^{-1} (desirable <150 mg · dL^{-1})
   e. Glucose: 110 mg · dL^{-1} (desirable <100 mg · dL^{-1})
   f. Homocysteine: 8 μmol · L^{-1} (desirable <12 μmol · L^{-1})
   g. Lipoprotein (a): 11 mg · dL^{-1} (desirable <20 mg · dL^{-1})

3. The patient has "combined" hyperlipidemia because both total triacylglycerol and LDL-C levels are higher than normal values for his age. This is sometimes referred to as "familial hyperlipidemia." In such a familial disorder, the diagnosis is based on (1) the combined hyperlipidemia in first-degree family members and (2) the elevated triacylglycerol and LDL-C concentrations. Familial hyperlipidemia represents the most common form of lipid disorder; it exists in 1 out of 100 Americans.

4. The patient's diet does not fall within recommended guidelines, with the following variables exceeding recommended levels: total fat intake (as % of total kCal) versus recommended 30% level; saturated fat versus recommended, 10% of total kCal; cholesterol versus recommended <300 mg · dL^{-1}; fiber versus recommended >30 g · d^{-1}. Daily caloric intake of 3100 kCal is high relative to energy expenditure and pro-

motes excess weight (fat) gain. The patient must reduce daily caloric intake by at least 500 kCal and increase caloric expenditure to a similar extent through moderate physical activity to promote consistent weight loss while preserving fat-free body mass.

5. Recommendations include lowering total cholesterol, LDL-C, and triacylglycerol levels, raising HDL-C levels, and reducing body weight (fat). To achieve these goals, the patient should follow the National Heart, Lung and Blood Institute guidelines for optimizing the blood lipid profile shown in the accompanying table. Translating these guidelines into specific recommendations includes the following: Eat (1) MUFA (up to 15% of total calories) from olive oil, peanuts, avocados, safflower and sunflower oils, cashew nuts; (2) 3 to 5 servings per day of fruits and vegetables; (3) 7 to 8 daily servings of whole grains, beans, and legumes; (4) only nonfat or low-fat dairy products, and chicken (without skin), fish, or lean meats limited to 6 oz per day. Fiber intake also needs to increase to 38 g per day, which should be accomplished by increasing fruit, whole grain, and vegetable intake.

National Cholesterol Education Program Diet Recommendations

Total fat	<30% total kCal
Saturated fat	8–10% total kCal
Polyunsaturated fat	Up to 10% total kCal
Monounsaturated fat	Up to 15% total kCal
Cholesterol	<300 mg/day
Carbohydrate	50–60% total kCal
Protein	10–20% total kCal
Calories	To achieve and maintain desired weight

6. Only after sufficient attempts at lifestyle changes that include dietary modification (see previous discussion) and initiating a regular exercise program (aerobic exercise such as daily walking, cycling, or swimming for 45 to 60 minutes at light-to-moderate intensity) should drug therapy be considered and only as an adjunct and not as a substitute for lifestyle modifications. The patient also requires medical clearance, including an exercise stress test, before starting an exercise program.

Modifiable risk factors include obesity, high-fat diet, sedentary lifestyle, smoking, and excessive alcohol intake. Along with an improved diet and a regular exercise program, he should enroll in a smoking cessation program and limit his alcohol intake. Meeting with a lifestyle management consultant should be encouraged.

TABLE 1.7   Cholesterol Content of Some Common Foods

Food	Quantity	Cholesterol (mg)	Food	Quantity	Cholesterol (mg)
Meat			**Dairy**		
Brains, pan fried	3 oz	1696	Egg salad	1 cup	629
Liver, chicken	3 oz	537	Custard, baked	1 cup	213
Caviar	3 oz	497	Egg, yolk	1 large	211
Liver, beef, fried	3 oz	410	Ice cream, soft	1 cup	153
Spare ribs, cooked	6 oz	198	serve, vanilla		
Shrimp, boiled	3 oz	166	Eggnog	1 cup	149
Tuna, light, water	1 can	93	Ice cream, rich	1 cup	88
pack			Pizza, cheese	1 slice	47
Chicken breast,	3 oz	91	Milk, whole	1 cup	34
fried, no skin			Cottage cheese,	1 cup	34
Halibut, smoked	3 oz	86	large curd		
Lamb chop,	1	84	Cheese, cheddar	1 oz	30
broiled			Milk, low fat, 2%	1 cup	18
Abalone, fried	3 oz	80	Chocolate milk	1 cup	13
Hamburger patty	3 oz	75	shake		
Corned beef	3 oz	73	Butter	1 pat	11
Chicken or turkey,	3 oz	70	Cottage cheese,	1 cup	10
light meat			low-fat 1%		
Lobster, cooked	3 oz	61	Yogurt, low-fat	1 cup	10
Clams	3 oz	57	with fruit		
Taco, beef	1	57	Buttermilk	1 cup	9
Swordfish, broiled	3 oz	50	(>1% fat)		
Bacon strips	3 pieces	36	Milk, skim	1 cup	5
Hot dog	1	29	Mayonnaise	1 Tbsp	5
Hot dog, beef	1	27			
French fries, McDonald's	Regular	13			

ering cholesterol appears to offer prudent heart disease protection. For individuals with heart disease, coronary blood flow improves (thus reducing myocardial ischemia during daily life) in 6 months or less when drug and diet therapy aggressively lower both total blood cholesterol and LDL cholesterol.[5] (For example, drugs called statins reduce cholesterol by up to 60 mg · dL^{-1}.) Studies with animals show that a diet high in cholesterol and saturated fatty acids raises serum cholesterol in "susceptible" animals. This diet combination eventually produces **atherosclerosis,** a degenerative process that forms cholesterol-rich deposits (**plaque**) on the inner lining of medium and large arteries, which narrow and eventually close. In humans, dietary cholesterol raises the ratio of total cholesterol to HDL cholesterol to adversely affect the cholesterol risk profile.[115] In addition, reducing saturated fatty acid and cholesterol intake generally lowers serum cholesterol, although for most people the effect remains modest. Similarly, increasing dietary intake of mono- and polyunsaturated fatty acids lowers blood cholesterol.[95]

Lowering cholesterol reduces heart attack risk and improves survival if a heart attack occurrs.[30,115] These research findings show the wisdom of reducing serum lipids through modifications that curtail intake of cholesterol-rich foods, increase physical activity, and control body weight. TABLE 1.8 presents recommendations of the American Heart Association (AHA, www.americanheart.org) for levels of triacylglycerol, total cholesterol, and LDL and HDL subfractions.

RECOMMENDED DIETARY LIPID INTAKE

Recommendations for dietary lipid intake for physically active individuals follow prudent recommendations for the general population. No firm standards for optimal lipid intake exist. Rather than providing a precise number for daily cholesterol intake, the AHA encourages Americans to focus more on replacing high-fat foods with fruits, vegetables, unrefined whole grains, fat-free and low-fat dairy products, fish, poultry, and lean meat.[55,61,93] Other new components of the AHA guidelines include a focus on weight control and the addition of two weekly servings of fish high in omega-3 fatty acids. The American Cancer Society (www.cancer.org) advocates a diet that contains only 20% of its calories from lipid to reduce risk of cancers of the colon and rectum, prostate, endometrium, and perhaps breast. More drastic lowering of total dietary fat intake toward the 10% level may produce even more pronounced cholesterol-lowering effects, accompanied by clinical improvement for patients with established coronary heart disease.[86]

The AHA has recommended a cholesterol intake of no more than 300 mg (0.01 oz) daily—almost the amount of cholesterol in an egg yolk—limiting intake to 100 mg per 1000 calories of food consumed. More desirable benefits occur by reducing daily cholesterol intake toward 150 to 200 mg. The main sources of dietary cholesterol include the same animal

TABLE 1.8   American Heart Association Recommendations and Classifications for Total Cholesterol and HDL- and LDL-Cholesterol and Triacylglycerol

Category	
Total cholesterol level*	
≥240	High blood cholesterol. A person with this level has more than twice the risk of heart disease a someone with cholesterol below 200.
200–239	Borderline high.
≤200	Desirable level that puts you at a lower risk for heart disease. Cholesterol level of 200 or higher raises risk.
HDL cholesterol level	
<40	Low HDL cholesterol. A major risk factor for heart disease.
40–59	Higher HDL levels are better.
≥60	High HDL cholesterol. An HDL of 60 mg · dL⁻¹ and above is considered protective against heart disease.
LDL cholesterol level	
>190	Very high; cholesterol-lowering drug therapies even if no heart disease and no risk factors.[†]
160–189	High; cholesterol-lowering drug therapies even if there is no heart disease but 2 or more risk factors are present.
130–159	Borderline high; cholesterol-lowering drug therapies if heart disease is present.
100–129	Near optimal; doctor may consider cholesterol-lowering drug therapies plus dietary modification if heart disease is present.
<100	Optimal; no therapy needed.
Triacyglycerol level	
<150	Normal
150–199	Borderline high
200–499	High
≥500	Very high

*All levels in mg · dL⁻¹.

[†]In men under age 35 and premenopausal women with LDL cholesterol levels of 190 to 219 mg · dL⁻¹, drug therapy should be delayed except in high-risk patients such as those with diabetes.

food sources rich in saturated fatty acids. Reducing intake of these foods not only reduces intake of preformed choesterol but also reduces, more importantly, intake of saturated fatty acids that stimulate endogenous cholesterol synthesis.

TABLE 1.9 presents three daily menus, each consisting of 2000 kCal but with different percentages of total lipid. *Meal Plan A,* typical of the North American diet, consists of 38% of total calories from lipid. *Meal Plan B* contains 29% lipid, a value recommended by most health professionals. *Meal Plan C,* with 10% lipid, may be desirable from a health perspective but is difficult to maintain, particularly for physically active individuals with high daily energy expenditures.

Ratio of Polyunsaturated to Saturated Fatty Acids

TABLE 1.10 lists examples of foods high and low in saturated fatty acids, foods high in monounsaturated and polyunsaturated fatty acids, and the ratio of polyunsaturated to saturated fatty acids (**P/S ratio**). One should attempt to maintain the P/S ratio at least at 1:1 and preferably at 2:1. Based on dietary surveys, the P/S ratio in the United States ranges between 0.43 and 1.0. The P/S ratio has some limitations and should not be used exclusively to guide lipid intake. For example, the ratio does not consider the potential cholesterol-lowering role of monounsaturated fatty acids if they replace the diet's satu-

---

TABLE 1.9   Three Different Daily Meal Plans, Each Consisting of 2000 Calories, but with Different Percentages of Total Fat

Plan A. 38% Fat Diet	Plan B. 29% Fat Diet	Plan C. 10% Fat Diet
Breakfast	**Breakfast**	**Breakfast**
1 apple Danish pastry	1 bagel	1/2 cup bran cereal with raisins
1/2 cup orange juice	1 tablespoon cream cheese	1 bagel
1 cup whole milk	1/2 cup orange juice	1 tablespoon cream cheese
	1 cup 1% milk	1/2 cup orange juice
Lunch		1 cup skimmed milk
2 slices of wheat bread	**Lunch**	1/2 grapefruit
2 oz turkey breast	2 slices of wheat bread	
1 oz Swiss cheese	2 oz of turkey breast	**Lunch**
1 teaspoon mayonnaise	1 teaspoon of mayonnaise	2 slices of wheat bread
1 small banana	1 small banana	2 oz turkey breast
1 small bag potato chips (15 chips)	Lettuce salad with 2 cups of fresh vegetables—broccoli, cauliflower, carrots, cucumbers, cherry tomatoes	1 teaspoon mayonnaise
		1 small banana
Snack	3 tablespoons reduced calorie salad dressing	Lettuce salad with 3 cups of fresh vegetables—broccoli, cauliflower, carrots, cucumbers, cherry tomatoes
1/2 cup vanilla ice cream		
	Snack	3 tablespoons fat-free salad dressing
Dinner	1 cup low-fat yogurt	
4 oz T-bone steak	1 fresh peach	**Snack**
1 large baked potato	6 cups of air-popped popcorn	1 cup nonfat yogurt
1 1/2 cup steamed broccoli		1 fresh peach
1 dinner roll	**Dinner**	6 cups of air-popped popcorn
1 teaspoon margarine	4 oz sirloin (grilled or broiled)	
2 tablespoons sour cream	1 large baked potato	**Dinner**
1 1/4 cup fresh strawberries	1 1/2 cup steamed broccoli	1 large baked potato
	1 dinner roll	1 1/2 cup steamed broccoli
Snack	1 tablespoon reduced-calorie margarine	2 dinner rolls
15 grapes		1 teaspoon margarine
2 chocolate chip cookies	2 tablespoons sour cream	1 1/4 cup fresh strawberries
Total calories: 1990	1 1/4 cup strawberries	1 cup skimmed milk
Total fat: 84 g; 38% of calories from fat		
Saturated fat: less than 10%	**Snack**	**Snack**
	30 grapes	30 grapes
	Total calories: 1971	1 cup skimmed milk
	Total fat: 63 g; 29% of calories from fat	**Total calories: 1990**
	Saturated fat: 7% of calories	**Total fat: 21 g; 10% of calories from fat**
		Saturated fat: less than 3%

---

rated fatty acids. Nevertheless, the P/S ratio provides useful information about the fatty acid content of food, provided the food source lists the fatty acid types.

Ratio of Saturated to Monounsaturated to Polyunsaturated Fatty Acids

The AHA takes a slightly different approach to healthful eating. Previous guidelines recommended a lipid intake less than 30% of total calories, with the percentage of lipid calories distributed in a ratio of 10:10:10 for saturated to monounsaturated to polyunsaturated fatty acids. Owing to difficulty determining the particular fat source percentage of a meal, the AHA now encourages Americans to focus more on replacing high-fat foods with fruits, vegetables, grains, fat-free and low-fat dairy products, fish, poultry, and lean meat.[55] Other new components of the AHA guidelines include a focus on weight control and the addition of two weekly servings of fish high in omega-3 fatty acids.

ROLE OF LIPID IN THE BODY

Four important functions of lipids in the body include:

1. Energy reserve
2. Protection of vital organs
3. Thermal insulation
4. Transport medium for fat-soluble vitamins and hunger suppressor

Energy Source and Reserve

Fat constitutes the ideal cellular fuel because each molecule carries large quantities of energy per unit weight, transports and stores easily, and provides a ready source of energy. In well-nourished individuals at rest, fat provides as much as 80 to 90% of the energy requirement. One gram of pure lipid contains about 9 kCal (38 kJ) of energy, more than *twice* the energy available to the body in an equal quantity of carbohydrate or protein. This occurs from the greater quantity of hydrogen in the lipid molecule. Chapter 4 points out that oxidation of hydrogen atoms provides the energy for bodily functions at rest

TABLE 1.10   Examples of Foods High and Low in Saturated Fatty Acids, Foods High in Monounsaturated and Polyunsaturated Fatty Acids, and the Polyunsaturated to Saturated Fatty Acid (P/S) Ratio of Common Fats and Oils

High saturated	%	Peanut oil	48
Coconut oil	91	Cashews, dry roasted	42
Palm kernel oil	82	Peanut butter	39
Butter	68	Bologna	39
Cream cheese	57	Beef, cooked	33
Coconut	56	Lamb, roasted	32
Hollandaise sauce	54	Veal, roasted	26
Palm oil	51	**High polyunsaturated**	**%**
Half & half	45	Safflower oil	77
Cheese, Velveeta	43	Sunflower oil	72
Cheese, mozzarella	41	Corn oil	58
Ice cream, vanilla	38	Walnuts, dry	51
Cheesecake	32	Sunflower seeds	47
Chocolate almond bar	29	Margarine, corn oil	45
Low saturated	**%**	Canola oil	32
Popcorn	0	Sesame seeds	31
Hard candy	0	Pumpkin seeds	31
Yogurt, nonfat	2	Tofu	27
Crackerjacks	3	Lard	11
Milk, skim	4	Butter	6
Cookies, fig bars	4	Coconut oil	2
Graham crackers	5	**P/S Ratio, Fats & Oils**	
Chicken breast, roasted	6	Coconut oil	0.2/1.0
Pancakes	8	Palm oil	0.2/1.0
Cottage cheese, 1%	8	Butter	0.1/1.0
Milk, chocolate, 1%	9	Olive oil	0.6/1.0
Beef, dried	9	Lard	0.3/1.0
Chocolate, mints	10	Canola oil	5.3/1.0
High monounsaturated	**%**	Peanut oil	1.9/1.0
Olives, black	80	Soybean oil	2.5/1.0
Olive oil	75	Sesame oil	3.0/1.0
Almond oil	70	Margarine, 100% corn oil	2.5/1.0
Canola oil	61	Cottonseed oil	2.0/1.0
Almonds, dry	52	Mayonnaise	3.7/1.0
Avocados	51	Safflower oil	13.3/1.0

Data from the Science and Education Administration, Home and Garden Bulletin 72, Nutritive value of foods. Washington, DC: US Government Printing Office, 1985, 1986; Agricultural Research Service, United States Department of Agriculture, Nutritive value of American foods in common units. Agricultural Handbook no. 456. Washington, DC: US Government Printing Office, 1975.

and during exercise. Recall that synthesis of a triacylglycerol molecule from glycerol and three fatty acid molecules creates three water molecules. In contrast, when glucose forms glycogen, 2.7 g of water stores with each gram. *Whereas fat exists as a relatively water-free, concentrated fuel, glycogen becomes hydrated and heavy relative to its energy content.*

FIGURE 1.14 illustrates the total mass (and energy content) from fat and various body fat depots in an 80-kg man. Approximately 15% of the body mass for men and 25% for women consists of fat. The potential energy stored in the fat molecules of a typical 80-kg young adult man translates to about 110,700 kCal (12,300 g body fat × 9.0 kCal · g^{-1}). Most of this energy—present as adipose tissue and intramuscular triacylglycerols and a small amount of plasma free fatty acids—is available for exercise. This amount of energy would fuel a run from New York City to Madison, Wisconsin (assuming an energy expenditure of about 100 kCal per mile).

Contrast this fact to the limited 2000-kCal reserve of stored carbohydrate that could only fuel a 20-mile run. Viewed from a different perspective, the body's energy reserves from carbohydrate could power high-intensity running for about 1.6 hours, whereas fat reserves would allow the person to continue for about 120 hours! As is the case for carbohydrate, fat used as a fuel "spares" protein to carry out its important functions of tissue synthesis and repair.

Protection and Insulation

Up to 4% of the body's fat protects against trauma to the heart, liver, kidneys, spleen, brain, and spinal cord. Fats stored just below the skin (subcutaneous fat) provide insulation, determining ability to tolerate extremes of cold exposure. Swimmers who excelled in swimming the English Channel showed only a slight fall in body temperature while resting in cold water and essentially no lowering effect while

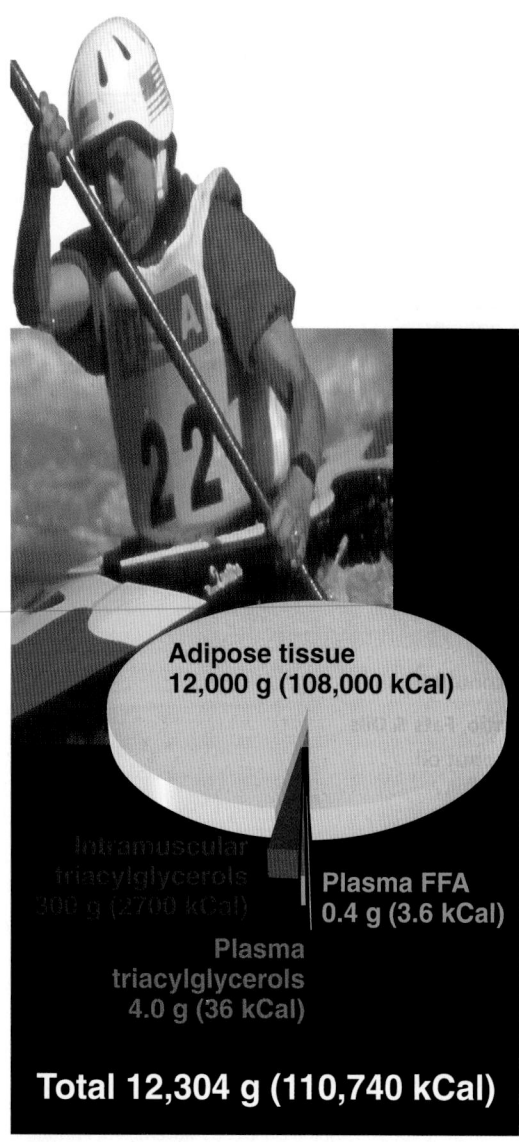

Adipose tissue
12,000 g (108,000 kCal)

Intramuscular
triacylglycerols
300 g (2700 kCal)

Plasma FFA
0.4 g (3.6 kCal)

Plasma
triacylglycerols
4.0 g (36 kCal)

Total 12,304 g (110,740 kCal)

FIGURE 1.14 ■ Distribution of fat energy in an average 80-kg man.

swimming.[91] In contrast, body temperature of leaner, non-Channel swimmers decreased markedly under rest and exercise conditions. The insulatory layer of fat probably affords little protection except in cold-related activities such as deep-sea diving or ocean or channel swimming or among Arctic inhabitants. Excess body fat hinders temperature regulation during heat stress, most notably during sustained exercise in air when the body's heat production can increase 20 times above the resting level. The insulation shield from subcutaneous fat retards the flow of heat from the body.

For large football linemen, excess fat storage provides additional cushioning to protect from the sport's normal hazards. Any possible protective benefit, however, must be evaluated against the liability imposed by the "dead weight" of excess fat and its effect on energy expenditure, thermal regulation, and exercise performance.

Vitamin Carrier and Hunger Depressor

Consuming about 20 g of dietary lipid daily provides a sufficient source and transport medium for the fat-soluble vitamins A, D, E, and K. Significantly reducing lipid intake depresses the body's level of these vitamins, which ultimately may lead to vitamin deficiency. Dietary lipid also facilitates absorption of vitamin A precursors from nonlipid plant sources like carrots and apricots. It takes about 3.5 hours after ingesting lipids to empty them from the stomach. Thus, some lipid in the diet can delay the onset of "hunger pangs" and contribute to satiety following the meal. This helps to explain why reducing diets containing a small amount of lipid sometimes prove initially more successful in blunting the immediate urge to eat than do more extreme fat-free diets.

Summary

1. Lipids, like carbohydrates, contain carbon, hydrogen, and oxygen atoms, but with a higher ratio of hydrogen to oxygen. For example, the lipid stearin has the formula $C_{57}H_{110}O_6$. Lipid molecules consist of one glycerol molecule and three fatty acid molecules.

2. Lipids, synthesized by plants and animals, are grouped into one of three categories: (1) simple lipids (glycerol plus three fatty acids), (2) compound lipids (phospholipids, glycolipids, and lipoproteins) composed of simple lipids combined with other chemicals, and (3) derived lipids like cholesterol, synthesized from simple and compound lipids.

3. Saturated fatty acids contain as many hydrogen atoms as chemically possible; thus, "saturated" describes this molecule with respect to hydrogen. Saturated fatty acids exist primarily in animal meat, egg yolk, dairy fats, and cheese. Dietary intakes high in saturated fatty acids elevate blood cholesterol and promote coronary heart disease.

4. Unsaturated fatty acids contain fewer hydrogen atoms attached to the carbon chain. Instead, double bonds connect carbon atoms and the fatty acid exists as either monounsaturated or polyunsaturated with respect to hydrogen. Heart disease protection occurs from increasing the diet's proportion of unsaturated fatty acids.

Summary *continued*

5. Dietary *trans* fatty acids may account for 30,000 deaths annually from heart disease. High intake of this fatty acid also increases risk for contracting type 2 diabetes.

6. Perhaps the most powerful cardioprotective benefit of fish oils relates to their antiarrhythmic effect on myocardial tissue. This protection against ventricular arrhythmias and sudden death is likely provided by the unique effects of these dietary fatty acids on the fatty acid content of the myocardial cell membranes.

7. Lowering blood cholesterol, especially that carried by LDL, reduces coronary heart disease risk.

8. Dietary lipid currently provides about 36% of total energy intake. Prudent advice recommends a 30% level or lower for dietary lipid, of which 70 to 80% should consist of unsaturated fatty acids.

9. Lipids provide the largest nutrient store of potential energy for biologic work. They also protect vital organs, provide insulation from the cold, and transport the fat-soluble vitamins A, D, E, and K.

Proteins

NATURE OF PROTEINS

The body of an average-sized adult contains between 10 and 12 kg of protein, primarily located within skeletal muscle mass. Structurally, proteins (from the Greek word meaning "of prime importance") resemble carbohydrates and lipids because they too contain atoms of carbon, oxygen, and hydrogen. Protein molecules also contain about 16% nitrogen, along with sulfur and occasionally phosphorus, cobalt, and iron. Just as glycogen forms from many simple glucose subunits linked together, the protein molecule polymerizes from its **amino acid** "building-block" constituents in endlessly complex arrays. **Peptide bonds** link amino acids in chains that take on diverse forms and chemical combinations. The hydrogen from the amino acid side chain of one amino acid combines with the hydroxyl group of the carboxylic (organic) acid end of another amino acid. Two joined amino acids produce a **dipeptide,** and linking three amino acids produces a **tripeptide,** and so on. A linear configuration of up to 100 amino acids produces a **polypeptide,** while combining more than 100 amino acids forms a **protein.** Three amino acids make up thyrotropin-releasing hormone, whereas the muscle protein myosin forms from the linkage of 4500 amino acid units. Single cells contain thousands of different protein molecules. In total, approximately 50,000 different protein-containing compounds exist in the body. The biochemical functions and properties of each protein depend on the sequence of specific amino acids.

Each of the 20 different amino acids required by the body has a positively charged amine group at one end and a negatively charged organic acid group at the other end. The amine group consists of two hydrogen atoms attached to nitrogen (NH_2), whereas the organic acid group (technically termed a *carboxylic acid group*) contains one carbon atom, two oxygen atoms, and one hydrogen atom (COOH). The remainder of

An Unlimited Potential to Synthesize Protein Compounds

The potential for combining the 20 amino acids creates an almost infinite number of possible proteins. For example, proteins formed from linking just three different amino acids could generate 20^3 or 8000 different proteins, and just 6 different amino acids yields 64 million proteins (20^6)!

the amino acid molecule may take several different forms, referred to as the amino acid's functional group, or **side chain.** *The side chain's unique structure dictates the amino acid's particular characteristics.* FIGURE 1.15 *(top)* shows the structure for the amino acid alanine.

KINDS OF PROTEINS

The body cannot synthesize eight amino acids (nine in children and some older adults), so they must be ingested preformed in foods. Isoleucine, leucine, lysine, methionine, phenylalanine, threonine, tryptophan, and valine make up these **essential amino acids.** The body also synthesizes cystine from methionine and tyrosine from phenylalanine. Infants cannot synthesize histidine, and children have reduced capability for synthesizing arginine. The body manufactures the remaining nine **nonessential** amino acids. The term *nonessential* does not mean they are unimportant; rather, they must be synthesized from other compounds already in the body at a rate to meet demands for normal growth and tissue repair.

Fortunately, animals and plants manufacture proteins that contain essential amino acids. No health or physiologic advantage exists from an amino acid derived from an animal

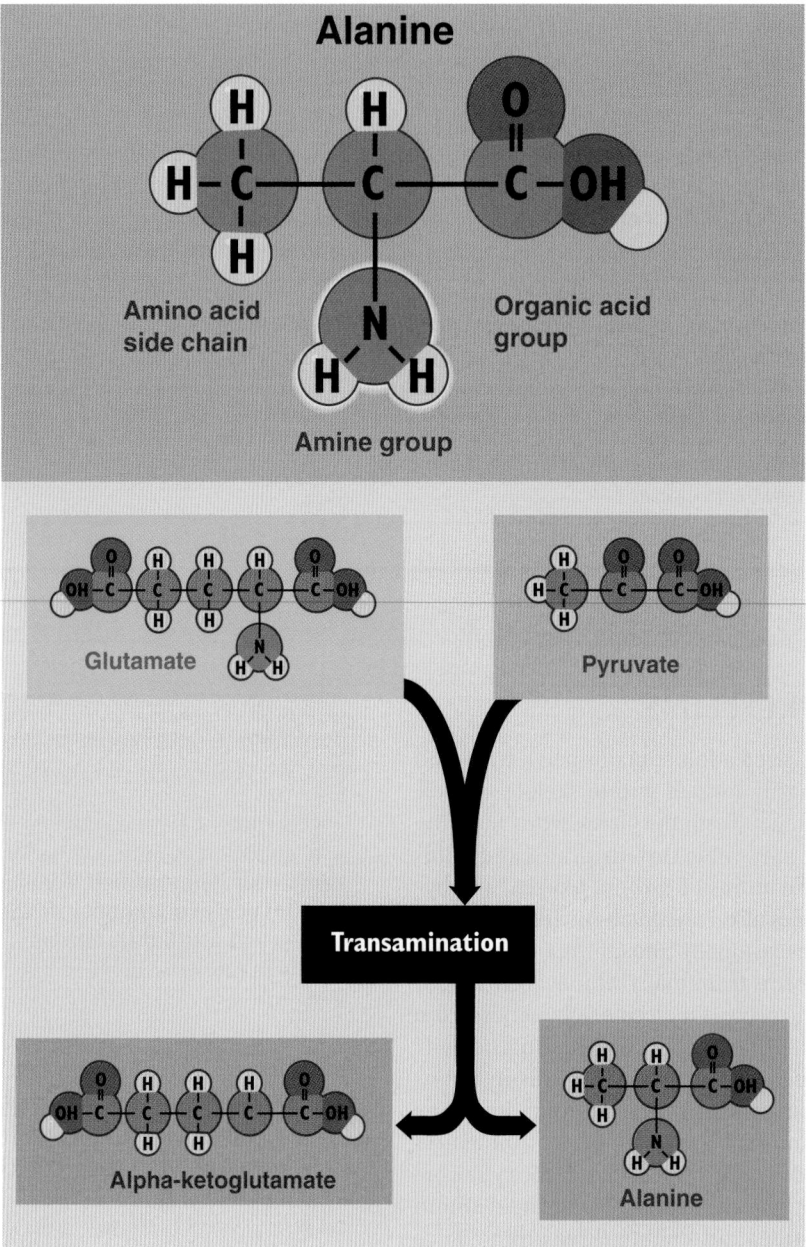

FIGURE 1.15 ■ *Top.* Chemical structure of the amino acid alanine. *Bottom.* Transamination occurs when an amine group from a donor amino acid transfers to an acceptor acid to form a new amino acid.

compared with the same amino acid from vegetable origin. Plants synthesize amino acids by incorporating nitrogen in the soil along with carbon, oxygen, and hydrogen from air and water. In contrast, animals do not possess broad capability for protein synthesis; they ingest most of their protein.

Synthesizing a specific protein requires the availability of appropriate amino acids. **Complete proteins,** or higher quality proteins, come from foods with all of the essential amino acids in the quantity and the correct ratio to maintain nitrogen balance and allow tissue growth and repair. An **incomplete protein,** or lower quality protein, lacks one or more essential amino acid. Incomplete protein diets eventually lead to protein malnutrition. This occurs whether or not the food sources contain adequate energy or protein quantity.

Protein Sources

Sources of complete protein include eggs, milk, meat, fish, and poultry. Among all food sources, eggs provide the optimal mixture of essential amino acids; hence, eggs receive the highest quality rating of 100 for comparison with other foods. TABLE 1.11 rates common sources of dietary protein.

TABLE 1.11	Rating of Protein Quality of Dietary Sources of Protein
Food	**Protein Rating**
Eggs	100
Fish	70
Lean beef	69
Cow's milk	60
Brown rice	57
White rice	56
Soybeans	47
Brewer's hash	45
Whole-grain wheat	44
Peanuts	43
Dry beans	34
White potato	34

TABLE 1.12	Good Food Sources of Protein	
Food	**Serving**	**Protein (g)**
Animal		
Tuna	3 oz	22
Turkey, light meat	4 oz	9
Fish	3 oz	17
Hamburger	4 oz	30
Egg, whole	1 large	6
Egg, white	1 large	4
Beef, lean	4 oz	24
Dairy		
Cottage cheese	0.5 cup	15
Yogurt, low fat	8 oz	11
Cheese	1 oz	8
Milk, skim	8 oz	8
Plant		
Peanuts	1 oz	7
Peanut butter	1 Tbsp	4
Pasta, dry	2 oz	7
Whole-wheat bread	2 slices	6
Baked beans	1 cup	14
Tofu	3.5 oz	11
Almonds, dried	12	3
Chick peas	0.5 cup	20
Lentils	0.5 cup	9

Presently, animal sources provide almost two thirds of the dietary protein, whereas 85 years ago protein consumption occurred equally from plant and animal origins. Reliance on animal sources for dietary protein largely accounts for the relatively high intake of cholesterol and saturated fatty acids in the world's major industrialized nations.

The **biologic value** of a food refers to its completeness for supplying essential amino acids. Higher quality protein foods come from animal sources, whereas vegetables (lentils, dried beans and peas, nuts, and cereals) remain incomplete in one or more essential amino acid; thus, these have a relatively lower biologic value. The animal protein collagen remains an exception because it lacks the essential amino acid tryptophan. This protein forms part of the connective tissue of animals. TABLE 1.12 lists examples of good food sources of protein.

The Vegetarian Approach

Eating a variety of plant foods (grains, fruits, and vegetables) supplies all of the essential amino acids, each providing a different quality and quantity of amino acids. Grains and legumes supply excellent protein content, but neither offers the full complement of essential amino acids. An exception may be well-processed, isolated soybean protein, termed *soy-protein isolates,* whose protein quality matches that of some animal proteins. Grains lack the essential amino acid lysine, while legumes contain lysine but lack the sulfur-containing essential amino acid methionine (found abundantly in grains). Tortillas and beans, rice and beans, rice and lentils, rice and peas, and peanuts and wheat (bread) serve as staples in many cultures because they provide **complementary protein** sources of all essential amino acids from the plant kingdom.

True vegetarians, or **vegans,** consume nutrients from only two sources—the plant kingdom and dietary supplements. Many physically active vegetarians are at somewhat greater risk for inadequate energy and nutrient intake because they eliminate meat and dairy products from the diet and increasingly rely on foods relatively low in energy, quality protein, and some micronutrients. Vegans make up less than 1% of the United States population, although between 5 and 7% of Americans consider themselves "almost" vegetarians. Nutritional diversity remains the key for these men and women. For example, a vegan diet provides all the essential amino acids if the recommended dietary allowance for protein contains 60% of protein from grain products, 35% from legumes, and 5% from green leafy vegetables. A 70-kg person obtains all essential amino acids by consuming about 56 g of protein from approximately $1\frac{1}{4}$ cups of beans, $\frac{1}{4}$ cup of seeds or nuts, 4 slices of whole-grain bread, 2 cups of vegetables (1 cup leafy green), and $2\frac{1}{2}$ cups from grain sources (brown rice, oatmeal, and cracked wheat).

A Potentially Healthful and Nutritious Way for Athletes to Eat

Well-balanced vegetarian and vegetarian-type diets provide abundant carbohydrate, crucial during intense, prolonged training. Such diets associate with reduced body weight and a lower incidence of certain chronic diseases.[8] They contain little or no cholesterol, are high in fiber, and are rich in fruit and vegetable sources of antioxidant vitamins and diverse phytochemicals.[53]

An Increasing Number of Near-Vegetarian Athletes

An increasing number of competitive and champion athletes consume diets composed predominately of nutrients from varied plant sources, including some dairy and meat products. Considering how much time it requires to train and prepare for competition, vegetarian athletes often encounter difficulty in planning, selecting, and preparing nutritious meals from predominantly plant sources without relying on supplementation.[7,112] The fact remains, however, that two thirds of the world's population subsist on largely vegetarian diets, with little reliance on animal protein.

Controlled clinical trials generally conclude that substituting soy protein for animal protein decreases blood pressure, plasma homocysteine levels, triacylglycerol, total cholesterol, and harmful oxidized LDL cholesterol, without reducing beneficial HDL cholesterol.[3,51,114] For example, daily consumption of as little as 20 g of soy protein instead of animal protein for 6 weeks favorably modified blood lipid profiles.[107] Genistein, a component of soy, also may offer protection against breast cancer.[59]

Obtaining ample higher quality protein becomes the strict vegetarian's main nutritional concern. Children on vegan diets should be monitored to ensure adequate vitamin D and calcium intake, which most Americans obtain from milk products. A **lactovegetarian diet** provides milk and related products such as ice cream, cheese, and yogurt. The lactovegetarian approach minimizes the problem of consuming sufficient higher quality protein and increases the intake of calcium, phosphorus, and vitamin B_{12} (produced by bacteria in the digestive tract of animals). Good meatless sources of iron include fortified ready-to-eat cereals, soybeans, and cooked farina; cereals, wheat germ, and oysters contain high zinc levels. Adding an egg to the diet (**ovolactovegetarian diet**) ensures intake of higher quality protein.

FIGURE 1.16 displays the contribution of various food groups to the protein content of the American diet. By far, the greatest protein intake comes from animal sources, with only about 30% derived from plant sources.

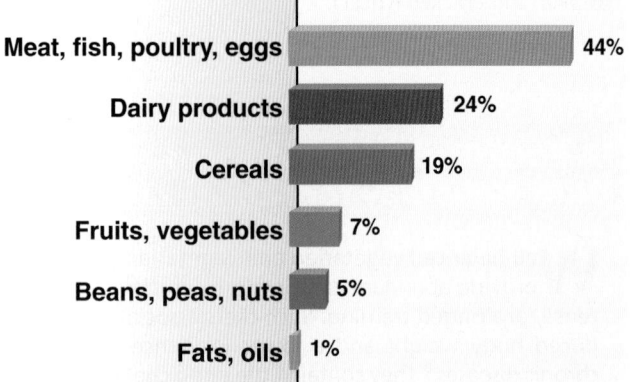

FIGURE 1.16 ■ Contribution from major food groups to the protein content of the typical American diet.

RECOMMENDED DIETARY PROTEIN INTAKE

Despite the beliefs of many coaches, trainers, and athletes, no benefit accrues from eating excessive protein. An intake exceeding three times the recommended level does *not* enhance work capacity during intensive training. *For athletes, muscle mass does not increase simply by eating high-protein foods or special amino acid mixtures.* If lean tissue synthesis resulted from the extra protein consumed by the typical athlete, then muscle mass would increase tremendously. For example, consuming an extra 100 g (400 kCal) of protein daily translates into a daily 500-g (1.1-lb) increase in muscle mass. This obviously does not happen. Excessive dietary protein ultimately is used directly for energy (following deamination) or recycled as components of other molecules, including stored fat in subcutaneous adipose tissue depots. Harmful side effects can occur when dietary protein intake significantly exceeds recommended values. A high protein catabolism strains liver and kidney functions owing to the elimination of urea and other compounds.

The Recommended Dietary Allowance

The **Recommended Dietary Allowance (RDA)** for protein, vitamins, and minerals represents a liberal standard for nutrient intake expressed as a daily average. These guidelines were initially developed in May 1942 by the Food and Nutrition Board of the National Research Council/National Academy of Science (www2.nas.edu/iom) to evaluate and plan for the nutritional adequacy of groups rather than of individuals. They have been revised 11 times.[34] RDA levels represent a liberal yet safe excess to prevent nutritional deficiencies in practically all healthy people. In the 11th edition (1999), RDA recommendations included 19 nutrients, energy intake, and the **Estimated Safe and Adequate Daily Dietary Intakes (ESADDI)** for seven additional vitamins and minerals and three electrolytes. The ESADDI should be viewed as more tentative and evolutionary than the RDA. ESADDI recommendations for certain essential micronutrients (e.g., vitamins biotin and pantothenic acid and trace elements copper, manganese, fluoride, selenium, chromium, and molybdenum) required sufficient scientific data to formulate an intake range considered adequate and safe, yet insufficient for a precise single RDA. Any intake within this range is considered acceptable for maintaining adequate physiologic function, and sufficient to prevent underexposure or overexposure. No RDA or ESADDI exists for sodium, potassium, and chlorine; instead, recommendations refer to a minimum requirement for health.

We emphasize that the RDA reflects an ongoing evaluation based on available data for the nutritional needs of a *population* over a prolonged period. Specific individual requirements can be determined only by laboratory measurements. Malnutrition occurs from cumulative weeks, months, and even years of inadequate nutrient intake. Also, someone who regularly consumes a diet containing nutrients below the RDA standards may not

TABLE 1.13	Average Daily Energy Allowance and Recommended Protein Intakes							
	Age (years) or Condition	Weight[a]		Height[a]		Average Energy Allowance (kCal)[b]		RDA for Protein
Category		(kg)	(lb)	(cm)	(in.)	kCal/kg	kCal·d^{-1c}	(g/day)
Infants	0.0–0.5	6	13	60	24	108	650	13
	0.5–1.0	9	20	71	28	89	850	14
Children	1–3	13	29	90	35	102	1300	16
	4–6	20	44	112	44	90	1800	24
	7–10	28	62	132	52	70	2000	28
Males	11–14	45	99	157	62	55	2500	45
	15–18	66	145	176	69	45	3000	59
	19–24	72	160	177	70	40	2900	58
	25–50	79	174	176	70	37	2900	63
	51+	77	170	173	68	30	2300	63
Females	11–14	46	101	157	62	47	2200	46
	15–18	55	120	163	64	40	2200	44
	19–24	58	128	164	65	38	2200	46
	25–50	63	138	163	64	36	2200	50
	51+	65	143	160	63	30	1900	50
Pregnant	1st trimester						0	60
	2nd trimester						+300	60
	3rd trimester						+500	60
Lactating	1st 6 months						+500	65
	2nd 6 months						+500	62

Source: National Research Council, Food and Nutrition Board.

[a]*Weights and heights represent median values.*

[b]*In the range of light-to-moderate activity the coefficient of variation equals ± 20%.*

[c]*Figure is rounded.*

become malnourished. Rather, the RDA represents a probability statement for adequate nutrition; as nutrient intake falls below the RDA, the statistical probability for malnourishment increases for that person. The chance increases progressively with lower nutrient intake. In Chapter 2, we discuss the **Dietary Reference Intakes,** which represent the current set of standards for recommended intake of nutrients and other food components.[32,110]

TABLE 1.13 lists the protein RDAs for adolescent and adult men and women. On average, 0.83 g of protein per kg body mass represents the recommended daily intake. To determine protein requirement for men and women ages 18 to 65, multiply body mass in kg by 0.83. Thus, for a 90-kg man, total protein requirement equals 75 g (90 × 0.83). The protein RDA holds even for overweight persons; it includes a reserve of about 25% to account for individual differences in protein requirement for about 98% of the population. Generally, the protein RDA (and the quantity of the required essential amino acids) decreases with age. In contrast, the protein RDA for infants and growing children of 2.0 to 4.0 g per kg body mass facilitates growth and development. Pregnancy requires that daily protein intake increase by 20 g, and nursing mothers should increase intake by 10 g. *A 10% increase in the calculated protein requirement, particularly for a vegetarian-type diet, ac-* *counts for dietary fiber's effect in reducing the digestibility of many plant-based protein sources.* Stress, disease, and injury usually increase the protein requirement.

Some Modifications Required for Recommended Protein Intake for Physically Active Persons

A continuing area of controversy concerns the necessity of a larger than normal protein requirement for still growing adolescent athletes, individuals involved in strength development programs that enhance muscle growth and endurance training regimens that increase protein breakdown, and athletes subjected to recurring tissue microtrauma, like wrestlers and football players.[14,46,75,89,106] Inadequate protein and energy intake can induce a loss of body protein, particularly from skeletal muscle, with concomitant performance deterioration. *A definitive answer remains elusive, but protein breakdown above the resting level occurs during intense endurance training and resistance training to a greater degree than previously believed.* Increased protein catabolism occurs to a greater extent when exercising with low carbohydrate reserves and/or low energy intakes. Unfortunately, research has not pinpointed protein requirements for individuals who train 4 to 6 hours daily by resistance exercise. Their protein needs may average only slightly more than those for sedentary individuals. In addition, despite increased protein use for energy during intense training, adaptations may augment the body's efficiency in using dietary protein to enhance amino acid balance.

Until research clarifies this issue, we recommend that athletes who train intensely should consume between 1.2 and 1.8 g of protein per kg of body mass daily. This protein intake falls within the range typically consumed by physically active men and women, thus obviating the need to consume supplementary protein.[40] With adequate protein intake, consuming animal sources of protein does not facilitate muscle strength or size gains with resistance training compared with protein intake from plant sources.[42] Chapter 7 presents a more complete discussion of protein balance and requirements in exercise and training.

ROLE OF PROTEIN IN THE BODY

Blood plasma, visceral tissue, and muscle represent the three major sources of body protein. No body "reservoirs" of this macronutrient exist. All protein contributes to tissue structures or exists as important constituents of metabolic, transport, and hormonal systems. Protein constitutes between 12 and 15% of the body mass, but the protein content of different cells varies considerably. A brain cell, for example, consists of only about 10% protein, while red blood cells and muscle cells include up to 20% of their total weight as protein. The protein content of skeletal muscle represents about 65% of the body's total protein. This quantity can increase somewhat with exercise training, depending on the nature of the training regimen, training duration, type of workout, and many other interrelated factors.

Amino acids provide the major building blocks for synthesizing the body's various tissues. They also incorporate nitrogen into RNA and DNA compounds, into the coenzyme electron carriers NAD^+ and FAD (see Chapter 5), into the heme components of the oxygen-binding hemoglobin and myoglobin compounds, into the catecholamine hormones epinephrine and norepinephrine, and into the neurotransmitter serotonin. Amino acids activate vitamins that play a key role in metabolic and physiologic regulation. **Anabolism** refers to tissue building processes; the amino acid requirement for anabolism can vary considerably. For example, tissue anabolism accounts for about one third of the protein intake during rapid growth in infancy and childhood. As growth rate declines, so does the percentage of protein retained for anabolic processes. Once a person attains optimal body size and growth stabilizes, a continual turnover still occurs for the tissue's existing protein component.

Proteins serve as primary constituents for plasma membranes and internal cellular material. Proteins in the cell nuclei (nucleoproteins) "supervise" cellular protein synthesis and transmission of hereditary characteristics. Collagenous **structural proteins** compose the hair, skin, nails, bones, tendons, and ligaments. Another classification, **globular proteins,** makes up the nearly 2000 different enzymes that modulate the rate of chemical reactions and regulate catabolism of fats, car-

bohydrates, and proteins for energy release. Blood plasma also contains the specialized proteins thrombin, fibrin, and fibrinogen required for blood clotting. Within red blood cells, the oxygen-carrying compound hemoglobin contains the large globin protein molecule.

Proteins play a role in regulating the acid–base quality of the body fluids. Buffering neutralizes excess acid metabolites formed during relatively intense exercise. The structural proteins actin and myosin play an essential role in muscle action; these proteins slide past each other as muscles shorten and lengthen during movement. Even in older adults, the body's protein-containing structures "turn over" on a regular basis; normal protein dynamics require adequate protein intake simply to replace the amino acids continually degraded in the turnover process.

DYNAMICS OF PROTEIN METABOLISM

Dietary protein primarily supplies amino acids for the various anabolic processes. In addition, some catabolism of protein for energy takes place. In well-nourished individuals at rest, protein breakdown contributes between 2% and 5% of the body's total energy requirement. During **catabolism,** protein first degrades into its amino acid components. The amino acid molecule then loses its nitrogen (amine group) in the liver by the process of **deamination.** This "freed" nitrogen forms **urea** (H_2NCONH_2), which the body then excretes. The remaining deaminated carbon compound can take one of three routes: it can be (1) synthesized to a new amino acid, (2) converted to carbohydrate or fat, or (3) catabolized directly for energy. Urea formed in deamination (including some ammonia) leaves the body in solution as urine. Excessive protein catabolism promotes fluid loss because urea must be dissolved in water for excretion.

In muscle, enzymes facilitate nitrogen removal from certain amino acids and subsequently pass this nitrogen to other compounds in the biochemical reactions of **transamination** (see Fig. 1.15 *bottom*). An amino group shifts from a donor amino acid to an acceptor acid (keto acid), the acceptor thus becoming a new amino acid. A specific transferase enzyme accelerates the transamination reaction. This allows amino acid formation from non–nitrogen-carrying organic compounds formed in metabolism (e.g., pyruvate). In both deamination and transamination, the resulting carbon skeleton of the non-nitrogenous amino acid residue further degrades during energy metabolism.

Fate of Amino Acids After Nitrogen Removal

After deamination, the remaining carbon skeletons of the α-keto acids such as pyruvate, oxaloacetate, or α-ketoglutarate follow three different biochemical routes that include the following (FIG. 1.17):

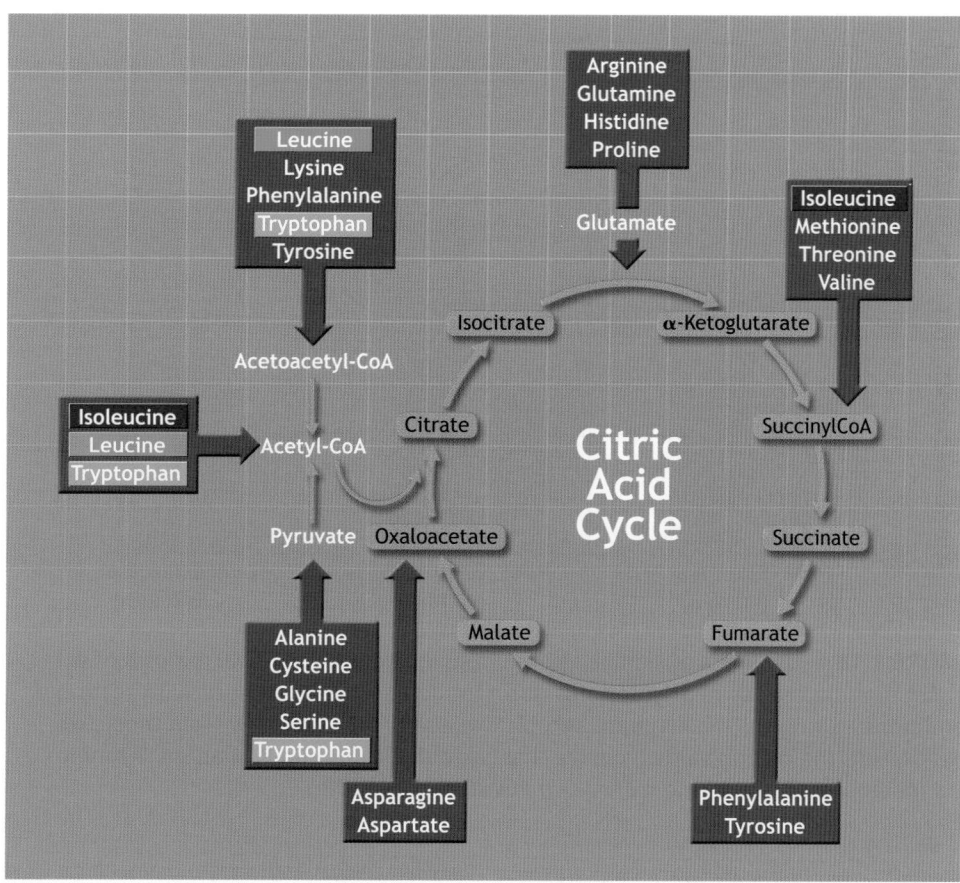

FIGURE 1.17 ■ Major metabolic pathways for amino acids following removal of the nitrogen group by deamination or transamination. Upon removal of their amine group, all amino acids form reactive citric acid cycle intermediates or related compounds. Some of the larger amino acid molecules (e.g., leucine, tryptophan, isoleucine) generate carbon-containing compounds that enter metabolic pathways at different sites. (Reprinted with permission from McArdle W, Katch F, and Katch V. *Exercise Physiology.* 6th ed. Baltimore: Lippincott Williams & Wilkins, 2007:39.)

1. *Gluconeogenesis:* 18 of the 20 amino acids serve as a source for glucose synthesis
2. *Energy source:* the carbon skeletons oxidize for energy because they form intermediates in citric acid cycle metabolism or related molecules
3. *Fat synthesis:* all amino acids provide a potential source of acetyl-CoA and thus furnish substrate to synthesize fatty acids

Nitrogen Balance

Nitrogen balance exists when nitrogen intake (protein) equals nitrogen excretion. In **positive nitrogen balance,** nitrogen intake exceeds nitrogen excretion, with the additional protein used to synthesize new tissues. Positive nitrogen balance occurs in growing children, during pregnancy, in recovery from illness, and during resistance exercise training, in which overloading muscle cells promotes protein synthesis. The body does not develop a protein reserve as it does with fat storage in adipose tissue or as carbohydrate stored as liver and muscle glycogen. Individuals who consume adequate protein have a higher content of muscle and liver protein than do individuals fed a subpar, low-protein diet. Also, labeling of protein (injecting protein with one or several of its carbon atoms "tagged") shows that some proteins become recruited for energy metabolism. Other proteins in neural and connective tissues remain relatively "fixed" as cellular constituents; they cannot be mobilized without harming tissue functions.

Greater nitrogen output than nitrogen intake (**negative nitrogen balance**) indicates protein use for energy and possible encroachment on amino acid reserves, primarily from skeletal muscle. Interestingly, a negative nitrogen balance occurs even when protein intake exceeds the recommended standard if the body catabolizes protein because it lacks other energy nutrients in the diet. For example, an individual engaged in arduous training may consume adequate or excess protein yet be deficient in energy as carbohydrate or lipid. In this scenario, protein becomes a primary energy fuel. This creates a negative protein (nitrogen) balance that reduces the body's lean tissue mass. The protein-sparing role of dietary lipid and carbohydrate discussed previously becomes important during tissue growth periods and high-energy output requirements of inten-

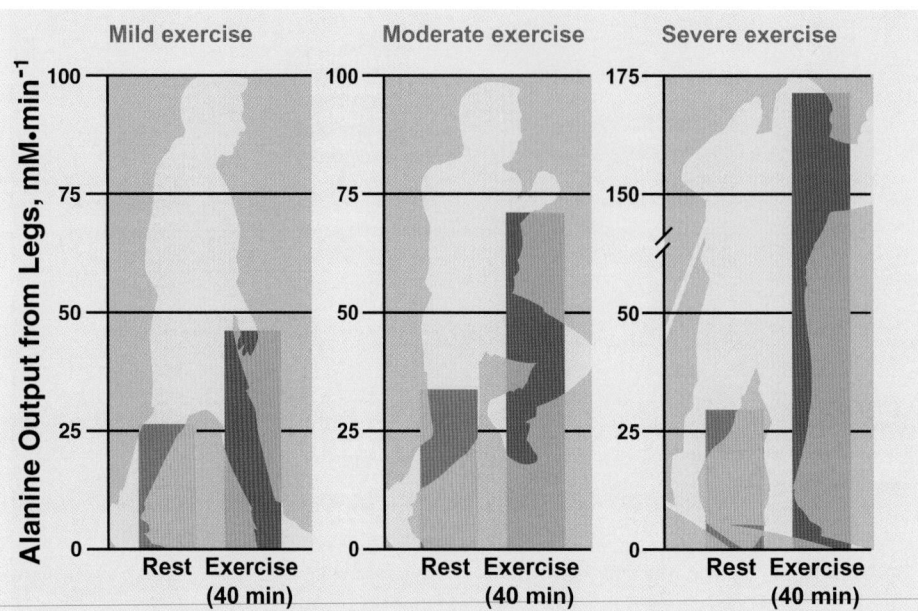

FIGURE 1.18 ■ Dynamics of alanine release from leg muscle during 40 minutes of exercise. Alanine release nearly doubles during mild exercise compared with resting conditions. During the most intense aerobic exercise the alanine flow from the active legs exceeds the resting value by more than sixfold. (From Felig P, Wahren J. Amino acid metabolism in exercising man. *J Clin Invest* 1971;50:2073.)

sive exercise training. Starvation produces the greatest negative nitrogen balance. *Starvation diets, or diets with reduced carbohydrate and/or energy, deplete glycogen reserves, which might trigger a protein deficiency with accompanying lean tissue loss.*

The Alanine–Glucose Cycle

Some body proteins do not readily metabolize for energy, but muscle proteins are more labile. Amino acids participate in energy metabolism when the exercise energy demand increases.[15,17,118] FIGURE 1.18 shows that alanine release (and possibly glutamine) from active leg muscles increases in proportion to exercise intensity.

A model indicates that alanine *indirectly* serves the energy requirements of exercise. Active skeletal muscle synthesizes alanine during transamination. This occurs from the glucose intermediate pyruvate (with nitrogen derived in part from the amino

acid leucine). Alanine deaminates after it leaves the muscle and enters the liver. Gluconeogenesis then converts the remaining carbon skeleton of alanine to glucose, which then enters the blood for use by active muscle. The residual carbon fragment from the amino acid that formed alanine oxidizes for energy within the muscle cell. FIGURE 1.19 summarizes the sequence of the **alanine–glucose cycle.** After 4 hours of continuous light exercise, the liver's output of alanine-derived glucose accounts for about 45% of the liver's total glucose release. *During prolonged exercise, the alanine–glucose cycle generates from 10 to 15% of the total exercise energy requirement.* Regular exercise training enhances the liver's synthesis of glucose using the carbon skeletons of noncarbohydrate compounds. This facilitates blood glucose homeostasis during prolonged exercise. Chapters 5 and 7 discuss protein's role as a potential energy fuel in exercise and protein requirements of physically active people.

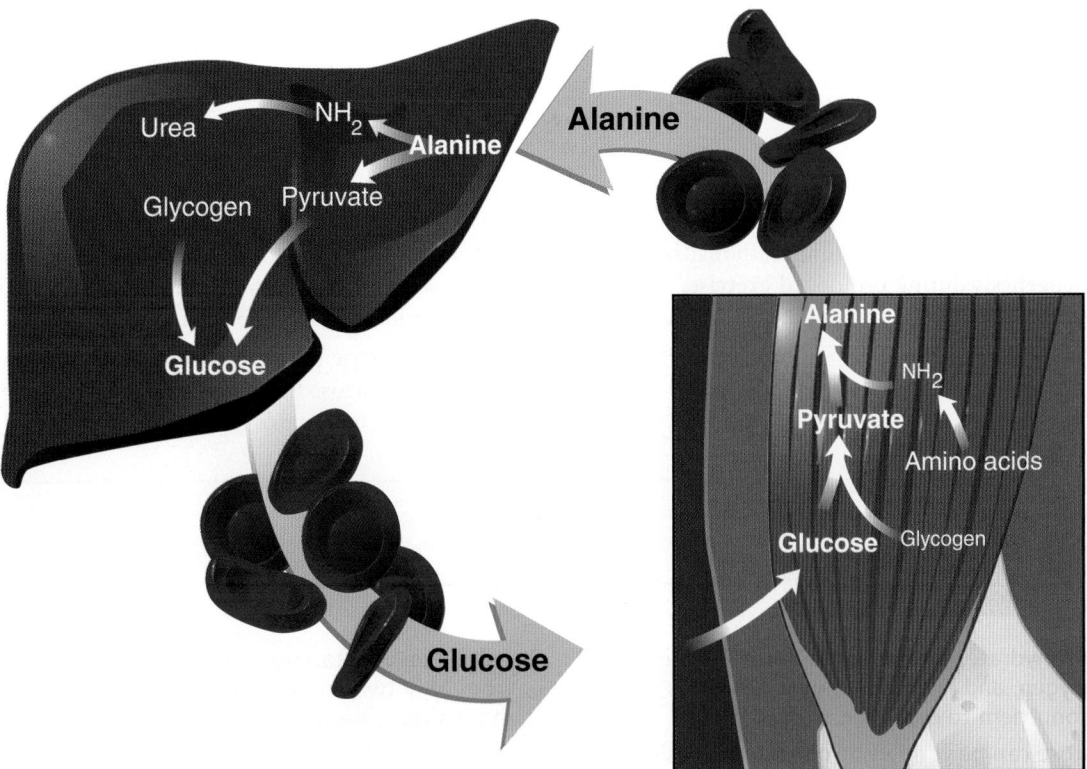

FIGURE 1.19 ▪ The alanine–glucose cycle. Alanine, synthesized in muscle from glucose-derived pyruvate via transamination, is released into the blood and converts to glucose and urea in the liver. Glucose release into the blood coincides with its subsequent delivery to the muscle for energy. During exercise, increased production and output of alanine from muscle helps to maintain blood glucose for nervous system and active muscle needs. Exercise training augments processes of hepatic gluconeogenesis. (From Felig P, Wahren J. Amino acid metabolism in exercising man. *J Clin Invest* 1971;50:2703.)

Summary

1. Proteins differ chemically from lipids and carbohydrates because they contain nitrogen in addition to sulfur, phosphorus, and iron.

2. Proteins form from subunits called amino acids. The body requires 20 different amino acids, each containing an amino radical (NH_2) and an organic acid radical called a carboxyl group (COOH). Amino acids contain a side-chain that defines the amino acid's particular chemical characteristics.

3. An almost infinite number of possible protein structures can form because of the diverse combinations possible for the 20 different amino acids.

4. The body cannot synthesize 8 of the 20 amino acids. These are the essential amino acids that must be consumed in the diet.

5. Animal and plant cells contain protein. Proteins with all the essential amino acids are called complete (higher qual-ity) proteins; the others are called incomplete (lower quality) proteins. Examples of higher quality, complete proteins include animal proteins in eggs, milk, cheese, meat, fish, and poultry.

6. The diets of many physically active persons and competitive athletes consist predominantly of nutrients from plant sources. Consuming a variety of plant foods provides all of the essential amino acids because each food source contains a different quality and quantity of them.

7. Proteins provide the building blocks for synthesizing cellular material during anabolic processes. Amino acids also contribute their "carbon skeletons" for energy metabolism.

8. The RDA, the recommended quantity for nutrient intake, represents a liberal yet safe level of excess to meet the nutritional needs of practically all healthy persons. For adults, the protein RDA equals 0.83 g per kg of body mass.

Summary *continued*

9. Proteins in nervous and connective tissue generally do not participate in energy metabolism. The amino acid alanine, however, plays a key role in providing carbohydrate fuel via gluconeogenesis during prolonged exercise. During strenuous exercise of long duration, the alanine–glucose cycle accounts for up to 40 to 50% of the liver's glucose release.

10. Protein catabolism accelerates during exercise because carbohydrate reserves deplete. Thus, individuals who train vigorously on a regular basis must maintain optimal levels of muscle and liver glycogen to minimize lean tissue loss and deterioration in performance.

11. Regular exercise training enhances the liver's capacity to synthesize glucose from the carbon skeletons of noncarbohydrate compounds.

Test Your Knowledge Answers

1. **False:** Carbohydrates do not contain nitrogen, only carbon, oxygen, and hydrogen atoms. Protein is the only macronutrient to contain nitrogen.

2. **True:** Glucose can be formed by gluconeogenesis, a process that synthesizes glucose (primarily in the liver) from carbon skeletons of specific amino acids as well as from nonprotein sources such as glycerol, pyruvate, and lactate.

3. **False:** Fibers exist exclusively in plants; they make up the structure of leaves, stems, roots, seeds, and fruit coverings. Because of its resistance to digestive enzymes, fiber cannot be absorbed by the body and used for energy. However, fiber does retain considerable water as it passes through the digestive tract and thus gives "bulk" to the food residues in the large intestine, often increasing stool weight and volume by 40 to 100% that aids gastrointestinal function.

4. **False:** For regular exercisers, carbohydrates should supply about 60% of total daily calories (400–600 g), predominantly as unrefined, fiber-rich fruits, grains, and vegetables.

5. **False:** About 25% of the population produces excessive insulin in response to an intake of rapidly absorbed carbohydrates (high glycemic rating). These insulin-resistant individuals increase their risk for obesity if they consistently eat such a diet. Weight gain occurs because abnormal quantities of insulin (1) promote glucose entry into cells and (2) facilitate the liver's conversion of glucose to triacylglycerol, which then becomes stored as body fat in adipose tissue. Also, excess calories, regardless of dietary source, contribute to obesity.

6. **False:** Carbohydrate and protein each contains 4.0 kCal per gram. In contrast, each gram of lipid contains more than twice the amount at 9.0 kCal.

7. **False:** Cholesterol, the most widely known derived lipid, exists only in animal tissue; it is never found in plants of any origin.

8. **True:** True vegetarians or vegans consume nutrients from only two sources, the plant kingdom and dietary supplements. This places vegans at a somewhat greater risk for inadequate energy and nutrient intake because they eliminate meat and dairy products from the diet and increasingly rely on foods relatively low in energy, quality protein, and certain micronutrients. Nutritional diversity remains the key for these men and women. For example, a vegan diet provides all the essential amino acids if 60% of protein intake comes from grain products, 35% from legumes, and 5% from green, leafy vegetables. Vitamin B_{12}, found only in the animal kingdom, must be obtained in supplement form.

9. **False:** For athletes, muscle mass does not increase simply by eating high-protein foods or special amino acid mixtures. If lean tissue synthesis resulted from extra protein, muscle mass would increase tremendously for individuals on the typical Western diet. For example, consuming an extra 100 g (400 kCal) of protein daily theoretically translates into a daily 500-g (1.1-lb) increase in muscle mass. This obviously does not happen. A proper resistance training program combined with a well-balanced diet increases muscle mass. Excessive dietary protein is used directly for energy or recycled as components of other molecules, including fat stored in the subcutaneous adipose tissue depots.

10. **False:** On average, 0.83 g of protein per kg body mass represents the recommended daily intake for both women and men. For a 90-kg man, the total daily protein requirement equals 75 g (90 × 0.83) while a 50-kg woman requires 41.5 g (50 × 0.83). The protein RDA even holds for overweight persons; it includes a reserve of about 25% to account for individual differences in protein requirement for about 98% of the population.

References

1. Agus MS, et al. Dietary composition and physiologic adaptations to energy restriction. *Am J Clin Nutr* 2000;71:901.
2. Albert CM, et al. Blood levels of long-chain n-3 fatty acids and risk of sudden death. *N Engl J Med* 2002;346:1113.
3. Anderson JW, et al. Meta-analysis of the effects of soy protein intake on serum lipids. *N Engl J Med* 1995;333:276.
4. Anderson JW, et al. Cholesterol-lowering effects of psyllium intake adjunctive to diet therapy in men and women with hypercholesterolemia: meta-analysis of 8 controlled trials. *Am J Clin Nutr* 2000;71:472.
5. Andrews TC, et al. Effect of cholesterol reduction on myocardial ischemia in patients with coronary disease. *Circulation* 1997;95:324.
6. Barnard RJ, et al. Diet-induced insulin resistance precedes other aspects of the metabolic syndrome. *J Appl Physiol* 1998;84:1311.
7. Barr SI, Rideout CA. Nutritional considerations for vegetarian athletes. *Nutrition* 2004;20:696.
8. Berkow SE, Barnard N. Vegetarian diets and weight status. *Nutr Rev* 2006;64:175.
9. Bingham SA, et al. Dietary fibre in food and protection against colorectal cancer in the European Prospective Investigation into Cancer and Nutrition (EPIC): an observational study. *Lancet* 2003;361:1496.
10. Braaten JT, et al. Oat B-glucan reduces blood cholesterol concentration in hypercholesterolemic subjects. *Eur J Clin Nutr* 1994;48:465.
11. Brown I, et al. Cholesterol-lowering effects of dietary fiber: a meta-analysis. *Am J Clin Nutr* 1999;69:30.
12. Buyken AE, et al. Glycemic index in the diet of European outpatients with type 1 diabetes: relations to glycated hemoglobin and serum lipids. *Am J Clin Nutr* 2001;73:574.
13. Caggiula AW, Mustak VA. Effects of dietary fat and fatty acids on coronary artery disease risk and total and lipoprotein cholesterol concentrations: epidemiologic studies. *Am J Clin Nutr* 1997;65(suppl):1597S.
14. Carraro F, et al. Effect of exercise and recovery on muscle protein synthesis in human subjects. *Am J Physiol* 1990;259:E470.
15. Carraro F, et al. Alanine kinetics in humans during low-intensity exercise. *Med Sci Sports Exerc* 1994;26:48.
16. Chandalia M, et al. Beneficial effects of high dietary fiber intake in patients with type 2 diabetes mellitus. *N Engl J Med* 2000;342:1392.
17. Christensen HN. Role of amino acid transport and counter transport in nutrition and metabolism. *Physiol Rev* 1990;70:43.
18. Connor WE. Do the n-3 fatty acids from fish prevent deaths from cardiovascular disease? *Am J Clin Nutr* 1997;66:188.
19. Connor WE. Importance of n-3 fatty acids in health and disease. *Am J Clin Nutr* 2000;71(suppl):171S.
20. Cowie DD, et al. Prevalance of diabetes and impaired fasting glucose in adults in the U.S. population: National Health and Nutrition Examination Survey 1999–2002. *Diabetes Care* 2006;29:1263.
21. Daly ME, et al. Dietary carbohydrates and insulin sensitivity: a review of the evidence and clinical implications. *Am J Clin Nutr* 1997;66:1072.
22. Daviglus ML, et al. Fish consumption and the 30-year risk of fatal myocardial infarction. *N Engl J Med* 1997;336:1046.
23. Davy BM, et al. High-fiber oat cereal compared with wheat cereal consumption favorably alters LDL-cholesterol subclass and particle numbers in middle-aged and older men. *Am J Clin Nutr* 2002;76:351.
24. Dewailly E, et al. N-3 Fatty acids and cardiovascular disease risk factors among the Inuit of Nunavik. *Am J Clin Nutr* 2001;74:474.
25. Dietschy JM. Theoretical considerations of what regulates low-density-lipoprotein and high-density-lipoprotein cholesterol. *Am J Clin Nutr* 1997;65(suppl):1581S.
26. Dreon DM, et al. Change in dietary saturated fat intake is correlated with change in mass of large low-density-lipoprotein particles in men. *Am J Clin Nutr* 1998;67:828.
27. Drexel H, et al. Plasma triglycerides and three lipoprotein cholesterol fractions are independent predictors of the extent of coronary arteriosclerosis. *Circulation* 1994;90:2230.
28. Engler MM, Engler MB. Omega-3 fatty acids: Role in cardiovascular health and disease. *J Cardiovasc Nurs* 2006;21:17.
29. Esmaillzadeh A, Azadbakht L. Whole-grain intake, metabolic syndrome, and mortality in older adults. *Am J Clin Nutr* 2006;83:1439.
30. Fernandez ML, et al. Guar gum effects on plasma low-density lipoprotein and hepatic cholesterol metabolism in guinea pigs fed low-and high-cholesterol diets: a dose-response study. *Am J Clin Nutr* 1995;61:127.
31. Finley CE, et al. Cardiorespiratory fitness, macronutrient intake and the metabolic syndrome: The Aerobics Center Longitudinal Study. *J Am Diet Assoc* 2006;106:673.
32. Food and Nutrition Board, Institute of Medicine. Dietary reference intakes: a risk assessment model for establishing upper intake levels for nutrients. Washington, DC: National Academy Press, 1998.
33. Food and Nutrition Board, Institute of Medicine. Dietary reference intakes for energy, carbohydrates, fiber, fat, protein and amino acids. Washington, DC: National Academy Press, 2002.
34. Food and Nutrition Board. Recommended Dietary Allowances. 11th ed. Washington, DC: National Academy of Sciences, 1999.
35. Ford ES, et al. Prevalence of the metabolic syndrome among US adults: findings from the Third National Health and Nutrition Examination Survey. *JAMA* 2002;287:356.
36. Frick MH, et al. Helsinki Heart Study: primary-prevention trial with gemfibrozil in middle-aged men with dyslipidemia. Safety of treatment, changes in risk factors, and incidence of coronary heart disease. *N Engl J Med* 1987;317:3217.
37. Friedman, MI. Fuel partitioning and food intake. *Am J Clin Nutr* 1998;67(suppl):513S.
38. Fuchs CF, et al. Dietary fiber and risk of colorectal cancer and adenoma in women. *N Engl J Med* 1999;440:169.
39. Fung TT, et al. Whole-grain intake and risk of type-2 diabetes: a prospective study in men. *Am J Clin Nutr* 2002;76:535.
40. Gaine PC, et al. Level of dietary protein impacts whole body protein turnover in trained males at rest. *Metabolism* 2006;55:501.
41. Harris WS. Fish oils and plasma lipid and lipoprotein metabolism: a critical review. *J Lipid Res* 1989;30:785.
42. Haub MD, et al. Effect of protein source on resistive-training-induced changes in body composition and muscle size in older men. *Am J Clin Nutr* 2002;76:511.
43. Heyward VH, et al. Anthropometric, body composition and nutritional profiles of bodybuilders during training. *J Appl Sports Sci Rev* 1989; 3:22.
44. Hickson JF, Wolinsky I. Research directions in protein nutrition for athletes. In: Wolinsky I, Hickson JF Jr, eds. Nutrition in exercise and sport. Boca Raton, FL: CRC Press, 1994.
45. Hickson JF, et al. Nutritional profile of football athletes eating from a training table. *Nutr Res* 1987;7:27.
46. Hickson JF, et al. Repeated days of body building exercise do not enhance urinary nitrogen excretions from untrained young males. *Nutr Res* 1990;10:723.
47. Howarth NC, et al. Dietary fiber and weight regulation. *Nutr Res* 2001;59:129.
48. Hu FB, et al. Dietary fat intake and the risk of coronary heart disease in women. *N Engl J Med* 1997;337:1491.
49. Hu FB, et al. Fish and omega-3 fatty acid intake on risk of coronary heart disease in women. 2002;287:1815.
50. Iso H, et al. Intake of fish and omega-3 fatty acids and risk of stroke in women. *JAMA* 2001;285:304.
51. Jenkins DJ, et al. Effects of high- and low-isoflavone soyfoods on blood lipids, oxidized LDL, homocysteine, and blood pressure in hyperlipidemic men and women. *Am J Clin Nutr* 2002;76:365.
52. Jenkins DJ, et al. Soluble fiber intake at a dose approved by the US Food and Drug Administration for a claim of health benefits: serum lipid risk factors for cardiovascular disease assessed in a randomized controlled crossover trial. *Am J Clin Nutr* 2002;75:834.
52. Key TJ, et al. Health effects of vegetarian and vegan diets. *Proc Nutr Soc* 2006;65:35.
54. Kobayashi IH, et al. Intake of fish and omega-3 fatty acids and risk of coronary heart disease among Japanese: The Japan Public Health Center-Based (JPHC) Study Cohort 1. *Circulation* 2006;113:195.
55. Krauss RM, et al. AHA dietary guidelines revision 2000: a statement for health care professionals from the Nutrition Committee of the American Heart Association. *Circulation* 2000;102:2284.

56. Krauss WE, et al. Effect of the amount and intensity of exercise on plasma lipoproteins. *N Engl J Med* 2002;347:1483.

57. Laidlaw M, Holub BJ. Effects of supplementation with fish-oil derived n-3 fatty acids and gamma-linoleic acid on circulating plasma lipids and fatty acid profiles in women. *Am J Clin Nutr* 2003;77:37.

58. Lakka HM, et al. The metabolic syndrome and total and cardiovascular disease mortality in middle-aged men. *JAMA* 2002;288:2709.

59. Lamartiniere CA. Protection against breast cancer with genistein: a component of soy. *Am J Clin Nutr* 2000;73:172.

60. Lambert EV, et al. Enhanced endurance in trained cyclists during moderate intensity exercise following 2 weeks adaptation to a high fat diet. *Eur J Appl Physiol* 1994;69:287.

61. Lauber RP, Sheard NF. The American Heart Association dietary guidelines for 2000: a summary report. *Nutr Rev* 2001;59:298.

62. Lemaitre RN, et al. n-3 Poly unsaturated fatty acids, fatal ischemic heart disease, and nonfatal myocardial infarction in obese adults. *Am J Clin Nutr* 2003;77:319.

63. LeMura LM, et al. Lipid and lipoprotein profiles, cardiovascular fitness, body composition, and diet during and after resistance, aerobic and combination training in young women. *Eur J Appl Physiol* 2000;82:451.

64. Liu S, et al. A prospective study of dietary glycemic load, carbohydrate intake, and risk of coronary heart disease in US women. *Am J Clin Nutr* 2000;71:1455.

65. Liu S, et al. Dietary glycemic load assessed by food-frequency questionnaire in relation to plasma high-density-lipoprotein cholesterol and fasting triacylglycerols in postmenopausal women. *Am J Clin Nutr* 2001;73:560.

66. Liu S, et al. Is intake of breakfast cereals related to total and cause-specific mortality in men? *Am J Clin Nutr* 2003;77:594.

67. Lopez-Garcia E, et al. Consumption of trans fatty acids is related to plasma biomarkers of inflammation and endothelial dysfunction. *J Nutr* 2005;135:562.

68. Ludwig DS, et al. Dietary fiber, weight gain, and cardiovascular disease risk factors in young adults. *JAMA* 1999;275:486.

69. Maclean CH, et al. Effects of omega-3 fatty acids on cancer risk: a systemic review. *JAMA* 2006;295:1900.

70. Marques-Lopes I, et al. Postprandial de novo lipogenesis and metabolic changes induced by a high-carbohydrate, low-fat meal in lean and overweight men. *Am J Clin Nutr* 2001;73:253.

71. McAuley KA, Mann JI. Nutritional determinants of insulin resistance. *J Lipid Res* 2007.

72. McIntosh M, Miller C. A diet containing food rich in soluble and insoluble fiber improves glycemic control and reduces hyperlipidemia among patients with type 2 diabetes. *Nutr Rev* 2001;59:52.

73. McKeown NM, et al. Whole-grain intake is favorably associated with metabolic risk factors for type 2 diabetes and cardiovascular disease in the Framingham Offspring Study. *Am J Clin Nutr* 2002;76:390.

74. Mensink RP, et al. Effects of dietary fatty acids and carbohydrates on the ratio of serum total to HDL cholesterol and on serum lipids and apolipoproteins: a meta-analysis of 60 controlled trials. *Am J Clin Nutr* 2003;77:1146.

75. Meridith CN, et al. Dietary protein requirements and body protein metabolism in endurance-trained men. *J Appl Physiol* 1989;66:2850.

76. Meyer KA, et al. Carbohydrates, dietary fiber, and incident type 2 diabetes in older women. *Am J Clin Nutr* 2000;71:921.

77. Mittendorfer B, Sidossis L. Mechanism for the increase in plasma triacylglycerol concentration after consumption of short-term, high-carbohydrate diets. *Am J Clin Nutr* 2001;73:892.

78. Montonen J, et al. Whole-grain and fiber intake and the incidence of type 2 diabetes. *Am J Clin Nutr* 2003;77:622.

79. Morris KL, Zemel MB. Glycemic index, cardiovascular disease, and obesity. *Nutr Rev* 1999;55:273.

80. Mozaffarian D. Trans fatty acids: effects on systemic inflammation and endothelial function. *Atheroscler Suppl* 2007.

81. Mozaffarian D, et al. Cereal, fruit, and vegetable fiber intake and risk of cardiovascular disease in elderly individuals. *JAMA* 2003;289:1659.

82. Mozaffarian D, et al. Trans fatty acids and cardiovascular disease. *N Eng J Med* 2006;354:1601.

83. National Institutes of Health. Third report of the National Cholesterol Education Program Expert Panel on Detection, Evaluation, and Treatment of High Blood Cholesterol in Adults (Adult Treatment Panel III). Bethesda, MD: National Institutes of Health; 2001. NIH publication 01-3670.

84. Nestle P, et al. The n-3 fatty acids eicosapentaenoic and docosahaenoic acid increase systemic arterial compliance in humans. *Am J Clin Nutr* 2002;76:326.

85. Noakes M, Clifton PM. Changes in plasma lipids and other cardiovascular risk factors during 3 energy-restricted diets differing in total fat and fatty acid composition. *Am J Clin Nutr* 2000;71:706.

86. Ornish D, et al. Intensive lifestyle changes for reversal of coronary heart disease. *JAMA* 1998;280:2001.

87. Parks EJ, Hellerstein MK. Carbohydrate induced hypertriacylglycerolemia: historical perspective and review of biological mechanisms. *Am J Clin Nutr* 2000;71:412.

88. Peters U, et al. Dietary fibre and colorectal adenoma in a colorectal cancer early detection programme. *Lancet* 2003;361:1491.

89. Phillips SM. Protein requirements and supplementation in strength sports. *Nutrition* 2004;20:689.

90. Poppitt SD, et al. Long-term effects of ad libitum low-fat, high-carbohydrate diets on body weight and serum lipids in overweight subjects with metabolic syndrome. *Am J Clin Nutr* 2002;75:11.

91. Pugh LGCE, Edholm OG. The physiology of channel swimmers. *Lancet* 1955;2:761.

92. Qi L, et al. Whole grain, bran, and cereal fiber intakes and markers of systemic inflammation in diabetic women. *Diabetes Care* 2006;29:207.

93. Raeini-Sarjaz M, et al. Comparison of the effect of dietary fat restriction with that of energy restriction on human lipid metabolism. *Am J Clin Nutr* 2001;73:262.

94. Rimm EB, et al. Vegetable, fruit, and cereal fiber intake and risk of coronary heart disease among men. *JAMA* 1996;275:447.

95. Roche HM, et al. Effect of long-term olive oil dietary intervention on postprandial triacylglycerol and factor VII metabolism. *Am J Clin Nutr* 1998;68:552.

96. Salmerón JE, et al. Dietary fiber, glycemic load, and risk of non-insulin-dependent diabetes mellitus in women. *JAMA* 1997;277:472.

97. Salmerón J.E, et al. Dietary fat intake and risk of type 2 diabetes in women. *Am J Clin Nutr* 2001;73:1019.

98. Schaefer EJ. Lipoproteins, nutrition, and heart disease. *Am J Clin Nutr* 2002;75:191.

99. Seal CJ. Whole grains and CVD risk. *Proc Nutr Soc* 2006;65:24.

100. Shahar E, et al. Dietary n-3 polyunsaturated fatty acids and smoking-related chronic obstructive pulmonary disease. *N Engl J Med* 1994;331:228.

101. Simonen P, et al. Introducing a new component of the metabolic syndrome; low cholesterol absorption. *Am J Clin Nutr* 2000;72:82.

102. Starc TJ, et al. Greater dietary intake of simple carbohydrate is associated with lower concentrations of high-density-lipoprotein cholesterol in hypercholesterolemic children. *Am J Clin Nutr* 1998;67:1147.

103. Stark KD, et al. Effect of fish-oil concentrate on serum lipids in postmenopausal women receiving and not receiving hormone replacement therapy in a placebo-controlled, double-blind trial. *Am J Clin Nutr* 2000;72:389.

104. Stefanick ML, et al. Effects of diet and exercise in men and postmenopausal women with low levels of HDL cholesterol and high levels of LDL cholesterol. *N Engl J Med* 1998;339:12.

105. Stender S, et al. High levels of industrial produced trans fat in popular fast foods. *N Eng J Med* 2006;354:1650.

106. Tarnopolosky MA, et al. Effect of bodybuilding exercise on protein requirements. *Can J Sport Sci* 1990;15:225.

107. Teixeira SR, et al. Effects of feeding 4 levels of soy protein for 3 and 6 wk on blood lipids and apolipoproteins in moderately hypercholesterolemic men. *Am J Clin Nutr* 2000;71:1077.

108. Terry PD, et al. Intakes of fish and marine fatty acids and the risk of cancers of the breast and prostate and of other hormone-related cancers: a review of the epidemiologic evidence. *Am J Clin Nutr* 2003;77:532.

109. Tiollotson JL, et al. Relation of dietary carbohydrates to blood lipids in the special intervention and usual care groups in the Multiple Risk Factor Intervention Trial. *Am J Clin Nutr* 1997;65(suppl):3214S.

110. Trumbo P, et al. Dietary reference intakes: vitamin A, vitamin K, arsenic, boron, chromium, iodine, manganese, molybdenum, nickel, silicon, vanadium, and zinc. *J Am Diet Assoc* 2001;101:294.

111. Van Wijk JPH, et al. Effects of different nutrient intakes on daytime triacylglycerolemia in healthy, normolipemic, free-living men. *Am J Clin Nutr* 2001;74:171.

112. Venderley AM, Campbell WW. Vegetarian diets: nutritional considerations for athletes. *Sports Med* 2006;36:293.

113. Vidon C, et al. Effects of isoenergetic high-carbohydrate compared with high-fat diets on human cholesterol synthesis and expression of key regulatory genes of cholesterol metabolism. *Am J Clin Nutr* 2001;73:878.

114. Wangen KE, et al. Soy isoflavones improve plasma lipids in normocholesterolemic and mildly hypercholesterolemic post menopausal women. *Am J Clin Nutr* 2001;73:225.

115. Weggemans RM, et al. Dietary cholesterol from eggs increases the ratio of total cholesterol to high-density lipoprotein cholesterol in humans: a meta-analysis. *Am J Clin Nutr* 2001;73:885.

116. Weiss R, et al. Obesity and the metabolic syndrome in children and adolescents. *N Engl J Med* 2004;350:2362.

117. Willett WC, Ascherio A. Trans fatty acids: are the effects only marginal? *Am J Public Health* 1994;84:722.

118. Williams BD, et al. Alanine and glutamine kinetics at rest and during exercise. *Med Sci Sports Exerc* 1998;30:1053.

119. Williams PT. High-density lipoprotein cholesterol and other risk factors for coronary heart disease in female runners. *N Engl J Med* 1996;334:1298.

120. Wolfe RR. Metabolic interactions between glucose and fatty acids in humans. *Am J Clin Nutr* 1998;67(suppl):519S.

121. Wolk A, et al. Long-term intake of dietary fiber and decreased risk of coronary heart disease among women. *JAMA* 1999;281:1998.

122. Woodside JV, Kromhout D. Fatty acids and CHD. *Proc Nutr Soc* 2005;64:554.

123. Wynder EL, et al. High fiber intake: indicator of a healthy lifestyle. *JAMA* 1996;275:486.

Chapter 2

The Micronutrients and Water

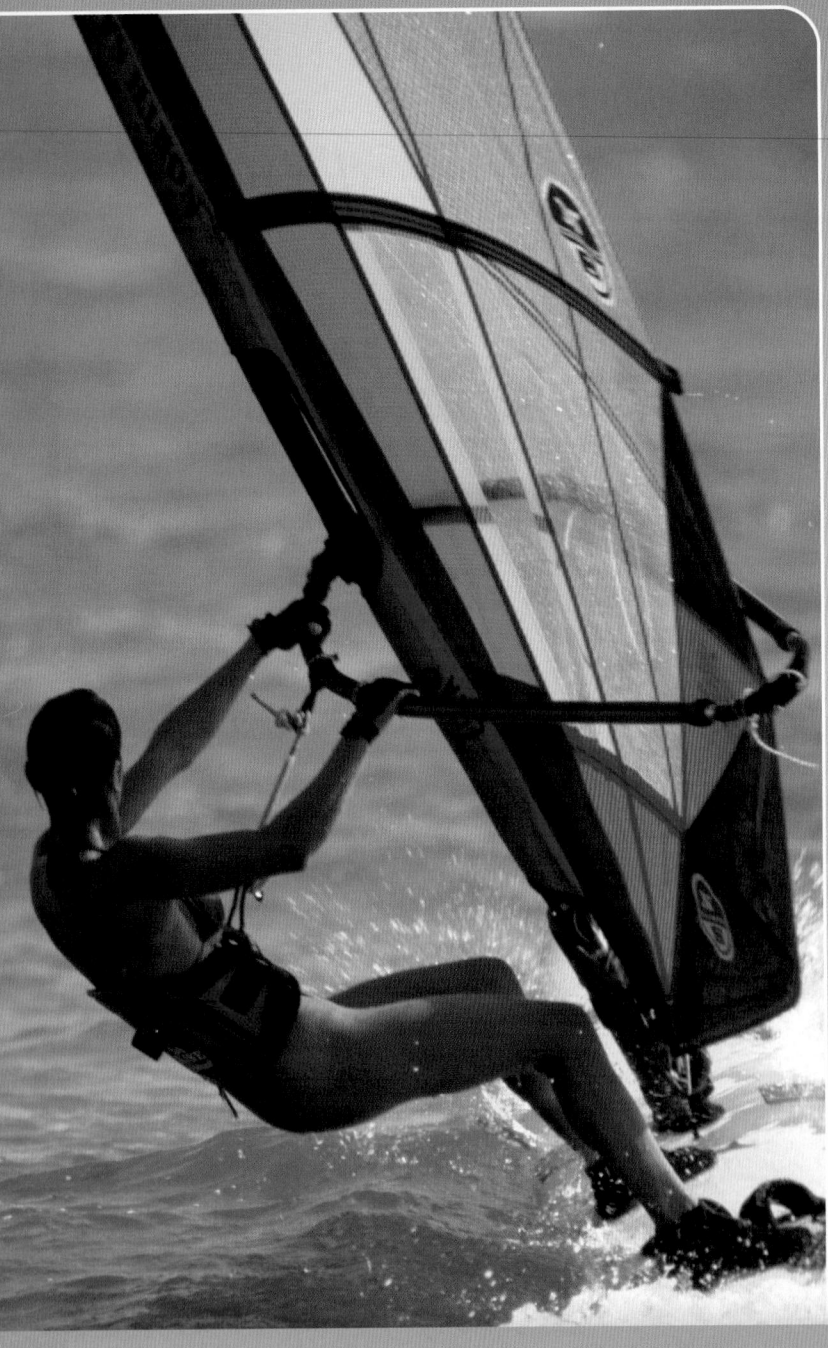

Outline

Vitamins

- The Nature of Vitamins
- Kinds of Vitamins
- Role of Vitamins in the Body
- Defining Nutrient Needs
- Beyond Cholesterol: Homocysteine and Coronary Heart Disease

Minerals

- The Nature of Minerals
- Kinds and Sources of Minerals
- Role of Minerals in the Body
- Calcium
- Phosphorus
- Magnesium
- Iron
- Sodium, Potassium, and Chlorine
- The Dash Eating Plan

Water

- Water in the Body
- Functions of Body Water
- Water Balance: Intake Versus Output
- Physical Activity and Environmental Factors Play an Important Role

Test Your Knowledge

Answer these 10 statements about vitamins, minerals, and water. Use the scoring key at the end of the chapter to check your results. Repeat this test after you have read the chapter and compare your results.

1. **T F** Vitamin supplementation above the Recommended Dietary Allowance (RDA) level does not improve exercise performance.
2. **T F** From a survival perspective, food is of greater importance than water.
3. **T F** Achieving the recommended intake of "major" minerals is more crucial to good health than achieving the recommended intake of "trace" minerals.
4. **T F** Plants provide a better source of minerals than do animal sources.
5. **T F** Sedentary adults require about 3.785 L (1 gal) of water each day to maintain optimal body functions.
6. **T F** Decreasing sodium in the diet represents the only important lifestyle approach to lowering high blood pressure.
7. **T F** None of the 13 vitamins required by the body is toxic if consumed in excess.
8. **T F** A telltale symptom of iron deficiency anemia is soft and brittle bones.
9. **T F** Stationary cycling is an excellent exercise to promote bone health.
10. **T F** Pharmacologic approaches to treating borderline hypertension are more effective than dietary approaches.

Effective regulation of all metabolic processes requires a delicate blending of food nutrients in the watery medium of the cell. Of special significance in this regard are the **micronutrients**—the small quantities of vitamins and minerals that facilitate energy transfer and tissue synthesis. For example, the body requires each year only about 350 g (12 oz) of vitamins from the 862 kg (1896 lb) of food consumed by the average adult. With proper nutrition from a variety of food sources, the physically active person or competitive athlete need not consume vitamin and mineral supplements; such practices usually prove physiologically and economically wasteful. Some micronutrients consumed in excess can adversely affect health and safety.

Vitamins

THE NATURE OF VITAMINS

Vitamins achieved importance centuries before scientists isolated and classified them. The Greek physician Hippocrates advocated ingesting liver to cure night blindness. He did not know the reason for the cure, but we now know that vitamin A, which helps to prevent night blindness, occurs plentifully in this organ meat. In 1897, Dutch physician Christiaan Eijkman (1858–1930; shared the 1929 Nobel Prize in Physiology or Medicine for his discovery of the antineuritic vitamin) observed that a regular diet of polished rice caused beriberi in fowl, while adding thiamine-rich rice polishings to table scraps cured the disease. In the early 19th century, adding oranges and lemons to the diet of British sailors paved the way for eradicating the dreaded disease scurvy because of the protective effects of the vitamin C contained in the fruits. In 1932, scientific experiments demonstrated that ascorbic acid (technically a liver metabolite) functioned in a manner essentially identical to vitamin C. Interestingly, most animal species synthesize ascorbic acid, except for humans, guinea pigs, and certain monkeys; thus, these species must consume vitamin C in their diet.

The formal discovery of vitamins, initially called "vital amines," revealed they were organic substances needed by the body in minute amounts. Vitamins, their amine role having been discredited, have no particular chemical structure in common and often are considered accessory nutrients because they neither supply energy nor contribute substantially to body mass. Except for vitamin D, the body cannot manufacture vitamins; hence, the diet or supplementation must supply them.

Some foods contain an abundant quantity of vitamins. For example, the green leaves and roots of plants manufacture vitamins during photosynthesis. Animals obtain vitamins from the plants, seeds, grains, and fruits they eat or from the meat of other animals that previously consumed these foods.

Several vitamins, notably vitamins A and D, niacin, and folate, become activated from their inactive precursor or **provitamin** form. **Carotenes,** the best known of the provitamins, comprise the yellow and yellow–orange pigment-precursors of vitamin A that give color to vegetables (carrots, squash, corn, pumpkins), and fruits (apricots, peaches).

KINDS OF VITAMINS

Thirteen different vitamins have been isolated, analyzed, classified, and synthesized; and RDA levels have been established for these. Vitamins are classified as either **fat soluble** or **water soluble.** The fat-soluble vitamins include vitamins A, D, E, and K. The water-soluble vitamins are vitamin C and the B-complex vitamins (based on their common source distribution and common functional relationships): thiamine (B_1), riboflavin (B_2), pyridoxine (B_6), niacin (nicotinic acid), pantothenic acid, biotin, folic acid (folacin or folate, its active form in the body), and cobalamin (B_{12}).

Fat-Soluble Vitamins

Fat-soluble vitamins dissolve and are stored in the body's fatty tissues without a need to consume them daily. Years may elapse before symptoms surface of a fat-soluble vitamin insufficiency. The liver stores vitamins A and D, whereas vitamin E distributes throughout the body's fatty tissues. Vitamin K is stored only in small amounts, mainly in the liver. Dietary lipid provides the source of fat-soluble vitamins; these vitamins, transported as part of lipoproteins in the lymph, travel to the liver for dispersion to various tissues. Consuming a true "fat-free" diet could certainly accelerate development of a fat-soluble vitamin insufficiency.

Fat-soluble vitamins should not be consumed in excess without medical supervision. Toxic reactions from excessive fat-soluble vitamin intake generally occur at a lower multiple of recommended intakes than those from water-soluble vitamins. For example, a daily moderate-to-large excess of vitamin A (as retinol but not in carotene form) and vitamin D produce serious toxic effects. Children are particularly susceptible; excess vitamin D, for example, can cause excessive calcium deposits and mental retardation. Consuming vitamin A in amounts not much greater than recommended values (RDA of 700 $\mu g \cdot d^{-1}$ for females and 900 $\mu g \cdot d^{-1}$ for males) precipitates bone fractures later in life. Also, high doses consumed early in pregnancy have been linked to a greater risk of birth defects. In young children, a large vitamin A accumulation (called hypervitaminosis A) causes irritability, swelling of the bones, weight loss, and dry, itchy skin. In adults, symptoms can include nausea, headache, drowsiness, hair loss, diarrhea, and loss of calcium from bones, causing osteoporosis and increased risk of fractures.[122] Excess vitamin A inhibits cells that produce new bone, stimulates cells that break down existing bone, and negatively affects the action of vitamin D, which helps the body maintain normal calcium levels. Discontinuing high vitamin A intakes reverses its adverse effects. A regular excess of vitamin D can precipitate kidney damage. Although "overdoses" from vitamins E and K are rare, intakes above the recommended levels yield no health benefits.

Water-Soluble Vitamins

The water-soluble vitamins act largely as **coenzymes**—small molecules combined with a larger protein compound (apoenzyme) to form an active enzyme that accelerates the interconversion of chemical compounds. Coenzymes participate directly in chemical reactions; when the reaction runs its course, coenzymes remain intact and participate in further reactions. Water-soluble vitamins, like their fat-soluble counterparts, consist of carbon, hydrogen, and oxygen atoms. They also contain nitrogen and metal ions, including iron, molybdenum, copper, sulfur, and cobalt.

Water-soluble vitamins disperse readily in body fluids without storage in the tissues to any appreciable extent. If the diet regularly contains less than 50% of the recommended values for these vitamins, marginal deficiencies could develop within about 4 weeks. Generally, even an excess intake of water-soluble vitamins becomes voided in the urine. Water-soluble vitamins exert their influence for 8 to 14 hours after ingestion; thereafter, their potency decreases. For maximum benefit, vitamin C supplements should be consumed at least every 12 hours. Increasing vitamin C intake for healthy persons from the recommended daily value of 75 mg for women and 90 mg for men to 200 mg (not in supplement form but in 2 to 4 daily servings of fruits and 3 to 5 servings of vegetables) may ensure optimal cellular saturation.[99] FIGURE 2.1 illustrates various food sources for vitamin C and its diverse biologic and biochemical functions. These include serving as an electron donor for eight enzymes and as a chemical reducing agent (antioxidant) in intracellular and extracellular reactions. Sweating, even during extreme physical activity, probably produces only a negligible loss of water-soluble vitamins.[12,65]

Vitamin Storage in the Body

The body does not readily excrete an excess of fat-soluble vitamins. In contrast, water-soluble vitamins continually leave the body because cellular water dissolves these compounds, which then leave via the kidneys. An exception is vitamin B_{12}, which stores more readily than the other water-soluble vitamins, and fat-soluble vitamin K. Because of their limited storage, water-soluble vitamins must be consumed regularly to prevent possible deficiency. A wide latitude exists because an average person would require 10 days without consuming thiamine before deficiency symptoms emerge; it takes about 30 to 40 days of lack of vitamin C before symptoms of deficiency appear. Because a broad array of vitamins is readily available in the foods consumed in a well-balanced diet, little chance occurs for long-term vitamin deficiency. Exceptions include conditions of starvation, alcoholism (which compromises nutrient intake), or significant deviations from prudent dietary recommendations.

ROLE OF VITAMINS IN THE BODY

FIGURE 2.2 summarizes many of the biologic functions of vitamins. These important nutrients contain no useful energy for the body, but instead serve as essential links and regula-

Food Sources

Source (Portion Size)	Vitamin C (mg)
Fruit	
Cantaloupe (1/4 Medium)	60
Fresh grapefruit (1/2 Fruit)	40
Honeydew melon (1/8 Medium)	40
Kiwi (1 Medium)	75
Mango (1 Cup, sliced)	45
Orange (1 Medium)	70
Papaya (1 Cup, cubes)	85
Strawberries (1 Cup, sliced)	95
Tangerines or tangelos (1 Medium)	25
Watermelon (1 Cup)	15
Juice	
Grapefruit (1/2 Cup)	35
Orange (1/2 Cup)	50
Fortified Juice	
Apple (1/2 Cup)	50
Cranberry juice cocktail (1/2 Cup)	45
Grape (1/2 Cup)	120
Vegetables	
Asparagus, cooked (1/2 Cup)	10
Broccoli, cooked (1/2 Cup)	60
Brussels sprouts, cooked (1/2 Cup)	50
Cabbage	
Red, raw, chopped (1/2 Cup)	20
Red, cooked (1/2 Cup)	25
Raw, chopped (1/2 Cup)	10
Cooked (1/2 Cup)	15
Cauliflower, raw or cooked (1/2 Cup)	25
Kale, cooked (1/2 Cup)	55
Mustard greens, cooked (1 Cup)	35
Pepper, red or green	
Raw (1/2 Cup)	65
Cooked (1/2 Cup)	50
Plantains, sliced, cooked (1 Cup)	15
Potato, baked (1 Medium)	25
Snow peas	
Fresh, cooked (1/2 Cup)	40
Frozen, cooked (1/2 Cup)	20
Sweet potato	
Baked (1 Medium)	30
Vacuum can (1 Cup)	50
Canned, syrup-pack (1 Cup)	20
Tomato	
Raw (1/2 Cup)	15
Canned (1/2 Cup)	35
Juice (6 Fluid oz)	35

Biologic and Biochemical Functions

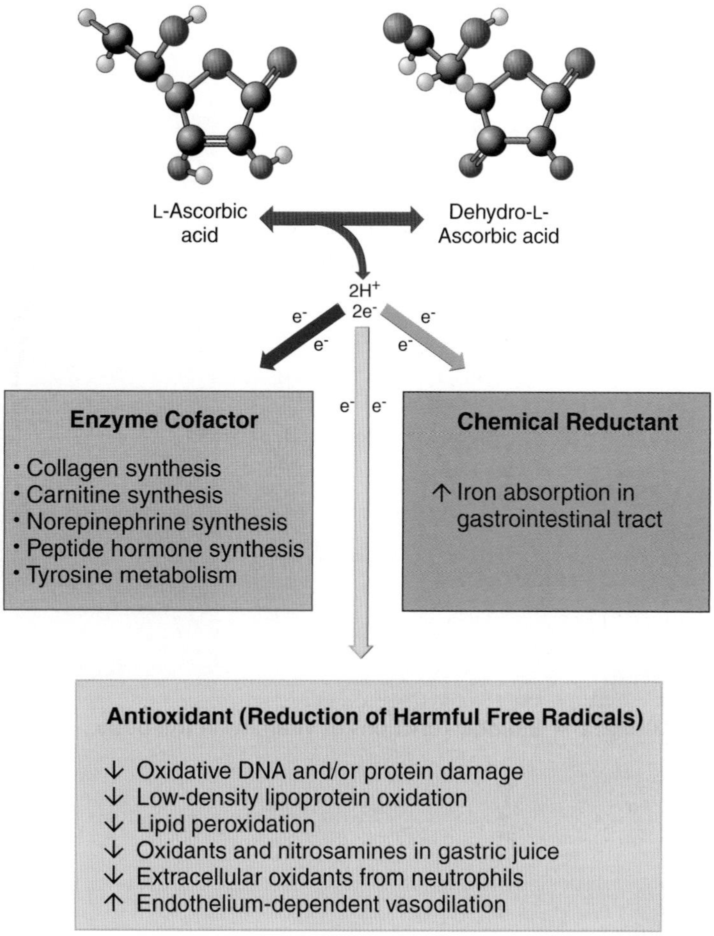

Vitamin C (L-ascorbic acid) oxidation releases donor electrons in pairs for biochemical reactions. The molecular diagrams show carbon atoms in black, oxygen in red, and hydrogen in white. Arrows indicate an increase or decrease in response.

FIGURE 2.1 ■ Various food sources for vitamin C and diverse biologic and biochemical functions. (Modified from Levine M, et al. Criteria and recommendations for vitamin C intake. *JAMA* 1999;281:1415.)

tors in numerous metabolic reactions that *release* energy from food. Vitamins also control processes of tissue synthesis and help to protect the integrity of the cells' unique plasma membrane. The water-soluble vitamins play important roles in energy metabolism (TABLE 2.1). *Vitamins participate repeatedly in metabolic reactions; thus, the vitamin needs of physically active people probably do not exceed those of sedentary counterparts.*

DEFINING NUTRIENT NEEDS

Controversy surrounding the RDAs caused the Food and Nutrition Board and scientific nutrition community to reexamine the usefulness of a single standard. This process, begun in 1997, led the National Academy's Institute of Medicine (in cooperation with Canadian scientists) to develop the **Dietary Reference Intakes** (www.nal.usda.gov/).

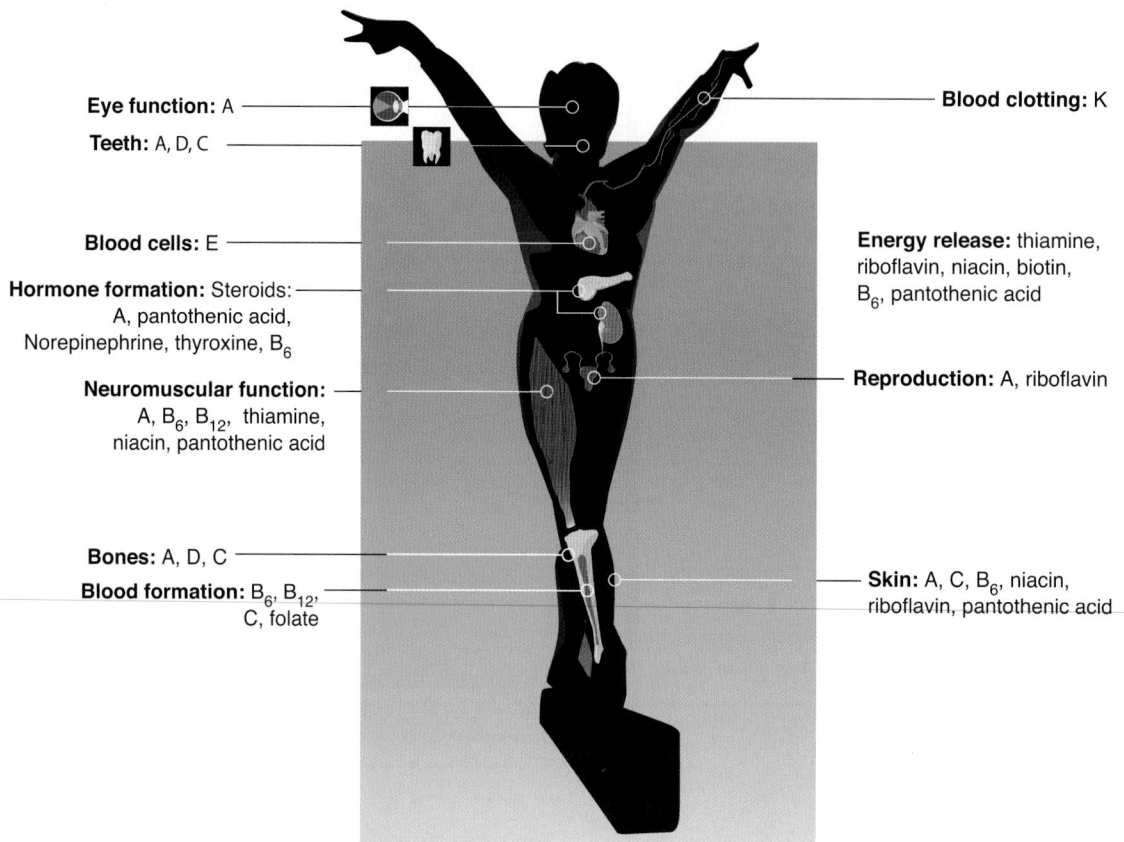

Eye function: A

Teeth: A, D, C

Blood cells: E

Hormone formation: Steroids: A, pantothenic acid, Norepinephrine, thyroxine, B_6

Neuromuscular function: A, B_6, B_{12}, thiamine, niacin, pantothenic acid

Bones: A, D, C

Blood formation: B_6, B_{12}, C, folate

Blood clotting: K

Energy release: thiamine, riboflavin, niacin, biotin, B_6, pantothenic acid

Reproduction: A, riboflavin

Skin: A, C, B_6, niacin, riboflavin, pantothenic acid

FIGURE 2.2 ■ Biologic functions of vitamins in the body.

Dietary Reference Intakes

Dietary Reference Intakes (DRIs) represent a radically new and more comprehensive approach to nutritional recommendations for individuals.[191] Think of the DRIs as the umbrella term that encompasses the array of new standards—RDAs, Estimated Average Requirements (EAR), Adequate Intakes (AI), and the Tolerable Upper Intake Levels (ULs)—for nutrient recommendations in planning and assessing diets for healthy persons.

Similarities of dietary patterns caused the inclusion of both Canada and the United States in the target population. Recommendations encompass not only daily intakes intended for health maintenance but also upper intake levels that reduce the likelihood of harm from excess nutrient intake. In addition to including values for energy, protein, and the micronutrients, DRIs also provide values for macronutrients and food components of nutritional importance, such as phytochemicals. Whenever possible, nutrient intakes are recommended in four categories instead of one. This concept of range places the DRIs more in line with the Estimated Safe and Adequate Daily Dietary Intakes (ESADDIs).

Unique Aspects of the DRIs

The DRIs differ from their predecessor RDAs by focusing more on promotoing health maintenance and risk reduction for nutrient-dependent diseases (e.g., heart disease, diabetes, hypertension, osteoporosis, various cancers, and age-related macular degeneration), rather than the traditional criterion of preventing the deficiency diseases scurvy, beriberi, or rickets.

Unlike its RDA predecessor, the DRI value also includes recommendations that apply to gender and life stages of growth and development based on age and, when appropriate, pregnancy and lactation. The goal of a complete revision every 5 years as with the RDAs was abandoned, with the new modification of making immediate changes in the DRI as new scientific data become available. The National Academy Press presents the reports to date on the DRIs (www.nap.edu/; search for Dietary Reference Intakes).

> **TABLE 2.1 Water-Soluble Vitamins and Energy Transfer**
>
> **Vitamin B₁ (thiamine):** Provides oxidizable substrate in citric acid cycle via oxidative decarboxylation of pyruvate to acetyl-CoA during carbohydrate breakdown; requirement related to total energy expenditure and total carbohydrate breakdown; needs may be somewhat higher in physically active people with large carbohydrate catabolism; membrane and nerve conduction; pentose synthesis; oxidative decarboxylation of α-keto acids in amino acid breakdown
>
> **Vitamin B₂ (riboflavin):** Hydrogen (electron) transfer during mitochondrial metabolism in respiratory chain; combines with phosphoric acid to form flavin adenine dinucleotide (FAD) and flavin adenine mononucleotide (FMN)
>
> **Vitamin B₆ (pyridoxine):** Important coenzyme in protein synthesis and glycogen metabolism; coenzyme in transamination reactions; formation of precursor compounds for heme in hemoglobin; coenzyme for phosphorylase, which facilitates glycogen release from liver
>
> **Vitamin B₁₂ (cyanocobalamin):** Important coenzyme in the transfer of single-carbon units in nucleic acid metabolism; influences protein synthesis; role in gastrointestinal, bone, and nervous tissue function
>
> **Niacin (nicotinamide and nicotinic acid):** Hydrogen (electron) transfer during glycolysis and mitochondrial metabolism; component of nicotine and nicotine adenine dinucleotide phosphate (NADP); role in fat and glycogen synthesis; amino acid tryptophan converted to niacin; excess niacin may depress fatty acid mobilization, which would facilitate carbohydrate depletion
>
> **Pantothenic acid:** Component of the citric acid cycle intermediate acetyl-CoA; involved in synthesis of cholesterol, phospholipids, hemoglobin, and steroid hormones
>
> **Folate (folic acid, folacin):** Coenzyme in amino acid metabolism and nucleic acid synthesis; essential for normal formation of red and white blood cells; protects against neural tube defects in fetus
>
> **Biotin:** Essential role in carbohydrate, fat, and amino acid metabolism; involved in carboxyl unit transport and CO_2 fixing in tissues; role in gluconeogenesis and fatty acid synthesis and oxidation
>
> **Vitamin C (ascorbic acid):** Antioxidant; may relate to exercise through its role in the synthesis of collagen and carnitine; enhances iron absorption and possibly heat acclimatization; facilitates iron availability; cofactor in some hydroxylation reactions (e.g., dopamine to noradrenaline)

The following definitions apply to the four different sets of values for the intake of nutrients and food components in the DRIs:

- **Estimated Average Requirement (EAR):** Average level of daily nutrient intake to meet the requirement of half of the healthy individuals in a particular life-stage and gender group. In addition to assessing nutritional adequacy of intakes of population groups, the EAR provides a useful value for determining the prevalence of inadequate nutrient intake by the proportion of the population with intakes below this value.
- **Recommended Dietary Allowance (RDA):** The average daily nutrient intake level sufficient to meet the requirement of nearly 98% of healthy individuals in a particular life-stage and gender group (FIG. 2.3). For most nutrients, this value represents the EAR plus two standard deviations of the requirement.
- **Adequate Intake (AI):** The AI provides an assumed adequate nutritional goal when no RDA exists. It represents a recommended average daily nutrient intake level based on observed or experimentally determined approximations or estimates of nutrient intake by a group (or groups) of apparently healthy persons and is used when an RDA cannot be determined. Low risk exists with intakes at or above the AI level.
- **Tolerable Upper Intake Level (UL):** The highest average daily nutrient intake level likely to pose no risk of adverse health effects to almost all individuals in the specified gender and life-stage group of the general population. As intake increases above the UL, the potential risk of adverse effects increases.

The DRI report indicates that fruits and vegetables yield about half as much vitamin A than previously believed. Thus, individuals who do not eat vitamin-A rich, animal-derived foods should upgrade their intake of carotene-rich fruits and vegetables. The report also sets a daily maximum intake level for vitamin A, in addition to boron, copper, iodine, iron, manganese, molybdenum, nickel, vanadium, and zinc. Specific recommended intakes are provided for vitamins A and K, chromium, copper, iodine, manganese, molybdenum, and

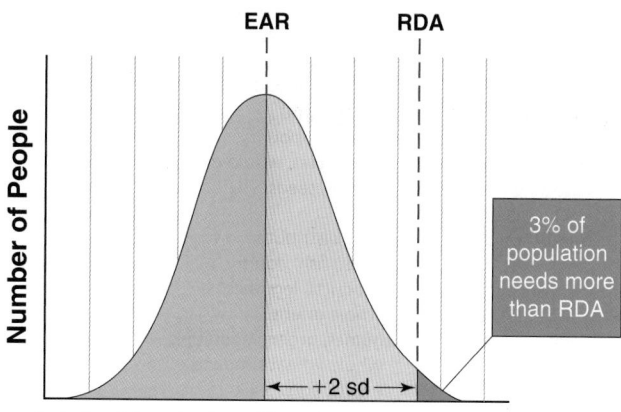

Intake Needed to Meet Requirements

FIGURE 2.3 ■ Theoretical distribution of the number of persons adequately nourished by a given nutrient intake. The recommended dietary allowance (RDA) is set at an intake level than would meet the nutrient needs 97% to 98% of the population (2 standard deviations [sd] above mean). EAR is the Estimated Average Requirement, which represents a nutrient intake value estimated to meet the requirement of half of the healthy individuals in a gender and life-stage group.

zinc. The report concludes that one can meet the daily requirement for the nutrients examined without supplementation. The exception is the mineral iron, for which most pregnant women need supplements to obtain their increased daily requirement.

TABLE 2.2 lists the major bodily functions, dietary sources, and symptoms of a deficiency or excess of the water-soluble and fat-soluble vitamins. TABLES 2.3 and 2.4 present the RDA, AI, and UL values for these vitamins. Well-balanced meals provide an adequate quantity of all vitamins, regardless of age

TABLE 2.2 Food Sources, Major Bodily Functions, and Symptoms of Deficiency or Excess of the Fat-soluble and Water-soluble Vitamins for Healthy Adults (19–50 Years of Age)

Vitamin	Dietary Sources	Major Bodily Functions	Deficiency	Excess
Fat soluble				
Vitamin A (retinol)	Provitamin A (β-carotene) widely distributed in green vegetables. Retinol present in milk, butter, cheese, fortified margarine	Constituent of rhodopsin (visual pigment). Maintenance of epithelial tissues. Role in mucopolysaccharide synthesis	Xerophthalmia (keratinization of ocular tissue), night blindness, permanent blindness	Headache, vomiting, peeling of skin, anorexia, swelling of long bones
Vitamin D	Cod-liver oil, eggs, dairy products, fortified milk, and margarine	Promotes growth and mineralization of bones. Increases absorption of calcium	Rickets (bone deformities) in children; osteomalacia in adults	Vomiting, diarrhea, loss of weight, kidney damage
Vitamin E (tocopherol)	Seeds, green leafy vegetables, margarines, shortenings	Functions as an antioxidant to prevent cell damage	Possible anemia	Relatively nontoxic
Vitamin K (phylloquinone)	Green leafy vegetables, small amounts in cereals, fruits, and meats	Important in blood clotting (involved in formation of prothombin)	Conditioned deficiencies associated with severe bleeding; internal hemorrhages	Relatively nontoxic; synthetic forms at high doses may cause jaundice
Water soluble				
Vitamin B$_1$ (thiamin)	Pork, organ meats, whole grains, nuts, legumes, milk, fruits, and vegetables	Coenzyme (thiamin pyrophosphate) in reactions involving the removal of carbon dioxide	Beriberi (peripheral nerve changes, edema, heart failure)	None reported
Vitamin B$_2$	Widely distributed in foods: meats, eggs, milk products, whole grain and enriched cereal products, wheat germ, green leafy vegetables	Constituent of two flavin nucleotide coenzymes involved in energy metabolism (FAD and FMN)	Reddened lips, cracks at mouth corner (cheilosis), eye lesions	None reported
Niacin	Liver, lean meats, poultry, grains, legumes, peanuts (can be formed from tryptophan)	Constituent of two coenzymes in oxidation-reduction reactions (NAD and NADP)	Pellagra (skin and gastrointestinal lesions, nervous mental disorders)	Flushing, burning and tingling around neck, face, and hands
Vitamin B$_6$	Meats, fish, poultry, vegetables, whole-grain, cereals, seeds	Coenzyme (pyridoxal phosphate) involved in amino acid and glycogen metabolism	Irritability, convulsions, muscular twitching, dermatitis, kidney stones	None reported
Pantothenic acid	Widely distributed in foods: meat, fish, poultry, milk products, legumes, whole grains	Constituent of coenzyme A, which plays a central role in energy metabolism	Fatigue, sleep disturbances, impaired coordination, nausea	None reported
Folate	Legumes, green vegetables, whole wheat products, meats, eggs, milk products, liver	Coenzyme (reduced form) involved in transfer of single-carbon units in nucleic acid and amino acid metabolism	Anemia, gastrointestinal disturbances, diarrhea, red tongue	None reported
Vitamin B$_{12}$	Muscle meats, fish, eggs, dairy products, (absent in plant foods)	Coenzyme involved in transfer of single-carbon units in nucleic acid metabolism	Pernicious anemia, neurologic disorders	None reported
Biotin	Legumes, vegetables, meats, liver, egg yolk, nuts	Coenzymes required for fat synthesis, amino acid metabolism, and glycogen (animal starch) formation	Fatigue, depression, nausea, dermatitis, muscular pains	None reported
Vitamin C (ascorbic acid)	Citrus fruits, tomatoes, green peppers, salad greens	Maintains intercellular matrix of cartilage, bone, and dentine; important in collagen synthesis	Scurvy (degeneration of skin, teeth, blood vessels, epithelial hemorrhages)	Relatively nontoxic; possibility of kidney stones

TABLE 2.3 Dietary Reference Intakes (DRIs): Recommended Intakes for Individuals: Vitamins

Life Stage Group	Vitamin A (μg/d)[a]	Vitamin C (mg/d)	Vitamin D (μg/d)[b,c]	Vitamin E (mg/d)[d]	Vitamin K (μg/d)	Thiamin (mg/d)	Riboflavin (mg/d)	Niacin (mg/d)[e]	Vitamin B₆ (mg/d)	Folate (μg/d)[f,i,j]	Vitamin B₁₂ (μg/d)	Pantothenic Acid (mg/d)	Biotin (mg/d)	Choline (mg/d)[g]
Infants														
0–6 mo	400*	40*	5*	4*	2.0*	0.2*	0.3*	2*	0.1*	65*	0.4*	1.7*	5*	125*
7–12 mo	500*	50*	5*	5*	2.5*	0.3*	0.4*	4*	0.3*	80*	0.5*	1.8*	6*	150*
Children														
1–3 y	300	15	5*	6	30*	0.5	0.5	6	0.5	150	0.9	2*	8*	200*
4–8 y	400	25	5*	7	55*	0.6	0.6	8	0.6	200	1.2	3*	12*	250*
Males														
9–13 y	600	45	5*	11	60*	0.9	0.9	12	1.0	300	1.8	4*	20*	375*
14–18 y	900	75	5*	15	75*	1.2	1.3	16	1.3	400	2.4	5*	25*	550*
19–30 y	900	90	5*	15	120*	1.2	1.3	16	1.3	400	2.4	5*	30*	550*
31–50 y	900	90	5*	15	120*	1.2	1.3	16	1.3	400	2.4	5*	30*	550*
51–70 y	900	90	10*	15	120*	1.2	1.3	16	1.3	400	2.4[h]	5*	30*	550*
>70 y	900	90	15*	15	120*	1.2	1.3	16	1.3	400	2.4[h]	5*	30*	550*
Females														
9–13 y	600	45	5*	11	60*	0.9	0.9	12	1.0	300	1.8	4*	20*	375*
14–18 y	700	65	5*	15	75*	1.0	1.0	14	1.2	400[f]	2.4	5*	25*	400*
19–30 y	700	75	5*	15	90*	1.1	1.1	14	1.3	400[f]	2.4	5*	30*	425*
31–50 y	700	75	5*	15	90*	1.1	1.1	14	1.3	400[f]	2.4	5*	30*	425*
51–70 y	700	75	10*	15	90*	1.1	1.1	14	1.5	400	2.4[h]	5*	30*	425*
>70 y	700	75	15*	15	90*	1.1	1.1	14	1.5	400	2.4[h]	5*	30*	425*
Pregnancy														
≤18 y	750	80	5*	15	75*	1.4	1.4	18	1.9	600[f]	2.6	6*	30*	450*
19–30 y	770	85	5*	15	90*	1.4	1.4	18	1.9	600[f]	2.6	6*	30*	450*
31–50 y	770	85	5*	15	90*	1.4	1.4	18	1.9	600[f]	2.6	6*	30*	450*
Lactation														
≤18 y	1200	115	5*	19	75*	1.4	1.6	17	2.0	500	2.8	7*	35*	550*
19–30 y	1300	120	5*	19	90*	1.4	1.6	17	2.0	500	2.8	7*	35*	550*
31–50 y	1300	120	5*	19	90*	1.4	1.6	17	2.0	500	2.8	7*	35*	550*

Sources: Dietary Reference Intakes for Calcium, Phosphorous, Magnesium, Vitamin D, and Fluoride (1997); Dietary Reference Intakes for Thiamin, Riboflavin, Niacin, Vitamin B₆, Folate, Vitamin B₁₂, Pantothenic Acid, Biotin, and Choline (1998); Dietary Reference Intakes for Vitamin C, Vitamin E, Selenium, and Carotenoids (2000); and Dietary Reference Intakes for Vitamin A, Vitamin K, Arsenic, Boron, Chromium, Copper, Iodine, Iron, Manganese, Molybdenum, Nickel, Silicon, Vanadium, and Zinc (2001). These reports may be accessed via www.nap.edu. Copyright 2001 by the National Academy of Sciences. All rights reserved.

*Note: This table (taken from the DRI reports, see www.nap.edu) presents Recommended Dietary Allowances (RDAs) in **bold type** and Adequate Intakes (AIs) in ordinary type followed by an asterisk (*). RDAs and AIs may both serve as goals for individual intake. RDAs are set to meet the needs of almost all (97 to 98 percent) individuals in a group. For healthy breastfed infants, the AI is the mean intake. The AI for other life stage and gender groups may cover needs of all individuals in the group, but lack of data or uncertainty in the data prevent being able to specify with confidence the percentage of individuals covered by this intake.*

[a]As retinol activity equivalents (RAEs). 1 RAE = 1 μg retinol, 12 μg β-carotene, 24 μg α-carotene, or 24 μg β-cryptoxanthin. To calculate RAEs from REs of provitamin A carotenoids in foods, divide the REs by 2. For preformed vitamin A in foods or supplements and for provitamin A carotenoids in supplements, 1 RE = 1 RAE.

[b]Calciferol. 1 mg calciferol = 40 IU vitamin D.

[c]In the absence of adequate exposure to sunlight.

[d]As a-tocopherol, a-Tocopherol includes RRR-α-tocopherol, the only form of α-tocopherol that occurs naturally in foods, and the 2R-stereoisometric forms of α-tocopherol (RRR-, RSR-, RRS-, and RSS-α-tocopherol) that occur in fortified foods and supplements. It does not include the 2S-stereoisomeric forms of α-tocopherol (SRR-, SSR-, SR-, and SSS-α-tocopherol), also found in fortified foods and supplements.

[e]As niacin equivalents (NE). 1 mg of niacin = 60 mg of tryptophan; 0-6 months = preformed niacin (not NE).

[f]As dietary folate equivalents (DFE). 1 DFE = 1 μg food folate = 0.6 μg of folic acid from fortified food or as a supplement consumed with food = 0.5 μg of a supplement taken on an empty stomach.

[g]Although AIs have been set for choline, there are few data to asses whether a dietary supply of choline is needed at all stages of the life cycle and it may be that the choline requirement can be met by endogenous synthesis at some of these stages.

[h]Because 10 to 30 percent of older people may malabsorb food-bound B₁₂, it is advisable for those older than 50 years to meet their RDA mainly by consuming foods fortified with B₁₂ or a supplement containing B₁₂.

[i]In view of evidence linking folate intake with neural tube defects in the fetus, it is recommended that all women capable of becoming pregnant consume 400 mg from supplements or fortified foods in addition to intake of food folate from a varied diet.

[j]It is assumed that women will continue consuming 400 μg from supplements or fortified food until their pregnancy is confirmed and they enter prenatal care, which ordinarily occurs after the end of the periconceptional period—the critical time for formation of the neural tube.

TABLE 2.4   Dietary Reference Intakes (DRIs): Tolerable Upper Intake Levels (UL^a): Vitamins

Life Stage Group	Vitamin A (μg/d)^b	Vitamin C (mg/d)	Vitamin D (μg/d)	Vitamin E (mg/d)^{c,d}	Vitamin K	Thiamin	Riboflavin	Niacin (mg/d)^d	Vitamin B$_6$ (mg/d)^d	Folate (μg/d)^d	Vitamin B$_{12}$	Pantothenic Acid	Biotin	Choline (g/d)	Carotenoids^e
Infants															
0–6 mo	600	ND^f	25	ND	ND	ND	ND	ND	ND	ND	ND	ND	ND	ND	ND
7–12 mo	600	ND	25	ND	ND	ND	ND	ND	ND	ND	ND	ND	ND	ND	ND
Children															
1–3 y	600	400	50	200	ND	ND	ND	10	30	300	ND	ND	ND	1.0	ND
4–8 y	900	650	50	300	ND	ND	ND	15	40	400	ND	ND	ND	1.0	ND
Males, Females															
9–13 y	1700	1200	50	600	ND	ND	ND	20	60	600	ND	ND	ND	2.0	ND
14–18 y	2800	1800	50	800	ND	ND	ND	30	80	800	ND	ND	ND	3.0	ND
19–70 y	3000	2000	50	1000	ND	ND	ND	35	100	1000	ND	ND	ND	3.5	ND
>70 y	3000	2000	50	1000	ND	ND	ND	35	100	1000	ND	ND	ND	3.5	ND
Pregnancy															
≤18 y	2800	1800	50	800	ND	ND	ND	30	80	800	ND	ND	ND	3.0	ND
19–50 y	3000	2000	50	1000	ND	ND	ND	35	100	1000	ND	ND	ND	3.5	ND
Lactation															
≤18 y	2800	1800	50	800	ND	ND	ND	30	80	800	ND	ND	ND	3.0	ND
19–50 y	3000	2000	50	1000	ND	ND	ND	35	100	1000	ND	ND	ND	3.5	ND

Sources: Dietary Reference Intakes for Calcium, Phosphorous, Magnesium, Vitamin D, and Fluoride (1997); Dietary Reference Intakes for Thiamin, Riboflavin, Niacin, Vitamin B$_6$, Folate, Vitamin B$_{12}$, Pantothenic Acid, Biotin, and Choline (1998); Dietary Reference Intakes for Vitamin C, Vitamin E, Selenium, and Carotenoids (2000); and Dietary Reference Intakes for Vitamin A, Vitamin K, Arsenic, Boron, Chromium, Copper, Iodine, Iron, Manganese, Molybdenum, Nickel, Silicon, Vanadium, and Zinc (2001). These reports may be accessed via www.nap.edu. Copyright 2001 by the National Academy of Sciences. All rights reserved.

^{a}UL = The maximum level of daily nutrient intake that is likely to pose no risk of adverse effects. Unless otherwise specified, the UL represents total intake from food, water, and supplements. Due to lack of suitable data, ULs could not be established for vitamin K, thiamin, riboflavin, vitamin B$_{12}$, pantothenic acid, biotin, or carotenoids. In the absence of ULs, extra caution may be warranted in consuming levels above recommended intakes.

^{b}As preformed vitamin A only.

^{c}As α-tocopherol; applies to any form of supplemental α-tocopherol.

^{d}The ULs for vitamin E, niacin, and folate apply to synthetic forms obtained from supplements, fortified foods, or a combination of the two.

^{e}β-Carotene supplements are advised only to serve as a provitamin A source for individuals at risk of vitamin A deficiency.

^{f}ND = Not determinable due to lack of data of adverse effects in this age group and concern with regard to lack of ability to handle excess amounts. Source of intake should be from food only to prevent high levels of intake.

and physical activity level. Indeed, individuals who expend considerable energy exercising generally need not consume special foods or supplements that increase vitamin intake above recommended levels. Also, at high levels of daily physical activity, food intake generally increases to sustain the added exercise energy requirements. Additional food through a variety of nutritious meals proportionately increases vitamin and mineral intakes. Chapter 7 summarizes recommendations from the DRI report on ranges for macronutrient and fiber intake and daily physical activity to optimize health and reduce chronic illness.

Several possible exceptions exist to the general rule that discounts a need for supplementation if one consumes a well-balanced diet. First, vitamin C and folate exist in foods that usually make up only a small part of most American's total caloric intake. The availability of these foods also varies by season. Second, different athletic groups have relatively low intakes of vitamins B$_1$ and B$_6$.[45,156] Their adequate intake occurs if the daily diet contains fresh fruit, grains, and uncooked or steamed vegetables. Individuals on meatless diets should consume a small amount of milk, milk products, or eggs because vitamin B$_{12}$ exists only in foods of animal origin. Consuming recommended quantities of folate is crucial to fetal nervous system development in the early stage of pregnancy.

Antioxidant and Disease Protection Role of Specific Vitamins

Most of the oxygen consumed during mitochondrial energy metabolism combines with hydrogen to produce water. Normally, electron "leakage" along the electron transport chain allows about 2 to 5% of oxygen to form oxygen-containing **free radicals** such as superoxide (O_2^-), hydrogen peroxide (H_2O_2), and hydroxyl (OH^-) radicals. *A free radical represents a highly chemically reactive atom, molecule, or molecular fragment that contains at least one unpaired electron in its outer orbital or valence shell.* (Paired electrons, by way of contrast, represent a far more stable state.) These are the same free radicals produced by external factors such as heat and ionizing radiation and carried in cigarette smoke, environmental pollutants, and even some medications. Once formed, free radicals search out other compounds to create new free radical molecules.

When superoxide forms, it dismutates to hydrogen peroxide. Normally, superoxide rapidly converts to O_2 and H_2O by the action of **superoxide dismutase,** an enzyme in the body's first line of antioxidant defense. An accumulation of free radicals increases the potential for cellular damage (**oxidative stress**) to many biologically important substances in processes that add oxygen to cellular components. These substances include the genetic material of DNA and RNA, proteins, and lipid-containing structures, particularly the polyunsaturated fatty acid-rich bilayer membrane that isolates the cell against noxious toxins and carcinogens. Oxygen radicals have strong affinity for the polyunsaturated fatty acids that make up the lipid bilayer of the cell membrane.

During unrestrained oxidative stress, the plasma membrane's fatty acids deteriorate. Membrane damage occurs through a chain-reaction series of events termed **lipid peroxidation.** These reactions, which incorporate oxygen into lipids, increase the vulnerability of the cell and its constituents. Free radicals also facilitate LDL cholesterol oxidation, thus leading to cytotoxicity and enhanced plaque formation in the coronary arteries.

A Harmful Process

Oxidative stress ultimately increases the likelihood of cellular deterioration associated with advanced aging, cancer, diabetes, coronary artery disease, exercise-related oxidative damage, and a general decline in central nervous system and immune functions.

No way exists to stop oxygen reduction and subsequent free radical production, but an elaborate natural defense against their damaging effects exists within the mitochondria and surrounding extracellular spaces. This defense includes the antioxidant scavenger enzymes catalase, glutathione peroxidase, superoxide dismutase, and metal-binding proteins. In addition, the nonenzymatic nutritive reducing agents vitamins A, C, and E; the vitamin A precursor β-carotene (one of the "carotenoids" in dark green and orange vegetables); the mineral selenium; and a supplement of a mixed fruit and vegetable juice concentrate serve important protective functions.[13,56,73,92,178] These antioxidant chemicals protect the plasma membrane by reacting with and removing free radicals. This quenches the harmful chain reaction. Many of these vitamins and minerals also blunt the damaging effects to cellular constituents of high serum homocysteine levels (see page 56).[115]

Maintaining a diet with appropriate quantities of antioxidant vitamins and other chemoprotective agents reduces the occurrence of cardiovascular disease, diabetes, osteoporosis, cataracts, premature aging, and diverse cancers, including those of the breast, distal colon, prostate, pancreas, ovary, and endometrium.[44,76,89,150,203] A normal to above normal intake of dietary vitamin E (in α- and γ-tocopherol forms[80]) and β-carotene and/or high serum levels of carotenoids may blunt the progression of coronary artery narrowing and reduce risk for heart attack and possibly diabetes in men and women.[52,63,71] Unfortunately, heart disease protection from vitamin E is not always observed in diverse populations, high-risk patients, and those with congestive heart failure.[83,119,184,199,211] For patients with vascular disease or diabetes mellitus, long-term vitamin E supplementation does not prevent cancer or major cardiovascular events and may increase the risk for heart failure.[106]

Examples of Health Benefits

Maintaining a diet with recommended levels of the antioxidant vitamins (particularly vitamin C) reduces risk for several types of cancer.[150] Protection against heart disease occurs with relatively high daily intakes from either foods or supplements of the B vitamins folate (400 μg) and vitamin B_6 (3 mg).[149] These two vitamins reduce blood levels of homocysteine, an amino acid that increases risk for heart attack and stroke. Good sources of folate include enriched whole-grain cereals, nuts and seeds, dark green, leafy vegetables, beans and peas, and orange juice.

Postmenopausal women whose diets contained the most vitamin E had 62% less chance of dying from coronary heart disease (CHD) than women who consumed the least vitamin E.[93] In elderly men, a high plasma concentration of vitamins C and E and β-carotene associates with a reduced development and progression of early atherosclerotic lesions.[52] One model for heart disease protection proposes that the antioxidant vitamins, particularly vitamin E (recommended intake of 15 mg · d^{-1}), inhibit oxidation of LDL cholesterol and its subsequent uptake into foam cells embedded in the arterial wall. The **oxidative modification hypothesis** maintains that the oxidation of LDL cholesterol—a process similar to butter turning rancid—contributes to the plaque-forming, artery-clogging atherosclerotic process.[34,100] Additional benefits of vitamin E in the diet include protection against prostate cancer (risk reduced by one third and death rate by 40%) and heart disease and stroke, perhaps by preventing blood clot formation from the anticoagulant properties of vitamin E quinone, a natural by-product of vitamin E metabolism. All evidence does not support a reduced colorectal cancer risk from increased intake of vitamin-rich fruits and vegetables.[121,183]

Nutritional guidelines now focus more on the consumption of a broad array of foods than on isolated chemicals within these foods. The current recommendation is to increase the consumption of fruits, vegetables, and whole grains and include lean meat or meat substitutes and low-fat dairy foods to gain substantial health benefits and reduce risk of early mortality. Disease protection from diet can be linked to the myriad of accessory nutrients and substances (e.g., the numerous "chemoprotectant" phytochemicals and zoochemicals) within the vitamin-containing foods in a healthful diet.[72] Three potential mechanisms for antioxidant health benefits include:

1. Influencing molecular mechanisms and gene expression
2. Providing enzyme-inducing substances that detoxify carcinogens
3. Blocking uncontrolled growth of cells

According to the director of the Division of Cancer Prevention and Control at the National Cancer Institute (NCI; www.cancer.gov/), more than 150 studies have clearly shown that groups of people who eat plenty of fruits and vegetables get less cancer at a number of cancer sites. The NCI encourages consumption of five or more servings (nine recommended for men) of fruits and vegetables daily, while the United States Department of Agriculture's (USDA's) *Dietary Guidelines* recommend two to four servings of fruits and three to five servings of vegetables daily. Rich dietary sources of three antioxidant vitamins include:

1. **β-Carotene:** (best known of the pigmented compounds, or carotenoids, that give color to yellow and green leafy vegetables) carrots; dark-green leafy vegetables such as spinach, broccoli, turnips, beet and collard greens; sweet potatoes; winter squash; apricots; cantaloupe; mangos; papaya
2. **Vitamin C:** citrus fruits and juices, cabbage, broccoli, turnip greens, cantaloupe, tomatoes, strawberries, apples with skin
3. **Vitamin E:** vegetable oils, wheat germ, whole-grain bread and cereals, dried beans, green leafy vegetables

EAT A VARIETY OF HEALTHFUL FOODS. Several randomized trials of supplements of β-carotene and vitamin A per se did not show a reduced incidence of cancer and cardiovascular disease.[69,140] Such findings have caused current nutritional guidelines to refocus more on the consumption of a broad array of foods rather than on isolated chemicals within these foods.[193] Current recommendations advise increased consumption of fruits, vegetables, and whole grains and include lean meat or meat substitutes and low-fat dairy foods to gain substantial health benefits and reduce risk of early mortality.

Disease protection from diet links to the myriad of accessory nutrients and substances within the vitamin-containing fruits, grains, and vegetables. Such nonvitamin substances include various plant phytochemicals such as isothiocyanates, potent stimulators of natural detoxifying enzymes in the body, present in broccoli, cabbage, cauliflower, and other cruciferous vegetables. Researchers at the National Eye Institute (www.nei.nih.gov) observed that persons with higher intakes of two specific antioxidants, lutein and zeaxanthin (found primarily in green leafy vegetables such as spinach, kale, and collard greens), experienced 70% less age-related macular degeneration than individuals with lower intakes. This disease results from deterioration of the macular cells in the center of

the retina, the light-sensitive layer in the back of the eye that enables us to see. Lycopene, a potent antioxidant substance in carotene-rich foods (and what makes tomatoes red, released largely by cooking) has been linked to reduced heart disease risk and reduced risk of developing several deadly forms of cancer (prostate, colon, and rectal).[8] Chapter 7 explores the possible interaction of exercise, free radical formation, and antioxidant vitamin requirements. The past decade has witnessed considerable research in the area of functional foods and **nutraceuticals**—the foods or parts of food that provide medical or health benefits, including prevention and/or treatment of diseases.

PERSONAL COMMITMENT TO GOOD NUTRITION

1. Eat cereals high in bran and whole grains to maximize fiber intake to lower heart disease risk and produce less weight gain.
2. Go meatless or at least reduce processed meat intake; instead replace with fish, poultry, or beans to reduce risk of colon, stomach, pancreatic, and possibly prostate cancer.
3. Eat at least 3 cups of legumes each day to optimize potassium, folate, iron, and protein intake and perhaps reduce risk of colon caner.
4. Decrease the intake of cheese to lower cholesterol-raising saturated fatty acids.
5. Smarten up on snacks and cut calories from muffins, chips, candies, scones, and assorted pastries. Switch to lower calorie density, nutrient-rich snacks such as fresh fruits and veggies.
6. Eat fish at least two times a week to reduce intake of saturated fat and increase omega-3 fats that may lower heart disease risk.

BEYOND CHOLESTEROL: HOMOCYSTEINE AND CORONARY HEART DISEASE

In 1969, an 8-year-old boy died of a stroke. Autopsy reveled that his arteries had the sclerotic look of the blood vessels of an elderly man, and his blood contained excess levels of the amino acid **homocysteine.** His rare genetic disorder, homocystinuria, causes premature hardening of the arteries and early death from heart attack or stroke. In the years following this observation, an impressive number of studies have shown an almost lockstep association between high homocysteine levels and both heart attack and all-cause mortality.[14,42,62,107,111,195,201] In the presence of other conventional CHD risks (e.g., smoking and hypertension), synergistic effects magnify the negative impact of homocysteine.[190,208] Elevated homocysteine levels also associate with increased risk of elevated osteoporetic fracture, cognitive impairment, Alzheimer's disease, and adverse outcomes and complications of pregnancy.[117,126,146,147,167,196]

All individuals produce homocysteine, but it normally converts to other nondamaging amino acids. Three B vitamins—folate, B_6, and B_{12}—facilitate the conversion. If the conversion slows from a genetic defect or vitamin deficiency, homocysteine levels increase and promote cholesterol's damaging effects on the arterial lumen. FIGURE 2.4 proposes a mechanism for homocysteine damage.[130,204] The homocysteine model points up the fact that CHD can mediate through multiple biologic pathways and helps to explain why some people contract heart disease despite low-to-normal LDL cholesterol levels.

Excessive homocysteine causes blood platelets to clump, fostering blood clots and deterioration of smooth muscle cells that line the arterial wall. Chronic homocysteine exposure can scar and thicken arteries and provides a fertile medium for circulating LDL cholesterol to initiate damage and encourage plaque formation. Persons with elevated homocysteine levels run a greater risk of death from heart disease than individuals with normal levels.

Some Question About the Strength of the Association

A recent report analyzed the data from 30 studies that encompassed almost 17,000 people who collectively suffered 5073 heart attacks and 1113 strokes.[185] After controlling for high blood pressure and stroke, a person who lowered homocysteine level by 25% reduced heart-attack risk by a modest 11% and stroke risk by19%. More definitive assessments of homocysteine and cardiovascular disease risk will emerge from prospective, randomized clinical trials currently under way that involve administering vitamins B_6 and B_{12} and folate to healthy persons and evaluating disease outcome over at least 5 years.

It remains uncertain what causes some persons to accumulate homocysteine, but evidence points to deficiency of B vitamins and lifestyle factors such as cigarette smoking, alcohol and coffee consumption, and high meat in-

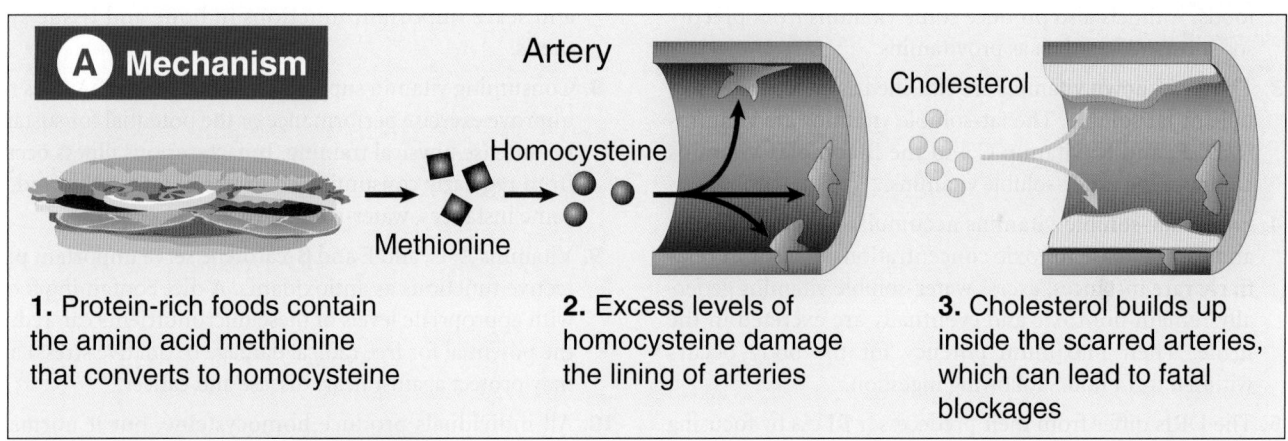

A. Mechanism

Artery

Homocysteine

Methionine

Cholesterol

1. Protein-rich foods contain the amino acid methionine that converts to homocysteine

2. Excess levels of homocysteine damage the lining of arteries

3. Cholesterol builds up inside the scarred arteries, which can lead to fatal blockages

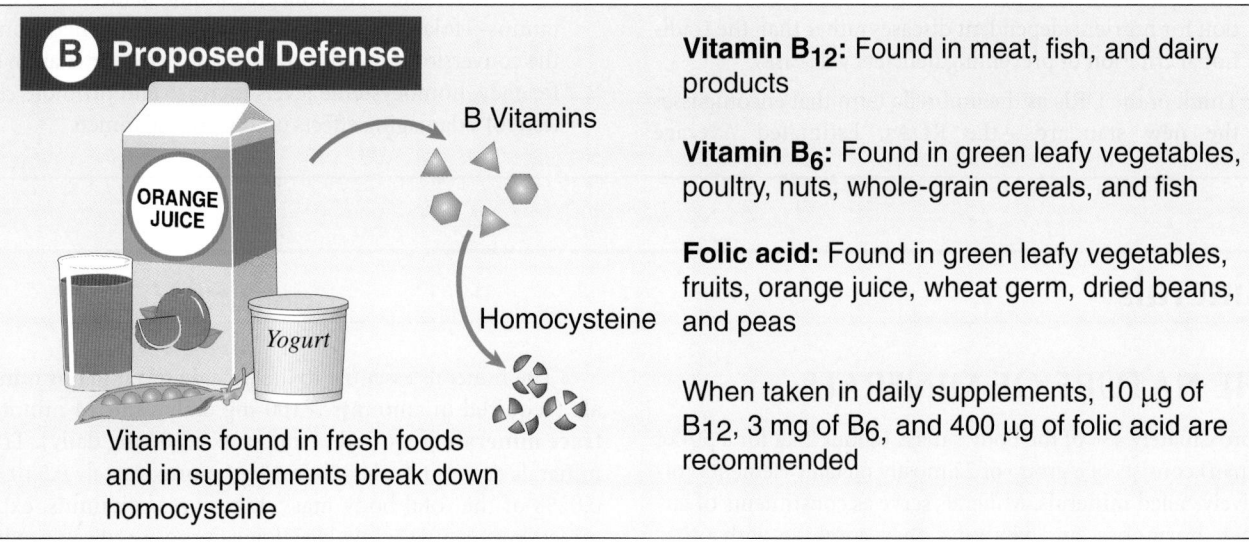

B. Proposed Defense

ORANGE JUICE

Yogurt

B Vitamins

Homocysteine

Vitamins found in fresh foods and in supplements break down homocysteine

Vitamin B_{12}: Found in meat, fish, and dairy products

Vitamin B_6: Found in green leafy vegetables, poultry, nuts, whole-grain cereals, and fish

Folic acid: Found in green leafy vegetables, fruits, orange juice, wheat germ, dried beans, and peas

When taken in daily supplements, 10 µg of B_{12}, 3 mg of B_6, and 400 µg of folic acid are recommended

FIGURE 2.4 ■ **A.** Proposed mechanism for how the amino acid homocysteine damages the lining of arteries and sets the stage for cholesterol infiltration into a blood vessel. **B.** Proposed defense against the possible harmful effects of elevated homocysteine levels.

take.[53,78,118,138,163,180] No clear standard for normal or desirable homocysteine levels currently exists. Research must show that normalizing homocysteine actually reduces risk of heart attack and stroke. In this regard, homocysteine-lowering therapy with the combination of folate and vitamins B_{12} and B_6 improved the outcome for heart disease patients undergoing coronary angioplasty.[165] Sufficient evidence supports consuming adequate B vitamins, particularly folate. Even small amounts of this vitamin (plentiful in enriched whole-grain cereals, nuts and seeds, dark green, leafy vegetables, beans and peas, and orange juice) provides a cost-efficient means to lower homocysteine levels (Fig. 2.4).[187] Folate fortifies all white flour, breads, pasta, grits, white rice, and cornmeal. Between 300 and 400 μg represents the current recommended daily folate intake.

Summary

1. Vitamins are organic substances that neither supply energy nor contribute to body mass. Vitamins serve crucial functions in almost all bodily processes; they must be obtained from food or dietary supplementation.

2. Plants manufacture vitamins during photosynthesis. Animals obtain vitamins from the plants they eat or from the meat of other animals that previously consumed these foods. Animals also produce some vitamins from precursor substances known as provitamins.

3. Thirteen known vitamins are classified as either water soluble or fat soluble. The fat-soluble vitamins are vitamins A, D, E, and K; vitamin C and the B-complex vitamins compose the water-soluble vitamins.

4. Excess fat-soluble vitamins accumulate in body tissues and can increase to toxic concentrations. Except in relatively rare instances, excess water-soluble vitamins generally remain nontoxic and eventually are excreted in the urine. Their maximum potency for the body occurs within 8 to 14 hours following ingestion.

5. The DRIs differ from their predecessor RDAs by focusing more on promoting health maintenance and risk reduction for nutrient-dependent diseases rather than the traditional criterion of preventing deficiency diseases.

6. Think of the DRIs as the umbrella term that encompasses the new standards—the RDAs, Estimated Average Requirements, Adequate Intakes, and the Tolerable Upper Intake Levels—for nutrient recommendations for use in planning and assessing diets for healthy people. DRI values include recommendations that apply to gender and life stages of growth and development based on age and, when appropriate, pregnancy and lactation.

7. Vitamins regulate metabolism, facilitate energy release, and serve important functions in bone and tissue synthesis.

8. Consuming vitamin supplements above the RDA does not improve exercise performance or the potential for sustaining intense physical training. In fact, serious illness occurs from regularly consuming an excess of fat-soluble and, in some instances, water-soluble vitamins.

9. Vitamins A, C, and E and β-carotene serve important protective functions as antioxidants. A diet containing foods with appropriate levels of these micronutrients can reduce the potential for free radical damage (oxidative stress) and may protect against heart disease and cancer.

10. All individuals produce homocysteine, but it normally converts to other nondamaging amino acids. Three B-vitamins—folate, B_6, and B_{12}—facilitate the conversion. If the conversion slows due to a genetic defect or vitamin deficiency, homocysteine levels increase and promote cholesterol's damaging effects on the arterial lumen.

Minerals

THE NATURE OF MINERALS

Approximately 4% of the body's mass (about 2 kg for a 50-kg woman) consists of a group of 22 mostly metallic elements collectively called **minerals.** Minerals serve as constituents of enzymes, hormones, and vitamins; they combine with other chemicals (e.g., calcium phosphate in bone, iron in the heme of hemoglobin) or exist singularly (free calcium in body fluids).

The minerals essential to life include seven **major minerals** (required in amounts >100 mg daily) and 14 minor or **trace minerals** (required in amounts <100 mg daily). Trace minerals account for less than 15 g (approximately 0.5 oz) or 0.02% of the total body mass. Like excess vitamins, excess minerals serve no useful physiologic purpose and can produce toxic effects. RDAs and recommended ranges of intakes have been established for many minerals; if the diet supplies these recommended levels, this ensures an adequate intake of the remaining minerals.

KINDS AND SOURCES OF MINERALS

TABLE 2.5 lists the major bodily functions, dietary sources, and symptoms of deficiency or excess of the minerals. TABLES 2.6 and 2.7 present the RDA, UL, and AI values for these minerals. Mineral supplements, like vitamin supplements, generally confer little benefit because the required minerals occur readily in food and water. Some supplementation may be necessary in geographic regions where the soil or water supply lacks a particular mineral. Iodine is required by the thyroid gland to synthesize thyroxine and triiodothyronine, hormones that accelerate resting metabolism. Adding iodine to the water supply or to table salt (iodized salt) easily prevents iodine deficiency. A common mineral deficiency in the United States results from a lack of iron in the diet. Between 30 and 50% of American women of child-bearing age suffer some form of dietary iron insufficiency. As discussed on page 76, upgrading one's diet with iron-rich foods or prudent use of iron supplements alleviates this problem.

ROLE OF MINERALS IN THE BODY

Whereas vitamins activate chemical processes without becoming part of the by-products of the reactions they catalyze, minerals often become incorporated within the structures and existing chemicals of the body. Minerals serve three broad roles in the body:

1. Minerals provide *structure* in forming bones and teeth.
2. In terms of *function,* minerals help to maintain normal heart rhythm, muscle contractility, neural conductivity, and acid–base balance.
3. Minerals *regulate* metabolism by becoming constituents of enzymes and hormones that modulate cellular activity.

FIGURE 2.5 lists minerals that participate in catabolic and anabolic cellular processes. Minerals activate reactions that release energy during carbohydrate, fat, and protein breakdown. In addition, minerals are essential for synthesizing biologic nutrients: glycogen from glucose, triacylglycerol from fatty acids and glycerol, and protein from amino acids. A lack of the essential minerals disrupts the fine balance between catabolism and anabolism. Minerals also form important components of hormones. Inadequate thyroxine production from iodine deficiency slows the body's resting metabolism. In extreme cases, this predisposes a person to develop obesity. The synthesis of insulin, the hormone that facilitates glucose uptake by cells, requires zinc (as do approximately 100 other enzymes), whereas the digestive acid hydrochloric acid forms from the mineral chlorine.

Mineral Bioavailability

The body varies considerably in its capacity to absorb and use the minerals in food. For example, spinach contains considerable calcium, but only about 5% of this calcium becomes absorbed. The same holds true for dietary iron, which the small intestine absorbs with efficiency averaging 5 to 10%. Factors that affect the **bioavailability** of minerals in food include:

1. **Type of food:** The small intestine readily absorbs minerals in animal products because plant binders and dietary fibers are unavailable to hinder digestion and absorption. Also, foods from the animal kingdom generally contain high mineral concentration (except for magnesium, which has a higher concentration in plants).
2. **Mineral–mineral interaction:** Many minerals have the same molecular weight and thus compete for intestinal absorption. This makes it unwise to consume an excess of any one mineral because it can retard another mineral's absorption.
3. **Vitamin–mineral interaction:** Various vitamins interact with minerals in a manner that affects mineral bioavailability. From a positive perspective, vitamin D facilitates calcium absorption and vitamin C improves iron absorption.
4. **Fiber–mineral interaction:** High fiber intake blunts the absorption of some minerals (e.g., calcium, iron, magnesium, phosphorus) by binding to them, causing them to pass unabsorbed through the digestive tract.

In the subsequent sections, we describe specific functions of the more important minerals related to physical activity.

CALCIUM

Calcium, the most abundant mineral in the body, combines with phosphorus to form bones and teeth. These two minerals represent about 75% of the body's total mineral content or about 2.5% of body mass. In its ionized form (about 1% of the body's 1200 g), calcium plays an important role in muscle action, blood clotting, nerve transmission, activation of several enzymes, synthesis of calcitriol (active form of vitamin D), and transport of fluids across cell membranes. Calcium also may contribute to easing premenstrual syndrome and polycystic ovary syndrome, preventing colon cancer, and optimizing blood pressure regulation,[40,112] although its role in reducing heart disease risk remains unclear.[2,77]

TABLE 2.5 **The Important Major and Minor (Trace) Minerals for Healthy Adults (19–50 Years of Age) and Their Dietary Requirements, Food Sources, Functions and the Effects of Deficiencies and Excesses**

Mineral	Dietary Sources	Major Bodily Functions	Deficiency	Excess
Major				
Calcium	Milk, cheese, dark green vegetables, dried legumes	Bone and tooth formation, blood clotting, nerve transmission	Stunted growth, rickets, osteoporosis, convulsions	Not reported in humans
Phosphorus	Milk, cheese, yogurt, meat, poultry, grains, fish	Bone and tooth formation, acid–base balance, helps prevent loss of calcium from bone	Weakness, demineralization	Erosion of jaw (phossy jaw)
Potassium	Leafy vegetables, cantaloupe, lima beans, potatoes, bananas, milk, meats, coffee, tea	Fluid balance, nerve transmission, acid–base balance	Muscle cramps, irregular cardiac rhythm, mental confusion, loss of appetite can be life-threatening	None if kidneys function normally; poor kidney function causes potassium buildup and cardiac arrhythmias
Sulfur	Obtained as part of dietary protein and is present in food preservatives	Acid–base balance, liver function	Unlikely to occur if dietary intake is adequate	Unknown
Sodium	Common salt	Acid–base balance, body water balance, nerve function	Muscle cramps, mental apathy, reduced appetite	High blood pressure
Chlorine (chloride)	Chloride is part of salt containing food; some vegetables and fruits	Important part of extracellular fluids	Unlikely to occur if dietary intake is adequate	Along with sodium contributes to high blood pressure
Magnesium	Whole grains, green leafy vegetables	Activates enzymes involved in protein synthesis	Growth failure, behavioral disturbances	Diarrhea
Minor				
Iron	Eggs, lean meats, legumes whole grains, green leafy vegetables	Constituent of hemoglobin and enzymes involved in energy metabolism	Iron deficiency anemia (weakness, reduced resistance to infection)	Siderosis; cirrhosis of the liver
Fluorine	Drinking water, tea, seafood	May be important in maintenance of bone structure	Higher frequency of tooth decay	Mottling of teeth, increased bone density
Zinc	Widely distributed in foods	Constituent of enzymes involved in digestion	Growth failure, small sex glands	Fever, nausea, vomiting, diarrhea
Copper	Meats, drinking water	Constituent of enzymes associated with iron metabolism	Anemia, bone changes (rare)	Rare metabolic condition (Wilson's disease)
Selenium	Seafood, meats, grains	Functions in close association with vitamin E	Anemia (rare)	Gastrointestinal disorders, lung irritations
Iodine (iodide)	Marine fish and shellfish, dairy products, vegetables, iodized salt	Constituent of thyroid hormones	Goiter (enlarged thyroid)	Very high intakes depress thyroid activity
Chromium	Legumes, cereals, organ meats, fats, vegetable oils, meats, whole grains	Constituent of some enzymes; involved in glucose and energy metabolism	Rarely reported in humans; impaired ability to metabolize glucose	Inhibition of enzymes Occupational exposures: skin and kidney damage

Osteoporosis: Calcium, Estrogen, and Exercise

Bone is a dynamic tissue matrix of collagen, minerals, and about 50% water. **Bone modeling** promotes continual increases in skeletal size and shape during youth. Bone also exists in a continual state of flux called **bone remodeling.** In the bone remodeling process, bone-destroying cells (osteoclasts) cause the breakdown (resorption) of bone while bone-forming osteoblast cells synthesize bone. This process is governed by an array of growth factors, gonadal hormones, and pituitary hormones. Calcium availability combined with regular physical activity affects the dynamics of bone remodeling. The plasma calcium level, regulated by hormonal action, is maintained either by calcium from food or calcium derived from the resorption of the bone mass. The two broad categories of bone include:

1. **Cortical bone:** dense, hard outer layer of bone such as the shafts of the long bones of the arms and legs
2. **Trabecular bone:** spongy, less dense, and relatively weaker bone most prevalent in the vertebrae and ball of the femur

A Mineral Whose Requirement Is Often Not Met

Growing children require more calcium per unit body mass than do adults, yet many adults remain deficient in calcium intake. As a general guideline, adolescents and young adults require 1300 mg of calcium daily (1000 mg for adults ages 19 to 50 and 1200 mg for those older than 50) or about as much calcium as in five 8-oz glasses of milk. Unfortunately, calcium remains one of the most frequent nutrients lacking in the diet of sedentary and physically active individuals, particularly adolescent girls. For an average adult, daily calcium intake ranges between 500 and 700 mg. *Female dancers, gymnasts, and endurance athletes are most prone to calcium dietary insufficiency.*[33,125]

TABLE 2.6   Dietary Reference Intakes (DRIs): Recommended Intakes for Individuals: Minerals

Life Stage Group	Calcium (mg/d)	Chromium (µg/d)	Copper (µg/d)	Flouride (mg/d)	Iodine (µg/d)	Iron (mg/d)	Magnesium (mg/d)	Manganese (mg/d)	Molybdenum (µg/d)	Phosphorus (mg/d)	Selenium (µg/d)	Zinc (mg/d)
Infants												
0–6 mo	210*	0.2*	200*	0.01*	110*	0.27*	30*	0.003*	2*	100*	15*	2*
7–12 mo	270*	5.5*	220*	0.5*	130*	11*	75*	0.6*	3*	275*	20*	3
Children												
1–3 y	500*	11*	340	0.7*	90	7	80	1.2*	17	460	20	3
4–8 y	800*	15*	440	1*	90	10	130	1.5*	22	500	30	5
Males												
9–13 y	1,300*	25*	700	2*	120	8	240	1.9*	34	1,250	40	8
14–18 y	1,300*	35*	890	3*	150	11	410	2.2*	43	1,250	55	11
19–30 y	1,000*	35*	900	4*	150	8	400	2.3*	45	700	55	11
31–50 y	1,000*	35*	900	4*	150	8	420	2.3*	45	700	55	11
51–70 y	1,200*	30*	900	4*	150	8	420	2.3*	45	700	55	11
>70 y	1,200*	30*	900	4*	150	8	420	2.3*	45	700	55	11
Females												
9–13 y	1,300*	21*	700	2*	120	8	240	1.6*	34	1,250	40	8
14–18 y	1,300*	24*	890	3*	150	15	360	1.6*	43	1,250	55	9
19–30 y	1,000*	25*	900	3*	150	18	310	1.8*	45	700	55	8
31–50 y	1,000*	25*	900	3*	150	18	320	1.8*	45	700	55	8
51–70 y	1,200*	20*	900	3*	150	8	320	1.8*	45	700	55	8
>70 y	1,200*	20*	900	3*	150	8	320	1.8*	45	700	55	8
Pregnancy												
≤18 y	1,300*	29*	1,000	3*	220	27	400	2.0*	50	1,250	60	13
19–30 y	1,000*	30*	1,000	3*	220	27	350	2.0*	50	700	60	11
31–50 y	1,000*	30*	1,000	3*	220	27	360	2.0*	50	700	60	11
Lactation												
≤18 y	1,300*	44*	1,300	3*	290	10	360	2.6*	50	1,250	70	14
19–30 y	1,000*	45*	1,300	3*	290	9	310	2.6*	50	700	70	12
31–50 y	1,000*	45*	1,300	3*	290	9	320	2.6*	50	700	70	12

Sources: Dietary Reference Intakes for Calcium, Phosphorous, Magnesium, Vitamin D and Fluoride (1997); Dietary Reference Intakes for Thiamin, Riboflavin, Niacin, Vitamin B6 Folate, Vitamin B12, Pantothenic Acid, Biotin, and Choline (1998); Dietary Reference Intakes for Vitamin C, Vitamin E, Selenium, and Carotenoids (2000); and Dietary Reference Intakes for Vitamin A, Vitamin K, Arsenic, Boron, Chromium, Copper, Iodine, Iron, Manganese, Molybdenum, Nickel, Silicon, Vanadium, and Zinc (2001). These reports may be accessed via www.nap.edu. Copyright 2001 by the National Academy of Sciences. Reprinted with permission.

Note: *This table presents Recommended Dietary Allowances (RDAs) in* **bold type** *and Adequate Intakes (AIs) in ordinary type followed by an asterisk (*). RDAs and AIs may both be used as goals for individual intake. RDAs are set to meet the needs of almost all (97 to 98 percent) individuals in a group. For healthy breastfed infants, the AI is the mean intake. The AI for other life stage and gender groups is believed to cover needs of all individuals in the group, but lack of data or uncertainty in the data prevent being able to specify with confidence the percentage of individuals covered by this intake.*

National Academy of Sciences Recommended Daily Calcium Intake

Age (y)	Amount (mg)
1–3	500
4–8	800
9–18	1300
19–50	1000
51 and older	1200

Over 75% of adults consume less than the RDA, and about 25% of women in the United States consume less than 300 mg of calcium daily. Inadequate calcium intake forces the body to draw on its bone calcium "reserves" to restore the deficit. Prolonging this restorative imbalance, either from inadequate calcium intake or low levels of calcium-regulating hormones, promotes one of two conditions:

1. **Osteoporosis:** literally meaning "porous bones," with bone density more than 2.5 standard deviations below normal for age and gender

TABLE 2.7   Dietary Reference Intakes (DRIs): Tolerable Upper Intake Levels (UL[a]): Minerals

Life Stage Group	Arsenic[b]	Boron (mg/d)	Calcium (g/d)	Chromium	Copper (μg/d)	Flouride (mg/d)	Iodine (μg/d)	Iron (mg/d)	Magnesium (mg/d)[c]	Manganese (mg/d)	Molybdenum (μg/d)	Nickel (mg/d)	Phosphorus (g/d)	Selenium (μg/d)	Silicon[d]	Vanadium (mg/d)[e]	Zinc (mg/d)
Infants																	
0–6 mo	ND	ND	ND	ND	ND	0.7	ND	40	ND	ND	ND	ND	ND	45	ND	ND	4
7–12 mo	ND	ND	ND	ND	ND	0.9	ND	40	ND	ND	ND	ND	ND	60	ND	ND	5
Children																	
1–3 y	ND	3	2.5	ND	1,000	1.3	200	40	65	2	300	0.2	3	90	ND	ND	7
4–8 y	ND	6	2.5	ND	3,000	2.2	300	40	110	3	600	0.3	3	150	ND	ND	12
Males, females																	
9–13 y	ND	11	2.5	ND	5,000	10	600	40	350	6	1,100	0.6	4	280	ND	ND	23
14–18 y	ND	17	2.5	ND	8,000	10	900	45	350	9	1,700	1.0	4	400	ND	ND	34
19–70 y	ND	20	2.5	ND	10,000	10	1,100	45	350	11	2,000	1.0	4	400	ND	1.8	40
>70 y	ND	20	2.5	ND	10,000	10	1,100	45	350	11	2,000	1.0	3	400	ND	1.8	40
Pregnancy																	
≤18 y	ND	17	2.5	ND	8,000	10	900	45	350	9	1,700	1.0	3.5	400	ND	ND	34
19–50 y	ND	20	2.5	ND	10,000	10	1,100	45	350	11	2,000	1.0	3.5	400	ND	ND	40
Lactation																	
≤18 y	ND	17	2.5	ND	8,000	10	900	45	350	9	1,700	1.0	4	400	ND	ND	34
19–50 y	ND	20	2.5	ND	10,000	10	1,100	45	350	11	2,000	1.0	4	400	ND	ND	40

Sources: Dietary Reference Intakes for Calcium, Phosphorous, Magnesium, Vitamin D and Fluoride (1997); Dietary Reference Intakes for Thiamin, Riboflavin, Niacin, Vitamin B₆, Folate, Vitamin B₁₂, Pantothenic Acid, Biotin, and Choline (1998); Dietary Reference Intakes for Vitamin C, Vitamin E, Selenium, and Carotenoids (2000); and Dietary Reference Intakes for Vitamin A, Vitamin K, Arsenic, Boron, Chromium, Copper, Iodine, Iron, Manganese, Molybdenum, Nickel, Silicon, Vanadium, and Zinc (2001). These reports may be accessed via www.nap.edu. Copyright 2001 by the National Academy of Sciences. Reprinted with permission.

[a]*UL = The maximum level of daily nutrient intake that is likely to pose no risk of adverse effects. Unless otherwise specified, the UL represents total intake from food, water, and supplements. Due to lack of suitable data, ULs could not be established for arsenic, chromium, and silicon. In the absence of ULs, extra caution may be warranted in consuming levels above recommended intakes.*

[b]*Although the UL was not determined for arsenic, there is no justification for adding arsenic to food or supplements.*

[c]*The ULs for magnesium represent intake from a pharmacologic agent only and do not include intake from food and water.*

[d]*Although silicon has not been shown to cause adverse effects in humans, there is no justification for adding silicon to supplements.*

[e]*Although vanadium in food has not been shown to cause adverse effects in humans, there is no justification for adding vanadium to food and vanadium supplements should be used with caution. The UL is based on adverse effects in laboratory animals and this data could be used to set a UL for adults but not children and adolescents.*

[f]*ND = not determinable due to lack of data of adverse effects in this age group and concern with regard to lack of ability to handle excess amounts. Source of intake should be from food only to prevent high levels of intake.*

2. **Osteopenia:** from the Greek words *osteo,* meaning bone and *penia,* meaning poverty—a midway condition whereby bones weaken, with increased fracture risk

Osteoporosis develops progressively as bone loses its calcium mass (bone mineral content) and calcium concentration (bone mineral density) and progressively becomes porous and brittle (FIG. 2.6). The stresses of normal living often cause bone to break.

Currently, osteoporosis afflicts more than 28 million Americans, of whom 80 to 90% are women, with another 18 million individuals with low bone mass (www.nof.org). Fifty percent of all women eventually develop osteoporosis. Men are not immune from osteoporosis, with about two million men in the Unites States currently suffering from this affliction. Among older individuals, particularly women above age 60, this disease has reached near-epidemic proportions. Osteoporosis accounts for more than 1.5 million fractures (the clinical manifestation of the disease) yearly, including about 700,000 spinal fractures, 300,000 hip fractures, 200,000 wrist fractures, and 300,000 fractures of other body parts. Nearly 15% of postmenopausal women will fracture a hip, and about 33% will suffer spine-shortening and often painful vertebral fractures. Of the women who suffer a bone fracture

Deficiency Begins at an Early Age

Inadequate dietary calcium affects about 50% of American children under age 5, 65% of teenage boys, and 85% of teenage girls. Part of this calcium lack occurs because Americans now drink far less milk than soft drinks, or about 23 gallons of milk a year versus 49 gallons of soft drinks.

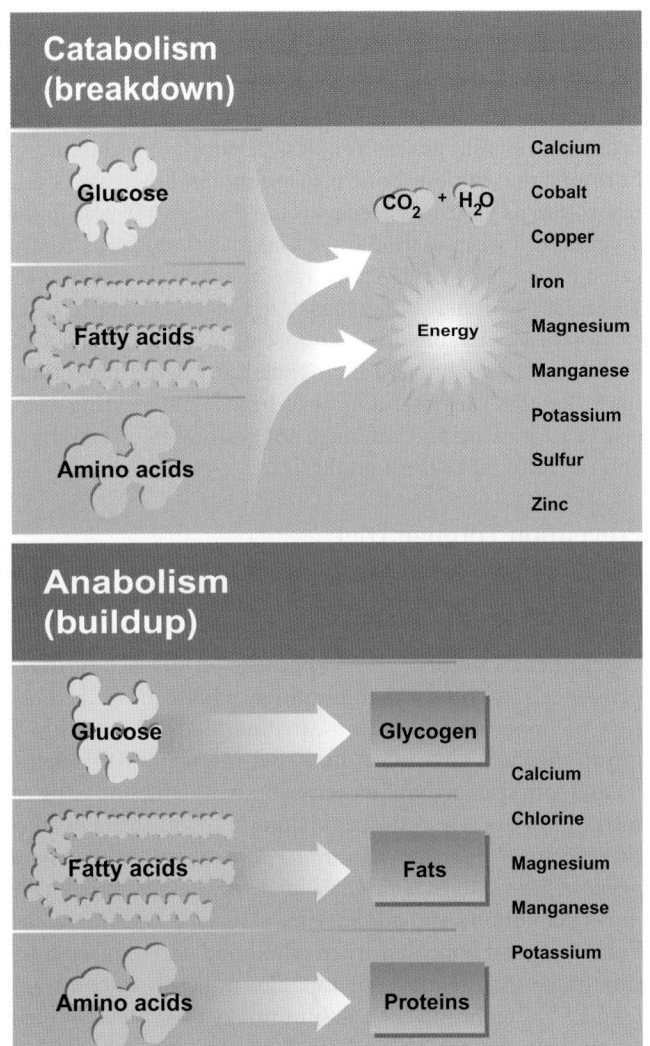

FIGURE 2.5 ■ Minerals function in the catabolism and anabolism of macronutrients.

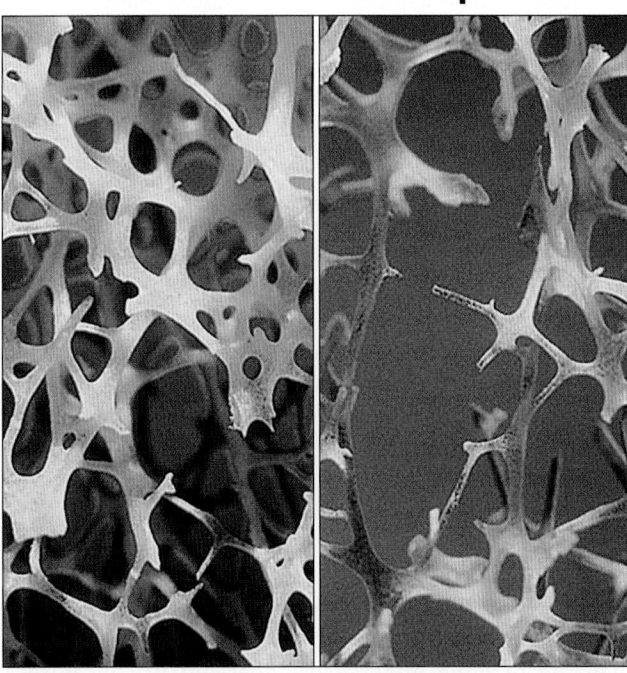

FIGURE 2.6 ■ Micrograph of normal bone *(left)* and osteoporotic bone *(right).* Osteoporotic bone shows these characteristics: loss of mineral matter, brittleness, cortex thinning (concomitant medullary diameter increase), increased porosity, imbalance between bone formation and resorption, disrupted bone architecture and cross-sectional geometry, microfracture accumulation, loss of mechanical integrity, and less tolerance to bending stress and thus more susceptibility to fracture.

after age 85, 25% die within 1 year. Estimates from the largest study to date indicate that nearly half of postmenopausal women aged 50 and older with no previous osteoporosis diagnosis have low bone mineral density, including 7% with os-

teoporosis.[172] This indicates that one of two women (lower risk among African American and Hispanic women) and one of eight men over age 50 will experience an osteoporosis-related fracture in their lifetime. The annual medical cost of hip fractures in the United States equals about $10 billion and may exceed $240 billion by the year 2040 (www.cdc.gov/ncipc/factsheetes/fallcost.htm).

Increased susceptibility to osteoporosis among older women coincides with the marked decrease in estrogen secretion that accompanies menopause.[28] Whether estrogen exerts its protective effects on bone by inhibiting bone resorption or decreasing bone turnover remains unknown (see page 72 for estrogen's possible actions). Men normally produce some estrogen, which largely explains their relatively low prevalence of osteoporosis. In addition, a portion of circulating testosterone converts to estradiol (a form of estrogen), which also promotes positive calcium balance. Most men maintain adequate testosterone levels throughout life. Risk factors for men include low testosterone levels, cigarette smoking, and use of medications such as steroids.

Bone Health Diagnostic Criteria Based on Variation (Standard Deviation) of Observed Bone Density. Values Compared with Values for Sex-Matched Young Adult Population

Normal	<1.0 SD below mean
Osteopenia	1.0–2.5 SD below mean
Osteoporosis	>2.5 SD below mean
Severe osteoporosis	>2.5 SD below mean plus one or more fragility fractures

A Progressive Disease

Between 60 and 80% of an individual's susceptibility to osteoporosis links to genetic factors, while 20 to 40% remains lifestyle related. Women normally show gains in bone mass throughout the third decade of life with proper nutrition (adequate calcium and vitamin D, which increases efficiency of calcium absorption) and regular moderate physical activity[96,159,186] (with a synergistic effect of both variables in children). However, adolescence serves as the prime bone building years to maximize bone mass; fully 90% of bone mass accumulates by about age 17.[5,124] In reality, osteoporosis for many women begins early in life because the average teenager consumes suboptimal calcium to support growing bones. This imbalance worsens into adulthood, particularly among women with genetic predisposition that limits their ability to compensate for low calcium intake by increasing calcium absorption.[49,54,105] By middle age, adult women generally consume only one third of the calcium required for optimal bone maintenance.

Beginning around age 50, the average man experiences a bone loss of about 0.4% each year, whereas the female begins to lose twice this amount at age 35. For men, the normal rate of bone mineral loss does not usually pose a problem until the eighth decade of life. Menopause makes women highly susceptible to osteoporosis because there is little or no release of estrogen from the ovaries. Muscle, adipose tissue, and connective tissue continue to produce estrogen, but only in limited quantities. The dramatic fall in estrogen production at menopause coincides with reduced intestinal calcium absorption, less calcitonin production (a hormone that inhibits bone resorption), and increased bone resorption as bone loss accelerates to 3 to 6% per year in the 5 years following menopause. The rate then drops to approximately 1% yearly. At this rate, the typical woman loses 15 to 20% of her bone mass in the first decade after menopause, and some women lose as much as 30% by age 70. Women can augment their genetically determined bone mass through purposeful increases in weight-bearing exercise (e.g., walking and running, not swimming or bicycling) and calcium intake throughout life.

Prevention Through Diet

FIGURE 2.7 illustrates that the variation in bone mass within a population results from a complex interaction among the various factors that affect bone mass rather than the distinct effect of each factor.[110,137,175] Because of this lack of independence among factors that influence bone mass, the portion of bone mass variation attributable to diet within a group may actually reflect how diet interacts with genetic factors, physical activity patterns, body weight, and drug or medication use (e.g., estrogen therapy). *Despite these interactive effects, adequate calcium intake throughout life remains a prime defense against bone loss with aging.* In fact, milk intake during childhood and adolescence associates with increased bone mass and bone density in adulthood and reduced fracture risk, independent of current milk or calcium intake.[81,160] Increasing the calcium intake of adolescent girls from their typical 80% of RDA level to the 110% level through supplementation increased total body calcium and spinal bone mineral density. A National Institutes of Health consensus panel in 2000 recommended that adolescent girls consume 1500 mg of calcium daily, an intake level that does not adversely affect zinc balance.[115] Furthermore, increasing daily calcium intake for middle-aged women, particularly for estrogen-deprived women after menopause, to between 1200 and 1500 mg improves the body's calcium balance and slows the rate of bone loss. Additionally, a positive link exists between consuming diverse fruits and vegetables and bone health.[133] The association between carbonated beverage intake and increased bone fracture risk most likely results from the beverage displacing milk consumption rather than the effects on urinary calcium excretion of one or more of the beverage's constituents.[66] Conversely, drinking tea may protect against osteoporosis. Although tea contains caffeine (about half to one-third less than the same volume of coffee), it also contains other nutrients such as flavonoids that positively influence bone accretion.[67]

TABLE 2.8 *(top)* indicates that good dietary calcium sources include milk and milk products, calcium-fortified orange juice, canned sardines and canned salmon with bones, almonds, and dark green leafy vegetables.

Important Risk Factors for Osteoporosis

1. Advanced age
2. White or Asian female
3. Slight build or tendency to be underweight
4. Anorexia nervosa or bulimia nervosa
5. Sedentary lifestyle
6. Postmenopause including early or surgically induced menopause
7. Low testosterone levels in men
8. High protein intake
9. Excess sodium intake
10. Cigarette smoking
11. Excessive alcohol use
12. Abnormal absence of menstrual periods (amenorrhea)
13. Calcium-deficient diet in years before and after menopause
14. Family history (genetic predisposition) of osteoporosis
15. High caffeine intake (possible)
16. Vitamin D deficiency, either through inadequate exposure to sunlight or dietary insufficiency (prevalent in about 40% of adults); aging skin loses much of its ability to synthesize vitamin D, even when exposed to sunlight

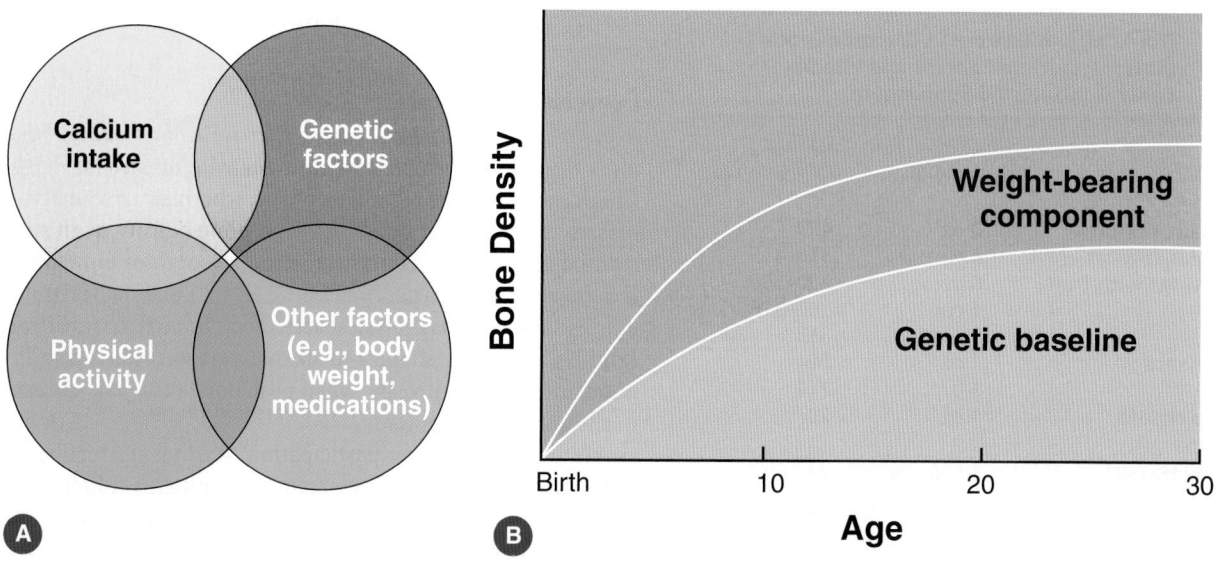

FIGURE 2.7 ■ **A.** The variation in bone mass within the population is likely a function of how the different factors that affect bone mass interact with each other. (Modified from Specker BL. Should there be dietary guidelines for calcium intake. *Am J Clin Nutr* 2000;71:663.) **B.** Weight-bearing exercise augments skeletal mass during growth above the genetic baseline. The degree of augmentation depends largely on the amount of mechanical loading to which a particular bone is subjected. (Modified from Turner CH. Site-specific effects of exercise: importance of interstitial fluid pressure. *Bone* 1999;24:161.)

Compliance Remains Critical to Provide Bone-Protective Benefits of Extra Calcium

Regular intake of calcium is crucial in providing bone-protective benefits. Several studies have cast doubts on the benefits of supplemental calcium for bone health. On further anlysis of the data it turned out that nearly 60% of the subjects failed to regularly take the supplements. For the 40% who consistently took calcium, a 30 to 40% reduction occurred in fracture risk. In essence, use of supplemental calcium does reduce fracture risk for aging women but it must be taken regularly.

Calcium supplements can correct dietary deficiencies regardless of whether extra calcium comes from fortified foods or commercial supplements (calcium citrate [less likely to cause stomach upset than other forms and also enhances iron absorption], calcium gluconate, calcium carbonate [can be constipating, especially for older people with low levels of stomach acid] or commercial products such as Tums).[127] Check the label for the amount of calcium, not the combined chemical, per dose. Calcium carbonate contains about 40% per dose, down to 21% in calcium citrate and 9% in calcium gluconate.

Because many calcium supplements, including those from refined sources, contain measurable lead, one should seek out brands that have been labeled as "tested for lead."[157] Adequate vitamin D facilitates calcium uptake, whereas excessive meat, salt, coffee, and alcohol consumption inhibit its absorption. The bottom of Table 2.8 indicates the calcium and vitamin D content of selected dietary supplements.

Beneficial Supplement When Sunlight Is Scarce

A daily vitamin D supplement of 200 IU is recommended for individuals who live and train in northern latitudes, primarily gymnasts and figure skaters who train indoors.[5]

In postmenopausal women, estrogen supplements or low-dose, slow-release fluoride-plus-calcium supplements can treat severe osteoporosis. Estrogen therapy increases bone density of the spine and hip during the first several years of hormone treatment in both middle-aged and frail elderly women.[21,103,113,198] However, this treatment is not without risk as discussed in Case Study: Personal Health and Exercise Nutrition.

TABLE 2.8 *(Top)* **Calcium Content in Common Foods** *(Bottom)* **Calcium Content and Vitamin D Content in Selected Supplements**

Food	Amount	Calcium Content (mg)
Yogurt, plain, nonfat	8 oz	450
Yogurt, plain, low fat	8 oz	350–415
Yogurt, low fat with fruit	8 oz	250–350
Milk, skim	1 cup	302–316
Milk, 2%	1 cup	313
Cheddar cheese	1 oz	204
Provolone	1 oz	214
Mozzarella cheese, part skim	1 oz	207
Ricotta cheese, part skim	1 cup	337
Swiss cheese	1 oz	272
Almonds	1/2 cup	173
Figs, dried	10	269
Orange juice, calcium fortified	1 cup	250
Orange	1 medium	56
Rhubarb, cooked with sugar	1/2 cup	174
Collards, turnip greens, spinach, cooked	1 cup	200–270
Broccoli, cooked	1 cup	178
Oatmeal with milk	1 cup	313
Salmon, canned with bones	3 1/2 oz	230
Sardines, canned with bones	3 1/2 oz	350
Halibut	one-half	95

Supplement	Elemental Calcium per Tablet (mg)	Vitamin D per Tablet (IU)
Calcium carbonate (generic)	600	200
Tums	200	0
Tums 500	500	0
Viactiv Soft Calcium chews	500	100
Citracal Caplets + D	315	200

MORE IS NOT NECESSARILY BETTER. The National Academy of Sciences (www.nationalacademies.org) has established an upper level intake of 2500 mg calcium per day—the equivalent of about 8 glasses of milk—for all age-groups. Indiscriminate use of calcium supplements, particularly calcium carbonate antacids, in excess of twice the recommended amount places an individual at risk for developing kidney stones. Another possible downside from excessively high calcium intakes concerns reduced zinc absorption and balance.[209] Individuals with high calcium intake should monitor the adequacy of dietary zinc intake (most readily available form of zinc occurs in red meats and poultry).

Exercise Is Helpful

Regular dynamic weight-bearing exercise helps to build bone mass and bone strength and slow the rate of skeletal aging. Children and adults, regardless of age, who maintain an active lifestyle show greater bone mass and bone density, with substantial improvements in mechanical strength of bone, than sedentary counterparts.[46,64,84,90,136,142,176] Benefits of regular exercise and everyday physical activity on bone mass accretion (and perhaps bone shape and size) are greatest during childhood and adolescent years, when peak bone mass can increase to the greatest extent (FIG. 2.7B).[4,79,91,101,102,104,131,193] For example, long-term soccer participation, starting at prepubertal age, relates to markedly increased bone mineral content and bone density at the femoral neck and lumber spine region.[20] Collegiate female gymnasts demonstrate greater whole-body, spine, femur, and upper limb bone mineral density and bone mineral content than controls.[144] These differences appear to reflect gymnastics activity rather than self-selection, because the athletes showed similar bone density values between dominant and nondominant arms in contrast to controls. For these athletes, bone mineral density increases during the competitive season and decreases in the off season.[173]

The benefits of regular exercise often accrue into the seventh and even eighth decade of life.[181,200] The decline in vigorous physical activity typically observed in advancing age closely parallels the age-related bone mass loss. In this regard, moderate levels of physical activity, including walking, associate with substantially lower risk of hip fracture in postmenopausal women.[47] Even prior exercise and sports experience provide a residual effect on an adult's bone mineral density. For example, former female gymnasts had greater bone mass as adults than females with no previous athletic experience.[86] Consciously restricting food intake blunts the bone-building benefits of regular physical activity.[116]

The osteogenic effect of exercise becomes particularly effective during the growth periods of childhood and adolescence (FIG. 2.8) and may reduce fracture risk later in life.[82] FIGURE 2.9 illustrates the beneficial effects of weight-bearing exercise. *Short intense bouts of mechanical loading of bone through dynamic exercise performed three to five times a week provides a potent stimulus to maintain or increase bone mass.* This form of exercise includes walking, running, dancing, rope skipping, high-impact jumping, winter sports, basketball, and gymnastics; high-intensity resistance exercises and circuit-resistance training also exert a positive effect. These exercises generate considerable impact load and/or intermittent force against the long bones of the body.[38,104,120,189] Activities providing relatively high impact on the skeletal mass (e.g., volleyball, basketball, gymnastics, judo, and karate) induce the greatest increases in bone mass, particularly at weight-bearing sites.[6,26,35,171] Even walking 1 mile daily benefits bone mass during and after menopause.

MECHANISM OF ACTION. Intermittent muscle forces acting on bones during physical activity modify bone metabolism at

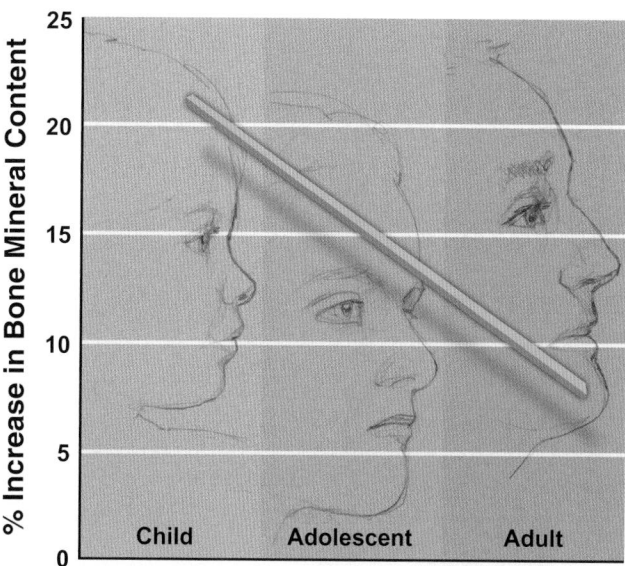

FIGURE 2.8 ■ Generalized curve for the association between age and the effects of regular bouts of intermittent, dynamic exercise on bone mass accretion.

the point of stress.[85,95,97] For example, the lower limb bones of older cross-country runners have greater bone mineral content than the bones of less active counterparts. Likewise, the playing arm of tennis players and the throwing arm of baseball players show greater bone thickness than their less-used, nondominant arm.

Prevailing theory considers that dynamic loading creates hydrostatic pressure gradients within a bone's fluid-filled network. Fluid movement within this network in response to pressure changes from dynamic exercise generates fluid shear stress on bone cells that initiates a cascade of cellular events to ultimately stimulate the production of bone matrix protein.[194] The mechanosensitivity of bone and its subsequent buildup of calcium depends on two main factors: (1) the magnitude of the applied force (strain magnitude) and (2) its frequency or number of cycles of application. Owing to the transient sensitivity of bone cells to mechanical stimuli, shorter, more frequent periods of mechanical strain facilitate bone mass accretion.[6,94,154,155] As the applied force and strain increase, the number of cycles required to initiate bone formation decreases.[27] Chemicals produced in bone itself also may contribute to bone formation. Alterations in bone's geometric configuration to long-term exercise enhance its mechanical properties.[9] FIGURE 2.10 illustrates the anatomic structure and cross-sectional view of a typical long bone and depicts the dynamics of bone growth and remodeling.

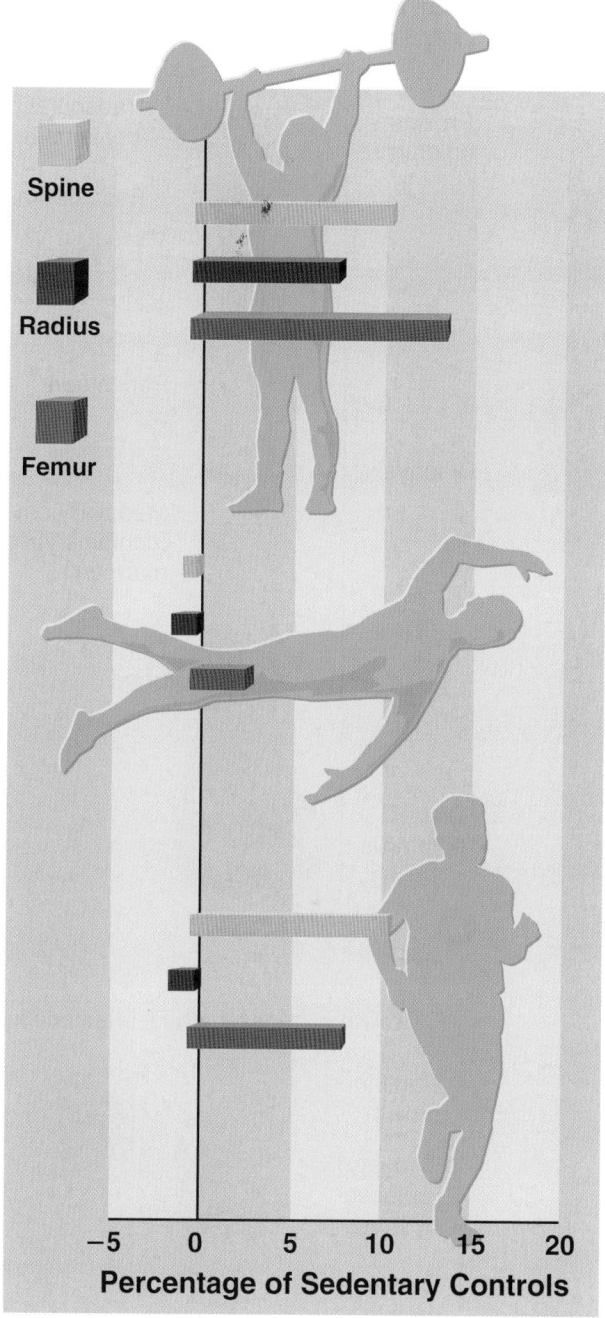

FIGURE 2.9 ■ Bone mineral density expressed as a percentage of sedentary control values at three skeletal sites for weightlifters, swimmers, and runners. (From Drinkwater BL. Physical activity, fitness, and osteoporosis. In: Bouchard C, et al., eds. *Physical Activity, Fitness, and Health.* Champaign, IL: Human Kinetics, 1994.)

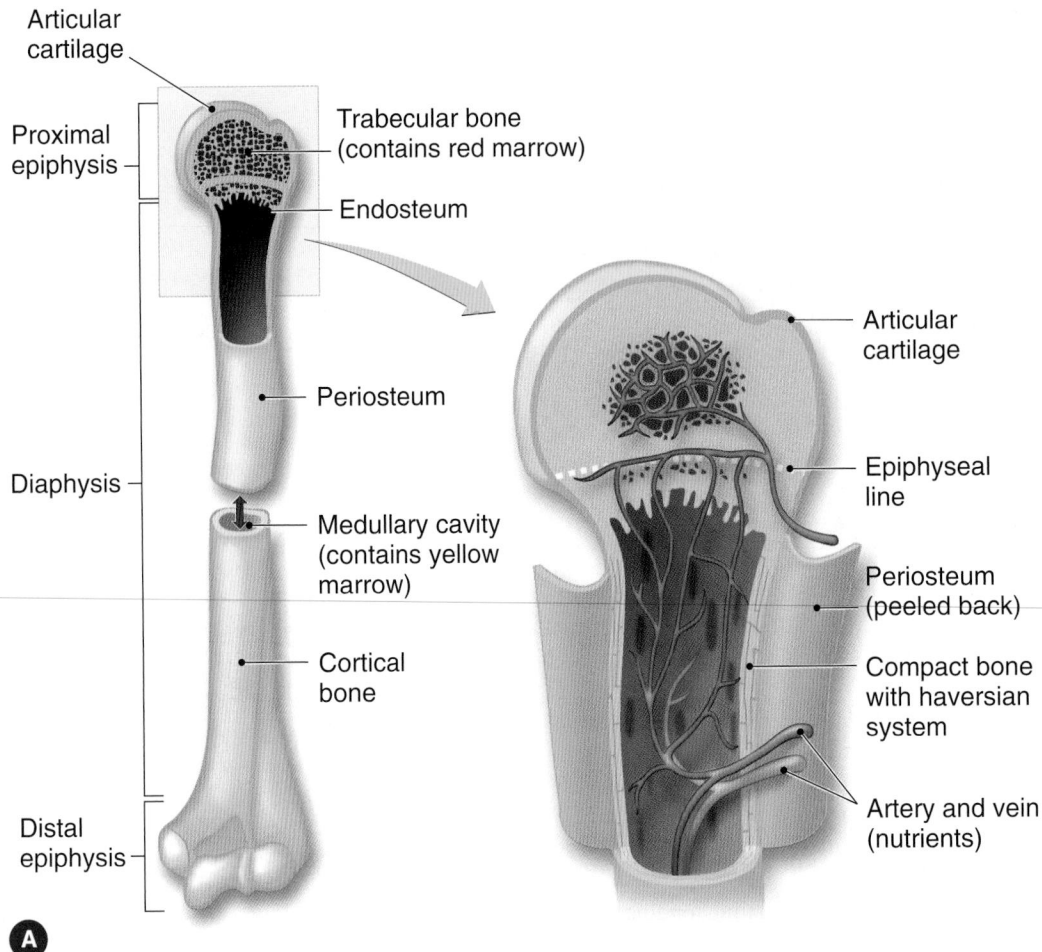

Articular cartilage

Proximal epiphysis

Trabecular bone (contains red marrow)

Endosteum

Periosteum

Diaphysis

Medullary cavity (contains yellow marrow)

Cortical bone

Distal epiphysis

Articular cartilage

Epiphyseal line

Periosteum (peeled back)

Compact bone with haversian system

Artery and vein (nutrients)

A

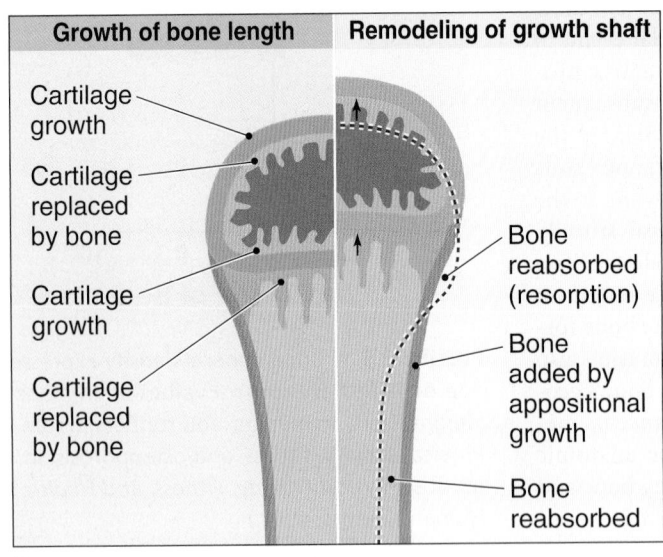

Growth of bone length	Remodeling of growth shaft

Cartilage growth

Cartilage replaced by bone

Cartilage growth

Cartilage replaced by bone

Bone reabsorbed (resorption)

Bone added by appositional growth

Bone reabsorbed

B

FIGURE 2.10 ■ **A.** Anatomic structure and longitudinal view of a typical long bone. **B.** Bone dynamics during growth and continual remodeling.

Case Study

Personal Health and Exercise Nutrition 2–1

Bone Health: Nutrition and Pharmacologic Therapy

Michelle became a near-vegan (consumes some fish) at age 12 years when she stopped eating meat and dairy products on urging from her mother, who had been a vegan her adult life. Now in her 20s and running regularly, Michelle remains a strict vegetarian. She plans to start a family in a year or so but is concerned that her diet may be inadequate in vitamins and minerals, particularly calcium, to ensure her and her baby's health. She also expresses concern she may be at high risk for osteoporosis because both her mother and grandmother have this disease. Michelle takes prednisone (a glucocorticoid drug) for psoriasis; she has normal estrogen levels.

Case Questions

1. What bone assessment tests should Michelle undergo?
2. Review possible treatments options for Michelle.
3. Give the long-term outlook for Michelle's bone health status.

Answers

1. Michelle should undergo a bone density test using dual-energy x-ray absorptiometry (DXA). If a DXA machine is unavailable, dual photon absorptiometry (measuring the spine, hip, and total body) and quantitative computed tomography (measuring the spine) can also evaluate bone density. If such devices are unavailable in her area, Michelle should contact a teaching hospital affiliated with a university.

> Michelle's bone mass is minus 2.6 Z-score values below the average for her age and classifies her as osteoporotic and a prime candidate for immediate treatment (see below).

DXA scans involve low-dose x-rays to capture images of the spine, hip, or entire body. A computer program compares the bone strength and risk of fracture with that of other people of the same age and sex in the United States and with young people at peak bone density.

Scoring bone mineral density (BMD) uses Z-scores that represent standard deviation units above or below the average for the group. A BMD score below average by 2.5 Z-score standard deviations scores indicates osteoporosis. The box on page 63 presents the scoring system for diagnosing bone health.

2. Michelle is a prime candidate for aggressive dietary and pharmacologic interventions based on her BMD test results.

DIETARY APPROACH

Michelle needs to ensure adequate calcium intake. The 1000-mg per day Adequate Intake (AI) level for calcium (see TABLE 2.6 in text) for a person of Michelle's age is based on an estimated 40% total for calcium absorption. However, calcium absorption efficiency varies among persons; individuals who absorb calcium with poor efficiency should consume more. In all likelihood, Michelle falls into the category of a "poor absorber" because her diet contains adequate calcium from such foods as cooked spinach (1 cup = 280 mg calcium), canned sardines (2 oz = 220 mg calcium), cooked turnip greens (1 cup = 200 mg calcium), and canned salmon (3 oz = 180 mg calcium).

Michelle should increase her calcium intake to at least 1500 mg per day (food and/or supplements) along with the pharmacologic intervention listed below as recommended by her physician. For some persons, calcium intake in excess of 2000 mg per day causes inordinately high blood and urinary calcium concentrations, irritability, headache, kidney failure, soft tissue calcification, kidney stones, and decreased absorption of other minerals ($2500 \text{ mg} \cdot \text{d}^{-1}$ represents the Tolerable Upper Intake value).

PHARMACOLOGIC APPROACH: ANTIRESORPTIVE MEDICATIONS

Currently, the U.S. Food and Drug Administration (FDA; www.fda.gov/) approves bisphosphonates (alendronate and risedronate), calcitonin, estrogens, parathyroid hormone, and raloxifene for the prevention and treatment of osteoporosis. These substances affect the bone remodeling cycle; they classify as antiresorptive medications. Bone remodeling progresses in two distinct stages: bone resorption and bone formation. During resorption, special osteoclast cells on the bone's surface dissolve bone tissue to create small cavities. During the formation stage, osteoblast cells fill the cavities with new bone tissue. Usually, bone resorption and bone formation occur in close sequence and remain balanced. A chronic negative balance in the bone-remodeling cycle causes bone loss that eventually leads to osteoporosis. Antiresorptive medications slow or stop the bone-re-

Case Study *continued*

sorbing portion of the remodeling cycle but do not slow the bone-forming stage. New bone formation occurs at a greater rate than resorption, and bone density may increase over time. Teriparatide, a form of parathyroid hormone, is an approved osteoporosis medication. It is the first osteoporosis medication to increase the rate of bone formation in the bone-remodeling cycle.

Possible medications for Michelle include:

a. Bisphosphonates. These compounds incorporate into the bone matrix to inhibit cells that break down bone. Only these medications have been shown to reduce hip fracture risk.

- Alendronate sodium (brand name Fosamax)
- Risedronate sodium (brand name Actonel)

Both drugs are approved for prevention (5 mg · d^{-1} or 35 mg once weekly) and treatment (10 mg · d^{-1} or 70 mg once weekly) of postmenopausal osteoporosis in women and for treatment in men. It is taken on an empty stomach, first thing in the morning, with 8 oz of water (no other liquid) at least 30 minutes before eating or drinking. The patient must remain upright during this 30-minute period. Alendronate sodium is also approved for treatment of glucocorticoid-induced osteoporosis, as occurs with the long-term use of such drugs as prednisone and cortisone, which Michelle had been taking for her psoriasis. Major side effects include nausea, heartburn, and irritation of the esophagus.

b. Selective estrogen receptor modulators (SERMs)

- Calcitonin (brand names Miacalcin, Calcimar). Calcitonin, a naturally occurring hormone, is involved in calcium regulation and bone metabolism. In postmenopausal women, calcitonin inhibits bone resorption, particularly in the presence of high levels of blood calcium, and in-

creases spinal bone density. Injectable calcitonin may cause an allergic reaction and flushing of the face and hands, increase urinary frequency, promote nausea, and produce a rash. Side effects for nasal administration of this drug are uncommon but may include nasal irritation, backache, nosebleed, and headaches.

- Raloxifene (brand name Evista). Used for prevention and treatment in women, increases bone density at spine, hip, and neck and reduces spinal fractures. Common side effects include hot flashes and leg cramps. Blood clots are a rare side effect.

c. Estrogen replacement therapy (ERT) and hormone replacement therapy (HRT) (multiple brand names.) ERT and HRT are approved to treat postmenopausal women. *Its use is not approved for premenopausal women with normal estrogen levels. Side effects may include vaginal bleeding, breast tenderness, mood disturbances, and gallbladder disease.*

A Word of Caution. A recent 8.5-year study of 16,808 healthy women aged 50 to 79 years showed that while combined estrogen and progestin therapy reduced incidence of bone fractures and colorectal cancer, dramatic increases occurred in blood clots, strokes, heart attacks, and breast cancer.[210] These findings caused researchers to halt the study 3 years early. Consequently, hormone treatment for osteoporosis should be viewed as a more dramatic approach requiring medical consultation and supervision.

3. The long-term outlook for bone health remains positive. Michelle can increase her bone mineral content over the next several years with nutritional and pharmacologic intervention. She should undergo bone density tests on a yearly basis to confirm treatment results.

The Female Triad: An Unexpected Problem for Women Who Train Intensely

A paradox exists between exercise and bone dynamics for highly active premenopausal women, particularly young athletes who have yet to attain peak bone mass. Women who train intensely and emphasize weight loss often engage in **disordered eating behaviors**—a serious ailment that in the extreme causes diverse and life-threatening complications (see Chapter 15).[22] This further decreases energy availability, reducing body mass and body fat to a point at which significant alterations occur in secretion of the pituitary gonadotropic hormones. This,

in turn, changes ovarian secretions, triggering irregular cycles (**oligomenorrhea;** six to nine menstrual cycles per year; 35 to 90 days between cycles) or cessation, a condition termed **secondary amenorrhea.** Chapter 13 more fully discusses the interactions between leanness, exercise, and menstrual irregularity.

A Clinical Definition

Clinicians define secondary amenorrhea as the cessation of monthly menstrual cycles for at least three consecutive months after establishing regular cycles.

The interacting, tightly bound continuum that generally begins with disordered eating (and a resultant energy drain) and leads to amenorrhea and then osteoporosis reflects the clinical entity labeled the **female athlete triad** (FIG. 2.11). Some researchers and physicians prefer the term **female triad** because this syndrome of disorders also afflicts physically active women in the general population who do not fit the typical competitive athlete profile.

associated with exercise-related amenorrhea, considered the "red flag" or most recognizable symptom for the triad's presence. Female athletes of the 1970s and 1980s believed that the loss of normal menstruation reflected appropriately hard training and was an inevitable consequence of athletic success. The prevalence of amenorrhea among female athletes in body weight–related sports (distance running, gymnastics, ballet, cheerleading, figure skating, body building) probably ranges between 25 and 75%, whereas no more than 5% of the nonathletic women of menstruating age experience this condition.

Excellent Web Resources

Some colleges and universities maintain web pages that deal directly with the female triad:

- www.bc.edu/bc_org/svp/uhs/eating/eating-female athletes.htm
- www.celebrate.uchc.edu/girls/body/triad.htlml
- www.vanderbilt.edu/AnS/psychologyhealth_psychology/ AthleteTriad.htm

Limited data exist as to the prevalence of the triad, mainly from a disagreement about how to define the disorder, although the combined prevalence of disordered eating, menstrual dysfunctiona, and low bone mineral density remains small among high school and collegiate athletes.[10,135] Many young women who play sports, particularly sports that emphasize leanness, likely suffer from at least one of the triad's irregularities, particularly disordered eating behaviors, which occur in 15 to 70% of female athletes based on informal surveys and detailed questionnaires.[10,88] FIGURE 2.12 illustrates the contributing factors

Six Principles for Promoting Bone Health Through Exercise

1. **Specificity:** Exercise provides a local osteogenic effect.
2. **Overload:** Progressively increasing exercise intensity promotes continued improvement.
3. **Initial values:** Individuals with the smallest total bone mass have the greatest potential for improvement.
4. **Diminishing returns:** As one approaches the biologic ceiling for bone density, further gains require greater effort.
5. **More not necessarily better:** Bone cells become desensitized in response to prolonged mechanical-loading sessions.
6. **Reversibility:** Discontinuing exercise overload reverses the positive osteogenic effects of exercise.

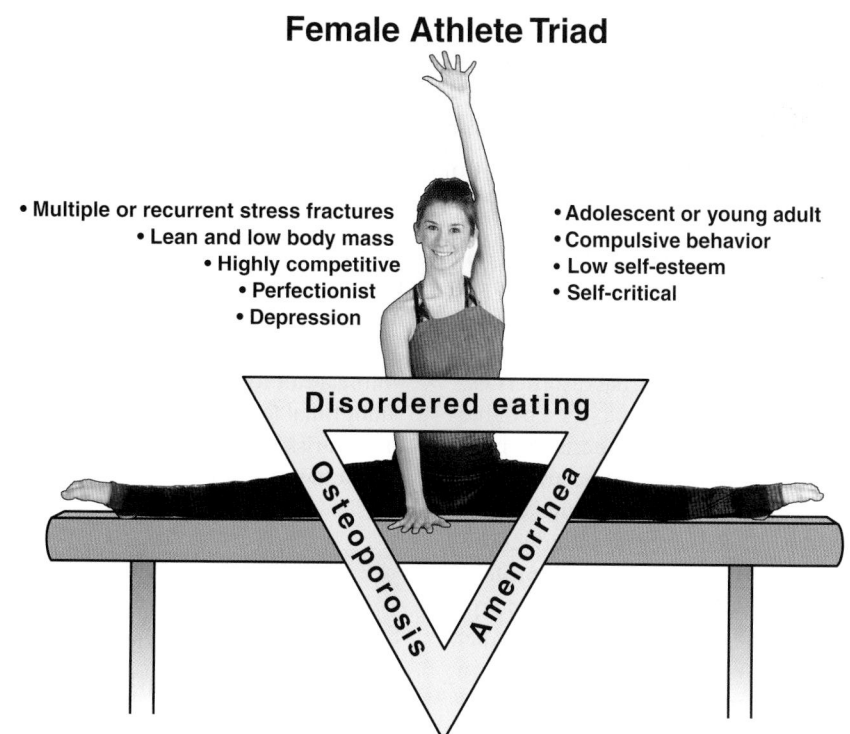

Female Athlete Triad

- Multiple or recurrent stress fractures
- Lean and low body mass
- Highly competitive
- Perfectionist
- Depression

- Adolescent or young adult
- Compulsive behavior
- Low self-esteem
- Self-critical

Disordered eating

Osteoporosis

Amenorrhea

FIGURE 2.11 ■ The female athlete triad: disordered eating, amenorrhea, and osteoporosis.

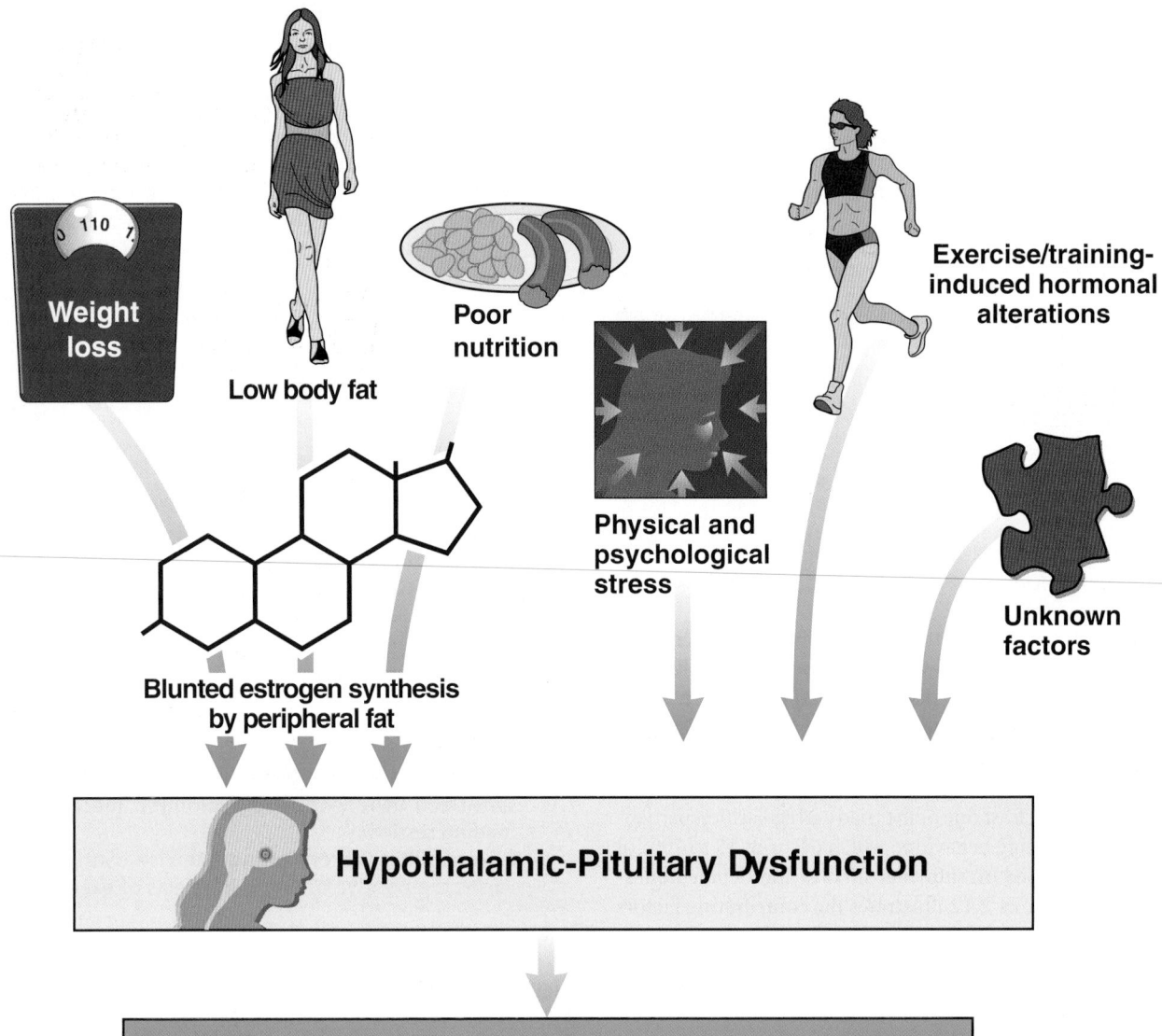

FIGURE 2.12 ■ Factors contributing to the development of exercise-related amenorrhea.

In general, bone density relates closely to (1) menstrual regularity and (2) total number of menstrual cycles. Cessation of menstruation removes estrogen's protective effect on bone, making calcium loss more prevalent, with a concomitant decrease in bone mass. The most severe menstrual disorders exert the greatest negative effect on bone mass.[188,207] Lowered bone density from extended amenorrhea often occurs at multiple sites, including the lumbar spine and bone areas subjected to increased force and impact loading during exercise.[139] Concurrently, the problem worsens in individuals undergoing an energy deficit and accompanying low protein, lipid, and energy intakes.[212] In such cases, a poor diet also provides inadequate calcium intake. Persistent amenorrhea that begins at an early age diminishes the benefits of exercise on bone mass and increases risk for musculoskeletal injuries (particularly repeated stress fractures) during exercise.[57,59] For example, a 5% bone mass loss increases stress fracture risk by nearly 40%. Reestablishing normal menses causes some regain in bone mass, but it does *not* reach levels achieved with normal menstruation.

Once bone mass is lost, it is not easily regained. Once a young adult loses bone mass, it may permanently remain at suboptimal levels throughout adult life, leaving women at increased risk for osteoporosis and stress fractures even years after competitive athletic participation.[36,123]

Estrogen's Three Roles in Bone Health

1. Increases intestinal calcium absorption
2. Reduces urinary calcium excretion
3. Facilitates calcium retention by bone

Professional organizations recommend that intervention begin within 3 months of the onset of amenorrhea. Successful treatment of athletic amenorrhea requires a nonpharmacologic, behavioral approach that includes the following four factors:[37]

1. Reduce training level by 10 to 20%
2. Gradually increase total energy intake
3. Increase body weight by 2 to 3%
4. Maintain daily calcium intake at 1500 mg

As with most medical ailments, prevention offers the most effective treatment for the female triad. Ideally, screening for the triad should begin in junior high school and high school at the preparticipation medical examination and in subsequent evaluations. Such screenings provide insight about behaviors and symptoms related to disordered eating and menstrual irregularity. In addition, coaches and athletic trainers should routinely monitor athletes for changes in menstrual patterns and eating behaviors. *The identification of any one ailment in the triad requires prompt screening for the other two disorders.* Chapter 15 more fully discusses various eating disorders, with emphasis on athletes and other physically active individuals.

Does Muscle Strength Relate to Bone Density?

Men and women who participate in strength and power activities have as much or more bone mass than endurance athletes.[153] Such findings have caused speculation about the possible relationship between muscular strength and bone mass. Laboratory experiments have documented greater maximum flexion and extension dynamic strength in postmenopausal women without osteoporosis than in their osteoporotic counterparts.[179] FIGURE 2.13 displays chest flexion and extension strength in normal and osteoporotic women. Unequivocal results emerged. The women with normal bone mineral density in the lumbar spine and femur neck exhibited 20% greater strength in 11 of 12 test comparisons for flexion; 4 of 12 comparisons for extension showed 13% higher values for women with normal bone density. Quite possibly, differences in maximum dynamic strength among postmenopausal women can serve a clinically useful role in screening for osteoporosis. Other data complement these findings; they indicate that regional lean tissue mass (often an indication of muscular strength) accurately predicts bone mineral density.[134] The lumbar spine and proximal femur bone mass of elite teenage weightlifters exceeds representative values for fully mature bone of reference adults.[25] In addition, a linear relation exists between increases in bone mineral density and total and exercise-specific weight lifted during a 1-year strength-training program.[29]

For female gymnasts, bone mineral density correlated moderately with maximal muscle strength and serum progesterone.[68] Despite oligomenorrhea and amenorrhea in many of these athletes, it is possible that they maintain bone mineral density levels that correlate to muscular strength in the axial

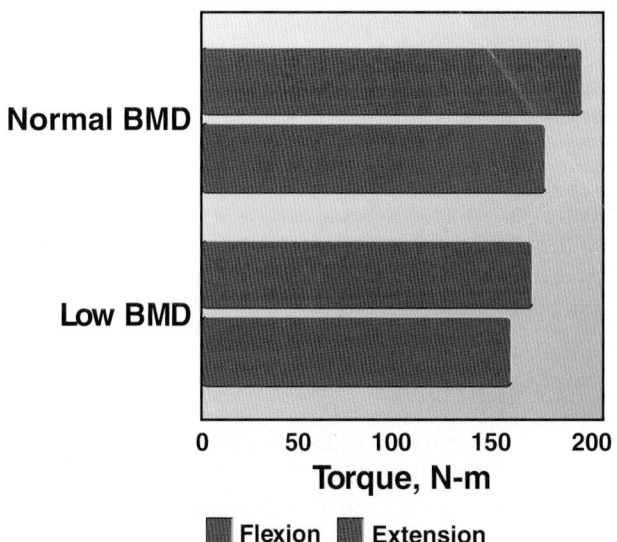

FIGURE 2.13 ■ Comparison of chest press extension and flexion strength in age- and weight-matched postmenopausal women with normal and low bone mineral density (BMD). Women with low BMD scored significantly lower on each measure of muscular strength than the reference group. (From Stock JL, et al. Dynamic muscle strength is decreased in postmenopausal women with low bone density. *J Bone Miner Res* 1987;2:338; Janey C, et al. Maximum muscular strength differs in postmenopausal women with and without osteoporosis. *Med Sci Sports Exerc* 1987;19:S61.)

(L2-L4) and appendicular skeleton. For adolescent female athletes, absolute knee extension strength was moderately associated with total body, lumbar spine, femoral neck, and leg bone mineral density.[38]

Women at high risk for osteoporosis and those with osteoporosis reduce their *factor of risk* for fracture (defined as the ratio of load on the spine to the bone's failure load) by (1) strengthening bones by maintaining or increasing their density and (2) reducing the magnitude of spinal forces by avoiding higher risk activities that increase spinal compression (e.g., heavy lifting activities).[128]

PHOSPHORUS

Phosphorus combines with calcium to form hydroxyapatite and calcium phosphate—compounds that give rigidity to bones and teeth. Phosphorus also serves as an essential component of the intracellular mediator, cyclic adenosine monophosphate (AMP), and the intramuscular high-energy compounds phosphocreatine (PCr) and adenosine triphosphate (ATP). ATP supplies the energy for all forms of biologic work. Phosphorus combines with lipids to form phospholipid compounds, integral components of the cells' bilayer plasma membrane. The phosphorus-containing phosphatase enzymes help to regulate cellular metabolism. Phosphorus also participates in buffering acid end products of energy metabolism. For this reason, some coaches and trainers recommend consuming special "phosphate drinks" to reduce the effects of acid production in strenuous exercise. "Phosphate loading" also has been proposed to facilitate oxygen release from hemoglobin at the cellular level. In Chapter 11, we discuss the usefulness of specific buffering drinks to augment intense exercise performance. Most studies confirm that the phosphorus intake of athletes generally attains recommended levels, with the possible exception of female dancers and gymnasts. Rich dietary sources of phosphorus include meat, fish, poultry, milk products, and cereals.

MAGNESIUM

About 400 enzymes that regulate metabolism contain magnesium. Magnesium plays a vital role in glucose metabolism by helping to form muscle and liver glycogen from blood-borne glucose. The 20 to 30 g of magnesium in the body also participates as a cofactor to break down glucose, fatty acids, and amino acids during energy metabolism. Furthermore, magnesium affects lipid and protein synthesis and contributes to proper functioning of the neuromuscular system. Magnesium also acts as an electrolyte, which, along with potassium and sodium, helps to maintain blood pressure. By regulating DNA and RNA synthesis and structure, magnesium regulates cell growth, reproduction, and the structure of plasma membranes. Because of its role as a Ca^{+2} channel blocker, inadequate magnesium could lead to hypertension and cardiac arrhythmias. Sweating generally produces only small losses of magnesium.

Conflicting data exist concerning the possible effects of magnesium supplements on exercise performance and the training response. In one study, magnesium supplementation did not affect quadriceps muscle strength or measures of fatigue in the 6-week period following a marathon.[189] Subsequent research showed that 4 weeks of 212 mg per day magnesium oxide supplement increased resting magnesium levels but did not affect anaerobic or aerobic exercise performance, compared with a placebo.[48] In contrast, untrained men and women who supplemented with magnesium increased quadriceps power compared with a placebo treatment during 7 weeks of resistance training.[15]

The magnesium intake of athletes generally attains recommended levels, although female dancers and gymnasts have low intakes.[125] Green leafy vegetables, legumes, nuts, bananas, mushrooms, and whole grains provide a rich source of magnesium. We do not recommend taking magnesium supplements because these often are mixed with dolomite $(CaMg[CO_3]_2)$, an extract from dolomitic limestone and marble, which often contains the toxic elements mercury and lead.

IRON

The body normally contains between 3 to 5 g (about 1/6 oz) of the trace mineral iron. Approximately 80% of this amount exists in functionally active compounds, predominantly combined with **hemoglobin** in red blood cells. This iron–protein compound increases the oxygen-carrying capacity of blood

approximately 65 times. FIGURE 2.14 displays the percentage composition of centrifuged whole blood for plasma and concentration of red blood cells (called the **hematocrit**), including average hemoglobin values for men and women.

Iron serves other important exercise-related functions besides its role in oxygen transport in blood. It is a structural component of **myoglobin** (about 5% of total iron), a compound with some similarities to hemoglobin, that aids in oxygen storage and transport within the muscle cell. Small amounts of iron also exist in **cytochromes,** the specialized substances that facilitate energy transfer within the cell. About 20% of the body's iron does not combine in functionally active compounds and exists as **hemosiderin** and **ferritin** stored in the liver, spleen, and bone marrow. These stores replenish iron lost from the functional compounds and provide the iron reserve during periods of insufficient dietary iron intake. Another plasma protein, **transferrin,** transports iron from ingested food and damaged red blood cells for delivery to tissues in need. *Plasma levels of transferrin generally reflect the adequacy of current iron intake.*

Physically active individuals should include normal amounts of iron-rich foods in their daily diet. Persons with inadequate iron intake or with limited rates of iron absorption or high rates of iron loss often develop a reduced concentration of hemoglobin in red blood cells. This extreme condition of iron insufficiency, called **iron deficiency anemia**, produces general sluggishness, loss of appetite, and reduced capacity to sustain even mild exercise. "Iron therapy" with this condition normalizes the hemoglobin content of the blood and improves exer-

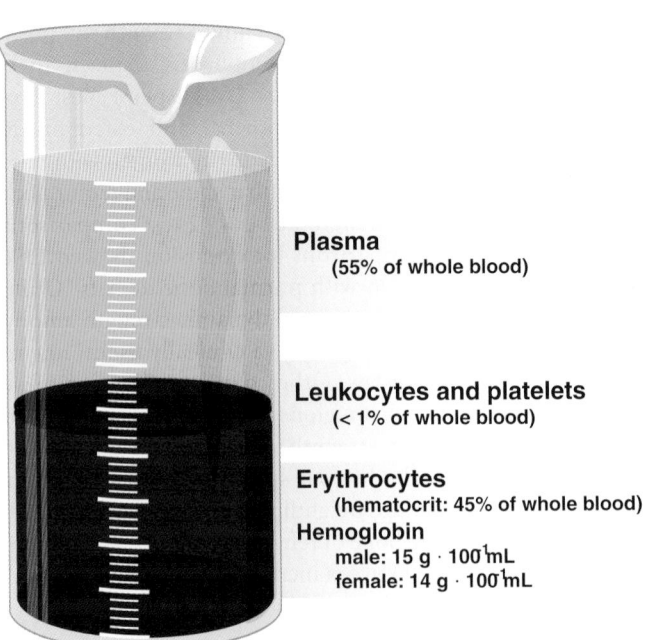

Plasma
(55% of whole blood)

Leukocytes and platelets
(< 1% of whole blood)

Erythrocytes
(hematocrit: 45% of whole blood)
Hemoglobin
male: 15 g · 100⁻¹mL
female: 14 g · 100⁻¹mL

FIGURE 2.14 ■ Percentage composition of centrifuged whole blood for plasma and red blood cell concentration (hematocrit). Also included are average values for hemoglobin for men and women per 100 mL of blood.

TABLE 2.9	Recommended Dietary Allowances for Iron	
	Age (years)	Iron (mg)
Children	1–10	10
Males	11–18	12
	191	10
Females	11–50	15
	51+	10
	Pregnant	30[a]
	Lactating	15[a]

Food and Nutrition Board, National Academy of Sciences-National Research Council, Washington, DC. Recommended dietary allowances, revised 2001.

[a]Generally, this increased requirement cannot be met by ordinary diets; therefore, the use of 30 to 60 mg of supplemental iron is recommended.

cise capacity. TABLE 2.9 lists recommendations for iron intake for children and adults.

Females: A Population at Risk

Insufficient iron intake represents the most common micronutrient insufficiency, affecting between 20 and 50% of the world's population.[11] In the United States, estimates place between 10 and 13% of premenopausal women as deficient in iron intake and between 3 and 5% are anemic by conventional diagnostic criteria.[41] Inadequate iron intake frequently occurs among young children, teenagers, and women of child-bearing age, including many physically active women. In addition, pregnancy can trigger a moderate iron-deficiency anemia from the increased iron demand for both mother and fetus.

Iron loss from the 30 to 60 mL of blood lost during a menstrual cycle ranges between 15 and 30 mg. This loss requires an additional 5-mg dietary iron daily for premenopausal females, which increases the average monthly iron requirement by about 150 mg. Thus, an additional 20 to 25 mg of iron becomes available to females each month (assuming typical iron absorption) for synthesizing red blood cells lost during menstruation. Dietary iron insufficiencies of the large number of American premenopausal women relate to a limited supply of iron in the typical diet, which averages about 6 mg of iron per 1000 kCal of food ingested.

Iron Source Is Important

Intestinal absorption of iron varies closely with iron need, yet considerable variation in bioavailability occurs because of diet composition. For example, the intestine usually absorbs between 2 and 10% of iron from plants (trivalent ferric or **nonheme** elemental **iron**), whereas iron absorption from animal sources (divalent ferrous or **heme iron**) increases to between 10 and 35%. The body absorbs about 15% of ingested iron, depending on one's iron status, form of iron ingested, and composition of the meal. For example, intestinal absorption

of nonheme (but not heme) iron increases when consuming diets with low iron bioavailability.[74] Conversely, iron supplementation reduces nonheme iron but not heme iron absorption from food.[158] Despite this partial adaptation in iron absorption, iron stores remain greater after supplementation than after placebo treatment. The presence of heme iron in food also increases iron absorption from nonheme sources. Consuming more meat maintains iron status more effectively in exercising women than supplementing with commercial iron preparations.[109]

Factors That Increase and Decrease Iron Absorption

Increase Iron Absorption

1. Stomach acid
2. Dietary iron in heme form
3. High body demand for red blood cells (blood loss, high altitude exposure, exercise training, pregnancy)
4. Presence of mean protein factor (MPF)
5. Vitamin C in small intestine

Decrease Iron Absorption

1. Phytic acid (in dietary fiber)
2. Oaxlic acid
3. Polyphenols (in tea or coffee)
4. Excess of other minerals (Zn, Mg, Ca), particularly taken as supplements
5. Reduced stomach acid
6. Antacid use

Of Concern to Vegetarians

The relatively low bioavailability of nonheme iron places women on vegetarian-type diets at increased risk for developing iron insufficiency. Female vegetarian runners have a poorer iron status than counterparts who consume the same quantity of iron from predominantly animal sources.[174] Including foods rich in vitamin C in the diet (see FIG. 2.1) upgrades the bioavailability of dietary iron. This occurs because ascorbic acid increases the solubility of nonheme iron, making it available for absorption at the alkaline pH of the small intestine. The ascorbic acid in a glass of orange juice, for example, significantly increases nonheme iron absorption from a breakfast meal.

The top panel of FIGURE 2.15 clearly illustrates the effect of exogenous vitamin C on nonheme iron absorption. Eight healthy men without iron deficiency were studied at rest after taking either 100 mg of ferric sodium citrate complex, 100 mg of ferric sodium citrate complex with 200 mg ascorbic acid, or no exogenous iron. The iron supplement alone caused an 18.4% increase in serum iron concentration compared with the control, no iron condition. Combining iron and vitamin C, however, induced a peak 72% increase in serum iron. Furthermore, taking the iron-only supplement followed by 1 hour of moderate exercise produced a 48.2% increase in serum iron concentration compared with only an 8.3% increase at

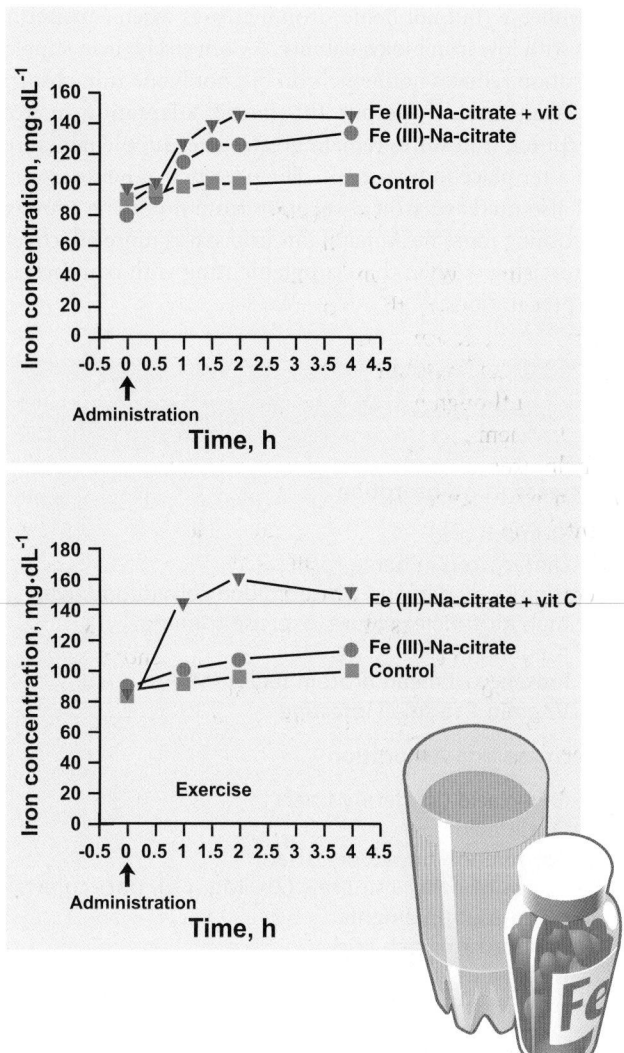

FIGURE 2.15 ■ *Top,* Serum iron concentrations following administration of a single dose of 100 mg ferric sodium citrate complex (Fe [III]-Na-citrate) or 100 mg of sodium citrate complex with 200 mg ascorbic acid (Fe [III]-Na-citrate + vit C) compared with controls at rest. *Bottom,* Serum iron concentrations following administration of a single dose of 100 mg of ferric sodium citrate complex (Fe [III]-Na-citrate) or 100 mg of sodium citrate complex with 200 mg ascorbic acid (Fe [III]-Na-citrate + vit C) compared with controls during moderate (60% $\dot{V}O_{2max}$) exercise. (From Schmid A, et al. Effect of physical exercise and vitamin C on absorption of ferric sodium citrate. *Med Sci Sports Exerc* 1996;28:1470.)

rest (FIG. 2.15, *bottom*). Combining exercise and iron supplementation plus vitamin C did not augment physical activity's effect on iron absorption. These data convincingly indicate that moderate exercise does not impair the body's absorption of supplemental iron; instead, it facilitates iron uptake to the same amount as vitamin C supplementation without exercise. These findings also provide a nutrition-based justification for moderate exercise following eating.

Heme iron sources include tuna (3 oz = 1.6 mg), chicken (4.0 oz breast = 1.8 mg), clams (3 oz = 2.6 mg), beef (3 oz = 2.7 mg), oysters (3 oz = 5.9 mg), and beef liver (3 oz = 6.6 mg); **nonheme iron sources** include oatmeal (1 cup nonfortified = 1.6 mg; fortified with nutrient added = 6.3 mg), spinach (½ cup cooked = 2.0 mg), soy protein (tofu, piece 2½ × 2¾ × 1 inch = 2.3 mg), dried figs (4 figs = 2.3 mg), beans (½ cup refried = 2.3 mg), raisins (½ cup = 2.5 mg), lima beans (½ cup = 2.5 mg), prune juice (1 cup = 3.0 mg), peaches (½ cup dried = 3.3 mg), and apricots (1 cup dried = 6.1 mg). Fiber-rich foods, coffee, and tea contain compounds that interfere with the intestinal absorption of iron (and zinc).

Are the Physically Active at Greater Risk for Iron Insufficiency?

Interest in endurance sports, combined with increased participation of women in these activities, has focused research on the influence of strenuous training on the body's iron status. The term **sports anemia** frequently describes reduced hemoglobin levels approaching clinical anemia (12 g · dL^{-1} of blood for women and 14 g · dL^{-1} for men) attributable to intense training.

Some maintain that exercise training creates an added demand for iron that often exceeds its intake. This would tax iron reserves and eventually depress hemoglobin synthesis and/or reduce iron-containing compounds within the cell's energy transfer system. Individuals susceptible to an "iron drain" could experience reduced exercise capacity because of iron's crucial role in oxygen transport and use.

Intense training theoretically increases iron demand from iron loss in sweat and from the loss of hemoglobin in urine from red blood cell destruction with increased temperature, spleen activity, circulation rates, and mechanical trauma from runners' feet pounding on the running surface (foot-strike hemolysis).[141,166] Gastrointestinal bleeding unrelated to age, sex, or performance time can also occur with long-distance running.[114,129] Such iron loss would stress the body's iron reserves required to synthesize 260 billion new red blood cells daily in the bone marrow of the skull, upper arm, sternum, ribs, spine, pelvis, and upper leg. Iron loss poses an additional burden to premenopausal women who have a greater iron requirement yet lower iron intake than men.

Real Anemia or Pseudoanemia?

Apparent suboptimal hemoglobin concentrations and hematocrits occur more frequently among endurance athletes, supporting the possibility of an exercise-induced anemia. On closer scrutiny, reductions in hemoglobin concentration appear transient, occurring in the early phase of training and then returning toward pretraining values. *The decrease in hemoglobin concentration generally parallels the disproportionately large expansion in plasma volume early in both endurance and resistance training.*[31,55,166,169] For example, just several days of training increases plasma volume by 20%, while the total volume of red blood cells remains unchanged.[58] Consequently, **total hemoglobin** (an important factor in endurance performance) remains the same or increases somewhat with training, yet hemoglobin *concentration* decreases in the expanding plasma volume.

Despite hemoglobin's apparent dilution, aerobic capacity and exercise performance normally improve with training. Some mechanical destruction of red blood cells may occur with vigorous exercise (including minimal iron loss in sweat[18]), but no evidence shows that these factors strain an athlete's iron reserves sufficiently to precipitate clinical anemia as long as iron intake remains at recommended levels. Applying stringent criteria for both anemia and insufficient iron reserves makes sports anemia much less prevalent among highly trained athletes than generally believed.[202] For male collegiate runners and swimmers, no indications of the early stages of anemia were noted despite large changes in training volume and intensity during different phases of the competitive season.[143] Data from female athletes indicate the prevalence of iron deficiency anemia did *not* differ in comparisons among specific athletic groups or with a nonathletic control group.[151] Recent research demonstrates a relatively high prevalence of nonanemic iron depletion among athletes in diverse sports and recreationally active men and women.[39,60,170]

Should the Physically Active Supplement with Iron?

Losing any iron with exercise training (coupled with poor dietary habits) in adolescent and premenopausal females, particularly among those in the low-weight or body-appearance sports, could strain an already limited iron reserve. This does not mean that all physically active individuals should take supplementary iron or that all indications of sports anemia result from dietary iron deficiency or iron loss caused by exercise. It does suggest, however, the importance of monitoring an athlete's iron status by periodic evaluation of hematologic characteristics and iron reserves, particularly athletes who choose to supplement with iron.[32] This is important because reversal of full-blown iron deficiency anemia can require up to 6 months of iron therapy.

An Objective Measure of Iron Reserves

Measuring serum ferritin concentration provides useful information about iron reserves. Depleted iron reserves occur when values are below 20 $\mu g \cdot L^{-1}$ for women and 30 $\mu g \cdot L^{-1}$ for men.

Hemoglobin concentration of 12 g per dL represents the cutoff for the clinical classification of anemia for women. Low values within the "normal" range could reflect **functional anemia** or **marginal iron deficiency**, a condition characterized by depleted iron stores, reduced iron-dependent protein production (e.g., oxidative enzymes) but relatively *normal* hemoglobin concentrations. The ergogenic effects of iron supplementation on aerobic exercise performance and training responsiveness have been noted for such groups of iron-defi-

cient athletes.[16,17,,51] For example, physically active but untrained women classified as iron depleted (serum ferritin, $\leq$ 16 $\mu g \cdot L^{-1}$) but not anemic (Hb $\geq$12 g $\cdot$ dL^{-1}) received either iron therapy (50 mg ferrous sulfate) or a placebo twice daily for 2 weeks.[70] All subjects then completed 4 weeks of aerobic training. The iron-supplemented group increased serum ferritin levels with only a small (nonsignificant) increase in hemoglobin concentration. The supplemented group also had twice the improvement in 15-km endurance cycling time (3.4 vs 1.6 min faster) than the women who consumed the placebo. The researchers concluded that women with low serum ferritin levels but hemoglobin concentrations above 12 g $\cdot$ dL^{-1}, although not clinically anemic, might still be functionally anemic and thus benefit from iron supplementation to help exercise performance. Similarly, iron-depleted but nonanemic women received either a placebo or 20 mg of elemental iron as ferrous sulfate twice daily for 6 weeks.[19] FIGURE 2.16 shows that the iron supplement attenuated the rate of decrease in maximal force measured sequentially during approximately 8 minutes of dynamic knee extension exercise.

These findings support current recommendations to use an iron supplement for physically active women with low serum ferritin levels. Iron supplementation exerts little effect on hemoglobin concentration and red blood cell volume in iron-deficient but nonanemic groups. Any improved exercise capacity most likely comes from increased muscle oxidative capacity, not oxygen transport capacity by the blood.

Steer Clear of Iron Supplements Unless an Insufficiency Exists

For healthy individuals whose diets contain the recommended iron intake, excess iron either through diet or supplementation does not increase hemoglobin, hematocrit, or other measures of iron status or exercise performance.[192] Potential harm exists from the overconsumption or overabsorption of iron, particularly with an excessive consumption of red meat and ready availability of iron and vitamin C supplements, which facilitate iron absorption.[50] Supplements should not be used indiscriminately because excessive iron can accumulate to toxic levels and contribute to diabetes, liver disease, and heart and joint damage. Excess iron intake may even augment the growth of latent cancers (e.g., colorectal cancer) and infectious organisms.[132] Controversy exists as to whether individuals with high levels of body iron stores have a higher CHD risk than individuals with iron levels in the low-to-normal range.[30,87,145] If risk exists, one explanation postulates that high serum iron catalyzes free radical formation, which augments the oxidation of LDL cholesterol, thus promoting atherosclerosis. Currently, the evidence supporting this hypothesis remains inconsistent and inconclusive.[168]

Approximately 1.5 million Americans have a genetic abnormality, **hereditary hemochromatosis,** that predisposes them to iron accumulation in the various body tissues. If undetected, this genetic abnormality produces excessive iron absorption and accumulation with early symptoms of chronic fatigue, abdominal pain, and menstrual dysfunction in fe-

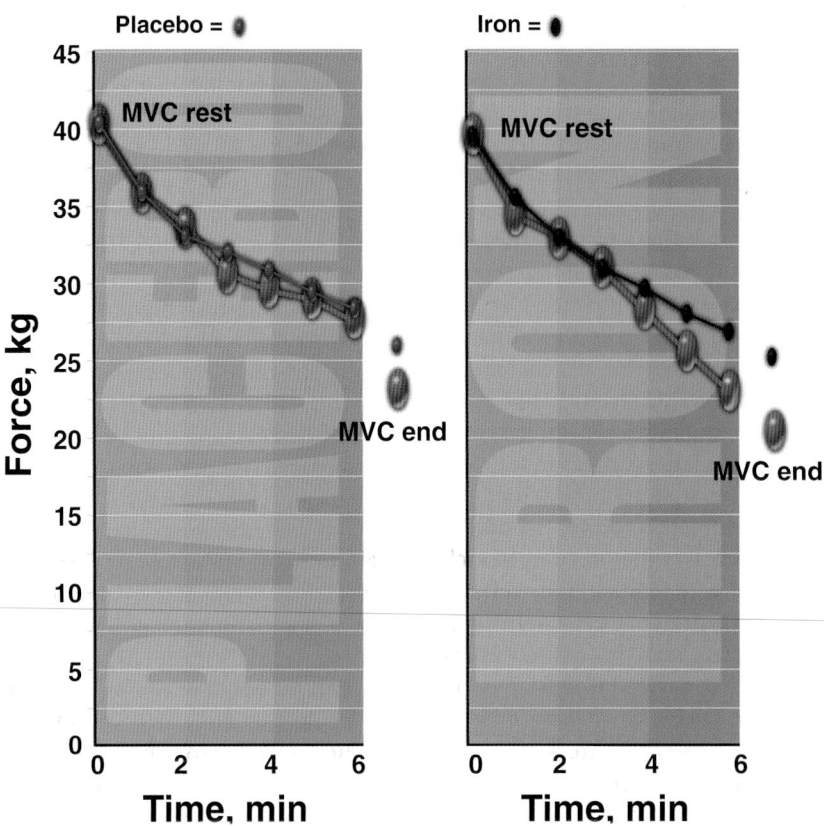

FIGURE 2.16 ■ Maximal voluntary static contractions (MVCs) over the first 6 minutes of a progressive fatigue test of dynamic knee extensions before (●) and after (●) supplementation with either a placebo or iron. MVC end represents the last MVC of the protocol and occurred at different times (average ~ 8 min) for each subject.

males. In the extreme, hemochromatosis leads to cirrhosis or cancer of the liver, heart and thyroid disease, diabetes, arthritis, and infertility. Early diagnosis and treatment can prevent the serious complications of hemochromatosis.

SODIUM, POTASSIUM, AND CHLORINE

Sodium, potassium, and chlorine, collectively termed **electrolytes,** remain dissolved in the body as electrically charged particles called ions. Sodium and chlorine represent the chief minerals contained in blood plasma and extracellular fluid. Electrolytes modulate fluid exchange within the body's fluid compartments, allowing a well-regulated exchange of nutrients and waste products between the cell and its external fluid environment. Potassium is the chief intracellular mineral.

The most important function of sodium and potassium ions concerns their role in establishing the proper electrical gradient across cell membranes. This difference in electrical balance between the cell's interior and exterior allows the transmission of nerve impulses, the stimulation and action of muscle, and proper gland functioning. Electrolytes also maintain plasma membrane permeability and regulate the acid and

base qualities of body fluids, particularly the blood. TABLE 2.10 lists values considered normal for electrolyte concentrations in serum and sweat, and the electrolyte and carbohydrate concentrations of common oral rehydration beverages.

How Much Sodium Is Enough?

With low-to-moderate sodium intake, the hormone **aldosterone** acts on the kidneys to conserve sodium. Conversely, high dietary sodium inhibits aldosterone release. Any excess sodium becomes excreted in the urine. Consequently, salt balance generally remains normal throughout a wide range of intakes. This does not occur in individuals who cannot adequately regulate excessive sodium intake. Abnormal sodium accumulation in body fluids increases fluid volume and elevates blood pressure to levels that pose a health risk. Such **sodium-induced hypertension** occurs in about one third of individuals with hypertension.

Sodium is widely distributed naturally in foods, so one can readily obtain the daily requirement without adding "extra" salt to foods. Sodium intake in the United States regularly exceeds the daily level recommended for adults of 2400 mg, or the amount of sodium in one heaping teaspoon of table salt (sodium makes up about 40% of salt). The typical Western

TABLE 2.10   Electrolyte Concentrations in Blood Serum and Sweat, and Carbohydrate and Electrolyte Concentrations of Some Common Beverages

	Na^+ (mEq·L^{-1})	K^+ (mEq·L^{-1})	Ca^{2+} (mEq·L^{-1})	Mg^{2+} (mEq·L^{-1})	Cl^- (mEq·L^{-1})	Osmolality (mOsm·L^{-1})	CHO (g·L^{-1})
Blood serum	140	4.5	2.5	1.5–2.1	110	300	—
Sweat	60–80	4.5	1.5	3.3	40–90	170–220	—
Coca Cola	3.0	—	—	—	1.0	650	107
Gatorade	23.0	3.0	—	—	14.0	280	62
Fruit juice	0.5	58.0	—	—	—	690	118
Pepsi Cola	1.7	trace	—	—	trace	568	81
Water	trace	trace	—	—	trace	10–20	—

diet contains about 4500 mg of sodium (8– 12 g of salt) each day with three quarters coming from processed food and restaurant meals. This represents 10 times the 500 mg of sodium the body actually needs. Reliance on table salt in processing, curing, cooking, seasoning, and preserving common foods accounts for the large sodium intake. Aside from table salt, common sodium-rich dietary sources include monosodium glutamate (MSG), soy sauce, condiments, canned foods, baking soda, and baking powder.

For decades, one low-risk, first line of defense in treating high blood pressure eliminated excess sodium from the diet. Reducing sodium intake possibly lowers sodium and body fluid, thereby lowering blood pressure. This effect is particularly apparent for **"salt sensitive"** individuals; reducing dietary sodium decreases their blood pressure.[75,177] Debate concerns the magnitude of this reduction for most hypertensives.[1,3,7,23,108] If dietary constraints prove ineffective in lowering blood pressure, drugs that induce a water loss (**diuretics**) become the next line of defense. Unfortunately, diuretics also produce losses in other minerals, particularly potassium. A potassium-rich diet (potatoes, bananas, oranges, tomatoes, and meat) becomes a necessity for a patient using diuretics.

THE DASH EATING PLAN

Research using **Dietary Approaches to Stop Hypertension** (DASH; www.nhlbi.nih.gov/health/public/heart/hbp/dash/) to treat hypertension shows that this diet lowers blood pressure in the general population and in persons with stage 1 hypertension to the same extent as pharmacologic therapy and often more than other lifestyle changes.[24,161] Two months of the diet reduced systolic pressure by an average of 11.4 mm Hg; diastolic pressure decreased by 5.5 mm Hg. Every 2-mm Hg reduction in systolic pressure lowers heart disease risk by 5% and stroke risk by 8%.

TABLE 2.11 shows the specifics of the DASH diet with its high content of fruits, vegetables, and dairy products and low-fat composition. Further good news emerges from the latest research from the DASH group indicating that the standard DASH diet combined with a daily salt intake of 1150 mg—

called the DASH-Sodium diet—produced greater blood pressure reductions than were achieved with the DASH diet only.[162,182] Blood pressure declined for both normotensive and hypertensive subjects, with the greatest benefits for subjects with high blood pressure. The DASH diet alone and sodium restriction alone both lowered blood pressure, but the greatest reductions emerged with the DASH–low sodium combination. The best scientific information currently recommends the following five lifestyle approaches to prevent hypertension:[43,205,206]

1. Regularly engage in moderate physical activity
2. Maintain normal body weight

TABLE 2.11   Dietary Approaches to Stop Hypertension (DASH)

Food Group	Example of 1 Serving	Servings
Vegetables	1/2 cup of cooked or raw chopped vegetables; 1 cup of raw leafy vegetables; or 6 oz of juice	8–12 daily
Fruit	1 medium apple, pear, orange, or banana; 1/2 grapefruit; 1/3 cantaloupe; 1/2 cup of fresh frozen or canned fruit; 1/4 cup of dried fruit; or 6 oz of juice	8–12 daily
Grains	1 slice of bread; 1/2 cup of cold, dry cereal; cooked rice or pasta	6–12 daily
Dairy	1 cup of no-fat or low-fat milk or 1 1/2 oz of low-fat or part-skim cheese	2–4 daily
Nuts, seeds, and beans	1/3 cup (1 1/2 oz) of nuts; 2 tablespoons of seeds; or 1/2 cup of cooked beans	4–7 weekly
Meat, poultry, or fish	3 oz chunk (roughly the size of a deck of cards)	1–2 daily
Oil or other fats	1 tsp. vegetable oil; butter; salad dressings; soft margarine	2–4 daily

3. Limit alcohol consumption
4. Reduce sodium intake and maintain an adequate intake of potassium
5. Consume a diet rich in fruits, vegetables, and low-fat dairy products and reduced in saturated fatty acids and total fat

TABLE 2.12 shows a sample DASH diet consisting of approximately 2100 kCal. This level of energy intake provides a stable body weight for a typical 70-kg person. More physically active and heavier individuals should boost portion size or the number of individual items to maintain weight. Individuals desiring to lose weight or who are lighter and/or sedentary should eat less, but not less than the minimum number of servings for each food group listed in Table 2.11.

Can Sodium Intake Be Too Low?

A low-sodium diet in conjunction with excessive perspiration, persistent vomiting, or diarrhea creates the potential to deplete the body's sodium content to critical levels, a condition termed **hyponatremia.** This condition causes a broad array of symptoms ranging from muscle cramps, nausea, vomiting, dizziness and, in the extreme, to shock, coma, and death. A minimal likelihood of hyponatremia exists for most persons because responses by the kidneys to low sodium status trigger sodium conservation. In addition, the availability of sodium in so many foods makes it improbable that sodium levels would fall to critically low levels.

Even when body weight loss from perspiration reaches 2 to 3% of body weight (about 5–7 lb), adding a bit of extra table salt to food usually restores sodium for most persons. Endurance athletes, basketball, baseball, soccer, and football players who routinely lose more than 4% of body weight following competition should consume salt-containing drinks before and after heavy sweating to ensure adequate sodium concentrations in the body. Chapter 10 discusses exercise, fluid intake, and risks of hyponatremia in greater detail.

TABLE 2.12 Sample 2100-kCal Dash Diet

Food	Amount
Breakfast	
Orange juice	6 oz
1% low-fat milk	8 oz (used with corn flakes)
Corn flakes (1 tsp. sugar)	1 cup (dry) [equals 2 servings of grains]
Banana	1 medium
Whole-wheat bread	1 slice
Soft margarine	1 tsp.
Lunch	
Low-fat chicken salad	3/4 cup
Pita bread	1/2 large
Raw-vegetable medley carrot and celery sticks	3–4 sticks each
Radishes	2
Lettuce	2 leaves
Part-skim mozzarella	1 1/2 slices (1.5 oz)
1% low-fat milk	8 oz
Fruit cocktail	1/2 cup
Dinner	
Herbed baked cod	3 oz
Scallion rice	1 cup [equals 2 servings of grain]
Steamed broccoli	1/2 cup
Stewed tomatoes	1/2 cup
Spinach salad (raw spinach)	1/2 cup
Cherry tomatoes	2
Cucumber	2 slices
Light Italian salad dressing	1 tbsp. (equals 1/2 fat serving)
Whole wheat dinner roll	1
Soft margarine	1 tsp.
Melon balls	1/2 cup
Snack	
Dried apricots	1 oz (1/4 cup)
Mixed nuts, unsalted	1.5 oz (1/3 cup)
Mini-pretzels, unsalted	1 oz (3/4 cup)
Diet ginger ale	12 oz (does not count as a serving of any food)

Summary

1. Approximately 4% of the body mass consists of 22 elements called minerals. Minerals become distributed in all body tissues and fluids.

2. Minerals occur freely in nature, in the waters of rivers, lakes, and oceans and in soil. The root system of plants absorbs minerals; they eventually become incorporated into the tissues of animals that consume plants.

3. Minerals function primarily in metabolism as constituents of enzymes. Minerals provide structure in the formation of bones and teeth and synthesize the biologic macronutrients glycogen, fat, and protein.

4. A balanced diet generally provides adequate mineral intake, except in some geographic locations lacking specific minerals (e.g., iodine).

5. Osteoporosis has reached almost epidemic proportions among older individuals, particularly women. Adequate calcium intake and regular weight-bearing exercise and/or resistance training provide an effective defense against bone loss at any age.

6. Paradoxically, women who train intensely but cannot match energy intake to energy output reduce body weight and body fat to the point that may adversely affect menstruation. These women often show advanced bone loss at an early age. Restoration of normal menstruation does not totally restore bone mass.

7. The association between muscular strength and bone density raises the likelihood of using strength testing of postmenopausal women as a clinically useful tool to screen for osteoporosis.

8. About 40% of American women of child-bearing age suffer from dietary iron insufficiency that could lead to iron-deficiency anemia. This condition negatively affects aerobic exercise performance and the ability to perform intense training.

9. For women on vegetarian-type diets, the relatively low bioavailability of nonheme iron increases the risk for developing iron insufficiency. Vitamin C (in food or supplement form) and moderate physical activity increase intestinal absorption of nonheme iron.

10. Regular physical activity generally does not create a significant drain on the body's iron reserves. If it does, women with the greatest iron requirement and lowest iron intake could increase their risk for anemia. Assessment of the body's iron status should evaluate hematologic characteristics and iron reserves.

11. The Dietary Approaches to Stop Hypertension (DASH) eating plan lowers blood pressure in some individuals to the same extent as pharmacologic therapy and often more than other lifestyle changes.

Water

WATER IN THE BODY

Water makes up from 40 to 70% of an individual's body mass, depending on age, sex, and body composition; it constitutes 65 to 75% of the weight of muscle and about 50% of the weight of body fat (adipose tissue). Consequently, differences in the relative percentage of total body water among individuals result largely from variations in body composition (i.e., differences in lean vs fat tissue).

FIGURE 2.17 depicts the fluid compartments of the body, the normal daily body water variation, and specific terminology to describe the various states of human hydration. The body contains two fluid "compartments." The first compartment, **intracellular,** refers to inside the cells; the second, **extracellular,** indicates fluids surrounding the cells. Extracellular fluid includes the blood plasma and the interstitial fluids, which primarily compose the fluid that flows in the microscopic spaces among the cells. Also included as interstitial fluid are lymph, saliva, and fluid in the eyes, fluids secreted by glands and the digestive tract, fluids that bathe the nerves of the spinal cord, and fluids excreted from the skin and kidneys. Blood plasma accounts for 20% of the extracellular fluid (3–4 L). Of the total body water, an average of 62% (26 L of the body's 42 L of water for an average-sized man) represents intracellular water and 38% comes from extracellular sources. These volumes do not remain static but represent averages from a dynamic exchange of fluid between compartments, particularly in physically active individuals.[164,197] Exercise training often increases the percentage of water distributed within the intracellular compartment from increases in muscle mass and its accompanying large water content. In contrast, an acute bout of exercise temporarily shifts fluid from the plasma to the interstitial and intracellular spaces from the increased hydrostatic (fluid) pressure within the active circulatory system.

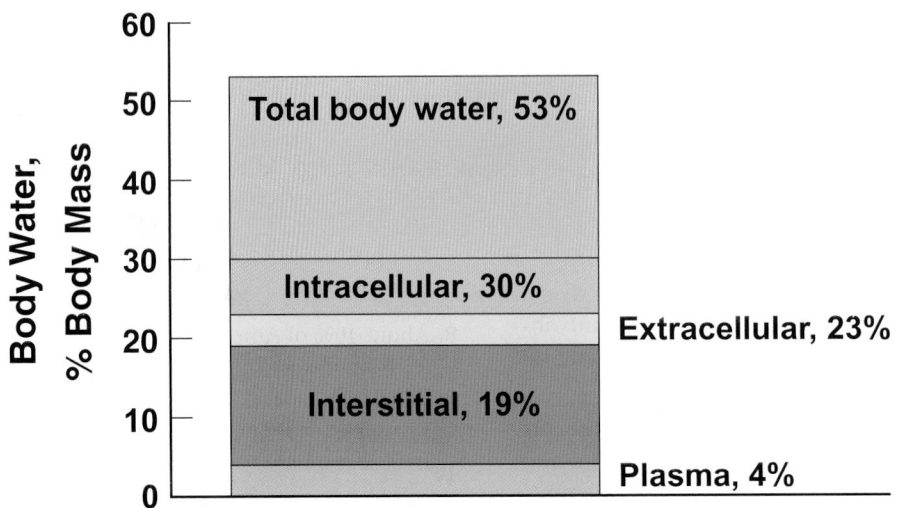

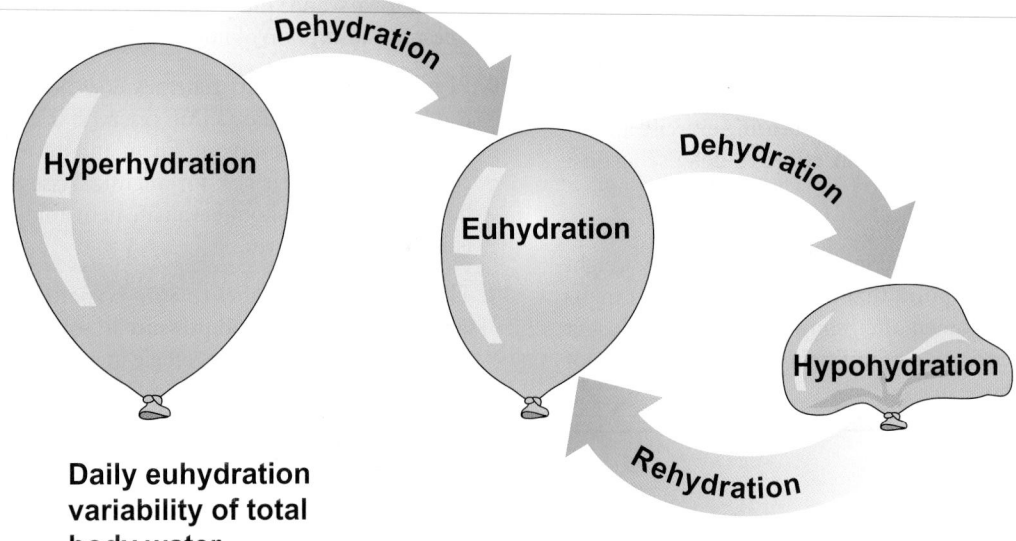

Daily euhydration variability of total body water

Temperature climate:
  0.165 L (±0.2% body mass)
Heat exercise conditions:
  0.382 L (±0.5% body mass)

Daily plasma volume variability

All conditions:
  0.027 L (±0.6% blood volume)

Hydration terminology

Euhydration: normal daily water variation
Hyperhydration: new steady-state condition of increased water content
Hypohydration: new steady-state condition of decreased water content
Dehydration: process of losing water either from the hyperhydrated state to euhydration, or from euhydration downward to hypohydration
Rehydration: process of gaining water from a hypohydrated state toward euhydration

FIGURE 2.17 ■ Fluid compartments, average volumes and variability, and hydration terminology. Volumes represent those for an 80-kg man. Approximately 60% of the body mass consists of water in striated muscle (80% water), skeleton (32% water), and adipose tissue (50% water). For a man and woman of similar body mass, the woman contains less total water because of her larger ratio of adipose tissue to lean body mass (striated muscle + skeleton). (Adapted from Greenleaf JE. Problem: thirst, drinking behavior, and involuntary dehydration. *Med Sci Sports Exerc* 1992;24:645.)

FUNCTIONS OF BODY WATER

Water is a ubiquitous, remarkable nutrient. Without water, death occurs within days. It serves as the body's transport and reactive medium; diffusion of gases always takes place across surfaces moistened by water. Nutrients and gases travel in aqueous solution; waste products leave the body through the water in urine and feces. Water, in conjunction with various proteins, lubricates joints and protects a variety of "moving" organs like the heart, lungs, intestines, and eyes. Because it is noncompressible, water gives structure and form to the body through the turgor provided for body tissues. Water has tremendous heat-stabilizing qualities because it absorbs considerable heat with only minor changes in temperature. This quality, combined with water's high heat of vaporization (energy required to change 1 g of a liquid into the gaseous state at the boiling point), facilitates maintenance of a relatively constant body temperature during (1) environmental heat stress and (2) the large increase in internal heat generated by exercise. Chapter 10 says more about the dynamics of thermoregulation during heat stress, particularly water's important role.

WATER BALANCE: INTAKE VERSUS OUTPUT

The body's water content remains relatively stable over time. Although considerable water output occurs in physically active individuals, appropriate fluid intake usually restores any imbalance in the body's fluid level. FIGURE 2.18 displays the sources of water intake and output.

Water Intake

A sedentary adult in a thermoneutral environment requires about 2.5 L of water each day. For an active person in a hot environment the water requirement often increases to between 5 and 10 L daily. Three sources provide this water: (1) liquids, (2) foods, and (3) metabolic processes.

Water from Liquids

The average individual normally consumes 1200 mL or 41 oz of water each day. Exercise and thermal stress can increase fluid intake five or six times above normal. At the extreme, an individual lost 13.6 kg (30 lb) of water weight during a 2-day, 17-hour, 55-mile run across Death Valley, California (lowest point in the Western Hemisphere at almost 300 feet below sea level; recognized as one of the hottest places on earth with the highest recorded temperature of 134°F). However, with proper fluid ingestion, including salt supplements, body

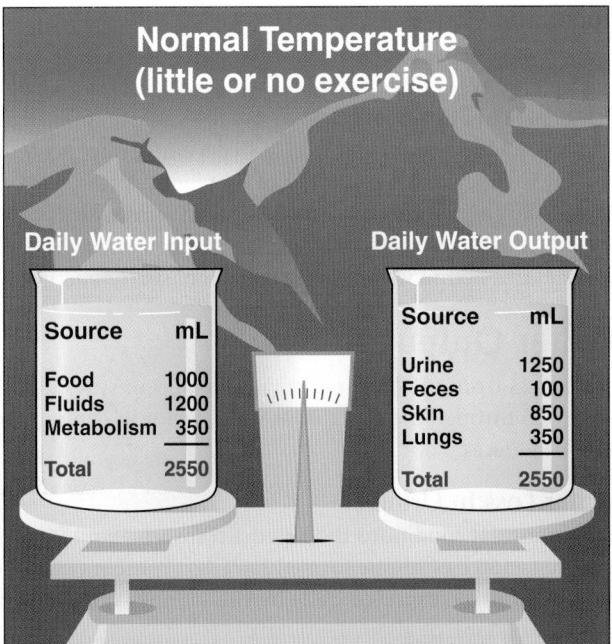

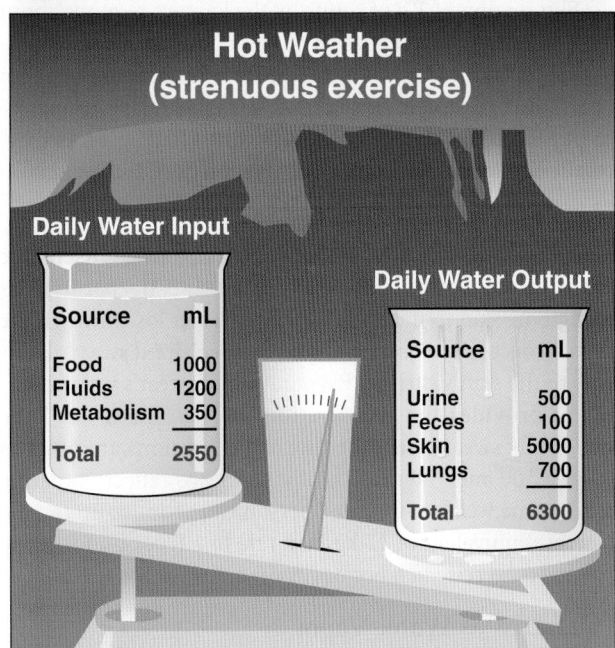

FIGURE 2.18 ■ Water balance in the body. *Top,* Little or no exercise in normal ambient temperature and humidity. *Bottom,* Moderate to heavy exercise in a hot, humid environment.

weight loss amounted to only 1.4 kg. In this example, fluid loss and replenishment represented between 3.5 and 4 gallons of liquid!

Water In Foods

Fruits and vegetables contain considerable water (e.g., lettuce, watermelon and cantaloupe, pickles, green beans, and broccoli); in contrast, butter, oils, dried meats, and chocolate, cookies, and cakes have a relatively low water content.

Metabolic Water

Carbon dioxide and water form when food molecules catabolize for energy. Termed **metabolic water,** this fluid provides about 14% of a sedentary person's daily water requirement. The complete breakdown of 100 g of carbohydrate, protein, and fat yields 55, 100, and 107 g of metabolic water, respectively. Additionally, each gram of glycogen joins with 2.7 g of water as its glucose units link together; subsequently, glycogen liberates this bound water during its catabolism for energy.

Water Output

Water loss from the body occurs in one of four ways: (1) in urine, (2) through the skin, (3) as water vapor in expired air, and (4) in feces.

Water Loss In Urine

Under normal conditions the kidneys reabsorb about 99% of the 140 to 160 L of filtrate formed each day; consequently, the volume of urine excreted daily by the kidneys ranges from 1000 to 1500 mL or about 1.5 quarts.

Elimination of 1 g of solute by the kidneys requires about 15 mL of water. Thus, a portion of water in urine becomes "obligated" to rid the body of metabolic by-products like urea, an end product of protein breakdown. Catabolizing large quantities of protein for energy (as occurs with a high-protein diet) actually accelerates the body's dehydration during exercise.

Water Loss Through the Skin

A small quantity of water, perhaps 350 mL, termed **insensible perspiration,** continually seeps from the deeper tissues through the skin to the body's surface. Water loss through the skin also occurs as sweat produced by specialized sweat glands beneath the skin's surface. Evaporation of sweat's water component provides the refrigeration mechanism to cool the body. Daily sweat rate under normal conditions amounts to between 500 and 700 mL. This by no means reflects sweating capacity; the well-acclimatized person can produce up to 12 L of sweat (equivalent of 12 kg) at a rate of 1 L per hour during prolonged exercise in a hot environment.

Water Loss as Water Vapor

Insensible water loss through small water droplets in exhaled air amounts to 250 to 350 mL per day. The complete moistening of all inspired air as it passes down the pulmonary airways accounts for this avenue of water loss. Exercise affects this source of water loss because inspired air requires humidification. For physically active persons, the respiratory passages release 2 to 5 mL of water each minute during strenuous exercise, depending on climatic conditions. Ventilatory water loss is least in hot, humid weather and greatest in cold temperatures (inspired cold air contains little moisture) or at altitude because inspired air volumes are larger than at sea-level conditions.

Water Loss in Feces

Intestinal elimination produces between 100 and 200 mL of water loss because water constitutes approximately 70% of fecal matter. The remainder comprises nondigestible material including bacteria from the digestive process and the residues of digestive juices from the intestine, stomach, and pancreas. With diarrhea or vomiting, water loss increases to between 1500 and 5000 mL.

PHYSICAL ACTIVITY AND ENVIRONMENTAL FACTORS PLAY AN IMPORTANT ROLE

The loss of body water represents the most serious consequence of profuse sweating. The severity of physical activity, environmental temperature, and humidity determine the amount of water lost through sweating. Exercise-induced increases in sweating also occur in the water enivronment, through activities such as vigorous swimming or water polo.[98] Relative humidity (water content of the ambient air) affects the efficiency of the sweating mechanism for temperature regulation. Ambient air becomes completely saturated with water vapor at 100% relative humidity. This blocks evaporation of fluid from the skin surface to the air, thus negating this important avenue for body cooling. Under such conditions, sweat beads on the skin and eventually rolls off, without providing an evaporative cooling effect. On a dry day, air can hold considerable moisture and fluid rapidly evaporates from the skin. Thus, the sweat mechanism functions at optimal efficiency and body temperature remains regulated within a narrow range. Importantly, plasma volume begins to decrease when sweating causes a fluid loss equal to 2 or 3% of body mass. Fluid loss from the vascular compartment strains circulatory function, which ultimately impairs exercise capacity and thermoregulation.

An Easy Yet Effective Method

Monitoring changes in body weight provides a convenient way to assess fluid loss during exercise and/or heat stress. Each 0.45 kg (1 lb) of body weight loss corresponds to 450 mL dehydration.

Summary

1. Water constitutes 40 to 70% of the total body mass; muscle contains 72% water by weight, whereas water represents only about 50% of the weight of body fat (adipose tissue).

2. Of the total body water, roughly 62% exists intracellularly (inside the cells) and 38% occurs extracellularly in the plasma, lymph, and other fluids outside the cell.

3. The normal average daily water intake of 2.5 L comes from liquid (1.2 L) and food (1.0 L) intake and metabolic water produced during energy-yielding reactions (0.3 L).

4. Daily water loss occurs in urine (1–1.5 L), through the skin as insensible perspiration (0.50–0.70 L), as water vapor in expired air (0.25–0.30 L), and in feces (0.10 L).

5. Food and oxygen exist in the body in aqueous solution, while nongaseous waste products always leave in a watery medium. Water also provides structure and form to the body and plays a crucial role in temperature regulation.

6. Exercise in hot weather greatly increases the body's water requirement. In extreme conditions, fluid needs increase five or six times above normal.

Test Your Knowledge Answers

1. **True:** Vitamin intake above the RDA does not improve exercise performance or the potential to sustain physical training. In fact, serious illness occurs from regularly consuming excess fat-soluble vitamins and, in some instances, water-soluble vitamins.

2. **False:** Although the body can conserve water, there is some loss every day. After only a few days, severe dehydration can result in death. In contrast, death from starvation takes much longer, perhaps 60 days or more.

3. **False:** The terms *major* and *trace* do not reflect nutritional importance; rather, they are classifications referring to the amount needed for (daily) functioning. In essence, each of the micronutrients, major or trace, is critical to the maintenance of optimal physiologic functioning and good health.

4. **False:** Most major and trace minerals occur freely in nature, mainly in the waters of rivers, lakes, and oceans, in topsoil, and beneath the earth's surface. Minerals exist in the root systems of plants and in the body structure of animals that consume plants and water containing minerals. Neither plant nor animal kingdom provides a "better" source for these micronutrients.

5. **False:** Adults need about 1 mL of water per kCal of energy expended each day. If the average woman expends 2400 kCal per day, she then requires about 2400 mL (2.4 L) of water on a daily basis. This volume transposes to about 0.63 gallons (2.4 L ÷ 3.785).

6. **False:** While sodium is an important contributor to increased blood pressure in some hypertensive individuals, weight (fat) loss, regular exercise, and a well-balanced diet are also important changes a person can make to lower blood pressure.

7. **False:** Fat-soluble vitamins should not be consumed in excess without medical supervision. Toxic reactions from excessive fat-soluble vitamin intake generally occur at a lower multiple of recommended intakes than water-soluble vitamins. An excess intake of certain water-soluble vitamins also causes untoward effects in certain individuals.

8. **False:** Iron deficiency anemia impairs the body's ability to transport oxygen and process it in energy transfer reactions. This condition produces general sluggishness, loss of appetite, and reduced capacity to sustain even mild exercise.

9. **False:** Short intense bouts of mechanical loading of bone through weight-bearing exercise performed three to five times a week provides a potent stimulus to maintain or increase bone mass. This form of exercise includes walking, running, dancing, rope skipping; high-intensity resistance exercises, and circuit-resistance training also exert a positive effect. Sport activities providing relatively high impact on the skeletal mass (e.g., volleyball, basketball, gymnastics, judo, and karate) also induce increases in bone mass, particularly at weight-bearing sites.

10. **False:** Research using Dietary Approaches to Stop Hypertension (DASH) to treat hypertension shows that this type of diet lowers blood pressure in the general population and in people with stage 1 hypertension to the same extent as pharmacologic therapy, and often more than other lifestyle changes.

References

1. Ajani UA, et al. Sodium intake among people with normal and high blood pressure. *Am J Prev Med* 2005;29(suppl 1):63.
2. Al-Delaimy WK, et al. A prospective study of calcium intake from diet and supplements and risk of ischemic heart disease among men. *Am J Clin Nutr* 2003;72:814.
3. Alderman MH. Evidence relating dietary sodium to cardiovascular disease. *J Am Coll Nutr* 2006;25:256S.
4. American College of Sports Medicine. Position stand on physical activity and bone health. *Med Sci Sports Exerc* 2004;36:1985.
5. American College of Sports Medicine, American Dietetic Association and Dietitians of Canada. Joint position statement. Nutrition and athletic performance. *Med Sci Sports Exerc* 2000;32:2130.
6. Andreoli A, et al. Effects of different sports on bone density and muscle mass in highly trained athletes. *Med Sci Sports Exerc* 2001;33:507.
7. Apple LJ, et al, A clinical trial of the effects of dietary patterns on blood pressure: DASH Collaborative Research Group. *N Engl J Med* 1997;336:1117.
8. Arab L, Steck S. Lycopene and cardiovascular disease. *Am J Clin Nutr* 2000;71:1691S.
9. Ashizawa N, et al. Tomographical description of tennis-loaded radius: reciprocal relation between bone size and volumetric BMD. *J Appl Physiol* 1999;86:1347.
10. Beals KA, Hill AK. The prevalence of disordered eating, menstrual dysfunction, and low bone mineral density among US collegiate athletes. *Int J Sport Nutr Exerc Metab* 2006;16:1.
11. Beard J, Stoltzfus R. Forward. *J Nutr* 2001;131(suppl):563S.
12. Beek EJ van der. Vitamin supplementation and physical exercise performance. *Sports Sci* 1991;9:77.
13. Bloomer RJ, et al. Oxidative stress response to aerobic exercise: comparison of antioxidant supplements. *Med Sci Sports Exerc* 2006; 38:1098.
14. Bostom AG, et al. Nonfasting plasma total homocysteine levels and all-cause and cardiovascular disease mortality in the elderly Framingham men and women. *Arch Intern Med* 1999;159:1077.
15. Brilla L, Haley T. Effect of magnesium supplementation on strength training in humans. *J Am Coll Nutr* 1992;11:326.
16. Brownlie IV T, et al. Marginal iron deficiency without anemia impairs aerobic adaptation among previously untrained women. *Am J Clin Nutr* 2002;75:734.
17. Brownlie IV T, et al. Tissue iron deficiency without anemia impairs adaptation in endurance capacity after aerobic training in previously untrained women. *Am J Clin Nutr* 2004;79:437.
18. Brune M, et al. Iron loss in sweat. *Am J Clin Nutr* 1986;43:438.
19. Brutsaert TD, et al. Iron supplementation improves progressive fatigue resistance during dynamic knee extensor exercise in iron-depleted, nonanemic women. *Am J Clin Nutr* 2003;77:441.
20. Cabet J, et al. High femoral bone mineral content and density in male football (soccer) players. *Med Sci Sports Exerc* 2001;33:1682.
21. Cauley JA, et al. Effects of estrogen plus progestin on risk of fracture and bone mineral density. *JAMA* 2003;290:1729.
22. Cobb KL, et al. Disordered eating, menstrual irregularity, and bone mineral density in female runners. *Med Sci Sports Exerc* 2003;35:711.
23. Cohen HW, et al. Sodium intake and mortality in the HNANES II follow-up study. *Am J Med* 2006;119:275.
24. Conlin PR, et al. The effect of dietary patterns on blood pressure control in hypertensive patients: results from the Dietary Approaches to Stop Hypertension (DASH) Trial. *Am J Hypertens* 2000;13:949.
25. Conroy BP, et al. Bone mineral density in elite junior Olympic weight lifters. *Med Sci Sports Exerc* 1993;25:1103.
26. Creighton DL, et al. Weight-bearing exercise and markers of bone turnover in female athletes. *J Appl Physiol* 2001;90:565.
27. Cullen DM, et al. Bone-loading response varies with strain magnitude and cycle number. *J Appl Physiol* 2001;91:1971.
28. Cummings SR, et al. Endogenous hormones and the risk of hip and vertebral fractures among older women. *N Engl J Med* 1998;339:733.
29. Cussler EC, et al. Weight lifted in strength training predicts bone change in postmenopausal women. *Med Sci Sports Exerc* 2003;35:10.
30. Derstine JL, et al. Iron status in association with cardiovascular disease risk in 3 controlled feeding studies. *Am J Clin Nutr* 2003;77:56.
31. Deruisseau KC, et al. Iron status of young males and females performing weight-training exercise. *Med Sci Sports Exerc* 2004;36:241.
32. Deugnier Y, et al. Increased body iron stores in elite road cyclists. *Med Sci Sports Exerc* 2002;34:876.
33. Deuster PA, et al. Nutritional survey of highly trained women runners. *Am J Clin Nutr* 1986;45:954.
34. Diaz MN, et al. Antioxidants and atherosclerotic heart disease. *N Engl J Med* 1997;337:408.
35. Dook JE, et al. Exercise and bone mineral density in mature female athletes. *Med Sci Sports Exerc* 1997;29:291.
36. Drinkwater BL, et al. Menstrual history as a determinant of current bone density in young athletes. *JAMA* 1990;263:545.
37. Dueck CA, et al. A diet and training intervention program for the treatment of athletic amenorrhea. *Int J Sports Nutr* 1996;6:134.
38. Duncan CS, et al. Bone mineral density in adolescent female athletes: relationship to exercise type and muscle strength. *Med Sci Sports Exerc* 2002;34:286.
39. Dvbnov G, Constantini NW. Prevalence of iron depletion and anemia in top-level basketball players. *Int J Sports Nutr Exerc Metab* 2004;14:30.
40. Dwyer JH, et al. Dietary calcium, calcium supplementation, and blood pressure in African American adolescents. *Am J Clin Nutr* 1998; 68: 648.
41. Eichner ER. Fatigue of anemia. *Nutr Revs* 2001;59:S17.
42. Eikelboom JW, et al. Homocyst(e)ine and cardiovascular disease: a critical review of epidemiologic evidence. *Ann Intern Med* 1999; 131:362.
43. Elmer PJ, et al. Effects of comprehensive lifestyle modification on diet, weight, physical fitness and blood pressure control: 18-month results of a randomized trial. *Ann Intern Med* 2006;144:127.
44. Erhardt JG, et al. Lycopene, β-carotene, and colorectal adenomas. *Am J Clin Nutr* 2003;78:1219.
45. Erp-Bart van AMJ, et al. Nationwide survey on nutritional habits in elite athletes. Part 1. Energy, carbohydrate, protein and fat intake. *Int J Sports Med* 1989;10(suppl 1):S3.
46. Faulkner RA, et al. Strength indices of the proximal femur and shaft in prepubertal female gymnasts. *Med Sci Sports Exerc* 2003;35:513.
47. Feskanich D, et al. Walking and leisure-time activity and risk of hip fracture in postmenopausal women. *JAMA* 2002;288:2300.
48. Finstad EW, et al. The effects of magnesium supplementation on exercise performance. *Med Sci Sports Exerc* 2001;33:493.
49. Fleet J. How well you absorb calcium is important for limiting hip fracture risk. *Nutr Rev* 2001;59:338.
50. Flemming DJ, et al. Dietary factors associated with the risk of high iron stores in the elderly Framingham Heart Study cohort. *Am J Clin Nutr* 2002;76:1375.
51. Friedmann B, et al. Effects of iron repletion on blood volume and performance capacity in young athletes. *Med Sci Sports Exerc* 2001;33:741.
52. Gale CR. Antioxidant vitamin status and carotid atherosclerosis in the elderly. *Am J Clin Nutr* 2001;74:402.
53. Ganji V, Kafi MR. Demographic, health, lifestyle, and blood vitamin determinants of serum total homocysteine concentrations in the third National Health and Nutrition Examination Survey. *Am J Clin Nutr* 2003;77:826.
54. Giguere Y, Rousseau F. The genetics of osteoporosis: "complexities and difficulties." *Clin Genet* 2000;57:161.
55. Gledhill N, et al. Haemoglobin, blood volume, cardiac function, and aerobic power. *Can J Appl Physiol* 1999;24:54.
56. Goldfarb AH, et el. Combined antioxidant treatment affects blood oxidative stress after eccentric exercise. *Med Sci Sports Exerc* 2005;37:234.
57. Goodman LR, Warren MP. The female athlete and menstrual function. *Curr Opin Obstet Gynecol* 2005;17:466.
58. Green HJ, et al. Training induced hypervolemia: lack of an effect on oxygen utilization during exercise. *Med Sci Sports Exerc* 1987;19:202.
59. Gremion G, et al. Oligo-amenorrheic long-distance runners may lose more bone in spine than in femur. *Med Sci Sports Exerc* 2001;33:15.

60. Gropper SS, et al. Iron status of female collegiate athletes involved in different sports. *Biol Trace Elem Res* 2006;109:1.

61. Gross TS, et al. Why rest stimulates bone formation: a hypothesis based on complex adaptive phenomenon. *Exerc Sport Sci Rev* 2004;32:9.

62. Haim M, et al. Serum homocysteine and long-term risk of myocardial infarction and sudden death in patients with coronary heart disease. *Cardiology* 2007;107:52.

63. Harats D, et al. Citrus fruit supplementation reduces lipoprotein oxidation in young men ingesting a diet high in saturated fat: presumptive evidence for an interaction between vitamins C and E in vivo. *Am J Clin Nutr* 1998;67:240.

64. Hawkins SA, et al. Five-year maintenance of bone mineral density in women master runners. *Med Sci Sports Exerc* 2003;35:137.

65. Haymes EM. Vitamin and mineral supplementation to athletes. *Int J Sports Nutr* 1991;1:146.

66. Heaney R, Rafferty K. Carbonated beverages and urinary calcium excretion. *Am J Clin Nutr* 2001:74:343.

67. Hegarty VM, et al. Tea drinking and bone mineral density in older women. *Am J Clin Nutr* 2000;71:1003.

68. Helge EW, Kanstrup I-L. Bone density in female elite gymnasts: impact of muscle strength and sex hormones. *Med Sci Sports Exerc* 2002;34:174.

69. Hennekens CH, et al. Lack of effect of long-term supplementation with beta carotene on the incidence of malignant neoplasm and cardiovascular disease. *N Engl J Med* 1996;334:1145.

70. Hinton PS, et al. Iron supplementation improves endurance after training in iron-depleted, nonanemic women. *J Appl Physiol* 2000;88:1103.

71. Hodis HN, et al. Serial coronary angiographic evidence that antioxidant vitamin intake reduces progression of coronary artery disease. *JAMA* 1995;273:1849.

72. Hu FB. Plant-based foods and prevention of cardiovascular disease: an overview. *Am J Clin Nutr* 2003;78(suppl):544S.

73. Huang H-Y, et al. Effects of vitamin C and vitamin E on in vivo lipid peroxidation: results of a randomized controlled trial. *Am J Clin Nutr* 2002;76:549.

74. Hunt JR, Roughead ZK. Adaptation of iron absorption in men consuming diets with high or low iron bioavailability. *Am J Clin Nutr* 2000;71:95.

75. Hunt SC, et al. Angiotensinogen genotype, sodium reduction, weight loss, and prevention of hypertension. Trials of Hypertension Prevention, Phase II. Hypertension 1998;32:393.

76. Hunter EJ, et al. Dietary carotenoids and vitamins A, C, and E and risk of breast cancer. *J Natl Cancer Inst* 1999;91:547.

77. Jacqmain M, et al. Calcium intake, body composition, and lipoprotein-lipid concentrations in adults. *Am J Clin Nutr* 1003;78:1448.

78. Jacques PF, et al. Determinants of plasma total homocysteine concentration in the Framingham Offspring cohort. *Am J Clin Nutr* 2001;73:613.

79. Janz KF, et al. Everyday activity predicts bone geometry in children: the Iowa Bone Development Study. *Med Sci Sports Exerc* 2004;36:1124.

80. Jiang Q, et al. γ-Tocopherol, the major form of vitamin E in the US diet, deserves more attention. *Am J Clin Nutr* 2001;74:714.

81. Kalkwarf HJ, et al. Milk intake during childhood and adolescence, adult bone density, and osteoporotic fractures in US women. *Am J Clin Nutr* 2003;77:257.

82. Karlsson MK, et al. Exercise during growth and young adulthood is associated with reduced fracture risk in old ages. *J Bone Miner Res* 2002;17(suppl 1):S297.

83. Keith ME, et al. A controlled clinical trial of vitamin E supplementation in patients with congestive heart failure. *Am J Clin Nutr* 2001; 73:219.

84. Kemmler W, et al. Exercise effects on fitness and bone mineral density in early postmenopausal women: 1-year EFOPS results. *Med Sci Sports Exerc* 2002;34:2115.

85. Kerr D, et al. Exercise effects on bone mass in postmenopausal women are site-specific and load-dependent. *J Bone Min Res* 1996; 11:218.

86. Kirchner EM, et al. Effect of past gymnastics participation on adult bone mass. *J Appl Physiol* 1996;80:226.

87. Klipstein-Grobusch K, et al. Dietary antioxidants and risk of myocardial infarction in the elderly: the Rotterdam Study. *Am J Clin Nutr* 1999;69:261.

88. Klungland Torstveit M, Sundgot-Borgen J. The female athlete triad: are elite athletes at increased risk? *Med Sci Sports Exerc* 2005;237:184.

89. Knekt P, et al. Antioxidant vitamins and coronary heart disease risk: a pooled analysis of 9 cohorts. *Am J Clin Nutr* 2004;80:1508.

90. Kohrt WM, et al. HRT preserves increases in bone mineral density and reductions in body fat after a supervised exercise program. *J Appl Physiol* 1998;84:1506.

91. Konyulsinrn D, et al. Good maintenance of exercise-induced bone gain with decreased training of female tennis and squash players: a prospective 5-year follow-up study of young and old starters and controls. *J Bone Miner Res* 2001;16:195.

92. Kritchevsky SB, et al. Provitamin A carotenoid intake and carotid artery plaques: the Atherosclerosis Risk in Communities Study. *Am J Clin Nutr* 1998;68:726.

93. Kushi LH, et al. Dietary antioxidant vitamins and death from coronary heart disease in postmenopausal women. *N Engl J Med* 1996;334:1156.

94. LaMothe JM, Zernicke RF. Rest-insertion combined with high-frequency loading enhances osteogenesis. *J Appl Physiol* 2004;96:1788.

95. Layne JE, Nelson ME. The effects of progressive resistance training on bone density: a review. *Med Sci Sports Exerc* 1999;31:25.

96. LeBoff MS, et al. Occult vitamin D deficiency in postmenopausal US women with acute hip fracture. *JAMA* 1999;281:1505.

97. Lee EJ, et al. Variations in bone status of contralateral and regional sites in young athletic women. *Med Sci Sports Exerc* 1995;27:1354.

98. Leiper JB, Maughan RJ. Comparison of water turnover rates in young swimmers in training and age-matched non-training individuals. *Int J Sport Nutr Exerc Metab* 2004;14:347.

99. Levine M, et al. Criteria and recommendations for vitamin C intake. *JAMA* 1999;281:1485.

100. Lin Y, et al. Estimating the concentration of β-carotene required for maximal protection of low-density lipoproteins in women. *Am J Clin Nutr* 1998;67:837.

101. Linden C, et al. A school curriculum-based exercise program increases bone mineral accrual and bone size in prepubertal girls: two-year data from the pediatric osteoporosis prevention (POP) study. *J Bone Miner Res* 2006;21:829.

102. Linden C, et al. Exercise, bone mass and bone size in prepubertal boys: one-year data from the pediatric osteoporosis prevention study. *Scand J Med Sci Sports* 2007;17:340.

103. Lindsay R, et al. Effect of lower doses of conjugated equine estrogens with and without dedroxyprogesterone acetate on bone in early postmenopausal women. *JAMA* 2002;287:2668.

104. Lima F, et al. Effect of impact load and active load on bone metabolism and body composition of adolescent athletes. *Med Sci Sports Exerc* 2001;33:1318.

105. Livshits G, et al. Genes play an important role in bone aging. *Hum Biol* 1998;10:421.

106. Lonn E, et al. Effects of long-term vitamin E supplementation on cardiovascular events and cancer: a randomized controlled trial. *JAMA* 2005;293:1338.

107. Loscalzo J. Homocysteine trials: clear outcomes for complex reasons. *N Engl J Med* 2006;354:1629.

108. Luft GS, Weinberger MH. Heterogeneous responses to changes in dietary salt intake: the salt-sensitivity paradigm. *Am J Clin Nutr* 1997;65(suppl):626S.

109. Lyle RM, et al. Iron status in exercising women: the effect of oral iron therapy vs increased consumption of muscle foods. *Am J Clin Nutr* 1992;56:1099.

110. Mackelvie KJ, et al. Lifestyle risk factors for osteoporosis in Asian and Caucasian girls. *Med Sci Sports Exerc* 2001;33:1818.

111. Malinow MR, et al. Plasma homocysteine levels and graded risk for myocardial infarction: findings in two populations at contrasting risk for coronary heart disease. *Atherosclerosis* 1996;126:27.

112. Martinez ME, et al. Physical activity, body mass index, and prostaglandin E2 levels in rectal mucosa. *J Natl Cancer Inst* 1999;91:950.

113. Mauck KF, Clarke BL. Diagnosis, screening, prevention, and treatment of osteoporosis. *Mayo Clin Proc* 2006;81:662.

114. McCabe ME, et al. Gastrointestinal blood loss associated with running a marathon. *Dig Dis Sci* 1986;31:1229.

115. McKenna AA, et al. Zinc balance in adolescent females consuming a low- or high-calcium diet. *Am J Clin Nutr* 1997;65:1460.

116. McLean JA, et al. Dietary restraint, exercise, and bone density in young women: are they related? *Med Sci Sports Exerc* 2001;33:1292.

117. McLean RR, et al. Homocysteine as a predictive factor of hip fracture in older persons. *N Engl J Med* 2004;350:2004.

118. Mennen LI, et al. Homocysteine, cardiovascular disease risk factors, and habitual diet in the French Supplementation with Antioxidant Vitamins and Minerals Study. *Am J Clin Nutr* 2002;76:1279.

119. Meydani M. Vitamin E and prevention of heart disease in high-risk patients. *Nutr Rev* 2000;58:278.

120. Meyer NL, et al. Bone mineral density of Olympic-level female winter sport athletes. *Med Sci Sports Exerc* 2004;36:1594.

121. Michaels KB, et al. Prospective study of fruit and vegetable consumption and incidence of colon and rectal cancers. *J Natl Cancer Inst* 2000;92:1740.

122. Michaëlsson K, et al. Serum retinol levels and the risk of fracture. *N Engl J Med* 2003;348:287.

123. Micklesfield LK, et al. Bone mineral density in mature, premenopausal ultramarathon runners. *Med Sci Sports Exerc* 1995;27:688.

124. Modlesky CM, Lewis RD. Does exercise during growth have a long-term effect on bone health? *Exerc Sport Sci Rev* 2002;30:171.

125. Moffatt RJ. Dietary status of elite female high school gymnasts: inadequacy of vitamin and mineral intake. *J Am Diet Assoc* 1984;84:1361.

126. Morris MS, et al. Hyperhomocysteinemia associated with poor recall in the third National Health and Sport Science Review Nutrition Examination Survey. *Am J Clin Nutr* 2001;73:927.

127. Mortensen L, Charles P. Bioavailability of calcium supplements and the effect of vitamin D: comparisons between milk, calcium carbonate, and calcium carbonate plus vitamin D. *Am J Clin Nutr* 1996;63:354.

128. Myers ER, Wilson SE. Biomechanics of osteoporosis and vertebral fracture. *Spine* 1997;22:25S.

129. Nachtigall D, et al. Iron deficiency in distance runners: a reinvestigation using ^{59}Fe-labeling and non-invasive liver iron quantification. *Int J Sports Med* 1996;17:473.

130. Nakayama MM, et al. T-786 mutation in the 59-flanking of the region of the endothelial nitric oxide synthase gene is associated with coronary spasm. *Circulation* 1999;99:2855.

131. Nelson DA, Bouxsein ML. Exercise maintains bone mass, but do people maintain exercise? *J Bone Miner Res* 2001;16:202.

132. Nelson RL. Iron and colorectal cancer risk: human studies. *Nutr Res* 2001;59:140.

133. New SA, et al. Dietary influences on bone mass and bone metabolism: further evidence of a positive link between fruit and vegetable consumption and bone health. *Am J Clin Nutr* 2000;71:142.

134. Nichols DL, et al. Relationship of regional body composition to bone mineral density in college females. *Med Sci Sports Exerc* 1995;27:178.

135. Nichols JF, et al. Prevalence of the female athlete triad syndrome among high school athletes. *Arch Pediatr Adolesc Med* 2006;160:137.

136. Nickols-Richardson SM, et al. Premenarcheal gymnasts possess higher bone mineral density than controls. *Med Sci Sports Exerc* 2000;32:62.

137. Nieves JN, et al. Calcium potentiates the effect of estrogen and calcitonin on bone mass: review and analysis. *Am J Clin Nutr* 1998;67:18.

138. Nygård O, et al. Major lifestyle determinants of plasma total homocysteine distribution: the Horland Homocysteine Study. *Am J Clin Nutr* 1998;67:263.

139. Obarzanek E, et al. Effects on blood lipids of a blood pressure-lowering diet: the Dietary Approaches to Stop Hypertension (DASH) Trial. *Am J Clin Nutr* 2001;74:80.

140. Omenn GS, et al. Effects of a combination of beta carotene and vitamin A on lung cancer and cardiovascular disease. *N Engl J Med* 1996;334:1150.

141. O'Toole ML, et al. Hemolysis during triathlon races: its relation to race distance. *Med Sci Sports Exerc* 1988;20:172.

142. Pescatello LS, et al. Daily physical movement and bone mineral density among a mixed racial cohort of women. *Med Sci Sports Exerc* 2002;34:1966.

143. Pizza FX, et al. Serum haptoglobin and ferritin during a competitive running and swimming season. *Int J Sports Med* 1997;18:233.

144. Proctor KL, et al. Upper-limb bone mineral density of female collegiate gymnasts versus controls. *Med Sci Sports Exerc* 2002;34:1830.

145. Ramakrishnan V, et al. Iron stores and cardiovascular disease risk factors in women of reproductive age in the United States. *Am J Clin Nutr* 2002;76:1256.

146. Ravaglia G, et al. Homocysteine and cognitive function in healthy elderly community dwellers in Italy. *Am J Clin Nutr* 2003;77:668.

147. Ravaglia G, et al. Homocysteine and folate as risk factors for dementia and Alzheimer disease. *Am J Clin Nutr* 2005;82:636.

148. Rencken ML, et al. Bone density at multiple skeletal sites in amenorrheic athletes. *JAMA* 1996;276:238.

149. Rimm EB, et al. Folate and vitamin B6 from diet and supplements in relation to risk of coronary heart disease among women. *JAMA* 1998;279:359.

150. Ripple MO, et al. Effect of antioxidants on androgen-induced AP-1 and NF-kB DNA-binding activity in prostate carcinoma cells. *J Natl Cancer Inst* 1999;91:1227.

151. Risser WL, et al. Iron deficiency in female athletes: its prevalence and impact on performance. *Med Sci Sports Exerc* 1988;20:116.

152. Robertson JO, et al. Fecal blood loss in response to exercise. *Br Med J* 1987;295:303.

153. Robinson TL, et al. Gymnasts exhibit higher bone mass than runners despite similar prevalence of amenorrhea and oligomenorrhea. *J Bone Miner Res* 1995;10:26.

154. Robling AG, et al. Recovery periods restore mechanosensitivity to dynamically loaded bone. *J Exp Biol* 2001;204:3389.

155. Robling AG, et al. Shorter, more frequent mechanical loading sessions enhance bone mass. *Med Sci Sports Med* 2002;34:196.

156. Rokitzk L, et al. Assessment of vitamin B6 status of strength and speed power athletes. *J Am Coll Nutr* 1994;13:87.

157. Ross EA, et al. Lead content of calcium supplements. *JAMA* 2000;284:1425.

158. Roughead ZK, Hunt JR. Adaptation in iron absorption: iron supplementation reduces nonheme-iron but not heme-iron absorption from food. *Am J Clin Nutr* 2000;72:946.

159. Rowlands AV, et al. Interactive effects of habitual physical activity and calcium intake on bone density in boys and girls. *J Appl Physiol* 2004;97:1203.

160. Rozen GS, et al. Calcium supplementation provides an extended window of opportunity for bone mass accretion after menarche. *Am J Clin Nutr* 2003;78:993.

161. Sacks FM, et al. Rationale and design of the dietary approaches to stop hypertension trial (DASH): a multicenter controlled feeding study of dietary patterns to lower blood pressure. *Ann Epidemiol* 1995;108:118.

162. Sacks FM, et al. Effects on blood pressure of reduced dietary sodium and the Dietary Approaches to Stop Hypertension (DASH) diet. DASH-Sodium Collaborative Research Group. *N Engl J Med* 2001;344:3.

163. Saw S-M, et al. Genetic, dietary, and other lifestyle determinants of plasma homocysteine concentrations in middle-aged and older Chinese men and women in Singapore. *Am J Clin Nutr* 2001;73:232.

164. Sawka MN, Coyle EF. Influence of body water and blood volume on thermoregulation and exercise performance in the heat. *Exerc Sport Sci Rev* 1999;27:167.

165. Schnyder G, et al. Effect of homocysteine lowering therapy with folic acid, vitamin B_{12} and vitamin B6 on clinical outcome after percutaneous coronary intervention. *JAMA* 2002;288:973.

166. Schumacher YO, et al. Hematological indices and iron status in athletes of various sports and performances. *Med Sci Sports Exerc* 2002;34:869.

167. Selhub J, et al. B vitamins, homocysteine and neurocognitive function in the elderly. *Am J Clin Nutr* 2000;71(suppl):614S.

168. Sempos CT, et al. Do body iron stores increase the risk of developing coronary heart disease? *Am J Clin Nutr* 2002;76:501.

169. Shoemaker JD, et al. Relationships between fluid and electrolyte hormones and plasma volume during exercise with training and detraining. *Med Sci Sports Exerc* 1998;30:497.

170. Sinclair LM, Hinton PS. Prevalence of iron deficiency with and without anemia in recreationally active men and women. *J Am Diet Assoc* 2005;105:975.

171. Singh R, et al. Maintenance of bone mass and mechanical properties after short-term cessation of high impact exercise in rats. *Int J Sports Med* 2002;23:77.

172. Siris E, et al. Identification and fracture outcomes of undiagnosed low bone mineral density in postmenopausal women: results from the National Osteoporosis Risk Assessment. *JAMA* 2001;286:2815.

173. Snow CM, et al. Bone gains and losses follow seasonal training and detraining in gymnasts. *Calcif Tissue Int* 2001;69:7.

174. Snyder AC, et al. Importance of dietary iron source on measures of iron status among female runners. *Med Sci Sports Exerc* 1989;21:7.

175. Specker BL. Should there be dietary guidelines for calcium intake? *North Am J Clin Nutr* 2000;71:663.

176. Stear SJ, et al. Effect of calcium and exercise intervention on the bone mineral status of 16–18-y-old adolescent girls. *Am J Clin Nutr* 2003;77:985.

177. Stamler J. The INTERSALT study: background, methods, findings, and implications. *Am J Clin Nutr* 1997;65(suppl):626S.

178. Steinberg FM, Chait A. Antioxidant vitamin supplementation and lipid peroxidation in smokers. *Am J Clin Nutr* 1998;68:319.

179. Stock JL, et al. Dynamic muscle strength is decreased in postmenopausal women with low bone density. *J Bone Miner Res* 1987;2:338.

180. Stolzenberg-Solomon RZ, et al. Association of dietary protein intake and coffee consumption on serum homocysteine concentrations in an older population. *Am J Clin Nutr* 1999;69:467.

181. Suominen H, Rahkila P. Bone mineral density of the calcaneus in 70- to 81-yr-old male athletes and a population sample. *Med Sci Sports Exerc* 1991;23:1227.

182. Svetkey LP, et al. Effects of dietary patterns on blood pressure: subgroup analysis of the dietary approaches to Stop Hypertension (DASH) Randomized Clinical Trial. *Arch Intern Med* 1999;159:285.

183. Terry P, et al. Fruit, vegetables, dietary fiber, and risk of colorectal cancer. *J Natl Cancer Inst* 2001;93:525.

184. The Heart Outcomes Prevention Evaluation Study Investigators. Vitamin E supplementation and cardiovascular events in high-risk patients. *N Engl J Med* 2000;342:154.

185. The Homocysteine Studies Collaboration. Homocysteine and risk of ischemic heart disease. *JAMA* 2002;288:2015.

186. Thomas MK, et al. Hypovitaminosis D in medical inpatients. *N Engl J Med* 1998;338:784.

187. Tice JA, et al. Cost-effectiveness of vitamin therapy to lower plasma homocysteine levels for the prevention of coronary heart disease: effect of grain fortification and beyond. *JAMA* 2001;286:936.

188. Tomten SE, et al. Bone mineral density and menstrual irregularities: a comparative study of cortical and trabecular bone structures in runners with alleged normal eating behavior. *Int J Sports Med* 1998;19:87.

189. Treblance S, et al. Failure of magnesium supplementation to influence marathon running performance or recovery in magnesium-replete subjects. *Int J Sports Nutr* 1992;2:154.

190. Troughton JA, et al. Homocysteine and coronary heart disease risk in the PRIME study. *Atherosclerosis* 2007;191:90.

191. Trumbo B, et al. Dietary reference intakes: vitamin K, arsenic, boron, chromium, copper, iodine, manganese, molybdenum, nickel, silicon, vanadium, and zinc. *Am Diet Assoc* 2001;101:294.

192. Tsalis G, et al. Effects of iron intake through food or supplement on iron status and performance of healthy adolescent swimmers during a training season. *Int J Sports Med* 2004;25:306.

193. Tucker KL. Eat a variety of healthful foods: old advice with new support. *Nutr Rev* 2001;59:156.

194. Turner CH, Robling AG. Designing exercise regimens to increase bone strength. *Exerc Sport Sci Rev* 2003;31:45.

195. Ueland PM, et al. The controversy over homocysteine and cardiovascular risk. *Am J Clin Nutr* 2000;72:324.

196. Van Meurs JB, et al. Homocysteine levels and the risk of osteoporetic fracture. *N Engl J Med* 2004;350:2033.

197. Von Duvillard SP, et al. Fluids and hydration in prolonged endurance performance. *Nutrition* 2004;20:651.

198. Villareal DT, et al. Bone mineral density response to estrogen replacement in frail elderly women: a randomized controlled trial. *JAMA* 2001;286:815.

199. Vivekananthan DP, et al. Use of antioxidant vitamins for the prevention of cardiovascular disease: meta-analysis of randomised trials. *Lancet* 2003;362:920.

200. Vincent KR, Braith RW. Resistance exercise and bone turnover in elderly men and women. *Med Sci Sports Exerc* 2002;34:17.

201. Vollset SE, et al. Plasma total homocysteine and cardiovascular and noncardiovascular mortality: the Hordaland Homocysteine Study. *Am J Clin Nutr* 2001;74:130.

202. Weight LM, et al. Sports anemia: a real or apparent phenomenon in endurance-trained athletes. *Int J Sports Med* 1992;13:344.

203. Weisburger JH. Approaches for chronic disease prevention based on current understanding of underlying mechanisms. *Am J Clin Nutr* 2000;71(suppl):1710S.

204. Welch GN, Loscalzo J. Homocysteine and atherothrombosis. *N Engl J Med* 1999;338:1042.

205. Whelton PK, et al. Sodium reduction and weight loss in the treatment of hypertension in older persons: a randomized controlled trial of nonpharmacologic interventions in the elderly (TONE). *JAMA* 1998;279:839.

206. Whelton PK, et al. Primary prevention of hypertension: clinical and public health advisory from the National High Blood Pressure Prevention Program. *JAMA* 2002;288:1882.

207. Winters K, et al. Bone density and cyclic ovarian function in trained runners and active controls. *Med Sci Sports Exerc* 1996;28:776.

208. Wood D. Established and emerging cardiovascular risk factors. *Am Heart J* 2001;141(2 Pt 2):549.

209. Wood RJ, Zheng JJ. High dietary calcium intakes reduce zinc absorption and balance in humans. *Am J Clin Nutr* 1997;65:1803.

210. Writing Group for the Women's Health Initiative Investigators. Risk and benefits of estrogen plus progestin in healthy postmenopausal women: principal results from the women's Health Initiative Randomized Controlled Trial. *JAMA* 2002;288:321.

211. Yusuf S, et al. Vitamin E supplementation and cardiovascular events in high-risk patients: the Heart Outcomes Prevention Evaluation Study investigators. *N Engl J Med* 2000;342:154.

212. Zanker CL, Cooke CB. Energy balance, bone turnover, and skeletal health in physically active individuals. *Med Sci Sports Exerc* 2004;36:1372.

Chapter 3

Digestion and Absorption of the Food Nutrients

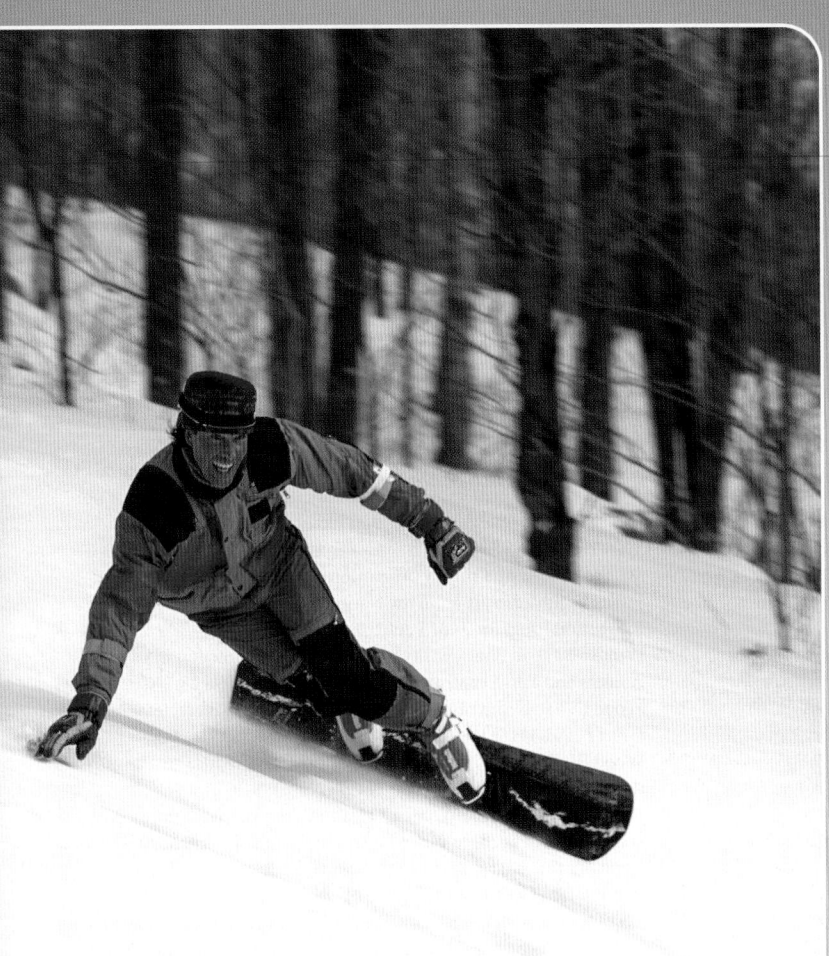

Outline

Test Your Knowledge

Answer these 10 statements about digestion and absorption of the food nutrients. Use the scoring key at the end of the chapter to check your results. Repeat this test after you have read the chapter and compare your results.

1. **T F** The digestion of food begins in the stomach.
2. **T F** The colon is another name for the large intestine.
3. **T F** The liver, gallbladder, and pancreas are all organs through which food nutrients must pass during digestion.
4. **T F** Glucose absorption requires energy, while the absorption of dietary fat occurs passively without expenditure of energy.
5. **T F** Active transport of a nutrient across the plasma membrane occurs by electrostatic transfer that does not require energy.
6. **T F** The main absorption of lipids takes place in the distal portion of the stomach.
7. **T F** Almost all nutrient digestion and absorption take place in the small intestine.
8. **T F** Glucose absorption takes place predominantly in the large intestine.
9. **T F** Hemorrhoids result largely from consuming a high-fiber diet.
10. **T F** Hydrolysis and condensation represent the two important tissue-building processes in the body.

P roper food intake provides an uninterrupted supply of energy and tissue-building chemicals to sustain life. For exercise and sports participants, the ready availability of specific food nutrients takes on added importance because physical activity increases energy expenditure and the need for tissue repair and synthesis. Nutrient uptake by the body involves complex physiologic and metabolic processes that usually progress unnoticed for a lifetime. Hormones and enzymes work nonstop in concert throughout the digestive tract, at proper levels of acidity–alkalinity, to facilitate the breakdown of complex nutrients into simpler subunits. Substances produced during digestion are absorbed through the razor-thin lining of the small intestine and pass into blood and lymph. Self-regulating processes within the digestive tract usually move food along at a slow enough rate to allow its complete absorption, yet rapid enough to ensure timely delivery of its nutrient components. Fibrous materials that resist digestion pass unabsorbed from one end of the body to the other.

The sections that follow outline the digestion and absorption of the various nutrients consumed in the diet. We present a brief discussion of some biology and chemistry basics related to digestive and absorptive processes and then describe the structures of the gastrointestinal tract, including the dynamics of digestion. We also discuss the different relationships among nutrition, exercise, and gastrointestinal tract disorders.

Biology and Chemistry Basics Related to the Digestion, Absorption, and Assimilation of the Food Nutrients

HYDROLYSIS AND CONDENSATION: THE BASIS FOR DIGESTION AND SYNTHESIS

In general, hydrolysis reactions digest or break down complex molecules into simpler subunits, and condensation reactions build larger molecules by bonding their subunits together.

Hydrolysis Reactions

Hydrolysis catabolizes complex organic molecules carbohydrates, lipids, and proteins into simpler forms that the body absorbs and assimilates. During this basic decomposition process, chemical bonds split by the addition of hydrogen ions (H^+) and hydroxyl ions (OH^-), the constituents of water, to the reaction by-products. Examples of hydrolytic reactions include the digestion of starches and disaccharides to monosaccharides, proteins to amino acids, and lipids to glycerol and fatty acids. A specific enzyme catalyzes each step in the breakdown process. For disaccharides, the enzymes are lactase (lactose), sucrase (sucrose), and maltase (maltose). The lipid enzymes (lipases) degrade the triacylglycerol molecule by adding water, cleaving the fatty acids from their glycerol backbone. During protein digestion, protease enzymes accelerate amino acid release when the addition of water splits the peptide linkages. The following equation represents the general form for all hydrolysis reactions:

$$AB + HOH \rightarrow A–H + B–OH$$

Water (HOH) added to substance AB decomposes the chemical bond that joins AB to produce the breakdown products A–H (H refers to hydrogen atom from water) and B–OH (OH refers to the remaining hydroxyl group from water). FIGURE 3.1A illustrates the hydrolysis reaction for the disaccharide

sucrose to its end product molecules of glucose and fructose. Also shown is the hydrolysis of a dipeptide (protein) into its two constituent amino acid units. Intestinal absorption occurs rapidly following hydrolysis of the carbohydrate, lipid, and protein macronutrients.

Condensation Reactions

The reactions illustrated for hydrolysis also occur in the opposite direction. In this reversible reaction, governed by specific enzymes, the compound AB synthesizes from A–H and

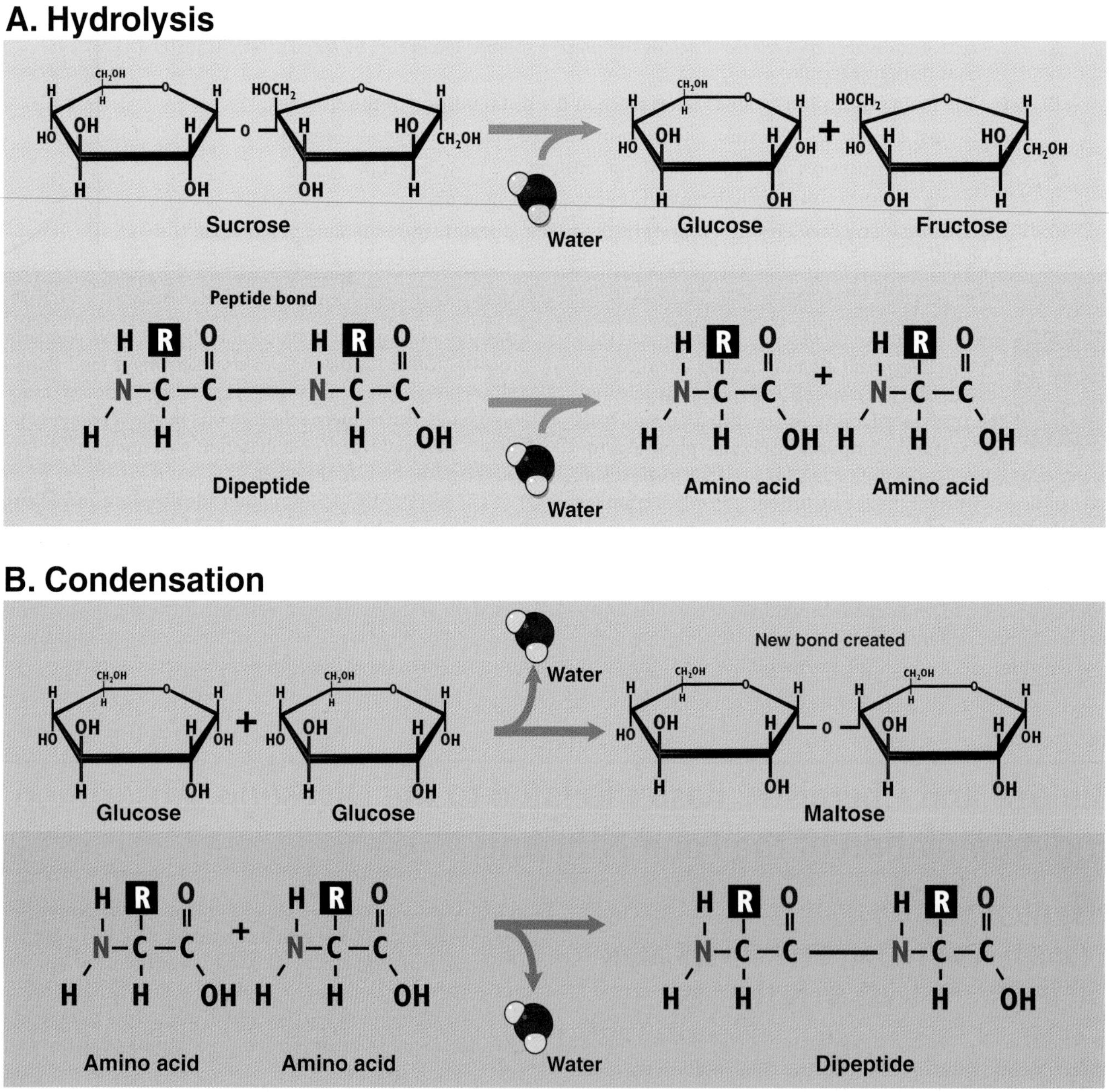

A. Hydrolysis

B. Condensation

FIGURE 3.1 ■ **A.** Hydrolysis chemical reaction of the disaccharide sucrose to the end product molecules glucose and fructose and a hydrolysis reaction of a dipeptide (protein) into two amino acid constituents. **B.** Condensation chemical reaction to synthesize maltose from two glucose units and creation of a protein dipeptide from two amino acid units. Note that the reactions in **B** illustrate the reverse of the hydrolysis reaction for the dipeptide. The symbol *R* represents the remainder of the molecule.

B–OH during **condensation** (also termed *dehydration synthesis*). A hydrogen atom is cleaved from one molecule and a hydroxyl group is removed from another. A water molecule forms in this building, or **anabolic,** process. The structural components of the nutrients bind together in condensation reactions to form more complex molecules and compounds. Figure 3.1B shows the condensation reactions for the synthesis of (1) maltose from two glucose units and (2) a more complex protein from two amino acid units. During protein synthesis, a hydroxyl removed from one amino acid and hydrogen from the other amino acid create a water molecule. The new bond for the protein is called a **peptide bond.** Water formation also occurs in synthesizing more complex carbohydrates from simple sugars. For lipids, water forms when glycerol and fatty acid components combine to form the triacylglycerol molecule.

ENZYMES: THE BIOLOGIC CATALYSTS

An **enzyme,** a highly specific protein catalyst, accelerates the forward and reverse rates of chemical reactions without being consumed or changed in the reaction. The great diversity of protein structures enables enzymes to perform highly specific functions. Enzymes only affect reactions that would normally take place but at a much slower rate. In a way, enzymes reduce the required **activation energy,** or energy input, to change the rate of the reaction. This occurs even though the equilibrium constants and total energy released (free energy change) per reaction remain unaltered. FIGURE 3.2 shows the effectiveness of a catalyst for initiating a chemical reaction compared with the uncatalyzed state. The horizontal axis represents the progress of the reaction; the vertical axis compares

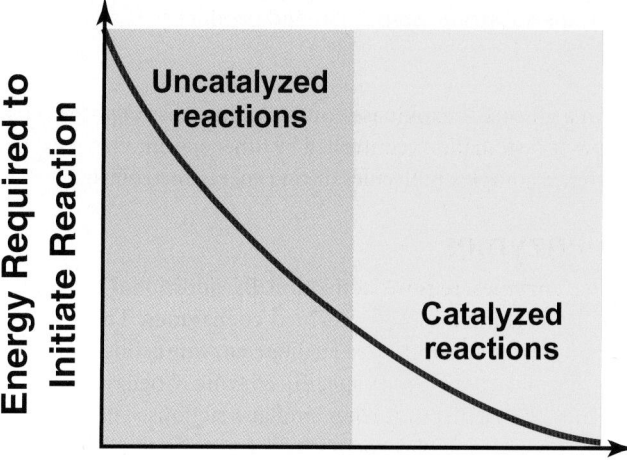

FIGURE 3.2 ■ The presence of a catalyst greatly reduces the activation energy required to initiate a chemical reaction compared with the energy required for an uncatalyzed reaction. For the reaction to proceed, the reactant must have a higher free-energy level than the product.

the energy required to initiate the reactions. Clearly, initiation (activation) of an uncatalyzed reaction requires considerably more energy than a catalyzed one.

Enzymes possess the unique property of not being altered by the reactions they affect. Consequently, the turnover of enzymes in the body remains relatively slow and specific enzymes are continually reused. A typical mitochondrion may contain up to 10 billion enzyme molecules, each carrying out millions of operations within a brief time. During strenuous exercise, enzyme activity rate increases tremendously within the cell because energy demands increase some 100 times above the resting level. The rate of a catalyzed reaction can be 10^6 to 10^{20} times faster than an uncatalyzed reaction under similar conditions. A single cell's fluids contain as many as 4000 different enzymes, each with a specific function that catalyzes a specific chemical reaction. For example, glucose breakdown to carbon dioxide and water requires 19 different chemical reactions, each catalyzed by a different enzyme. Enzymes make contact at precise locations on the surfaces of cell structures; they also operate within the structure itself. Many enzymes function outside the cell—in the bloodstream, digestive mixture, or fluids of the small intestine.

Except for older enzyme names such as renin, trypsin, and pepsin, the suffix *-ase* appends to the enzyme based on its mode of operation or substance with which it interacts. For example, hydrolase adds water during hydrolysis reactions, protease interacts with protein, oxidase adds oxygen to a substance, isomerase rearranges atoms within a substrate to form structural isomers such as glucose and fructose, and ribonuclease splits apart ribonucleic acid (RNA). Enzymes do not all operate at the same rate; some operate slowly, others more rapidly.

Enzymes work cooperatively among their binding sites. While one substance "turns on" at a particular site, its neighbor "turns off" until the process completes. The operation then reverses, with one enzyme becoming inactive and the other active. Enzymes also act along small regions of the **substrate** (any substance acted upon by an enzyme), each time working at a different rate than previously. Some enzymes delay beginning their work. The precursor digestive enzyme trypsinogen manufactured by the pancreas in inactive form serves as a good example. Trypsinogen enters the small intestine, where, on activation by intestinal enzyme action, it becomes the active enzyme trypsin, which digests complex proteins into simple amino acids. **Proteolytic action** describes this process. Without the delay in activity, trypsinogen would literally digest the pancreatic tissue that produced it.

The temperature and hydrogen ion concentrations (acidity–alkalinity) of the reactive medium dramatically affect enzyme activity. Each enzyme performs its maximum activity at a specific pH. The optimum pH of an enzyme usually reflects the pH of the body fluids in which it bathes. For some enzymes, optimal activity requires a relatively high acidity level (e.g., the protein-digesting enzyme pepsin is optimally active in the hydrochloric acid of the gut); for others, the optimal pH occurs on the alkaline side of neutrality, as trypsin does in the pancreatic juice. Increases in temperature generally accelerate enzyme reactivity. As temperature rises above 40 to 50°C, the protein enzymes permanently denature and activity ceases.

How Many Enzymes Do Humans Process?

Identification of the number of known enzymes increased rapidly by the late 1950s because of the advent of new biochemical procedures; however, the *naming* of enzymes by individual workers had proved unsatisfactory. The same enzymes often were known by several different names, and the same name was sometimes given to very different enzymes. Many names conveyed little or no idea of the nature of the reactions catalyzed, and similar names were sometimes attributed to enzymes of quite different types. To correct such limitations, the General Assembly of the International Union of Biochemistry (IUB) decided in August, 1955 to establish an International Commission on Enzymes Nomenclature. As of June 26, 2007, the number of known enzymes in the human body exceeds 4000 (www.expasy.org/enzyme/).

Year	Number of enzymes
1961	712
1964	875
1972	1770
1978	2122
1984	2477
1992	3196
2007 (June 26)	4037

Mode of Enzyme Action

A unique characteristic of an enzyme's three-dimensional globular protein structure is its interaction with its specific substrate. Interaction works similarly to a key fitting a lock. The enzyme turns on when its **active site,** usually a groove, cleft, or cavity on the protein's surface, joins in a "perfect fit" with the substrate's active site (FIG. 3.3). By forming an **enzyme-substrate complex,** the splitting of chemical bonds produces a new product with new bonds. This frees the enzyme to act on additional substrate. Figure 3.3 depicts the interaction sequence of the enzyme maltase as it disassembles maltose into its component glucose building blocks.

The **"lock and key mechanism"** describes the enzyme–substrate interaction. This interactive process ensures that the correct enzyme "mates" with its specific substrate to perform a particular function. Once the enzyme and substrate join, the enzyme changes shape as it molds to the substrate. Even if an enzyme links with a substrate, unless the specific conformational change occurs in the enzyme's shape, it will not interact chemically with the substrate.

The lock and key mechanism offers a protective function so only the correct enzyme activates the targeted substrate. Consider the enzyme hexokinase, which accelerates a chemical reaction by linking with a glucose molecule. When this linkage occurs, a phosphate molecule transfers from adenosine triphosphate (ATP) to a specific binding site on one of glucose's carbon atoms. Once the two binding sites join to

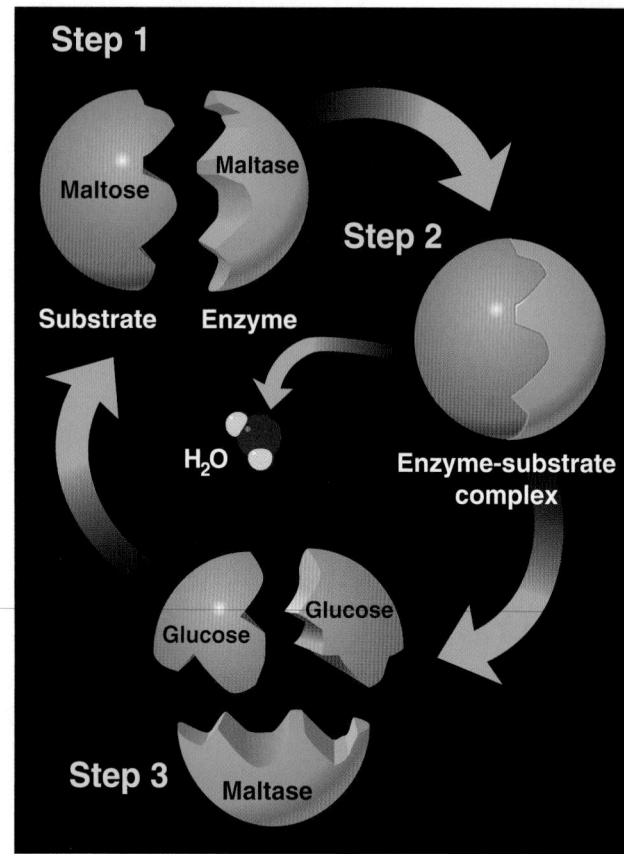

FIGURE 3.3 ■ Sequence of steps in the "lock and key" mechanism of an enzyme with its substrate. The example shows how two monosaccharide molecules of glucose form when the enzyme maltase interacts with its disaccharide substrate maltose. *Step 1,* The active site of the enzyme and substrate line up to achieve a perfect fit, forming an enzyme–substrate complex. *Step 2,* The enzyme catalyzes (greatly speeds up) the chemical reaction with the substrate. *Step 3,* An end product forms.

form a glucose–hexokinase complex, the substrate begins its stepwise degradation (controlled by other specific enzymes) to form less complex molecules during energy metabolism.

Coenzymes

Some enzymes require activation by additional ions and smaller organic molecules termed **coenzymes.** These complex, nonprotein substances facilitate enzyme action by binding the substrate with its specific enzyme. Coenzymes then regenerate to assist in further similar reactions. The metallic ions iron and zinc play coenzyme roles, as do the B vitamins or their derivatives. Oxidation-reduction reactions use the B vitamins riboflavin and niacin, while other vitamins serve as transfer agents for groups of compounds in metabolic processes (see Chapter 2, Table 2.2). Some advertisements imply that taking vitamin supplements provides immediate usable energy for exercise. Although vitamins "make the reactions go," they contain no chemical energy available to power biologic work.

A coenzyme requires less specificity in its action than an enzyme because the coenzyme affects a number of different reactions. It acts as a "cobinder," or it can serve as a temporary carrier of intermediary products in the reaction. For example, the coenzyme **nicotinamide adenine dinucleotide (NAD$^+$)** forms NADH to transport the hydrogen atoms and electrons that split from food fragments during energy metabolism. The electrons then pass to special transporter molecules in another series of chemical reactions that ultimately deliver the electrons to molecular oxygen.

TRANSPORT OF NUTRIENTS ACROSS CELL MEMBRANES

Literally thousands of chemicals, including ions, vitamins, minerals, acids, salts, water, gases, hormones, and carbohydrate, protein, and lipid components, continually traverse the cell's bilayer plasma membrane during exchange between the cell and its surroundings. Plasma membranes remain highly permeable to some substances but not others. Such selective permeability allows cells to maintain reasonable consistency in chemical composition. Disrupting the equilibrium triggers immediate adjustments to restore constancy in the cell's "internal milieu." This occurs by two processes: (1) **passive transport** of substances through the plasma membrane (requires no energy), and (2) **active transport** through the plasma membrane, which requires metabolic energy to "power" the exchange of materials.

Passive Transport Processes

Simple diffusion, facilitated diffusion, osmosis, and filtration represent the four types of passive transport. FIGURE 3.4 shows an example of each.

Simple Diffusion

In the cellular environment, **simple diffusion** involves the free and continuous net movement of molecules in aqueous solution across the plasma membrane. In Figure 3.4, note that molecules of water, small lipids, and gases move unim-

A. Simple Diffusion

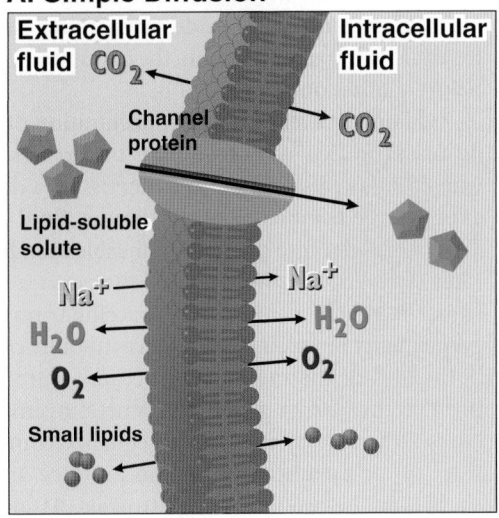

B. Facilitated Diffusion

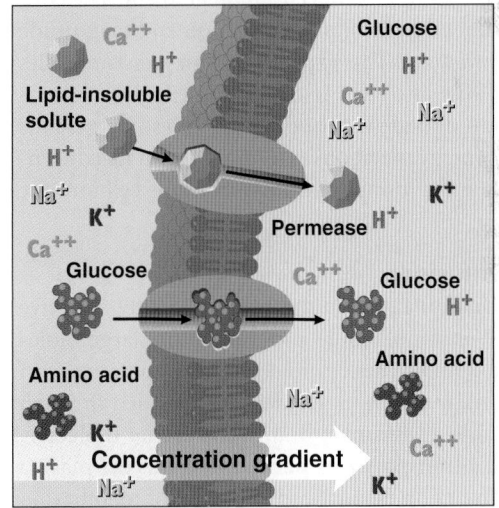

C. Osmosis

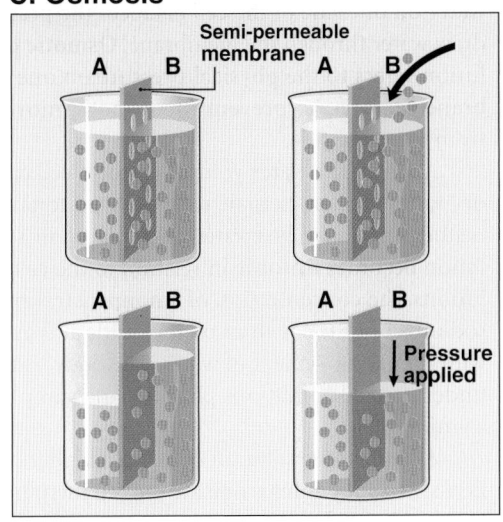

D. Filtration

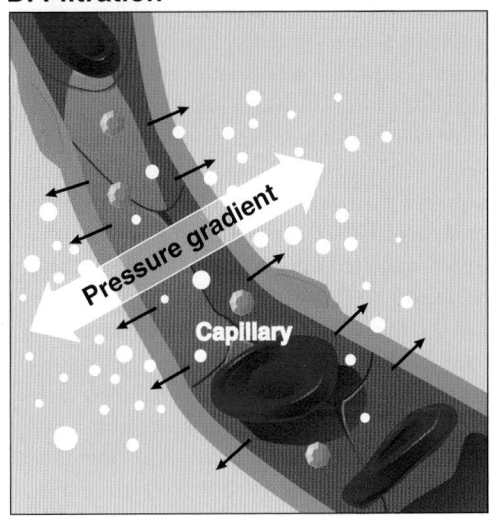

FIGURE 3.4 ■ **A.** Simple diffusion. **B.** Facilitated diffusion. **C.** Osmosis. **D.** Filtration.

peded from outside the cell through the lipid bilayer into the intracellular fluid. In simple diffusion, a substance moves from an area of higher concentration to lower concentration until it evenly disperses. Only the kinetic energy of the molecules themselves, with no expenditure of stored cellular energy, powers this passive process. When sugar and water mix, for example, the sugar molecules dissolve and evenly disperse by their continuous, random movement. Hot water speeds diffusion because higher temperature increases molecular movement and thus the diffusion rate. If the particles remain within a closed system, they eventually distribute evenly throughout, and the net movement of particles ceases.

Simple diffusion across plasma membranes occurs for water molecules, dissolved gases (oxygen, carbon dioxide, and nitrogen), small uncharged polar molecules such as urea and alcohol, and various lipid-soluble molecules. These substances diffuse quickly because the plasma membrane consists of sheetlike, fluid structures composed mainly of lipids. This structure allows relatively small, uncomplicated molecules to easily traverse the membrane. For example, when a molecule of oxygen diffuses from its normal higher concentration outside the cell toward a lower concentration on the cell's inside, it moves down (or along) its concentration gradient. The concentration gradient determines the direction and magnitude of molecular movement. This explains how oxygen molecules continuously diffuse into cells. In contrast, the higher concentration of carbon dioxide within the cell causes this gaseous end product of energy metabolism to move down its concentration gradient and continually diffuse from the cell into the blood.

Facilitated Diffusion

Facilitated diffusion involves the passive, highly selective binding of lipid-insoluble molecules (and other large molecules) to a lipid-soluble carrier molecule. This contrasts with simple diffusion, by which molecules pass unaided through the semipermeable plasma membrane. The carrier molecule, a protein called a transporter or **permease,** spans the plasma membrane. Its function facilitates the transfer of membrane-insoluble chemicals (hydrogen, sodium, calcium, and potassium ions, and glucose and amino acid molecules) down their concentration gradients across the cell's plasma membrane.

Glucose transport into the cell provides an excellent example of facilitated diffusion. Glucose, a large lipid-insoluble, uncharged molecule, would not pass readily into the cell without its specific permease. More specifically, if simple diffusion were the only means of glucose entrance into a cell, its maximum rate of uptake would be nearly 500 times slower than glucose transport by facilitated diffusion. Facilitated diffusion allows glucose molecules to first attach to a binding site on a specific permease in the plasma membrane. A structural change then occurs in the permease that creates a "passageway" enabling the glucose molecule to penetrate the permease to enter the cytoplasm. Fortunately, facilitated diffusion of glucose keeps this important energy fuel readily available. Also, glucose transport does not require cellular energy. Consequently, facilitated diffusion serves as an energy-con-

serving mechanism that spares cellular energy for other vital functions.

Osmosis

Osmosis represents a special case of diffusion. Osmosis moves water (the solvent) through a selectively permeable membrane. This occurs because of a difference in the concentration of water molecules on both sides of the membrane, which is more permeable to water than to the solute. This passive process distributes water throughout the intracellular, extracellular, and plasma fluid body compartments.

In the example in Figure 3.4C, a semipermeable membrane separates compartments A and B. When an equal number of solute particles appear on sides A and B, the same water volume exists in both compartments. By adding a solute to an aqueous solution, the concentration of the solution increases by the amount of solute added. Adding more solute increases the concentration of particles while correspondingly decreasing the concentration of water molecules. In the example, adding nondiffusable solute to side B forces water from side A to move through the semipermeable membrane to side B. The volume of water then becomes greater on side B than side A. More water flows into an area containing more particles, leaving less water on the side with fewer solute particles. Eventually, by osmotic action, the concentration of solute particles equalizes on sides A and B.

Osmolality refers to the concentration of particles in solution, expressed as osmolal units of particles or ions formed when a solute dissociates. In living tissue, a difference always exists in the osmolality of the various fluid compartments. This occurs because the semipermeable membrane that separates different solutions retards the passage of many solute substances such as ions and intracellular proteins. Selective permeability maintains a difference in solute concentration on both sides of the membrane. Because water diffuses freely through the plasma membrane, a net movement of water occurs as the system attempts to equalize osmolality on both sides of the membrane. This can produce dramatic volume changes in the two fluid compartments. At some point, water no longer enters the cell because the hydrostatic pressure of water on one side of the cell balances the pressure tending to draw water through the membrane. **Osmotic pressure** of a solution refers to the physical pressure on one side of a membrane required to prevent the osmotic movement of water from the other side.

Altering the water volume inside a cell changes its shape or "tone," a characteristic referred to as tonicity. When a cell neither loses nor gains water when placed in a solution the solution becomes **isotonic** in relation to the cell. In isotonic solutions, the concentration of a nonpenetrating solute such as sodium chloride equalizes on the inside and outside of the cell, with no net movement of water. The body's extracellular fluid under normal conditions provides an example of an isotonic solution.

A **hypertonic** solution contains a higher concentration of nonpenetrating solutes outside the cell membrane than inside. When this occurs, water migrates out of the cell by osmosis, the cell now shrinking in size. Edema, an excess accumulation of water in body tissues, can be countered by infusing hypertonic solutions into the bloodstream. In contrast, ingesting highly concentrated beverages with salt or slowly absorbed fructose sugar creates an intestinal osmotic environment that causes water to move into the intestinal lumen. This sets the stage for intestinal cramping and impedes the rehydration process.

When the concentration of nondiffusible solutes outside the cell becomes diluted compared with the cell's interior, the extracellular solution becomes **hypotonic.** In such cases, the cell fills with water by osmosis and appears bloated. If the condition goes uncorrected, cells actually burst (lyse). Administering hypotonic solutions during dehydration returns the tissues to isotonic conditions.

For a membrane permeable to the solute and water (e.g., sugar in water), the solute and solvent molecules diffuse until the sugar molecules distribute equally. In contrast, for a membrane impermeable to the solute, osmotic pressure draws water in the direction that equalizes the solute concentration on both sides of the membrane. Water movement continues until solute concentration equalizes or until the hydrostatic pressure on one side of the membrane counteracts the force exerted by osmotic pressure. FIGURE 3.5 illustrates the osmotic effect on cells placed in isotonic, hypertonic, and hypotonic solutions.

Filtration

In **filtration,** water and its solutes flow passively from a region of higher hydrostatic pressure to one of lower pressure. The filtration mechanism allows plasma fluid and its solutes to move across the capillary membrane to literally bathe the tissues. Filtration moves the plasma filtrate (the fluid portion of the blood with no significant amount of proteins) through the kidney tubules during the production of urine.

Active Transport Processes

Energy-requiring **active transport** comes into play when a substance cannot move across the cell membrane by one of the four passive transport processes. Each active transport process requires the expenditure of cellular energy from ATP.

Sodium–Potassium Pump

FIGURE 3.6 illustrates the operation of the **sodium–potassium pump,** one of the active transport mechanisms for moving substances through semipermeable membranes. Energy from ATP "pumps" ions "uphill" against their electrochemical gradients through the membrane by a specialized carrier enzyme (sodium–potassium ATPase) that serves as the pumping mechanism. Recall that substances usually diffuse along their concentration gradients, from an area of higher to lower concentration. In the living cell, diffusion alone cannot provide optimal distribution of cellular chemicals. Instead, charged sodium and potassium ions and large amino acid molecules, insoluble in the lipid bilayer, must move against their concentration gradients to fulfill normal functions. Sodium ions, for example, exist in relatively low concentration inside the cell; thus, extracellular Na^+ tends to continually diffuse into the

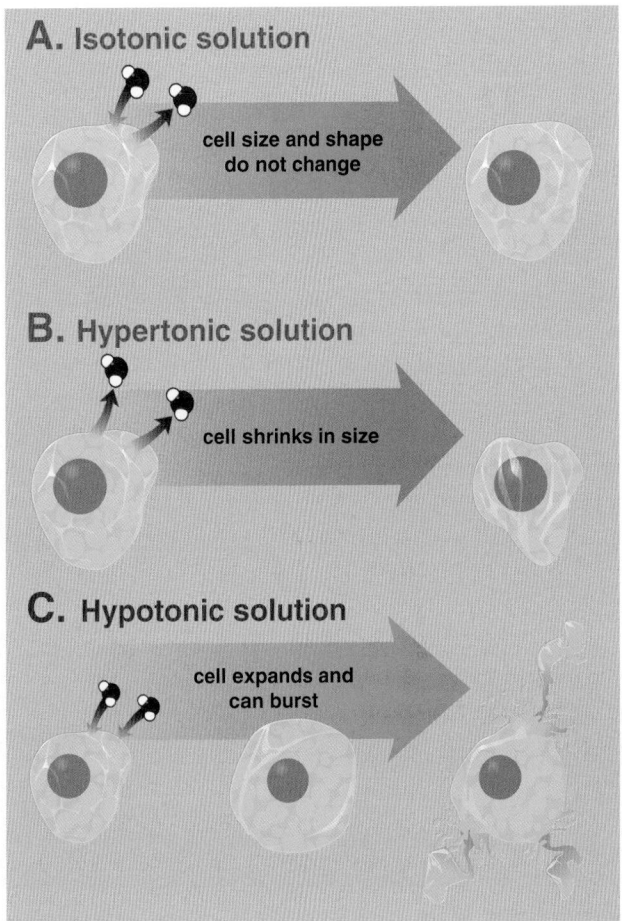

FIGURE 3.5 ■ **A.** *Isotonic solution.* The cell retains its shape because of equal concentrations of solute inside and outside the cell. **B.** *Hypertonic solution.* The cell shrinks (crenates) because the outside of the cell has a higher concentration of nondiffusible solutes than the inside. **C.** *Hypotonic solution.* The concentration of nondiffusible solutes outside the cell is diluted compared to the concentration within the cell. The cell takes on water by osmosis, which can burst (lyse) the cell.

cell. In contrast, potassium ions exist in higher concentration inside the cell and intracellular K^+ tends to diffuse toward the extracellular space. Consequently, to achieve proper Na^+ and K^+ concentrations about the plasma membrane for normal nerve and muscle functions, both ions continually move against their normal concentration gradients. This concentrates Na^+ extracellularly, whereas K^+ builds up within the cell. Countering the normal tendency of solutes to diffuse by means of the sodium–potassium pump provides the biologic way to establish normal electrochemical gradients for nerve and muscle stimulation.

Coupled Transport

Active transport absorbs nutrients through epithelial cells of the digestive tract and reabsorbs important plasma chemicals filtered by the kidneys. Absorption of intestinal glucose, for example, takes place by a form of active transport called **cou-**

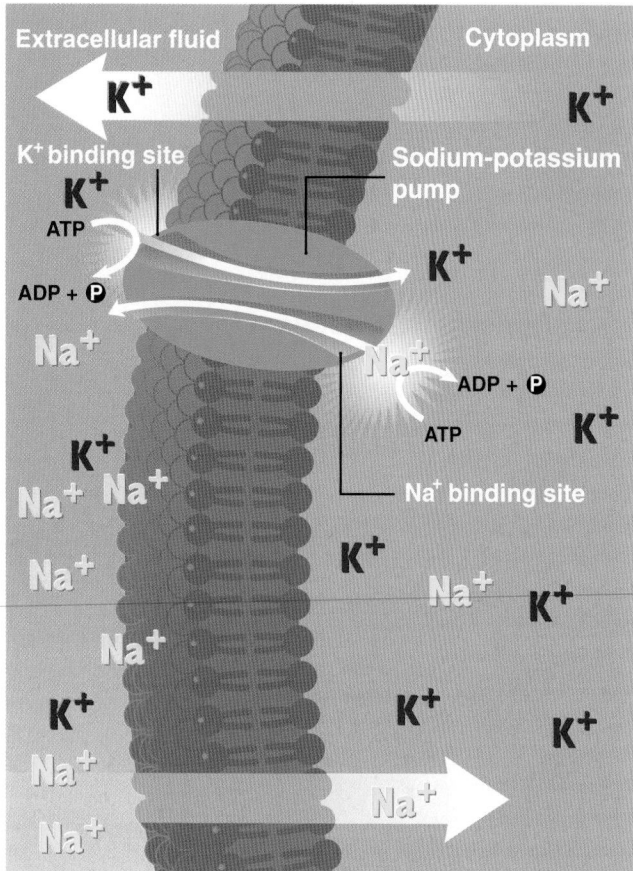

FIGURE 3.6 ■ The dynamics of the sodium–potassium pump. (ATP, adenosine triphosphate; ADP, adenosine diphosphate; P, phosphate.)

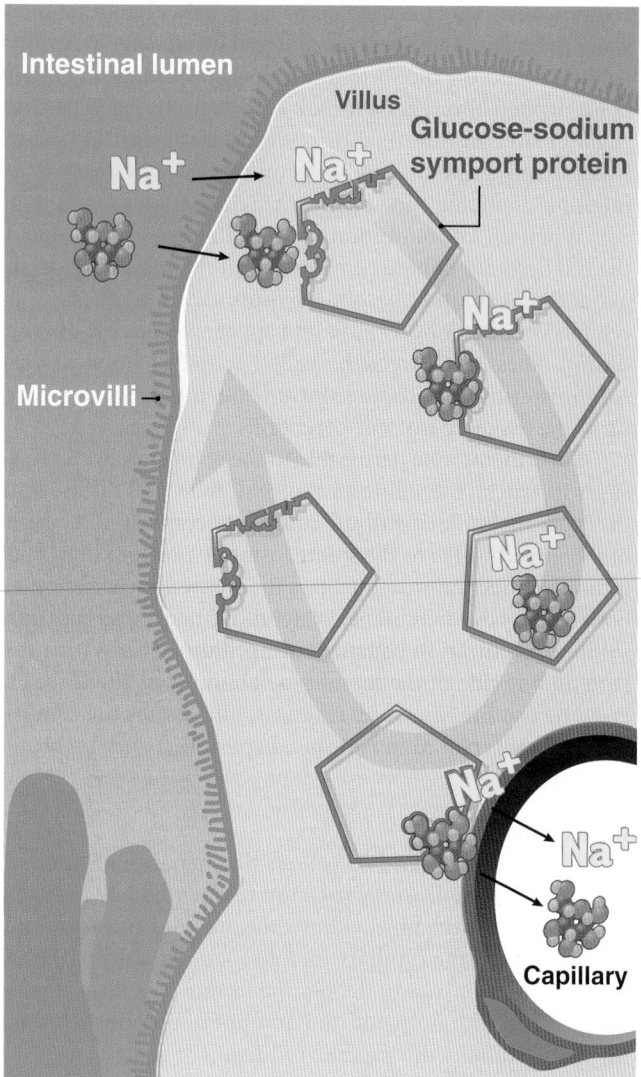

FIGURE 3.7 ■ Coupled transport. A molecule of glucose and a sodium ion move together in the same direction through the plasma membrane in a symport protein.

pled transport. FIGURE 3.7 shows molecules of glucose and Na^+ coupling together before they enter an intestinal villus; they move in the same direction when "pumped" through the plasma membrane to the cell's inside and subsequently into the bloodstream. Amino acids also join with Na^+ for active absorption through the small intestine. A cotransporter, or **symport,** refers to the simultaneous transport of two chemicals in the same direction; each symport has its own specialized permease with a specific binding site for each substance. Coupled transport occurs in one direction only. When the glucose–sodium and amino acid–sodium symports move from the intestine to the blood, they cannot move back and reenter the intestine.

Bulk Transport

Bulk transport moves a large number of particles and macromolecules through cell membranes by an energy-requiring process. Bulk transport occurs in two ways: exocytosis and endocytosis.

EXOCYTOSIS. Exocytosis transfers hormones, neurotransmitters, and mucous secretions from intracellular to extracellular fluids. Exocytosis involves three distinct phases. First, the substance for transfer encloses within a membranous, saclike pouch, with the

pouch then migrating to the plasma membrane; once fused to the membrane, its contents eject into the extracellular fluids.

ENDOCYTOSIS. In the transfer process of **endocytosis,** the cell's plasma membrane surrounds the substance, which then pinches away and moves into the cytoplasm.

ACID–BASE CONCENTRATION AND pH

Maintaining the acid–base balance of body fluids, a critical component of homeostasis, provides optimal functioning of digestion and overall physiologic regulation.

Acid

An **acid** refers to any substance that dissociates (ionizes) in solution and releases hydrogen ions (H^+). Acids taste sour, turn litmus indicators red, react with bases to form salts, and cause some metals to liberate hydrogen. Examples of acids in the body include hydrochloric, phosphoric, carbonic, citric, lactic, and carboxylic acids.

Base

A **base** refers to any substance that picks up or accepts H^+ to form hydroxide ions (OH^-) in water solutions. Basic or alkaline solutions taste bitter, are slippery to the touch, turn litmus indicators blue, and react with acids to form salts. Examples of bases in the body include sodium and calcium hydroxide and aqueous solutions of ammonia that form ammonium hydroxide.

pH

The **pH** provides a quantitative measure of the acidity or alkalinity (basicity) of a liquid solution. Specifically, pH refers to the concentration of protons or H^+; it computes as the logarithm of 1.0 divided by the H^+ concentration $[H^+]$ as follows:

$$pH = \log 1 \div [H^+]$$

where $[H^+]$ equals the molar concentration of H^+.

Solutions with relatively more OH^- than H^+ have a pH above 7.0 and are called basic, or alkaline. Conversely, solutions with more H^+ than OH^- have a pH below 7.0 and are termed acidic. Chemically pure (distilled) water has a neutral pH of 7.0 with equal amounts of H^+ and OH^-. The pH scale shown in FIGURE 3.8, devised in 1909 by the Danish chemist Sören Sörensen (1868–1939), ranges from 1.0 to 14.0. An inverse relation exists between pH and the concentration of H^+. Because of the logarithmic nature of the pH scale, a one-unit change in pH corresponds to a tenfold change in H^+ concentration. For example, lemon juice and gastric juice (pH = 2.0) have 1000 times greater H^+ concentration than black coffee (pH = 5.0), whereas hydrochloric acid (pH = 1.0) has approximately 1,000,000 times the H^+ concentration of blood (pH = 7.4).

The pH of body fluids ranges from a low of 1.0 for the digestive acid hydrochloric acid to a slightly basic pH between 7.35 and 7.45 for arterial and venous blood (and most other body fluids). The term **alkalosis** refers to an increase in pH above the normal average of 7.4; this results directly from a decrease in $[H^+]$ (increase in pH). Conversely, **acidosis** refers to an increase in $[H^+]$ concentration (decrease in pH). The body regulates the diverse yet highly specific pH of various body fluids within narrow limits because metabolism remains highly sensitive to the H^+ concentration of the reacting medium.

Enzymes and pH

Many chemical processes in the body occur only at a specific pH. An enzyme that works at one pH inactivates when the pH of its surroundings change. For example, the lipid-digesting enzyme gastric lipase functions effectively in the stomach's highly acidic environment, but ceases to function within the slightly alkaline small intestine. The same occurs for salivary amylase, the enzyme that initiates starch break-

down in the mouth. The pH of the salivary fluids ranges between 6.4 and 7.0. When passed to the stomach (pH 1.0–2.0), salivary amylase ceases its digestive function because the stomach acids digest it as with any other protein. As a general rule, extreme changes in pH irreversibly damage enzymes. For this reason, the body maintains its acid–base balance within narrow limits.

Buffers

The term **buffering** designates reactions that minimize changes in H^+ concentration. Chemical and physiologic mechanisms that prevent H^+ changes are termed **buffers.** Inability of the buffer system to neutralize deviations in $[H^+]$ disrupts effective body function, and coma or death ensues. Three mechanisms regulate the acid–base quality of the internal environment: (1) chemical buffers, (2) pulmonary ventilation, and (3) kidney function.

Chemical Buffers

The chemical buffering system consists of a weak acid and a base or salt of that acid. For example, the bicarbonate buffer consists of the weak carbonic acid and its salt sodium bicarbonate. Carbonic acid forms when the bicarbonate binds H^+. As long as $[H^+]$ remains elevated, the reaction produces the weaker acid because the excess H^+ binds in accordance with the general reaction:

$$H^+ + Buffer \rightarrow H\text{--}Buffer$$

The strong stomach acid hydrochloric acid (HCl) combines with sodium bicarbonate to form the much weaker carbonic acid (H_2CO_3). This produces only a slight reduction in pH. When stomach acid remains elevated from inadequacy of the buffer response during digestion, many individuals seek "outside help" by ingesting neutralizing agents or antacids to provide buffering relief. If the concentration of H^+ decreases and body fluids become more alkaline, the buffering reaction moves in the opposite direction. This releases H^+ and acidity increases as follows:

$$H^+ + Buffer \leftarrow H\text{--}Buffer$$

The body continually produces other acids in addition to digestive juices. Most carbon dioxide generated in energy metabolism reacts with water to form the relatively weak carbonic acid ($CO_2 + H_2O \rightarrow H_2CO_3$), which then dissociates to H^+ and HCO_3^-. Sodium bicarbonate buffers lactic acid, a stronger acid produced during anaerobic metabolism, to form sodium lactate and carbonic acid; in turn, carbonic acid dissociates and increases the $[H^+]$ of extracellular fluids. Other organic acids such as fatty acids dissociate and liberate H^+, as do sulfuric and phosphoric acids produced during protein breakdown. The buffering of hydrochloric acid by sodium bicarbonate occurs as follows:

$$HCl + NaHCO_3 \rightarrow NaCl + H_2CO_3 \rightarrow H^+ + HCO_3^-$$

Concentration in moles per liter   Examples

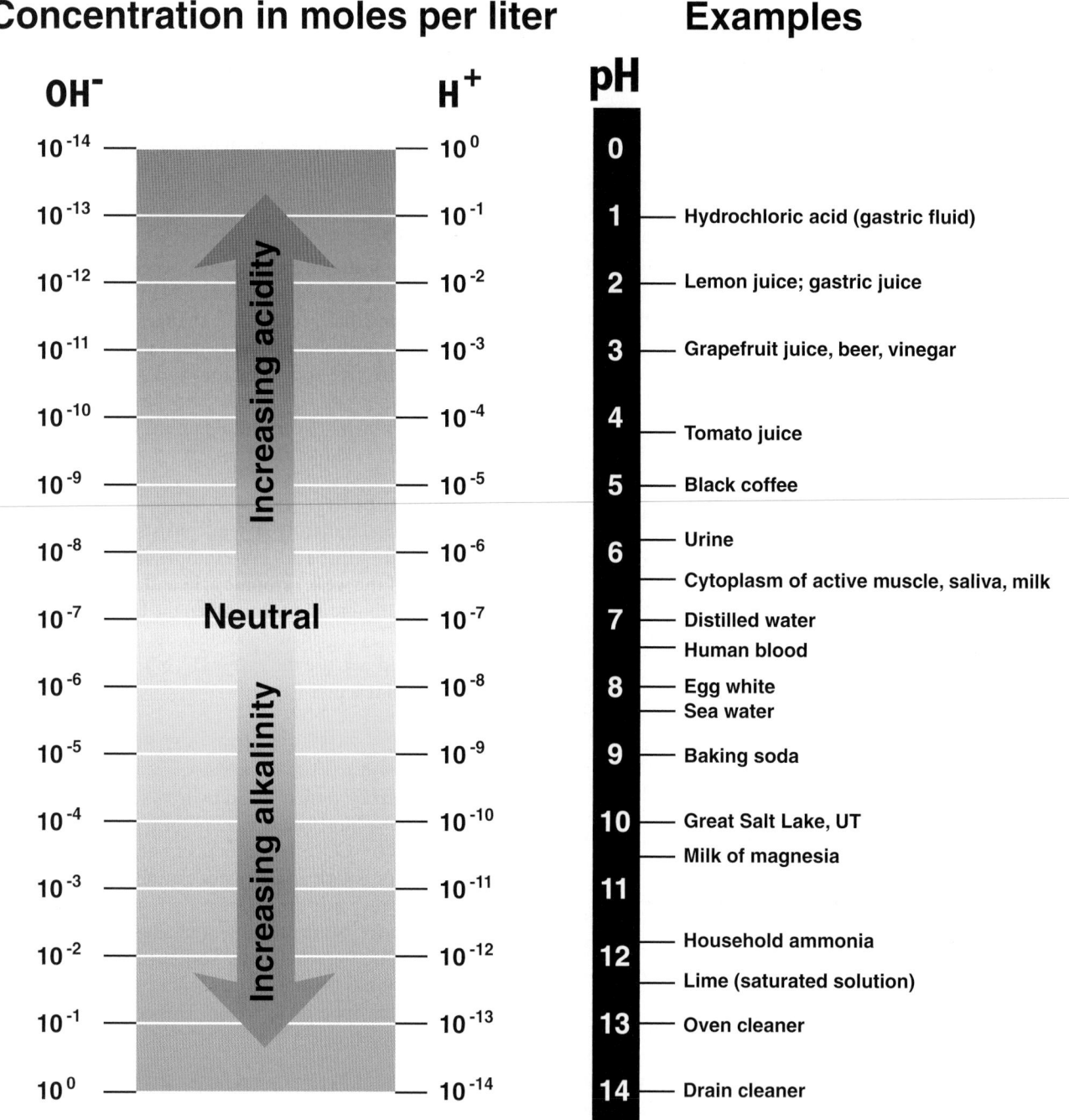

FIGURE 3.8 ■ The pH scale quantifies the acidity or alkalinity (basicity) of a liquid solution. Blood pH remains regulated at the slightly alkaline pH of 7.4. Values for blood pH rarely fall below 6.9, even during the most vigorous exercise.

Other available chemical buffers include the phosphate buffers phosphoric acid and sodium phosphate. These chemicals act similarly to the bicarbonate buffering system. Phosphate buffers regulate acid–base quality of the kidney tubules and intracellular fluids that contain high concentrations of phosphates. The protein-containing hemoglobin compound within red blood cells and other plasma proteins buffers carbonic acid.

Ventilatory Buffer

Any increase in $[H^+]$ in body fluids stimulates the respiratory center in the brain to increase pulmonary ventilation. This ad-justment causes greater than normal amounts of carbon dioxide to leave the blood. Carbon dioxide combines with water to form carbonic acid for transport dissolved in the blood. Thus, reducing the body's carbon dioxide content acts directly as a buffer by lowering carbonic acid concentration. This causes body fluids to become more alkaline. Conversely, ventilation below normal levels causes carbon dioxide (and carbonic acid) buildup, and the body fluids become more acidic.

Renal Buffer

The kidneys continually excrete H^+ to maintain long-term

acid–base stability of body fluids. The renal buffer controls acidity by adjusting the concentration of bicarbonate ions, ammonia, and hydrogen ions secreted into the urine. At the same time, it reabsorbs alkali, chloride, and bicarbonate.

Summary

1. Hydrolysis (catabolism) of complex organic molecules performs critical functions in digestion and energy metabolism. Condensation (anabolism) reactions synthesize complex biomolecules for tissue maintenance and growth.

2. Enzymes, highly specific protein catalysts, facilitate the interaction of substances to accelerate chemical reactions.

3. Coenzymes consist of nonprotein substances to assist enzyme action by binding a substrate to its specific enzyme.

4. Four passive processes transport nutrients throughout the body: simple diffusion, facilitated diffusion, osmosis, and filtration. Physical laws govern each of these processes, which do not require the input of chemical energy.

5. In active transport, substances move against their concentration gradients; metabolic energy "powers" the exchange of materials. Active transport absorbs nutrients from the digestive tract and reabsorbs plasma chemicals filtered by the kidneys.

6. Osmolality refers to the concentration of particles in a solution, expressed as osmolal units of particles or ions formed when a solute dissociates in solution.

7. Chemical and physiologic buffer systems normally regulate the acid–base quality of the body fluids within narrow limits.

8. Bicarbonate, phosphate, and protein chemical buffers serve as the rapid first line of defense to stabilize acid–base regulation. These buffers consist of a weak acid and the salt of that acid. Under acid conditions, buffering action converts a strong acid to a weaker acid and a neutral salt.

9. Lungs and kidneys help to regulate pH when a "stressor" affects the chemical buffer system. Changes in alveolar ventilation rapidly alter the free H^+ in extracellular fluids. With increased acidity, the renal tubules act as the body's final sentinels by secreting H^+ into the urine and reabsorbing bicarbonate.

Digestion and Absorption of Food Nutrients

The physiology of human digestion had its origins when the Italian physiologist Spallanzani (1729–1799) first observed that gastric juice dissolved bread and animal tissues. However, pioneer American physician William Beaumont's classic experiments on Alexis St. Martin over an 8-year period (1825–1833) first detailed the human digestive processes. Beaumont discovered the function of the stomach's gastric juice and the time required for the digestion of different foods.

OVERVIEW OF DIGESTION

The Beginning of Digestion: Taste and Smell

Digestion begins with smell and taste. Different foods emit a variety of odors; interestingly, the sense of smell has evolved over time to recognize more than 10,000 different odors. For example, the smell of baking biscuits or the aroma of vanilla bean coffee stimulates nerve cells within the nose. In the mouth, taste (including texture and temperature) combines with the odors to produce a *perception* of flavor. It is flavor, sensed mainly through smell, that tells us whether we are eating an onion or an apple, or garlic or a fudge brownie. Holding your nose while eating a Belgian chocolate, for example, makes it difficult to identify the substance, even though one can distinguish the food's sweetness or bitterness. In fact, familiar flavors are sensed largely by odor, and the combination of two aromatic substances could create a third odor sensation unlike the odor of either of the original ones. In 2004, Linda B. Buck (1947–) of the Fred Hutchinson Cancer Research Center, Seattle, WA, shared the Nobel Prize in Physiology or Medicine for her pioneering research that explained the odorant receptors and the organization of the olfactory system. The research identified approximately 1000 different genes that promote an equivalent number of olfactory receptor types (nobelprize.org/nobel_prizes/medicine/laureates/2004/illpres/index.html). In essence, the research provided the molecular details about the sense of smell. The sight, smell, thought of, taste, and perhaps the sounds of different foods, such as crunching or smashing, trigger responses that prepare the digestive tract to receive the food—the mouth begins to salivate and stomach secretions begin to flow.

Digestion: Physical and Chemical Processes

The breakdown of food into absorbable nutrients involves physical and chemical process. The physical process starts with chewing, by which the food substances degrade into smaller pieces. Muscular contractions of the gastrointestinal tract continue this process; the pulverized food mixes with various watery secretions as smooth muscle actions move the mixture called chyme through the digestive tract. Enzymes and other chemicals help to complete the breakdown process and promote absorption by the small intestine.

THE GASTROINTESTINAL TRACT

FIGURE 3.9A depicts the structures of the **gastrointestinal (GI) tract;** this includes the esophagus, gallbladder, liver, stomach, pancreas, small intestine, large intestine, rectum, and anus. The GI tract, also called the alimentary canal, essentially consists of a 7- to 9-m long tube that runs from the mouth to the anus. This serpentlike tube supplies the body with water and

nutrients. FIGURE 3.9B shows the highly specialized connective tissue **mesentery** that weaves around and supports the approximately 2-kg mass of intestinal organs. This membrane contains a diffuse network of capillaries that transports absorbed nutrients. FIGURE 3.9C shows that the mesenteric blood vessels eventually converge to become the large **hepatic portal vein** that delivers nutrient-rich blood to the liver. The nutrients undergo processing in the liver and then return to the general circulation for transport throughout the body.

Mouth and Esophagus

The journey of a bite of food begins in the mouth. Crushing forces of up to 90 kg cut, grind, mash, and soften the food. **Mechanical digestion** increases the surface area of the food particles, making them easier to swallow and more accessible to enzymes and other digestive substances that start the degradation process. With swallowing, the bolus of food moves past the pharynx at the back of the mouth and enters the **esophagus,** the 25-cm portion of the GI tract that connects the pharynx to the stomach. Two layers of muscle tissue encircle the

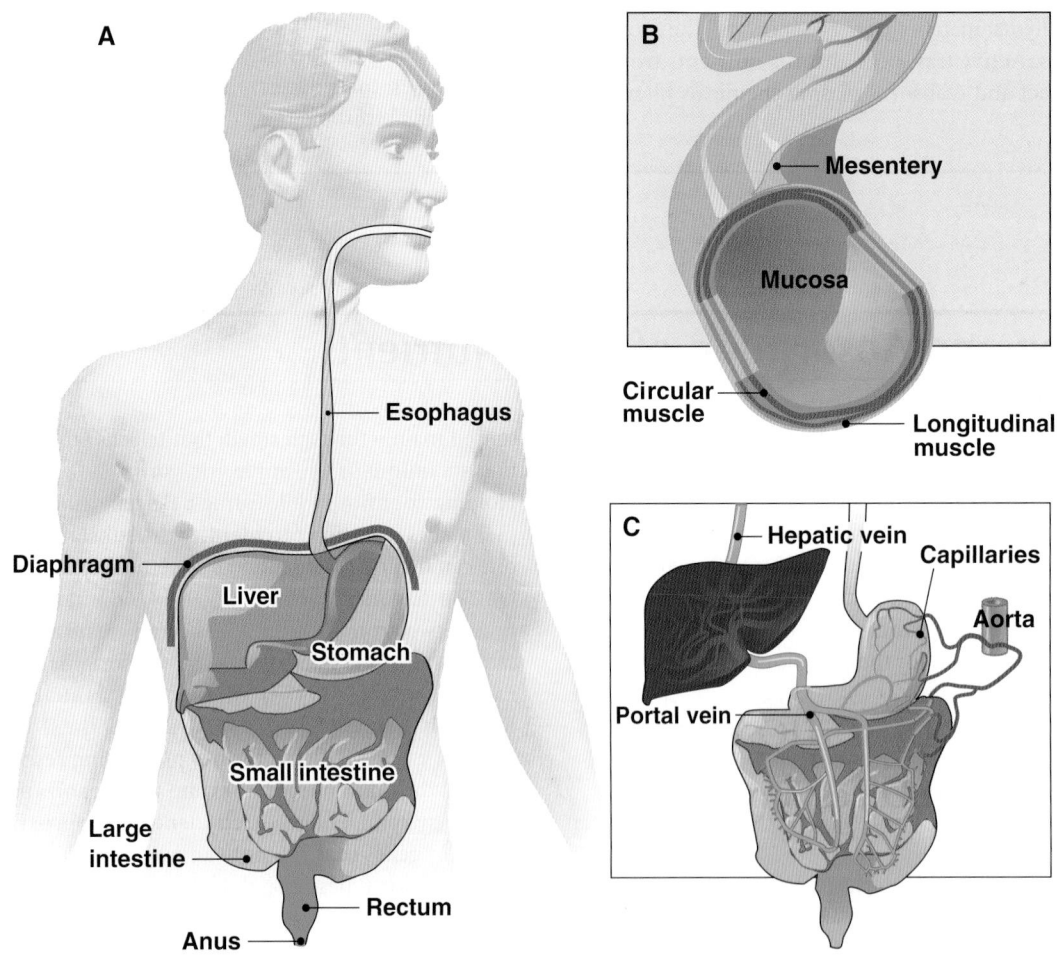

FIGURE 3.9 ■ **A.** Structures of the gastrointestinal (GI) tract. **B.** Mesentery, which weaves around and gives support to the intestinal organs. **C.** The large portal vein collects blood from the mesenteric area and transports it to the liver for processing before the blood returns to the general circulation.

length of the esophagus; the inner layer consists of circular bands of muscle, while the outer tissue layer runs longitudinally. The esophagus constricts when the circular muscles reflexly contract and the longitudinal muscles relax; the reverse causes the esophagus to bulge. These powerful waves of rhythmic contraction and relaxation, called **peristalsis,** propel the small round food mass down the esophagus (see FIG. 3.10A).

Peristalsis involves progressive and recurring waves of smooth muscle contractions that compress the alimentary tube in a squeezing action, causing its contents to mix and move forward. This intrinsic means of food propulsion can occur in the microgravity of space flight and even when a person turns upside down. The end of the esophagus contains a one-way ring or valve of smooth muscle called the **esophageal sphincter,** which relaxes to allow the food mass entry into the **stomach,** the next section of the GI tract. This sphincter then constricts to help prevent the stomach contents from regurgitating back into the esophagus (gastric reflux). The stomach serves as a temporary holding tank for the partially digested food before moving it into the small intestine.

Sphincters That Control the Passage of Food

A sphincter is a circular muscle arrangement acting as a valve to regulate passage or flow of material through the GI tract. Several sphincters exist throughout the length of the GI tract; they respond to stimuli from nerves, hormones, and hormonelike substances and an increase in pressure around them. TABLE 3.1 lists the important sphincters, their location in the digestive tract, and the factors that control them.

Stomach

FIGURE 3.11 shows structural details of the approximately 25-cm long, J-shaped stomach, the most distensible portion of the GI tract; the inset details the stomach wall, showing the gastric glands. The **parietal cells** of the gastric glands secrete hydrochloric acid—stimulated by gastrin, acetylcholine, and histamine—and powerful enzyme-containing digestive juices that continually degrade the nutrients after they leave the esophagus and enter the stomach (**www.vivo.colostate.edu/ hbooks/pathphys/digestion/stomach/parietal.htm**). Alkaline mucus, secreted from mucous neck cells, protects the mucosal lining of the gastric tissue. The buffering action of bicarbonate in alkaline pancreatic juice and alkaline secretions from glands in the submucosa of the duodenum (the first portion of the small intestine) normally protect the duodenum portion of the stomach from its highly acidic contents. The chief cells produce pepsinogen, the inactive form of the protein-digesting enzyme pepsin. Simple sugars are the easiest nutrients to digest, followed by proteins, and then lipids. With the exception of alcohol and aspirin, little absorption takes place in the stomach.

The stomach's volume averages about 1.5 L; however, it can hold a volume ranging from as little as 50 mL when nearly "empty" to about 6.0 L when fully distended after an excessively large meal. Regardless of its volume, the stomach contents mix with chemical substances to produce **chyme,** a slushy, acidic mixture of food and digestive juices.

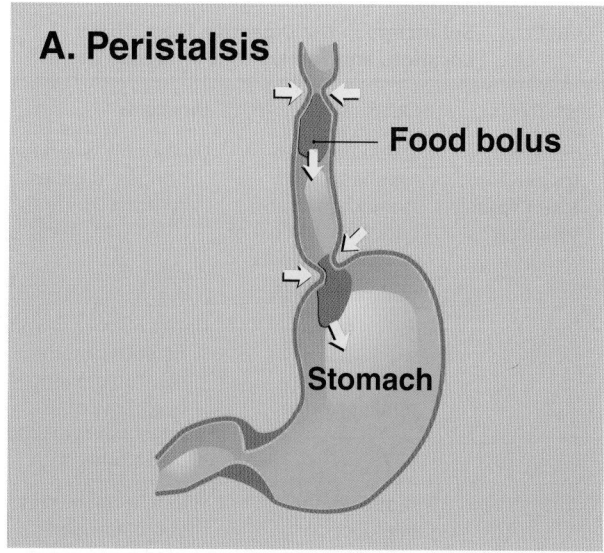

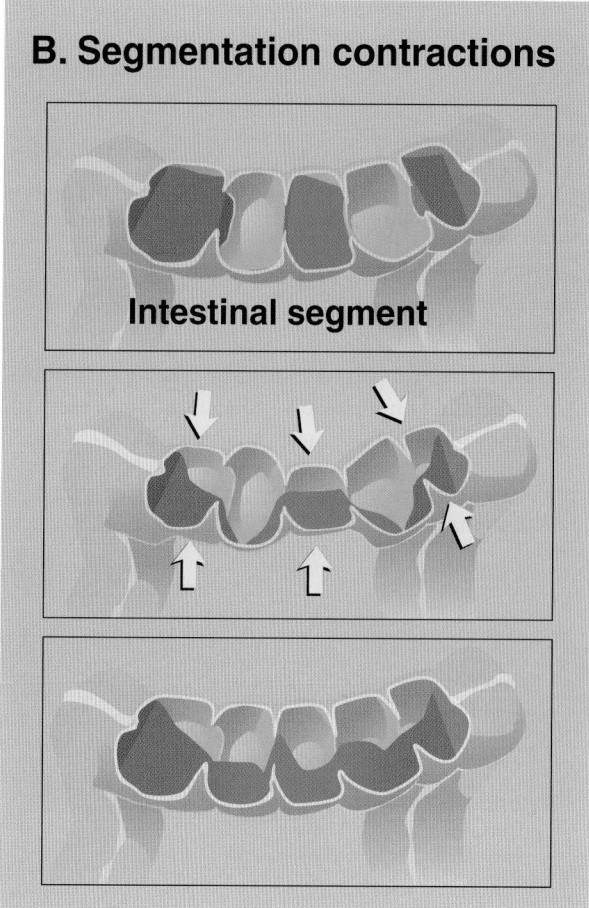

FIGURE 3.10 ■ Propulsion of nutrients through the GI tract. **A.** Peristalsis involves the reflex-controlled alternate contraction and relaxation of adjacent segments of the GI tract, which causes one-directional flow of food (with some mixing). **B.** Segmentation contractions involve the alternate contraction and relaxation of nonadjacent segments of the intestine. This localized intestinal rhythmicity propels food forward and then backward, causing food to mix with digestive juices.

TABLE 3.1	Sphincters in the Digestive Tract, Their Location, and Factors that Influence Them	
Sphincter	**Location**	**Comments**
Esophageal (upper and lower cardiac sphincter)	Junction between esophagus and stomach; prevents back flow (reflux) of stomach contents into esophagus	Opens only when esophageal muscles contract
Pyloric	Junction between stomach and first part of small intestine	Under hormonal and nervous system control; prevents back flow of intestinal contents into stomach
Oddi	End of common bile duct	When hormone CCK stimulates gallbladder to contract during digestion, this sphincter relaxes to allow bile to flow down the common bile duct and enter the intestinal duodenum
Ileocecal	Terminus of small intestine	Opens in the presence of intestinal contents
Anal (two sphincters)	Terminus of large intestine	Under voluntary control

After eating, the stomach usually takes 1 to 4 hours to empty, depending on the relative concentration of each nutrient and the volume of the meal. A large meal takes longer to clear the stomach than a smaller one. When eaten singularly, carbohydrates leave the stomach most rapidly, followed by proteins, and then lipids. The stomach may retain a high-fat meal for up to 6 hours before its chyme empties into the **small intestine.** Furthermore, food in liquefied form and fluids per se pass from the stomach most rapidly, whereas solids undergo a liquefaction phase. The nervous system, through hormonal regulation, largely controls the time and rate of stomach emptying via peristaltic waves that traverse the stomach toward the opening of the small intestine. A self-regulating feedback control also occurs between the stomach and small intestine. Excessive distension of the stomach from volume overload sends signals that cause the sphincter at the intestinal entrance to relax to allow more chyme to enter. Conversely, distension of the first portion of the intestine or the presence of excessive protein, lipid, or highly concentrated or acidic solutions, reflexly slows gastric emptying. A unique life-sustaining stomach function is its secretion of **intrinsic factor,** a polypeptide required for vitamin B_{12} absorption by the terminal portion of the small intestine.

Small Intestine

Approximately 90% of digestion (and essentially all lipid digestion) occurs in the first two sections of the 3-m long small intestine. This coiled structure consists of three sections: the **duodenum** (first 0.3 m), **jejunum** (next 1–2 m, where most digestion occurs), and **ileum** (last 1.5 m). Absorption takes place through millions of specialized protruding structures of the intestinal mucosa. These fingerlike protrusions called **villi** move in wavelike fashion. Most nutrient absorption through villi occurs by active transport that uses a carrier molecule and expends ATP energy. FIGURE 3.12 shows that highly vas-

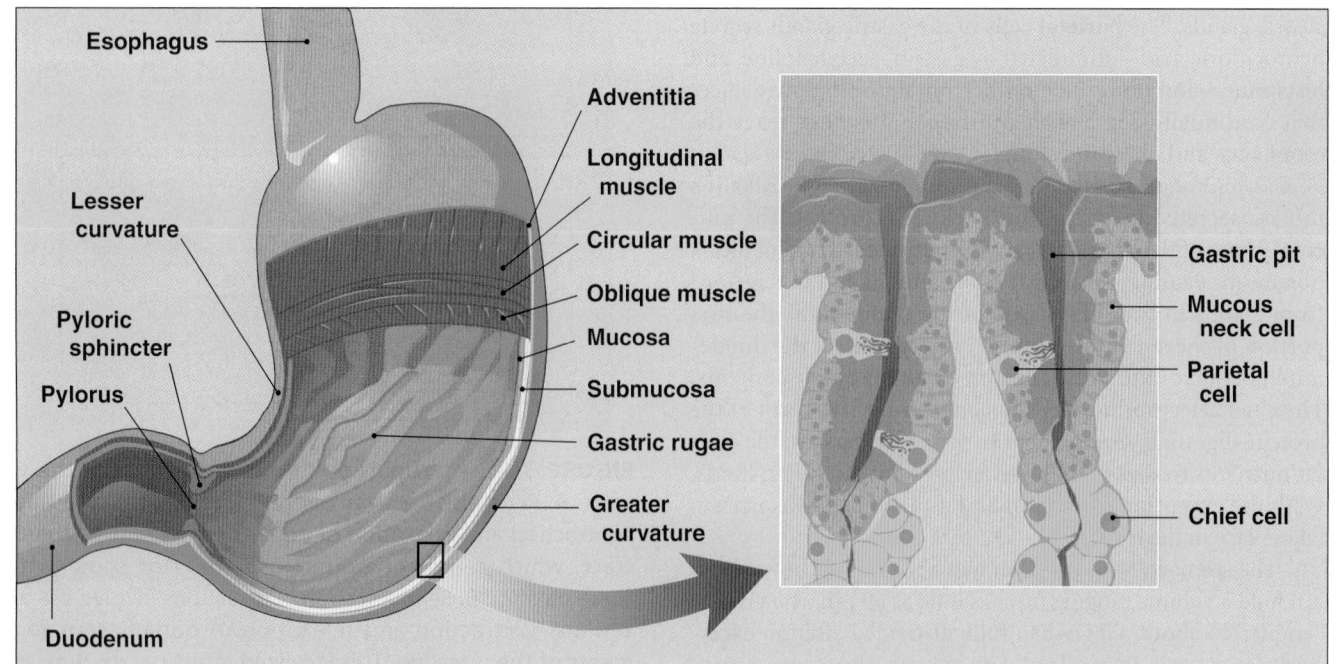

FIGURE 3.11 ■ Structure of the stomach and gastric glands. The parietal cells primarily secrete hydrochloric acid, neck cells secrete mucus, and chief cells produce pepsinogen.

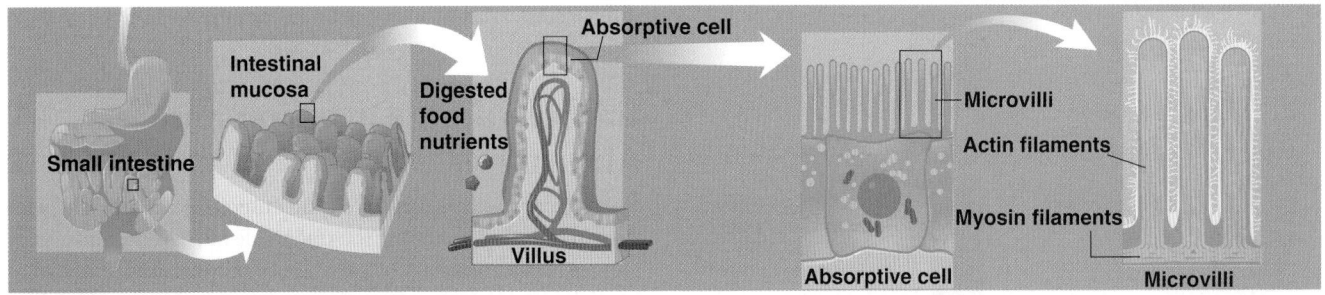

FIGURE 3.12 ■ Microscopic structure of the small intestine. Tiny villi and microvilli projections (termed *brush border*) greatly increase the surface area of the mucosal cell's plasma membrane for nutrient absorption.

cularized surfaces of villi contain small projections known as **microvilli.** These structures (1) contain the digestive enzymes embedded within its cell membranes and (2) absorb the smaller digested units of carbohydrates, proteins, and lipids, electrolytes (80% absorbed), alcohol, vitamins, and minerals.

Villi increase the absorptive surface of the intestine by up to 600-fold compared with a flat-surfaced tube of the same dimensions. If spread out, the 300-m² surface area of the small intestine would cover the area of a tennis court or about 150 times the external surface of the body! This large surface greatly augments the speed and capacity for nutrient absorption. Each villus contains small lymphatic vessels called **lacteals** that absorb most digested lipids from the intestine. They transport via the lymphatic vessels that drain into the large veins near the heart.

Intestinal Contractions

It usually takes 1 to 3 days after eating food before the GI tract eliminates it. The movement of chyme through the small intestine takes 3 to 10 hours. Peristaltic contractions are much weaker in the small intestine than in the esophagus and stomach. The major contractile activity of the intestines occurs by segmentation contractions. These intermittent oscillating contractions and relaxations of the intestinal wall's circular smooth muscle augment mechanical mixing of intestinal chyme with bile, pancreatic juice, and intestinal juice. Figure 3.10B shows that segmentation contractions give the small intestine section of the GI tract a "sausage-link" look because the alternating contraction and relaxation occur in nonadjacent segments of this structure. Thus, instead of propelling food directly forward as in peristalsis (Fig. 3.10A), the food moves slightly backward before advancing. This gives the digestive juices additional time to blend with the food mass before it reaches the large intestine. The propulsive movements of segmentation contractions continue to churn and mix the chyme before it passes the pyloric sphincter and enters the large intestine.

During digestion, **bile,** produced in the liver and stored and secreted by the **gallbladder,** increases the lipid droplets' solubility and digestibility through **emulsification.** The lipid content of the intestinal chyme stimulates the gallbladder's pulsatile release of bile into the duodenum. In a manner similar to the action of many household detergents, bile salts break apart fat into numerous smaller droplets that do not coalesce.

This renders fatty acid end products insoluble in water so the small intestine can absorb them. Some bile components are excreted in the feces, but the intestinal mucosa reabsorbs most of the bile salts; they return in the hepatic portal blood to the liver, where they become components in the resynthesis of new bile.

The **pancreas** secretes between 1.2 and 1.6 L of alkali-containing juice (digestive enzymes in an inactive form plus sodium bicarbonate) to help buffer the hydrochloric acid from the stomach that remains in the intestinal chyme. At a higher pH, pancreatic enzymes, released by neural and hormonal mechanisms, degrade the larger protein, carbohydrate, and lipid nutrients into smaller subunits for further digestion and absorption. The intestinal lining cannot withstand the highly acidic gastric juices from the stomach. Consequently, neutralizing this acid provides crucial protection against duodenal damage, which in extreme form triggers tissue ulceration or ulcers.

Large Intestine

FIGURE 3.13 depicts the components of the **large intestine,** the final digestive structure for absorbing water and electrolytes from the chyme it receives and storing digestive residues as fecal matter. This terminal 1.2-m (4-ft) portion of the GI tract, also known as the **colon** or **bowel,** contains no villi. Its major anatomic sections include the ascending colon, transverse colon, descending colon, sigmoid colon, rectum, and anal canal. Of the 8- to 12-L volume of food, fluid, and gastric secretions that enter the GI tract daily, only about 750 mL pass into the large intestine. Here, bacteria ferment the remaining undigested food residue devoid of all but about 5% of useful nutrients. Intestinal bacteria (through their own metabolism) synthesize small amounts of vitamins K and biotin, which then become absorbed. Bacterial fermentation also produces about 500 mL of gas (flatus) each day. This gas consists of hydrogen, nitrogen, methane, hydrogen sulfide, and carbon dioxide. A small amount produces no outward effects, but excessive flatus can trigger severe abdominal distress as usually occurs from consuming large quantities of beans or dairy products. These foods leave partially digested sugars that contribute to larger than normal intestinal gas production. Mucus, the only significant secretion of the large intestine, protects the intestinal wall and helps to hold fecal matter together.

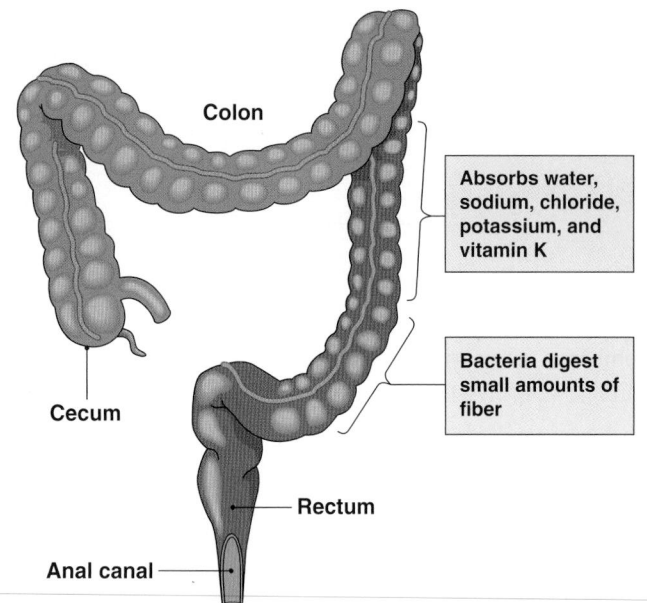

FIGURE 3.13 ■ The large intestine, a 5-foot long tube, includes the cecum, colon, rectum, and anal canal. As chyme fills the cecum, a local reflex signals the ileocical valve to close, preventing material from reentering the ileum and small intestine.

THE DIGESTIVE PROCESS

Digestion occurs almost entirely under involuntary control, in harmony with exquisite neural and hormonal regulation, to help maintain relative constancy in the internal environment. Polypeptides and polysaccharides degrade into simpler subunits to enter the epithelial cells of the intestinal villi for absorption into the blood. Fats, emulsified by bile, hydrolyze into their fatty acid and monoglyceride subunits for absorption by the intestinal villi. Within the epithelial cells of the villi, triacylglycerols resynthesize and combine with protein for secretion into the lymphatic fluid. The autonomic nervous system controls the entire GI tract: the parasympathetic system generally increases gut activity, while the sympathetic system exerts an inhibitory effect. Even without neural control, intrinsic autoregulatory mechanisms eventually return gut function to near-normal levels.

FIGURE 3.14 presents an overview of digestive processes throughout the GI tract. The diagram lists the major enzymes and hormones that act on proteins, lipids, and carbohydrates during their journey from the mouth through the GI tract.

Hormones That Control Digestion

Four hormones that regulate digestion are gastrin, secretin, cholecystokinin (CCK), and gastric inhibitory peptide (TABLE 3.2). Hormonelike compounds, many of which occur in the small intestine and brain (e.g., vasoactive intestinal peptide, bombesin, substance P, and somatostatin), control other important aspects of GI function. These different compounds diffuse from cells or nerve endings throughout the GI tract to exert their influence on nearby cells.

Carbohydrate Digestion and Absorption

Starch hydrolysis begins once food enters the mouth. The **salivary glands,** located along the underside of the jaw, continually secrete lubricating mucus substances that combine with food particles during chewing. The enzyme **salivary α-amylase** (ptyalin) attacks starch and reduces it to smaller linked glucose molecules and the simpler disaccharide form maltose. When the food–saliva mixture enters the more acidic stomach, some additional starch breakdown occurs, but this quickly ceases because salivary amylase deactivates at the low pH of gastric juice.

Food entering the alkaline environment of the duodenum portion of the small intestine encounters **pancreatic amylase,** a powerful enzyme released from the pancreas. This enzyme, in conjunction with other enzymes, completes the hydrolysis of starch into smaller branched chains of glucose molecules (4–10 glucose linkages, called dextrins and oligosaccharides); the disaccharides cleave into simple monosaccharides. Enzyme action on the surface of the cells of the intestinal lumen's brush border completes the final stage of carbohydrate digestion to simple monosaccharide form. For example, **maltase** breaks down maltose to its glucose components, **sucrase** reduces sucrose to the simple sugars glucose and fructose, and **lactase** degrades lactose to glucose and galactose. Active transport (common protein carriers) in the intestinal villi and microvilli (see Fig. 3.12) absorbs the monosaccharides. Glucose and galactose absorption occurs by a sodium-dependent, carrier-mediated active transport process. The electrochemical gradient created with sodium transport (see Figs. 3.6 and 3.7) augments the absorption of these monosaccharides.

The maximum rate of glucose absorption from the small intestine ranges between 50 and 80 g · h^{-1} for a person who weighs 70 kg. If we assume that high-intensity aerobic exercise (20 kCal · min^{-1}) derives 80% of its energy from carbohydrate breakdown, then roughly 4 g of carbohydrate (1 g carbohydrate = 4.0 kCal) are catabolized each minute (240 g · h^{-1}). Even under optimal conditions for intestinal absorption, carbohydrate intake during prolonged intense exercise cannot balance its utilization rate. Fructose is not absorbed via active transport, but in combination with a carrier protein by the much slower method of facilitated diffusion.

If disease affects intestinal enzymes or the villi themselves, the GI tract can indeed become "upset" and may take several weeks to resume normal functioning. For example, carbohydrates cannot completely break down when the digestive enzyme level is altered. A person recovering from diarrhea (or intestinal infection) often experiences transient **lactose intolerance** and should avoid milk products that contain lactose. Reestablishing appropriate lactase concentration allows a person to consume this sugar once again without undesirable consequences. About 70% of the world's population suffer from reduced intestinal lactase levels to the point that it affects the digestion of milk sugar.

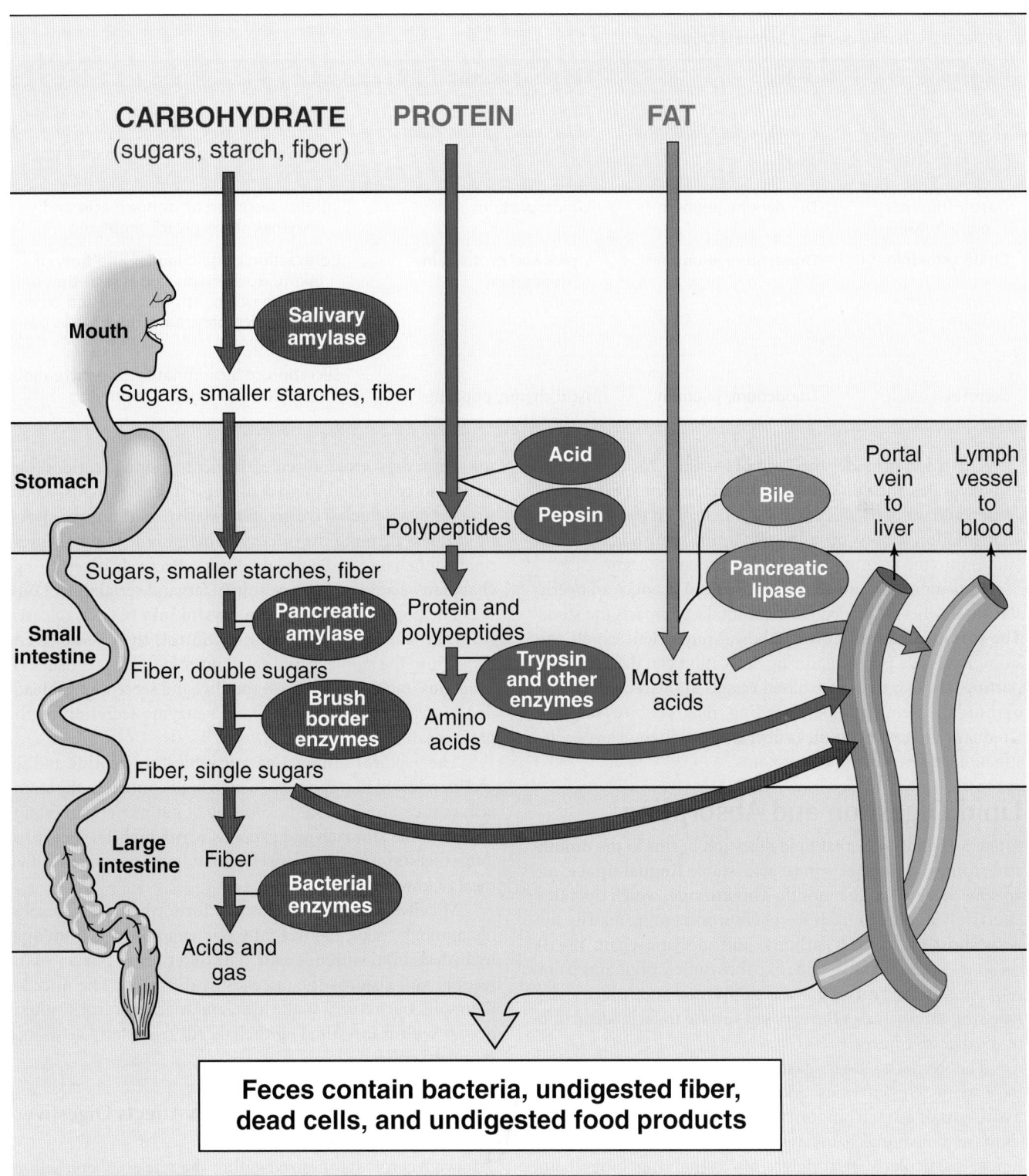

FIGURE 3.14 ■ Overview of human digestion.

The epithelial cells of the small intestine secrete monosaccharides into the bloodstream for transport by capillaries to the hepatic portal vein, which empties directly to the liver. The liver removes the greatest portion of glucose and essentially all of the absorbed fructose and galactose. Peripheral tissues, under the influence of insulin, absorb any remaining blood glucose.

Circulatory transport from the GI tract occurs via the **hepatic portal circulation.** Blood drained from the small intestine does not pass directly to the heart. Instead, intestinal blood travels to the liver, which processes its nutrients before they finally enter the general circulation. The hepatic portal circulation also drains blood from portions of the stomach and pancreas.

TABLE 3.2	**Hormones that Regulate Digestion**		
Hormone	**Origin**	**Secretion Stimulus**	**Action**
Gastrin	Pyloric areas of stomach and upper duodenum	Food in stomach (protein, caffeine, spices, alcohol); nerve input	Stimulates flow of stomach enzymes and acid; stimulates action of lower esophageal sphincter; slows gastric emptying
Gastric inhibitory peptide (GIP)	Duodenum, jejunum	Lipids; proteins	Inhibits secretion of stomach acid and enzymes; slows gastric emptying
Cholecystokinin (CCK)	Duodenum, jejunum	Lipids and proteins in duodenum	Contraction of gallbladder and flow of bile to duodenum; causes secretion of enzyme-rich pancreatic juice and bicarbonate-rich pancreatic fluid; slows gastric emptying
Secretin	Duodenum, jejunum	Acid chyme; peptones	Secretion of bicarbonate-rich pancreatic fluid and slows gastric emptying

The colon provides the "end of the line" for undigested carbohydrates, including fibrous substances. Some further digestion and water reabsorption occur here; then peristaltic and segmentation actions push the remaining semisolid contents (stool) into the rectum for expulsion through the anus.

Consuming too much dietary fiber can produce an overly soft stool, whereas inadequate fiber intake compacts the stool. The pressure exerted during a bowel movement expels the stool. Excessive pressure during defecation can damage supporting tissues and expose blood vessels in the rectum (**hemorrhoids**). Hemorrhoidal bleeding may require surgery. Gradually increasing the diet's fiber content often relieves constipation and hemorrhoid symptoms.

Lipid Digestion and Absorption

FGURE 3.15 illustrates that lipid digestion begins in the mouth and stomach by the action of acid-stable **lingual lipase,** an enzyme secreted in the mouth. This enzyme, which operates effectively in the stomach's acid environment, primarily digests short-chain (4–6 carbons) and medium-chain (8–10 carbons) saturated fatty acids like those in coconut and palm oil. Chewing food mixes lipase with the food and reduces particle size; this increases the exposed surface to facilitate action of the digestive juices.

The stomach secretes **gastric lipase,** its own lipid-digesting enzyme. This enzyme works with lingual lipase to continue hydrolysis of a small amount of triacylglycerol that contains short- and medium-chain fatty acids. The major breakdown of lipids, particularly triacylglycerols containing long-chain (12–18 carbons) fatty acids, occurs in the small intestine. When chyme enters the small intestine, mechanical mixing and bile act on the triacylglycerols (bound together as large lipid globules) and emulsify them into a fine immersion of oil droplets in an aqueous suspension. Bile contains no digestive enzymes; its action breaks up the fat droplets and thereby increases surface contact between lipid molecules and the water-soluble enzyme **pancreatic lipase.** Pancreatic lipase exerts a strong effect on the surface of the fat droplets to hydrolyze

some triacylglycerol molecules further to monoglycerides (one fatty acid connected to glycerol) and free fatty acids. These simpler fats, which have greater polarity than unhydrolyzed lipids, pass through the microvilli membrane to enter intestinal epithelial cells. Pancreatic lipase effectively digests long-chain fatty acids common in animal fats and certain plant oils.

The peptide hormone **cholecystokinin (CCK),** released from the wall of the duodenum, controls the release of enzymes into the stomach and small intestine. CCK regulates GI functions, including stomach motility and secretion, gallbladder contraction and bile flow, and enzyme secretion by the pancreas.

The peptide hormones **gastric inhibitory peptide** and **secretin,** released in response to a high lipid content in the stomach, reduce gastric motility. Slowing of gut movement retains chyme in the stomach and explains why a high-fat meal prolongs digestion and gives a feeling of fullness compared with a meal of lower lipid content.

Micelles (fat–bile salt clusters) form when water-insoluble monoglyceride and free fatty acid end products from lipid hydrolysis bind with bile salts. The outer brush border of intestinal villi absorbs the micelles by diffusion. The micelles then split, bile returns to the liver, and triacylglycerol synthesis occurs within intestinal epithelial cells from fatty acids and monoglycerides.

Fatty Acid Carbon Chain Length Affects Digestive and Metabolic Processes

Triacylglycerols synthesized within the intestinal epithelium take one of two routes (hepatic portal system or lymphatic system), depending on their chain length. Most **medium-chain triacylglycerol** becomes absorbed directly into the portal vein (hepatic portal system) bound to albumin as glycerol and medium-chain free fatty acids. Because medium-chain triacylglycerols bypass the lymphatic system, they enter the bloodstream rapidly for transport to the liver for subsequent use by various tissues in energy metabolism. Medium-chain triacylglycerol supplementation has clinical application for patients

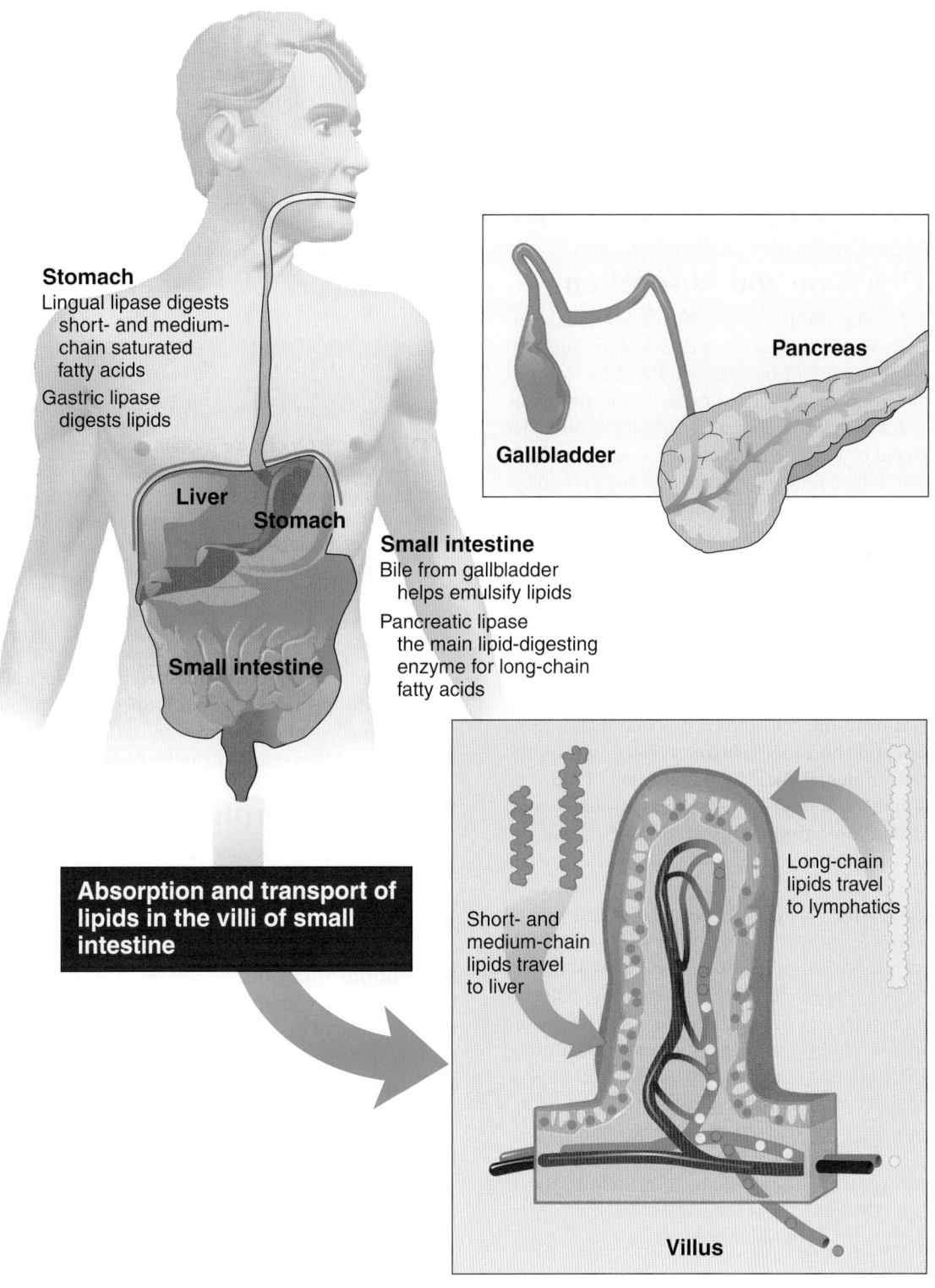

Stomach

Lingual lipase digests short- and medium-chain saturated fatty acids

Gastric lipase digests lipids

Liver

Stomach

Small intestine

Bile from gallbladder helps emulsify lipids

Pancreatic lipase the main lipid-digesting enzyme for long-chain fatty acids

Gallbladder

Pancreas

Absorption and transport of lipids in the villi of small intestine

Short- and medium-chain lipids travel to liver

Long-chain lipids travel to lymphatics

Villus

FIGURE 3.15 ■ Digestion of dietary lipids.

with tissue-wasting disease or with intestinal malabsorption difficulties. Chapter 12 discusses the proposed use of medium-chain triacylglycerols as an energy aid in endurance exercise.

Once absorbed inside the epithelial cells, long-chain fatty acids (more than 12 carbons in the fatty acid chain) re-form into triacylglycerols. These combine with a small amount of phospholipid, protein, and cholesterol to form small fatty droplets called **chylomicrons.** The chylomicrons move slowly upward via the second route, the lymphatic system. They eventually empty into the venous blood of the systemic circulation in the neck region via the thoracic duct. Through the action of the enzyme **lipoprotein lipase,** which lines capillary walls, the chylomicrons in the bloodstream readily hydrolyze to provide free fatty acids and glycerol for use by peripheral tissues. The liver then takes up the remaining cholesterol-containing remnant particles of the chylomicron. It generally takes 3 to 4 hours before ingested long-chain triacylglycerols enter the blood.

Protein Digestion and Absorption

The digestive efficiency for protein, particularly animal protein normally remains high, with less than 3% of this ingested macronutrient appearing in the feces. Indigestible components of this macronutrient include fibrous connective tissue of meat, some coverings of grains, and particles of nuts that remain unaffected by digestive enzymes. In essence, protein digestion liberates the building blocks of ingested proteins to produce the final end products—simple amino acids and dipeptides and tripeptides—for absorption across the intestinal mucosa. Specific enzymes within the stomach and small intestine promote protein hydrolysis.

The powerful enzyme **pepsin** initiates protein digestion chiefly to short-chain polypeptides in the stomach (see Fig. 3.14). Pepsin (actually a group of protein-digesting enzymes) represents the active form of its precursor pepsinogen. Pepsin's release from the cells of the stomach wall is controlled by the peptide hormone **gastrin,** secreted in response to external environmental cues (sight and smell of food) or internal cues (thought of food or stomach distension by food contents). Gastrin also stimulates secretion of gastric hydrochloric acid, a harsh acid that lowers the pH of gastric contents to about 2.0. The acidification of ingested food achieves the following: (1) activates pepsin, (2) kills pathogenic organisms, (3) improves absorption of iron and calcium, (4) inactivates hormones of plant and animal origin, and (5) denatures food proteins, making them more vulnerable to enzyme action. Pepsin, particularly effective in the stomach's acidic medium, easily degrades meat's collagenous connective tissue fibers. Once these fibers dismantle, other enzymes digest the remaining animal protein.

Stomach enzymes and acids attack the long, complex protein strands to hydrolyze about 15% of the ingested proteins. Uncoiling the three-dimensional shape of protein breaks it into smaller polypeptide and peptide units. Pepsin inactivates at the relatively high pH of the duodenum as the chyme passes into the small intestine.

The final steps in protein digestion occur in the small intestine. Here the peptide fragments dismantle further by alkaline enzyme action from the pancreas—most notably **trypsin** from its inactive precursor **trypsinogen**—into tripeptides, dipeptides, and single (free) amino acids. Free amino acid absorption occurs by active transport (coupled to the transport of sodium) and delivery to the liver via the hepatic portal vein. In contrast, dipeptides and tripeptides move into the intestinal epithelial cells by a single membrane carrier that uses an H^+ gradient for active transport. Once inside the cytoplasm, the dipeptides and tripeptides hydrolyze into their amino acid constituents and flow into the bloodstream.

One important function of the small intestine is to absorb amino acids and protein in more complex form. When amino acids reach the liver, one of three events occurs:

1. Conversion to glucose (glucogenic amino acids)
2. Conversion to fat (ketogenic amino acids)
3. Direct release into the bloodstream as plasma proteins such as albumin or as free amino acids

Let Nature Do It

The normal process for protein digestion argues against the widespread practice advocated in body building and strength magazines of ingesting a "predigested," hydrolyzed simple amino acid supplement to facilitate amino acid availability. The advertising hype does not justify the purchase of these products.

Free amino acids are synthesized into biologically important proteins, peptides (e.g., hormones), and amino acid derivatives such as phosphocreatine and choline, the essential component of the neurotransmitter acetylcholine.

Vitamin Absorption

Vitamin absorption occurs mainly by the passive process of diffusion in the jejunum and ileum portions of the small intestine. Absorption and storage by the body constitutes a basic difference between the fat-soluble and water-soluble vitamins.

Fat-Soluble Vitamins

Up to 90% of fat-soluble vitamins are absorbed with dietary lipids (as part of dietary fat containing micelles) throughout various sections of the small intestine. Once absorbed, chylomicrons and lipoproteins transport these vitamins to the liver and fatty tissues.

Water-Soluble Vitamins

The diffusion process absorbs water-soluble vitamins except for vitamin B_{12}. This vitamin combines with intrinsic factor that the stomach produces, which the intestine absorbs by endocytosis. Water-soluble vitamins do not remain in tissues to any great extent. Instead, they pass into urine when their concentration in plasma exceeds renal capacity for reabsorption. Consequently, food intake must regularly replenish water-soluble vitamins. Ingested B vitamins in food exist as part of coenzymes; digestion then releases vitamins to their free vitamin form. This coenzyme breakdown occurs first in the stomach and then along sections of small intestine, where absorption proceeds. Ingestion of a variety of vitamin-laden nutrients, not their absorption, becomes the limiting factor in proper vitamin nutrition for healthy men and women.

Absorption Sites for Water-Soluble Vitamins

- **Vitamin C:** Approximately 90% of absorption takes place in the distal portion of the small intestine. Excess vitamin C intake above about 1500 mg daily decreases kidney reabsorption efficiency, with large amounts voided in the urine.
- **Thiamine:** Absorption occurs mainly in the jejunum of the small intestine. Alcoholics, individuals on extremely low-calorie diets, and the confined elderly often show symptoms of thiamine deficiency (beriberi, depression, mental confusion, loss of muscle coordination). Symptoms often become evident within 10 days because of the body's small thiamine reserve.
- **Riboflavin:** Absorption occurs mainly in the proximal portion of the small intestine.
- **Niacin:** Some absorption takes place in the stomach, but most occurs in the small intestine.
- **Pantothenic acid:** This vitamin exists as part of coenzyme A. Absorption occurs readily throughout the small intestine when the vitamin releases from its coenzyme.
- **Biotin:** Absorption occurs mainly in the upper one third to one half of the small intestine.
- **Folate:** Absorption occurs in the small intestine with the help of a specialized intestinal enzyme system (conjugase).
- **Vitamin B$_6$** (pyridoxine): Absorption occurs mainly in the intestinal jejunum.
- **Vitamin B$_{12}$:** A salivary enzyme initially acts on this vitamin in the stomach. The vitamin then combines with intrinsic factor, a glycoprotein secreted by the gastric glands, before it enters the small intestine. The pancreatic enzyme trypsin then liberates vitamin B$_{12}$ from the intrinsic factor. The small intestine absorbs up to 70% in the ileum.

Mineral Absorption

Both extrinsic (dietary) and intrinsic (cellular) factors control the eventual fate of ingested minerals. Intestinal absorption increases to preserve the small micronutrient quantities when dietary intake of a particular mineral falls below the required level. The converse holds when mineral supplies exceed their limit, allowing little need for further increased absorption. Overall, the body does not absorb minerals very well. For most persons, this simply means that minerals exist in fairly generous amounts in a well-balanced normal diet. Thus, the body has little need to stockpile minerals. A possible exception exists for iron and calcium, two minerals that tend to be insufficient in the typical diet of American females.

Mineral availability in the body depends on its chemical form. For example, heme iron has an absorptive capacity of about 15% compared with nonheme iron absorption, which ranges between 2 and 10%. Variation in mineral absorption also exists between the sexes. Men absorb calcium better than women, yet total calcium absorption rarely exceeds 35% of the amount ingested, with the remaining two thirds excreted in the feces. Of the calcium absorbed, half is voided in the urine. For phosphorus, about two thirds is excreted daily in the urine. Poor absorption also occurs for magnesium (20–30%) and the trace minerals zinc (14–40%) and chromium (less than 2%). Determination of absorption rates for the other minerals requires further research. FIGURE 3.16 presents a generalized schema for major and trace mineral absorption, including the common pathways for their excretion.

Absorption of calcium, phosphorus, magnesium, and the trace minerals occurs mainly in the small intestine. The following six intrinsic factors affect mineral absorption:

1. Bioavailability
2. Transit time from the source (diet) to the absorption site
3. Quantity of digestive juices
4. pH of intestinal lumen contents
5. Presence of receptor sites in the intestine's mucosal lining and brush border
6. Availability of substances that combine with the minerals during movement from the gut (via diffusion, facilitated diffusion, and/or active transport) and across cell membranes

Metallic minerals combine with a specific protein transporter (e.g., iron binds with transferrin) or a general protein carrier such as albumin, which binds with many minerals. Peptide and amino acid complexes also carry a small amount of each mineral in the blood. Although dietary fiber negatively affects absorption of certain minerals, consuming 30 to 40 g of fiber daily does not impair absorption.

Water Absorption

The major absorption of ingested water and water contained in foods occurs by the passive process of osmosis in the small intestine. FIGURE 3.17 shows that in addition to the 2.0 L of water ingested daily by the typical sedentary adult, saliva, gastric secretions, bile, and pancreatic and intestinal secretions contribute an additional 7 L. This means that the intestinal tract absorbs about 9 L of water each day. Seventy-two percent of this water becomes absorbed in the proximal small intestine and 20% from its distal segment; the large intestine absorbs the remaining 8%.

The continuous secretion and absorption of water within the GI tract makes it difficult to quantify the body's net water uptake. The intestinal mucosa absorbs electrolytes and the components of macronutrient hydrolysis. This makes the intestinal medium progressively more hypotonic than the opposite side of the lumen membrane. This creates an osmotic gradient that forces water to move from the intestine to maintain isotonicity between the two fluid "compartments." In contrast, ingesting fluid hypertonic to plasma (greater than 280 mOsm $\cdot$ L^{-1}) causes water secretion into the intestinal lumen. This retards net water absorption and increases the potential for GI distress. This can occur when consuming salt

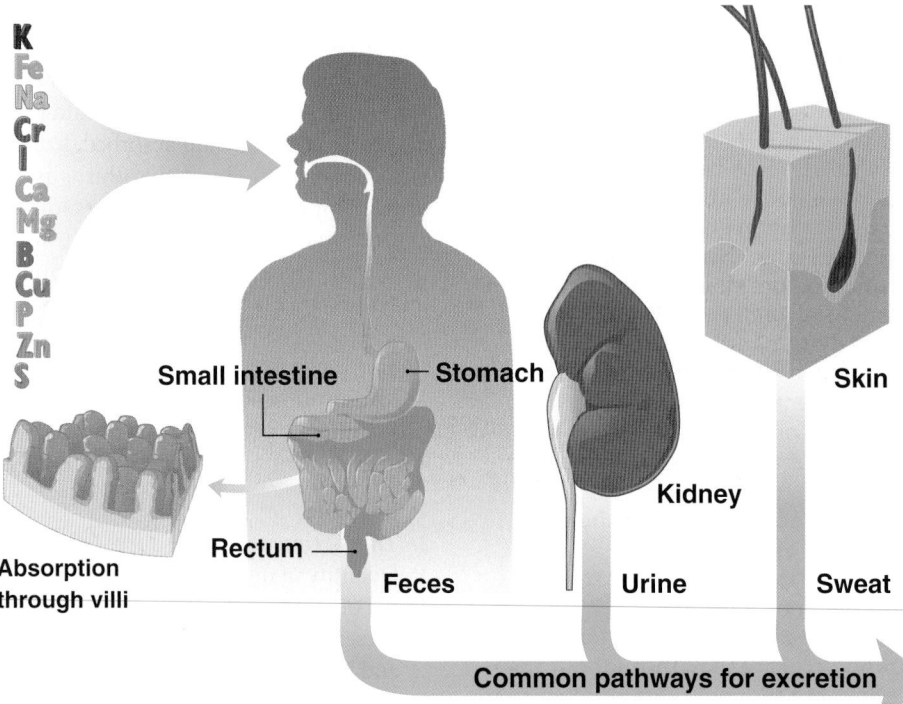

FIGURE 3.16 ▪ Absorption of minerals and their common excretion pathways.

tablets, concentrated mixtures of simple amino acids, or a "sports drink" with a high percentage of simple sugars and minerals (see Chapter 10).

NUTRITION, EXERCISE, AND GASTROINTESTINAL TRACT DISORDERS

Many factors influence GI function. The brain exerts a strong influence through diverse neurochemical connections with different digestive organs. Emotional state affects nearly all of the GI tract to some degree. For example, many individuals experience intestinal cramping or a queasy stomach before a "big date" or "big game." Some individuals get an "upset stomach" at the sight of their own blood, and it is well known that emotional stress contributes to the production of gastric mucosal abnormalities. In contrast, other GI tract disorders, originally thought linked to emotional distress such as peptic ulcer disease, are probably caused by infection and other physical ailments (see p. 114). Recent evidence suggests that most GI tract problems can be treated with a healthful diet, exercise, and maintenance of a healthy body weight.

Regular, moderate physical activity promotes several health benefits for the GI tract. Regular exercise, for example, enhances gut emptying, with a concomitant reduction in the incidence of liver disease, gallstones, colon cancer, and constipation. Conversely, individuals who engage in frequent, intense exercise report GI symptoms such as self-limited food poisoning, gastroesophageal reflux disease (GERD), hiatal her-

nia, irritable bowel syndrome (IBS), and viral gastroenteritis. These symptoms, reported by between 20 and 50% of high-performance athletes, occur (1) more frequently in women than men, (2) common in younger athletes, and (3) less frequently among athletes in sports such as cycling that incorporate gliding movements.

More serious medical conditions such as Crohn's disease (ongoing disorder that inflames the ileum), ulcerative colitis, appendicitis, mesenteric adenitis, and invasive diarrhea, are far less common and generally present dramatically with abdominal pain, nausea, vomiting, and bloody diarrhea.

Constipation

Constipation: a delay in stool movement through the colon, results when the large intestine absorbs excessive water, producing hard, dry stools. A diet high in fat and low in water and fiber represents the most common cause. Some fibers (see Chapter 1) such as pectin in fruits and gums in beans dissolve easily in water and take on a soft, gel-like texture in the colon. Other fibers, such as cellulose, in wheat bran pass essentially unchanged on their journey through the colon. The bulking action and softer texture of water-soluble and insoluble fibers help to prevent hard, dry stools that pass tortuously through the GI system.

Diarrhea (Lower Intestinal Motility Disorder)

Diarrhea: loose, watery stools that occur more than three times a day occur because digestive products move through the large intestine too rapidly for sufficient water reabsorp-

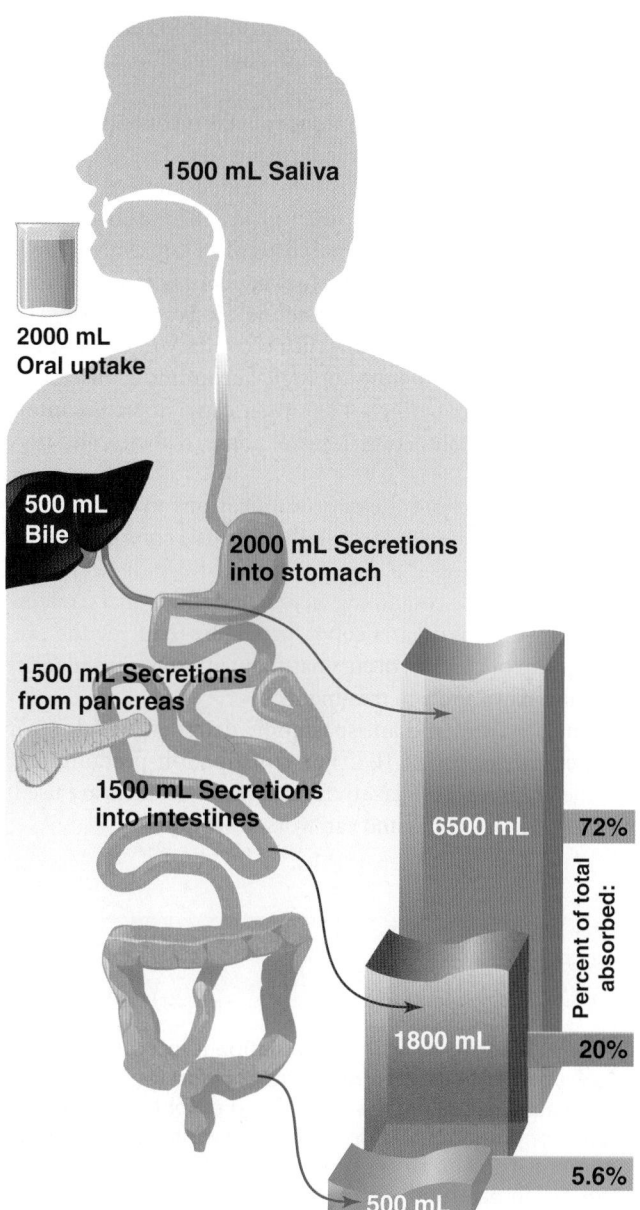

FIGURE 3.17 ■ Estimated daily volumes of water that enter the small and large intestines of a sedentary adult and the volumes absorbed by each component of the intestinal tract. (From Gisolfi CV, Lamb DR, eds. *Perspectives in Exercise and Sports Medicine: Fluid Homeostasis During Exercise.* Indianapolis: Benchmark Press, 1990.)

tion. The condition represents a symptom of increased peristalsis (perhaps caused by stress), intestinal irritation or damage, medication side effects, and intolerance to gluten (a protein in some wheat products).

Distance runners and female athletes are most susceptible to diarrhea and IBS. Possible causative factors include fluid and electrolyte imbalance and altered colonic motility. Fortunately, acute exercise-induced diarrhea, also known as "runner's trots," is considered physiologic diarrhea that does not produce dehydration or electrolyte imbalances and tends to improve with fitness level. In healthy athletes, acute diar-

rhea is either induced by running, food poisoning, traveler's diarrhea, or viral gastroenteritis and is typically self-limited.

Prolonged diarrhea can produce dehydration, particularly in children and those of small body size. In general, a diet of broth, tea, toast, and other low-fiber foods, and the avoidance of lactose, fructose, caffeine, and sugar alcohols, help to reduce diarrhea. Potassium-rich foods are also helpful.

Diverticulosis

Common in older individuals, the colon develops small pouches that bulge outward through weak spots, a condition known as **diverticulosis** (see FIG. 3.18). This condition afflicts about half of all Americans aged 60 to 80 years and almost everyone over 80 years of age. In about 10 to 25 % of these people, the pouches become infected or inflamed (diverticulitis). Diverticulosis and diverticulitis are common in industrialized countries where individuals typically consume low-fiber diets; it rarely occurs in countries where people routinely eat high-fiber, vegetable-based diets (e.g., Asia and Africa).

Gastroesophageal Reflux Disease and Heartburn

Heartburn occurs when the sphincter between the esophagus and stomach relaxes (involuntarily), allowing the stomach's contents to flow back into the esophagus. Unlike the stomach, the esophagus has no protective mucous lining so acid backflow can damage it and quickly cause pain. For many people,

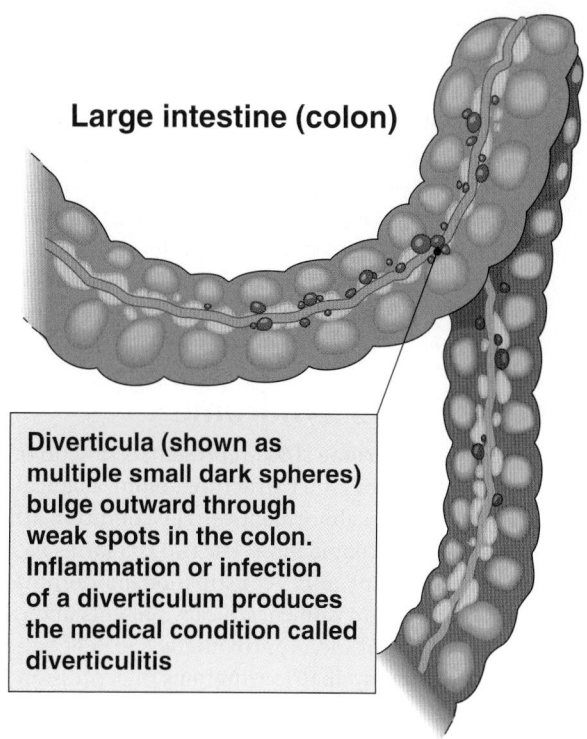

FIGURE 3.18 ■ Diverticulosis is common among older people, particularly those who consume a diet with inadequate fiber.

chronic heartburn represents a more serious disorder called **gastroesophageal disease** or **GERD**.

GERD occurs in approximately 60% of athletes and more frequently during exercise than at rest. Exercise not only exacerbates GERD, but it also contributes to reflux in healthy volunteers. Although the precise causative mechanisms are not well defined, either the isolated effects of exercise or the combined effects of several physiologic alterations with exercise contribute to acid reflux during physical activity. Suggested mechanisms related to exercise include gastric dysmotility, relaxation of the lower esophageal sphincter, enhanced pressure gradient between the stomach and esophagus, gastric distension, delayed gastric emptying (especially in a dehydrated state), enhanced intra-abdominal pressure in football, weight-lifting, and cycling and increased mechanical stress by the bouncing of organs related to GI function.

Athletes involved in predominantly anaerobic sports such as weight-lifting experience the most frequent heartburn and gastric reflux; compared with weight-lifters, runners have mild symptoms and moderate reflux and cyclists have mild symptoms and mild reflux.

Exercise-related GERD symptoms include substernal chest pressure, pain or burning that mimics angina, sour taste, eructation (the voiding of gas or a small quantity of acid fluid from the stomach through the mouth), nausea, and vomiting. A subset of athletes may present with atypical cough, hoarseness, and wheezing—symptoms that mimic either exercise-induced bronchospasm or vocal cord dysfunction.

Effective lifestyle modifications remain the treatment of choice for athletes with GERD. These include avoidance of (1) trying to sleep within 4 hours of the evening meal, (2) postprandial exercise, and (3) excessive consumption of foods such as chocolate, peppermint, onions, high-fat foods, alcohol, tobacco, coffee, and citrus products that relax the lower esophageal sphincter. Sleeping on two pillows to enhance gravity-associated esophageal clearance often reduces GERD symptoms. Athletes treated with calcium-channel blockers for migraine headaches or to control hypertension should be counseled on the propensity for these drugs to worsen GERD symptoms. GERD coupled with obesity are key risk factors for esophageal cancer.

Irritable Bowel Syndrome

Irritable Bowel Syndrome (IBS) represents a functional GI tract disorder devoid of either structural, biomechanical, radiologic, or laboratory abnormalities. The condition afflicts up to 20% of the adult population. The two IBS forms include "diarrhea-predominant" and "constipation-predominant." IBS, twice as common in women, typically presents in the second or third decade of life. Approximately 50% of patients with IBS also report psychiatric symptoms of depression and anxiety.

Causes of IBS include eight factors: (1) increased GI motor reactivity to various stimuli such as stress, (2) food, (3) cholecystokinin (a peptide hormone responsible for stimulating fat and protein digestion), (4) impaired transit of bowel gas, (5) visceral hypersensitivity, (6) impaired reflex control that delays gas transit, (7) autonomic dysfunction, and (8) altered immune activation.

The most common symptoms of IBS include these four factors: (1) cramping abdominal pain relieved by defecation, (2) altered stool frequency, (3) form (mucus, watery, hard, or loose), and passage (strain, urgency, a sense of incomplete evacuation), and (4) abdominal distension especially following meals. Athletes with IBS rarely experience nocturnal symptoms and do not manifest systemic signs of illness. The diagnosis for IBS includes diarrhea secondary to celiac sprue (a genetic, inheritable immunologic autoimmune disease of the small bowel that afflicts 4700 Americans) or lactose intolerance, thyroid dysfunction, laxative abuse, diabetes, and psychiatric illnesses.

Four lifestyle and dietary modifications that effectively counter IBS include: (1) stress reduction, (2) consumption of small meals during the day, (3) a high-fiber diet, and (4) avoidance of foods containing lactose and candy that contains sorbitol (6-carbon sugar alcohol formed by reducing the carbonyl group of glucose; occurs naturally in fruits). Regular exercise also plays a role in treating IBS.

Antidiarrheal and antispasmodic drugs effectively treat diarrhea-predominant IBS. For constipation-predominant IBS, dietary fiber, bulk laxatives, and stool softeners are used, but their efficacy varies and can worsen symptoms.

Helicobacter pylori Bacterium: Half of the World Infected

Over half of the world's population is infected with a type of bacterium, *Helicobacter pylori* (or *H. pylori*), that causes ulcers in the stomach and esophagus, a long-term condition that associates with gastric cancer development. The end result of *H. pylori* infection promotes the rise in destructive compounds (superoxide radicals) that attack cells of the stomach's protective mucosal lining. Within a few days of infection, gastritis and eventually peptic ulcer occur. The classic sign of a peptic ulcer is a gnawing, burning pain in the upper abdomen. Other symptoms include a dull, gnawing ache that comes and goes over several days, and pain that occurs 2 to 3 hours following a meal (previously relieved by eating) and responds to antacid medications. Other symptoms can include weight loss, poor appetite, excessive burping, bloating, and vomiting. It may not be *H. pylori* itself that causes peptic ulcer, but inflammation of the mucosal lining in peptic ulcer that represents a response to *H. pylori*. Researchers believe that *H. pylori* is transmitted orally by means of fecal matter contained in tainted food or water. Possible transmission could also occur from the stomach to the mouth through gastroesophageal reflux (a small amount of the stomach's contents is involuntarily forced into the esophagus) or belching—common symptoms of gastritis. The bacterium can then be transmitted through oral contact.

Gas

Swallowing air while eating or drinking commonly produces stomach **gas.** A person can take in an excess of air while eating or drinking rapidly, chewing gum, and smoking. Burping or belching is the most common way for most of the swallowed air to leave the stomach. Any remaining gas moves into the small intestine and becomes partially absorbed. A small amount of air travels into the large intestine for release through the rectum. Rectal gas is seldom a symptom of serious disease. Flatus (lower tract intestinal gas) composition depends to a great extent on nutrient intake (carbohydrates produce the most gas, fats and protein the least) and the colon's bacterial population. In the large intestine, bacteria partially break down undigested carbohydrate to produce hydrogen, carbon dioxide, and in about 30% of the population, methane gas. These gases eventually exit through the rectum. The amount and type of gastrointestinal bacteria largely determines variation in the quantity of colonic gas production among individuals.

Carbohydrates that commonly cause gas production include raffinose and stachyose (found in beans), fructose (found in soft drinks and fruit drinks), lactose, and sorbitol (artificial sweetener). Other gas-producing starches include potatoes, corn, noodles, and wheat products. Rice contains the only starch that does not cause abdominal or colonic gas. The fiber in oat bran, beans, peas, and most fruits causes gas. In contrast, fiber in wheat bran and some vegetables passes essentially unchanged through the intestinal tract, producing little if any abdominal gas.

Functional Dyspepsia

Functional dyspepsia refers to chronic pain in the upper abdomen without obvious physical cause. It produces vague GI symptoms, including gnawing or burning in the stomach, epigastric pain, nausea, vomiting, belching, bloating, indigestion, and generalized abdominal discomfort. The three most common causes for dyspepsia include peptic ulcer disease, GERD, and gastritis (inflammation of the lining of the stomach that leads to pain). Other less common causes include diabetes, thyroid disease, lactose intolerance, frequent dehydration, repeated stress of sports competition, excessive use of nonsteroidal anti-inflammatory drugs (NSAIDs) and alcohol and caffeine products. Dietary supplements with amino acids and creatine may further exacerbate mucosal injury and eventually lead to blood loss and anemia.

Lifestyle modifications to treat GERD represent the treatment of choice for dyspepsia. Also, avoidance of NSAIDs, caffeine, tobacco, gas-producing foods, and dairy products in individuals with lactose intolerance generally helps to alleviate most symptoms.

ACUTE GASTROENTERITIS: BACTERIAL AND VIRAL INDUCED

Only a few GI illnesses associate with travel, yet athletes show particular susceptibility to travel-induced **acute gastroenteritis** from bacterial and viral causes. Acute gastroenteritis typically presents with fever, nausea, vomiting, diarrhea, and cramping. Acute outbreaks have occurred in athletic populations during competitions where athletes from different countries congregate and share food, bathroom facilities, and sleeping quarters. Athletes with acute gastroenteritis, particularly those involved in contact sports, should not participate in practices and competition until they have been adequately treated, are without fever, and are hemodynamically stable. To prevent contamination and spread of the illness, the fundamental importance of good hygiene (especially frequent washing of hands with hot water and soap) must be practiced.

Case Study

Personal Health and Exercise Nutrition 3–1

Fundamentals of Nutritional Assessment: Applying Analysis Skills

Nutritional assessment evaluates an individual's nutritional status and nutrient requirements on the basis of interpretation of clinical information from different sources. Examples include diet history, medical history, review of symptoms, and physical examination, including anthropometric and laboratory data. Purposes of nutritional assessment include defining current nutritional status, determining levels of nutritional support, and monitoring changes in nutrient intake from a particular intervention program.

Nutritional deficiency usually develops over time, starting at a young age and then progressing in stages. An overt deficiency often remains unrecognized until the condition passes the individual's "clinical horizon" and moves into a disease state or becomes manifested by acute trauma (e.g., heart attack or type 2 diabetes complications). Nutritional assessment during any developmental stage of deficiency provides the basis for identifying a problem area and planning a prudent intervention.

Assessing Dietary Intake

Several different methods commonly provide dietary information:

24-HOUR DIETARY RECALL

This approach, usually a qualitative assessment by the individual or by another person, involves informal oral questioning about food and beverage intake during the previous 24 hours. The person recalls all foods and beverages consumed, starting from the last meal, and includes the approximate portion size and specifics of food preparation. This method is relatively easy, particularly when administered by a registered dietitian. Particular problems involve inaccuracy in quantity assessment and method of food preparation. This frequently produces gross underestimation of hidden fats (and hence calories) in such foods as sauces and dressings. Repeat 24-hour recalls that span several days provide a more accurate and reliable estimate of a typical day.

FOOD DIARY

With the food diary method, the individual records all foods and beverages at the time consumed (or as close to the time as possible). This approach also enables the recording of food by brand, weight, and portion size. Typically, the person maintains a food diary for 2 to 7 days. Assessment includes at least one weekend day because most people eat differently on the weekend than during a typical schoolday or workday. The method can become tedious; individuals when confronted with having to record everything eaten often change what they eat or eat nothing to avoid the hassle.

FOOD FREQUENCY ASSESSMENT

A food frequency questionnaire lists a variety of foods, and the individual estimates the frequency of consuming each item. This method does not itemize a specific day's intake; instead it provides a general picture of the typical food consumption pattern.

DIET HISTORY

A diet history yields general information about an individual's dietary patterns. Factors include eating habits (number of meals per day, who prepares meals, and patterns of food preparation), food preferences, eating locations, and typical food choices in different situations.

Analyzing Dietary Intake

A combination of methods proves more valid than a single method in developing a comprehensive dietary assessment. For a general picture of the adequacy of a person's dietary intake, compare the food record with an established guide for diet planning such as MyPyramid (see Chapter 7). Evaluate the energy and macronutrient and micronutrient content of the diet through food labels and food composition tables. The most comprehensive food database is the USDA Nutrient Database for Standard Reference Release 13, available at www.nal.usda.gov/fnic/foodcomp/Data/SR13/sr13.html. With most computer programs for diet analysis, one enters each food and the exact size of the portion consumed. Based on the input data, the program calculates the nutrients consumed for each day or provides an average over several days. In essence, a dietary analysis program compares nutrient intake to recommended values.

Medical History

PERSONAL MEDICAL HISTORY

Medical history includes immunizations, hospitalizations, surgeries, and acute and chronic injuries and illness—each of these has nutritional implications. History of prescriptions and the use of vitamin and mineral supplements, laxatives, topical medications, and herbal remedies (herbs and other supplements not typically identified as medications) also provide valuable information.

FAMILY MEDICAL AND SOCIAL HISTORY

Medical histories that include information about health/nutrition/exercise status of parents, siblings, children, and spouse reveal risk for chronic diseases that may have a genetic or social connection. Moreover, sociocultural relationships regarding food choices help in understanding individual eating patterns and practices. Information about duration and frequency of use of alcohol, tobacco, illicit drugs, and caffeine help to formulate a more effective treatment plan and assess risk for chronic diseases.

Physical Examination

Nutrition-oriented aspects of the physical examination focus on the mouth, skin, head, hair, eyes, mouth, fingernails, extremities, abdomen, skeletal musculature, and fat stores. Dry skin, cracked lips, or lethargy may indicate nutritional deficiencies. The accompanying table lists specific signs of vitamin or mineral deficiencies. Malnutrition often results from low calorie intake and protein deficiency. This produces a condition known as *marasmus,* which is characterized by severe tissue wasting, loss of subcutaneous fat, and usually dehydration. Marasmus typically occurs in individuals with anorexia nervosa (see Chapter 15).

ANTHROPOMETRIC DATA

Use of anthropometric data permits nutritional classification of individuals by categories ranging from undernourished to obese. Interpreting nutritional status involves comparing an individual with reference data from large numbers of healthy people of similar age and gender.

A typical nutritional assessment collects the following anthropometric data:

1. Height
2. Body weight
3. BMI (BW, kg $\div$ Ht^2,m): Normal BMI ranges between 19 and 25; individuals with a BMI of 25.1 to 29.9 are considered overweight, and BMIs of 30 and above classify as obese. BMI may not accurately reflect actual body fat content, but it has become a clinically acceptable "first approximation" measure of excess body weight.
4. Waist girth: Excess fat located in the abdominal area coincides with greater health risk. It most often occurs in individuals with type 2 diabetes, dyslipidemia, hypertension, and cardiovascular disease.

Clinical Signs and Symptoms of Nutritional Inadequacy

Organ	Sign/Symptom	Probable Cause
Skin	Pallor	Iron folate, vitamin B$_{12}$ deficiency
	Ecchymosis (purplish patch)	Vitamin K deficiency
	Pressure ulcers/delayed healing	Protein malnutrition
	Hair hyperkeratosis (excess eruption)	Vitamin A deficiency
	Petechiae (minute hemorrhagic spots)	Vitamin A, C, or K deficiency
	Purpura (hemorrhage into skin)	Vitamin C or K deficiency
	Rash/eczema/scaling	Zinc deficiency
Hair	Dyspigmentation, easy pluckability	Protein malnutrition
Head	Temporal muscle wasting	Protein-energy malnutrition
Eyes	Night blindness, xerosis (pathologic dryness)	Vitamin A deficiency
Mouth	Bleeding gum	Vitamin C, riboflavin deficiency
	Tongue fissuring (splitting), raw tongue, tongue atrophy (wasting)	Niacin, riboflavin deficiency
Heart	Tachycardia	Thiamin deficiency
Genital/ urinary	Delayed puberty	Protein-energy malnutrition
Extremities	Bone softening	Vitamin D, calcium, phosphorous
	Bone/joint aches	Vitamin C deficiency
	Edema	Protein deficiency
	Muscle wasting	Protein-energy malnutrition
	Ataxia	Vitamin B$_{12}$ deficiency
Neurologic	Tetany (muscle twitches, cramps)	Calcium, magnesium deficiency
	Paresthesia (abnormal sensation)	Thiamin deficiency
	Loss of reflexes, wrist/foot drop	Thiamin, vitamin B$_{12}$ deficiency
	Dementia	Niacin deficiency

Case Study *continued*

The easily measured waist girth provides an independent predictor of disease risk and correlates reasonably well with the more difficult assessment of total abdominal fat. For individuals whose BMI exceeds 35, waist girth provides little additional risk information because a BMI this large already indicates severe risk. Waist girth becomes particularly useful for individuals with a family history of diabetes and who exhibit borderline excess weight. Waist girths above 102 cm (40 inches) in men and 88 cm (35 inches) in women indicate increased disease risk.

5. Percentage weight change—If personal history information reveals a body weight change, compute percentage weight change as follows:

Percentage weight change = (usual weight − current weight ÷ usual weight) × 100

6. Triceps skinfold (TSF)—In nutritional assessment, TSF indicates excess energy stored as subcutaneous fat. A TSF above the 95th percentile for age and gender indicates obesity.

LABORATORY DATA

Measures of nutrients or their by-products in body cells or fluids (blood or urine) often detect nutrient deficiencies or excesses. Typical laboratory measures include serum albumin to indicate total body protein status and liver and renal disease; serum transferrin to assess protein balance and iron status; serum prealbumin to show protein status and liver disease; and concentrations of sodium, potassium, chloride, phosphorus, and magnesium to reflect overall mineral status. Other valuable laboratory tests that diagnose selected clinical conditions related to nutrition include iron and hemoglobin, zinc, cholesterol, triacylglycerol, the different lipid subfractions (HDL, LDL, and VLDL), and glucose.

Applying Critical Analysis Skills

1. Keep a food diary of everything you eat for 3 days including one weekend day. Prepare a form that contains the following headings:

Food or Beverage	Kind/How Prepared	Amount
_____	_____	_____
_____	_____	_____

2. Record your food as you eat without relying on memory at a later time. Increase accuracy with the following guidelines:

a. Be specific when recording food intake; record size, type (chicken leg vs thigh), and amount (oz, tsp.).
b. Record the method of preparation (i.e., baked vs fried; peeled vs not peeled; skinless vs with skin).
c. Include items like butter, ketchup, and salad dressing.
d. Include all deserts and toppings.
e. If you eat out, indicate where.
f. If you eat mixed dishes, break them down into component ingredients. For example, a chicken sandwich might be listed as 2 slices of white bread, 1 tablespoon of mayonnaise, and 3 ounces of skinless chicken breast.

3. Construct the following form to assess the adequacy of your diet versus MyPyramid:

Food	Quantity	MyPyramid Group	Number of Servings
_____	_____	_____	_____
_____	_____	_____	_____

4. Answer the following questions:

a. How many servings from each MyPyramid food group did you consume?
b. Does your diet meet MyPyramid guidelines (see Chapter 7). If not, what changes must you make to bring your diet more in line with these guidelines?
c. Compare and contrast your nutrient intake with DRIs for your age and gender on pages 53–54 and 61–62.
d. Suppose you consumed two (about 200 kCal each) plain doughnuts extra each day (above your current energy balance). How much extra weight would you gain in 6 months? How much in 12 months? 36 months? What specific additional energy expenditure (with specific exercise examples) would you need to offset this weight gain?
e. List and discuss specific changes you need to make in your energy and nutrient intake to improve your health profile.

Evans-Stoner N. Nutritional assessment: a practical approach. Nurs Clin North Am 1997;32:637.

Johansson L, et al. Under- and over-reporting of energy intake related to weight status and lifestyle in a nationwide sample. Am J Clin Nutr 1998;68:266.

Mascarenas MR, et al. Nutritional assessment in pediatrics. Nutrition 1998;14:105.

Summary

1. Digestion hydrolyzes complex molecules into simpler substances for absorption. Self-regulating processes within the digestive tract largely control the liquidity, mixing, and transit time of the digestive mixture.

2. Physically altering food in the mouth makes it easier to swallow, while at the same time increasing its accessibility to enzymes and other digestive substances. Swallowing transfers the food mixture to the esophagus, where peristaltic action forces it into the stomach.

3. In the stomach, food contents mix as hydrochloric acid and enzymes continue the breakdown process. Little absorption occurs in the stomach except for some water and alcohol and aspirin.

4. The enzyme salivary α-amylase degrades starch to smaller linked glucose molecules and simpler disaccharides in the mouth. In the duodenum of the small intestine, pancreatic amylase continues carbohydrate hydrolysis into smaller chains of glucose molecules and simple monosaccharides.

5. Enzyme action on the surfaces of the intestinal lumen's brush border completes the final stage of carbohydrate digestion to simple monosaccharides.

6. Lipid digestion begins in the mouth and stomach by action of lingual lipase and gastric lipase, respectively. The major lipid breakdown occurs in the small intestine by the emulsifying action of bile and the hydrolytic action of pancreatic lipase.

7. Medium-chain triacylglycerol rapidly absorbs into the portal vein bound to glycerol and medium-chain free fatty acids.

8. Once absorbed by the intestinal mucosa, long-chain fatty acids reform into triacylglycerols. They then form small fatty droplets called chylomicrons. These substances move slowly through the lymphatic system to eventually empty into the venous blood of the systemic circulation.

9. The enzyme pepsin initiates protein digestion in the stomach. The final steps in protein digestion occur in the small intestine, most notably under the action of the enzyme trypsin.

10. Vitamin absorption occurs mainly by the passive process of diffusion in the jejunum and ileum portions of the small intestine.

11. The large intestine serves as the final path for water and electrolyte absorption, including storage of undigested food residue (feces).

12. Many factors influence gastrointestinal (GI) function. The brain exerts a strong influence on the GI tract through diverse neurochemical connections with digestive organs.

13. Individuals who engage in frequent, high-intensity exercise report GI symptoms that include self-limited food poisoning, gastroesophageal reflux disease (GERD), hiatal hernia, irritable bowel syndrome (IBS), and viral gastroenteritis.

14. The most common GI tract disorders include constipation, diarrhea, diverticulosis, GERD, IBS, and excessive gas production.

Test Your Knowledge Answers

1. **False:** For many foods, digestion begins during cooking when protein structures break down, starch granules swell, and vegetables fibers soften. But for the most part, food breakdown begins in the mouth, where mechanical digestion increases the surface area of the food particles, making them easier to swallow and more accessible to enzymes and other digestive substances that start the breakdown process. For example, the enzyme salivary α-amylase (ptyalin) attacks starch and reduces it to smaller linked glucose molecules and the simpler disaccharide form maltose. Lipid digestion also begins in the mouth by the action of lingual lipase.

2. **True:** The colon is the division of the large intestine extending from the cecum to the rectum. It comprises the ascending colon (portion between the ileocecal orifice and the right colic flexure), descending colon (portion that extends from the left colic flexure to the pelvic brim), transverse colon (portion between the right and left colic flexures), and sigmoid colon (S-shaped final portion of colon that is continuous with the rectum).

3. **False:** The liver, pancreas, and gallbladder play key roles in the process of digesting and assimilating food nutrients, but they are not structures through which the nutrients pass directly during the digestive process.

4. **True:** Glucose and galactose absorb from the small intestine into the blood against a concentration gradient; thus energy must be expended to power absorption of additional glucose across the intestinal mucosa. Absorption occurs by a sodium-dependent, carrier-mediated active transport process. The electrochemical gradient created with sodium transport augments absorption of these monosaccharides. In contrast, the low concentration of fat in intestinal cells allows for passive absorption of these molecules.

5. **False:** Active transport of nutrients across cell membranes requires the expenditure of cellular energy from ATP. This process occurs when a substance cannot be transported by one of the four passive transport processes.

6. **False:** With the exception of some water and alcohol and aspirin, no nutrient absorption takes place in any portion of the stomach.

7. **True:** Approximately 90% of digestion (and essentially all lipid digestion) and absorption occurs in the first two sections of the 3-m long small intestine. This coiled structure consists of three sections: the duodenum (first 0.3 m), jejunum (next 1–2 m, where most of digestion occurs), and ileum (last 1.5 m).

8. **False:** Starch hydrolysis begins as food enters the mouth. The salivary glands continually secrete lubricating mucous substances that combine with food particles during chewing. The enzyme salivary α-amylase (ptyalin) attacks starch and reduces it to smaller linked glucose molecules and the disaccharide maltose. When the food–saliva mixture enters the more acidic stomach, some additional starch breakdown occurs, but this quickly ceases because salivary amylase deactivates under the low pH of stomach's gastric juices.

9. **False:** Consuming excessive dietary fiber produces an overly soft stool, whereas inadequate fiber intake compacts the stool, making it more difficult to expel through the rectum. Extreme pressure during defecation can damage supporting tissues and expose blood vessels in the rectum (hemorrhoids). Gradually increasing the diet's fiber content often relieves constipation and hemorrhoid symptoms.

10. **False:** In genzeral, hydrolysis reactions digest or break down complex molecules into simpler subunits, and condensation reactions build larger molecules by bonding their subunits together. Hydrolysis catabolizes complex organic molecules—carbohydrates, lipids, and proteins—to simpler forms that the body absorbs and assimilates. During this basic decomposition process, chemical bonds are split by addition of hydrogen ions (H^+) and hydroxyl ions (OH^-), the constituents of water, to the reaction byproducts. Examples of hydrolytic reactions include the digestion of starches and disaccharides to monosaccharides, proteins to amino acids, and lipids to glycerol and fatty acids. In contrast to hydrolysis reactions, reactions of condensation occur in the opposite direction and bind together the structural components of the nutrients to form more complex molecules and compounds.

General References

Boyle M. *Personal Nutrition*. 4th ed. Belmont, CA: Wadsworth Publishing, 2001.

Brody T. *Nutritional Biochemistry*. 2nd ed. New York: Academic Press, 1999.

Brown J. *Nutrition Now*. 5th ed. Belmont, CA: Wadsworth Publishing, 2007.

Campbell MK, Farrell SO. *Biochemistry*. 5th ed. Philadelphia: WB Saunders, 2005.

Emken EA. Metabolism of dietary stearic acid relative to other fatty acids in human subjects. *Am J Clin Nutr* 1994;60(suppl):1023S.

Fox SI. *Human Physiology*. 10th ed. New York: McGraw-Hill, 2007.

Groff JL, Gropper SS. *Advanced Nutrition and Human Metabolism*. 4th ed. Belmont, CA: Thomson Learning, 2004.

Guyton AC, et al. *Textbook of Medical Physiology*. 11th ed. Philadelphia: WB Saunders, 2005.

Kraut J. How do enzymes work? *Science* 1988;242:533.

Mahan LK, Escott-Stump S. *Krause's Food, Nutrition, & Diet Therapy*. Philadelphia: WB Saunders, 2004.

Marieb EN. *Essentials of Human Anatomy and Physiology*. 8th ed. Menlo Park, CA: Pearson Education: Benjamin Cummings, 2005.

Powers HJ. Riboflavin (vitamin B-2) and Health. *Am J Clin Nutr* 2003;77:1352.

Shils ME, et al. *Modern Nutrition in Health and Disease*. 10th ed. Baltimore: Lippincott Williams & Wilkins, 2005.

Vander AJ, et al. *Human Physiology: the Mechanisms of Body Function*. 8th ed. New York: McGraw-Hill, 2001.

Whitney EN, et al. *Understanding Nutrition*. Stamford, CT: Thomson/Wadsworth, 2007.

Stanfield CL, Germann WJ. *Principles of Human Physiology*. 3rd ed. Menlo Park, CA: Pearson Education: Benjamin Cummings, 2006.

Stipanuk M. *Biochemical, Physiological and Molecular Aspects of Human Nutrition*. 2nd ed. Philadelphia: WB Saunders, 2006.

Additional Readings

Bi L, Triadafilopoulos G. Exercise and gastrointestinal function and disease: an evidence-based review of risks and benefits. *Clin Gastroenterol Hepatol* 2003;1:345.

Casey E, et al. Training room management of medical conditions: sports gastroenterology. *Clin Sports Med* 2005;24:525.

Chan MA, et al. Influence of carbohydrate ingestion on cytokine responses following acute resistance exercise. *Int J Sport Nutr Exerc Metab* 2003;13:454.

Collings KL, et al. Esophageal reflux in conditioned runners, cyclists, and weightlifters. *Med Sci Sports Exerc* 2003;35:730.

Jeanes YM, et al. The absorption of vitamin E is influenced by the amount of fat in a meal and the food matrix. *Br J Nutr* 2004;92:575.

Lancaster GI, et al. Effect of pre-exercise carbohydrate ingestion on plasma cytokine, stress hormone, and neutrophil degranulation responses to continuous, high-intensity exercise. *Int J Sport Nutr Exerc Metab* 2003;13:436.

Lustyk MK, Jarrett ME, Bennett JC, et al. Does a physically active lifestyle improve symptoms in women with irritable bowel syndrome? *Gastroenterol Nurs* 2001;24:129.

Moses FM. The effect of exercise on the gastrointestinal tract. *Sports Med* 1990;9:159.

Peters HP, et al. Potential benefits and hazards of physical activity and exercise on the gastrointestinal tract. *Gut* 2001;48:435.

Rao KA, et al. Objective evaluation of small bowel and colonic transit time using pH telemetry in athletes with gastrointestinal symptoms. *Br J Sports Med* 2004;38:482.

Sanchez LD, et al. Ischemic colitis in marathon runners: a case-based review. *J Emerg Med* 2006;30:321.

Van Nieuwenhoven MA, et al. Gastrointestinal profile of symptomatic athletes at rest and during physical exercise. *Eur J Appl Physiol* 2004;91:429.

Vuorilehto K, et al. Indirect electrochemical reduction of nicotinamide coenzymes. *Bioelectrochemistry* 2004;65:1.

Wade TJ, et al. Rapidly measured indicators of recreational water quality are predictive of swimming-associated gastrointestinal illness. *Environ Health Perspect* 2006;114:24.

Williams C, Serratosa L. Nutrition on match day. *J Sports Sci* 2006;24:687.

Part 2

Nutrient Bioenergetics in Exercise and Training

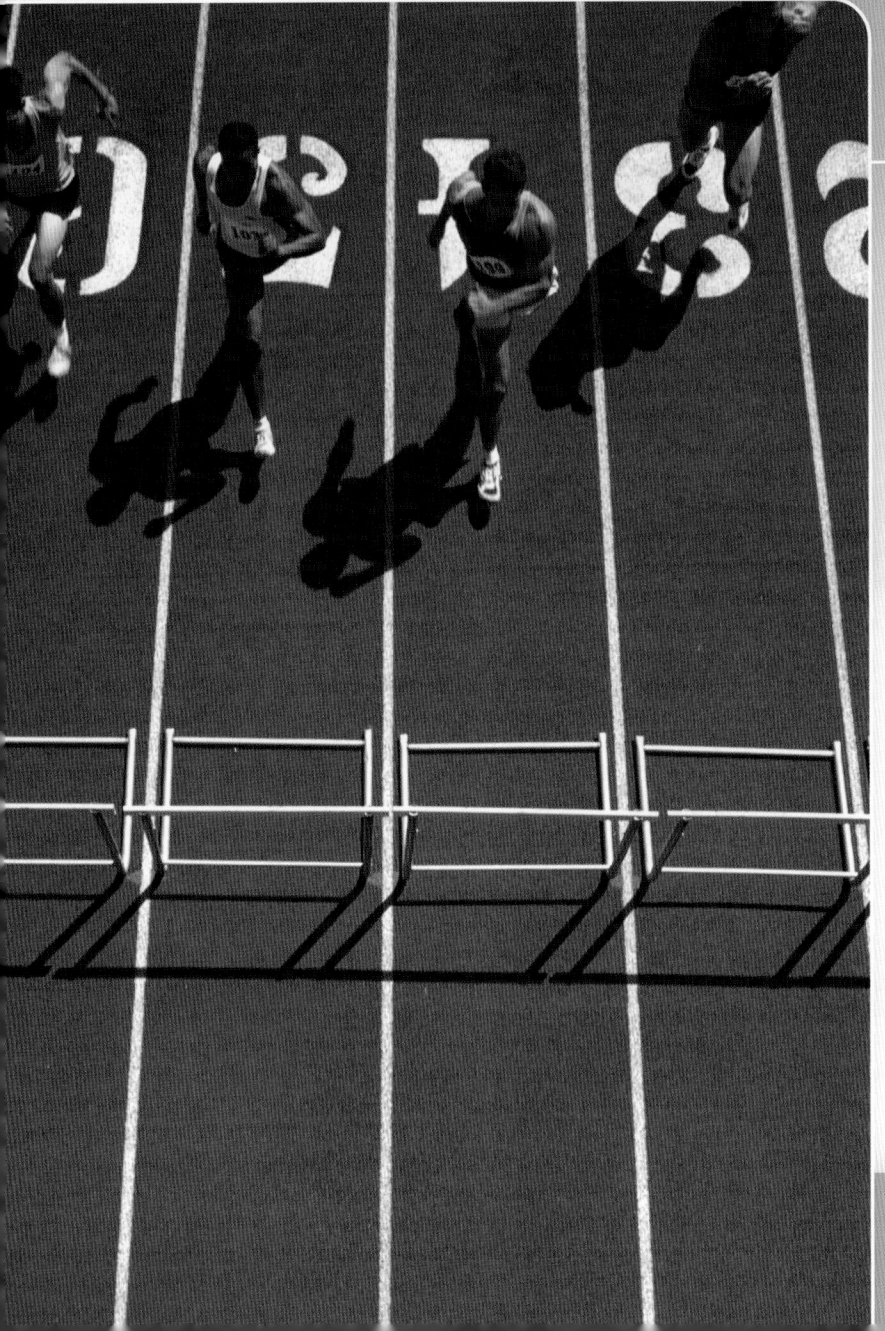

Chapter 4

Nutrient Role in Bioenergetics

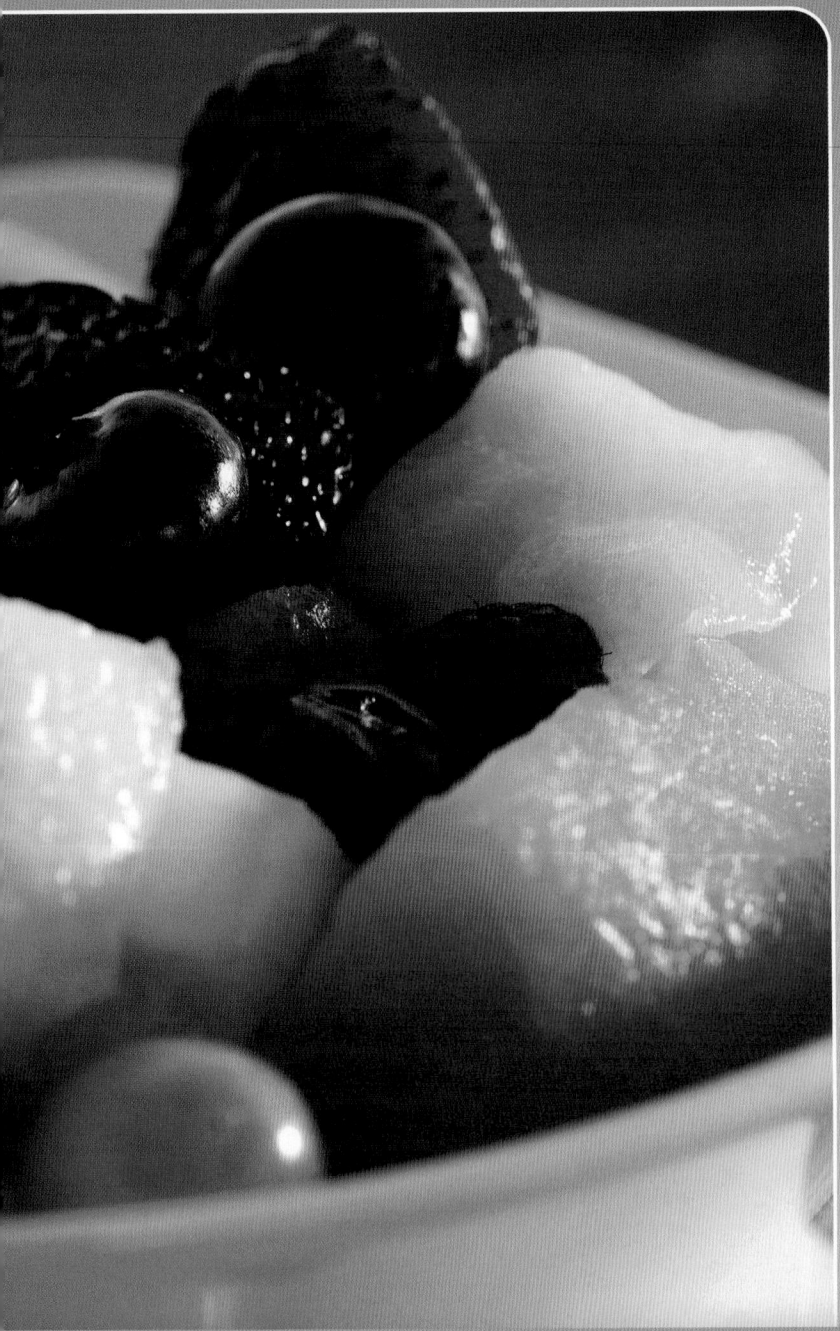

Test Your Knowledge

Answer these 10 statements about nutrient bioenergetics. Use the scoring key at the end of the chapter to check your results. Repeat this test after you have read the chapter and compare your results.

1. **T F** Carbohydrates are used for energy and stored as glycogen in the liver and muscles. They also readily convert to fat for storage in adipose tissue.
2. **T F** Lipids are used for energy and stored as fat. Fatty acids also readily convert to carbohydrate.
3. **T F** An enzyme is an inorganic, nonprotein compound that catalyzes chemical reactions in the body.
4. **T F** Excessive protein intake does not contribute to body fat accumulation because of lack of the enzymes to facilitate this conversion.
5. **T F** ATP forms only from the breakdown of the glycerol and fatty acid components of the triacylglycerol molecule.
6. **T F** The first law of thermodynamics refers specifically to the process of photosynthesis.
7. **T F** Oxidation and reduction refer to the conversion of oxygen into useful energy.
8. **T F** Energy is defined as the ability to perform work.
9. **T F** The main role for oxygen in the body is to combine with ADP in the synthesis of ATP.
10. **T F** The total net energy yield from the complete breakdown of a molecule of glucose is 40 ATPs.

U nderstanding each macronutrient's role in energy metabolism becomes crucial to optimizing the interaction between food intake and storage and exercise performance. No nutritional "magic bullets" exist per se, yet the quantity and blend of the daily diet's macronutrients profoundly affect exercise capacity, training response, and overall health.

A useful analogy shows how a car and the human body both obtain energy to make them "go." In an automobile engine, igniting the proper mixture of gasoline fuel with oxygen provides the energy required to drive the pistons. Gears and linkages harness the energy to turn the wheels; increasing or decreasing energy release either speeds up or slows down the engine. Similarly, the human body continuously extracts the energy from its fuel nutrients and harnesses it to perform its many complex biologic functions. Besides expending considerable energy for muscle action during physical activity, the body also expends energy for other "quieter" forms of biologic work including:

- Digestion, absorption, and assimilation of food nutrients
- Glandular function that secretes hormones at rest and exercise
- Maintenance of electrochemical gradients along cell membranes for proper neuromuscular function
- Synthesis of new chemical compounds such as thick and thin protein structures in skeletal muscle tissue that enlarge with resistance training

NUTRITION–ENERGY INTERACTION

Bioenergetics refers to the flow of energy within a living system. The body's capacity to extract energy from food nutrients and transfer it to the contractile elements in skeletal muscle determines capacity to swim, run, bicycle, and ski long distances at high intensity. Energy transfer occurs through thousands of complex chemical reactions using a balanced mixture of macro- and micronutrients and a continual supply and use of oxygen. The term **aerobic** describes such oxygen-requiring energy reactions. In contrast, **anaerobic** chemical reactions generate energy rapidly for short durations without oxygen. Rapid anaerobic energy transfer maintains a high standard of performance in maximal short-term efforts such as sprinting in track and swimming or repeated stop-and-go sports like soccer, basketball, lacrosse, water polo, volleyball, field hockey, and football, including the high power outputs generated during resistance training. The following point requires emphasis: *Anaerobic and aerobic breakdown of ingested food nutrients provides the energy source for synthesizing the chemical fuel that powers* all *forms of biologic work.*

Introduction to Energy Transfer

ENERGY: THE CAPACITY FOR WORK

Extracting energy from the stored macronutrients and ultimately transferring it to the contractile proteins of skeletal muscle greatly influences exercise performance. But unlike the physical properties of matter, energy cannot be defined in concrete terms of size, shape, or mass. Rather, motion plays a part in all forms of energy. This suggests a dynamic state related to change; thus, the presence of energy emerges only when a change occurs. Within this context, energy relates to the performance of work—as work increases so does energy transfer.

The First Law of Thermodynamics

The **first law of thermodynamics** describes one of the most important principles related to work within biologic systems. The basic tenet states that energy is neither created nor destroyed, but instead transforms from one state to another without being used up. In essence, this law describes the immutable principle of the **conservation of energy** that applies to both living and nonliving systems, first validated by chemists in the late 1890s. For example, the large amount of chemical energy "trapped" within the structure of fuel oil readily converts to heat energy in the home oil burner. In the body, chemical energy stored within the macronutrients' bonds does not immediately dissipate as heat. Rather, a large portion is conserved as chemical energy before changing into mechanical energy (and then ultimately to heat energy) by the musculoskeletal system. FIGURE 4.1 illustrates the interconversions for the six different forms of energy.

The Body Does Not Produce Energy

The first law of thermodynamics dictates that the body does not produce, consume, or use up energy; it merely transforms energy from one state to another as physiologic systems undergo continual change.

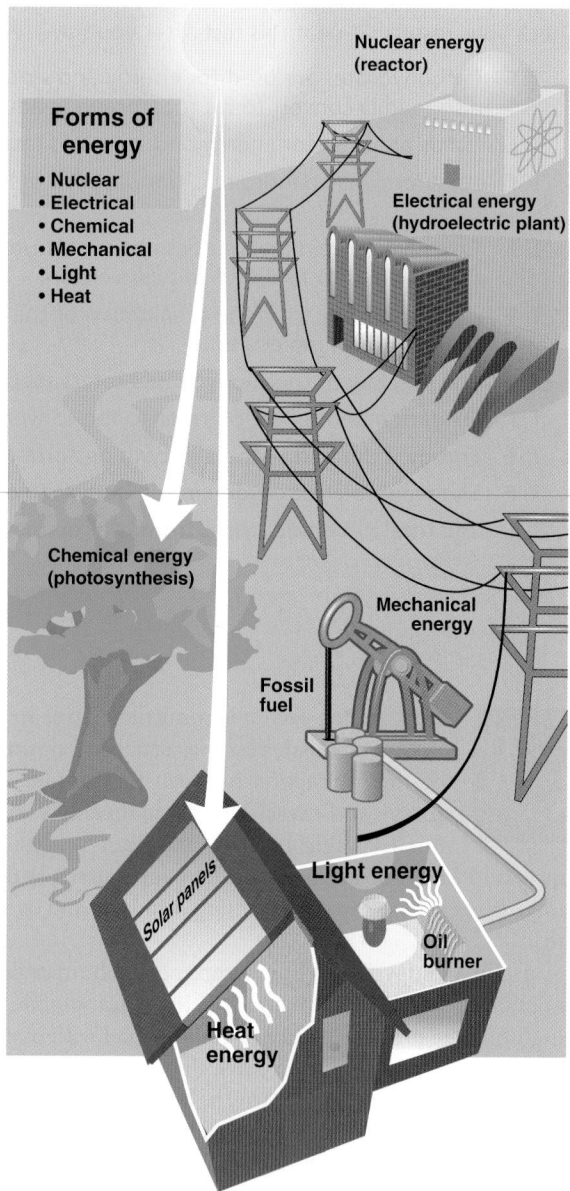

FIGURE 4.1 ■ Interconversions of the six forms of energy.

Photosynthesis and Respiration

Photosynthesis and respiration provide the most fundamental examples of energy conversion in living cells.

Photosynthesis

In the sun, nuclear fusion releases part of the potential energy stored in the nucleus of the hydrogen atom. This energy, in the form of gamma radiation, converts to radiant energy.

FIGURE 4.2 depicts **photosynthesis**. The plant pigment chlorophyll (contained in chloroplasts, the large organelles located in the leaf's cells) absorbs radiant (solar) energy to synthesize glucose from carbon dioxide and water while oxygen flows to the environment. Animals subsequently use glucose and oxygen during respiration. Plants also convert carbohydrates to lipids and proteins. Animals then ingest plant nutrients to serve their own energy needs. In essence, solar energy coupled with photosynthesis powers the animal world with food and oxygen.

Cellular Respiration

FIGURE 4.3 shows that the reactions of **respiration** are the reverse of photosynthesis, as animals recover the plant's stored energy for use in biologic work. During respiration, the chemical energy stored in glucose, lipid, or protein molecules is extracted in the presence of oxygen. A portion of energy re-

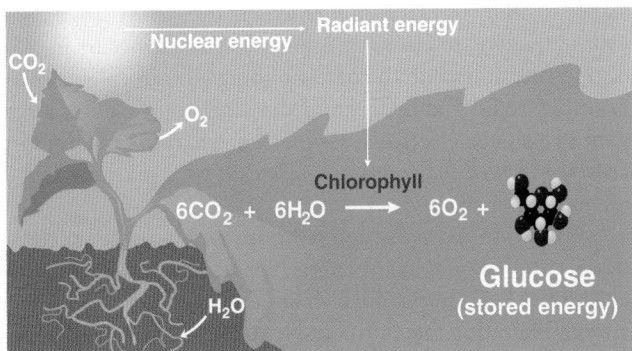

FIGURE 4.2 ■ Photosynthesis serves as the plant's mechanism for synthesizing carbohydrates, lipids, and proteins. In this example, a glucose molecule forms from the union of carbon dioxide and water.

mains in other chemical compounds that the body uses in diverse energy-requiring processes; the remaining energy flows as heat to the environment.

Biologic Work in Humans

Figure 4.3 also illustrates that biologic work takes one of three forms: (1) **mechanical work** of muscle contraction, (2) **chemical work** for synthesizing cellular molecules, and (3) **transport work** that concentrates diverse substances in the intracellular and extracellular fluids.

Mechanical Work

Mechanical work generated by muscle contraction provides the most obvious example of energy transformation. A muscle fiber's protein filaments directly convert chemical energy into mechanical energy. However, this does not represent the only form of mechanical work. In the cell nucleus, for example, contractile elements literally tug at the chromosomes to facilitate cell division. Specialized structures such as cilia also perform mechanical work in many cells.

Chemical Work

All cells perform chemical work for maintenance and growth. Continuous synthesis of cellular components occurs as other components break down. The extreme of muscle tissue synthesis from chronic overload in resistance training vividly illustrates this form of biologic work.

Transport Work

The biologic work of concentrating substances in the body (transport work) progresses much less conspicuously than mechanical or chemical work. Cellular materials normally flow from an area of high concentration to one of lower concentration. This passive process of diffusion requires no energy. For proper physiologic functioning, certain chemicals require transport uphill, against their normal concentration gradients from an area of lower to one of higher concentration. Active transport describes this energy-requiring process (see Chapter 3). Secretion and reabsorption in the kidney

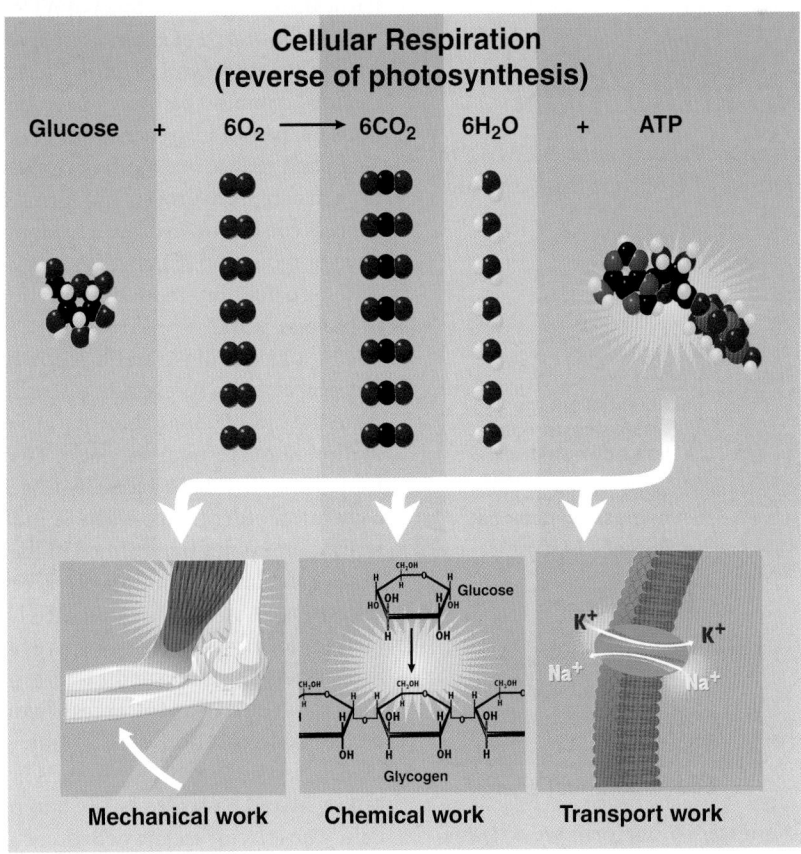

FIGURE 4.3 ■ Respiration harvests the potential energy in food to form adenosine triphosphate (ATP). The energy in ATP powers all forms of biologic work.

tubules use active transport mechanisms, as does neural tissue in establishing the proper electrochemical gradients about its plasma membranes. These "quiet" forms of biologic work require continual expenditure of stored chemical energy.

Potential and Kinetic Energy

Potential energy and kinetic energy constitute the total energy of any system. FIGURE 4.4 shows potential energy as energy of position similar to water at the top of a hill before it flows downstream.

In this example, energy changes proportionally to the water's vertical drop—the greater the vertical drop, the greater is the potential energy at the top. Other examples of potential energy include bound energy within the internal structure of a battery, a stick of dynamite, or a macronutrient before release of its stored energy through metabolism. *Releasing potential energy transforms it into kinetic energy of motion.* In some cases, bound energy in one substance directly transfers to other substances to increase their potential energy. Energy transfers of this type provide the necessary energy for the body's chemical work of biosynthesis. Specific building-block atoms of carbon, hydrogen, oxygen, and nitrogen join other atoms and molecules to synthesize important biologic compounds (e.g., cholesterol, enzymes, and hormones). Some newly created compounds serve structural needs of bone or the lipid-containing plasma membrane that encapsulates each cell. Other synthesized compounds such as adenosine triphosphate (ATP) and phosphocreatine (PCr) serve the cell's energy needs.

OXIDATION AND REDUCTION

Literally thousands of simultaneous chemical reactions occur in the body that involve transfer of electrons from one sub-

stance to another. *Oxidation reactions transfer oxygen atoms, hydrogen atoms, or electrons.* A loss of electrons occurs in oxidation reactions, with a corresponding gain in valence. For example, removing hydrogen from a substance yields a net gain of valence electrons. *Reduction reactions involve any process in which the atoms in an element gain electrons with a corresponding decrease in valence.*

Oxidation and reduction reactions are always characteristically **coupled,** so that any energy released by one reaction incorporates into the products of another reaction. In essence, energy-liberating reactions couple to energy-requiring reactions. The term **reducing agent** describes the substance that donates or loses electrons as it oxidizes. The substance being reduced or gaining electrons is called the electron acceptor or **oxidizing agent.** The term **redox** reaction describes a coupled oxidation–reduction reaction.

An excellent example of an oxidation reaction involves electron transfer within the mitochondria. Here, special carrier molecules transfer oxidized hydrogen atoms and their removed electrons for delivery to oxygen, which becomes reduced. The carbohydrate, lipid, and protein nutrient substrates provide the source of hydrogen. Dehydrogenase (oxidase) enzymes tremendously speed up redox reactions. Two hydrogen-accepting dehydrogenase coenzymes are the vitamin B–containing nicotinamide adenine dinucleotide (NAD^+), derived from the B vitamin niacin, and flavin adenine dinucleotide (FAD), derived from another B vitamin, riboflavin. Transferring electrons from NADH and $FADH_2$ harnesses energy in the form of ATP (see p. 133).

The transport of electrons by specific carrier molecules constitutes the **respiratory chain.** **Electron transport** represents the final common pathway in aerobic (oxidative) metabolism. For each pair of hydrogen atoms, two electrons flow down the chain and reduce one atom of oxygen. The process ends when oxygen accepts hydrogen and forms water. The coupled redox process constitutes hydrogen oxidation coupled to subsequent oxygen reduction. Chemical energy trapped or conserved in cellular oxidation–reduction reactions powers various forms of biologic work.

FIGURE 4.5 illustrates a redox reaction during vigorous physical activity. As exercise intensifies, hydrogen atoms strip from the carbohydrate substrate at a greater rate than their oxidation in the respiratory chain. To continue energy metabolism, the nonoxidized excess hydrogens must be "accepted" by a chemical other than oxygen. A molecule of pyruvate, an intermediate compound formed in the initial phase of carbohydrate catabolism, temporarily accepts a pair of hydrogens (electrons). A new compound called **lactic acid** (in the body as **lactate**) forms when reduced pyruvate accepts additional hydrogens. As illustrated in the figure, more intense exercise produces a greater flow of excess hydrogens to pyruvate, and lactate concentration rises rapidly within the active muscle. During recovery, excess hydrogens in lactate oxidize (electrons removed and passed to NAD^+) to re-form a pyruvate molecule. The enzyme lactate dehydrogenase (LDH) facilitates this reaction.

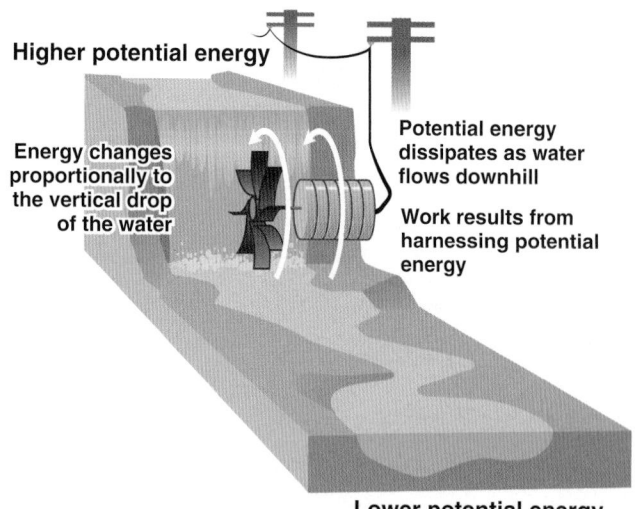

Higher potential energy

Energy changes proportionally to the vertical drop of the water

Potential energy dissipates as water flows downhill

Work results from harnessing potential energy

Lower potential energy

FIGURE 4.4 ■ Potential energy to perform work transforms into kinetic energy.

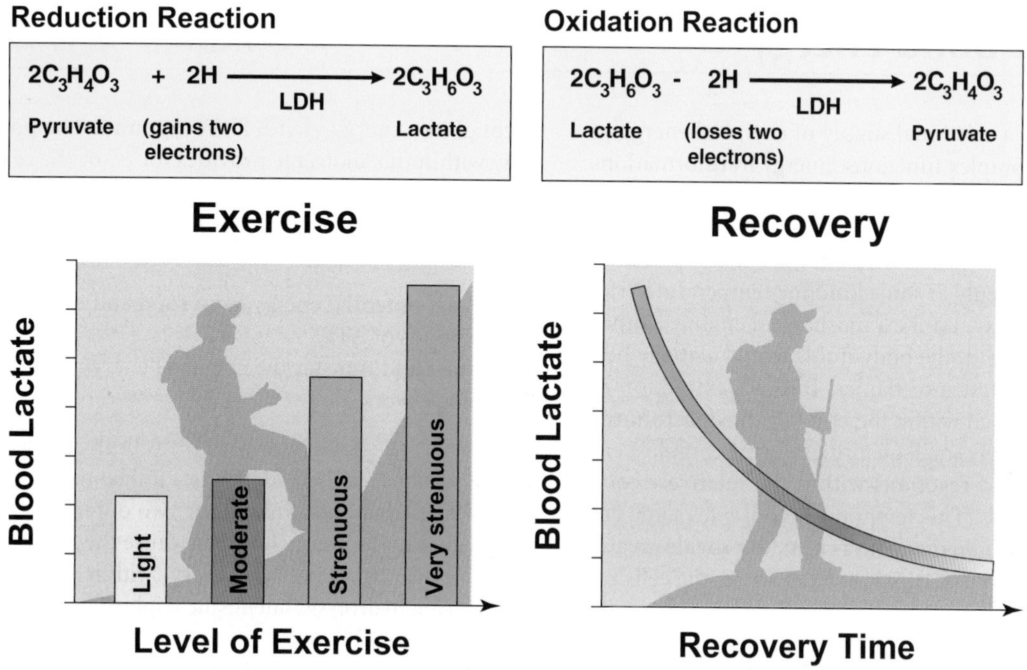

Reduction Reaction

$$2C_3H_4O_3 + 2H \xrightarrow{\text{LDH}} 2C_3H_6O_3$$

Pyruvate   (gains two   Lactate
            electrons)

Oxidation Reaction

$$2C_3H_6O_3 - 2H \xrightarrow{\text{LDH}} 2C_3H_4O_3$$

Lactate   (loses two   Pyruvate
           electrons)

Exercise

Recovery

FIGURE 4.5 ■ Example of a redox (oxidation–reduction) reaction. During progressively strenuous exercise when the oxygen supply becomes inadequate, some pyruvate formed in energy metabolism gains two hydrogens (gains two electrons) and becomes *reduced* to a new compound, lactate. In recovery, when oxygen supply becomes adequate, lactate loses two hydrogens (two electrons) and *oxidizes* back to pyruvate. LDH, lactate dehydrogenase.

Summary

1. Energy, defined as the ability to perform work, appears only when a change occurs.

2. Energy exists in either potential or kinetic form. Potential energy refers to energy associated with a substance's structure or position; kinetic energy refers to energy of motion. Potential energy can be measured when it transforms to kinetic energy.

3. There are six forms of interchangeable energy states—chemical, mechanical, heat, light, electrical, and nuclear—and each can convert or transform to another form.

4. In photosynthesis, plants transfer the energy of light into the potential energy of carbohydrates, lipids, and proteins. Respiration releases stored energy in plants and couples it to other chemical compounds for biologic work.

5. Biologic work takes one of three forms: chemical (biosynthesis of cellular molecules), mechanical (muscle contraction), or transport (transfer of substances among cells).

6. Oxidation–reduction (redox) reactions couple so oxidation (a substance loses electrons) coincides with the reverse reaction of reduction (a substance gains electrons). Redox reactions power the body's energy-transfer processes.

Phosphate Bond Energy

The body demands a continual supply of chemical energy to perform its many complex functions. Energy transformations in the body largely depend on (1) oxidation–reduction reactions and (2) chemical reactions that conserve and liberate the energy in ATP. Energy derived from the oxidation of food does not release suddenly at some kindling temperature (FIG. 4.6A) because the body, unlike a mechanical engine, cannot use heat energy. If it did, the body fluids would actually boil and tissues would burst into flames. Instead, extraction of chemical energy trapped within the bonds of the macronutrients releases in relatively small quantities during complex, enzymatically controlled reactions within the relatively cool, watery medium of cells. This temporarily conserves some energy that otherwise would dissipate as heat, to provide greater efficiency in energy transformations. In a sense, the cells receive energy as needed.

The story of how the body maintains its continuous energy supply begins with **adenosine triphosphate,** the body's special carrier for free energy.

ADENOSINE TRIPHOSPHATE: THE ENERGY CURRENCY

The energy in food does not transfer directly to the cells for biologic work. Instead, "macronutrient energy" funnels through the energy-rich ATP compound. The potential energy within this molecule provides for *all* of the cell's energy-requiring processes. In essence, this energy receiver–energy donor role of ATP represents the cells' two major energy-transforming activities:

1. Extract potential energy from food and conserve it within the bonds of ATP
2. Extract and transfer the chemical energy in ATP to power biologic work

FIGURE 4.7 shows how ATP forms from a molecule of adenine and ribose (called adenosine) linked to three phosphate molecules. The bonds linking the two outermost phosphates are termed **high-energy bonds** because they represent a considerable quantity of potential energy within the ATP molecule.

During hydrolysis, adenosine triphosphatase catalyzes the reaction when ATP joins with water. In the degradation of one mole of ATP to **adenosine diphosphate (ADP),** the outermost phosphate bond splits and liberates approximately 7.3 kilocalories (kCal) of free energy (i.e., energy available for work).

$$ATP + H_2O \xrightarrow{\text{ATPase}} ADP + P - 7.3 \text{ kCal per mole}$$

The free energy liberated in ATP hydrolysis reflects the energy difference between the reactant and end products. This reaction generates considerable energy, so we refer to ATP as a

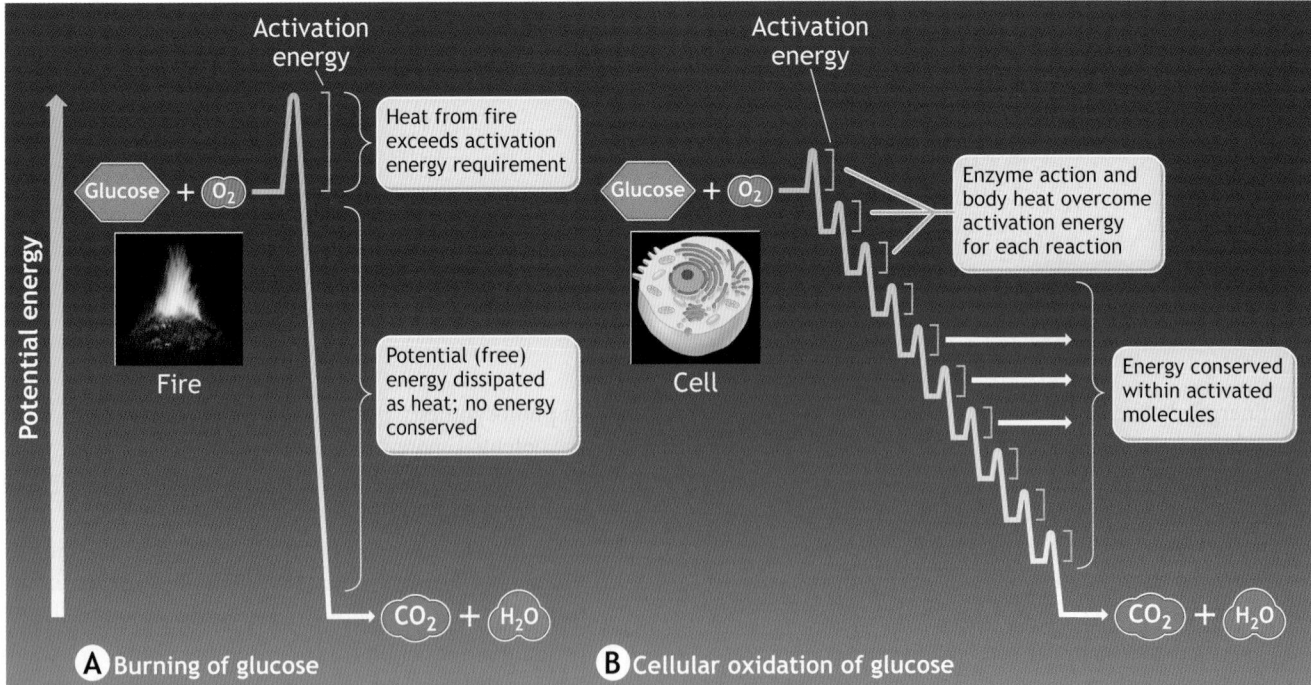

FIGURE 4.6 ■ **A.** The heat generated by fire exceeds the activation energy requirement of a macronutrient (e.g., glucose), causing all of the molecule's potential energy to release suddenly at kindling tempreature and dissipate as heat. **B.** Human energy dynamics involve release of the same amont of potential energy from carbohydrate in small quantities when bonds split during enzymatically controlled reactions. The formation of new molecules conserves energy.

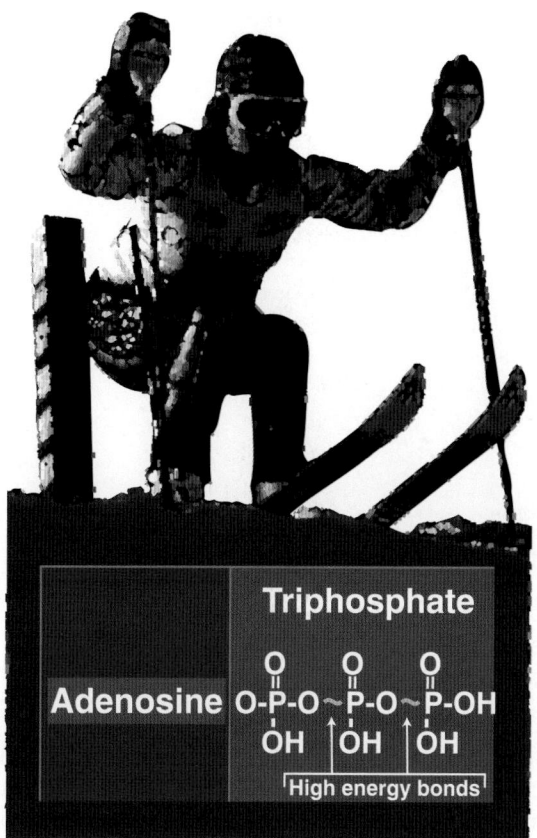

FIGURE 4.7 ■ Simplified illustration of ATP, the energy currency of the cell. The symbol ∼ represents the high-energy bonds.

high-energy phosphate compound. Infrequently, additional energy releases when another phosphate splits from ADP. In some reactions of biosynthesis, ATP donates its two terminal phosphates simultaneously to synthesize cellular material. Adenosine monophosphate, or AMP, becomes the new molecule with a single phosphate group.

The energy liberated during ATP breakdown transfers directly to other energy-requiring molecules. In muscle, for example, this energy activates specific sites on the contractile elements, causing the muscle fiber to shorten. *Because energy from ATP powers all forms of biologic work, ATP constitutes the cell's "energy currency."* FIGURE 4.8 illustrates the general role of ATP as energy currency.

The splitting of an ATP molecule takes place immediately and without oxygen. The cell's capability for ATP breakdown generates energy for rapid use; this would not occur if energy metabolism required oxygen at all times. Anaerobic energy release can be thought of as a back-up power source called upon when the body requires energy in excess of what can be generated aerobically. For this reason, any form of physical activity can take place immediately without instantaneously consuming oxygen; examples include sprinting for a bus, lifting a weight, driving a golf ball, spiking a volleyball, doing a pushup, or jumping up in the air. The well-known practice of holding one's breath during a short sprint swim or run provides a clear example of ATP splitting without reliance on atmospheric

oxygen. Withholding air (oxygen), although inadvisable, can be done during a 60-yard sprint on the track, lifting a barbell, opening and closing your hand as fast as possible for 20 seconds, or dashing up multiple flights of stairs. In each case, energy metabolism proceeds uninterrupted because the energy for performing the activity comes almost exclusively from intramuscular anaerobic sources.

Diverse Ways to Produce ATP

The body maintains a continuous ATP supply through different metabolic pathways: some are located in the cell's cytosol while others operate within the mitochondria. For example, the cytosol contains pathways for ATP synthesis from the anaerobic breakdown of PCr, glucose, glycerol, and the carbon skeletons of deaminated amino acids. Reactions that harness cellular energy to generate ATP aerobically—the citric acid cycle, β-oxidation of fatty acids, and respiratory chain—reside within the mitochondria.

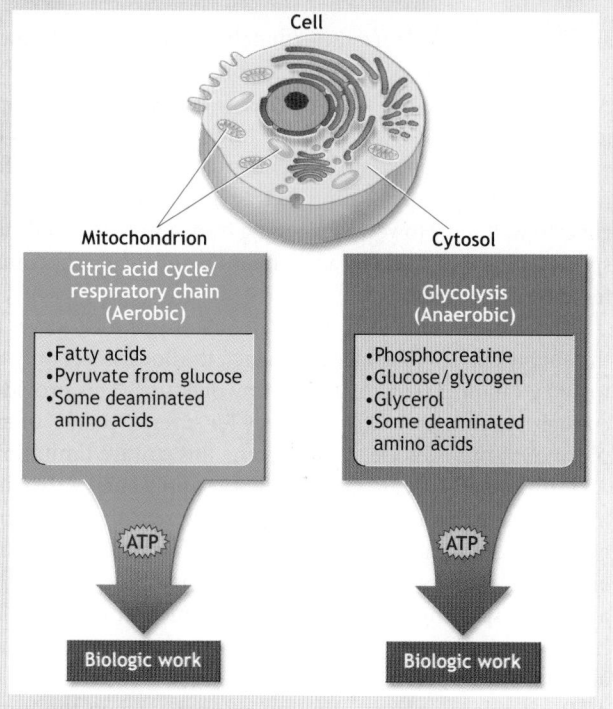

PHOSPHOCREATINE: THE ENERGY RESERVOIR

Cells store only a small quantity of ATP and must therefore continually resynthesize it at its rate of use. This provides a biologically useful mechanism for regulating energy metabolism. By maintaining only a small amount of ATP, its relative concentration (and corresponding concentration of ADP) changes rapidly, increasing a cell's energy demands. Any increase in energy requirement (i.e., disturbance in the cell's current state) immediately disrupts the balance between ATP

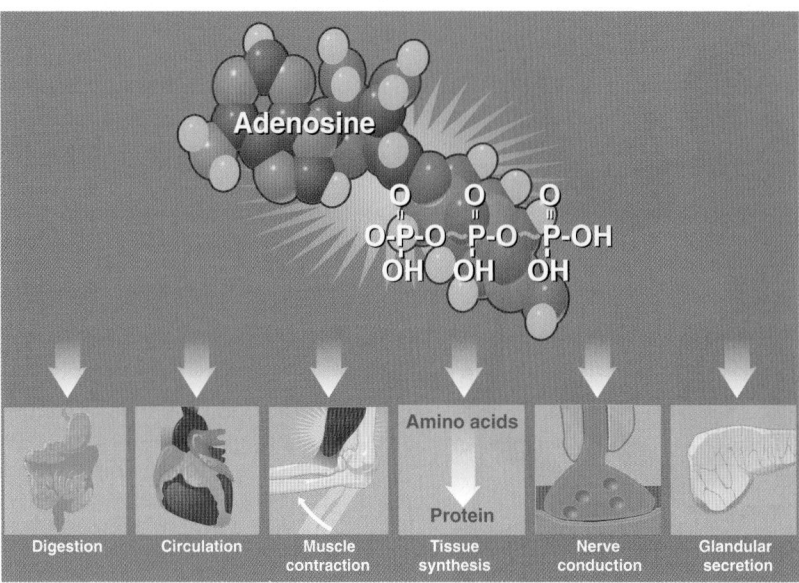

FIGURE 4.8 ■ ATP, the energy currency, powers all forms of biologic work. The symbol $\sim$ represents the high-energy bonds.

and ADP. An imbalance immediately stimulates breakdown of other stored energy-containing compounds to resynthesize ATP. This helps to explain why energy transfer increases rapidly when exercise begins. As one might expect, increases in energy transfer depend on exercise intensity. Energy transfer increases about fourfold in the transition from sitting in a chair to walking. However, changing from a walk to an all-out sprint almost immediately accelerates the rate of energy transfer about 120 times!

As pointed out above, a limited quantity of ATP serves as the energy currency for all cells. In fact, the body stores only 80 to 100 g (about 3.0 oz) of ATP at any one time. This provides enough intramuscular stored energy for several seconds of explosive, all-out exercise. To overcome this storage limitation, ATP resynthesis occurs continually to supply energy for biologic work. Fatty acids and glycogen represent the major energy sources for maintaining continual ATP resynthesis. Some energy for ATP resynthesis, however, comes directly from the anaerobic splitting of a phosphate from another intracellular high-energy phosphate compound **phosphocreatine (PCr)**, also known as creatine phosphate or CP. PCr is similar to ATP—it releases a large amount of energy when the bond splits between creatine and phosphate molecules. FIGURE 4.9 schematically illustrates the release and use of phosphate-bond energy in ATP and PCr. The term **high-energy phosphates** describes these stored intramuscular compounds.

In each reaction, the arrow points in both directions, indicating a reversible reaction. In other words, phosphate (P) and creatine (Cr) join again to re-form PCr. This also applies to ATP, for ADP plus P re-forms ATP. Cells store approximately four to six times more PCr than ATP. *The onset of intense exercise triggers PCr hydrolysis for energy; it does not require oxygen and reaches a maximum in about 10 seconds.*[36] Thus, PCr serves as a "reservoir" of high-energy phosphate bonds. PCr's speed for ADP phosphorylation considerably ex-

ceeds anaerobic energy transfer from stored muscle glycogen owing to the high activity rate of the creatine phosphokinase reaction.[14] If maximal effort continues beyond 10 seconds, the energy for continual ATP resynthesis must originate from the less rapid catabolism of the stored macronutrients.[10] Chapter 12 discusses the potential for exogenous creatine supplementation to increase intracellular levels of PCr and enhance short-term, all-out exercise performance.

Intramuscular High-Energy Phosphates

Energy release from the intramuscular energy-rich phosphates ATP and PCr sustains all-out exercise for approximately 5 to 8 seconds. Thus, in a 100-m sprint in world record time of 9.74 s by Jamaican Asafa Powell (Sept. 9, 2007), the body cannot maintain maximum speed throughout this duration. During the last few seconds of the race, the runners actually slow down, with the winner often slowing down least! If all-out effort continues beyond 8 seconds or if moderate exercise continues for much longer periods, ATP resynthesis requires an additional energy source other than PCr. If resynthesis does not happen, the "fuel" supply diminishes and high-intensity movement ceases. As we discuss later, the foods we eat and store for ready access provide chemical energy to continually recharge cellular supplies of ATP and PCr.

Transfer of Energy by Chemical Bonds

Human energy dynamics involve transferring energy by means of chemical bonds. Potential energy releases by the splitting of bonds and is conserved by the formation of new bonds. Some energy lost by one molecule transfers to the chemical structure of other molecules without appearing as heat. In the

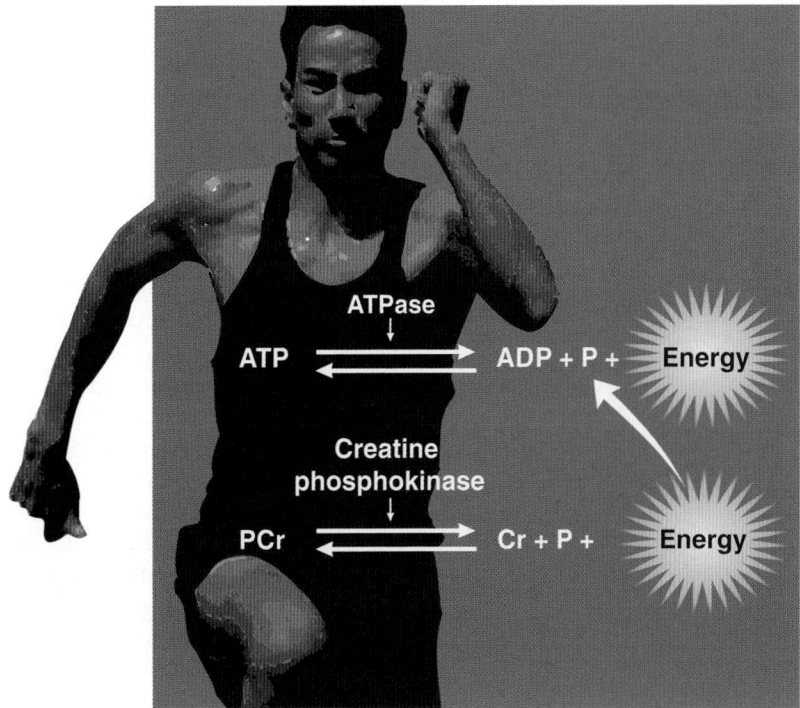

FIGURE 4.9 ■ ATP and PCr provide anaerobic sources of phosphate-bond energy. The energy liberated from the hydrolysis (splitting) of PCr rebonds ADP and P to form ATP.

body, biologic work occurs when compounds relatively low in potential energy become "juiced up" from transfer of energy via high-energy phosphate bonds.

ATP serves as the ideal energy-transfer agent. In one respect, phosphate bonds of ATP "trap" a relatively large portion of the original food molecule's potential energy. ATP also readily transfers this energy to other compounds to raise them to a higher activation level. **Phosphorylation** refers to energy transfer through phosphate bonds.

CELLULAR OXIDATION

Most of the energy for ATP phosphorylation comes from oxidation ("biologic burning") of the carbohydrate, lipid, and protein macronutrients consumed in the diet. Recall that a molecule reduces when it accepts electrons from an electron donor. In turn, the molecule that gives up electrons is oxidized. Oxidation reactions (donating electrons) and reduction reactions (accepting electrons) remain coupled because every oxidation coincides with a reduction. *In essence, cellular oxidation–reduction constitutes the mechanism for energy metabolism.* This process often involves the transfer of hydrogen atoms (contains one electron and one proton in its nucleus) rather than free electrons. Thus, a molecule that loses hydrogen oxidizes and one that gains hydrogen reduces. For example, the stored carbohydrate, fat, and protein molecules continually provide hydrogen atoms. The mitochondria, the cell's "energy factories," contain carrier molecules that remove electrons from hydrogen (oxidation) and eventually pass them to oxygen (reduction). Synthesis of the high-energy phosphate ATP occurs during oxidation–reduction reactions.

Electron Transport

FIGURE 4.10 illustrates the general scheme for hydrogen oxidation and accompanying electron transport to oxygen. During cellular oxidation, hydrogen atoms are not merely turned loose in the cell fluid. Rather, highly specific **dehydrogenase coenzymes** catalyze hydrogen's release from the nutrient substrate. The coenzyme part of the dehydrogenase (usually the niacin-containing coenzyme NAD^+) accepts pairs of electrons (energy) from hydrogen. While the substrate oxidizes and loses hydrogen (electrons), NAD^+ gains one hydrogen and two electrons and reduces to NADH; the other hydrogen appears as H^+ in the cell fluid.

The riboflavin-containing coenzyme **FAD** serves as the other important electron acceptor in oxidizing food fragments. FAD catalyzes dehydrogenations and accepts pairs of electrons. Unlike NAD^+, however, FAD becomes $FADH_2$ by accepting both hydrogens. *The NADH and $FADH_2$ formed in the breakdown of food are energy-rich molecules that carry electrons with a high energy transfer potential.*

Misleading Information from the Supplement Purveyors

The coenzymes NAD^+ and FAD are derived from the water-soluble vitamins niacin and riboflavin, respectively. Unfortunately, vitamin manufacturers often misleadingly link the consumption of these vitamins above recommended levels to increased energy capacity. To the contrary, once sufficient amounts of these coenzymes are available in the body, any excess vitamins are voided in the urine.

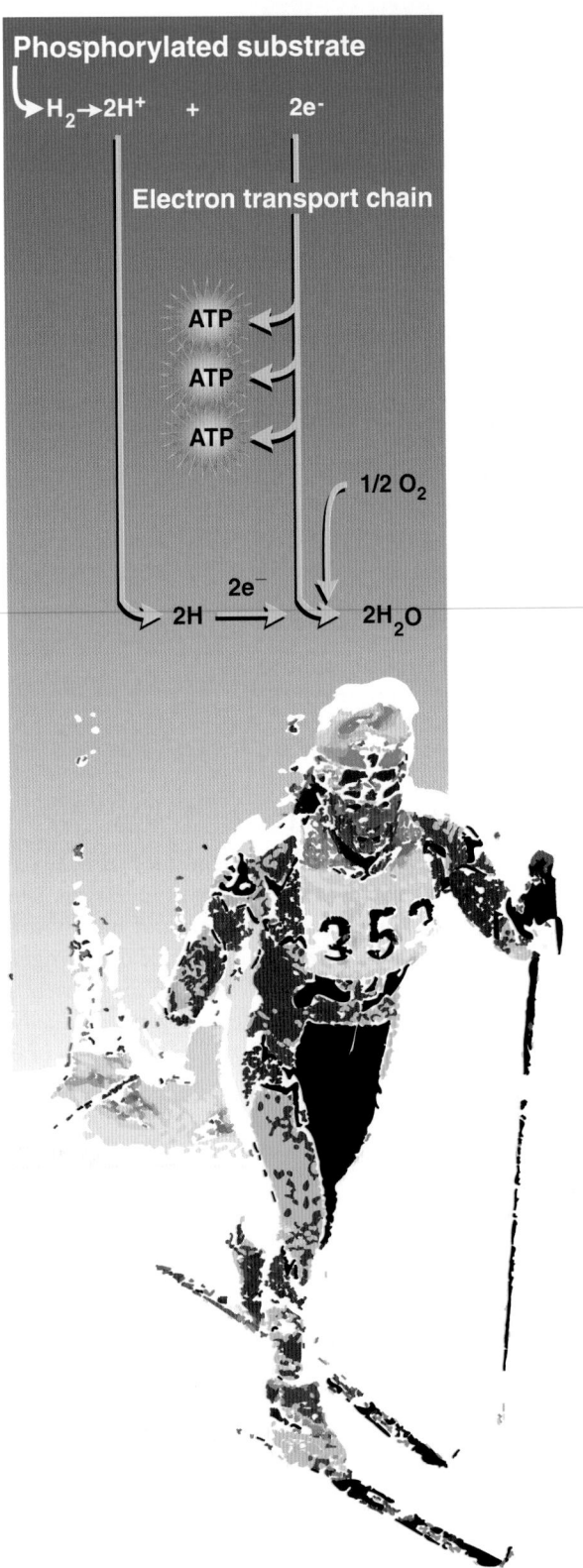

FIGURE 4.10 ■ General scheme for oxidation (removing electrons) of hydrogen and accompanying electron transport. In this process, oxygen becomes reduced (gain of electrons) and water forms. ATP, adenosine triphosphate.

The **cytochromes,** a series of iron–protein electron carriers, then pass in "bucket brigade" fashion pairs of electrons carried by NADH and $FADH_2$ on the inner membranes of mitochondria. The iron portion of each cytochrome exists in either its oxidized (ferric or Fe^{3+}) or reduced (ferrous or Fe^{2+}) ionic state. By accepting an electron, the ferric portion of a specific cytochrome reduces to its ferrous form. In turn, ferrous iron donates its electron to the next cytochrome, and so on down the line. By shuttling between these two iron forms, the cytochromes transfer electrons to their ultimate destination, where they reduce oxygen to form water. The NAD^+ and FAD then recycle for subsequent use in energy metabolism.

Electron transport by specific carrier molecules constitutes the respiratory chain; this serves as the final common pathway where the electrons extracted from hydrogen pass to oxygen. For each pair of hydrogen atoms, two electrons flow down the chain and reduce one atom of oxygen to form water. Of the five specific cytochromes, only the last one, cytochrome oxidase (cytochrome aa_3, with a strong affinity for oxygen) discharges its electron directly to oxygen. The right panel of FIGURE 4.11 shows the route for hydrogen oxidation, electron transport, and energy transfer in the respiratory chain. The respiratory chain releases free energy in relatively small amounts. In several of the electron transfers, energy conservation occurs by forming high-energy phosphate bonds.

Oxidative Phosphorylation

Oxidative phosphorylation synthesizes ATP by transferring electrons from NADH and $FADH_2$ to oxygen. This primary process represents the cell's way of extracting and trapping chemical energy in the high-energy phosphates. *More than 90% of ATP synthesis takes place in the respiratory chain by oxidative reactions coupled with phosphorylation.*

In a way, oxidative phosphorylation can be likened to a waterfall divided into several separate cascades by the intervention of water wheels at different heights. The left panel of Figure 4.11 depicts water wheels harnessing the energy of falling water. Similarly, electrochemical energy generated via electron transport in the respiratory chain is harnessed and transferred (or coupled) to ADP. Three distinct coupling sites during electron transport transfer the energy in NADH to ADP to re-form ATP (Fig. 4.11, *right panel*). The theoretical value for ATP production from the oxidation of hydrogen and subsequent phosphorylation occur as follows:

$$\text{NADH} + \text{H}^+ + 3\ \text{ADP} + 3\ \text{P} + 1/2\ \text{O}_2 \rightarrow$$
$$\text{NAD}^+ + \text{H}_2\text{O} + 3\ \text{ATP}$$

Note in the above reaction that three ATPs form for each NADH plus H^+ oxidized. Biochemists have recently adjusted their accounting transpositions regarding conservation of energy in the resynthesis of an ATP molecule in aerobic pathways. While it is true that energy provided by oxidation of NADH and $FADH_2$ resynthesizes ADP to ATP, additional energy (H^+) is also required to transport the newly formed ATP molecule across the mitochondrial membrane into the cell's cytoplasm in exchange for ADP and P, which then move into

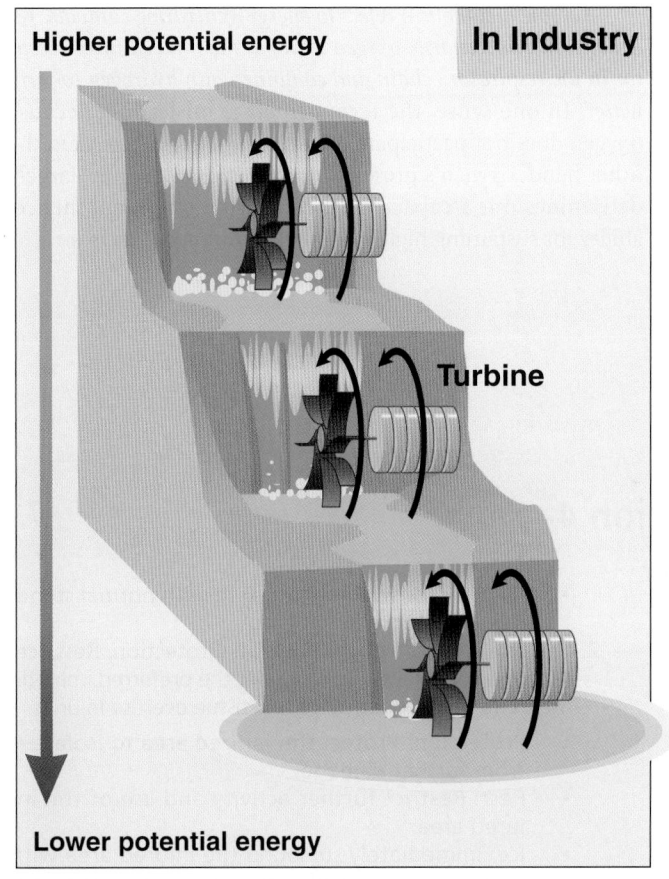

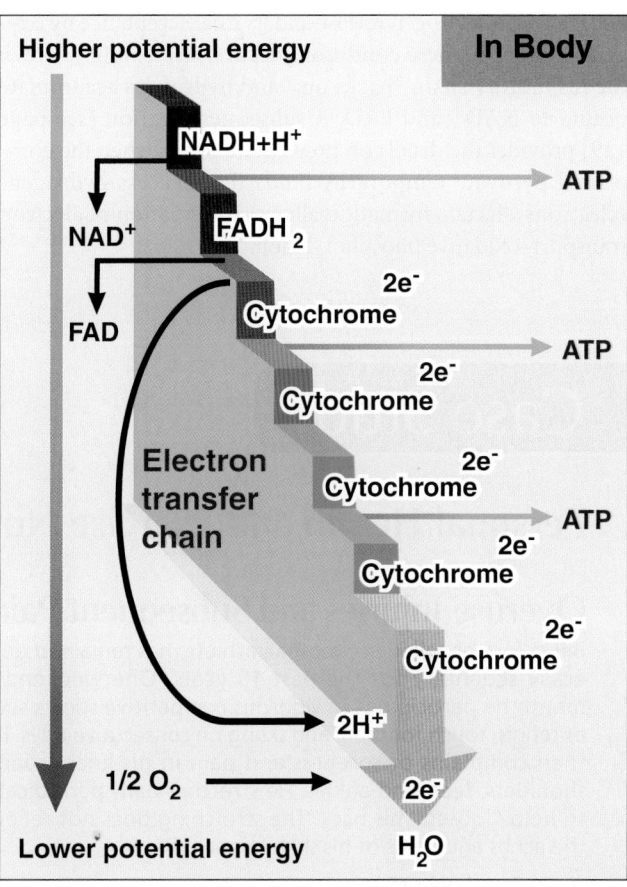

FIGURE 4.11 ■ Examples of harnessing potential energy. *Left,* In industry, energy from falling water becomes harnessed to turn the waterwheel, which in turn performs mechanical work. *Right,* In the body, the electron transfer chain removes electrons from hydrogens for ultimate delivery to oxygen. In oxidation–reduction, much of the chemical energy stored within the hydrogen atom does not dissipate to kinetic energy, but instead is conserved within ATP.

mitochondria. This added energy of transport reduces the *net* ATP yield for glucose metabolism. Actually, on average, only 2.5 ATP molecules form from oxidation of one NADH molecule. This decimal value for ATP does not indicate formation of one-half ATP molecule but rather indicates the average number of ATP produced per NADH oxidation with the energy for mitochondrial transport subtracted. When $FADH_2$ donates hydrogen, then on average only 1.5 molecules of ATP form for each hydrogen pair oxidized.

Efficiency of Electron Transport and Oxidative Phosphorylation

The formation of each mole of ATP from ADP conserves approximately 7 kCal of energy. Because 2.5 moles of ATP come from oxidizing 1 mole of NADH, about 18 kCal (7 kCal per mole × 2.5) are conserved as chemical energy. A relative efficiency of 34% occurs for harnessing chemical energy by electron transport–oxidative phosphorylation, since the oxidation of one mole of NADH liberates a total of 52 kCal (18 kCal ÷ 52 kCal × 100). The 66% remaining energy dissipates as heat. Considering that a steam engine transforms its

fuel into useful energy at only about 30% efficiency, the value of 34% for the human body represents a remarkably high efficiency rate.

ROLE OF OXYGEN IN ENERGY METABOLISM

Three prerequisites exist for continual resynthesis of ATP during coupled oxidative phosphorylation from macronutrient catabolism. Satisfying the following three conditions causes hydrogen and electrons to shuttle uninterrupted down the respiratory chain to oxygen during energy metabolism:

1. Availability of the reducing agent NADH (or $FADH_2$) in the tissues
2. Presence of an oxidizing agent (oxygen) in the tissues
3. Sufficient concentration of enzymes and mitochondria in the tissues to ensure that energy transfer reactions proceed at their appropriate rate

In strenuous exercise, inadequate oxygen delivery (condition 2) or its rate of use (condition 3) creates a relative imbalance between hydrogen release and its final acceptance by oxygen. If either of these conditions occurs, electron flow down the respiratory chain "backs up," and hydrogens accumulate bound to NAD^+ and FAD. A subsequent section (see page 139) provides the details on how lactate forms when the compound pyruvate temporarily binds these excess hydrogens (electrons); lactate formation allows continuation of electron transport–oxidative phosphorylation.

Aerobic metabolism refers to energy-generating catabolic reactions. In this scenario, oxygen serves as the final electron acceptor in the respiratory chain and combines with hydrogen to form water. In one sense, the term *aerobic* is misleading because oxygen does not participate directly in ATP synthesis. On the other hand, oxygen's presence at the "end of the line" largely determines one's capacity for ATP production and, hence, ability for sustaining high-intensity, endurance exercises.

Case Study

Personal Health and Exercise Nutrition 4–1

Overuse Injuries and Subsequent Pain

Bill, a former collegiate football athlete, has remained generally sedentary for the past 10 years. One weekend a month he participates in vigorous competitive sports such as tennis, touch football, and skiing on consecutive days. He then complains of soreness and pain in his knees, back, shoulders, feet, and ankles. He stretches daily periodically to help "loosen" his back. The stretching does not relieve the aches and pains of his skeletal maladies.

Past Medical History

Bill does not smoke, has no history of major disease, and maintains desirable body weight (although he weighs 10 pounds more than in college) and normal blood pressure. All blood work done yearly at a local hospital falls within normal range. He is healthy, but more sedentary than he desires.

Diagnosis

Weekend warrior with signs and symptoms of overuse injuries.

Case Questions

1. Track progression of an overuse injury.
2. Give immediate first aid procedures for treating an overuse injury.
3. Describe how to prevent overuse injuries.

Answers

1. Overuse injuries result from repetitive use of muscles, tendons, and joints in the same way without sufficient rest. Such repeated muscle actions often occur in strenuous sports, but they also take place during any repeated motions such as cutting wood, digging in the ground, or raking leaves.

   Pain that worsens with activity often progresses as follows:

   - Initially, dull pain, discomfort, and general fatigue occurs.
   - Pain becomes sharper and pinpointed to a defined area (hip, knee, or elbow).
   - Pain lingers, often accompanied by some swelling tissue inflammation.
   - Pain and/or swelling become severe enough to interfere with further activity.

   - Pain and/or swelling interfere with normal standing, walking, and sleeping.

2. The five-letter acronym **P-R-I-C-E** (Protection, Rest, Ice, Compression, Elevation) describes the preferred immediate treatment sequence for soft tissue overuse injuries.

   - Protection: Protect the injured area to isolate it from further damage.
   - Rest: Restrict further activity and use of the injured area.
   - Ice: Immediately surround the injured area with an ice pack secured with elastic wrap and continue application for 24 to 72 hours depending on injury severity. Vasoconstriction from the ice helps to reduce bleeding, swelling, and pain. The standard ice application interval lasts 15 to 20 minutes. Reapply ice hourly or when pain persists. Do not apply ice or compression at bedtime unless the pain interferes with sleep.
   - Compression: Compress the injured area firmly but not with excessive pressure. Begin the wrap distal to the injury and proceed toward and over the injured area.
   - Elevation: If applicable, raise the injured area above heart level to minimize the hydrostatic effect of gravity on venous pooling and fluid efflux into injured tissues. Maintain limb elevation as long as practical. During sleep, elevate the injured limb with blankets or pillows.

3. Overuse injuries often take longer to heal than other injuries. Prevention thus becomes an important consideration. Bill can reduce overuse injuries by doing the following:

   (1) Allow at least 48 hours between activities.
   (2) Decrease exercise (ease up while playing).
   (3) Decrease the duration of activity (refrain from doing too much at one time).
   (4) Gradually increase training level. Bill should join a gym to upgrade his fitness.
   (5) Make sure the exercise equipment is up-to-date and in good working order.
   (6) Consider the participant's age. Bill needs to acknowledge his bodily changes as he ages and adjust workouts accordingly.

Summary

1. Energy within the chemical structure of carbohydrate, fat, and protein molecules does not suddenly release in the body at some kindling temperature. Rather, energy release occurs slowly in small amounts during complex enzymatically controlled reactions, thus enabling more efficient energy transfer and conservation.

2. About 34% of the potential energy in food nutrients transfers to the high-energy compound adenosine triphosphate (ATP).

3. Splitting the terminal phosphate bond of ATP liberates free energy to power all forms of biologic work.

4. ATP serves as the body's energy currency, although its quantity amounts to only about 3.0 ounces.

5. Phosphocreatine (PCr) interacts with adenosine diphosphate (ADP) to form ATP. This nonaerobic, high-energy reservoir replenishes ATP rapidly.

6. Phosphorylation refers to energy transfer by phosphate bonds, in which ADP and creatine continually recycle into ATP and PCr.

7. Cellular oxidation occurs on the inner lining of the mitochondrial membranes; it involves transferring electrons from NADH and $FADH_2$ to oxygen. This process results in the release and coupled transfer of chemical energy to form ATP from ADP plus a phosphate ion.

8. During aerobic ATP resynthesis, oxygen serves as the final electron acceptor in the respiratory chain and combines with hydrogen to form water.

Energy Release from Macronutrients

The energy released in macronutrient breakdown serves one crucial purpose—to phosphorylate ADP to re-form the energy-rich compound ATP (FIG. 4.12). Macronutrient catabolism favors the generation of phosphate-bond energy, yet the specific pathways of degradation differ depending on the nutrients metabolized. In the sections that follow, we show how ATP resynthesis occurs from the extraction of potential energy in the food macronutrients.

FIGURE 4.13 outlines the basic macronutrient fuel sources that supply substrate for oxidation and subsequent ATP formation. These sources consist primarily of the following:

1. Glucose derived from liver glycogen
2. Triacylglycerol and glycogen molecules stored within muscle cells
3. Free fatty acids derived from triacylglycerol (in liver and adipocytes) that enter the bloodstream for delivery to active muscle
4. Intramuscular and liver-derived carbon skeletons of amino acids

A small amount of ATP also forms from (1) anaerobic reactions in the cytosol in the initial phase of glucose or glycogen breakdown and (2) the phosphorylation of ADP by PCr under enzymatic control by creatine phosphokinase.

ENERGY RELEASE FROM CARBOHYDRATE

The *primary function of carbohydrate is to supply energy for cellular work.* The complete breakdown of one mole of glucose (180 g) to carbon dioxide and water yields a maximum of 686 kCal of chemical free energy available for work. In the body, however, complete glucose breakdown conserves only some of this energy in the form of ATP.

$$C_6H_{12}O_6 + 6O_2 \rightarrow 6CO_2 + 6H_2O + 686 \text{ kCal per mole}$$

Synthesizing one mole of ATP from ADP and phosphate ion requires 7.3 kCal of energy. Therefore, coupling all of the energy in glucose oxidation to phosphorylation could theoretically form 94 moles of ATP per mole of glucose (686 kCal ÷ 7.3 kCal • mole^{-1}). In muscle, however, the phosphate bonds conserve only 34%, or 233 kCal, of energy, with the remainder dissipated as heat. Consequently, glucose breakdown regenerates 32 moles of ATP (233 kCal ÷ 7.3 kCal • mole^{-1}), with an accompanying free energy gain of 233 kCal.

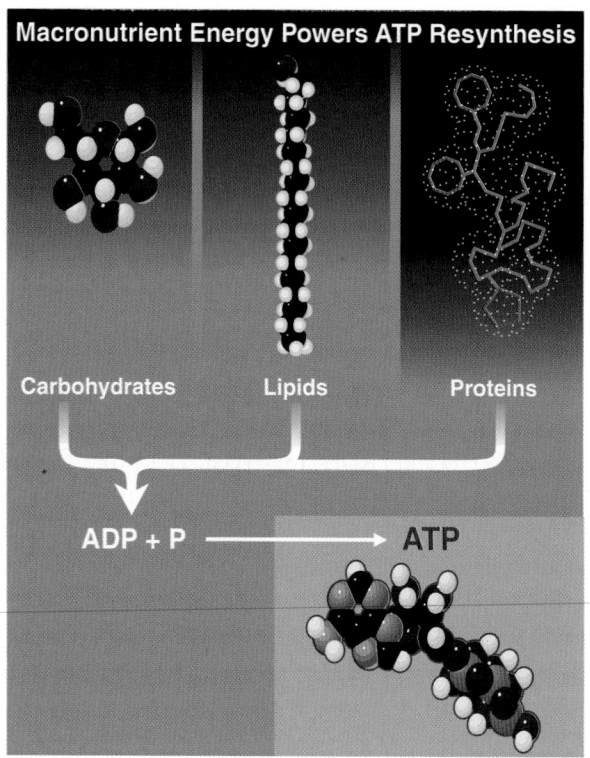

FIGURE 4.12 ■ The potential energy in the macronutrients powers ATP resynthesis. ADP, adenosine diphosphate; P, phosphate.

Anaerobic versus Aerobic

Glucose degradation occurs in two stages. In stage one, glucose breaks down relatively rapidly to two molecules of pyruvate. Energy transfers occur without oxygen (anaerobic). In stage two of glucose catabolism, pyruvate degrades further to carbon dioxide and water. Energy transfers from these reactions require electron transport and accompanying oxidative phosphorylation (aerobic).

Glycolysis: Anaerobic Energy from Glucose Catabolism

The first stage of glucose degradation within cells involves a series of chemical reactions collectively termed **glycolysis** (also termed the Embden-Meyerhof pathway for its two biochemist discoverers). This series of reactions, summarized in FIGURE 4.14, occurs in the watery medium of the cell outside of the mitochondrion. In a sense, the reactions represent a more primitive form of energy transfer well developed in amphibians, reptiles, fish, and marine mammals. In humans, the cells' capacity for glycolysis becomes crucial during physical activities that require maximal effort for up to 90 seconds.

In the first reaction of Figure 4.14, ATP acts as a phosphate donor to phosphorylate glucose to glucose 6-phosphate. In most tissues of the body, phosphorylation "traps" the glucose molecule in the cell. (Liver and, to a small extent, kidney cells

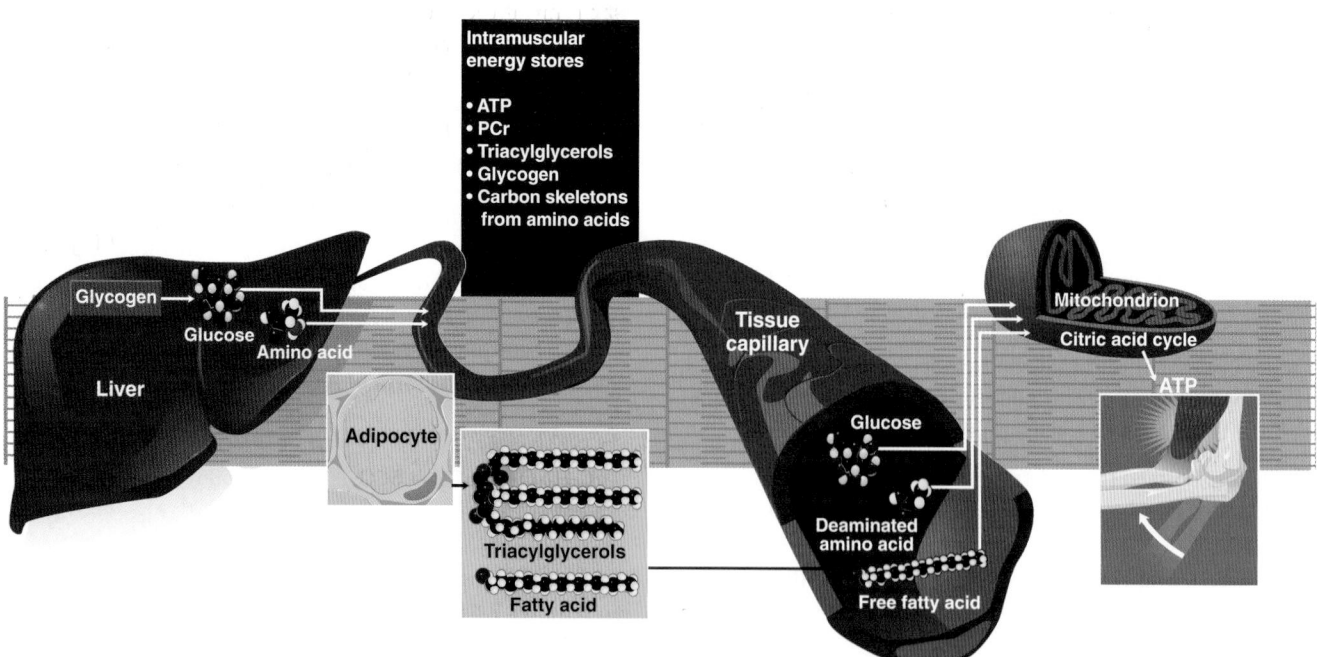

FIGURE 4.13 ■ Basic macronutrient fuel sources that supply substrates for regenerating ATP. The liver provides a rich source of amino acid and glucose, while adipocytes generate large quantities of energy-rich fatty acid molecules. Once released, the bloodstream delivers these compounds to the muscle cell. Most of the cells' energy transfer takes place within the mitochondria. Mitochondrial proteins carry out oxidative phosphorylation in the inner membranous walls of this architecturally elegant complex. The intramuscular energy sources consist of the high-energy phosphates ATP and PCr and triacylglycerols, glycogen, and amino acids.

Importance of Carbohydrates in Energy Metabolism

1. Carbohydrates are the only macronutrient whose stored energy generates ATP anaerobically. This becomes important in maximal exercise that requires rapid energy release above levels supplied by aerobic metabolic reactions. In this case, most of the energy for ATP resynthesis comes from stored intramuscular glycogen.
2. During light and moderate aerobic exercise, carbohydrates supply about one third of the body's energy requirements.
3. Processing fat through the metabolic mill for energy requires some carbohydrate catabolism.
4. Aerobic breakdown of carbohydrate for energy occurs more rapidly than energy generation from fatty acid breakdown. Thus, depleting glycogen reserves significantly reduces exercise power output. In prolonged high-intensity aerobic exercise such as marathon running, athletes often experience nutrient-related fatigue—a state associated with muscle and liver glycogen depletion.
5. The central nervous system requires an uninterrupted stream of carbohydrate to function properly. Under normal conditions, the brain uses blood glucose almost exclusively as its fuel. In poorly regulated diabetes, during starvation, or with a prolonged low carbohydrate intake, the brain adapts after about 8 days and metabolizes relatively large amounts of fat (as ketones) for alternative fuel.

contain the enzyme **glucose 6-phosphatase,** which splits the phosphate from glucose 6-phosphate, thus freeing glucose for transport across the cell membrane for delivery throughout the body.) In the presence of **glycogen synthase,** glucose joins (become polymerized) with other glucose molecules to form glycogen. In energy metabolism, however, glucose 6-phosphate changes to fructose 6-phosphate. At this stage, no energy extraction occurs, yet energy incorporates into the original glucose molecule at the expense of one ATP molecule. In a sense, phosphorylation "primes the pump" for energy metabolism to proceed. The fructose 6-phosphate molecule gains an additional phosphate from ATP and changes to fructose 1,6-diphosphate under control of **phosphofructokinase (PFK).** The activity level of PFK probably places a limit on the rate of glycolysis during maximum-effort exercise. Fructose 1,6-diphosphate then splits into two phosphorylated molecules, each with three carbon chains; these further decompose to pyruvate in five successive reactions. Fast-twitch muscle fibers contain relatively large quantities of PFK; this makes them ideally suited for generating rapid anaerobic energy from glycolysis.

Glycogen Catabolism

Glycogenolysis describes the cleavage of glucose from stored glycogen (glycogen → glucose). The **glycogen phosphorylase** enzyme in skeletal muscle regulates and limits glycogen's

breakdown for energy. **Epinephrine,** a sympathetic nervous system hormone, influences the activity of this enzyme to cleave one glucose component at a time from the glycogen molecule.[4,9] The glucose residue then reacts with a phosphate ion to produce glucose 6-phosphate, bypassing step one of the glycolytic pathway. Thus, when glycogen provides a glucose molecule for glycolysis, a net gain of 3 ATPs occurs rather than the 2 ATPs that occur during this first phase of glucose breakdown (see next section).

Substrate-Level Phosphorylation in Glycolysis

Most of the energy generated in the cytoplasmic reactions of glycolysis does not result in ATP resynthesis but instead dissipates as heat. In reactions 7 and 10, however, the energy released from the glucose intermediates stimulates the direct transfer of phosphate groups to ADPs while generating four ATP molecules. *Because two molecules of ATP were lost in the initial phosphorylation of the glucose molecule, glycolysis generates a net gain of two ATP molecules.* These specific energy transfers from substrate to ADP by phosphorylation do not require oxygen. Rather, energy transfers directly via phosphate bonds in the anaerobic reactions called **substrate-level phosphorylation.** Energy conservation during glycolysis operates at an efficiency of about 30%.

Glycolysis generates only about 5% of the total ATP formed during the glucose molecule's complete breakdown. However, the high concentration of glycolytic enzymes and the speed of these reactions provide significant energy for intense muscle action. The following represent examples of activities that rely heavily on ATP generated by glycolysis: sprinting at the end of the mile run, performing all-out from start to finish in the 50- and 100-m swim, routines on gymnastics apparatus, and sprint running races up to 200 m.

The Anaerobic Macronutrient

Anaerobic energy transfer from the macronutrients occurs *only* from carbohydrate breakdown during glycolytic reactions.

Hydrogen Release in Glycolysis

During glycolysis, two pairs of hydrogen atoms are stripped from the substrate (glucose) and their electrons passed to NAD^+ to form NADH (FIG. 4.14). *Because two molecules of NADH form in glycolysis, five molecules of ATP (2.5 per NADH) generate aerobically by subsequent electron transport–oxidative phosphorylation.*

Lactate Formation

Sufficient oxygen bathes the cells during light-to-moderate levels of energy metabolism. Consequently, the hydrogens (electrons) stripped from the substrate and carried by NADH oxidize within the mitochondria to form water when they join with oxygen. In a biochemical sense a "steady state," or more precisely a "steady rate," exists because hydrogen oxidizes at about the same *rate* that it becomes available. Biochemists fre-

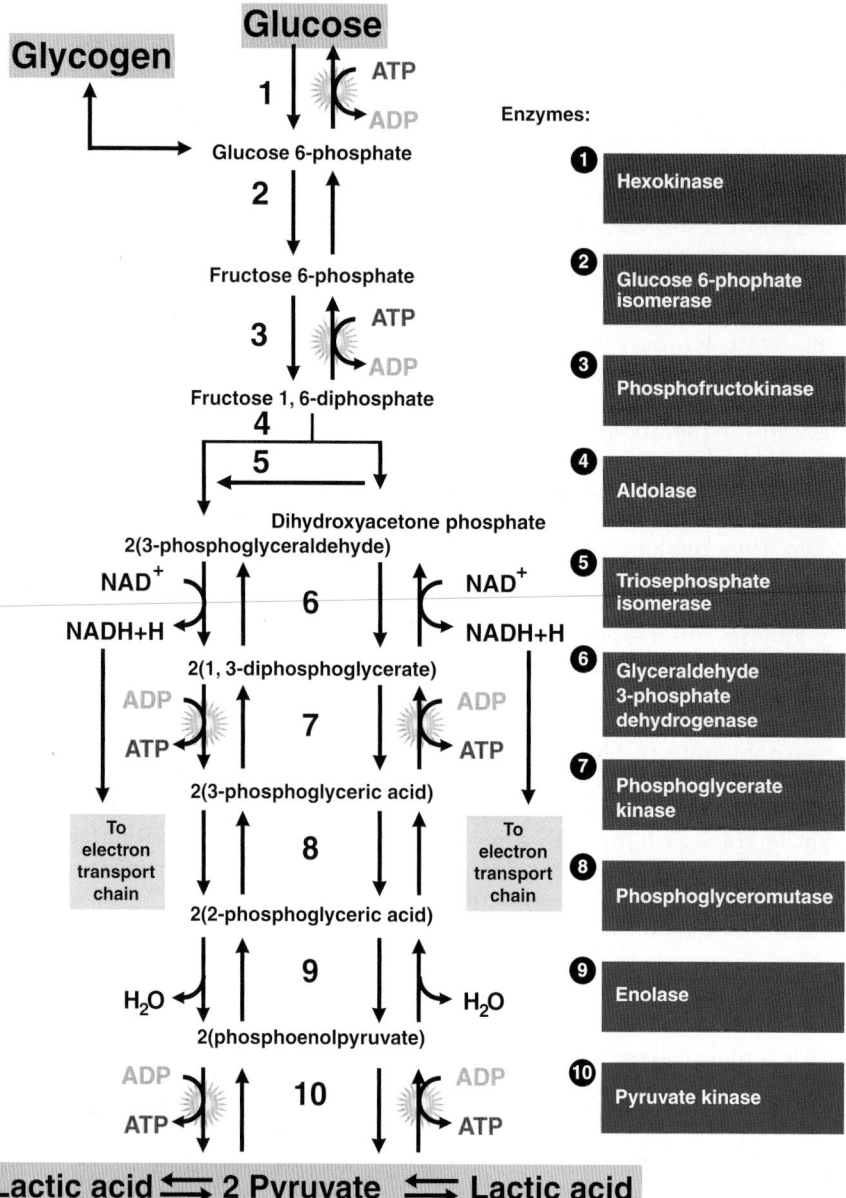

FIGURE 4.14 ■ Glycolysis, a series of 10 enzymatically controlled chemical reactions, creates two molecules of pyruvate from the anaerobic breakdown of glucose. Lactic acid (lactate) forms when NADH oxidation does not keep pace with its formation in glycolysis. ATP, adenosine triphosphate; ADP, adenosine diphosphate; NAD, nicotinamide adenine dinucleotide.

quently refer to this relatively steady dynamic condition as **aerobic glycolysis,** with pyruvate becoming the end product.

In strenuous exercise, when energy demands exceed either the oxygen supply or its rate of use, the respiratory chain cannot process all of the hydrogen joined to NADH. Continued release of anaerobic energy in glycolysis depends on NAD^+ availability for oxidizing 3-phosphoglyceraldehyde (see reaction 6 in Fig. 4.14); otherwise, the rapid rate of glycolysis "grinds to a halt." Under **anaerobic glycolysis,** NAD^+ re-forms as pairs of "excess" nonoxidized hydrogens combine temporarily with pyruvate to form lactate in an additional step, catalyzed by **lactate dehydrogenase,** in the reversible reaction shown in FIGURE 4.15.

The temporary storage of hydrogen with pyruvate represents a unique aspect of energy metabolism because it pro-

vides a ready "reservoir" to temporarily store the end products of anaerobic glycolysis. Also, once lactic acid forms in the muscle, it diffuses into the blood for buffering to sodium lactate and removal from the site of energy metabolism. In this way, glycolysis continues to supply additional anaerobic energy for ATP resynthesis. This avenue for extra energy remains temporary; blood and muscle lactate levels increase, and ATP regeneration cannot keep pace with its utilization rate. Fatigue soon sets in, and exercise performance diminishes. Increased acidity from lactate accumulation (and perhaps the effect of the lactate anion itself) mediates fatigue by inactivating various enzymes involved in energy transfer and inhibiting some aspect of the muscle's contractile machinery.[3,13,18]

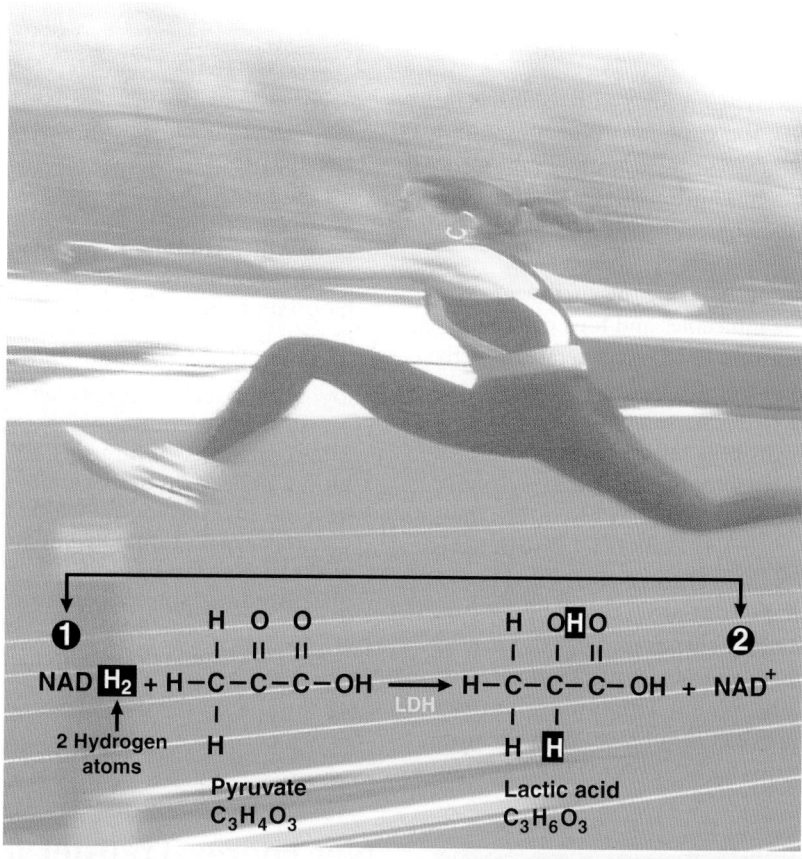

FIGURE 4.15 ■ *(1)* Lactic acid forms when excess hydrogens from NADH combine temporarily with pyruvate. *(2)* This frees up NAD$^+$ to accept additional hydrogens generated in glycolysis. LDH, lactate dehydrogenase; NAD, nicotinamide adenine dinucleotide.

Some Blood Lactate at Rest

Even at rest, energy metabolism in red blood cells forms some lactate. This occurs because the red blood cells contain no mitochondria and thus must derive their energy from anaerobic glycolysis.

Lactate should not be viewed as a metabolic "waste product." To the contrary, it provides a valuable source of chemical energy that accumulates in the body during heavy exercise. When sufficient oxygen once again becomes available during recovery, or when exercise pace slows, NAD$^+$ scavenges hydrogens attached to lactate; these hydrogens subsequently oxidize to synthesize ATP. Consequently, much circulating blood lactate becomes an energy source as it readily reconverts to pyruvate. In addition, the liver cells conserve the potential energy in the lactate and pyruvate molecules formed during exercise, as the carbon skeletons of these molecules become synthesized to glucose in the **Cori cycle** (FIG. 4.16). The Cori cycle not only removes lactate, but it also uses the lactate substrate to resynthesize blood glucose and muscle glycogen (gluconeogenesis in the liver) depleted in intense exercise.[34]

Citric Acid Cycle: Aerobic Energy from Glucose Catabolism

Anaerobic glycolysis releases only about 10% of the energy within the original glucose molecule. Thus, extracting the remaining energy requires an additional metabolic pathway. This occurs when pyruvate *irreversibly* converts to acetyl-CoA, a form of acetic acid. Acetyl-CoA enters the second stage of carbohydrate breakdown, termed the **citric acid cycle,** also known as the **Krebs cycle** in honor of chemist Hans Krebs (1900–1981), who shared the 1953 Nobel Prize in Physiology or Medicine for his discovery of the citric acid cycle.

As shown schematically in FIGURE 4.17, the citric acid cycle degrades the acetyl-CoA substrate to carbon dioxide and hydrogen atoms within the mitochondria. Hydrogen atoms then oxidize during electron transport–oxidative phosphorylation with subsequent ATP regeneration. FIGURE 4.18 shows pyruvate preparing to enter the citric acid cycle by joining with the vitamin B (pantothenic acid)-derivative coenzyme A (A stands for acetic acid) to form the 2-carbon compound acetyl-CoA. This process releases two hydrogens and transfers their electrons to NAD$^+$, forming one molecule of carbon dioxide as follows:

$$\text{Pyruvate} + \text{NAD}^+ + \text{CoA} \rightarrow$$
$$\text{Acetyl-CoA} + CO_2 + \text{NADH} + H^+$$

The acetyl portion of acetyl-CoA joins with oxaloacetate to form citrate (citric acid), the same 6-carbon compound found in citrus fruits, which then proceeds through the citric acid cycle. The citric acid cycle continues its operations because it retains the original oxaloacetate molecule to join with a new acetyl fragment that then enters the cycle.

Each acetyl-CoA molecule entering the citric acid cycle releases two carbon dioxide molecules and four pairs of hydrogen atoms. One molecule of ATP also regenerates directly by substrate-level phosphorylation from citric acid cycle reactions (see reaction 7 in Fig. 4.18). As summarized at the bottom of Figure 4.18, four hydrogens release when acetyl-CoA forms from the two pyruvate molecules created in glycolysis, and 16 hydrogens are released in the citric acid cycle. The most important function of the citric acid cycle generates electrons (H^+) for passage in the respiratory chain to NAD^+ and FAD.

Oxygen does not participate directly in citric acid cycle reactions. The major portion of the chemical energy in pyruvate transfers to ADP through the aerobic process of electron transport–oxidative phosphorylation within the folding, or cristae, of the inner mitochondrial membrane. With adequate oxygen, including enzymes and substrate, NAD^+ and FAD re-

An Important Macronutrient Component of Blood

Blood sugar usually remains regulated within narrow limits for two main reasons: (1) glucose serves as a primary fuel for nerve tissue metabolism, and (2) glucose represents the sole energy source for red blood cells, which contain no mitochondria. At rest and during exercise, liver glycogenolysis maintains normal blood glucose levels, usually at 100 mg · dL^{-1} (5.5 mM). In prolonged, intense exercise such as marathon running, blood glucose concentration eventually falls below normal levels because liver glycogen depletes, and active muscle continues to catabolize the available blood glucose. Symptoms of significantly reduced blood glucose (**hypoglycemia:** <45 mg of glucose per deciliter [dL] of blood) include weakness, hunger, and dizziness. This ultimately impairs exercise performance and can contribute to central nervous system fatigue associated with prolonged exercise. Sustained and profound hypoglycemia triggers unconsciousness and produces irreversible brain damage.

generation takes place and citric acid cycle metabolism proceeds unimpeded.

Net Energy Transfer from Glucose Catabolism

FIGURE 4.19 summarizes the pathways for energy transfer during glucose breakdown in skeletal muscle that culminate in the production of 32 moles of ATP. Two ATPs (net gain) are formed from substrate-level phosphorylation in glycolysis. The remaining ATPs are accounted for as follows:

1. Four extramitochondrial hydrogens (2 NADH) generated in glycolysis yield 5 ATPs during oxidative phosphorylation.
2. Four hydrogens (2 NADH) released in the mitochondrion as pyruvate degrades to acetyl-CoA yield 5 ATPs.
3. Two guanosine triphosphatates (GTP; a molecule similar to ATP) are produced in the citric acid cycle via substrate level phosphorylation.
4. Twelve of the 16 hydrogens (6 NADH) released in the citric acid cycle yield 15 ATPs (6 NADH × 2.5 ATP per NADH = 15 ATP).
5. Four hydrogens joined to FAD (2 FADH_2) in the citric acid cycle yield 3 ATPs.

Thirty-four ATPs represents the total ATP yield from the complete breakdown of glucose. *Because 2 ATPs initially phosphorylate glucose, 32 ATP molecules equal the net ATP yield from complete glucose breakdown in skeletal muscle. Four ATP molecules form directly from substrate-level phosphorylation (glycolysis and citric acid cycle), whereas 28 ATP molecules regenerate during oxidative phosphorylation.* Chapter 5 explains the specifics of carbohydrate's role in energy release under anaerobic and aerobic exercise conditions.

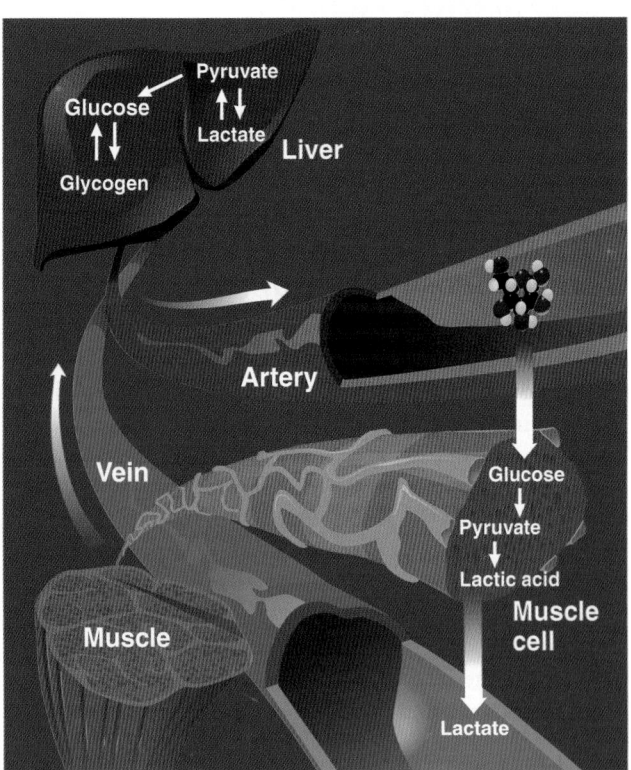

FIGURE 4.16 ■ In the Cori cycle, lactic acid from muscle enters the venous system and converts to lactate. Lactate then enters the liver for conversion to pyruvate and synthesis to glucose for subsequent delivery to muscle. This gluconeogenic process helps to maintain carbohydrate reserves.

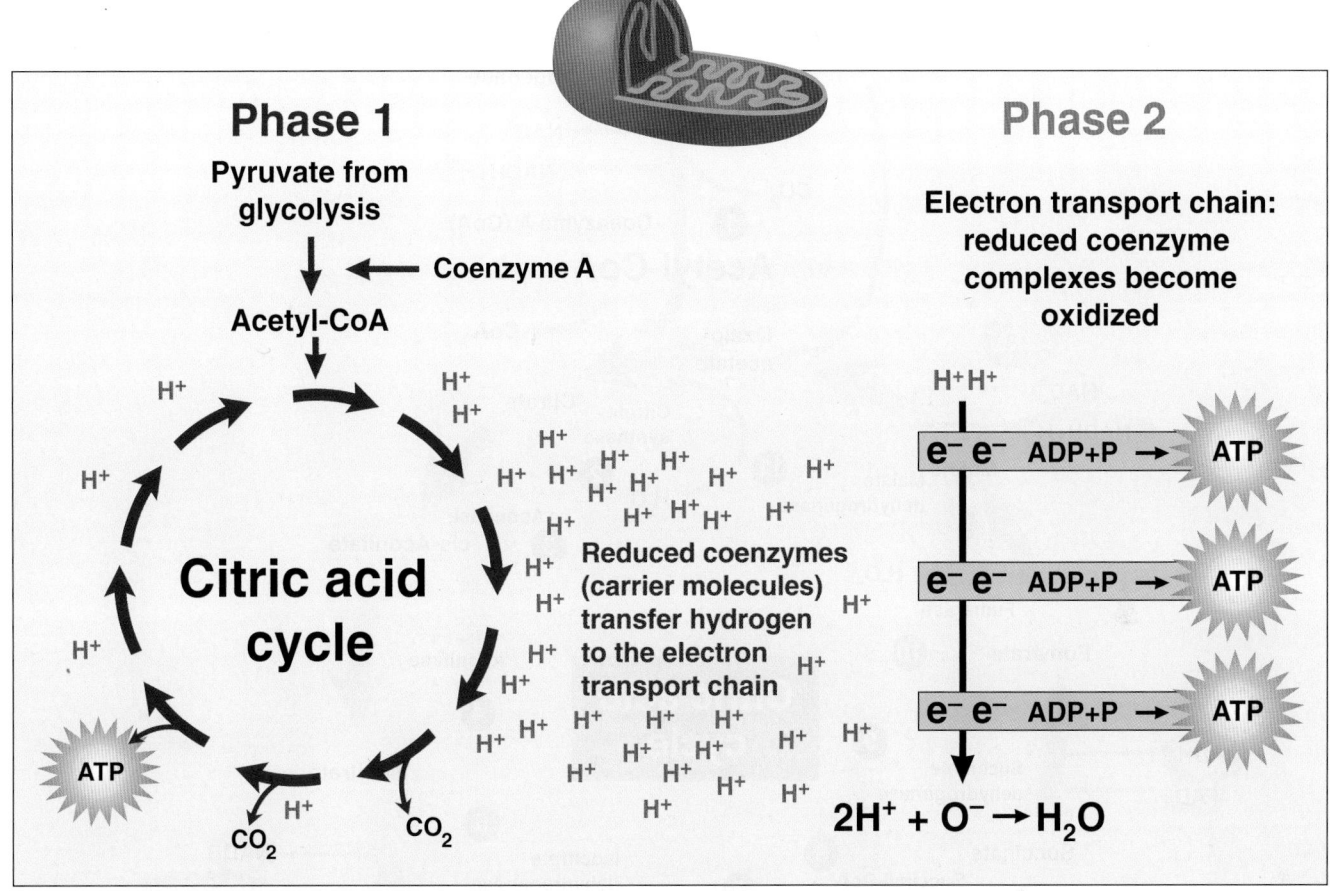

FIGURE 4.17 ■ Hydrogen formation and subsequent oxidation during aerobic energy metabolism. *Phase 1.* In the mitochondria, the citric acid cycle generates hydrogen atoms during acetyl-CoA breakdown. *Phase 2.* Significant quantities of ATP regenerate when these hydrogens oxidize via the aerobic process of electron transport–oxidative phosphorylation (electron transport chain). ADP, adenosine diphosphate; P, phosphate.

ENERGY RELEASE FROM FAT

Stored fat represents the body's most plentiful source of potential energy. Relative to carbohydrate and protein, stored fat provides almost unlimited energy. The fuel reserves in a typical young adult male equal between 60,000 and 100,000 kCal from triacylglycerol in fat cells (**adipocytes**) and about 3000 kCal from intramuscular triacylglycerol (12 mmol · kg^{-1} muscle). In contrast, the carbohydrate energy reserve generally amounts to less than 2000 kCal. Three energy sources for fat catabolism include:

1. Triacylglycerol stored directly within the muscle fiber in close proximity to the mitochondria (more in slow-twitch than fast-twitch muscle fibers)
2. Circulating triacylglycerol in lipoprotein complexes that hydrolyze on the surface of a tissue's capillary endothelium catalyzed by lipoprotein lipase
3. Circulating free fatty acids mobilized from triacylglycerol in adipose tissue that serve as blood-borne energy carriers

Before energy release from fat, hydrolysis (**lipolysis** or fat breakdown) splits the triacylglycerol molecule into glycerol

and three water-insoluble fatty acid molecules. The enzyme **hormone-sensitive lipase** catalyzes triacylglycerol breakdown as follows:

$$\text{Triacylglycerol} + 3\,H_2O \xrightarrow{\text{lipase}} \text{Glycerol} + 3\,\text{Fatty acids}$$

An intracellular mediator, **adenosine 3′,5′-cyclic monophosphate,** or **cyclic AMP,** activates hormone-sensitive lipase and thus regulates fat breakdown.[31] Cyclic AMP in both adipocytes and muscle cells becomes activated by the various fat-mobilizing hormones—epinephrine, norepinephrine, glucagon, and growth hormone—which themselves cannot enter the cell.[30] Lactate, ketones, and insulin inhibit cyclic-AMP activation.[7]

Adipocytes: Site of Fat Storage and Mobilization

FIGURE 4.20 outlines the dynamics of fat storage and fat mobilization. All cells store some fat; however, adipose tissue serves as an active and major supplier of fatty acid molecules. Adipocytes specialize in synthesizing and storing triacylglyc-

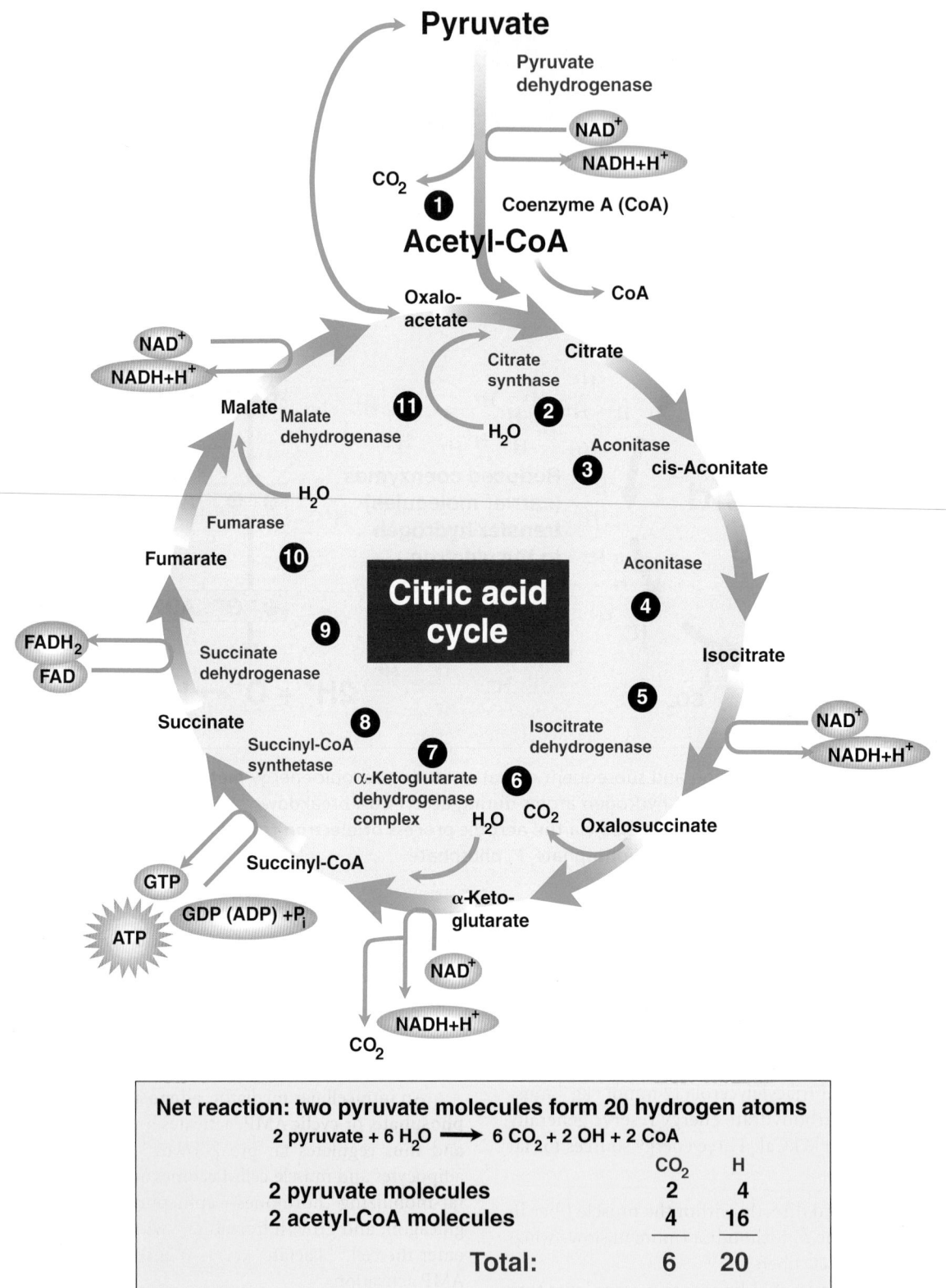

Pyruvate

Pyruvate
dehydrogenase

NAD$^+$

NADH+H$^+$

CO$_2$

1

Coenzyme A (CoA)

Acetyl-CoA

CoA

Oxalo-
acetate

Citrate

NAD$^+$

NADH+H$^+$

Citrate
synthase

Malate Malate
dehydrogenase

11

H$_2$O

2

cis-Aconitate

Aconitase

3

H$_2$O

Fumarase

Fumarate

10

Aconitase

**Citric acid
cycle**

4

Isocitrate

FADH$_2$

FAD

9

Succinate
dehydrogenase

5

NAD$^+$

NADH+H$^+$

Succinate

8

Succinyl-CoA
synthetase

7

α-Ketoglutarate
dehydrogenase
complex

6

H$_2$O CO$_2$

Isocitrate
dehydrogenase

Oxalosuccinate

GTP

GDP (ADP) +P$_i$

ATP

Succinyl-CoA

α-Keto-
glutarate

NAD$^+$

NADH+H$^+$

CO$_2$

Net reaction: two pyruvate molecules form 20 hydrogen atoms

2 pyruvate + 6 H$_2$O ⟶ 6 CO$_2$ + 2 OH + 2 CoA

	CO$_2$	H
2 pyruvate molecules	2	4
2 acetyl-CoA molecules	4	16
Total:	6	20

FIGURE 4.18 ■ Schematic illustration and quantification for hydrogen (H) and carbon dioxide (CO$_2$) release in the mitochondrion during the breakdown of one pyruvate molecule. All values have been doubled when computing the net gain of H and CO$_2$ from pyruvate breakdown because glycolysis produces two molecules of pyruvate from one molecule of glucose. Note the formation of guanosine triphosphate (GTP), a molecule similar to ATP, from guanosine diphosphate (GDP) by substrate level phosphorylation in reaction 8. P$_i$, phosphate; ADP, adenosine diphosphate; ATP, adenosine triphosphate; NAD, nicotinamide adenine dinucleotide; FAD, flavin adenine dinucleotide; GDP, guanosine diphosphate; GTP, guanosine triphosphate.

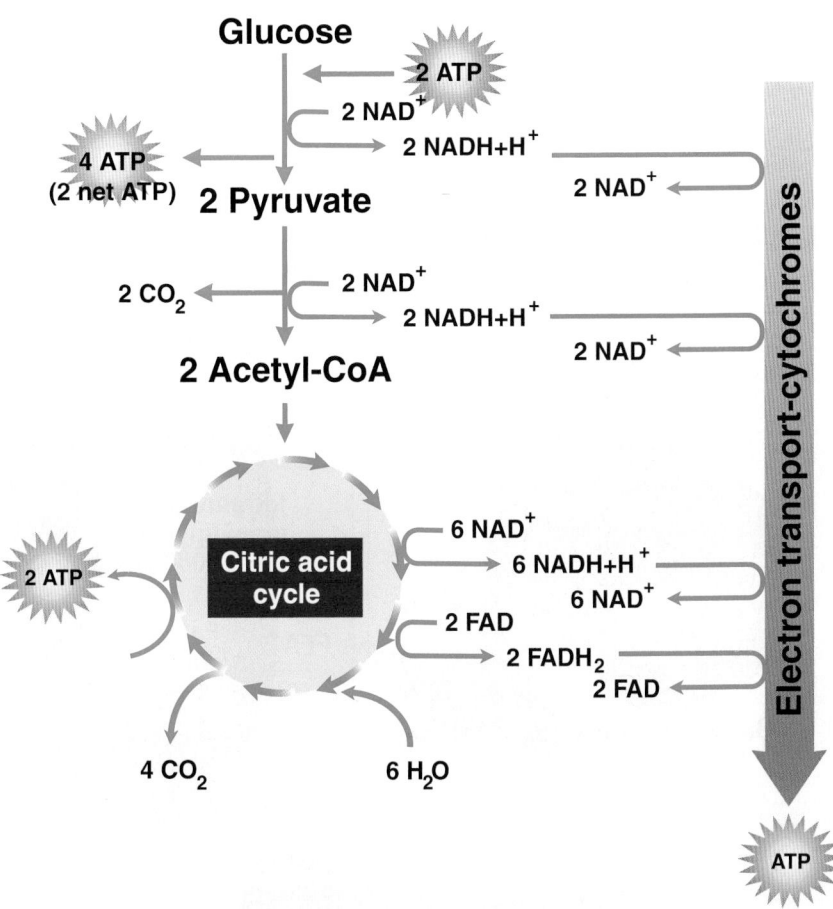

Glucose

2 ATP

2 NAD$^+$

2 NADH+H$^+$

4 ATP
(2 net ATP) **2 Pyruvate**

2 NAD$^+$

2 CO$_2$

2 NAD$^+$

2 NADH+H$^+$

2 NAD$^+$

2 Acetyl-CoA

Electron transport-cytochromes

Citric acid cycle

2 ATP

6 NAD$^+$

6 NADH+H$^+$

6 NAD$^+$

2 FAD

2 FADH$_2$

2 FAD

4 CO$_2$

6 H$_2$O

ATP

Net ATP from glucose metabolism		
Source	Reaction	Net ATP
Substrate phosphorylation	Glycolysis	2
2 H$_2$ (4 H$^+$)	Glycolysis	5
2 H$_2$ (4 H$^+$)	Pyruvate → Acetyl-CoA	5
Substrate phosphorylation	Citric acid cycle	2
6 H$_2$ (12 H$^+$)	Citric acid cycle	15
2 H$_2$ (H H$^+$)	Citric acid cycle	3
	Total:	32 ATP

FIGURE 4.19 ■ Net yield of 32 ATP molecules from energy transfer during the complete oxidation of one glucose molecule through glycolysis, the citric acid cycle, and electron transport.

erol. Triacylglycerol fat droplets occupy up to 95% of the adipocyte cell's volume. Once hormone-sensitive lipase stimulates fatty acids to diffuse from the adipocyte into the circulation, nearly all bind to plasma albumin for transport as **free fatty acids** (**FFAs**) to active tissues.[8,29] Hence, FFAs are not truly "free" entities. At the muscle site, FFAs release from the albumin–FFA complex for transport across the plasma membrane (by diffusion and/or a protein-mediated carrier system). Once inside the muscle cell, FFAs either re-esterify to form intracellular triacylglycerols or they bind with intramuscular proteins and enter the mitochondria for energy metabo-

lism (by action of **carnitine–acyl-CoA transferase**). Medium- and short-chain fatty acids do not depend on carnitine–acyl-CoA transferase transport, and most diffuse freely into the mitochondrion.

The water-soluble glycerol molecule formed during lipolysis readily diffuses from the adipocyte into the circulation. As a result, plasma glycerol levels often reflect the level of the body's triacylglycerol breakdown.[26] When delivered to the liver, glycerol serves as a gluconeogenic precursor for glucose synthesis. This relatively slow process explains why glycerol supplementation contributes little as an energy substrate during exercise.[21]

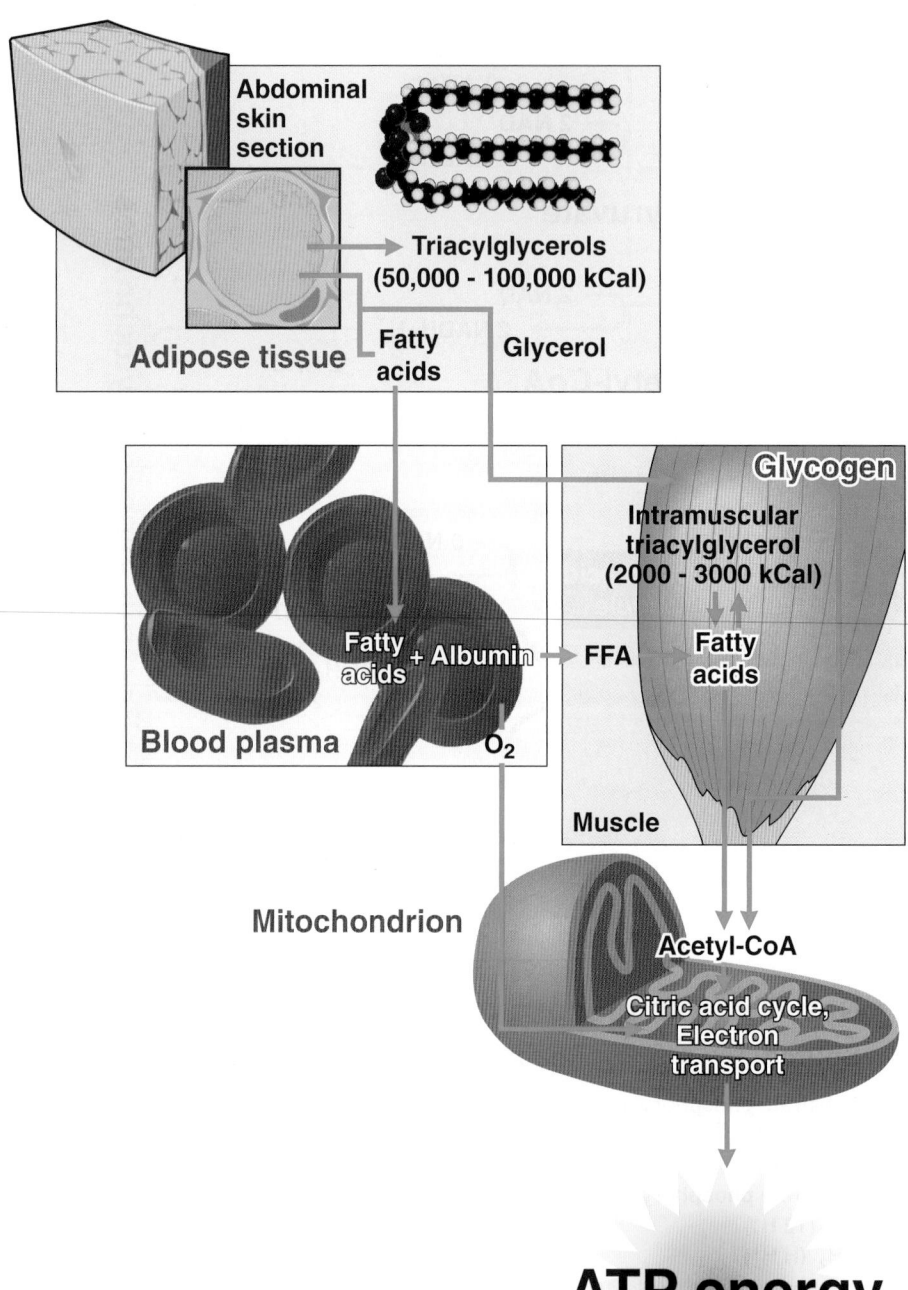

FIGURE 4.20 ■ Dynamics of fat mobilization and storage. Hormone-sensitive lipase stimulates triacylglycerol breakdown into glycerol and fatty acid components. After their release from adipocytes, the blood transports free fatty acids (FFAs) bound to plasma albumin. Fats stored within the muscle fiber also degrade to glycerol and fatty acids to provide energy. ATP, adenosine triphosphate.

Hormonal Effects

Epinephrine, norepinephrine, glucagon, and growth hormone augment lipase activation and subsequent lipolysis and FFA mobilization from adipose tissue. Plasma concentrations of these lipogenic hormones increase during exercise to continu- ally supply active muscles with energy-rich substrate. An intra- cellular mediator cyclic AMP, activates hormone-sensitive li- pase and thus regulates fat breakdown. The various lipid-mobilizing hormones, which themselves do not enter the cell, activate cyclic AMP.[30] Circulating lactate, ketones, and particularly insulin inhibit cyclic AMP activation.[8] Exercise training-induced increases in the activity level of skeletal muscle and adipose tissue lipases, including biochemical and vascular adaptations in the muscles themselves, enhance fat use for energy during moderate exercise.[6,16,17,19,25] Paradoxically, excess body fat decreases fatty acid availability and oxidation during exercise.[20]

Fat breakdown or synthesis depends on the availability of fatty acid molecules. After a meal, when energy metabolism remains relatively low, digestive processes increase FFA and triacylglycerol delivery to cells; this in turn stimulates triacylglycerol synthesis. In contrast, moderate exercise increases fatty acid use of energy, which reduces their cellular concentration. The decrease in intracellular FFAs stimulates triacylglycerol breakdown into glycerol and fatty acid components. Concurrently, hormonal release triggered by exercise stimulates adipose tissue lipolysis to further augment FFA delivery to active muscle.

Breakdown of Glycerol and Fatty Acids

FIGURE 4.21 summarizes the pathways for the breakdown of the glycerol and fatty acid fragments of the triacylglycerol molecule.

Glycerol

The anaerobic reactions of glycolysis accept glycerol as 3-phosphoglyceraldehyde, which then degrades to pyruvate to form ATP by substrate-level phosphorylation. Hydrogen atoms pass to NAD^+, and the citric acid cycle oxidizes pyruvate. Glycerol also provides carbon skeletons for glucose synthesis. This gluconeogenic role of glycerol becomes important when depletion of glycogen reserves occurs from dietary restriction of carbohydrates or in long-term exercise or intense training.

Fatty Acids

Almost all fatty acids contain an even number of carbon atoms, ranging from 2 to 26. The first step in transferring the potential energy in a fatty acid to ATP (a process termed *fatty acid oxidation*) cleaves 2-carbon acetyl fragments split from the long chain of the fatty acid. The process of converting an FFA to multiple acetyl-CoA molecules is called **beta (β)-oxidation** because the second carbon on a fatty acid is termed the "beta carbon." ATP phosphorylates the reactions, water is added, hydrogens pass to NAD^+ and FAD, and the acetyl fragment joins with coenzyme A to form acetyl-CoA. *β-oxidation provides the same two-carbon acetyl unit as acetyl generated from glucose breakdown.* β-oxidation continues until the entire fatty acid molecule degrades to acetyl-CoA for direct entry into the citric acid cycle. The hydrogens released during fatty acid catabolism oxidize through the respiratory chain. *Note that fatty acid breakdown relates directly with oxygen uptake.* β-oxidation proceeds only when oxygen joins with hydrogen. Under anaerobic conditions, hydrogen remains with NAD^+ and FAD, bringing a halt to fat catabolism.

Energy Transfer from Fat Catabolism

The breakdown of a fatty acid molecule progresses as follows:

1. β-oxidation produces NADH and $FADH_2$ by cleaving the fatty acid molecule into 2-carbon acetyl fragments.
2. Citric acid cycle degrades acetyl Co-A into carbon dioxide and hydrogen atoms.
3. Hydrogen atoms oxidize by electron transport–oxidative phosphorylation.

The rich hydrogen content of each of the triacylglycerol's three fatty acid molecules allows the complete oxidation of one triacylglycerol molecule to generate about 12 times more ATPs than produced from oxidation of one glucose molecule. Depending on a person's state of nutrition, level of training, and the intensity and duration of physical activity, intra- and extracellular lipid molecules usually supply between 30 and 80% of the energy for biologic work.[26,35] When high-intensity, long-duration exercise depletes glycogen reserves, fat serves as the *primary* fuel for exercise and recovery.[17]

FATS BURN IN A CARBOHYDRATE FLAME

Interestingly, fatty acid breakdown depends in part on a continual background level of carbohydrate breakdown. Recall that acetyl-CoA enters the citric acid cycle by combining with oxaloacetate to form citrate. This oxaloacetate is generated from pyruvate during carbohydrate breakdown (under the control of pyruvate carboxylase), which adds a carboxyl group to the pyruvate molecule. Carbohydrate depletion de-

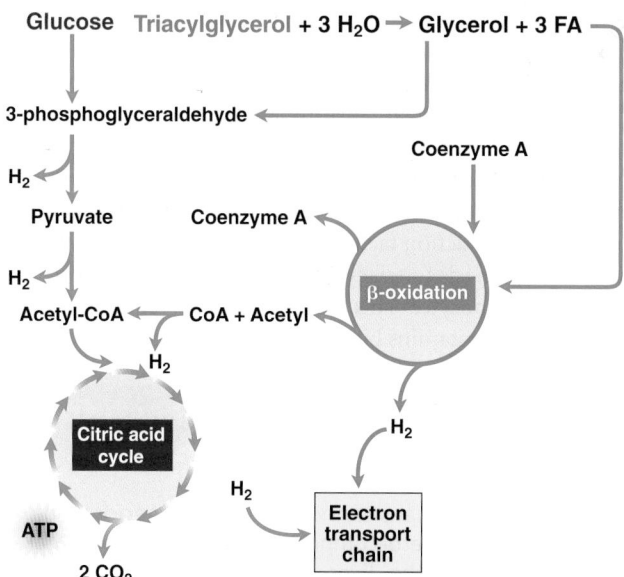

FIGURE 4.21 ■ General scheme for the breakdown of the glycerol and fatty acid fragments of triacylglycerol. Glycerol enters the energy pathways during glycolysis. The fatty acid fragments prepare to enter the citric acid cycle through β-oxidation. The electron transport chain accepts hydrogens released during glycolysis, β-oxidation, and citric acid cycle metabolism. ATP, adenosine triphosphate; FA, fatty acids.

creases pyruvate production during glycolysis. Diminished pyruvate reduces levels of citric acid cycle intermediates (oxaloacetate and malate), which slows citric acid cycle activity (SEE FIG. 4.22).[2,24,28,32,37] Citric acid cycle degradation of fatty acids depends on sufficient oxaloacetate availability to combine with the acetyl-CoA formed during β-oxidation. When the carbohydrate level decreases, the oxaloacetate level may become inadequate. In this sense, "fats burn in a carbohydrate flame."

A Slower Rate of Energy Release From Fat

A rate limit exists for fatty acid use by active muscle.[38] Aerobic training enhances this limit, but the power generated solely by fat breakdown still represents only about half that achieved with carbohydrate as the chief aerobic energy source. Thus, depleting muscle glycogen decreases a muscle's maximum aerobic power output. Just as the hypoglycemic condition coincides with a "central" or neural fatigue, muscle glycogen depletion probably causes "peripheral" or local muscle fatigue during exercise.[23]

Gluconeogenesis provides a metabolic option for synthesizing glucose from noncarbohydrate sources, but it cannot replenish or even maintain glycogen stores unless one regularly consumes carbohydrates. Appreciably reducing carbohydrate availability seriously limits energy transfer capacity. Glycogen depletion could occur in prolonged exercise (marathon running), consecutive days of heavy training, inadequate energy intake, dietary elimination of carbohydrates (as advocated with high-fat, low-carbohydrate "ketogenic" diets), or diabetes. Diminished aerobic exercise intensity occurs even though large amounts of fatty acid substrate circulate to muscle. During extreme carbohydrate depletion, the acetate fragments produced in β-oxidation accumulate in the extracellular fluids because they cannot readily enter the citric acid cycle. The liver converts these compounds to ketone bodies (4-carbon long acidic derivatives, acetoacetic acid and β-hydroxybutyric acid together with acetone), some of which pass in the urine. If ketosis persists, the acid quality of the body fluids can increase to potentially toxic levels.

LIPOGENESIS

Lipogenesis describes the formation of fat, mostly in the cytoplasm of liver cells. It occurs as follows: ingested excess glucose or protein not used immediately to sustain metabolism converts into stored triacylglycerol. For example, when muscle and liver glycogen stores fill, as occurs after a large carbohydrate-containing meal, insulin release from the pancreas causes a 30-fold increase in glucose transport into adipocytes. Insulin initiates the translocation of a latent pool of GLUT 4 transporters from the adipocyte cytosol to the plasma membrane. GLUT 4 action facilitates glucose transport into the cytosol for synthesis to triacylglycerols and subsequent storage within the adipocyte.[5] This lipogenic process requires ATP energy and the B vitamins biotin, niacin, and pantothenic acid.

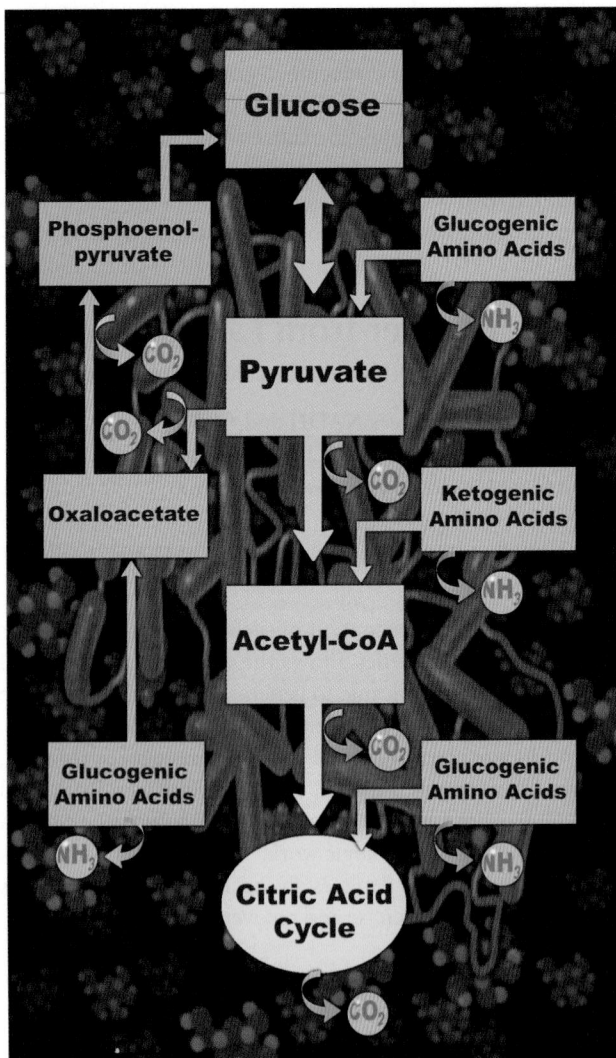

FIGURE 4.22 ■ Glucogenic and ketogenic amino acids. Carbon skeletons from amino acids that form pyruvate or directly enter the citric acid cycle are glucogenic because these carbon compounds can form glucose. Carbon skeletons that form acetyl-CoA are ketogenic because they cannot form glucose molecules but rather synthesize fat.

Potential for Glucose Synthesis from Triacylglycerol Components

Although humans cannot convert fatty acids to glucose, the glycerol component of triacylglycerol breakdown provides the liver with substrate for glucose synthesis. This provides the body with an important, albeit limited, option for maintaining blood glucose for neural and red blood cell functions. It also helps to minimize the muscle-wasting effects of low blood glucose in stimulating excessive muscle protein degradation to gluconeogenic constituents to sustain plasma glucose levels.

Lipogenesis begins with carbons from glucose and the carbon skeletons from amino acid molecules that metabolize to acetyl-CoA (see section on protein metabolism). Liver cells bond together the acetate parts of the acetyl-CoA molecules in a series of steps to form the16-carbon saturated fatty acid palmitic acid. Palmitic acid can then lengthen to an 18- or 20-carbon chain fatty acid in either the cytosol or the mitochondria. Ultimately, three fatty acid molecules join (esterify) with one glycerol molecule (produced during glycolysis) to yield one triacylglycerol molecule. Triacylglycerol releases into the circulation as a very-low-density lipoprotein (VLDL); cells may use VLDL for ATP production or store it in adipocytes along with other fats from dietary sources.

ENERGY RELEASE FROM PROTEIN

Chapter 1 emphasized that protein plays a role as an energy substrate during endurance-type activities and heavy training. The amino acids (primarily the branched-chain amino acids leucine, isoleucine, valine, glutamine, and aspartate) first convert to a form that readily enters pathways for energy release. This conversion requires nitrogen (amine) removal from the amino acid molecule. The liver serves as the main site for **deamination,** but skeletal muscle also contains enzymes that remove nitrogen from an amine group of an amino acid and pass it to other compounds during **transamination.** In this way, the "carbon skeleton" by-products of donor amino acids participate directly in energy metabolism within muscle. Enzyme levels for transamination increase with exercise training to further facilitate protein's use as an energy substrate.

Once an amino acid loses its nitrogen-containing amine group, the remaining compound (usually a component of the citric acid cycle's reactive compounds) contributes to ATP formation. Some amino acids are **glucogenic** and when deaminated yield intermediate products for glucose synthesis via gluconeogenesis (Fig. 4.22). For example, pyruvate forms in the liver as alanine loses its amine group and gains a double-bond oxygen; pyruvate can then be synthesized to glucose. This gluconeogenic method serves as an important adjunct to the Cori cycle to provide glucose during prolonged exercise. Regular exercise training enhances the liver's capacity for gluconeogenesis from alanine.[33,34] Other amino acids such as glycine are **ketogenic** and when deaminated yield the intermediate acetyl-CoA or acetoacetate. These compounds cannot be synthesized to glucose, but instead are synthesized to fat or are catabolized for energy in the citric acid cycle.

Protein Conversion to Fat

Surplus dietary protein (like carbohydrate) readily converts to fat. The amino acids absorbed by the small intestine after protein's digestion are transported in the circulation to the liver. FIGURE 4.23 illustrates that carbon skeletons derived from these amino acids after deamination convert to pyruvate. Pyruvate then enters the mitochondrion for conversion to acetyl-CoA for either (1) catabolism in the citric acid cycle or (2) fatty acid synthesis.

Protein Breakdown Facilitates Water Loss

When protein provides energy, the body must eliminate the nitrogen-containing amine group and other solutes from protein breakdown. This requires excretion of "obligatory" water because the waste products of protein catabolism leave the body dissolved in fluid (urine). For this reason, excessive protein catabolism increases the body's water needs.

THE METABOLIC MILL

The citric acid cycle plays a much more important role than simply degrading pyruvate produced during glucose catabolism. Fragments from other organic compounds formed from fat and protein breakdown provide energy during citric acid cycle metabolism. Figure 4.23 illustrates that deaminated residues of excess amino acids enter the citric acid cycle at various intermediate stages, whereas the glycerol fragment of triacylglycerol catabolism gains entrance via the glycolytic pathway. Fatty acids become oxidized in β-oxidation to acetyl-CoA. This compound then enters the cycle directly.

The "metabolic mill" depicts the citric acid cycle as the vital link between food (macronutrient) energy and the chemical energy of ATP. The citric acid cycle also serves as a "metabolic hub" to provide intermediates that cross the mitochondrial membrane into the cytosol to synthesize bionutrients for maintenance and growth. For example, excess carbohydrates provide glycerol and acetyl fragments to synthesize triacylglycerol. Acetyl-CoA also functions as the branch point for synthesizing cholesterol, bile, and many hormones, as well as ketone bodies and fatty acids. Fatty acids *cannot* contribute to glucose synthesis because the conversion of pyruvate to acetyl-CoA does not reverse (notice the one-way arrow in Fig. 4.23). Many of the carbon compounds generated in citric cycle reactions also provide the organic starting points for synthesizing nonessential amino acids.

REGULATION OF ENERGY METABOLISM

Under normal conditions, electron transfer and subsequent energy release tightly couple to ADP phosphorylation. In general, without the availability of ADP for phosphorylation to ATP, electrons do not shuttle down the respiratory chain to oxygen. Compounds that either inhibit or activate enzymes at key control points in the oxidative pathways modulate regulatory control of glycolysis and the citric acid cycle.[1,11,12,15,22] Each pathway has at least one enzyme considered "rate-limiting" because it controls the speed of that pathway's reactions. By far, cellular ADP concentration exerts the greatest effect on the rate-limiting enzymes that control the energy metabolism

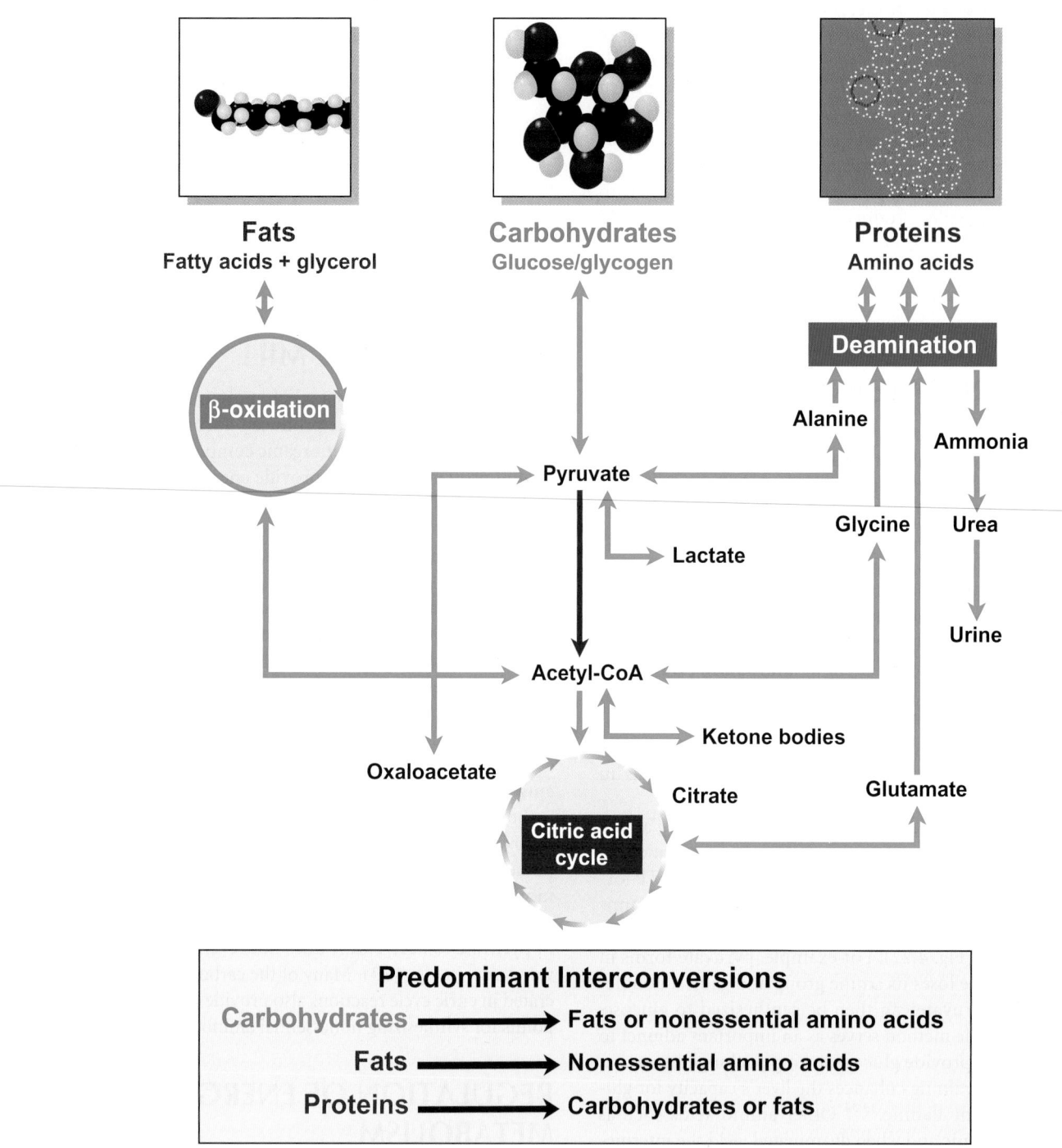

FIGURE 4.23 ■ The "metabolic mill" shows important interconversions among carbohydrates, fats, and proteins. Note that all interconversions are possible except that fatty acids cannot contribute to glucose synthesis (note one-way *red arrow*).

of carbohydrates, fats, and proteins. This mechanism for respiratory control makes sense because any increase in ADP signals a need for energy to restore ATP levels. Conversely, high levels of cellular ATP indicate a relatively low energy requirement. From a broader perspective, ADP concentrations function as a cellular feedback mechanism to maintain a relatively constant level (homeostasis) of energy currency available for biologic work. Other rate-limiting modulators include cellular levels of phosphate, cyclic AMP, calcium, NAD^+, citrate, and pH.

Summary

1. Food macronutrients provide the major sources of potential energy to rejoin ADP and phosphate ion to form ATP.

2. The complete breakdown of 1 mole of glucose liberates 689 kCal of energy. Of this, ATP bonds conserve about 224 kCal (34%), with the remainder dissipated as heat.

3. During glycolytic reactions in the cell's cytosol, a net of two ATP molecules forms during anaerobic substrate-level phosphorylation.

4. Pyruvate converts to acetyl-CoA during the second stage of carbohydrate breakdown within the mitochondrion. Acetyl-CoA then progresses through the citric acid cycle.

5. Hydrogen atoms released during glucose breakdown oxidize via the respiratory chain; the energy generated couples to ADP phosphorylation.

6. The complete breakdown of a glucose molecule in skeletal muscle theoretically yields a net total of 32 ATP molecules.

7. A biochemical "steady state" or "steady rate" exists when hydrogen atoms oxidize at their rate of formation.

8. During intense exercise, when hydrogen oxidation does not keep pace with its production, lactate forms as pyruvate temporarily binds hydrogen. This allows progression of anaerobic glycolysis for an additional time period.

9. The complete breakdown of a triacylglycerol molecule yields about 460 molecules of ATP. Fatty acid catabolism requires oxygen; the term *aerobic* describes such reactions.

10. Protein serves as a potentially important energy substrate. After nitrogen removal from the amino acid molecule during deamination, the remaining carbon skeletons enter various metabolic pathways to produce ATP aerobically.

11. Numerous interconversions take place among the food nutrients. Fatty acids represent a noteworthy exception because they cannot be synthesized to glucose.

12. Fats require a certain level of carbohydrate breakdown for their continual catabolism for energy in the metabolic mill. To this extent, "fats burn in a carbohydrate flame."

13. Compounds that either inhibit or activate enzymes at key control points in the oxidative pathways modulate control of glycolysis and the citric acid cycle. Cellular ADP concentration exerts the greatest effect on the rate-limiting enzymes that control energy metabolism.

Test Your Knowledge Answers

1. **True:** Carbohydrates provide energy (4 kCal per g) for the body to resynthesize ATP. They convert to glycogen in glycogenesis for storage in muscle and liver. Once the glycogen reserves become filled, any excess energy from carbohydrate readily converts to stored body fat, primarily in adipose tissue.

2. **False:** Lipids provide energy (9 kCal per g) for ATP resynthesis. They store as fat in adipose tissue for future energy needs. Fatty acids cannot contribute to glucose formation because of the unavailability of the enzyme to convert acetyl-CoA (from fatty acid breakdown) to pyruvate for glucose synthesis.

3. **False:** An enzyme is a highly specific and large organic protein catalyst that accelerates the rate of chemical reactions without being consumed or changed in the reactions.

4. **False:** As in the case of carbohydrates and lipids, excess energy from dietary protein readily converts to fat for storage in adipose tissue. Thus, high-protein diets, if they constitute excess caloric intake, result in positive energy balance and a gain in body fat.

5. **False:** The catabolism of all three macronutrients, carbohydrates, lipids, and proteins, results in ATP formation. On a relative basis, fat and carbohydrate provide their carbon skeletons for ATP synthesis more readily than protein, which primarily serves an anabolic role.

6. **False:** The first law of thermodynamics states that energy is neither created nor destroyed but instead transforms from one form to another without being used up. In essence, the law dictates that the body does not produce, consume, or use up energy; it merely transforms energy from one form into another as physiologic systems undergo continual change.

7. **False:** Oxidation reactions transfer oxygen atoms, hydrogen atoms, or electrons. A loss of electrons occurs in oxidation reactions with a corresponding gain in valence. Reduction reactions involve any process in which atoms gain electrons with a corresponding decrease in valence. Oxidation and reduction reactions always couple, so the energy released by one reaction becomes incorporated into the products of the other reaction.

8. **True:** The term *energy* suggests a dynamic state related to change; thus energy emerges only when a

Test Your Knowledge Answers *continued*

change occurs. Potential energy and kinetic energy constitute the total energy of a system. Potential energy refers to energy associated with a substance's structure or position, while kinetic energy refers to energy of motion. Potential energy can be measured when it transforms to kinetic energy. There are six forms of energy—chemical, mechanical, heat, light, electrical, and nuclear—and each can convert or transform to another form.

9. **False:** In essence, cellular oxidation–reduction constitutes the biochemical mechanism that underlies energy metabolism. The mitochondria, the cell's "energy factories," contain carrier molecules that remove electrons from hydrogen (oxidation) and eventually pass them to oxygen (reduction). ATP synthesis occurs during oxidation–reduction reactions. Aerobic metabolism refers to energy-gener-

ating catabolic reactions in which oxygen serves as the final electron acceptor in the respiratory chain and combines with hydrogen to form water. In one sense, the term *aerobic* seems misleading because oxygen does not participate directly in ATP synthesis. On the other hand, oxygen's presence at the end of the line largely determines the capacity for ATP production.

10. **False:** Thirty-four ATP molecules represents the total (gross) ATP yield from the complete breakdown of a glucose molecule. Because 2 ATPs initially phosphorylate glucose, 32 ATP molecules equal the net ATP yield from glucose breakdown in skeletal muscle. Four ATP molecules form directly from substrate-level phosphorylation (glycolysis and citric acid cycle), whereas 28 ATP molecules regenerate during oxidative phosphorylation.

References

1. Balban RS. Regulation of oxidative phosphorylation in the mammalian cell. *Am J Physiol* 1990;258:C377.
2. Campbell MK. Biochemistry. Philadelphia, WB Saunders, 1991.
3. Carins SP, et al. Role of extracellular $[Ca^{2+}]$ in fatigue of isolated mammalian skeletal muscle. *J Appl Physiol* 1998;84:1395.
4. Chasiotis D. Role of cyclic AMP and inorganic phosphate in the regulation of muscle glycogenolysis during exercise. *Med Sci Sports Exerc* 1988;20:545.
5. Christ-Roberts CY, et al. Exercise training increases glycogen synthase activity and GLUT4 expression but not insulin signaling in overweight nondiabetic and type 2 diabetic subjects. *Metabolism* 2004;53:1233.
6. Coggan AR, et al. Isotopic estimation of CO_2 production during exercise before and after endurance training. *J Appl Physiol* 1993;75:70.
7. Fox SI. Human physiology. 7th ed. New York: McGraw-Hill, 2002.
8. Donsmark M, et al. Hormone-sensitive lipase as mediator of lipolysis in contracting skeletal muscle. *Exerc Sport Sci Rev* 2005;33:127.
9. Febbario MA, et al. Effect of epinephrine on muscle glycogenolysis during exercise in trained men. *J Appl Physiol* 1998;84:465.
10. Greehnaff PL, Timmons JA. Interaction between aerobic and anaerobic metabolism during intense muscle contraction. *Exerc Sport Sci Rev* 1998;26:1.
11. Hardie DG. AMP-activated protein kinase: a key system mediating metabolic responses to exercise. *Med Sci Sports Med* 2004;36:28.
12. Hawley JA, Zierath JR. Integration of metabolic and mitogenic signal transduction in skeletal muscle. *Exerc Sport Sci Rev* 2004;32:4.
13. Hogan MC, et al. Increased [lactate] in working dog muscle reduces tension development independent of pH. *Med Sci Sports Exerc* 1995; 27:371.
14. Hultman E, et al. Energy metabolism and fatigue. In: Taylor AW, et al, eds. *Biochemistry of Exercise VII*. Champaign, IL: Human Kinetics, 1990.
15. Jacobs I, et al. Effects of prior exercise or ammonium chloride ingestion on muscular strength and endurance. *Med Sci Sports Exerc* 1993;25:809.
16. Jorgensen SB, et al. Role of AMPK in skeletal muscle metabolic regulation and adaptation in relation to exercise. *J Physiol* 2006;574(pt 1):17.
17. Kiens B. Skeletal muscle lipid metabolism in exercise and insulin resistance. *Physiol Rev* 2006;86:205.
18. Mainwood GW, Renaud JM. The effect of acid-base on fatigue of skeletal muscle. *Can J Physiol Pharmacol* 1985;63:403.
19. Messonnierl L, et al. Are the effects of training on fat metabolism involved in the improvement of performance during high intensity exercise? *Eur J Appl Physiol* 2005;94:434.
20. Mittendorfer B, et al. Excess body fat in men decreases plasma fatty acid availability and oxidation during endurance exercise. *Am J Physiol Endocrinol Metab* 2004;286:E354.
21. Murray R, et al. Physiological responses to glycerol ingestion during exercise. *J Appl Physiol* 1991;71:144.
22. Myburgh KH. Can any metabolites partially alleviate fatigue manifestations at the cross-bridge? *Med Sci Sports Exerc* 2004;36:20.
23. Nybo L. CNS fatigue and prolonged exercise: effect of glucose supplementation. *Med Sci Sports Exerc* 2003;35:589.
24. Richter EA. Interaction of fuels in muscle metabolism during exercise. In: *Integration of Medical and Sports Sciences*. Basal: Karger, 1992.
25. Richterova B, et al. Effect of endurance training on adrenergic control of lipolysis in adipose tissue of obese women. *J Clin Endocrinol Metab* 2004;89:1325.
26. Romijn JA, et al. Regulations of endogenous fat and carbohydrate metabolism in relation to exercise intensity and duration. *Am J Physiol* 1993;265:E380.
27. Rose AJ, Richter EA. Skeletal muscle glucose uptake during exercise: how is it regulated? *Physiology* 2005;20:260.
28. Sahlin K, Broberg S. Tricarboxylic acid cycle intermediates in human muscle during prolonged exercise. *Am J Physiol* 1990;259:C834.
29. Seip RL, Semenkovich CF. Skeletal muscle lipoprotein lipase: molecular regulation and physiological effects in relation to exercise. *Exerc Sport Sci Rev* 1998;26:191.
30. Shepherd RE, Bah MD. Cyclic AMP regulation of fuel metabolism during exercise: regulation of adipose tissue lipolysis during exercise. *Med Sci Sports Exerc* 1988;20:531.
31. Stefanick ML, Wood PD. Physical activity, lipid and lipoprotein metabolism, and lipid transport. In: Bouchard C, et al., eds. *Physical Activity, Fitness, and Health*. Champaign, IL: Human Kinetics, 1994.
32. Stryer L. *Biochemistry*. 4th ed. San Francisco: WH Freeman, 1995.
33. Sumida KD, Donovan CM. Enhanced hepatic gluconeogenic capacity for selected precursors after endurance training. *J Appl Physiol* 1995;79:1883.

34. Sumida KD, et al. Enhanced gluconeogenesis from lactate in perfused livers after endurance training. *J Appl Physiol* 1993;74:782.

35. Thompson DL, et al. Substrate use during and following moderate- and low-intensity exercise: implications for weight control. *Eur J Appl Physiol* 1998;78:43.

36. Trump ME, et al. Importance of muscle phosphocreatine during intermittent maximal cycling. *J Appl Physiol* 1996;80:1574.

37. Turcoatte LP, et al. Impaired plasma FFA oxidation imposed by extreme CHO deficiency in contracting rat skeletal muscle. *J Appl Physiol* 1994;77:517.

38. Vusse van der GJ, et al. *Lipid Metabolism in Muscle: Handbook of Physiology,* Section 12: Exercise—regulation and integration of multiple systems. New York: Oxford Press, 1996.

General References

Alberts B, et al. *Essential Cell Biology: An Introduction to the Molecular Biology of the Cell.* 2nd ed. New York: Garland Publishers, 2003.

Berg JM, et al. *Biochemistry,* 6th ed. San Francisco: WH Freeman, 2006.

Bodner GM. Metabolism. Part 1. Glycolysis, or the Embden-Meyerhof pathway. *J Chem Educ* 1986;63:566.

Bodner GM. The tricarboxylic acid (TA), citric acid, Krebs cycle. *J Chem Educ* 1986;63:673.

Brooks GA, et al. *Exercise Physiology: Human Bioenergetics and its Applications.* New York: McGraw-Hill, 2005.

Campbell MK, Farrell SO. *Biochemistry.* 5th ed. London: Thomson Brooks/Cole, 2005.

Fox SI. *Human Physiology.* 9th ed. New York: McGraw-Hill, 2005.

Hammes, GG. Physical Chemistry for the Biological Sciences. New York: Wiley, 2007.

Guyton AC, Hall JE. *Textbook of Medical Physiology.* 11th ed. Philadelphia: WB Saunders, 2005.

Hargreaves M. Interactions between muscle glycogen and blood glucose during exercise. *Exerc Sport Sci Rev* 1997;25:21.

Ivy J. *Nutrient Timing: The Future of Sports Nutrition.* North Bergan, NJ: Basic Health Publications, 2005.

Marieb EN. *Essentials of Human Anatomy and Physiology.* 8th ed. San Francisco: Benjamin Cummings, 2006.

Nelson DL, Cox MM. *Lehninger's Principles of Biochemistry* 4th ed. New York: Worth Publishers, 2004.

Nicklas BJ. Effects of endurance exercise on adipose tissue metabolism. *Exerc Sport Sci Rev* 1997;25:77.

Shils ME, et al. *Modern Nutrition in Health and Disease.* 10th ed. Baltimore: Lippincott Williams & Wilkins, 2005.

Stryer L. *Biochemistry.* 4th ed. San Francisco: WH Freeman, 1995.

Watson JD, Berry A. *DNA: The Secret of Life.* New York: Knopf, 2003.

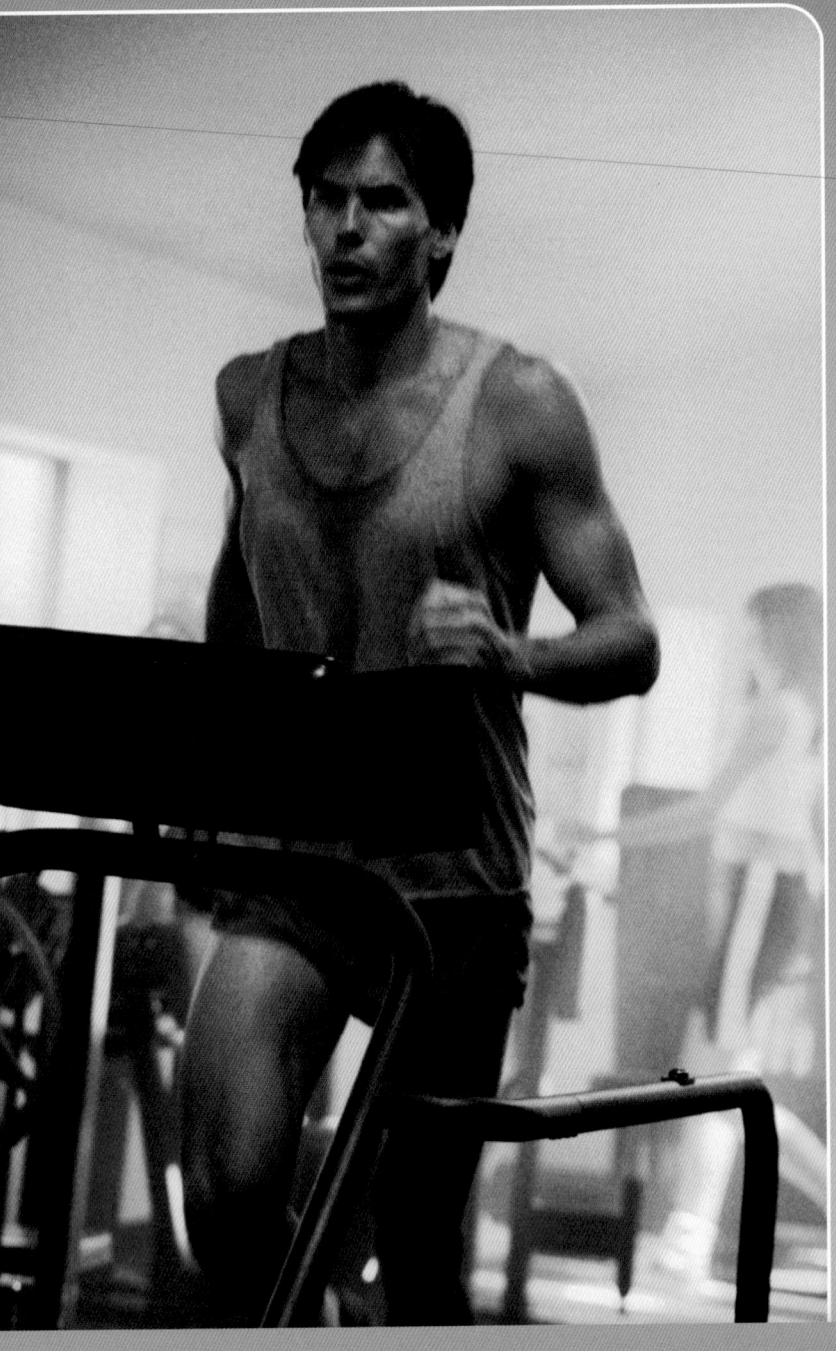

Chapter 5

Macronutrient Metabolism in Exercise and Training

Test Your Knowledge

Test Your Knowledge

Answer these 10 statements about macronutrient metabolism in exercise and training. Use the scoring key at the end of the chapter to check your results. Repeat this test after you have read the chapter and compare your results.

1. **T F** Anaerobic sources supply the predominant energy for short-term, powerful movement activities.
2. **T F** Lipid provides the primary energy macronutrient for ATP resynthesis during high-intensity aerobic exercise.
3. **T F** As blood flow increases with light and moderate exercise, more free fatty acids leave adipose tissue depots for delivery to active muscle.
4. **T F** Carbohydrate provides the preferential energy fuel during high-intensity anaerobic exercise.
5. **T F** Severely lowered liver and muscle glycogen levels during prolonged exercise induce fatigue, despite sufficient oxygen availability to muscles and an almost unlimited potential energy from stored fat
6. **T F** A diet low in lipid content reduces fatty acid availability, which negatively affects endurance capacity in high-intensity aerobic exercise.
7. **T F** A decrease in blood sugar during prolonged exercise concomitantly increases fat catabolism for energy.
8. **T F** Exercise training enhances the ability to oxidize carbohydrate but not fat during exercise.
9. **T F** Because protein provides the building block molecules for tissue synthesis, its catabolism occurs only minimally (2% of total energy) during exercise.
10. **T F** Consuming a high-fat diet in the 7- to 10-day period before a bout of heavy exercise significantly improves exercise performance.

G as exchange in the lungs along with biochemical and biopsy techniques, magnetic resonance imaging, and labeled nutrient tracers provide insight into contributions of the stored macronutrients and high-energy phosphates to exercise bioenergetics. The needle biopsy technique samples small quantities of active muscle to assess intramuscular nutrient kinetics throughout exercise. Such data provide an objective basis for recommending meal plans during exercise training, and specific nutritional modifications before, during, and in recovery from strenuous competition. *The fuel mixture that powers exercise generally depends on the intensity and duration of effort, and the exerciser's fitness and nutritional status.*

The Energy Spectrum of Exercise

FIGURE 5.1 depicts the relative contributions of anaerobic and aerobic energy sources during various durations of maximal exercise. In addition, TABLE 5.1 lists the approximate percentage of total energy for adenosine triphosphate (ATP) resynthesis from each energy transfer system for different competition running events. The data represent estimates from all-out running experiments in the laboratory, but they can relate to other activities by drawing the appropriate time relationships. A 100-m sprint run equates to any all-out activity lasting about 10 seconds, while an 800-m run lasts approximately 2 minutes. Maximal exercise for 1 minute includes the 400-m dash in track, the 100-m swim, and multiple full-court presses at the end of a basketball game.

The sources for energy transfer exist along a continuum. At one extreme, intramuscular high-energy phosphates ATP and phosphocreatine (PCr) supply most energy for exercise. The ATP–PCr and lactic acid systems provide about half of the energy required for intense exercise lasting 2 minutes; aerobic reactions provide the remainder. For top performance in all-out 2-minute exercise, a person must possess a well-developed capacity for *both* aerobic and anaerobic metabolism. Intense exercise of intermediate duration performed for 5 to 10 minutes, like middle-distance running and swimming or basketball, requires a greater demand for aerobic energy transfer. Performances of longer duration—marathon running, distance swimming and cycling, recreational jogging, and hiking and backpacking—require a fairly steady energy supply derived aerobically without reliance on lactate formation.

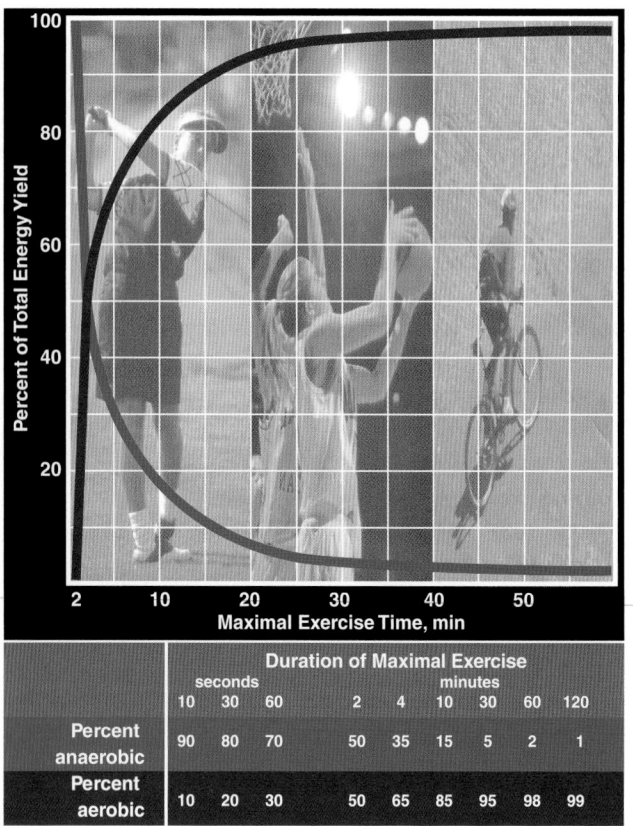

FIGURE 5.1 ■ Relative contributions of aerobic (*red*) and anaerobic (*blue*) energy metabolism during maximal physical effort of varying durations. Note that 2 minutes of maximal effort requires about 50% of the energy from both aerobic and anaerobic processes. At a world-class 4-minute per mile pace, approximately 65% of the energy comes from aerobic metabolism, with the remainder generated from anaerobic processes. For a marathon, on the other hand, the energy derived from aerobic processes almost totally powers the run.

Generally, anaerobic sources supply most of the energy for fast movements or during increased resistance to movement at a given speed. When movement begins at either fast or slow speed, the intramuscular high-energy phosphates provide immediate anaerobic energy for muscle action. After a few seconds, the glycolytic pathway (intramuscular glycogen breakdown in glycolysis) generates an increasingly greater proportion of energy for ATP resynthesis. Intense exercise continued beyond 30 seconds places a progressively greater demand on the relatively slower aerobic energy metabolism of the stored macronutrients. For example, power output during 30 seconds of maximal exercise (e.g., sprint cycling or running) is about twice the power output generated exercising all-out for 5 minutes at one's maximal oxygen uptake. Some activities rely predominantly on a single energy transfer system, whereas more than one energy system energizes most physical activities, depending on their intensity and duration. Higher intensity and shorter duration activities place greater demand on anaerobic energy transfer.

Two main macronutrient sources provide energy for ATP resynthesis during exercise: (1) liver and muscle glycogen and (2) triacylglycerols within adipose tissue and active muscle. To a lesser degree, amino acids within skeletal muscle donate carbon skeletons (minus nitrogen) to processes of energy metabolism. FIGURE 5.2 provides a generalized overview of the relative contribution to energy metabolism of carbohydrate, fat, and protein for adequately nourished individuals during rest and various exercise intensities. This illustration does not depict the considerable alterations in metabolic mixture (increases in fat and protein breakdown) during prolonged, intense exercise with accompanying depletion of liver and muscle glycogen. The following sections discuss the specific energy contribution of each macronutrient during exercise and the adaptations in substrate use with training.

TABLE 5.1   **Estimated Percentage Contribution of Different Fuels to ATP Generation in Various Running Events**

| | Percentage Contribution to ATP Generation | | | | |
| | Glycogen | | | | |
Event	Phosphocreatine	Anaerobic	Aerobic	Blood Glucose (Liver Glycogen)	Triacylglycerol (Fatty Acids)
100 m	50	50	—	—	—
200 m	25	65	10	—	—
400 m	12.5	62.5	25	—	—
800 m	6	50	44	—	—
1500 m	[a]	25	75	—	—
5000 m	[a]	12.5	87.5	—	—
10,000 m	[a]	3	97	—	—
Marathon	—	—	75	5	20
Ultramarathon (80 km)	—	—	35	5	60
24-h race	—	—	10	2	88

From Newsholme EA, et al. Physical and mental fatigue. Br Med Bull 1999;48:477.

[a]*In such events, phosphocreatine will be used for the first few seconds and, if it has been resynthesized during the race, in the sprint to the finish.*

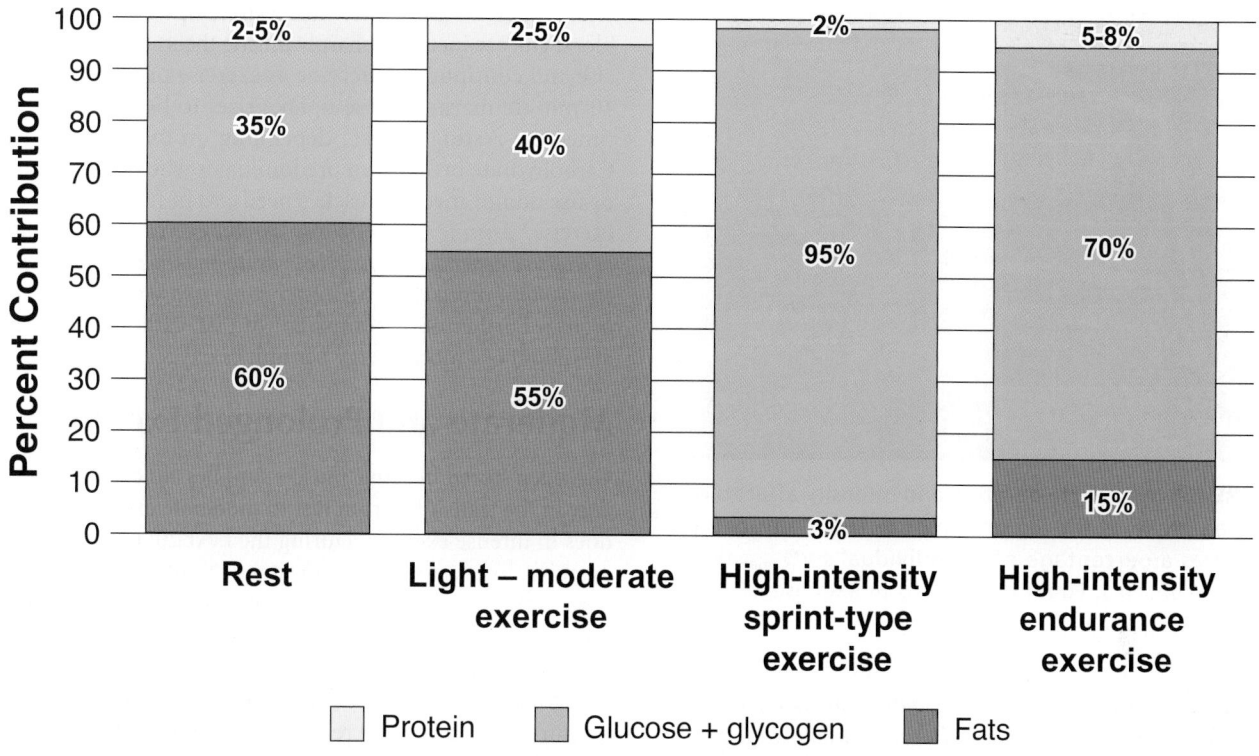

FIGURE 5.2 ■ Generalized illustration of the contribution of the carbohydrate (green), fat (orange), and protein (yellow) macronutrients to energy metabolism at rest and during various intensities of exercise.

Carbohydrate Mobilization and Use During Exercise

The liver markedly increases its release of glucose for use by active muscle as exercise progresses from low to high intensity.[8,53] Simultaneously, glycogen stored within muscle serves as the predominant carbohydrate energy source during the early stages of exercise and as exercise intensity increases.[19,39,46,48] Compared with fat and protein catabolism, carbohydrate remains the preferential fuel during high intensity aerobic exercise because it rapidly supplies ATP during oxidative processes. In anaerobic effort (reactions of glycolysis), carbohydrate becomes the *sole* contributor of ATP.

An Intricate Look at Fuel Utilization in Exercise

Biochemical and biopsy techniques and labeled nutrient tracers assess the energy contribution of nutrients during diverse forms of physical activity. For example, needle biopsies permit serial sampling of specific muscles to assess the kinetics of intramuscular nutrient metabolism with little interruption during exercise. Data from such research indicate that the intensity and duration of effort and the fitness and nutritional status of the exerciser largely determine the fuel mixture in exercise.[11,24]

Carbohydrate availability in the metabolic mixture during exercise helps regulate fat mobilization and its use for energy.[13,14] For example, increasing carbohydrate oxidation by

ingesting rapidly absorbed (high-glycemic) carbohydrates before exercise (with associated hyperglycemia and hyperinsulinemia) blunts long-chain fatty acid oxidation by skeletal muscle and free fatty acid (FFA) liberation from adipose tissue during exercise. Perhaps increased carbohydrate availability (and resulting increased catabolism) inhibits long-chain fatty acid transport into the mitochondria, thus controlling the metabolic mixture in exercise. It also appears that the concentration of blood glucose provides feedback regulation of the liver's glucose output; an increase in blood glucose inhibits hepatic glucose release during exercise.[22]

INTENSE EXERCISE

With strenuous exercise, neural–humoral factors increase hormonal output of epinephrine, norepinephrine, and glucagon and decrease insulin release. These actions stimulate **glycogen phosphorylase** to augment glycogen breakdown (glycogenolysis) in the liver and active muscles. In the early minutes of exercise when oxygen use fails to meet energy demands, stored muscle glycogen becomes the primary energy contributor because it provides energy without oxygen. As exercise duration progresses, blood-borne glucose from the liver increases its contribution as a metabolic fuel. Blood glucose, for example, can supply 30% of the total energy required by active muscle, with *most* of the remaining carbohydrate energy supplied by

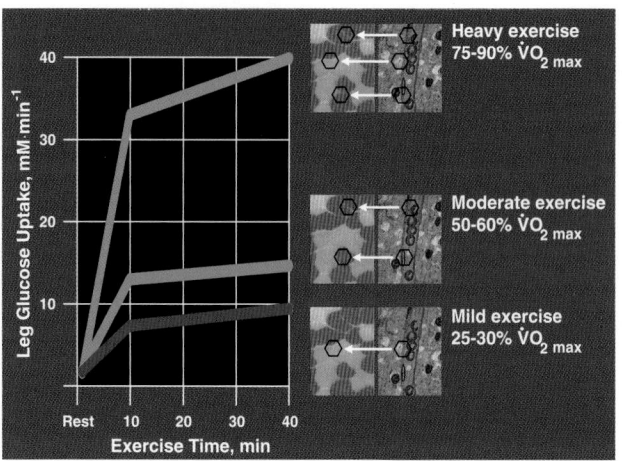

FIGURE 5.3 ■ Exercise duration and intensity affect blood glucose uptake by the leg muscles. Exercise intensity is expressed as a percentage of an individual's $\dot{V}O_{2max}$. (From Felig P, Wahren J. Fuel homeostasis in exercise. *N Engl J Med* 1975;293:1078.)

cles. FIGURE 5.3 illustrates that muscle uptake of circulating blood glucose increases sharply during the initial stage of exercise and continues to increase as exercise progresses. By the 40-minute mark, glucose uptake rises to between 7 and 20 times the resting uptake, depending on exercise intensity. Carbohydrate breakdown predominates when oxygen supply or use do not meet a muscle's needs, as in intense anaerobic exercise.[6] *During high-intensity aerobic exercise, the advantage of selective dependence on carbohydrate metabolism lies in its two times more rapid energy transfer compared with that of fat or protein.* Furthermore, compared with fat, carbohydrate generates about 6% more energy per unit of oxygen consumed.

Moderate and Prolonged Exercise

Glycogen stored in active muscle supplies almost all of the energy in the transition from rest to moderate exercise, just as it does in intense exercise. During the next 20 minutes or so of exercise, liver and muscle glycogen supply between 40 and 50% of the energy requirement; the remainder is provided by fat breakdown (intramuscular triacylglycerols, which may contribute up to 20% of the total exercise energy expenditure,[37] including a small use of protein). (The nutrient energy mixture depends on the relative intensity of submaximal exercise. In light exercise, fat remains the main energy substrate [see Fig. 5.9]). As exercise continues and muscle glycogen stores diminish, blood glucose from the liver becomes the major supplier of carbohydrate energy. Still, fat provides an

intramuscular glycogen.[15,41] *Carbohydrate availability in the metabolic mixture controls its use. In turn, carbohydrate intake dramatically affects its availability.*

One hour of high-intensity exercise decreases liver glycogen by about 55%, and a 2-hour strenuous workout just about depletes glycogen in the liver and specifically exercised mus-

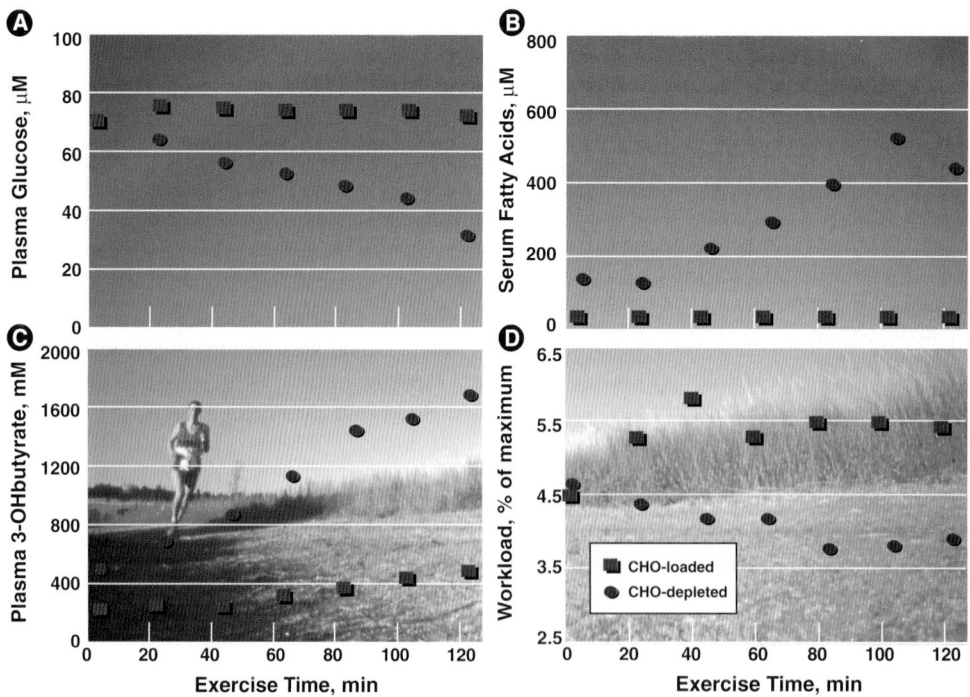

FIGURE 5.4 ■ Dynamics of nutrient metabolism in the glycogen-loaded and glycogen-depleted states. During exercise with limited carbohydrate (CHO) availability, blood glucose levels *(A)* progressively decrease, while fat metabolism *(B)* progressively increases compared with similar exercise when glycogen loaded. In addition, protein use for energy *(C)*, as indicated by plasma levels of 3-OH butyrate, remains considerably higher with glycogen depletion. After 2 hours, exercise capacity *(D)* decreases to about 50% of maximum in exercise begun in the glycogen-depleted state. (From Wagenmakers AJM, et al. Carbohydrate supplementation, glycogen depletion, and amino acid metabolism. *Am J Physiol* 1991;260:E883.)

increasingly larger percentage of the total energy metabolism. Eventually, plasma glucose concentration decreases because the liver's glucose output fails to keep pace with its use by muscles. During 90 minutes of strenuous exercise, blood glucose may actually decrease to **hypoglycemic levels** (less than 45 mg of glucose per 100 mL [dL] blood).[16]

FIGURE 5.4 (page 158) depicts the metabolic profile during prolonged exercise in the glycogen-depleted and glycogen-loaded states. With glycogen depletion, blood glucose levels fall as submaximal exercise progresses. Concurrently, the level of fatty acids circulating in the blood increases dramatically compared with the same exercise with adequate glycogen reserves. Protein also provides an increased contribution to the energy pool. With carbohydrate depletion, exercise intensity (expressed as a percentage of maximum) progressively decreases after 2 hours to about 50% of the starting exercise intensity. The reduced power output level comes directly from the relatively slow rate of aerobic energy release from fat oxidation, which now becomes the primary energy source.[20,49]

Carbohydrate and fat breakdown use identical pathways for acetyl-CoA oxidation. Thus, metabolic processes that precede the citric acid cycle (e.g., β-oxidation, fatty acid activation, and intracellular and mitochondrial transport) most likely account for the relatively slow rate of fat versus carbohydrate oxidation. FIGURE 5.5 lists these possible rate-limiting factors.

Nutrient-Related Fatigue

Severely lowered levels of liver and muscle glycogen during exercise induce fatigue, despite sufficient oxygen availability to muscles and almost unlimited potential energy from stored fat. Endurance athletes commonly refer to this extreme sensation of fatigue as "bonking" or "hitting the wall." The image of hitting the wall suggests an inability to continue exercising, which in reality is not the case, although pain becomes apparent in the active muscles and exercise intensity decreases markedly. Because of the absence of the phosphatase enzyme in skeletal muscle (which releases glucose from liver cells), the relatively inactive muscles retain all of their glycogen. Controversy exists about why carbohydrate depletion during prolonged exercise coincides with reduced exercise capacity. Part of the answer relates to three factors:

1. Use of blood glucose as energy for the central nervous system
2. Muscle glycogen's role as a "primer" in fat metabolism
3. Slower rate of energy release from fat catabolism than from carbohydrate breakdown

REGULAR EXERCISE IMPROVES CAPACITY FOR CARBOHYDRATE METABOLISM

Aerobically trained muscle exhibits a greater capacity to oxidize carbohydrate than untrained muscle. Consequently, considerable amounts of pyruvate move through the aerobic energy pathways

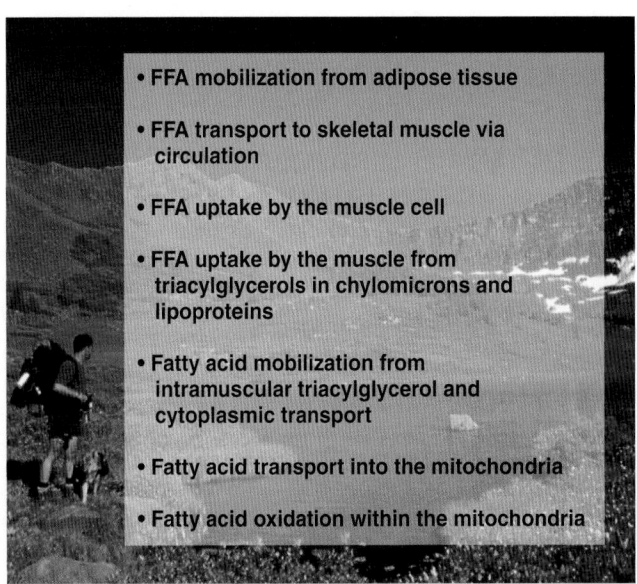

- FFA mobilization from adipose tissue
- FFA transport to skeletal muscle via circulation
- FFA uptake by the muscle cell
- FFA uptake by the muscle from triacylglycerols in chylomicrons and lipoproteins
- Fatty acid mobilization from intramuscular triacylglycerol and cytoplasmic transport
- Fatty acid transport into the mitochondria
- Fatty acid oxidation within the mitochondria

FIGURE 5.5 ■ Processes that potentially limit the magnitude of fat oxidation during aerobic exercise. FFA, free fatty acid.

during intense endurance exercise following training.[18] A trained muscle's augmented mitochondrial oxidative capacity and increased glycogen storage helps to explain its enhanced capacity for carbohydrate breakdown. During submaximal exercise, the endurance-trained muscle exhibits *decreased* reliance on muscle glycogen and blood glucose as fuel sources and greater fat use. This training adaptation represents a desirable response because it conserves the body's limited glycogen reserves.

Gender Differences in Substrate Use During Exercise

Available data support the notion of gender differences in carbohydrate metabolism in exercise. During submaximal exercise at equivalent percentages of $\dot{V}O_{2max}$ (i.e., same relative workload), women derive a *smaller* proportion of total energy from carbohydrate oxidation than men.[23] This gender difference in substrate oxidation does not persist into recovery.[21]

Gender Differences in Training Effects on Substrate Use

With similar endurance-training protocols, both women and men show a decrease in glucose flux for a given submaximal power output.[9,17] But at the same relative workload after training, women display an exaggerated shift toward fat catabolism, whereas men do not.[24] This suggests that endurance training induces greater glycogen-sparing at a given relative submaximal exercise intensity for women than for men. This gender difference in substrate metabolism's response to training may reflect differences in sympathetic nervous system adaptation to regular exercise (i.e., a more-blunted catecholamine response for women). The sex hormones estrogen and progesterone may affect metabolic mixture indirectly via interactions with the catecholamines or directly by augmenting lipolysis and/or constraining glycolysis.[5] Five potential sites for endocrine regulation of substrate use include:

1. Substrate availability (via effects on nutrient storage)
2. Substrate mobilization from body tissue stores
3. Substrate uptake at tissue site of use
4. Substrate uptake within tissue itself
5. Substrate trafficking among storage, oxidation, and recycling

Any glycogen-sparing metabolic adaptations to training could benefit a woman's performance during high-intensity endurance competition.

EFFECT OF DIET ON GLYCOGEN STORES AND ENDURANCE CAPACITY

We emphasized above that active muscle relies on ingested carbohydrate as a readily available energy nutrient. Diet composition profoundly affects glycogen reserves. FIGURE 5.6 shows the results from a classic experiment in which dietary manipulation varied muscle glycogen concentration. In one condition, caloric intake remained normal in six subjects for 3 days when lipid supplied most ingested calories (less than 5% as carbohydrate). In the second condition, the 3-day diet contained the recommended daily percentages of carbohydrate, lipid, and protein. With the third diet, carbohydrates supplied 82% of the calories. The needle biopsy technique determined glycogen content of the quadriceps femoris muscle; it averaged 0.63 g of glycogen per 100 g wet muscle with the high-fat diet, 1.75 g for the normal diet, and 3.75 g for the high-carbohydrate diet.

Endurance capacity during cycling exercise varied considerably depending on each person's diet for the 3 days before the exercise test. With the normal diet, exercise lasted an average of 114 minutes, but only 57 minutes with the high-fat diet. Endurance capacity of subjects fed the high-carbohydrate diet averaged more than three times greater than that with the high-fat diet. In all instances, the point of fatigue coincided with the same low level of muscle glycogen. This clearly demonstrated the importance of muscle glycogen to maintain high-intensity exercise lasting more than 1 hour. These results emphasize the important role that diet plays in establishing appropriate energy reserves for long-term exercise and strenuous training.

A carbohydrate-deficient diet rapidly depletes muscle and liver glycogen; it subsequently affects performance in all-out, short-term (anaerobic) exercise and in prolonged high-intensity endurance (aerobic) activities. These observations pertain to both athletes and physically active individuals who modify

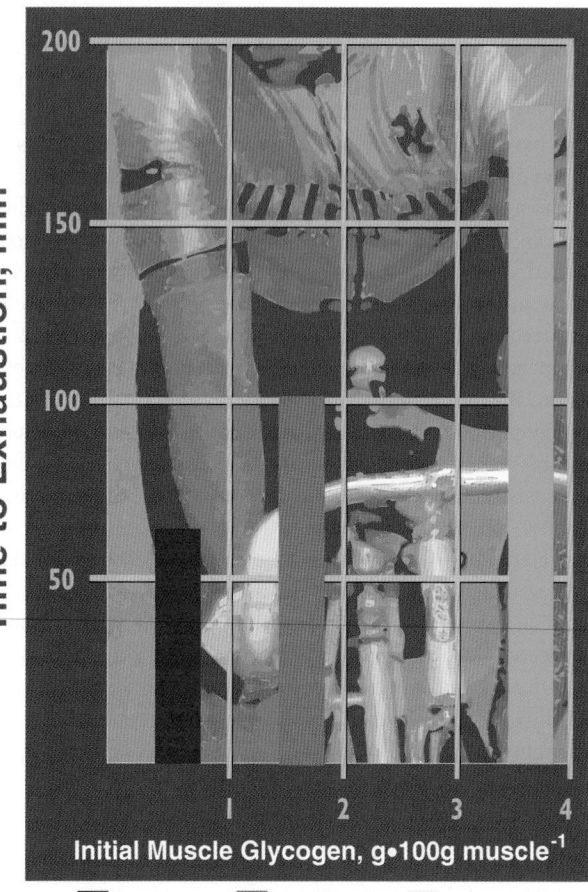

FIGURE 5.6 ■ Effects of a low-carbohydrate (CHO) diet, mixed diet, and high-CHO diet on glycogen content of the quadriceps femoris muscle and duration of endurance exercise on a bicycle ergometer. With a high-CHO diet, endurance time increases 3 times more than with a low-CHO diet. (Adapted from Bergstrom J, et al. Diet, muscle glycogen and physical performance. *Acta Physiol Scand* 1967; 71:140.)

their diets by reducing carbohydrate intake below recommended levels (see Chapter 1). Reliance on starvation diets or potentially harmful low-carbohydrate, high-fat diets or low-carbohydrate, high-protein diets remains counterproductive for weight control, exercise performance, optimal nutrition, and good health. A low-carbohydrate diet makes it extremely difficult from the standpoint of energy supply to engage in vigorous physical activity.[2,12,31,37] Because of carbohydrate's important role in central nervous system function and neuromuscular coordination, training and competing under conditions of low glycogen reserves also increases the likelihood of injury. More is said in Chapter 8 concerning optimizing carbohydrate availability before, during, and in recovery from intense exercise training and competition.

Fat Mobilization and Use During Exercise

Depending on nutritional and fitness status of the individual and the exercise intensity and duration, intracellular and extracellular fat supplies between 30 and 80% of exercise energy requirement.[3,27,42,52] Three lipid sources supply the major energy for light-to-moderate exercise:

1. Fatty acids released from the triacylglycerol storage sites in adipocytes and delivered relatively slowly to muscles as FFAs bound to plasma albumin
2. Circulating plasma triacylglycerol bound to lipoproteins as very-low-density lipoproteins and chylomicrons
3. Triacylglycerol within the active muscle itself

Fat use for energy in light and moderate exercise varies closely with blood flow through adipose tissue (a threefold increase is not uncommon) and through active muscle. Adipose tissue releases more FFAs to active muscle as blood flow increases with exercise. Hence, somewhat greater quantities of fat from adipose tissue depots participate in energy metabolism. The energy contribution from intramuscular triacylglycerol ranges between 15 and 35%, with endurance-trained men and women using the largest quantity, and substantial impairment in use among the obese and type 2 diabetics.[26,27,29,38,47]

Initiation of exercise produces a transient initial drop in plasma FFA concentration from the increased uptake by active muscles and the time lag in the release and delivery from adipocytes. Subsequently, increased FFA release from adipose tissue (and concomitant suppression of triacylglycerol formation) occurs through hormonal–enzymatic stimulation by sympathetic nervous system activation and decreased insulin levels. Subcutaneous abdominal adipocytes represent a particularly lively area for lipolysis compared with fat cells in the gluteal–femoral region. When exercise transitions to a high intensity, FFA release from adipose tissue fails to increase much above resting levels, which eventually produces a decrease in plasma FFAs. This, in turn, increases muscle glycogen usage, with a concurrent large increase in intramuscular triacylglycerol oxidation (see Fig. 5.9).[40]

On a relative basis, considerable fatty acid oxidation occurs during low-intensity exercise. For example, fat combustion almost totally powers light exercise at 25% of aerobic capacity. Carbohydrate and fat combustion contribute energy equally during moderate exercise. Fat oxidation gradually increases as exercise extends to an hour or more and glycogen depletes. Toward the end of prolonged exercise (with glycogen reserves low), circulating FFAs supply nearly 80% of the total energy required. FIGURE 5.7 shows this phenomenon for a subject who exercised continuously for 6 hours. A steady decline occurred in carbohydrate combustion (reflected by the respiratory quotient [RQ]; see Chapter 6) during exercise with an accompanying increase in fat combustion. Toward the end of exercise, 84% of the total energy for exercise came from fat breakdown! This experiment, conducted nearly 75 years ago, illustrates fat oxidation's important contribution in prolonged exercise with glycogen depletion.

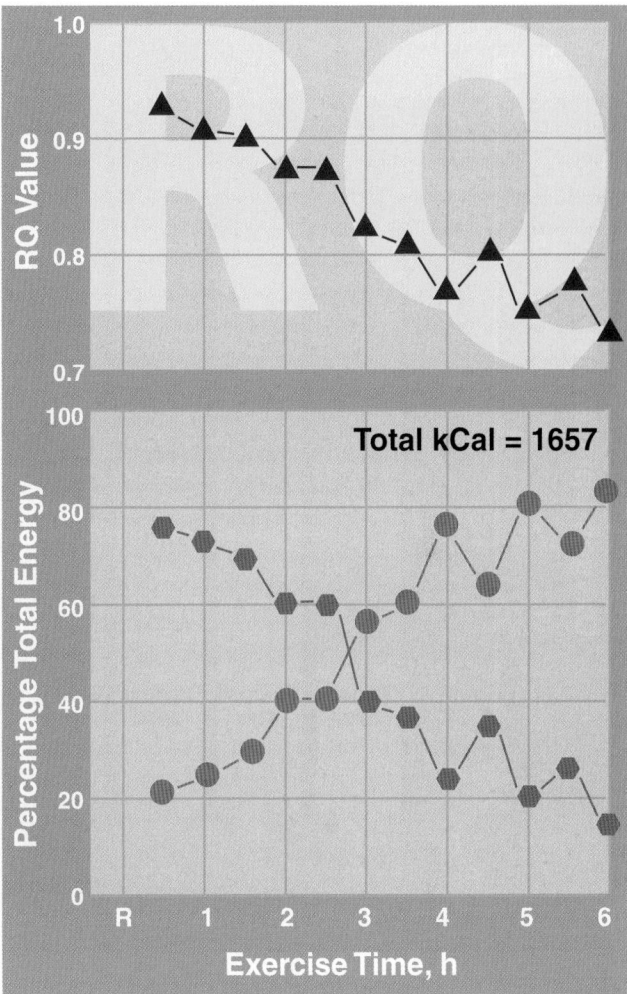

FIGURE 5.7 ■ *Top:* Reduction in respiratory quotient *(RQ)* at an oxygen uptake of 2.36 L · min⁻¹ during 6 hours of continuous exercise. *Bottom:* Percentage of energy derived from carbohydrate (CHO) *(purple)* and fat *(orange)* (1 kCal = 4.2 kJ; R, rest). (Modified from Edwards HT, et al. Metabolic rate, blood sugar and utilization of carbohydrate. *Am J Physiol* 1934;108:203.)

The hormones epinephrine, norepinephrine, glucagon, and growth hormone activate hormone-sensitive lipase. This causes lipolysis and mobilization of FFAs from adipose tissue. Exercise increases plasma levels of lipogenic hormones, so the active muscles receive a continual supply of energy-rich fatty acid substrate. Increased activity of skeletal muscle and adipose tissue lipases, including biochemical and vascular adaptations within the muscle, help to explain the training-induced enhanced use of fats for energy during moderate-intensity exercise.[10,11,33,34,43]

Augmented fat metabolism in prolonged exercise probably results from a small drop in blood sugar, accompanied by a decrease in insulin (a potent inhibitor of lipolysis) and increased glucagon output by the pancreas as exercise progresses.

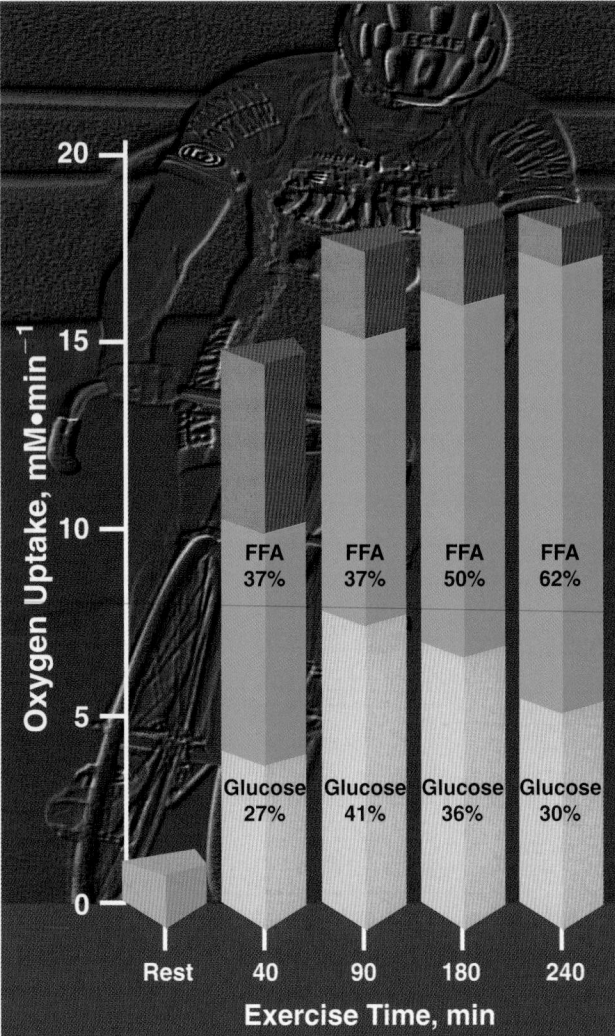

FIGURE 5.8 ■ Uptake of oxygen and nutrients by the legs during prolonged exercise. *Green* and *yellow* areas represent the proportion of total oxygen uptake caused by oxidation of free fatty acids (FFAs) and blood glucose oxidation, respectively. *Orange* areas indicate the oxidation of non–blood-borne fuels (muscle glycogen and intramuscular fat and proteins). (From Ahlborg G, et al. Substrate turnover during prolonged exercise in man. *J Clin Invest* 1974;53:1080.)

These changes ultimately reduce glucose metabolism to further stimulate FFA liberation for energy. FIGURE 5.8 shows that FFA uptake by working muscle rises during 1 to 4 hours of moderate exercise. In the first hour, fat supplies about 50% of the energy, while in the third hour, fat contributes up to 70% of the total energy requirement. *With carbohydrate depletion, exercise intensity decreases to a level governed by the body's ability to mobilize and oxidize fat.* Interestingly, prior exercise also partitions the trafficking of dietary fat fed in recovery toward a direction that favors its oxidation rather than storage. This may partly explain the protection against weight gain offered by regular physical activity.[28,51]

Consuming a high-fat diet for a protracted period produces enzymatic adaptations that enhance capacity for fat oxidation during exercise.[30,35,44,54] We discuss the effectiveness of this dietary manipulation to improve endurance performance in Chapter 8.

EXERCISE INTENSITY MAKES A DIFFERENCE

The contribution of fat to the metabolic mixture in exercise differs depending on exercise intensity. For moderately trained subjects, the exercise intensity that maximizes fat burning ranges between 55 and 72% of $\dot{V}O_{2max}$.[1] FIGURE 5.9 illustrates the dynamics of fat use by trained men who cycled at 25 to 85% of their aerobic capacity. During light-to-mild exercise (40% of maximum or less), fat provided the main energy source, predominantly as plasma FFAs from adipose tissue depots. Increasing exercise intensity produced an eventual *crossover* in the balance of fuel use. The total energy from fat breakdown (from all sources) remained essentially unchanged, while blood glucose and muscle glycogen supplied the added energy for more intense exercise. No difference existed in total energy from fats during exercise at 85% of maximum and exercise at 25% of maximum. *Such data highlight the important role that carbohydrate, particularly muscle glycogen, plays as the major fuel source during high-intensity aerobic exercise.*

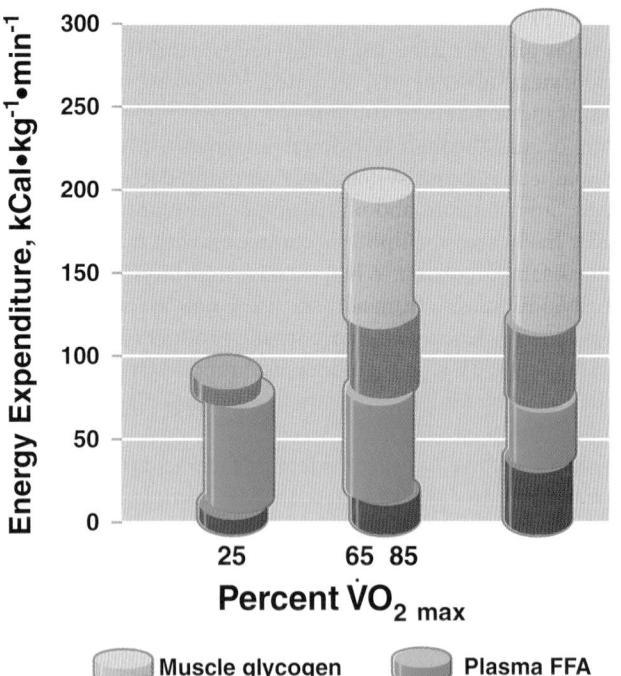

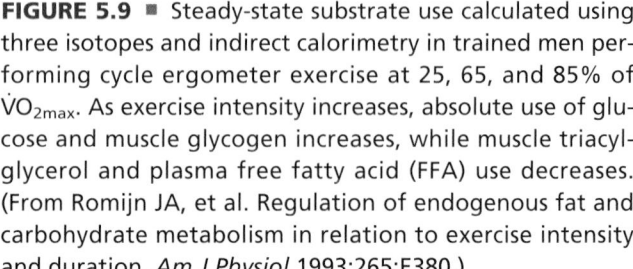

FIGURE 5.9 ■ Steady-state substrate use calculated using three isotopes and indirect calorimetry in trained men performing cycle ergometer exercise at 25, 65, and 85% of $\dot{V}O_{2max}$. As exercise intensity increases, absolute use of glucose and muscle glycogen increases, while muscle triacylglycerol and plasma free fatty acid (FFA) use decreases. (From Romijn JA, et al. Regulation of endogenous fat and carbohydrate metabolism in relation to exercise intensity and duration. *Am J Physiol* 1993;265:E380.)

NUTRITIONAL STATUS PLAYS A ROLE

The dynamics of fat breakdown or its synthesis depend on availability of the "building block" fatty acid molecules. After a meal, when energy metabolism is low, digestive processes increase FFA and triacylglycerol delivery to cells. Increased fat delivery, in turn, promotes triacylglycerol synthesis through esterification. In contrast, with moderate exercise, increased use of fatty acids for energy reduces their concentration in the active cells, thus stimulating triacylglycerol breakdown into its glycerol and fatty acid components. Concurrently, hormonal release in exercise stimulates adipose tissue lipolysis, which further augments FFA delivery to active muscle. Long-duration exercise in the fasted state places heavy demands on FFA use as an energy substrate.[32]

> ## More Fat Burned During Submaximal Effort
>
> Adaptions producing enhanced responsiveness of adipocytes to lipolysis allow the trained person to exercise at a higher absolute level of submaximal exercise before experiencing the fatiguing effects of glycogen depletion.

EXERCISE TRAINING AND FAT METABOLISM

Regular aerobic exercise profoundly improves ability to oxidize long-chain fatty acids, particularly from triacylglycerol stored within active muscle, during mild- to moderate-intensity exercise.[25,26,33,36] FIGURE 5.10 shows the increase in fat catabolism during submaximal exercise following aerobic training, with a corresponding decrease in carbohydrate breakdown. Even for endurance athletes, the improved capacity for fat oxidation cannot sustain the level of aerobic metabolism generated when oxidizing glycogen for energy. Consequently, well-

> ## Six Fat-Burning Adaptations with Aerobic Training
>
> 1. Facilitated rate of lipolysis and reesterfication within adipocytes.
> 2. Proliferation of capillaries in trained muscle to create a greater total number and density of these microvessels.
> 3. Improved transport of FFAs through the plasma membrane (sarcolemma) of the muscle fiber.
> 4. Augmented transport of fatty acids within the muscle cell by the action of carnitine and carnitine acyl transferase.
> 5. Increased size and number of muscle mitochondria.
> 6. Increased quantity of enzymes involved β-oxidation, citric acid cycle metabolism, and the electron-transport chain within specifically trained muscle fibers.

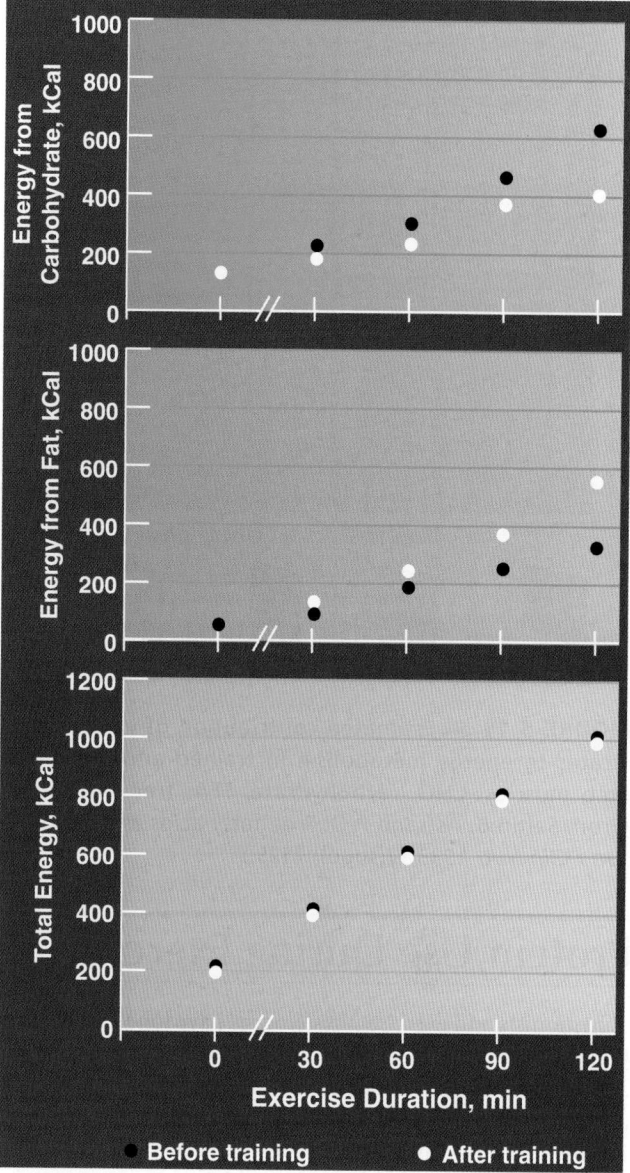

FIGURE 5.10 ■ Training enhances catabolism of fat. During constant-load prolonged exercise, energy from fat oxidation significantly increases following aerobic training, while corresponding decreases occur in carbohydrate breakdown. Carbohydrate-sparing adaptations can occur in two ways: *(a)* release of fatty acids from adipose tissue depots (augmented by a reduced level of blood lactate) and *(b)* greater intramuscular fat stores in the endurance-trained muscle. (From Hurley BF, et al. Muscle triglyceride utilization during exercise: effect of training. *J Appl Physiol* 1986;5:62.)

nourished endurance athletes rely almost totally on oxidation of stored glycogen in near-maximal, sustained aerobic effort.

FIGURE 5.11 displays the contribution of various energy substrates to exercise metabolism of trained and untrained limb muscles. The important point concerns the greater uptake of FFAs (and concurrent conservation of limited glycogen reserves) by the trained limb during moderate exercise through six mechanisms shown in the shaded box at the left.

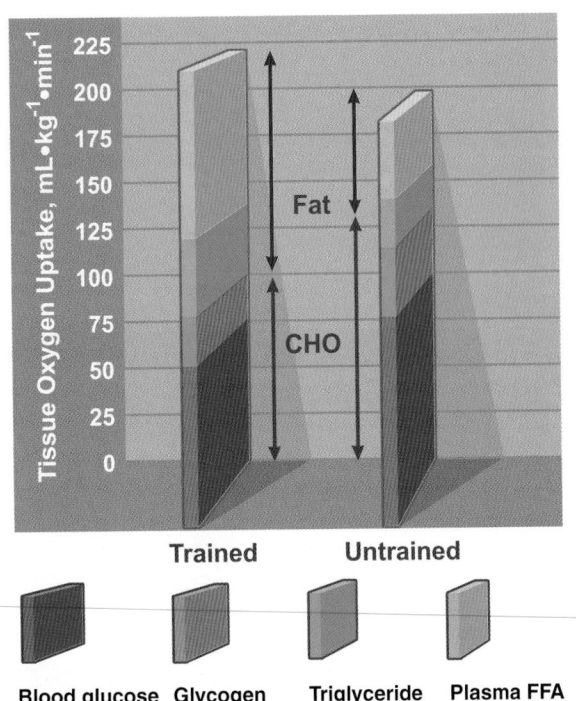

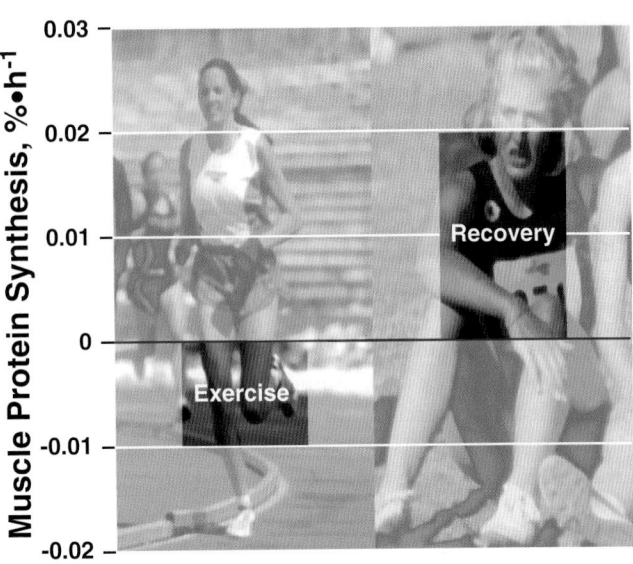

FIGURE 5.11 ■ Estimated contribution of various substrates to energy metabolism in trained and untrained limb muscles. CHO, carbohydrate; FFA, free fatty acid. (From Saltin B, Åstrand P-O. Free fatty acids and exercise. *Am J Clin Nutr* 1993;57(suppl):752S.)

FIGURE 5.12 ■ Protein synthesis stimulation during recovery from aerobic exercise. Values refer to differences between the exercise group and the control group who received the same diet for each time interval. (From Carraro F, et al. Whole body and plasma protein synthesis in exercise and recovery in human subjects. *Am J Physiol* 1990; 258:E821.)

Protein Use During Exercise

Nutritionists and exercise physiologists have long maintained that the protein RDA represents a liberal "margin of safety" to account for amino acids catabolized during exercise and amino acids required for protein synthesis following exercise. For the past 100 years, three reasons stand out as to why protein constitutes a limited fuel in exercise:

1. Protein's primary role provides amino-acid building blocks for tissue synthesis
2. Early studies show only minimal protein breakdown during endurance exercise as reflected by urinary nitrogen excretion
3. Theoretical computations and experimental evidence of protein requirements for muscle tissue synthesis with resistance training

More recent research on protein balance in exercise presents a compelling argument that protein serves as energy fuel to a much greater extent than previously believed, depending on energy expenditure and nutritional status.[4,7,45,50] *This applies primarily to the branched-chain amino acids (for the way the side chain branches from the molecule's amine core) leucine, valine, and isoleucine oxidized in skeletal muscle rather than in the liver.* As shown in Figure 5.4, endurance exercise in a carbohydrate-depleted state caused considerably more protein catabolism than protein breakdown with ample carbohydrate reserves.

Energy Intake Must Balance Energy Output

If energy intake does not match energy expenditure in intense training, even *twice* the protein RDA intake may not maintain nitrogen balance. Thus, dieting could negatively affect training regimens geared to increase muscle mass or maintain muscular strength and power.

Whereas protein breakdown generally increases only modestly with exercise, muscle protein synthesis rises markedly following both endurance and resistance-type exercise. FIGURE 5.12 shows that the rate of muscle protein synthesis (determined from labeled leucine incorporation into muscle) increased between 10 and 80% in the 4 hours following aerobic exercise. It then remained elevated for at least 24 hours. Thus, two factors justify reexamining protein intake recommendations for those involved in exercise training: (1) increased protein breakdown during long-term exercise and heavy training and (2) increased protein synthesis in recovery from exercise. Chapter 7 further discusses the adequacy of the protein RDA for those who undertake intense training.

Case Study

Personal Health and Exercise Nutrition 5–1

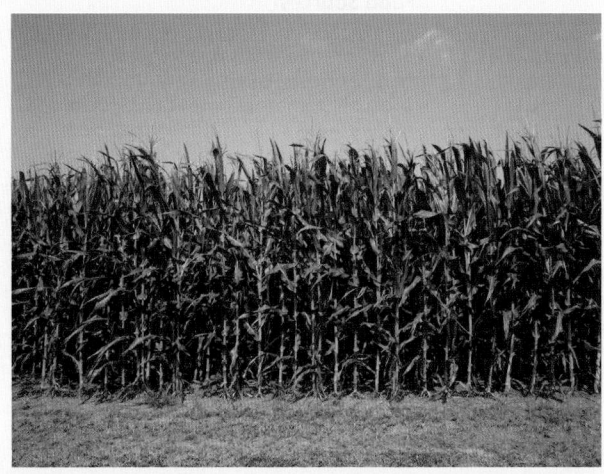

Know What You Eat: Benefits of Phytochemicals

Background
Based on years of research in the field of nutrition, current consensus suggests that an optimum diet should:

1. Supply an individual's needs for energy (calories) and macronutrients and micronutrients
2. Support health and promote successful aging
3. Provide pleasure, both individual and social, and reinforce personal and cultural identity

Within this framework, the following represent five major characteristics of an optimum diet that most scientists from diverse disciplines would agree with:

1. Contain foods of sufficient variety from all the major food groups
2. Contain as much fresh food as possible
3. Contain as few processed foods as possible
4. Contain an abundance of fruits and vegetables
5. Contain foods that provide health benefits beyond basic nutrition

Foods that provide health benefits beyond basic nutrition have been termed *functional foods*. Beneficial substances in these foods include both *zoochemicals* (health-promoting compounds from the animal kingdom) and *phytochemicals* (health-promoting compounds from the plant kingdom). Much research has focused on phytochemicals because of their protective role in fighting chronic disease. Foods such as garlic, soybeans, cruciferous vegetables, legumes, onions, citrus fruits, tomatoes, whole grains, and diverse herbs and spices are excellent sources of chemoprotective phytochemicals. Specific phytochemicals with health benefits include allium compounds, isoflavones, saponins, indoles, isothiocyanates, dithiolthione, ellagic acid, polyacetylenes, flavonoids, carotenoids, phytates, lignins, glucarates, phthalides, and terpenoids.

Know Your Phytochemicals
Many different plants contain healthful phytochemicals. For example, carotenoids, polyphenols, and saponins exert strong antioxidant effects; sulfides and isothiocyanates stimulate enzymes that deactivate carcinogens; phytosterols and saponins alter the harmful effects of excess cholesterol; phytoestrogens possess a chemical structure similar–that of hormones and act by blocking deleterious effects of excessive hormone production. The accompanying table lists the more important phytochemicals, their biologic activity, and food sources.

Case Study *continued*

Know Your Phytochemicals

Phytochemical	Activity and Effects	Food Sources
Carotenoids (α-carotene, β-carotene, β-cryptoxanthin, luten, lycopene, zeaxanthin)	Vitamin-A precursors; antioxidants; increase cell-to-cell communication; decrease risk of macular degeneration	Yellow-orange fruits and vegetable (e.g., apricots, carrots, cantaloupe, broccoli, tomatoes, sweet potatoes); leafy greens such as spinach; dairy products, eggs, and margarine
Flavonoids (quercetin, kaempferol, myricetin), flavones (apigenin), flavonols (catechins)	Decrease capillary fragility and permeability; block carcinogens and slow growth of cancer cells	Fruits, vegetables, berries, citrus fruits, onions, purple grapes, tea, red wine
Phytoestrogens (isoflavones—genistein, biochanin A, daidzein, and lignins)	Metabolized to estrogen-like compounds in the GI tract; induce cancer cell death (apoptosis); slow cancer cell growth; reduce risk of breast, ovarian, colon, and prostate cancer; inhibit cholesterol synthesis; may reduce risk of osteoporosis	Isoflavones in soybeans and soy products; lignins in flax, rye, some berries, and some vegetables
Phytosterols (β-sitosterol, stigmasterol, campesterol)	Decrease cholesterol absorption; inhibit proliferation of colonic cells	Vegetable oils, nuts, seeds, cereals, legumes
Saponins (soyasaponins, soyasapogenols)	Bind bile acids and cholesterol in the GI tract to reduce absorption; toxic to tumor cells; antioxidant effects	Soybeans, modified margarines
Glucosinolates (glucobrassicin, isothiocyanates [sulphorophane], indoles [indole-3-carbinol])	Increase enzyme activity that deactivates carcinogens; favorably alter estrogen metabolism; affect regulation of gene expression	Cruciferous vegetables (broccoli, Brussels sprouts, cabbage), horseradish, mustard greens
Sulfides and thiols (dithiolthiones and allium compounds like diallyl sulfides, allyl methyl trisulfides)	Increase activity of enzymes that deactivate carcinogens; decrease conversion of nitrates to nitrites in intestines; may lower cholesterol, prevent blood clotting, and normalize blood pressure	Sulfides in onions, garlic, leeks, scallions; dithiolthiones in cruciferous vegetables
Inositol phosphates (phytate, inositol, pentaphosphate)	Bind metal ions and prevent them from generating free radicals; protect against cancer	Cereals, soybeans, soy-based foods, cereal grains, nuts, and seeds (especially abundant in sesame seeds and soybeans)
Phenolic acids (caffeic and ferulic acids, ellagic acid)	Anticancer properties; prevent formation of stomach carcinogens	Blueberries, cherries, apples, oranges, pears, potatoes
Protease inhibitors	Bind to trypsin and chymotrypsin; decrease cancer cell growth and inhibit malignant changes in cells; inhibit hormone binding; may aid DNA repair to slow cancer cell division; prevent tumors from releasing proteases that destroy neighboring cells	Soybeans; other legumes, cereals, vegetables
Tannins	Antioxidant effects; may inhibit activation of carcinogens and slow cancer promotion	Grapes, tea, lentils, red and white wine, black-eyed peas
Capsaicin	Modulates blood clotting	Hot peppers
Coumarin (phenolic)	Promotes enzyme function to protect against cancer	Citrus fruits
Curcumin (phenolic)	Inhibits enzymes that activate carcinogens; antiinflammatory and antioxidant properties	Turmeric, mustard
Monoterpene (limonene)	Triggers enzyme production to detoxify carcinogens; inhibits cancer promotion and cell proliferation; favorably affects blood clotting and cholesterol levels	Citrus fruit peels and oils, garlic

From Grosvenor MB, Smolin LA. Nutrition. From Science to Life. Philadelphia: Harcourt College Publishers, 2002.

Summary

1. The major pathway for ATP production differs depending on exercise intensity and duration.

2. For all-out, short-duration efforts (100-m dash, lifting heavy weights), the intramuscular stores of ATP and PCr (immediate energy system) provide the required energy for exercise.

3. For intense exercise of longer duration (1–2 min), the anaerobic reactions of glycolysis (short-term energy system) provide the energy.

4. When exercise progresses beyond several minutes, the aerobic system predominates with oxygen uptake capacity becoming the important factor (long-term energy system).

5. Muscle glycogen and blood glucose serve as primary fuels during intense anaerobic exercise beyond 10-seconds duration. Glycogen stores also play an important energy metabolism role in sustained high levels of aerobic exercise such as marathon running, distance cycling, and endurance swimming.

6. Trained muscle exhibits an augmented capacity to catabolize carbohydrate aerobically for energy because of increased oxidative capacity of the mitochondria and increased glycogen storage.

7. Women derive a smaller proportion of the total energy from carbohydrate oxidation than do men during submaximal exercise at equivalent percentages of aerobic capacity. Following aerobic exercise training, women show a more exaggerated shift toward fat catabolism than men.

8. A carbohydrate-deficient diet rapidly depletes muscle and liver glycogen and profoundly affects both anaerobic capacity and prolonged, high-intensity aerobic physical effort.

9. Fat contributes about 50% of the energy requirement during light and moderate exercise. The role of stored fat (intramuscular and derived from adipocytes) becomes even more important at the latter stages of prolonged exercise. In this situation, the fatty acid molecules (mainly as circulating FFAs) provide more than 80% of the exercise energy requirements.

10. With carbohydrate depletion, exercise intensity decreases to a level determined by how well the body mobilizes and oxidizes fat.

11. Aerobic training increases long-chain fatty acid oxidation, particularly the fatty acids derived from triacylglycerols within active muscle during mild- to moderate-intensity exercise.

12. Enhanced fat oxidation spares glycogen, permitting trained individuals to exercise at a higher absolute level of submaximal exercise before experiencing the fatiguing effects of glycogen depletion.

13. A high-fat diet stimulates adaptations that augment fat use, yet reliable research has not yet demonstrated consistent exercise or training benefits from such dietary modifications.

14. Protein serves as an energy fuel to a much greater extent than previously thought, depending on nutritional status and the intensity of exercise training or competition. This applies particularly to branched-chain amino acids that oxidize within skeletal muscle rather than within the liver.

15. Reexamining the current protein RDA seems justified for those who engage in intense exercise training. Protein intake must account for the increased protein breakdown during exercise and the augmented protein synthesis in recovery.

Test Your Knowledge Answers

1. **True:** Anaerobic sources supply most of the energy for fast, powerful movements, or during increased resistance to movement at a given speed. When movement begins at either fast or slow speed, the intramuscular high-energy phosphates (ATP and PCr) provide immediate anaerobic energy for muscle action. After a few seconds, the glycolytic pathway (intramuscular glycogen breakdown via glycolysis) generates an increasingly greater proportion of energy for ATP resynthesis.

2. **False:** Liver and muscle glycogen provide the main macronutrient energy sources for ATP resynthesis during high-intensity aerobic exercise. The liver markedly increases its release of glucose as exercise progresses from low to high intensity. Concurrently, glycogen stored within the active muscles serves as the predominant energy source during the early stages of exercise and in high-intensity aerobic exercise. Compared with fat and protein catabolism, carbohydrate remains the preferential fuel during intense aerobic exercise because it more rapidly supplies ATP in oxidative processes. More specifically, dependence on carbohydrate during high-intensity aerobic exercise lies in its two-times more rapid rate of energy transfer than with fat and protein. Furthermore, carbohydrate generates about 6% more energy per unit oxygen consumed than fat.

3. **True:** Depending on nutritional and fitness status of the individual and exercise intensity and duration, fat supplies between 30 and 80% of the exercise energy requirement. Fat use in light and moderate exercise varies closely with blood flow through adipose tissue and blood flow through active muscle. Adipose tissue releases more FFAs for delivery to active muscle as blood flow increases with exercise. Hence, somewhat greater quantities of fat from adipose tissue depots participate in energy metabolism.

4. **True:** In predominantly anaerobic effort, carbohydrate becomes the sole macronutrient contributor of energy for ATP resynthesis. Carbohydrate breakdown in glycolysis provides the only available means for rapid anaerobic energy. This anaerobic energy is unavailable via the breakdown of fatty acids and amino acids, which provide energy only through aerobic metabolism.

5. **True:** Controversy exists as to why carbohydrate depletion during prolonged exercise coincides with a reduced exercise capacity, commonly termed "bonking" or "hitting the wall." Part of the answer relates to the use of blood glucose as energy for the central nervous system, muscle glycogen's role as a "primer" in fat metabolism, and the slower rate of energy release from fat than from carbohydrate breakdown. In essence, with carbohydrate deple-tion, exercise intensity decreases to a level governed by the body's ability to mobilize and oxidize fat.

6. **False:** A carbohydrate-deficient diet, not a diet deficient in fat, rapidly depletes muscle and liver glycogen This diet subsequently impairs performance in all-out, short-term (anaerobic) exercise and in prolonged high-intensity endurance (aerobic) activities. These observations pertain to both athletes and physically active individuals who modify their diets by reducing carbohydrate intake below recommended levels.

7. **True:** Carbohydrate availability during exercise helps to regulate fat mobilization and its use for energy. Augmented fat metabolism in prolonged exercise probably results from a small drop in blood sugar, accompanied by a decrease in insulin (a potent inhibitor of lipolysis) and increased glucagon output by the pancreas as exercise progresses. These changes ultimately reduce glucose metabolism to further stimulate FFA liberation for energy. Toward the end of prolonged exercise (with glycogen reserves low), circulating FFAs supply nearly 80% of the total energy requirement.

8. **False:** Regular aerobic exercise profoundly improves the ability to oxidize long-chain fatty acids, particularly from triacylglycerol stored within active muscle, during mild- to moderate-intensity exercise. These adaptations allow the trained person to exercise at a higher absolute level of submaximal exercise before experiencing the fatiguing effects of glycogen depletion. Even for endurance athletes, however, improved capacity for fat oxidation cannot sustain the high level of aerobic metabolism generated when oxidizing glycogen for energy.

9. **False:** Protein serves as an energy fuel to a much greater extent than previously thought, depending on nutritional status and exercise intensity. This applies particularly to branched-chain amino acids that oxidize within skeletal muscle rather than within the liver. The use of protein for energy most frequently occurs in a glycogen-depleted state as amino acids donate their carbon skeletons for the synthesis of glucose by the liver.

10. **False:** Individuals consuming a high-carbohydrate diet perform significantly better after 7 weeks of training than individuals consuming a high-fat diet. A high-fat diet stimulates adaptive responses that augment fat use, but reliable research has yet to demonstrate consistent exercise or training benefits from such dietary modifications. Furthermore, one should carefully consider recommending a diet consisting of up to 60% total calories from lipid in terms of detrimental health risks, particularly those associated with cardiovascular disease.

References

1. Achten J, et al. Determination of the exercise intensity that elicits maximal fat oxidation. *Med Sci Sports Exerc* 2002;34:92.
2. Ball D, et al. The acute reversal of diet-induced metabolic acidosis does not restore endurance capacity during high-intensity exercise in man. *Eur J Appl Physiol* 1996;73:105.
3. Bergman BC, Brooks GA. Respiratory gas-exchange ratios during graded exercise in fed and fasted trained and untrained men. *J Appl Physiol* 1999;86:479.
4. Bowtell JL, et al. Modulation of whole body protein metabolism, during and after exercise, by variation of dietary protein. *J Appl Physiol* 1998;85:1744
5. Braun B, Horton T. Endocrine regulation of exercise substrate utilization in women compared to men. *Exerc Sport Sci Rev* 2001;29:149.
6. Burgomaster KA, et al. Effect of short-term sprint interval training on human skeletal muscle carbohydrate metabolism during exercise and time-trail performance. *J Appl Physiol* 2006;86:205.
7. Carraro F, et al. Alanine kinetics in humans during low-intensity exercise. *Med Sci Sports Exerc* 1994;26:48.
8. Coggan AR. Plasma glucose metabolism during exercise: effect of endurance training in humans. *Med Sci Sports Exerc* 1997;29:620,
9. Coggan AR, et al. Endurance training increases plasma glucose turnover and oxidation during moderate-intensity exercise in men. *J Appl Physiol* 1990;68:990.
10. Coggan AR, et al. Plasma glucose kinetics in subjects with high and low lactate thresholds. *J Appl Physiol* 1992;73:1873.
11. Coggan AR, et al. Isotopic estimation of CO_2 production before and after endurance training. *J Appl Physiol* 1993;75:70.
12. Costill DL, et al. Effects of repeated days of intensified training on muscle glycogen and swimming performance. *Med Sci Sports Exerc* 1988;20:249.
13. Coyle EF, et al. Fatty acid oxidation is directly regulated by carbohydrate metabolism during exercise. *Am J Physiol* 1997;273(*Endocrinol Metab* 36):E268.
14. De Gliszinski I, et al. Effects of carbohydrate ingestion of adipose tissue lipolysis during long-lasting exercise in trained men. *J Appl Physiol* 1998;84:1627.
15. Felig P, Wahren J. Fuel homeostasis in exercise. *N Engl J Med* 1975;293:1078.
16. Felig P, et al. Hypoglycemia during prolonged exercise in normal men. *N Engl J Med* 1982;306:895.
17. Friellander AL, et al. Training induced alterations in carbohydrate metabolism in women: women respond differently than men. *J Appl Physiol* 1998;85:1175.
18. Fujimoto T, et al. Skeletal muscle glucose uptake response to exercise in trained and untrained men. *Med Sci Sports Exerc* 2003;35:777.
19. Hargreaves M. Interactions between muscle glycogen and blood glucose during exercise. *Exerc Sport Sci Rev* 1997;25:21.
20. Hawley JA. Effect of increased fat availability on metabolism and exercise capacity. *Med Sci Sports Exerc* 2002;34:1485.
21. Horton TJ, et al. Fuel metabolism in men and women during and after long-duration exercise. *J Appl Physiol* 1998;85:1823.
22. Howlett K, et al. Effect of increased blood glucose availability on glucose kinetics during exercise. *J Appl Physiol* 1998;84:1423.
23. Jansson E. Sex differences in metabolic response to exercise. In: Saltin B, ed. *Biochemistry of Exercise*, VI. Champaign, IL: Human Kinetics, 1986.
24. Jansson E, Kaijser L. Substrate utilization and enzymes in skeletal muscle of extremely endurance-trained men. *J Appl Physiol* 1987;62:999.
25. Jeukendrup AE, et al. Exogenous glucose oxidation during exercise in endurance-trained and untrained subjects. *J Appl Physiol* 1997;83:835.
26. Kiens B. Effect of endurance training on fatty acid metabolism: local adaptations. *Med Sci Sports Exerc* 1997;29:640.
27. Kiens B. Skeletal muscle lipid metabolism in exercise and insulin resistance. *Physiol Rev* 2006;86:205.
28. King G, et al. Relationship of leisure-time physical activity and occupational activity to the prevalence of obesity. *Int J Obes* 2001;25:606.
29. Klein S, et al. Fat metabolism during low intensity exercise in endurance-trained and untrained men. *Am J Physiol* 1993;267:E708.
30. Lambert EV, et al. Enhanced endurance in trained cyclists during moderate intensity exercise following a 2 week adaptation to a high fat diet. *Eur J Appl Physiol* 1994;69:26.
31. Macdermid PW, Stannard SR. A whey-supplemented, high-protein diet versus a high-carbohydrate diet: effects on endurance cycling performance. *Int J Sport Nutr Exerc Metab* 2006;16:65.
32. Martin WH. Effect of acute and chronic exercise on fat metabolism. *Exerc Sport Sci Rev* 1996;24:203.
33. Martin WH III, et al. Effect of endurance training on plasma free fatty acid turnover and oxidation during exercise. *Am J Physiol* 1993;265: E708.
34. Messonnierl, et al. Are the effects of training on fat metabolism involved in the improvement of performance during high intensity exercise. *Eur J Appl Physiol* 2005;94:434.
35. Mudio DM. Effect of dietary fat on metabolic adjustments to maximal $\dot{V}O_2$ and endurance in runners. *Med Sci Sports Exerc* 1994;26:81.
36. Nicklas BJ. Effects of endurance exercise on adipose tissue metabolism. *Exerc Sport Sci Revs* 1997;25:77.
37. Peters SJ, Leblanc PJ. Metabolic aspects of low carbohydrate diets and exercise. *Nutr Metab* (Lond) 2004;1:7.
38. Roepstorff C, et al. Intramuscular triacylglycerol in energy metabolism during exercise in humans. *Exer Sport Sci Rev* 2005;33:182.
39. Romijn JA, et al. Regulation of endogenous fat and carbohydrate metabolism in relation to exercise intensity and duration. *Am J Physiol* 1993;265:E380.
40. Romijn JA, et al. Relationship between fatty acid delivery and fatty acid oxidation during strenuous exercise. *J Appl Physiol* 1995;79:1939.
41. Sherman WM. Metabolism of sugars and physical performance. *Am J Clin Nutr* 1995;62(suppl):228S.
42. Spirit LL. Regulation of skeletal muscle fat oxidation during exercise in humans. *Med Sci Sports Exerc* 2002;34:1477.
43. Stallknecht B, et al. Effect of training on epinephrine-stimulated lipolysis determined by microdialysis in human adipose tissue. *Am J Physiol* 1995;265:E1059.
44. Stellingwerff T, et al. Decreased PDH activation and glycogenolysis during exercise following fat adaption with carbohydrate restoration. *Am J Physiol Endocrinol Metab* 2006;298:E380.
45. Tarnopolosky MA, et al. Effect of bodybuilding exercise on protein requirements. *Can J Sport Sci* 1990;15:225.
46. Turcotte LP. Muscle fatty acid uptake during exercise: possible mechanisms. *Exerc Sport Sci Rev* 2000;1:4.
47. van Loon LJC. Use of intramuscular triacylglycerol as a substrate source during exercise in humans. *J Appl Physiol* 2004;97:1170.
48. Venables MC, et al. Determinants of maximal fat oxidation during exercise in healthy men and women. *J Appl Physiol* 2005;98:160.
49. Vusse, van der GJ, et al. Lipid metabolism in muscle. *Handbook of Physiology*, Section 12: Exercise—regulation and integration of multiple systems. New York: Oxford Press, 1996.
50. Wagenmakers AJM. Muscle amino acid metabolism at rest and during exercise: role in human physiology and metabolism. *Exerc Sport Sci Rev* 1998;26:287.
51. Wier L, et al. Determining the amount of physical activity needed for long-term weight control. *Int J Obes* 2001;25:613.
52. Winder WW. Malonyl-CoA: regulator of fatty acid oxidation in muscle during exercise. *Exerc Sport Sci Rev* 1998;26:117.
53. Wolfe RR., et al. Role of changes in insulin and glucagon in glucose homeostasis in exercise. *J Clin Invest* 1986;77:900.
54. Zderic TW, et al. High-fat diet elevates resting intramuscular triglyceride concentration and whole body lipolysis during exercise. *Am J Physiol Endocrinol Metab* 2004;286:E217.

Chapter 6

Measurement of Energy in Food and During Physical Activity

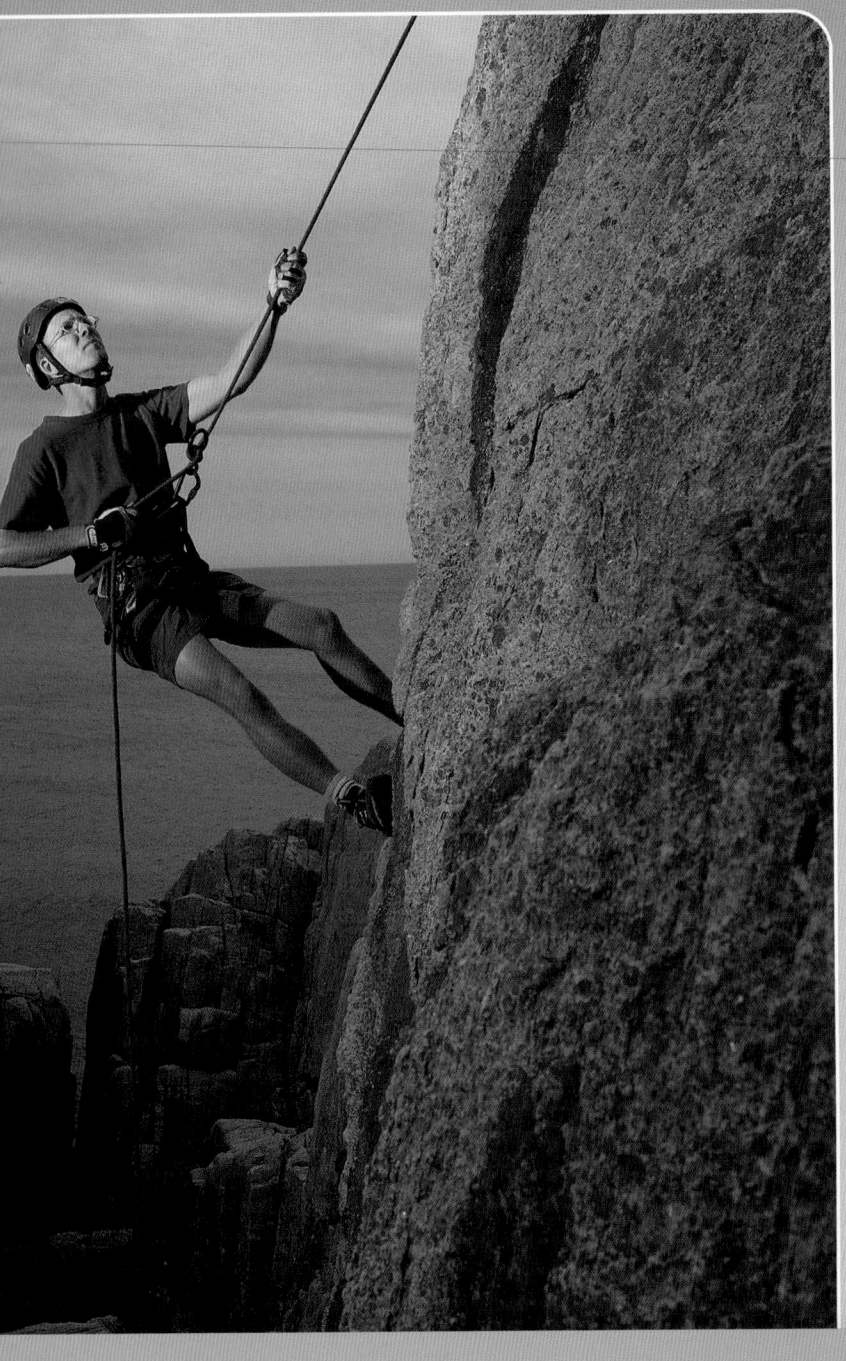

Test Your Knowledge

Answer these 10 statements about the measurement of energy in food and during physical activity. Use the scoring key at the end of the chapter to check your results. Repeat this test after you have read the chapter and compare your results.

1. **T F** The calorie is a unit of energy measurement.
2. **T F** The bomb calorimeter operates on the principle of indirect calorimetry by measuring the oxygen consumed as the food burns completely.
3. **T F** Heat of combustion refers to a food's ability to release carbon dioxide in relation to oxygen consumed as it burns completely.
4. **T F** The heat of combustion for all carbohydrates averages 5.0 kCal per gram.
5. **T F** The heat of combustion for lipid averages 6.0 kCal per gram.
6. **T F** The heat of combustion for protein averages 7.0 kCal per gram.
7. **T F** The doubly labeled water technique provides a way to evaluate sweat loss during intense exercise.
8. **T F** In terms of net energy release in the body, each of the three macronutrients releases about 4.0 kCal per gram.
9. **T F** Celery would become a "fattening" food if consumed in excess.
10. **T F** The respiratory quotient (RQ) for carbohydrate equals 1.00.

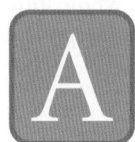 ll biologic functions require energy. The carbohydrate, lipid, and protein macronutrients contain the energy that ultimately powers biologic work, making energy the common denominator for classifying both food and physical activity.

Measurement of Food Energy

THE CALORIE—A UNIT OF ENERGY MEASUREMENT

In nutritional terms, one calorie expresses the quantity of heat necessary to raise the temperature of 1 kg (1 L) of water 1°C (specifically, from 14.5 to 15.5°C). Thus, **kilogram calorie** or kilocalorie **(kCal)** more accurately defines calorie. (Note the use of the letter k to designate a kilocalorie, as compared to a small calorie (c) that indicates the quantity of heat necessary to raise the temperature of 1 g of water 1°C.) For example, if a particular food contains 300 kCal, then releasing the potential energy trapped within this food's chemical structure increases the temperature of 300 L of water 1°C.

Different foods contain different amounts of potential energy. One-half cup of peanut butter with a caloric value of 759 kCal contains the equivalent heat energy to increase the temperature of 759 L of water 1°C. A corresponding unit of heat using Fahrenheit degrees is the British thermal unit or BTU. One BTU represents the quantity of heat necessary to raise the temperature of 1 lb (weight) of water 1°F from 63 to 64°F. *A clear distinction exists between temperature and heat. Temperature reflects a quantitative measure of an object's hotness or coldness. Heat describes energy transfer (exchange) from one body or system to another.* The following conversions apply:

1 cal = 4.184 J
1 kCal = 1000 cal = 4186 J = 4.184 kJ
1 BTU = 778 ft lb = 252 cal = 1055 J

The joule, or **kilojoule (kJ),** reflects the standard international unit (SI unit) for expressing energy. To convert kilocalories to kilojoules, multiply the kilocalorie value by 4.184. The kilojoule value for 1/2 cup of peanut butter, for example, would equal 759 kCal × 4.184, or 3176 kJ. The **megajoule (MJ)** equals 1000 kJ; its use avoids unmanageably large numbers. The name joule honors British scientist Sir Prescott Joule (1818–1889), who studied how vigorous stirring of a paddle wheel warmed water. Joule determined that the movement of the paddle wheel added energy to the water, raising the water temperature in direct proportion to the work done.

GROSS ENERGY VALUE OF FOODS

Laboratories use **bomb calorimeters** similar to one illustrated in FIGURE 6.1 to measure the total heats of combustion (see below) values of the various food macronutrients. Bomb calorimeters operate on the principle of **direct calorimetry**, measuring the heat liberated as the food burns completely.

Figure 6.1 shows food within a sealed chamber charged with oxygen at high pressure. An electrical current moving through the fuse at the tip ignites the food–oxygen mixture. As the food burns, a water jacket surrounding the bomb absorbs the heat (energy) liberated. Because the calorimeter is fully insulated from the outside environment, the increase in water temperature *directly* reflects the heat released during a food's oxidation (burning).

Heat of combustion refers to the heat liberated by oxidizing a specific food; it represents the food's total energy value. For example, a teaspoon of margarine releases 100 kCal of heat energy when burned completely in a bomb calorimeter. This equals the energy required to raise 1.0 kg (2.2 lb) ice water to its boiling point. The oxidation pathways of food in the intact organism and the bomb calorimeter differ, but the energy liberated in the complete breakdown of a food remains the same, regardless of the combustion pathways.

Carbohydrates

The heat of combustion for carbohydrate varies depending on the arrangement of atoms in the particular carbohydrate molecule. For glucose, heat of combustion equals 3.74 kCal per

gram, about 12% less than for glycogen (4.19 kCal) and starch (4.20 kCal). *For 1 g of carbohydrate, a value of 4.2 kCal generally represents the average heat of combustion.*

Lipids

The heat of combustion for lipid varies with the structural composition of the triacylglycerol molecule's fatty acid components. For example, 1 g of either beef or pork fat yields 9.50 kCal, whereas oxidizing 1 g of butterfat liberates 9.27 kCal. The average energy value for 1 g of lipid in meat, fish, and eggs equals 9.50 kCal. In dairy products, the energy equivalent amounts to 9.25 kCal per gram, and 9.30 kCal in vegetables and fruits. *The average heat of combustion for lipid equals 9.4 kCal per gram.*

Proteins

Two factors affect energy release from protein combustion: (1) type of protein in the food and (2) relative nitrogen content of the protein. Common proteins in eggs, meat, corn (maize), and beans (jack, lima, navy, soy) contain approximately 16% nitrogen, and have a corresponding heat of combustion that averages 5.75 kCal per gram. Proteins in other foods have a somewhat higher nitrogen content; most nuts and seeds contain 18.9% nitrogen, and whole-kernel wheat, rye, millets, and barley contain 17.2%. Other foods contain a slightly lower nitrogen percentage; for example, whole milk has 15.7% and bran 15.8%. *The heat of combustion for protein averages 5.65 kCal per gram.*

Comparing Macronutrient Energy Values

The average heats of combustion for the three macronutrients (carbohydrate, 4.2 kCal · g^{-1}; lipid, 9.4 kCal · g^{-1}; protein, 5.65 kCal · g^{-1}) demonstrates that the complete oxidation of lipid in the bomb calorimeter liberates about 65% more energy per gram than protein oxidation and 120% more energy than carbohydrate oxidation. Recall from Chapter 1 that a lipid molecule contains more hydrogen atoms than either carbohydrate or protein molecules. The common fatty acid palmitic acid, for example, has the structural formula $C_{16}H_{32}O_2$. The ratio of hydrogen atoms to oxygen atoms in fatty acids always greatly exceeds the 2:1 ratio in carbohydrates. Simply stated, lipid molecules have more hydrogen atoms available for cleavage and subsequent oxidation for energy than carbohydrates and proteins.

One can conclude from the previous discussion that lipid-rich foods have a higher energy content than foods relatively fat free. One cup of whole milk contains 160 kCal, whereas the same quantity of skim milk contains only 90 kCal. If a person who normally consumes 1 quart of whole milk each day switches to skim milk, the total calories ingested each year would decrease by the equivalent calories in 25 pounds of body fat! In 3 years, all other things remaining constant, body fat loss would approximate 75 pounds. Such a theoretical comparison merits serious consideration because of the al-

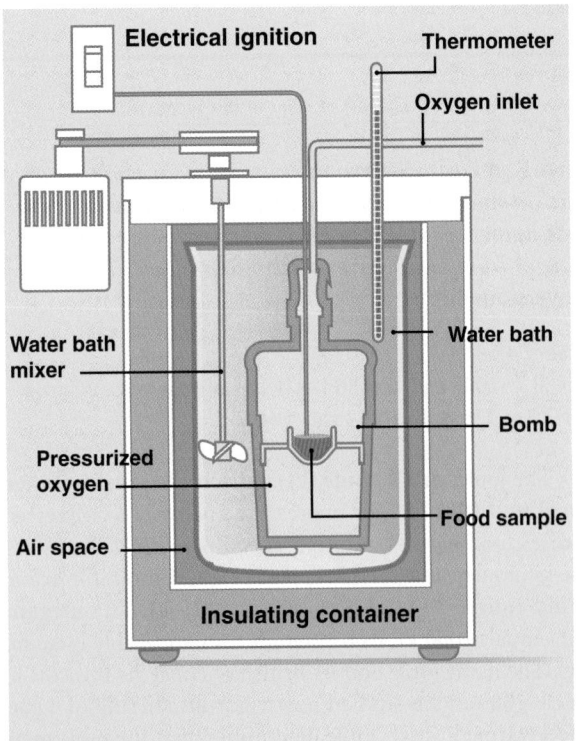

FIGURE 6.1 ■ A bomb calorimeter directly measures the energy value of food.

Electrical ignition
Thermometer
Oxygen inlet
Water bath mixer
Water bath
Bomb
Pressurized oxygen
Food sample
Air space
Insulating container

most identical nutritional composition between whole milk and skim milk except for fat content. Drinking an 8-oz glass of skim milk rather than whole milk also significantly reduces saturated fatty acid intake (0.4 vs 5.1 g) and cholesterol (0.3 vs 33 mg).

Interchangeable Expression for Energy and Work

1 foot-pound (ft-lb) = 0.13825 kilogram-meters (kg-m)
1 kg-m = 7.233 ft-lb = 9.8066 joules
1 kilocalorie (kCal) = 3.0874 ft-lb = 426.85 kg-m = 4.186 kilojoules (kJ)
1 joule (J) = 1 Newton-meter (Nm)
1 kilojoule (kJ) = 1000 J = 0.23889 kCal

NET ENERGY VALUE OF FOODS

Differences exist in the energy value of foods when comparing the heat of combustion determined by direct calorimetry (**gross energy value**) to the **net energy value** actually available to the body. This pertains particularly to proteins, because the body cannot oxidize the nitrogen component of this nutrient. Rather, nitrogen atoms combine with hydrogen to form urea (NH_2CONH_2) for excretion in the urine. Elimination of hydrogen in this manner represents a loss of approximately 19% of the protein molecule's potential energy. This hydrogen loss reduces protein's heat of combustion in the body to approximately 4.6 kCcal per gram instead of 5.65 kCal per gram released during oxidation in the bomb calorimeter. In contrast, *identical* physiologic fuel values exist for carbohydrates and lipids (which contain no nitrogen) compared with their respective heats of combustion in the bomb calorimeter.

Coefficient of Digestibility

The efficiency of the digestive process influences the ultimate caloric yield from macronutrients. Numerically defined as the **coefficient of digestibility,** digestive efficiency represents the percentage of ingested food digested and absorbed to serve the body's metabolic needs. The food remaining unabsorbed in the intestinal tract becomes voided in the feces. Dietary fiber reduces the coefficient of digestibility: A high-fiber meal has less total energy absorbed than does a fiber-free meal of equivalent caloric content. This difference occurs because fiber moves food more rapidly through the intestine, reducing absorption time. Fiber also may cause mechanical erosion of the intestinal mucosa, which then becomes resynthesized through energy-requiring processes.

TABLE 6.1 shows different digestibility coefficients, heats of combustion, and net energy values for nutrients in the various food groups. *The relative percentage of macronutrients completely digested and absorbed averages 97% for carbohydrate, 95% for lipid, and 92% for protein.* Little difference exists in digestive efficiency between obese and lean individuals. However, considerable variability exists in efficiency percent-

ages for any food within a particular category. Proteins in particular have variable digestive efficiencies, ranging from a low of about 78% for high-fiber legumes to a high of 97% for protein from animal sources. Some advocates promote the use of vegetables in weight loss diets because of plant protein's relatively low coefficient of digestibility. Those on a vegetarian-type diet should consume adequate and diverse protein food sources to obtain all essential amino acids (see Chapter 1).

From the data in Table 6.1, the average net energy values can be rounded to simple whole numbers referred to as **Atwater general factors** (http://www.sportsci.org/news/history/atwater/atwater.html).

Atwater General Factors

- 4 kCal per gram for carbohydrate
- 9 kCal per gram for lipid
- 4 kCal per gram for protein

These values, named for Wilbur Olin Atwater (1844–1907), the 19th-century chemist who pioneered human nutrition and energy balance studies, represent the energy available to the body from ingested foods. Except when requiring exact energy values for experimental or therapeutic diets, the Atwater general factors accurately estimate the *net metabolizable energy* of typically consumed foods. For alcohol, 7 kCal (29.4 kJ) represents each g (mL) of pure (200 proof) alcohol ingested. In terms of metabolizable energy available to the body, alcohol's efficiency of use equals that of other carbohydrates.[15]

ENERGY VALUE OF A MEAL

The Atwater general factors can determine the caloric content of any portion of food (or an entire meal) from the food's composition and weight. TABLE 6.2 illustrates the method for calculating the kCal value of 100 g (3.5 oz) of chocolate-chip ice cream. Based on laboratory analysis, this ice cream contains approximately 3% protein, 18% lipid, and 23% carbohydrate, with the remaining 56% being essentially water. Thus, each gram of ice cream contains 0.03 g protein, 0.18 g lipid, and 0.23 g carbohydrate. Using these compositional values and the Atwater factors, the following represents the kCal value per gram of the chocolate-chip ice cream: Net kCal values show that 0.03 g of protein contains 0.12 kCal (0.03 × 4.0 kCal · g^{-1}), 0.18 g lipid contains 1.62 kCal (0.18 × 9 kCal · g^{-1}), and 0.23 g carbohydrate contains 0.92 kCal (0.23 × 4.0 kCal · g^{-1}). Combining the separate values for the nutrients yields a total energy value for each gram of chocolate-chip ice cream of 2.66 kCal (0.12 + 1.62 + 0.92). A 100-g serving yields a caloric value 100 times as large or 266 kCal. The percentage of total calories derived from lipid equals 60.9% (162 lipid kCal ÷ 266 total kCal). Similar computations estimate the caloric value for any food serving. Of course, increasing or decreasing portion sizes (or adding lipid-rich sauces or

TABLE 6.1 Factors for Digestibility, Heats of Combustion, and Net Physiologic Energy Values[a] of Dietary Protein, Lipid, and Carbohydrate

Food Group	Digestibility (%)	Heat of Combustion (kCal·g^{-1})	Net Energy (kCal·g^{-1})
Protein			
Meats, fish	97	5.65	4.27
Eggs	97	5.75	4.37
Dairy products	97	5.65	4.27
Animal food (Average)	97	5.65	4.27
Cereals	85	5.80	3.87
Legumes	78	5.70	3.47
Vegetables	83	5.00	3.11
Fruits	85	5.20	3.36
Vegetable food, (Average)	85	5.65	3.74
Total protein, Average	**92**	**5.65**	**4.05**
Lipid			
Meat and eggs	95	9.50	9.03
Dairy products	95	9.25	8.79
Animal food	95	9.40	8.93
Vegetable food	90	9.30	8.37
Total lipid, Average	**95**	**9.40**	**8.93**
Carbohydrate			
Animal food	98	3.90	3.82
Cereals	98	4.20	3.11
Legumes	97	4.20	4.07
Vegetables	95	4.20	3.99
Fruits	90	4.00	3.60
Sugars	98	3.95	3.87
Vegetable food	97	4.15	4.03
Total carbohydrate, Average	**97**	**4.15**	**4.03**

From Merrill AL, Watt BK. *Energy values of foods: basis and derivation. Agricultural handbook no. 74, Washington, DC: U.S. Department of Agriculture, 1973.*

[a]*Net physiologic energy values computed as the coefficient of digestibility times the heat of combustion adjusted for energy loss in urine.*

creams or using fruits or calorie-free substitutes) affects caloric content accordingly.

Computing the caloric value of foods is time-consuming and laborious. Various governmental agencies in the United States and elsewhere have evaluated and compiled nutritive values for thousands of foods. The most comprehensive data bank resources include the U.S. Nutrient Data Bank (USNDB) maintained by the U.S. Department of Agriculture's (USDA) Consumer Nutrition Center,[10] and a computerized data bank maintained by the Bureau of Nutritional Sciences of Health and Welfare Canada.[8] Many commercial software programs make use of the original USDA nutritional databases, which are available for download to the public for a nominal fee. (The USDA Nutrient Database for Standard Reference Release 11 can be viewed or downloaded from www.nal.usda.gov/fnic/food comp/Data/SR11/ae11.html; access the Nutrient Data Laboratory at www.nal.usda.gov/fnic/foodcomp/; and access the Food and Nutrition Information Center, National Agricultural Library, Agricultural Research Service of the USDA at www.nalusda.gov/fnic/).

Appendix A presents energy and nutritive values for common foods, including specialty and fast-food items. Compute nutritive values for specialty dishes such as chicken or beef tacos from standard recipes; actual values vary considerably depending on the method of preparation. Examination of Appendix A reveals large differences among the energy values of various foods. Consuming an equal number of calories from diverse foods often requires increasing or decreasing the quantity of a particular food. For example, to consume 100 kCal from each of six common foods—carrots, celery, green peppers, grapefruit, medium-sized eggs, and mayonnaise—one must eat 5 carrots, 20 stalks of celery, 6.5 green peppers, 1 large grapefruit, 1¼ eggs, but only 1 tablespoon of mayonnaise. Consequently, an average sedentary adult woman would need to consume 420 celery stalks, 105 carrots, 136 green peppers, or 26 eggs, yet only 1½ cup of mayonnaise or 8 oz of salad oil, to meet her daily 2100-kCal energy needs. These examples dramatically illustrate that foods high in lipid content contain considerably more calories than foods low in lipid with correspondingly higher water content.

TABLE 6.2	**Method for Calculating the Caloric Value of a Food from Its Composition of Macronutrients**

Food: ice cream (chocolate with chocolate chips)

Weight: ¾ cup = 100 g

	Composition		
	Protein	Lipid	Carbohydrate
Percentage	3%	18%	23%
Total grams	3	18	23
In 1 g	0.03	0.18	0.23
Calories per gram	0.12	1.62	0.92

$(0.04 \times 4.0 \text{ kCal}) + (0.18 \times 9.0 \text{ kCal}) + (0.23 \times 4.0 \text{ kCal})$

Total calories per gram: $0.12 + 1.62 + 0.92 = 2.66$ kCal

Total calories per 100 g: $2.66 \times 100 = 266$ kCal

Percentage of calories from lipid: $(18 \text{ g} \times 9.0 \text{ kCal} \cdot \text{g}^{-1})$

$\div 266 \text{ kCal} \times 100 = 60.9\%$

Note that a calorie reflects food energy *regardless* of the food source. Thus, from a standpoint of energy, 100 kCal from mayonnaise equals the same 100 kCal in 20 celery stalks. The more one eats of any food, the more calories one consumes. However, a small quantity of fatty foods represents a considerable quantity of calories; thus, the term "fattening" often describes these foods. An individual's caloric intake equals the sum of *all* energy consumed from either small or large food portions. Indeed, celery becomes a "fattening" food if consumed in excess! Chapter 7 considers variations in daily energy intake among sedentary and active individuals, including diverse groups of athletes.

Case Study

Personal Health and Exercise Nutrition 6–1

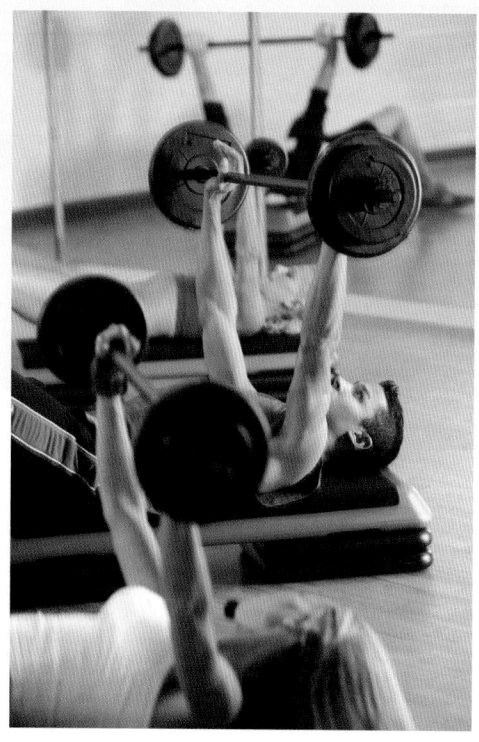

Nutrient Timing to Optimize Muscle Response to Resistance Training

An evidence-based nutritional approach can enhance the quality of resistance training and facilitate muscle growth and strength development. This easy-to-follow new diminsion to sports nutrition emphasizes not only the specific type and mixture of nutrients but also the timing of nutrient intake. Its goal is to blunt the catabolic state (release of hormones glucagon, epinephrine norephinephrine, cortisol) and activate the natural muscle-building hormones (testosterone, growth hormone, IGF-1, insulin) to facilitate recovery from exercise and maximize muscle growth. Three phases for optimizing specific nutrient intake are proposed:

1. The **energy phase** (1) enhances nutrient intake to spare muscle glycogen and protein, (2) enhances muscular endurance, (3) limits immune system suppression, (4) reduces muscle damage, and (5) facilitates recovery in the postexercise period. Consuming a carbohydrate/protein supplement in the immediate pre-exercise period and during exercise extends muscular endurance; the ingested protein promotes

Case Study *continued*

protein metabolism, thus reducing demand for muscle's release of amino acids. Carbohydrates consumed during exercise suppress cortisol release. This blunts the suppressive effects of exercise on immune system function and reduces branched-chain amino acids generated by protein breakdown for energy.

> The recommended *energy phase* supplement profile contains the following nutrients: 20 to 26 g of high-glycemic carbohydrates (glcose, sucrose, maltodextrin), 5 to 6 g whey protein (rapidly digested, high-quality protein separated from milk in the cheese-making process), 1 g leucine, 30 to 120 mg vitamin C, 20 to 60 IU vitamin E, 100 to 250 mg sodium, 60 to 100 mg potassium, and 60 to 220 mg magnesium.

2. The **anabolic phase** consistes of the 45-minute postexercise metabolic window—a period that enhances insulin sensitivity for muscle glycogen replenishment and muscle tissue repair and synthesis. This shift from catabolic to anabolic state occurs largely by blunting the action of cortisol and increasing the anabolic, muscle-building effects of insulin by consuming a standard high-glycemic carbohydrate/protein supplement in liquid form (e.g., whey protein and high-glycemic carbohydrates). In essence, the high-glycemic carbohydrate consumed post exercise serves as a nutrient activator to stimulate insulin release, which in the presence of amino acids increases muscle tissue synthesis and decreases protein degradation.

> The recommended *anabolic phase* supplement profile contains the following nutrients: 40 to 50 g of high-glycemic carbo-hydrates (glucose, sucrose, maltodextrin), 13 to 15 g whey protein, 1 to 2 g leucine, 1 to 2 g glutamine, 60 to 120 mg vitamin C, and 80 to 400 IU vitamin E.

3. The **growth phase** extends from the end of the anabolic phase to the beginning of the next workout. It represents the time period to maximize insulin sensitivity and maintain an anabolic state to accentuate gains in muscle mass and muscle strength. The first several hours *(rapid segment)* of this phase helps maintain increased insulin sensitivity and glucose uptake to maximize glycogen replenishment. It also aims to speed elimination of metabolic wastes via increases in blood flow and stimulation of tissue repair and muscle growth. The next 16 to 18 hours *(sustained segment)* maintains a positive nitrogen balance. This occurs with a relatively high daily protein intake (between 0.91 and 1.2 g of protein per pound of body weight) that fosters sustained but slower muscle tissue synthesis. An adequate carbohydrate intake emphasizes glycogen replenishment.

> The recommended *growth phase* supplement profile contains the following nutrients: 14 g whey protein, 2 g casein, 3 g leucine, 1 g glutamine, and 2 to 4 g high-glycemic carbohydrates.

Ivy J, Portman R. Nutrient Timing: The Future of Sports Nutrition. North Bergen, NY: Basic Health Publications Inc., 2004.

Summary

1. A kilocalorie (kCal) represents a measure of heat that expresses the energy value of food.

2. Burning food in the bomb calorimeter directly quantifies the food's energy content.

3. The heat of combustion represents the amount of heat liberated by the complete oxidation of a food in the bomb calorimeter. Average gross energy values equal 4.2 kCal per gram for carbohydrate, 9.4 kCal per gram for lipid, and 5.65 kCal per gram for protein.

4. The coefficient of digestibility indicates the proportion of food consumed that the body digests and absorbs.

5. Coefficients of digestibility average 97% for carbohydrates, 95% for lipids, and 92% for proteins. Thus, the net

energy values (known as Atwater general factors) are 4 kCal per gram of carbohydrate, 9 kCal per gram of lipid, and 4 kCal per gram of protein.

6. The Atwater calorific values allow one to compute the caloric content of any meal from the food's carbohydrate, lipid, and protein content.

7. The calorie represents a unit of heat energy regardless of food source. From an energy standpoint, 500 kCal of chocolate ice cream topped with whipped cream and hazelnuts is no more fattening than 500 kCal of watermelon, 500 kCal of cheese and pepperoni pizza, or 500 kCal of a bagel with salmon, onions, and sour cream.

Measurement of Human Energy Expenditure

ENERGY RELEASED BY THE BODY

Direct calorimetry and **indirect calorimetry** and the **doubly labeled water technique** represent the most common approaches to accurately quantifying the energy generated by the body (energy expenditure) during rest and physical activity.

Direct Calorimetry

Heat represents the ultimate fate of all of the body's metabolic processes. The early experiments of French chemist Antoine Lavoisier (1743–1794) and his contemporaries (www.science world.wolfram.com/biography/Lavoisier.html) in the 1770s provided the impetus to directly measure energy expenditure during rest and physical activity. The idea, similar to that used in the bomb calorimeter depicted in Figure 6.1, provides a convenient though elaborate way to directly measure heat production in humans.

The human calorimeter illustrated in FIGURE 6.2 consists of an airtight chamber with an oxygen supply where a person lives and works for an extended period.[1] A known water volume at a specified temperature circulates through a series of coils at the top of the chamber. This water absorbs the heat produced and radiated by the individual while in the calorimeter. Insulation protects the entire chamber, so any change in water temperature relates directly to the individual's energy metabolism. For adequate ventilation, the person's exhaled air continually passes from the room through chemicals that remove moisture and absorb carbon dioxide. Oxygen added to the air recirculates through the chamber. Direct

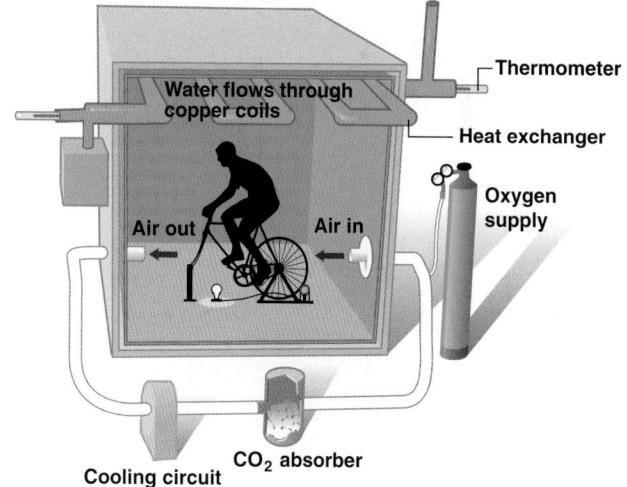

FIGURE 6.2 ■ A human calorimeter directly measures energy metabolism (heat production). In the Atwater-Rosa calorimeter, a thin copper sheet lines the interior wall to which heat exchangers attach overhead and through which water passes. Water cooled to 2°C moves at a high flow rate, rapidly absorbing the heat radiated from the subject during exercise. As the subject rests, warmer water flows at a slower flow rate. In the original bicycle ergometer shown in the schematic, the rear wheel contacts the shaft of a generator that powers a light bulb. In a later version of the ergometer, copper made up part of the rear wheel. The wheel rotated through the field of an electromagnet, producing an electric current for accurately determining power output.

measurement of heat production in humans has considerable theoretical implications, yet its application is limited. Accurate measurements of heat production in the calorimeter require considerable time, expense, and formidable engineering expertise. Thus, use of the calorimeter remains inapplicable for energy determinations for most sport, occupational, and recreational activities.

Indirect Calorimetry

All energy-releasing reactions in the body ultimately depend on oxygen use. Measuring a person's oxygen uptake during aerobic exercise provides an indirect yet accurate estimate of energy expenditure. Indirect calorimetry remains relatively simple to operate and less expensive to maintain and staff than direct calorimetry.

Caloric Transformation for Oxygen

Studies with the bomb calorimeter show that approximately 4.82 kCals release when a blend of carbohydrate, lipid, and protein burns in 1 L of oxygen. Even with large variations in the metabolic mixture, this calorific value for oxygen varies only slightly (generally within 2–4%). Assuming the metabolism of a mixed diet, a rounded value of 5.0 kCal per liter of oxygen consumed designates the appropriate conversion factor for estimating energy expenditure under steady-rate conditions of aerobic metabolism. An energy-oxygen equivalent of 5.0 kCal per liter provides a convenient yardstick for transposing any aerobic physical activity to a caloric (energy) frame of reference. In fact, indirect calorimetry through oxygen-uptake measurement serves as the basis to quantify the energy (caloric) stress of most physical activities (refer to Appendix B).

Closed-circuit spirometry and open-circuit spirometry represent the two common methods of indirect calorimetry.

Closed-Circuit Spirometry

FIGURE 6.3 illustrates the technique of closed-circuit spirometry developed in the late 1800s and still used in hospitals and some laboratories dedicated to human nutrition research to estimate resting energy expenditure. The subject breathes 100% oxygen from a prefilled container (spirometer). The equipment consists of a "closed system" because the person rebreathes only the gas in the spirometer. A canister of soda lime (potassium hydroxide) in the breathing circuit absorbs the carbon dioxide in exhaled air. A drum attached to the spirometer revolves at a known speed and records oxygen uptake from changes in the system's volume.

Oxygen uptake measurement using closed-circuit spirometry becomes problematic during exercise. The subject must remain close to the bulky equipment, the circuit's resistance to the large breathing volumes in exercise is considerable, and the speed of carbon dioxide removal becomes inadequate during heavy exercise. For these reasons, open-circuit spirom-

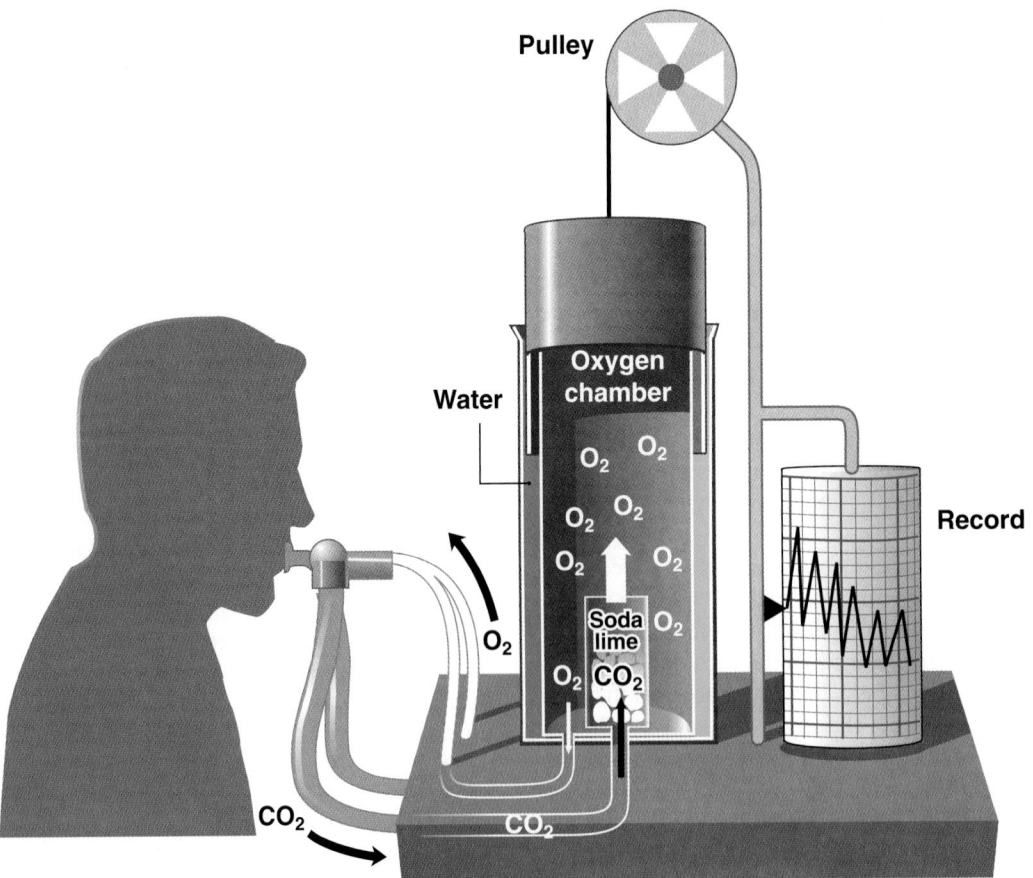

FIGURE 6.3 ■ The closed-circuit method uses a spirometer prefilled with 100% oxygen. As the subject breathes from the spirometer, soda lime removes the expired air's carbon dioxide content.

etry remains the most widely used procedure to measure exercise oxygen uptake.

Open-Circuit Spirometry

With open-circuit spirometry, a subject inhales ambient air with a constant composition of 20.93% oxygen, 0.03% carbon dioxide, and 79.04% nitrogen. The nitrogen fraction also includes a small quantity of inert gases. The changes in oxygen and carbon dioxide percentages in expired air compared with those in inspired ambient air indirectly reflect the ongoing process of energy metabolism. Thus, analysis of two factors—volume of air breathed during a specified time period and composition of exhaled air—provides a useful way to measure oxygen uptake and infer energy expenditure.

Four common indirect calorimetry procedures measure oxygen uptake during various physical activities:

1. Portable spirometry
2. Bag technique
3. Computerized instrumentation
4. Doubly labeled water technique

PORTABLE SPIROMETRY. German scientists in the early 1940s perfected a lightweight, portable system (first devised by German respiratory physiologist Nathan Zuntz [1847–1920] at the turn of the 20th century) to determine indirectly the energy expended during physical activity.[11] Activities included war-related operations such as traveling over different terrain with full battle gear, operating transportation vehicles including tanks and aircraft, and physical tasks that soldiers encounter during combat operations. The subject carried like a backpack the 3-kg box-shaped apparatus shown in FIGURE 6.4. Ambient inspired air passed through a two-way valve, and the expired air exited through a gas meter. The meter measured total expired air volume and collected a small gas sample for later analysis of oxygen and carbon dioxide content. Subsequent determination was made of oxygen uptake and energy expenditure for the measurement period.

Carrying the portable spirometer allows considerable freedom of movement for estimating energy expenditure in diverse activities such as mountain climbing, downhill skiing, sailing, golf, and common household activities (Appendix B). The equipment becomes cumbersome during vigorous activity. Also, the meter under-records airflow volume during intense exercise when breathing is rapid.[13]

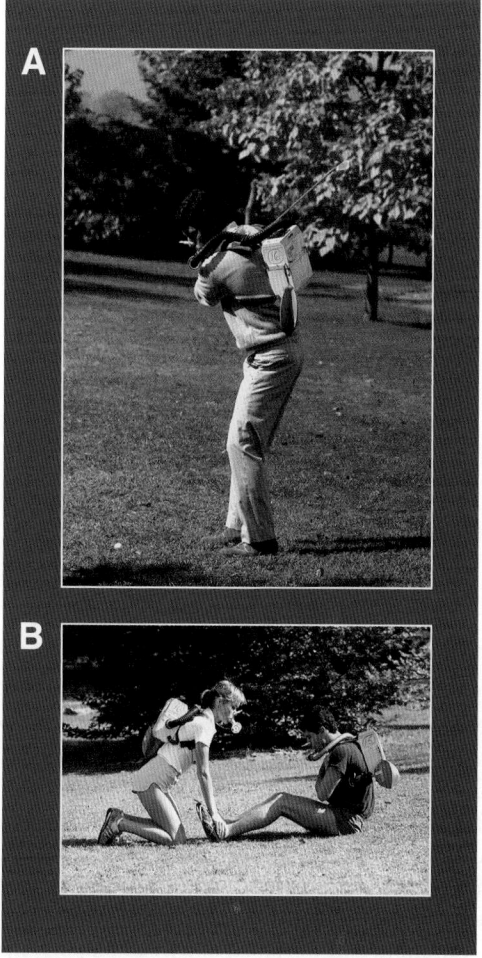

FIGURE 6.4 ■ Portable spirometer to measure oxygen uptake by the open-circuit method during **(A)** golf and **(B)** calisthenics exercise.

Bag Technique. FIGURE 6.5 depicts the bag technique. A subject rides a stationary bicycle ergometer, wearing headgear containing a two-way, high-velocity, low-resistance breathing valve. He breathes ambient air through one side of the valve and expels it out the other side. The air then passes into either large canvas or plastic Douglas bags (named for distinguished British respiratory physiologist Claude G. Douglas [1882–1963]) or rubber meteorologic balloons or directly through a gas meter that continually measures expired air volume. The meter collects a small sample of expired air for analysis of oxygen and carbon dioxide composition. Assessment of oxygen uptake (as with all indirect calorimetric techniques) uses an appropriate calorific transformation for oxygen to compute energy expenditure.[7]

COMPUTERIZED INSTRUMENTATION. With advances in computer and microprocessor technology, the exercise scientist can rapidly measure metabolic and physiologic responses to exercise, although questions have recently been raised concerning accuracy of a widely used computerized breath-by-breath system.[6]

A computer interfaces with at least three instruments: a system that continuously samples the subject's expired air, a flow-measuring device that records air volume breathed and

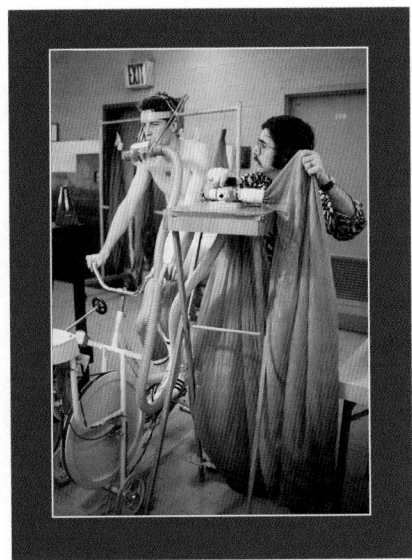

FIGURE 6.5 ■ Measurement of oxygen uptake during open-circuit spirometry (bag technique) during stationary cycle ergometer exercise.

oxygen and carbon dioxide analyzers that measure the composition of the expired gas mixture. The computer performs metabolic calculations based on electronic signals it receives from the instruments. A printed or graphic display of the data appears throughout the measurement period. More advanced systems include automated blood pressure, heart rate, and temperature monitors and preset instructions to regulate speed, duration, and workload of a treadmill, bicycle ergometer, stepper, rower, swim flume, or other exercise apparatus. FIGURE 6.6 depicts a modular computerized systems approach for collecting, analyzing, and displaying metabolic and physiologic responses during exercise.

Newer portable systems include wireless telemetric transmission of data for metabolic measurement—pulmonary ventilation and oxygen and carbon dioxide analysis—during a broad range of exercise, sport, and occupational activities.[3] The lightweight and miniaturized components include a voice-sensitive chip that provides feedback on pacing, duration of exercise, energy expenditure, heart rate, and pulmonary ventilation. The unit's microprocessor stores several hours of exercise data for later downloading to a computer. Telemetry provides "real-time" data on a host computer.

DOUBLY LABELED WATER TECHNIQUE. The doubly labeled water technique provides a useful way to estimate total daily energy expenditure of children and adults in free-living conditions without the normal constraints imposed by other indirect procedures.[5,18,21] The technique does not furnish sufficient refinement for accurate estimates of an individual's energy expenditure, but is more applicable for group estimates.[16] Because of the expense involved in using doubly labeled water, relatively few subjects participate in research studies. Its accuracy allows doubly labeled water to serve as a criterion for validating other methods (e.g., physical activity questionnaires and physical activity records) for estimating total daily energy expenditure of groups over prolonged time periods.[2,4,13]

The subject consumes a quantity of water containing a known concentration of the stable isotopes of hydrogen (^2H or deuterium) and oxygen (^{18}O or oxygen-18)—hence the term *doubly labeled water*. The isotopes distribute throughout all body fluids. Labeled hydrogen leaves the body as water (^2H_2O) in sweat, urine, and pulmonary water vapor, while labeled oxygen leaves as water ($H_2{}^{18}O$) and carbon dioxide ($C^{18}O_2$) produced during macronutrient oxidation in energy metabolism. An isotope ratio mass spectrometer determines the differences between the two isotopes' elimination relative to the body's normal "background" levels. This procedure estimates total carbon dioxide production during the measurement period. Oxygen consumption (uptake) is easily estimated based on carbon dioxide production and an assumed (or measured) RQ value of 0.85 (see page 181).

Under normal circumstances, a control baseline value for ^{18}O and ^2H is determined by analyzing the subject's urine or saliva before ingesting the doubly labeled water. The ingested isotopes require about 5 hours to distribute throughout the body water. The initial enriched urine or saliva sample is then measured and measured every day (or week) thereafter for the study's duration (usually up to 2 or 3 weeks). The progressive decrease in the sample concentrations of the two isotopes permits computation of carbon dioxide production rate.[17] Accuracy of the doubly labeled water technique versus energy expenditure with oxygen consumption in controlled settings averages between 3 and 5%. This magnitude of error probably increases in field studies, particularly among physically active individuals.[20]

The doubly labeled water technique provides an ideal way to assess total energy expenditure of groups over prolonged time periods, including bed rest and during extreme activities such as climbing Mt. Everest, cycling the Tour de France, rowing, and endurance running and swimming.[9,14,19] Major drawbacks of the method include the cost of enriched ^{18}O and the expense of spectrometric analysis of the two isotopes.

Direct Versus Indirect Calorimetry

Energy metabolism studied simultaneously with direct and indirect calorimetry provides convincing evidence for validity of the indirect method to estimate human energy expenditure. At the turn of the century, Atwater and Rosa compared direct and indirect calorimetric methods for 40 days with three men who lived in calorimeters similar to the one in Figure 6.2. Their daily caloric outputs averaged 2723 kCal when measured directly by heat production and 2717 kCal when computed indirectly using closed-circuit measures of oxygen consumption. Other experiments with animals and humans based on moderate exercise also have demonstrated close agreement between the two methods; the difference averaged mostly less than ±1%. In the Atwater and Rosa experiments, the ±0.2% method error represents a remarkable achievement given that these experiments relied on hand-made instruments.

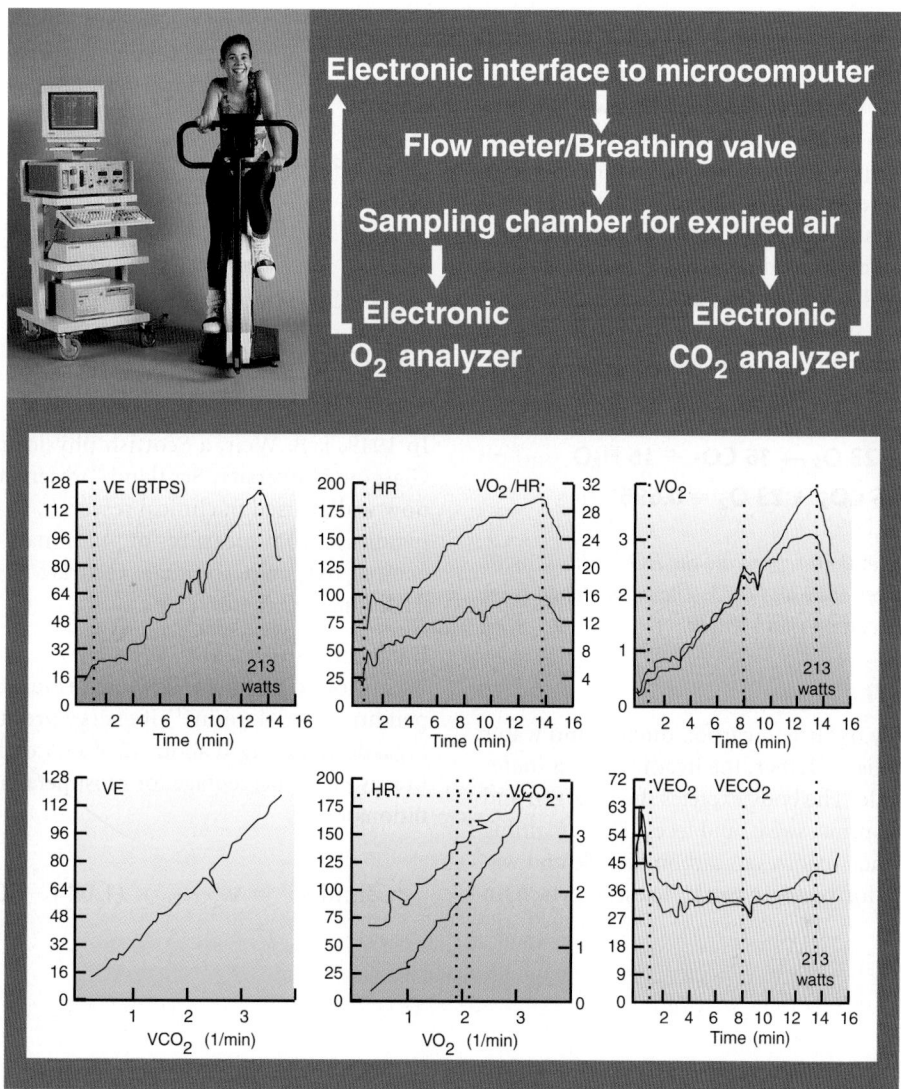

FIGURE 6.6 ■ Computer systems approach to the collection, analysis, and output of physiologic and metabolic data.

THE RESPIRATORY QUOTIENT

Research in the early part of the 19th century discovered a way to evaluate the metabolic mixture in exercise from measures of gas exchange in the lungs.[12] Because of inherent chemical differences in the composition of carbohydrates, lipids, and proteins, complete oxidation of a molecule's carbon and hydrogen atoms to the carbon dioxide and water end products requires different amounts of oxygen. Thus, the substrate metabolized determines the quantity of carbon dioxide produced relative to oxygen consumed. The **respiratory quotient (RQ)** refers to this ratio of metabolic gas exchange as follows:

$$RQ = CO_2 \text{ produced} \div O_2 \text{ consumed}$$

The RQ provides a convenient guide to approximate the nutrient mixture catabolized for energy during rest and aerobic exercise. Also, because the caloric equivalent for oxygen differs somewhat, depending on the macronutrients oxidized, precisely determining the body's heat production or energy expenditure requires knowledge of both the RQ and the oxygen uptake.

RQ for Carbohydrate

The complete oxidation of one glucose molecule requires six oxygen molecules and produces six molecules of carbon dioxide and water as follows:

$$C_6H_{12}O_6 + 6\,O_2 \rightarrow 6\,CO_2 + 6\,H_2O$$

Gas exchange during glucose oxidation produces a number of carbon dioxide molecules equal to the oxygen molecules consumed; therefore, the RQ for carbohydrate equals 1.00.

$$RQ = 6\,CO_2 \div 6O_2 = 1.00$$

RQ for Lipid

The chemical composition of lipids differs from that of carbohydrates in that lipids contain considerably fewer oxygen atoms in proportion to carbon and hydrogen atoms. (Note the 2:1 ratio of hydrogen to oxygen in carbohydrate matches the ratio in water, whereas fatty acids have a much larger ratio.) Consequently, catabolizing fat for energy requires considerably more oxygen consumed relative to carbon dioxide produced. Palmitic acid, a typical fatty acid, oxidizes to carbon dioxide and water, producing 16 carbon dioxide molecules for every 23 oxygen molecules consumed. The following equation summarizes this exchange to compute RQ:

$$C_{16}H_{32}O_2 + 23\ O_2 \rightarrow 16\ CO_2 + 16\ H_2O$$
$$RQ = 16\ CO_2 \div 23\ O_2 = 0.696$$

Generally, a value of 0.70 represents the RQ for lipid, with variation ranging between 0.69 and 0.73. The value depends on the oxidized fatty acid's carbon chain length.

RQ for Protein

Proteins do not simply oxidize to carbon dioxide and water during energy metabolism. Rather, the liver first deaminates the amino acid molecule. The body excretes the nitrogen and sulfur fragments in the urine, sweat, and feces. The remaining "keto acid" fragment then oxidizes to carbon dioxide and water to provide energy for biologic work. These short-chain keto acids, as with fat catabolism, require more oxygen consumed in relation to carbon dioxide produced to achieve complete combustion. The protein albumin oxidizes as follows:

$$C_{72}H_{112}N_2O_{22}S + 77\ O_2 \rightarrow 63\ CO_2 + 38\ H_2O$$
$$+ SO_3 + 9\ CO(NH_2)_2$$
$$RQ = 63\ CO_2 \div 77\ O_2 = 0.818$$

The general value 0.82 characterizes the RQ for protein.

Estimating Energy Expenditure by Use of the Weir Method

In 1949, J. B. Weir, a Scottish physician/physiologist from Glasgow University, Scotland, presented a simple method, now widely used in clinical research, to estimate caloric expenditure from measures of pulmonary ventilation and the expired oxygen percentage, accurate to within ± 1% of the traditional RQ method.

Basic Equation

Weir showed that the following formula calculates caloric expenditure (kCal · min^{-1}) if energy production from protein breakdown averaged about 12.5% of total energy expenditure (a reasonable percentage for most persons under typical conditions):

$$kCal \cdot min^{-1} = \dot{V}_{E(STPD)} \times (1.044 - [0.0499 \times \%\ O_{2E}])$$

TABLE 6.3	Weir Factors for Different Expired Oxygen Percentages (%O_{2E})						
%O_{2E}	Weir Factor	%O_{2E}	Weir Factor	%O_{2E}	Weir Factor	%O_{2E}	Weir Factor
14.50	.3205	15.80	.2556	17.10	.1907	18.30	.1308
14.60	.3155	15.90	.2506	17.20	.1807	18.40	.1268
14.70	.3105	16.00	.2456	17.30	.1857	18.50	.1208
14.80	.3055	16.10	.2406	17.40	.1757	18.60	.1168
14.90	.3005	16.20	.2366	17.50	.1658	18.70	.1109
15.00	.2955	16.30	.2306	17.60	.1707	18.80	.1068
15.10	.2905	16.40	.2256	17.70	.1608	18.90	.1009
15.20	.2855	16.50	.2206	17.80	.1558	19.00	.0969
15.30	.2805	16.60	.2157	17.90	.1508	19.10	.0909
15.40	.2755	16.70	.2107	18.00	.1468	19.20	.0868
15.50	.2705	16.80	.2057	18.10	.1308	19.30	.0809
15.60	.2556	16.90	.2007	18.20	.1368	19.40	.0769
15.70	.2606	17.00	.1957				

From Weir JB. J Physiol 1949;109:1. If %$_{O2}$ expired does not appear in the table, compute individual Weir factors as 1.044 − 0.0499 × %O_{2E}.

where $\dot{V}_{E(STPD)}$ represents expired ventilation per minute (corrected to STPD conditions), and %O_{2E} represents expired oxygen percentage. The value in parenthesis (1.044 - [0.0499 × O_{2E}]) represents the "Weir factor." TABLE 6.3 displays Weir factors for different %O_{2E} values.

To use the table, find the %O_{2E} and corresponding Weir factor. Compute energy expenditure in kCal · min^{-1} by multiplying the Weir factor by $\dot{V}_{E(STPD)}$.

Example

During a steady-rate jog on a treadmill, $\dot{V}_{E(STPD)}$ = 50 L · min^{-1} and O_{2E} = 16.0%. Energy expenditure by the Weir method computes as follows:

$$kCal \cdot min^{-1} = \dot{V}_{E(STPD)} \times (1.044 - [0.0499 \times \%O_{2E}])$$
$$= 50 \times (1.044 - [0.0499 \times 16.0])$$
$$= 50 \times 0.2456$$
$$= 12.3$$

RQ for a Mixed Diet

During activities ranging from complete bed rest to moderate aerobic exercise (walking or slow jogging), the RQ seldom reflects the oxidation of pure carbohydrate or pure fat. Instead, metabolism of a mixture of these two nutrients occurs, with an RQ intermediate between 0.70 and 1.00. *For most purposes, we assume an RQ of 0.82 from the metabolism of a mixture of 40% carbohydrate and 60% fat, applying the caloric equivalent of 4.825 kCal per liter of oxygen for the energy transformation.* Using 4.825, a value of 4% represents the maximum error possible when estimating energy metabolism from steady-rate oxygen uptake.

TABLE 6.4 presents the energy expenditure per liter of oxygen uptake for different nonprotein RQ values, including their corresponding percentages and grams of carbohydrate and fat used for energy. The nonprotein value assumes that the metabolic mixture comprises *only* carbohydrate and fat. Interpret the table as follows:

Suppose oxygen uptake during 30 minutes of aerobic exercise averages 3.22 L · min^{-1} with carbon dioxide production of 2.78 L min^{-1}. The RQ, computed as $\dot{V}_{CO_2} \div \dot{V}_{O_2}$ (2.78 ÷ 3.22), equals 0.86. From Table 6.4, this RQ value (left column) corresponds to an energy equivalent of 4.875 kCal per liter of oxygen uptake or an exercise energy output of 13.55 kCal · min^{-1} (2.78 L O_2 · min^{-1} × 4.875 kCal). Based on a nonprotein RQ, 54.1% of the calories come from the combustion of carbohydrate and 45.9% from fat. The total calories expended during the 30-minute exercise equals 406 kCal (13.55 kCal · min^{-1} × 30).

Oxygen Uptake and Body Size

To adjust for the effects of variations in body size on oxygen consumption (i.e., bigger people usually consume more oxygen), researchers frequently express oxygen consumption in terms of body mass (termed **relative oxygen consumption**), as milliliters of oxygen per kilogram of body mass per minute (mL · kg^{-1} · min^{-1}). At rest, this averages about 3.5 mL · kg^{-1} · min^{-1} **(1 MET)**, or 245 mL · min^{-1} **(absolute oxygen consumption)** for a 70-kg person. Other means of relating oxygen consumption to aspects of body size and body composition include milliliters of oxygen per kilogram of fat-free body mass per minute (mL · kg FFM^{-1} · min^{-1}) and sometimes as milliliters of oxygen per square centimeter of muscle cross-sectional area per minute (mL · cm MCSA^{-2} · min^{-1}).

THE RESPIRATORY EXCHANGE RATIO

Application of the RQ assumes that oxygen and carbon dioxide exchange measured at the lungs reflects the actual gas exchange from macronutrient metabolism in the cell. This assumption remains reasonably valid for rest and during steady-rate (mild to moderate) aerobic exercise when no lactate accumulation takes place. However, factors can spuriously alter the exchange of oxygen and carbon dioxide in the lungs so the ratio of gas exchange no longer reflects only the substrate mixture in cellular energy metabolism. Respiratory physiologists term the ratio of carbon dioxide produced to oxygen consumed under such conditions the **respiratory exchange ratio (R or RER)**. This ratio computes in exactly the same manner as RQ.

For example, carbon dioxide elimination increases during hyperventilation because the breathing response increases to disproportionately high levels compared with actual metabolic demand. By overbreathing, normal carbon dioxide level in blood decreases as this gas "blows off" in expired air. A corresponding increase in oxygen uptake does not occur with this additional carbon dioxide elimination; thus, the rise in respiratory exchange ratio cannot be attributed to the oxidation of foodstuff. In such cases, R usually increases above 1.00.

Exhaustive exercise presents another situation that causes R to rise above 1.00. In such cases, sodium bicarbonate in the blood buffers or "neutralizes" the lactate generated during anaerobic metabolism to maintain proper acid–base balance in the following reaction:

$$HLa + NaHCO_3 \rightarrow NaLa + H_2CO_3 \rightarrow H_2O + CO_2 \rightarrow Lungs$$

Buffering of lactate produces carbonic acid, a weaker acid. In the pulmonary capillaries, carbonic acid degrades to carbon dioxide and water components, and carbon dioxide readily exits through the lungs. The R increases above 1.00 because buffering adds "extra" carbon dioxide to the expired air, in excess of the quantity normally released during energy metabolism.

Relatively low values for R occur following exhaustive exercise when carbon dioxide remains in cells and body fluids to replenish the bicarbonate that buffered the accumulating lactate. This action reduces the expired carbon dioxide without affecting oxygen uptake. This causes the R to dip below 0.70.

TABLE 6.4   **Thermal Equivalents of Oxygen for the Nonprotein Respiratory Quotient (RQ), Including Percentage Kilocalories and Grams Derived from Carbohydrate and Lipid**

Nonprotein RQ	kCal per L O_2	Percentage kCal derived from		Grams per L O_2	
		Carbohydrate	Lipid	Carbohydrate	Lipid
0.707	4.686	0.0	100.0	0.000	0.496
0.71	4.690	1.1	98.9	0.012	0.491
0.72	4.702	4.8	95.2	0.051	0.476
0.73	4.714	8.4	91.6	0.090	0.460
0.74	4.727	12.0	88.0	0.130	0.444
0.75	4.739	15.6	84.4	0.170	0.428
0.76	4.750	19.2	80.8	0.211	0.412
0.77	4.764	22.8	77.2	0.250	0.396
0.78	4.776	26.3	73.7	0.290	0.380
0.79	4.788	29.9	70.1	0.330	0.363
0.80	4.801	33.4	66.6	0.371	0.347
0.81	4.813	36.9	63.1	0.413	0.330
0.82	4.825	40.3	59.7	0.454	0.313
0.83	4.838	43.8	56.2	0.496	0.297
0.84	4.850	47.2	52.8	0.537	0.280
0.85	4.862	50.7	49.3	0.579	0.263
0.86	4.875	54.1	45.9	0.621	0.247
0.87	4.887	57.5	42.5	0.663	0.230
0.88	4.889	60.8	39.2	0.705	0.213
0.89	4.911	64.2	35.8	0.749	0.195
0.90	4.924	67.5	32.5	0.791	0.178
0.91	4.936	70.8	29.2	0.834	0.160
0.92	4.948	74.1	25.9	0.877	0.143
0.93	4.961	77.4	22.6	0.921	0.125
0.94	4.973	80.7	19.3	0.964	0.108
0.95	4.985	84.0	16.0	1.008	0.090
0.96	4.998	87.2	12.8	1.052	0.072
0.97	5.010	90.4	9.6	1.097	0.054
0.98	5.022	93.6	6.4	1.142	0.036
0.99	5.035	96.8	3.2	1.186	0.018
1.00	5.047	100.0	0.0	1.231	0.000

MEASUREMENT OF HUMAN ENERGY GENERATING CAPACITIES

We all possess the capability for anaerobic and aerobic energy metabolism, although the capacity for each form of energy transfer varies considerably among individuals. FIGURE 6.7 shows the involvement of the anaerobic and aerobic energy transfer systems for different durations of all-out exercise. At the initiation of either high- or low-speed movements, the intramuscular phosphagens ATP and PCr provide immediate and nonaerobic energy for muscle action. After the first few seconds of movement, the glycolytic energy system (initial phase of carbohydrate breakdown) provides an increasingly greater proportion of total energy. Continuation of exercise

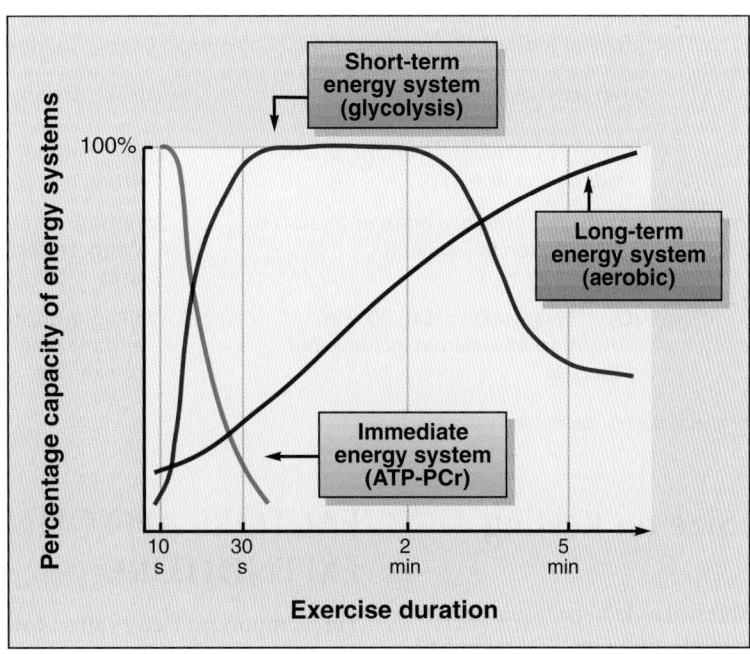

FIGURE 6.7 ▪ Three energy systems and their percentage contribution to total energy output during all-out exercise of different durations.

places a progressively greater demand on aerobic metabolic pathways for ATP resynthesis.

Some physical activities require the capacity of more than one energy transfer system, whereas other activities rely predominantly on a single system. All activities activate each energy system to some degree depending on exercise intensity and duration. Of course, greater demand for anaerobic energy transfer occurs for higher intensity and shorter duration activities.

Both direct and indirect calorimetric techniques estimate the power and capacity of the different energy systems during activity. TABLE 6.5 lists some of the direct and indirect physiologic performance tests in common use for such purposes.

ENERGY EXPENDITURE DURING REST AND PHYSICAL ACTIVITY

Three factors determine total daily energy expenditure (FIG. 6.8):

1. Resting metabolic rate, which includes basal and sleeping conditions plus the added energy cost of arousal
2. Thermogenic influence of food consumed
3. Energy expended during physical activity and recovery

Basal Metabolic Rate

For each individual, a minimum energy requirement sustains the body's functions in the waking state. Measuring oxygen consumption under the following three standardized conditions quantifies this requirement called the **basal metabolic rate (BMR):**

1. No food consumed for at least 12 hours before measurement. The **postabsorptive state** describes this condition

2. No undue muscular exertion for at least 12 hours before measurement
3. Measured after the person has been lying quietly for 30 to 60 minutes in a dimly lit, temperature-controlled (thermoneutral) room

Regular Exercise Slows a Decrease in Metabolism with Age

Increases in body fat and decreases in fat-free body mass (FFM) largely explain the 2% decline in BMR per decade through adulthood. Regular physical activity blunts the age-related decrease in BMR. An accompanying 8% increase in resting metabolism occurred when 50- to 65-year old men increased FFM with intense resistance training. Also, an 8-week aerobic conditioning program for older adults, increased resting metabolism by 10% without any change in FFM—indicating that endurance and resistance exercise training can offset the decrease in resting metabolism usually observed with aging.

Maintaining controlled conditions provides a standardized way to study the relationship among energy expenditure and body size, gender, and age. The BMR also establishes an important energy baseline for implementing a prudent program of weight control by food restraint, exercise, or combination of both. In most instances, basal values measured in the laboratory remain only marginally lower than values for the resting metabolic rate measured under less stringent conditions, for example, 3 to 4 hours after a light meal without physical activity. The terms basal and resting metabolism often are applied interchangeably.

TABLE 6.5   Common Direct (Physiologic) and Indirect (Performance) Tests of Human Energy Generating Capacities.

Energy System	Direct (physiologic) Measures	Indirect (performance test) Measures
Immediate (anaerobic) system	Changes in ATP/PCr levels for all-out exercise, ≤ 30 s	Stair-sprinting; power jumping; power lifting
Short-term (anaerobic) system	Lactate response/glycogen depletion to all-out exercise, ≤ 3 min	Sprinting; all-out cycle ergometry (e.g., Wingate Test), running and swimming tests
Long-term (aerobic) system	$\dot{V}O_{2max}$[a] assessment; 4 to 20 min duration of maximal incremental exercise	Walk/jog/run/step/cycle tests; submaximal and maximal tests; heart rate response to exercise

[a]*Highest oxygen uptake achieved per minute during maximal endurance exercise*

Influence of Body Size on Resting Metabolism

FIGURE 6.9 shows that BMR (expressed as kCal per square meter of body surface area per hour; $kCal \cdot m^{-2} \cdot h^{-1}$) averages 5 to 10% lower in females compared with males at all ages. A female's larger percentage body fat and smaller muscle mass relative to body size helps explain her lower metabolic rate per unit surface area. From ages 20 to 40, average values for BMR equal 38 $kCal \cdot m^{-2} \cdot h^{-1}$ for men and 36 $kCal \cdot m^{-2} \cdot h^{-1}$ for women.

FACTORS AFFECTING ENERGY EXPENDITURE

Three important factors affect **total daily energy expenditure (TDEE):** (1) physical activity, (2) dietary-induced thermogenesis, and (3) climate. Pregnancy also affects TDEE, mainly through its effect of increasing the energy cost of many modes of physical activity.

Components of Daily Energy Expenditure

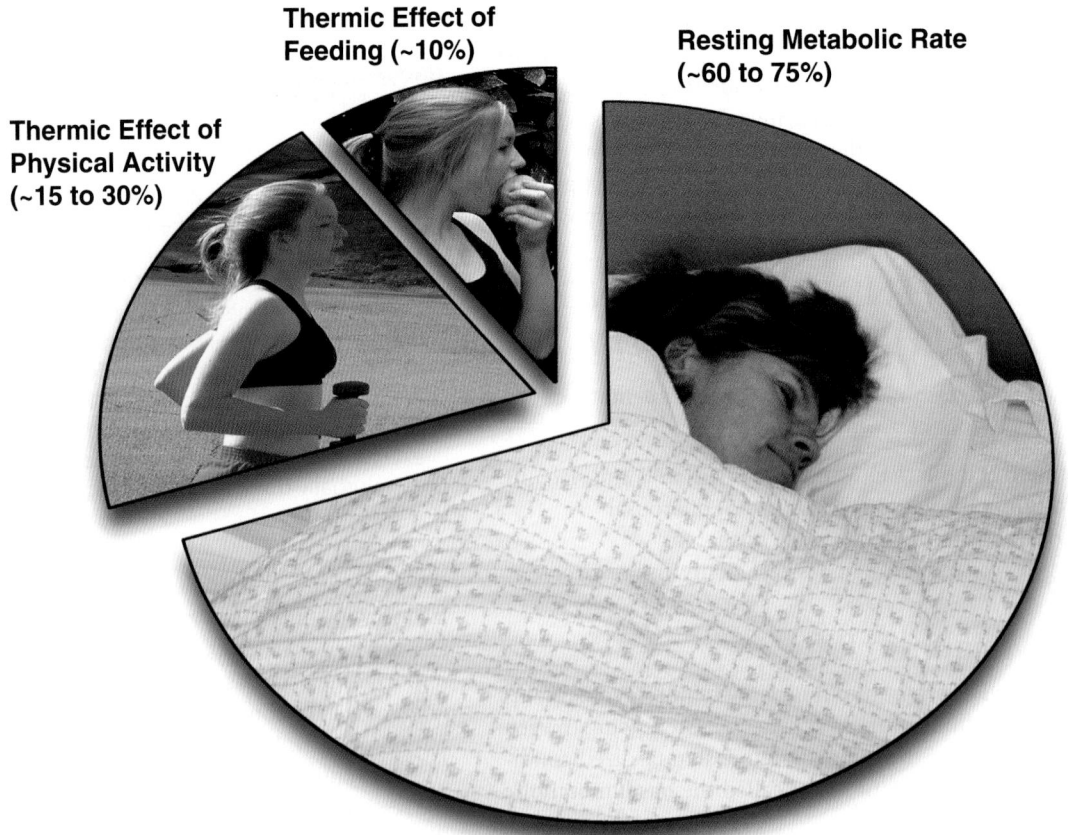

Thermic Effect of Feeding (~10%)

Thermic Effect of Physical Activity (~15 to 30%)

Resting Metabolic Rate (~60 to 75%)

FIGURE 6.8 ■ Components of daily energy expenditure.

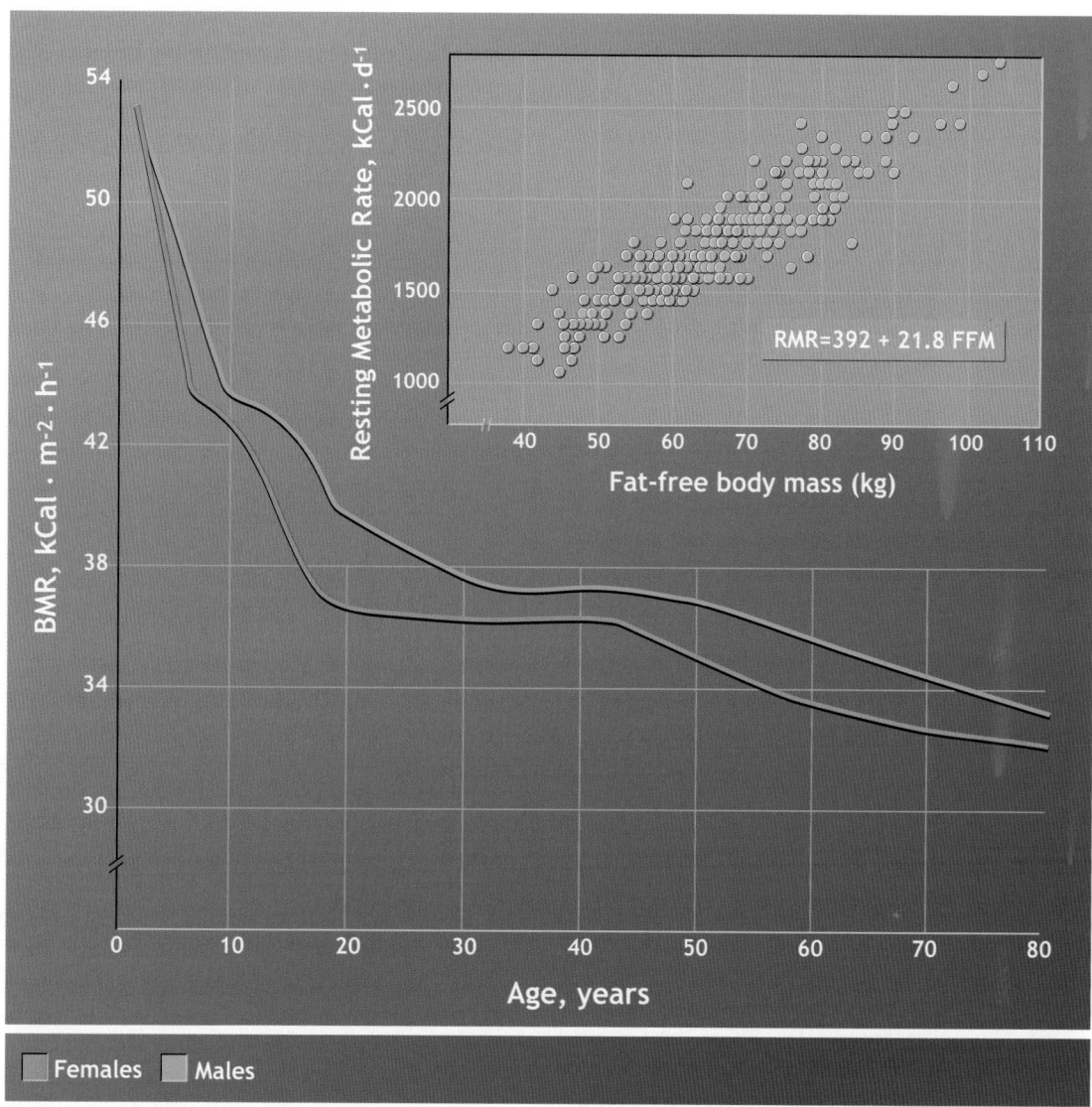

FIGURE 6.9 ■ Basal metabolic rate (BMR) as a function of age and gender. (Data from Altman PL, Dittmer D. *Metabolism*. Bethesda, MD: Federation of American Societies for Experimental Biology, 1968.) Inset graph shows the strong relationship between fat-free body mass and daily resting metabolic rate for men and women. (From Ravussin E, et al. Determination of 24-h energy expenditure in man: methods and results using a respiratory chamber. *J Clin Invest* 1968;78:1568.)

Physical Activity

Physical activity profoundly affects human energy expenditure. World-class athletes nearly double their daily caloric outputs with 3 or 4 hours of intense training. Most people can sustain metabolic rates that average 10 times the resting value during "big muscle" exercises such as fast walking and hiking, running, cycling, and swimming. *Physical activity generally accounts for between 15 and 30% TDEE.*

Dietary-Induced Thermogenesis

Consuming food increases energy metabolism from the energy-requiring processes of digesting, absorbing, and assimilating nutrients. **Dietary-induced thermogenesis (DIT;** also termed **thermic effect of food**) typically reaches maximum within 1 hour after eating depending on food quantity and type. The magnitude of DIT ranges between 10 and 35% of

the ingested food energy. A meal of pure protein, for example, elicits a thermic effect often equaling 25% of the meal's total energy content.

Take a Walk After Eating

Individuals with poor control over body weight often have a depressed thermic response to eating, an effect most likely related to a genetic predisposition. This can contribute to considerable body fat accumulation over a period of years. Exercising after eating augments an individual's normal thermic response to food intake. This supports the wisdom of "going for a brisk walk" following a meal.

Climate

Environmental factors influence resting metabolic rate. The resting metabolism of people who live in tropical climates, for example, averages 5 to 20% higher than counterparts in more temperate regions. Exercise performed in hot weather also imposes a small additional metabolic load; it causes about a 5% elevation in oxygen uptake compared with the same work performed in a thermoneutral environment. The increase in metabolism comes from a direct thermogenic effect of elevated core temperature plus additional energy required for sweat gland activity and altered metabolism.

Pregnancy

Maternal cardiovascular dynamics follow normal response patterns during pregnancy. Moderate exercise generally presents no greater physiologic stress to the mother other than imposed by the additional weight gain and possible encumbrance of fetal tissue. Pregnancy does not compromise the absolute value for aerobic capacity ($L \cdot min^{-1}$). As pregnancy progresses, increases in maternal body weight add considerably to exercise effort during weight-bearing walking, jogging, and stair climbing and may also reduce the economy of physical effort.

ENERGY EXPENDITURE DURING PHYSICAL ACTIVITY

An understanding of resting energy metabolism provides an important frame of reference to appreciate the potential of humans to increase daily energy output. According to numerous surveys, *physical inactivity* (e.g., watching television or playing computer games, lounging around the home, and other sedentary activities) accounts for about one third of a person's waking hours. This means that regular physical activity has the potential to considerably boost the TDEE of large numbers of men and women. Actualizing this potential depends on the intensity, duration, and type of physical activity performed.

Researchers have measured the energy expended during diverse activities such as brushing teeth, house cleaning, mowing the lawn, walking the dog, driving a car, playing ping-pong, bowling, dancing, swimming, rock climbing, and physical activity during space flight within the space vehicle and outside during work tasks (extravehicular activity [EVA]). Consider an activity such as rowing continuously at 30 strokes per minute for 30 minutes. If the amount of oxygen consumed averaged $2.0 \, L \cdot min^{-1}$ during each minute of rowing, then in 30 minutes the rower would consume 60 L of oxygen. A reasonably accurate estimate of the energy expended in rowing can be made because 1 L of oxygen generates about 5 kCal of energy. In this example, the rower expends 300 kCal (60 L × 5 kCal) during the exercise. This value represents **gross energy expenditure** for the exercise period. The **net energy expenditure** attributable solely to rowing equals gross energy expenditure (300 kCal) minus the energy requirement for rest for an equivalent time.

One can estimate TDEE by determining the time spent in daily activities (using a diary) and determining the activity's corresponding energy requirement. Listings of energy expen-diture for a wide range of physical activities are available in Appendix B or can be found on the Internet at various sites (e.g., www.caloriesperhour.com/index_burn.html).

Energy Cost of Recreational and Sport Activities

TABLE 6.6 illustrates the energy cost among diverse recreational and sport activities. Notice, for example, that volleyball requires about 3.6 kCal per minute (216 kCal per hour) for a person who weighs 71 kg (157 lb). The same person expends more than twice this energy, or 546 kCal per hour, swimming the front crawl. Viewed somewhat differently, 25 minutes spent swimming expends about the same number of calories as playing 1 hour of recreational volleyball. Energy expenditure increases proportionately if the pace of the swim increases or volleyball becomes more intense.

Effect of Body Mass

Body weight plays an important contributing role in exercise energy requirements. This occurs because the energy expended during **weight-bearing exercise** increases directly with the body weight transported. *Such a strong relationship exists that one can predict energy expenditure during walking or running from body weight with almost as much accuracy as measuring oxygen consumption under controlled laboratory conditions.* In non–weight-bearing or **weight-supported exercise** (e.g., stationary cycling), little relationship exists between body weight and exercise energy cost.

From a practical standpoint, walking and other weight-bearing exercises require a substantial calorie burn for heavier people. Notice in Table 6.6 that playing tennis or volleyball requires considerably greater energy expenditure for a person weighing 83 kg than for someone 20 kg lighter. Expressing caloric cost of weight-bearing exercise in relation to body mass as kCal per kilogram of body weight per minute ($kCal \cdot kg^{-1} \cdot min^{-1}$) greatly reduces the difference in energy expenditure among individuals of different body weights. The absolute energy cost of the exercise ($kCal \cdot min^{-1}$), however, remains greater for the heavier person.

AVERAGE DAILY RATES OF ENERGY EXPENDITURE

A committee of the United States Food and Nutrition Board (www.lom.edu/cms/3708.aspx) proposed various norms to represent average rates of energy expenditure for men and women in the United States. These values apply to people with occupations considered between sedentary and active and who participate in some recreational activities (i.e., weekend swimming, golf, and tennis). TABLE 6.7 shows that between 2900 and 3000 kCal for males and 2200 kCal for females between the ages of 15 and 50 years represent the average daily energy expenditures. As shown in the lower part of the table, the typical person spends about 75% of the day in sedentary activities. This predominance of physical *inactivity* has prompted some sociologists to refer to the modern-day American as *homo sedentarius*. Compelling evidence

TABLE 6.6 Gross Energy Cost (kCal) for Selected Recreational and Sports Activities in Relation to Body Mass

kg	50	53	56	59	62	65	68	71	74	77	80	83
lb	110	117	123	130	137	143	150	157	163	170	176	183
ACTIVITY												
Volleyball	12.5	2.7	2.8	3.0	3.1	3.3	3.4	3.6	3.7	3.9	4.0	4.2
Aerobic dancing	6.7	7.1	7.5	7.9	8.3	8.7	9.2	9.6	10.0	10.4	10.8	11.2
Cycling, leisure	5.0	5.3	5.6	5.9	6.2	6.5	6.8	7.1	7.4	7.7	8.0	8.3
Tennis	5.5	5.8	6.1	6.4	6.8	7.1	7.4	7.7	8.1	8.4	8.7	9.0
Swimming, slow crawl	6.4	6.8	7.2	7.6	7.9	8.3	8.7	9.1	9.5	9.9	10.2	10.6
Touch football	6.6	7.0	7.4	7.8	8.2	8.6	9.0	9.4	9.8	10.2	10.6	11.0
Running, 8-min mile	10.8	11.3	11.9	12.5	13.11	3.6	14.2	14.8	15.4	16.0	16.5	17.1
Skiing, uphill racing	13.7	14.5	15.3	16.2	17.0	17.8	18.6	19.5	20.3	21.1	21.9	22.7

Copyright © from Fitness Technologies, Inc. 5043 Via Lara lane. Santa Barbara, CA. 93111

Note: Energy expenditure computes as the number of minutes of participation multiplied by the kCal value in the appropriate body weight column. For example, the kCal cost of 1 hour of tennis for a person weighing 150 lb (68 kg) equals 444 kCal (7.4 kCal × 60 min).

supports this descriptor because at least 60% of American adults do not obtain enough physical activity to provide health benefits. In fact, more than 25% of adults receive no additional physical activity at all in their leisure time. Physical activity decreases with age, and sufficient activity becomes less common among women than men, particularly among those with lower incomes and less formal education. Unfortunately, nearly half of youths aged 12 to 21 are not vigorously active on a regular basis.

THE METABOLIC EQUIVALENT (MET)

Values for oxygen consumption and kCal commonly express differences in exercise intensity. As an alternative, a conven-

TABLE 6.7 Average Rates of Energy Expenditure for Men and Women Living in the United States[a]

	AGE, y	BODY MASS, kg	lb	STATURE, cm	in	ENERGY EXPENDITURE, kCal
Males	15–18	66	145	176	69	3000
	19–24	72	160	177	70	2900
	25–50	79	174	176	70	2900
	51+	77	170	173	68	2300
Females	15–18	55	120	163	64	2200
	19–24	58	128	164	65	2200
	25–50	63	138	163	64	2200
	50+	65	143	160	63	1900

AVERAGE TIME SPENT DURING THE DAY	
ACTIVITY	**TIME (h)**
Sleeping and lying down	8
Sitting	6
Standing	6
Walking	2
Recreational activity	2

Data from Food and Nutrition Board, National Research Council: Recommended Dietary Allowances, revised. Washington, DC: National Academy of Sciences.

[a]*The information in this table was designed for the maintenance of practically all healthy people in the United States.*

TABLE 6.8 FIVE-LEVEL CLASSIFICATION OF PHYSICAL ACTIVITY BASED ON EXERCISE INTENSITY

LEVEL	KCAL · MIN^{-1}	ENERGY EXPENDITURE[a] L · MIN^{-1}	mL · KG^{-1}· MIN^{-1}	METs
Men				
Light	2.0–4.9	0.40–0.99	6.2–15.2	1.6–3.9
Moderate	5.0–7.4	1.00–1.49	15.3–22.9	4.0–5.9
Heavy	7.5–9.9	1.50–1.99	23.0–30.6	6.0–7.9
Very Heavy	10.0–12.4	2.00–2.49	30.7–38.3	8.0–9.9
Unduly Heavy	≥12.5	≥2.50	≥38.4	≥10.0
Women				
Light	1.5–3.4	0.30–0.69	5.4–12.5	1.2–2.7
Moderate	3.5–5.4	0.70–1.09	12.6–19.8	2.8–4.3
Heavy	5.5–7.4	1.10–1.49	19.9–27.1	4.4–5.9
Very Heavy	7.5–9.4	1.50–1.89	27.2–34.4	6.0–7.5
Unduly Heavy	≥9.5	≥1.90	≥34.5	≥7.6

[a]L · min^{-1} based on 5 kCal per liter of oxygen; mL · kg^{-1} · min^{-1} based on 65-kg man and 55-kg woman; one MET equals the average resting oxygen consumption (250 mL · min^{-1} for men, 200 mL · min^{-1} for women).

ient way to express exercise intensity classifies physical effort as multiples of resting energy expenditure with a unit-free measure. To this end, scientists have developed the concept of **METs**, an acronym derived from the term **M**etabolic **E**quivalen**T**. One **MET** represents an adult's average seated, resting oxygen consumption or energy expenditure − about 250 mL O_2 · min^{-1}, 3.5 mL O_2 · kg^{-1} · min^{-1}, 1 kCal · kg^{-1} · h^{-1}, or 0.017 kCal · kg^{-1} · min^{-1} (1 kCal · kg^{-1}· h^{-1} ÷ 60 min· h^{-1} = 0.017). Using this frame of reference, a two-**MET** activity requires twice the resting metabolism, or about 500 mL of oxygen per minute; a 3-**MET** intensity level requires three times as much energy as expended at rest, and so on.

The MET provides a convenient way to rate exercise intensity with respect to a resting baseline, that is, multiples of rest-

ing energy expenditure. Conversion from MET to kCal · min^{-1} necessitates knowledge of body mass and use of the conversion: 1.0 kCal · kg^{-1} · h^{-1} = 1 MET. For example, if a person weighing 70 kg bicycled at 10 mph, listed as a 10-MET activity, the corresponding kCal expenditure calculates as follows:

$$10.0 \text{ METs} = 10.0 \text{ kCal} \cdot \text{kg}^{-1} \cdot \text{h}^{-1} \times 70 \text{ kg} \div 60 \text{ min}$$

$$= 700 \text{ kCal} \div 60 \text{ min}$$

$$= 11.7 \text{ kCal} \cdot \text{min}^{-1}$$

TABLE 6.8 presents a five-level classification scheme of physical activity based on energy expenditure and corresponding MET levels for untrained men and women.

Summary

1. Direct calorimetry and indirect calorimetry are two methods for determining the body's rate of energy expenditure. Direct calorimetry measures actual heat production in an appropriately insulated calorimeter. Indirect calorimetry infers energy expenditure from measurements of oxygen uptake and carbon dioxide production, using closed-circuit spirometry, open-circuit spirometry, or the doubly labeled water technique.

2. The doubly labeled water technique estimates energy expenditure in free-living conditions without the normal constraints of laboratory procedures. Although serving as a gold standard for other long-term energy expenditure estimates, drawbacks include the cost of enriched ^{18}O and the expense of spectrometric analysis of the two isotopes.

3. The complete oxidation of each macronutrient requires a different quantity of oxygen uptake compared to carbon dioxide production. The ratio of carbon dioxide produced to oxygen consumed, termed the *respiratory quotient*, or *RQ*, provides key information about the nutrient mixture catabolized for energy. The RQ equals 1.00 for carbohydrate, 0.70 for fat, and 0.82 for protein.

4. For each RQ value, a corresponding caloric value exists for each liter of oxygen consumed. This RQ–kCal relationship provides an accurate estimate of exercise expenditure during steady-rate exercise.

5. The RQ does not indicate specific substrate use during non–steady rate exercise because of nonmetabolic carbon dioxide production in the buffering of lactate.

Summary *continued*

6. The respiratory exchange ratio (R) reflects pulmonary exchange of carbon dioxide and oxygen under various physiologic and metabolic conditions; R does not fully mirror the macronutrient mixture catabolized.

7. Basal metabolic rate (BMR) reflects the minimum energy required for vital functions in the waking state. BMR relates inversely to age and gender, averaging 5 to 10% lower in women than men.

8. Total daily energy expenditure (TDEE) represents the sum of energy required in basal and resting metabolism, thermogenic influences (particulary the thermic effect of food), and energy generated in physical activity.

9. Body mass, stature, and age, or estimates of fat-free body mass (FFM), provide for accurate estimates of resting daily energy expenditure.

10. Physical activity, dietary-induced thermogenesis, and environmental factors (and to a lesser extent pregnancy) significantly affect TDEE.

11. Energy expenditure can be expressed in gross or net terms. Gross (total) values include the resting energy requirement, whereas net energy expenditure reflects the energy cost of the activity that excludes resting metabolism over an equivalent time interval.

12. Daily rates of energy expenditure classify different occupations and sports professions. Within any classification, variability exists from energy expended in recreational and on-the-job pursuits. Heavier individuals expend more energy in most physical activities than lighter counterparts simply from the energy cost of transporting the additional body mass.

13. Different classification systems rate the strenuousness of physical activities. These include rating based on energy cost expressed in $kCal \cdot min^{-1}$, oxygen requirement in $L \cdot min^{-1}$, or multiples of the resting metabolic rate (METs).

Test Your Knowledge Answers

1. **True:** In nutritional terms, one calorie expresses the quantity of heat needed to raise the temperature of 1 kg (1 L) of water 1°C (specifically, from 14.5 to 15.5°C). Thus, kilogram-calorie or kilocalorie (kCal) more accurately defines a calorie.

2. **False:** Laboratories use the bomb calorimeter to measure the total energy value of the various food macronutrients. Bomb calorimeters operate on the principle of direct calorimetry, measuring the heat liberated as the food burns completely.

3. **False:** Heat of combustion refers to the heat liberated by oxidizing a specific food; it represents the food's total energy value as measured by the bomb calorimeter. The oxidation pathways of food in the intact organism and bomb calorimeter differ, yet the energy liberated in the complete breakdown of food remains the same regardless of the combustion pathways.

4. **False:** The heat of combustion for carbohydrate varies depending on the arrangement of atoms in the particular carbohydrate molecule. On average, for 1 g of carbohydrate, a value of 4.2 kCal generally represents the average heat of combustion.

5. **False:** The heat of combustion for lipid varies with the structural composition of the triacylglycerol molecule's fatty acid components. The average heat of combustion for lipid equals 9.4 kCal per gram.

6. **False:** The coefficient of digestibility represents the percentage of an ingested macronutrient actually digested and absorbed by the body. The quantity of food remaining unabsorbed in the intestinal tract becomes voided in the feces. The relative percentage digestibility coefficients average 97% for carbohydrate, 95% for lipid, and 92% for protein.

7. **False:** The doubly labeled water technique estimates total daily energy expenditure of children and adults in free-living conditions without the normal constraints imposed by other procedures of indirect calorimetry. It involves the ingestion of stable isotopes of hydrogen and oxygen, which distribute throughout all body fluids. Differences between elimination rates of the two isotopes relative to the body's normal "background" level estimates total carbon dioxide production from energy metabolism during the measurement period.

8. **False:** The average net energy values can be rounded to simple whole numbers and are referred to as Atwater general factors, which are as follows: 4 kCal per gram for carbohydrate, 9 kCal per gram for lipid, 4 kCal per gram for protein.

9. **True:** The more one eats of any food, the more calories one consumes. An individual's caloric intake equals the sum of all energy consumed from either small or large quantities of foods. Thus, celery becomes a "fattening" food if consumed in excess. Achieving this excess involves consuming a considerable quantity of celery. For example, the typical

Test Your Knowledge Answers   *continued*

sedentary woman needs to consume 420 celery stalks, yet only 8 oz of salad oil, to meet her daily 2100 kCal energy needs.

10. **True:** Inherent chemical differences in the composition of carbohydrates, lipids, and proteins means that the complete oxidation of a molecule's carbon and hydrogen atoms to carbon dioxide and water

end products requires different amounts of oxygen. Gas exchange during glucose oxidation produces six carbon dioxide molecules for six oxygen molecules consumed. Therefore, the RQ (CO_2 produced ÷ O_2 consumed) for carbohydrate equals 1.00. (RQ = 6 CO_2 ÷ 6 O_2 = 1.00).

References

1. Atwater WO, Rosa EB. Description of a new respiration calorimeter and experiments on the conservation of energy in the human body. US Department of Agriculture, Office of Experiment Stations, bulletin no. 63. Washington, DC: Government Printing Office, 1899.
2. Conway JM, et al. Comparison of energy expenditure estimates from doubly labeled water, a physical activity questionnaire, and physical activity records. *Am J Clin Nutr* 2002;75:519.
3. Crandall CG, et al. Evaluation of the Cosmed K2 portable telemetric oxygen uptake analyzer. *Med Sci Sports Exerc* 1994;26:108.
4. Ekelund U, et al. Energy expenditure assessed by heart rate and doubly labeled water in young athletes. *Med Sci Sports Exerc* 2002;34:1360.
5. Ekelund U, et al. Physical activity but not energy expenditure is reduced in obese adolescents: a case-controlled study. *Am J Clin Nutr* 2002;76:935.
6. Gore JC, et al. CPX/D underestimates $\dot{V}O_2$ in athletes compared with an automated Douglas log system. *Med Sci Sports Exerc* 2003;35:1341.
7. Gunn SM, et al. Determining energy expenditure during some household and garden tasks. *Med Sci Sports Exerc* 2002;34:895.
8. Health and Welfare Canada. Nutrient value of some common foods. Ottawa, Canada: Health Services and Promotion Branch, Health and Welfare Canada, 1988.
9. Hill RJ, Davies PS. Energy intake and energy expenditure in elite lightweight female rowers. *Med Sci Sports Exerc* 2002;34:1823.
10. Katch FI. U.S. government raises serious questions about reliability of U.S. Department of Agriculture's food composition tables. *Int J Sports Nutr* 1995;5:62.
11. Koffranyi E, Michaelis HF. Ein tragbarer Apparat zur Bestimmung des Gasstoffwechsels. *Arbeitsphysiologie* 1940;11:148.
12. Krogh A, Lindhard J. The relative value of fat and carbohydrate as sources of muscular energy. *Biochem J* 1920;14:290.
13. Montoye HJ, et al. *Measuring Physical Activity and Energy Expenditure.* Boca Raton, FL: Human Kinetics, 1996.
14. Mudambo KS, et al. Adequacy of food rations in soldiers during exercise in hot, day-time conditions assessed by double labeled water and energy balance methods. *Eur J Appl Physiol* 1997;76:346.
15. Rumpler WW, et al. Energy value of moderate alcohol consumption by humans. *Am J Clin Nutr* 1996;64:108.
16. Speakman JR. The history and theory of the doubly labeled water technique. *Am J Clin Nutr* 1998;68(suppl):932S.
17. Speakman JR, et al. Revised equations for calculating CO_2 production from doubly labeled water in humans. *Am J Physiol* 1993;61:1200.
18. Starling RD, et al. Energy requirements and physical activity in free-living older women and men: a doubly labeled water study. *J Appl Physiol* 1998;85:1063.
19. Stroud MA, et al. Energy expenditure using isotope-labeled water ($^2H^{18}O$), exercise performance, skeletal muscle enzyme activities and

plasma biochemical parameters in humans during 95 days of endurance exercise with inadequate energy intake. *Eur J Appl Physiol* 1997;76:243.
20. Westerterp KR, et al. Comparison of doubly labeled water with respirometry at low-and high-activity levels. *J Appl Physiol* 1988;65:53.
21. Withers RT, et al. Energy metabolism in sedentary and active 49- to 70-yr-old women. *J Appl Physiol* 1998;84:1333.

Additional References:

ACSM's Resource Manual for Guidelines for Exercise Testing and Prescription. 7th ed. Baltimore: Williams & Wilkins, 2006.

Ainsworth BE, et al. Compendium of physical activities: classification of energy costs of human physical activities. *Med Sci Sports Exerc* 1993;25:71.

Atwater WO, Woods CD. The chemical composition of American food materials. USDA bulletin no. 28. Washington, DC: USDA, 1896.

Boyle M, Long, S. *Personal nutrition.* Belmont, CA: Wadsworth Publishing, 2006.

Brody T. *Nutritional Biochemistry.* New York: Academic Press, 1998.

Brooks GA, et al. *Exercise Physiology: Human Bioenergetics and its Applications.* 4th ed. New York: McGraw-Hill, 2005.

Durnin JVGA, Passmore R. *Energy, Work and Leisure.* London: Heinemann, 1967.

Gibson RS. *Principles of Nutritional Assessment.* New York: Oxford University Press, 1990.

Guyton AC. *Textbook of Medical Physiology.* 10th ed. Philadelphia: WB Saunders, 2000.

Hamilton EM, et al. *Nutrition: Concepts and Controversies.* New York: West Publishing, 1999.

Health and Welfare Canada. *Nutrient value of some common foods.* Ottawa, Canada: Health Services and Promotion Branch, Health and Welfare, 1988.

Keys A, et al. Basal metabolism and age of adult men. *Metabolism* 1973;22:579.

Mahan IK, Escott-Stump S. *Krause's Food, Nutrition, & Diet Therapy.* Philadelphia: WB Saunders, 2000.

McCance A, Widdowson EM. *The Composition of Foods.* 5th ed. London: Royal Society of Chemistry. Ministry of Agriculture, Fisheries and Food, 1991.

Pennington JAT, Church HN. *Bowes and Church's Food Values of Portions Commonly Used.* 15th ed. Philadelphia: Lippincott, 1993.

Poehlman ET, et al. Resting metabolic rate and post prandial thermogenesis in highly trained and untrained males. *Am J Clin Nutr* 1988;47:793.

Segal KR, et al. Thermic effects of food and exercise on lean and obese men of similar lean body mass. *Am J Physiol* 1987;252: E110.

Shils ME, et al. *Modern Nutrition in Health and Disease.* 10th ed. Baltimore: Lippincott Williams & Wilkins, 2005.

U.S. Department of Agriculture. Composition of foods: raw, processed, and prepared. no. 8. Washington, DC: U.S. Department of Agriculture, 1963–1987.

Part **3**

Optimal Nutrition for the Physically Active Person: Making Informed and Healthful Choices

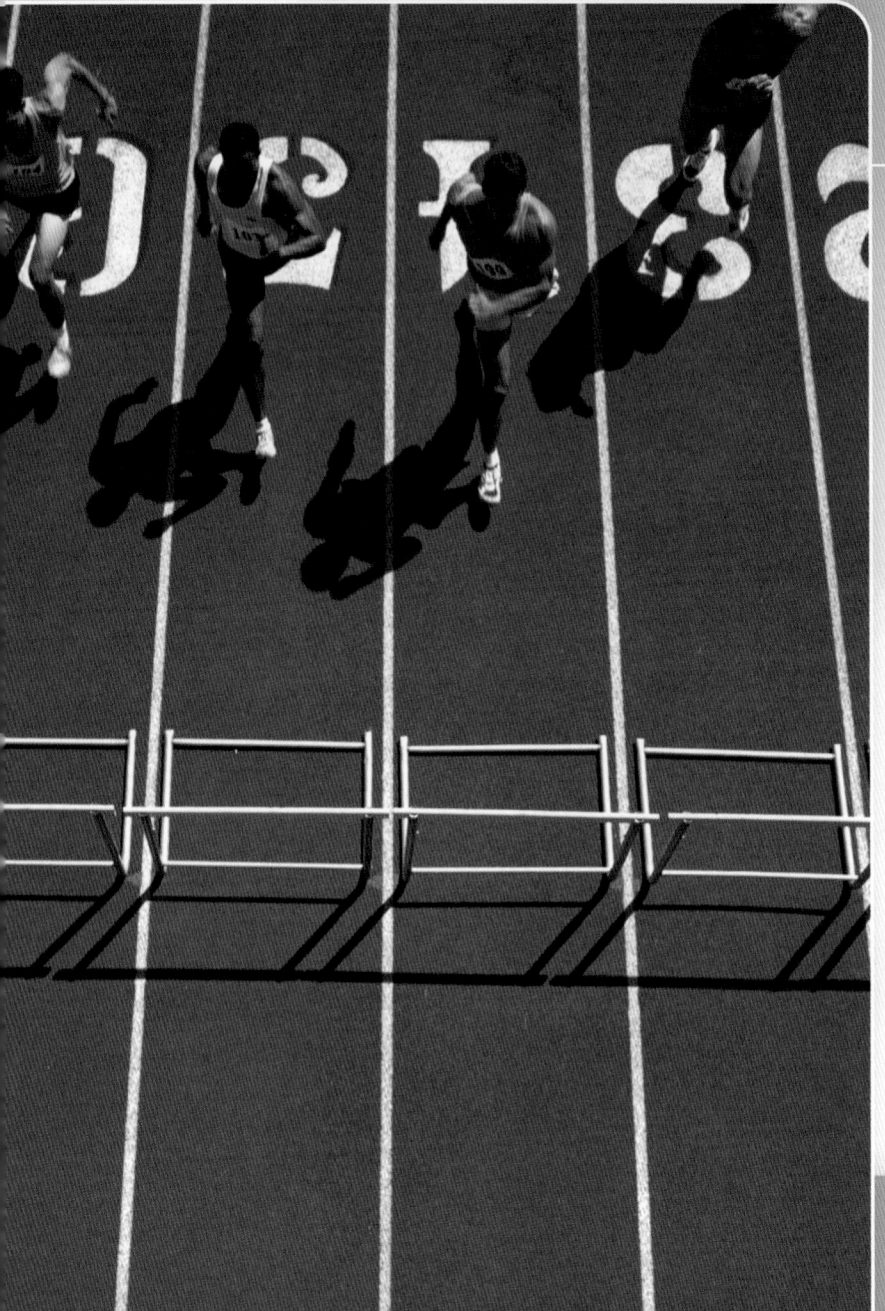

Outline

Chapter 7

Nutritional Recommendations for the Physically Active Person

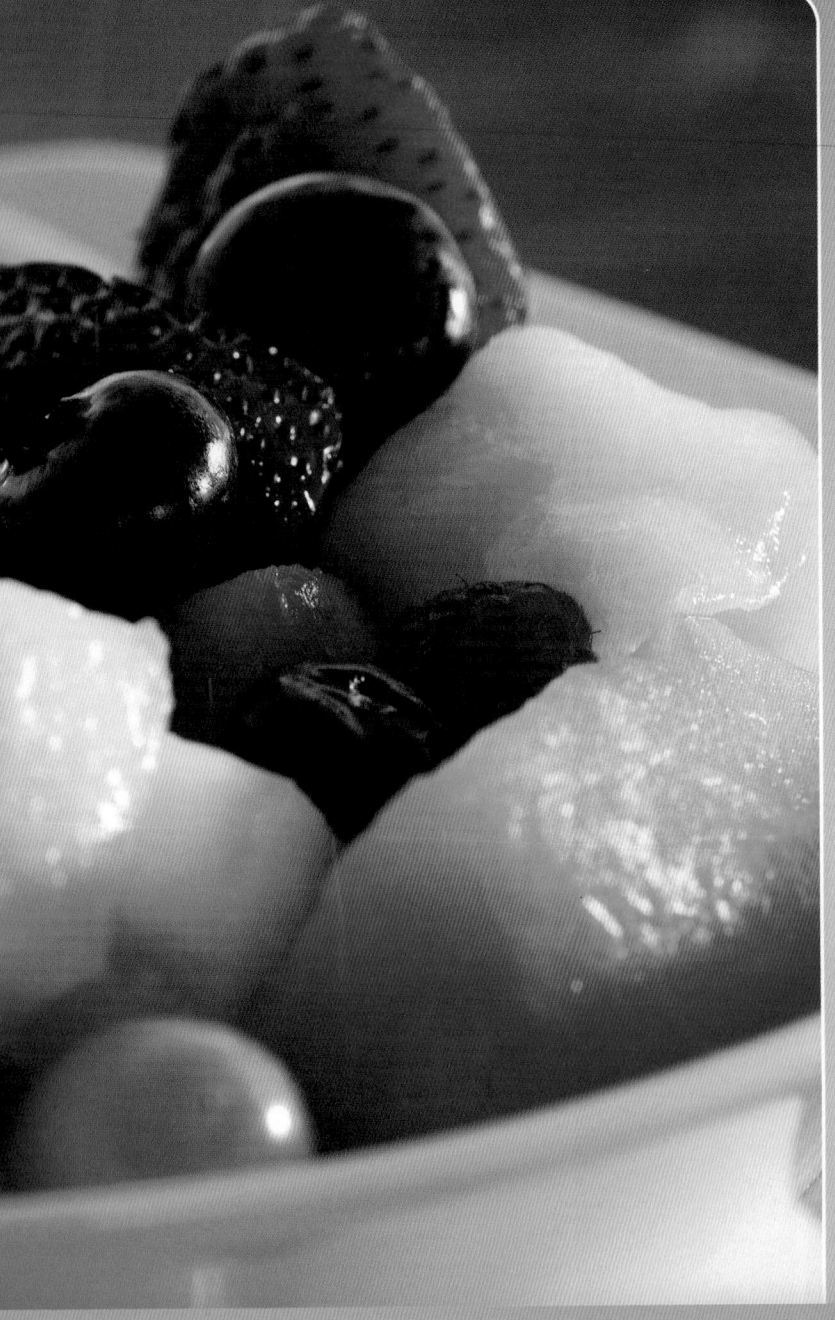

- A Unique Case for Vitamin C

- Megavitamins

Exercise, Free Radicals, and Antioxidants: The Potentially Protective Micronutrients for Physically Active People

- Increased Metabolism and Free Radical Production

Exercise, Infectious Illness, Cancer, and the Immune Response

- Upper Respiratory Tract Infections

- Glutamine and the Immune Response

Minerals and Exercise Performance

- Mineral Losses in Sweat

- Trace Minerals and Exercise

Exercise and Food Intake

- Physical Activity Makes a Difference

- High-Risk Sports for Marginal Nutrition

Eat More, Weigh Less

Test Your Knowledge

Answer these 10 statements about optimal nutrition for the physically active person. Use the scoring key at the end of the chapter to check your results. Repeat this test after you have read the chapter and compare your results.

1. **T F** Humans differ from machines in that they do not conform to the laws of thermodynamics, at least in terms of energy balance.

2. **T F** One pound of stored body fat contains approximately 3500 kCal of energy.

3. **T F** A major problem with MyPyramid is that it lumps all foods within a food category together (e.g., bread, cereal, rice and pasta group) without distinguishing between healthful and not so healthful foods within that category.

4. **T F** Recent government guidelines for good nutrition emphasize specific numeric goals for different individual nutrients.

5. **T F** Physically active individuals require additional micronutrients above recommended values to support their increased level of energy expenditure.

6. **T F** Serious weight trainers benefit from taking high doses of amino acid supplements to increase muscle mass.

7. **T F** To promote good health, lipid intake should not exceed 10% of total caloric intake.

8. **T F** High-carbohydrate (60–70% total caloric intake), high-fiber (30–50 g per day) diets do not promote good health because they deprive an individual of needed quantities of lipid.

9. **T F** Athletes who train intensely require vitamin and mineral intake above recommended values for optimal physical performance and training responsiveness.

10. **T F** Saturated fatty acids provide an excellent source of antioxidant vitamins.

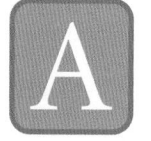

An optimal diet supplies required nutrients in adequate amounts for tissue maintenance, repair, and growth without excess energy intake. Proper nutrition helps (1) improve athletic performance, (2) optimize programs of physical conditioning, (3) improve recovery from fatigue, and (4) avoid injury.[5] Dietary recommendations for physically active men and women must account for the energy requirements of a particular activity or sport and its training demands, including in-

dividual dietary preferences. Although no "one" food or diet exists for optimal health and exercise performance, careful planning and evaluation of food intake should follow sound nutritional guidelines. The physically active person must obtain sufficient energy and macronutrients to replenish liver and muscle glycogen, provide amino acid building blocks for tissue growth and repair, and maintain a desirable body weight. Lipid intake must also provide essential fatty acids and fat-soluble vitamins. Supplementing with vitamins and minerals is unnecessary provided a well-balanced diet provides for the body's energy needs. TABLE 7.1 outlines the recommendations of a joint position statement from the American College of Sports Medicine, American Dietetic Association, and Dietitians of Canada about how qualified health, exercise, and nutrition professionals can counsel individuals who engage regularly in physical activity.

THE ENERGY BALANCE EQUATION

The concept of energy balance most typically applies to body weight maintenance and weight loss, as discussed in Chapter 14. Proper attainment of energy balance also becomes an important goal for physically active people, particularly during intense training or multiple daily workouts when maintaining energy balance with proper nutrient intake optimizes exercise performance and the training response.

No Circumventing It!

The human body functions in accord with the laws of thermodynamics. If total calories from food exceed daily energy expenditure, excess calories accumulate as fat in adipose tissue.

One must consider the rationale underlying the **energy balance equation** when replenishing the body's macronutrient energy reserves in training or in planning to favorably modify body weight and body composition. *In accord with the first law of thermodynamics, the energy balance equation dictates that body mass remains constant when caloric intake equals caloric expenditure.* FIGURE 7.1 depicts factors that contribute to daily energy balance and imbalance. The middle example shows what happens all too frequently when energy input exceeds energy output and the calories consumed in excess of daily requirements become stored as fat in adipose tissue. Weight gain occurs with a long-term positive energy imbalance that often results from subtle regulatory alterations between energy intake and energy expenditure. *Thirty-five hundred "extra" kCal through either increased energy intake or decreased energy output approximates 1 lb (0.45 kg) of stored body fat.* The lower example illustrates what occurs when energy output exceeds energy input. In this case, the body obtains the required calories from its energy stores, resulting in reduced body weight and body fat. Little fluctuation occurs in body weight if an equilibrium exists in which energy input (calories in food) balances energy output (calories expended in daily activities), as shown in the top panel of the figure. This situation most typically applies to physically active individuals who must regularly replenish the energy to power exercise through nutrient-rich food sources as outlined in sections that follow.

PRINCIPLES OF GOOD EATING

Key principles of good eating include *variety*, *balance*, and *moderation*. This does not mean one must give up enjoyable foods to eat healthfully. To the contrary, a healthful diet requires some simple planning that does not demand a lifetime of deprivation and misery. In reality, eliminating enjoyable foods often proves detrimental in the long run and creates a diet program doomed to failure.

TABLE 7.1   Six Ways that Exercise Nutritionists Can Help Physically Active Individuals and Competitive Athletes

1. Educate athletes about energy requirements for their sport and the role of food in fueling the body. Discourage unrealistic weight and body composition goals and emphasize the importance of adequate energy intake for good health, prevention of injury, and exercise performance.
2. Assess the body size and composition of an athlete for the determination of an appropriate weight and composition for the sports in which he or she participates. Provide the athlete with nutritionally sound techniques for maintaining an appropriate body weight and composition without the use of fad or severe diets. Undue pressure on athletes for weight loss or the maintenance of a lean body build can increase the risk of restrictive eating behaviors and, in extreme cases, lead to a clinical eating disorder.
3. Assess the athlete's typical dietary and supplement intake during training, competition, and the off-season. Use this assessment to provide appropriate recommendations for energy and nutrient intakes for the maintenance of good health, appropriate body weight and composition, and optimal sport performance throughout the year. Give specific guidelines for making good food and fluid selections while traveling and eating away from home.
4. Assess the fluid intake and weight loss of athletes during exercise and make appropriate recommendations regarding total fluid intake and fluid intake before, during, and after exercise. Help athletes to determine appropriate types and amounts of beverages to use during exercise, especially if the athlete is exercising in extreme environments.
5. For athletes such as the vegetarian athlete with special nutrition concerns, provide appropriate nutritional guidelines to ensure adequate intakes of energy, protein, and micronutrients.
6. Carefully evaluate any vitamin/mineral or herbal supplements, ergogenic aids, or performance-enhancing drugs an athlete wants to use. These products should be used with caution and only after careful review of their legality and the current literature pertaining to the ingredients listed on the product label; these products should not be recommended until after evaluating the athlete's health, diet, nutrition needs, current supplement and drug use, and energy requirements.

From American College of Sports Medicine, American Dietetic Association, and Dietitians of Canada. Joint position statement. Nutrition and athletic performance. Med Sci Sports Exerc 2000;32:2130.

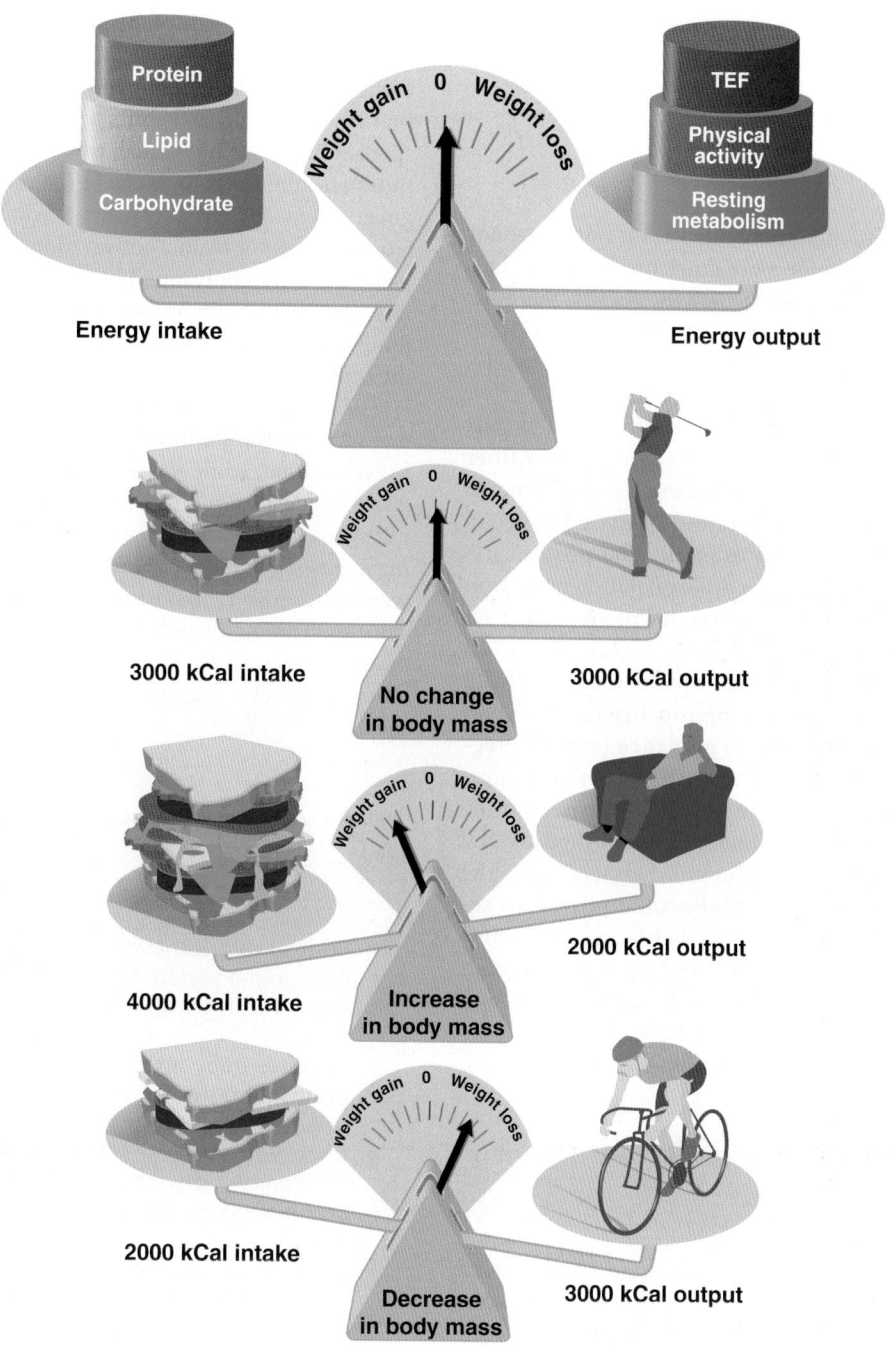

FIGURE 7.1 ■ The energy balance equation (*TEF* = thermic effect of food).

Variety

Choosing foods from a variety of sources creates a diet that contains sufficient amounts of all required nutrients. For example, each vegetable form contains a unique set of phytochemicals (see Case Study 5-1, p. 165), so consuming a variety of vegetables provides a broad array of these beneficial food constituents. A diverse diet also makes mealtime more interesting and something to look forward to.

Balance

Balance in one's diet indicates the intake of nutrients from the major food groups and thus enables the person to benefit from the variety of accessory chemicals unique to each food. Prolonged intake of a diet that inordinately focuses on one food group often creates nutritional deficiency, despite intake of sufficient energy. For example, if a person dislikes milk or milk products (yogurt, ice cream, and cheese), the likelihood of calcium deficiency increases because this food group constitutes the major source of calcium.

Moderation

Eating moderately requires appropriate planning to maintain a balanced nutrient intake throughout the day. For example, if one meal contains high-fat foods, other meals during the day must contain less fat. A good action plan moderates rather than eliminates the intake of certain foods. In this way one can enjoy all types of foods during the day.

MyPYRAMID: ESSENTIALS OF GOOD NUTRITION

In the typical American diet, energy-dense but nutrient-poor foods frequently substitute for more nutrient-rich foods. This pattern of food intake increases the risk for obesity, marginal micronutrient intakes, low high-density lipoprotein (HDL) and high low-density lipoprotein (LDL) cholesterol, and elevated homocysteine levels.[71]

In April 2005 the federal government unveiled its latest attempt to personalize the approach to choose a healthier lifestyle that balances nutrition and exercise. **MyPyramid** replaces the 1992 Food Guide Pyramid criticized as broad and vague; it recommended, for example, that people eat 6 to 12 servings of grains, but gave no explanation as to who should eat 6 and who should eat 12 and did not identify a serving size. The new color-coded MyPyramid (FIG. 7.2) offers a fresh look and a complementary website (www.mypyramid.gov) to provide personalized and supplementary materials on food intake guidance (e.g., the recommended number of cups of vegetables) based on age, sex, and level of daily exercise. The pyramid is based on the 2005 *Dietary Guidelines for Americans* published by the Department of Health and Human Services and the Department of Agriculture.[67,78] MyPyramid provides a series of vertical color bands of varying widths, with the combined bands for fruits (red band) and vegetables (green band) occupying the greatest width, followed by grains, and the narrowest bands for fats, oils, meats, and sugars. A personalized pyramid can be obtained on the website.

The Beverage Pyramid

The Beverage Guidance Panel, a group of academics and nutritionists formed to help consumers to make wise and healthful choices about what they drink, has devised the Beverage Pyramid similar to the MyPyramid offered by the U.S. Department of Agriculture. Shaped like a pitcher, the chart lists the most preferable drink—water—at its base with the least-preferable drinks—sodas and fruit juices—at the top. Recommendations for servings (and kCals) are based on consuming 2000 kCal per day (see figure in Case Study 10-1 on page 310).

For example, a 40-year-old man who exercises less than 30 minutes a day should consume about 2200 kCal daily; this includes 7 ounces of grains, 3 cups of vegetables, 2 cups of fruit, 3 cups of low-fat milk, and 6 ounces of lean meat. He can also consume 6 teaspoons of oil and another 290 kCal of fats and sweets. A new addition to MyPyramid includes a figure

walking up the left side of the pyramid to emphasize at least 30 minutes of moderate to vigorous daily physical activity (The authors of this text recommend 60 minutes). Critics maintain that the new approach shifts too much of the burden of responsibility to the individual, who must have access to a computer and the skills to navigate the relatively "complicated" government site. Also, much of what is contained in the Guidelines is not readily conveyed in the pyramid. For example, the pyramid only hints about the necessity for eating fewer fats, sugars, and salt, and the concept of replacing unhealthy food (fast food, junk food, sodas) with more desirable food is difficult to discern.

The latest *Dietary Guidelines for Americans,* revised every 5 years, with the sixth edition evidence-based revisions published in 2006, while formulated for the general population, also provide a sound framework for meal planning for physically active individuals. *The principle message advises consuming a varied but balanced diet.* To maintain a healthful body weight, attention must focus on portion size and number of calories. The major point is to consume a diet rich in fruits and vegetables, cereals and whole grains, nonfat and low-fat dairy products, legumes, nuts, fish, poultry, and lean meats.[8,24,38,62,85]

Sound Advice from the *Dietary Guidelines for Americans*

- Control caloric intake to manage body weight
- Consume a variety of foods within and among the basic food groups while staying within energy needs
- Increase daily intake of fruits, vegetables, whole grains, and nonfat or low-fat milk and milk products
- Choose fats wisely for good health. Limit saturated fats (dairy, fatty meats, and other animal products) and trans fats (packaged baked goods and fried foods).
- Choose carbohydrates wisely for good health. Select fiber-rich foods: whole fruits rather than juices, whole grains (wheat bread, oatmeal, brown rice) rather than refined grains.
- Choose and prepare foods with little salt. Reduce daily salt intake to 2300 mg or less.
- If you drink alcoholic beverages, do so in moderation. Up to one drink per day for women, two for men.
- Be physically active every day. At least 30 minutes of moderate activity a day, although children and adolescents need at least 60 minutes a day for healthy growth.
- Keep food safe to eat. Wash and cook foods properly to avoid food-borne illnesses. Refrigerate perishable items promptly.

The complete report appears at www.health.gov/ dietary guidelines/dga2005/report/

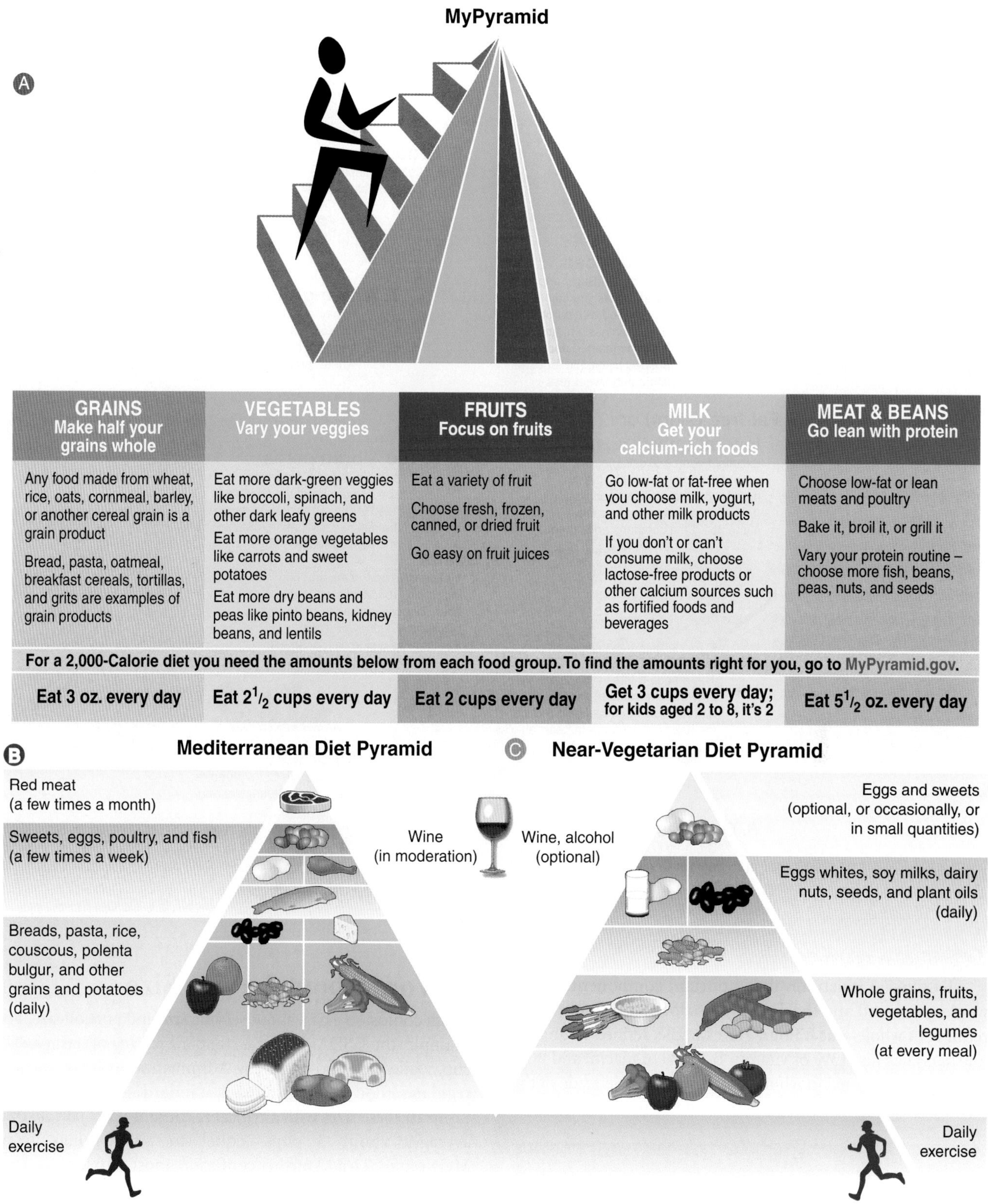

MyPyramid

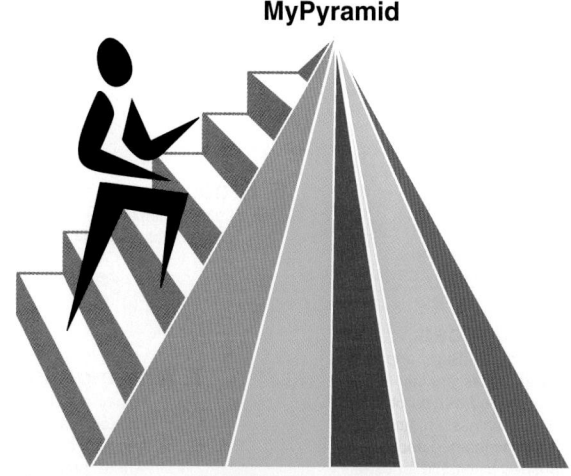

GRAINS Make half your grains whole	VEGETABLES Vary your veggies	FRUITS Focus on fruits	MILK Get your calcium-rich foods	MEAT & BEANS Go lean with protein
Any food made from wheat, rice, oats, cornmeal, barley, or another cereal grain is a grain product Bread, pasta, oatmeal, breakfast cereals, tortillas, and grits are examples of grain products	Eat more dark-green veggies like broccoli, spinach, and other dark leafy greens Eat more orange vegetables like carrots and sweet potatoes Eat more dry beans and peas like pinto beans, kidney beans, and lentils	Eat a variety of fruit Choose fresh, frozen, canned, or dried fruit Go easy on fruit juices	Go low-fat or fat-free when you choose milk, yogurt, and other milk products If you don't or can't consume milk, choose lactose-free products or other calcium sources such as fortified foods and beverages	Choose low-fat or lean meats and poultry Bake it, broil it, or grill it Vary your protein routine – choose more fish, beans, peas, nuts, and seeds

For a 2,000-Calorie diet you need the amounts below from each food group. To find the amounts right for you, go to MyPyramid.gov.

| Eat 3 oz. every day | Eat 2½ cups every day | Eat 2 cups every day | Get 3 cups every day; for kids aged 2 to 8, it's 2 | Eat 5½ oz. every day |

B ### Mediterranean Diet Pyramid

Red meat
(a few times a month)

Sweets, eggs, poultry, and fish
(a few times a week)

Breads, pasta, rice, couscous, polenta bulgur, and other grains and potatoes (daily)

Wine
(in moderation)

Daily exercise

C ### Near-Vegetarian Diet Pyramid

Wine, alcohol
(optional)

Eggs and sweets
(optional, or occasionally, or in small quantities)

Eggs whites, soy milks, dairy nuts, seeds, and plant oils (daily)

Whole grains, fruits, vegetables, and legumes (at every meal)

Daily exercise

FIGURE 7.2 ■ **A.** MyPyramid: A more comprehensive and personalized guide to sound nutrition. **B.** Mediterranean Diet Pyramid. **C.** Near-Vegetarian Diet Pyramid.

Ten Super Foods You Should Eat

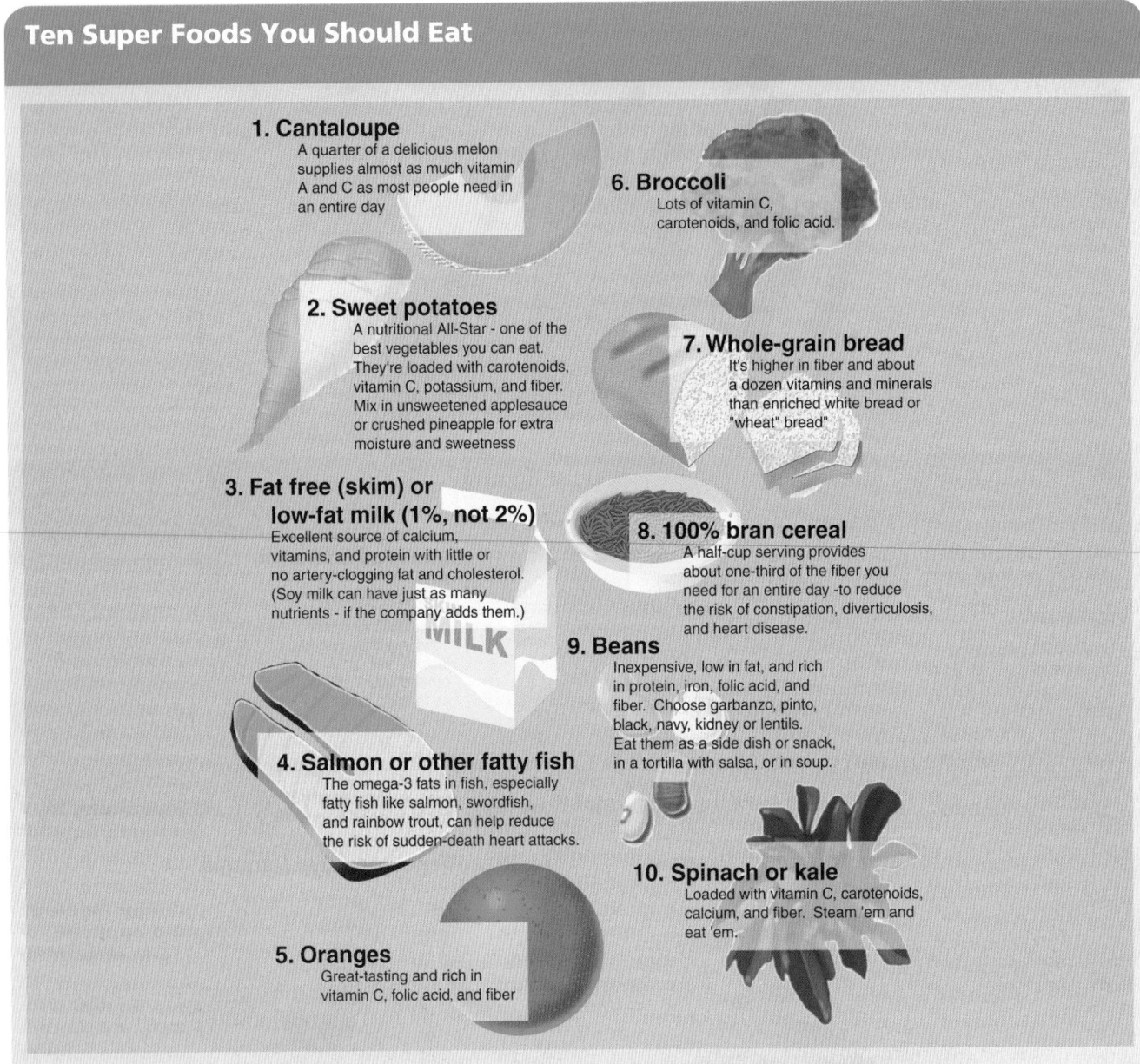

1. Cantaloupe
A quarter of a delicious melon supplies almost as much vitamin A and C as most people need in an entire day

2. Sweet potatoes
A nutritional All-Star - one of the best vegetables you can eat. They're loaded with carotenoids, vitamin C, potassium, and fiber. Mix in unsweetened applesauce or crushed pineapple for extra moisture and sweetness

3. Fat free (skim) or low-fat milk (1%, not 2%)
Excellent source of calcium, vitamins, and protein with little or no artery-clogging fat and cholesterol. (Soy milk can have just as many nutrients - if the company adds them.)

4. Salmon or other fatty fish
The omega-3 fats in fish, especially fatty fish like salmon, swordfish, and rainbow trout, can help reduce the risk of sudden-death heart attacks.

5. Oranges
Great-tasting and rich in vitamin C, folic acid, and fiber

6. Broccoli
Lots of vitamin C, carotenoids, and folic acid.

7. Whole-grain bread
It's higher in fiber and about a dozen vitamins and minerals than enriched white bread or "wheat" bread"

8. 100% bran cereal
A half-cup serving provides about one-third of the fiber you need for an entire day -to reduce the risk of constipation, diverticulosis, and heart disease.

9. Beans
Inexpensive, low in fat, and rich in protein, iron, folic acid, and fiber. Choose garbanzo, pinto, black, navy, kidney or lentils. Eat them as a side dish or snack, in a tortilla with salsa, or in soup.

10. Spinach or kale
Loaded with vitamin C, carotenoids, calcium, and fiber. Steam 'em and eat 'em.

FIGURE 7.3 illustrates the important components of the whole grain seed and the nutrient loss for 13 nutrients in the refining of whole-wheat flour. For example, refined flour (yellow bars) has just 13% of vitamin B$_6$, 20% of niacin, and 30% of the iron contained in whole-wheat form. The left side of the figure describes the whole grain seed and its nutritional value.

A Big Plus for Whole Grains

According to the government's 2005 *Dietary Guidelines*, prudent nutrition includes eating "at least 3 ounces of whole-grain cereals, breads, crackers, rice, or pasta every day." Increasing one's intake of whole grains can lower risk of stroke, diabetes, obesity, constipation, and particularly heart disease.[64]

A Word About Serving Size

Much confusion exists about serving size and portion size. For example, the USDA defines a standard *serving* of pasta as 1/2 cup, while the Food and Drug Administration (FDA), which regulates food labels, claims a standard serving is 1 cup. Contrast these sizes with a typical restaurant pasta *portion* that averages about 3 cups—equal to six servings from MyPyramid. To add further confusion, most people consider a serving to be the amount of food they typically consume (actually a portion) when, for the government's purpose, it represents a far smaller standard unit of measure. Within the perspective of "real-world" standards and government standards, the USDA recommendation to consume 6 to 11 servings of grains or breads daily seems an unattainable goal. Keep in mind that one serving by government standards represents a relatively small portion size: a 6-oz glass of fruit or vegetable juice; 1 medium-sized orange, banana, or apple; 1 cup of salad

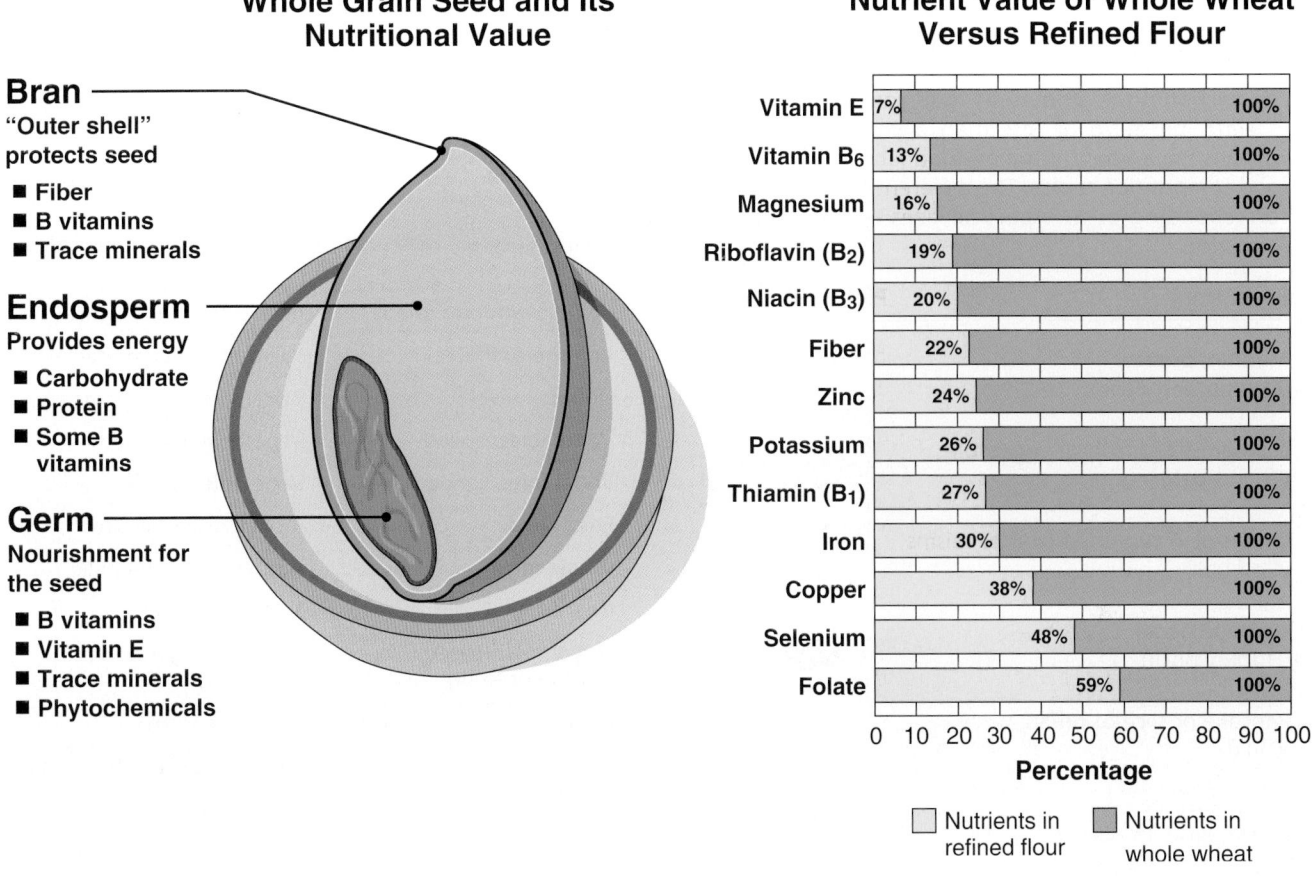

FIGURE 7.3 ■ Whole grains provide a rich nutritional package.

greens, about the size of your fist; 1 egg; 1 cup of milk or yogurt; 1 slice of bread; 2 tablespoons of peanut butter, about the size of a ping-pong ball; $^1/_2$ cup of chopped fruits and vegetable—3 medium asparagus spears, 8 carrot sticks, 1 ear of corn, or $^1/_4$ cup of dried fruit like raisins; 3 oz of meat, fish, or poultry, about the size of a deck of playing cards; 1 teaspoon of butter or mayonnaise, the size of a fingertip; or 2 oz of cheese, the size equivalent of two thumbs.

The *Dietary Guidelines for Americans* recommends diet and lifestyle choices to promote health, support physically active lives, and reduce chronic disease risks. It also includes advice to exercise moderately for 30 minutes (e.g., walking, jogging, bicycling, and lawn, garden, and house work) "most, preferably all, days of the week." The Guidelines advise children to exercise moderately for 60 minutes daily. They acknowledge that good nutrition and regular exercise provide an important approach to ensure good health and combat the obesity epidemic in the United States. The Guidelines separate fruits and vegetables from grains and emphasize whole grain consumption. Interestingly, the Guidelines recommend replacing foods in the diet with more nutrient-dense options, yet no consistant standards or criteria exist for such categorization.[30]

USING THE DIETARY GUIDELINES

Proper use of the *Dietary Guidelines* produces nutritional practices that reduce the incidence of obesity, hypertension,

heart disease, and type 2 diabetes. Implementation involves making changes in typical food choices to adhere more closely to guideline recommendations. TABLE 7.2 lists examples of food substitutions that apply the *Dietary Guidelines*.

American Heart Association Recommendations

Dietary guidelines from the American Heart Association (AHA; www.americanheart.org/) for the general public over the age of 2 years (formerly known as the "Step 1" diet) address the growing rates of obesity, hypertension, and type 2 diabetes in the United States.[77,83] Because of the strong association between excess body weight and cardiovascular disease, the recommendations also emphasize achieving and maintaining a healthful body weight. Lifestyle modifications include increasing the level of regular physical activity and eliminating all tobacco. These guidelines are essentially similar to guidelines from other agencies (including the USDA). They place great emphasis on the adoption of healthy eating patterns and lifestyle behaviors instead of targeting specific numeric goals as in the number of grams to consume for dietary fat. TABLE 7.3 outlines four major goals and associated guidelines for the general population; TABLE 7.4 presents specific dietary recommendations for the general population and for those men and women at higher disease risk (formerly known as the "Step 2" diet).

Picture Portions

A portion is the amount of food you actually eat. It may be more or less than a standard serving, which is the amount listed on food labels and listed in food composition tables. The different food items and corresponding picture portion sizes can be used for reference.

Food Item	Picture Portion
Medium potato (Computer mouse)	
Medium-sized fruit or vegetable (Tennis ball)	
One-fourth cup dried fruit or raisins (Golf ball)	
Average bagel (Hockey puck)	
Pancake or slice of bread (DVD)	
Cup of fruit (Baseball)	
Cup of lettuce (Four leaves)	
Three ounces cooked meat or poultry (Cassette tape)	
Three ounces grilled fish (Your checkbook)	
One ounce cheese (Four dice)	
One teaspoon butter or margarine (Postage stamp)	
One tablespoon salad dressing (Thumb tip)	
Two tablespoons peanut butter (Ping pong ball)	
One cup cooked dry beans (Tennis ball)	
One ounce nuts or candies (One small handful)	
One ounce chips or pretzels (One large handful)	

TABLE 7.2 **Examples of Appropriate Substitutions to Bring Existing Eating Behaviors More in Line with the** *Dietary Guidelines*

If you eat this	Try this
White bread	Whole-wheat or whole grain bread
Breakfast cereal with sugar	Low-sugar cereal; shredded wheat
Cole slaw/potato salad	Bean salad with yogurt
Chips/salty snacks	Low salt, baked pretzels
Donuts	Bran muffin; corn bread
Vegetables, boiled	Vegetables steamed
Vegetables, canned	Vegetables frozen
Fried foods	Broiled or barbecued
Whole milk	Nonfat or low-fat milk
Ice cream	Sherbet or frozen yogurt
Mayonnaise-based salad dressing	Oil and vinegar or diet dressings
Cookies	Air-popped corn
Salted foods	Flavor foods with herbs and or lemons

The principle message advises consuming a varied but balanced diet. To maintain a healthful body weight, attention must focus on portion size and number. Importance is placed on consuming a diet rich in fruits and vegetables, cereals and whole grains, nonfat and low-fat dairy products, legumes, nuts, fish, poultry, and lean meats.[8,38,59,86]

From the American Heart Association (AHA)

The AHA guidelines (Guide to the Primary Prevention of Cardiovascular Diseases) to prevent heart attacks and strokes, lists secondhand smoke for the first time as a risk factor. They also recommend screening for risk factors beginning at age 20 and every 5 years thereafter to asses smoking habits, family medical history, and blood pressure. Men should maintain a waistline of 40 inches or less and women 35 inches or less. Persons 40 years of age and older should be screened for additional risk factors such as cholesterol levels. The new guidelines drop passages that recommended hormone supplements and antioxidant vitamins to reduce cardiovascular risk. Also, a daily dose of aspirin, previously recommended for individuals who have already suffered a heart attack or stroke, is now suggested for those whose risk assessment indicates at least a 10% risk of a heart attack in the next decade.

TABLE 7.3   Nutritional Guidelines for the General Population

Population Goals	Major Guidelines
Overall healthy eating pattern	• Consume a varied diet that includes foods from each of the major food groups with an emphasis on fruits, vegetables, whole grains, low-fat or nonfat dairy products, fish, legumes, poultry, and lean meats. • Monitor portion size and number to ensure adequate, not excess, intake.
Appropriate body weight BMI ≤25[a]	• Match energy intake to energy needs. • When weight loss is desirable, make appropriate changes to energy intake and expenditure (physical activity). • Limit foods with a high sugar content, and those with a high caloric density.
Desirable cholesterol profile	• Limit foods high in saturated fat, *trans* fat, and cholesterol. • Substitute unsaturated fat from vegetables, fish, legumes, and nuts.

Desirable blood pressure
  Systolic <140 mm Hg
  Diastolic <90 mm Hg
	• Maintain a healthy body weight.
	• Consume a varied diet with an emphasis on vegetables, fruits, and low-fat or nonfat dairy products.
	• Limit sodium intake.
	• Limit alcohol intake.

Modified from Krauss RM, et al. AHA dietary guidelines revision 2000: a statement for healthcare professionals from the Nutrition Committee of the American Heart Association. Circulation 2000;102:2284.

[a]BMI, body mass index (kg·m^{-2}).

TABLE 7.4   Specific Dietary Recommendations for the General Population and For Men and Women at Higher Disease Risk

For the General Population	For Populations at Higher Risk[a]
1. Restrict total fat to ≤30% of total calories. 2. Restrict saturated fat to ≤10% of total calories. 3. Limit the total intake of cholesterol-raising fatty acids (saturated and *trans*) to ≤10% of calories. 4. Limit cholesterol intake to ≤300 mg·day. 5. Replace cholesterol-raising fatty acids with whole grains and unsaturated fatty acids from fish, vegetables, legumes, and nuts. 6. Limit sodium intake to ≤2400 mg·day (≤6.0 g/day of salt). 7. If alcohol is consumed, limit intake to 2 drinks/day for men, 1 drink/day for women. 8. Eat at least 2 servings of fish per week. 9. Eat 5 or more servings of vegetables and fruits per day. 10. Eat 6 or more servings of grain products per day. 11. Emphasize daily intake of low-fat or nonfat dairy products.	***Elevated LDL-cholesterol or preexisting cardiovascular disease*** 1. Restrict saturated fat to ≤7% of total calories. 2. Limit cholesterol intake to ≤200 mg·day. 3. Weight loss when appropriate. 4. Include soy protein with isoflavones. ***Dyslipidemia characterized by low HDL-cholesterol, elevated triglycerides, and small, dense LDL-cholesterol*** 1. Replace saturated fat calories with unsaturated fat. 2. Limit carbohydrate intake, especially sugars and refined carbohydrates. 3. Weight loss when appropriate. 4. Increase physical activity. ***Diabetes mellitus and insulin resistance*** 1. Restrict saturated fat to ≤7% of total calories. 2. Limit cholesterol intake to ≤200 mg·day. 3. When selecting carbohydrates, choose those with high fiber content.

Modified from Krauss RM, et al. AHA dietary guidelines revision 2000: a statement for healthcare professionals from the Nutrition Committee of the American Heart Association. Circulation 2000;102:2284.

[a]Elevated LDL, low-density lipoprotein cholesterol; low HDL, high-density lipoprotein cholesterol.

AN EXPANDING EMPHASIS ON HEALTHFUL EATING AND REGULAR PHYSICAL ACTIVITY

Scientists have responded to the rapidly rising number of adults and children who are overweight or obese and the increasing incidence of comorbidities associated with the overweight condition. In September, 2002, the Institute of Medicine (www.iom.edu/), the medical division of the National Academies, issued guidelines as part of their *Dietary Reference Intakes* (see Chapter 2).[11,35] They recommend that Americans spend at least *1 hour* (about 400–500 kCal) over the course of each day in moderately intense physical activity (brisk walking, swimming, or cycling) to maintain health and normal body weight. This amount of regular physical activity—based on an assessment of the amount of exercise healthy persons engage in each day—represents twice as much as previously recommended in 1996 in a report from the United States Surgeon General! The advice agrees with the 2003 recommendations by the World Health Organization (WHO; www.who.int) and the Food and Agriculture Organization of the United Nations (and most recently, the International Association for the Study of Obesity[134]), and recent research findings that point to the health and weight-loss benefits of longer duration weekly physical activity.[56,62] The advice represents a bold increase in exercise duration considering that (1) 30 minutes of similar type exercise on most days significantly decreases disease risk, and (2) more than 60% of the U.S. population fails to incorporate even a moderate level of exercise into their lives and 25% do no exercise at all.

The team of 21 experts also recommended for the first time a range for macronutrient intake plus how much dietary fiber to consume in the daily diet. These recommendations are intended for professional nutritionists and the general public. To meet daily energy and nutrient needs while minimizing risk for chronic diseases such as heart disease and type 2 diabetes, adults should consume between 45 and 65% of total calories from carbohydrates. This relatively wide range provides for flexibility, in recognition that both the high-carbohydrate, low-fat diet of Asian peoples and the higher-fat diet of peoples from the Mediterranean region, with its high monounsaturated fatty acid olive oil content, contribute to good health. The maximum intake of added sugars—the caloric sweeteners added to manufactured foods and beverages such as soda, candy, fruit drinks, cakes, cookies, and ice cream—is placed at 25% of total calories. This relatively high 25% level represented the threshold above which a significant decline would occur for several important micronutrients such as vitamin A and calcium. Acceptable lipid intake ranges between 20 and 35% of caloric intake, a range at the lower end of most recommendations and at the upper end of the 30% limit set by the AHA, American Cancer Society, and National Institutes of Health. The panel noted that very low fat intake combined with high intake of carbohydrate tends to lower HDL cholesterol and raise triacylglycerol levels. Conversely, high intake of dietary fat (and accompanying increased caloric intake) con-

tributes to obesity and its related medical complications. Moreover, high-fat diets usually link with an increased saturated fatty acid intake, raising plasma LDL cholesterol concentrations, which further potentiates coronary heart disease risk. "As low as possible" saturated fat intake was recommended; the panel also recognized that no safe level existed for *trans* fatty acid intake.

Recommended protein intake ranges between 10 and 35% of calories, which remains consistent with prior recommendations. For the first time, age-based recommendations are provided for all of the essential amino acids contained in dietary protein. TABLE 7.5 presents an example of the macronutrient composition for a 2500-kCal diet based on these new guidelines.

The panel's recommendations for dietary fiber intake are discussed in Chapter 1. Particularly important is the consumption of water-soluble fibers (pectin from fruits and oat and rice bran); these reduce plasma cholesterol levels and slow digestion to increase satiety and decrease the risk of overeating.

TABLE 7.5 **Possible Macronutrient Composition of a 2500-kCal Diet Based on Recommendations of Expert Panel of the Institute of Medicine, National Academies**

	Composition of 2500-kCal Intake		
	Carbohydrate	Lipid	Protein
Percentage	60	15	25
kCal	1500	375	625
Grams	375	94	69
Ounces	13.2	3.3	2.4

One Size Does Not Fit All

Clearly, no one food or meal provides optimal nutrition and associated health-related benefits. Perhaps the following statement best summarizes the metabolic, epidemiologic, and clinical trial evidence over the past several decades regarding diet and lifestyle behaviors and coronary heart disease[58]:

"Substantial evidence indicates that diets using non-hydrogenated unsaturated fats as the predominant form of dietary fat, whole grains as the main form of carbohydrates, an abundance of fruits and vegetables, and adequate omega-3 fatty acids can offer significant protection against coronary heart disease. Such diets, together with regular physical activity, avoidance of smoking, and maintenance of a healthy body weight, may prevent the majority of cardiovascular disease in Western populations."

MEDITERRANEAN AND VEGETARIAN DIET PYRAMIDS

The illustrations in Figure 7.2B and C present modifications of the basic pyramid for application to individuals whose diet consists largely of (1) fruits, nuts, vegetables, legumes, and all manner of unrefined grains, and protein derived from fish, beans, and chicken, with dietary fat composed mostly of monounsaturated fatty acids with mild ethanol consumption (**Mediterranean Diet Pyramid**) or (2) foods from the plant kingdom (**Near Vegetarian Diet Pyramid**). A Mediterranean-type diet—possibly mediated via several plant foods in the diet—substantially reduces the rate of recurrence after a first myocardial infarction, perhaps from its association with increased total antioxidant capacity and low LDL-cholesterol levels.[28,120] Its high monounsaturated fatty acid content (generally olive oil with its associated phytochemicals[145]) also staves off age-related memory loss, heart disease, cancer, and overall mortality rate in healthy, elderly people.[82,144,150] Dietary focus of all three pyramids on fruits and vegetables, particularly cruciferous and green leafy vegetables and citrus fruit and juice, also reduces risk for ischemic stroke[69] and may enhance the beneficial effects of cholesterol-lowering drugs.[70]

Good for the Nervous System

People who follow a Mediterranean-style meal plan (diet) are 40% less likely to develop Alzheimer's disease compared to individuals who do not follow this diet. The diet includes eating diverse vegetables, legumes, fruits, cereals, and fish, while limiting intake of meat and dairy products, drinking moderate amounts of alcohol and emphasizing monounsaturated fats over saturated fats, a dietary focus that also reduces heart disease risk.

PERSONAL ASSESSMENT

An objective assessment of energy and nutrient intake provides the frame of reference for judging the adequacy of one's diet in relation to recommended guidelines. Such determinations from careful daily food intake records provide a reasonably close estimate compared with more direct measurements. Appendix C outlines the *Three-Day Dietary Survey* procedure to assess a diet's adequacy.

Diet Quality Index

The revised **Diet Quality Index** appraises the "healthfulness" of one's diet; it gives a score based on a composite of the eight food- and nutrient-based recommendations of the National Academy of Sciences. This index, presented in FIGURE 7.4, offers a simple scoring schema based on the risk gradient associated with diet and the major diet-related chronic diseases. It evaluated the diets of participants in three national surveys

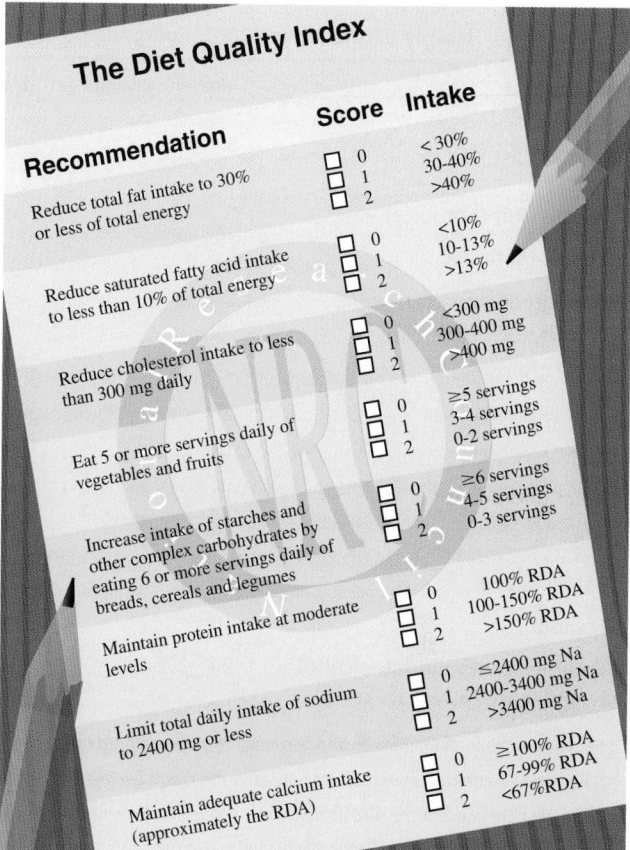

FIGURE 7.4 ■ The revised Diet Quality Index assesses risk for chronic diseases associated with overall dietary pattern. A score of 0 indicates that a respondent's diet meets the desired dietary goal for the item; a score of 1 means the intake falls within 30% of the goal; and an intake that fails to fall within 30% of the goal receives a score of 2. Scores are then added (range from 0 to 16), with the lower score indicating a better quality of diet. (From National Research Council, Committee on Diet and Health. Diet and health implications for reducing chronic disease risk. Washington, DC: National Academy Press, 1989.)

conducted in the United States between 1965 and 1989–1991.[121] Respondents who meet or exceed a given dietary goal receive a score of 0; a score of 1 applies to an intake that falls within 30% of a dietary goal; the score becomes 2 when intake fails to fall within 30% of the goal. The scores for all eight categories are then totaled. The index ranges from 0 to 16, with the lower score representing a higher quality diet. A score of *4 or less* reflects a more healthful diet, while an index of *10 or higher* pinpoints a less healthful diet needing improvement.

The Healthy Eating Index

The USDA designed the **Healthy Eating Index (HEI)** presented in TABLE 7.6 for nutrition promotion activities and to monitor changes in diet quality over time. This 100-point analytic tool evaluates how well a person's diet conforms to such

TABLE 7-6 **Healthy Eating Index—2005: Components and Standards for Scoring**[a]

Component	Maximum points	Standard for maximum score	Standard for minimum score of zero
Total fruit (includes 100% juice)	5	≥0.8 cup equiv. per 1000 kCal	No fruit
Whole fruit (not juice)	5	≥0.4 cup equiv. per 1000 kCal	No whole fruit
Total vegetables	5	≥1.1 cup equiv. per 1000 kCal	No vegetables
Dark green and orange vegetables and legumes[b]	5	≥0.4 cup equiv. per 1000 kCal	No dark green and orange vegetables and legumes
Total grains	5	≥3.0 oz equiv. per 1000 kCal	No grains
Whole grains	5	≥1.5 oz equiv. per 1000 kCal	No whole grains
Milk[c]	10	≥1.3 oz equiv. per 1000 kCal	No milk
Meat and beans	10	≥2.5 oz equiv. per 1000 kCal	No meat or beans
Oils[d]	10	≥12 grams per 1000 kCal	No oil
Saturated fat	10	≤7% of energy[e]	≤15% of energy
Sodium	10	≤0.7 gram per 1000 kCal	≥2.0 grams per 1000 kCal
Calories from solid fat, alcohol, and added sugar (SoFAAS)	20	≤20% of energy	≥50% of energy

[a]Intakes between the minimum and maximum levels are scored proportionately, except for saturated fat and sodium, see note e.

[b]Legumes are counted as vegetables only after meat and beans standard is met.

[c]Includes all milk products, such as fluid milk, yogurt, and cheese.

[d]Includes nonhydrogenated vegetable oil and oils in fish, nuts, and seeds.

[e]Saturated fat and sodium get a score of 8 for the intake levels that reflect the 2005 Dietary Guidelines for Americans,[67,78] <10% of calories from saturated fat and 1.1 grams of sodium/1000 kCal, respectively.

recommendations as MyPyramid and *Dietary Guidelines for Americans* based on dietary balance, moderation, and variety.[47,153] Total scores can range from a "poor" diet (HEI score, 65) to a "good" diet (HEI score, >85), with 65 to 74 and 75 to 84 in between. HEI scores for each component of the index are defined as "poor" (score, <5), "needs improvement" (score between 5 and 8), and "good" (score, >8).

MACRONUTRIENT NEEDS FOR THE PHYSICALLY ACTIVE

Many physically active individuals receive either inadequate or incorrect information concerning prudent dietary practices. *Research in exercise nutrition, although far from complete, indicates that teenagers, adults, and competitive athletes, who exercise regularly to keep fit do not require additional nutrients beyond those obtained by consuming a nutritionally well-balanced diet.*

What the Physically Active Actually Eat

Inconsistencies exist among studies that relate diet quality to physical activity level and/or physical fitness. Some studies have shown a positive association between healthier diets and higher physical activity levels, whereas others have not. Part

of the inconsistency results from use of relatively crude and imprecise self-reported measures of physical activity, small sample size, and unreliable dietary assessments.[31,44,48,94] TABLE 7.7 contrasts the nutrient and energy intakes with national dietary recommendations of a large population-based cohort of nearly 7,059 men and 2,453 women classified as low, moderate, and high for cardiorespiratory fitness who participated in the Aerobics Center Longitudinal Study. The four most significant findings of this study indicate:

1. A progressively lower body mass index was found for both men and women with increasing levels of physical fitness.
2. Remarkably small differences in energy intake in relation to physical fitness classification was found for women (= 94 kCal per day) and men (= 82 kCal per day), with the moderate fitness group consuming the fewest calories for both sexes.
3. A progressively higher dietary fiber intake and lower cholesterol intake were noted across fitness categories.
4. Men and women with higher fitness levels generally consumed diets that more closely approached dietary recommendations (with respect to dietary fiber, percentage of energy from total fat, percentage of energy from saturated fat, and dietary cholesterol) than peers of lower fitness.

FIGURE 7.5 lists the recommended intakes for protein, lipid, and carbohydrate and food sources for these macronu-

TABLE 7.7 Average Values for Nutrient Intake Based on 3-day Diet Records by Levels of Cardiorespiratory Fitness in 7059 Men and 2453 Women

	Men		
Variable	Low Fitness[a,b] (N = 786)	Moderate Fitness[c] (N = 2457)	High Fitness (N = 4716)
Demographic and health data			
Age (y)	$47.3 \pm 11.1^{a,b}$	47.3 ± 10.3^{c}	48.1 ± 10.5
Apparently healthy (%)	$51.5^{a,b}$	69.1^{c}	77.0
Current smokers (%)	$23.4^{a,b}$	15.8^{c}	7.8
BMI (kg·m^{-2})	$30.7 \pm 5.5^{a,b}$	27.4 ± 3.7^{c}	25.1 ± 2.7
Nutrient data			
Energy (kCal)	2378.6 ± 718.6^{a}	2296.9 ± 661.9^{c}	2348.1 ± 664.3
Kcal·kg^{-1}·d^{-1}	25.0 ± 8.1^{a}	26.7 ± 8.4^{c}	29.7 ± 9.2
Carbohydrate (% kCal)	43.2 ± 9.4^{b}	44.6 ± 9.1^{c}	48.1 ± 9.7
Protein (% kCal)	18.6 ± 3.8	18.5 ± 3.8	18.1 ± 3.8
Total fat (% kCal)	36.7 ± 7.2^{b}	35.4 ± 7.1^{c}	32.6 ± 7.5
SFA (% kcal)	11.8 ± 3.2^{b}	11.3 ± 3.2^{c}	10.0 ± 3.2
MUFA (% kCal)	$14.5 \pm 3.2^{a,b}$	13.8 ± 3.1^{c}	12.6 ± 3.3
PUFA (% kCal)	$7.4 \pm 2.2^{a,b}$	7.5 ± 2.2	7.4 ± 2.3
Cholesterol (mg)	349.5 ± 173.2^{b}	314.5 ± 147.5^{c}	277.8 ± 138.5
Fiber (g)	21.0 ± 9.5^{b}	22.0 ± 9.7^{c}	26.2 ± 11.9
Calcium (mg)	$849.1 \pm 371.8^{a,b}$	860.2 ± 360.2^{c}	924.4 ± 386.8
Sodium (mg)	4317.4 ± 1365.7	4143.0 ± 1202.3	4133.2 ± 1189.4
Folate (μg)	336.4 ± 165.2^{b}	359.5 ± 197.0^{c}	428.0 ± 272.0
Vitamin B6 (mg)	2.4 ± 0.9^{b}	2.4 ± 0.9^{c}	2.8 ± 1.1
Vitamin B12 (μg)	6.6 ± 5.5^{a}	6.8 ± 6.0	6.6 ± 5.8
Vitamin A (RE)	$1372.7 \pm 1007.3^{a,b}$	1530.5 ± 1170.4^{c}	1766.3 ± 1476.0
Vitamin C (mg)	117.3 ± 80.4^{b}	129.2 ± 108.9^{c}	166.0 ± 173.2
Vitamin E (AE)	11.5 ± 9.1^{b}	12.1 ± 8.6^{c}	13.7 ± 11.4
	Women		
Variable	Low Fitness[a,b] (N = 233)	Moderate Fitness[c] (N = 730)	High Fitness (N = 1490)
Demographic and health data			
Age (y)	47.5 ± 11.2^{b}	46.7 ± 11.6	46.5 ± 11.0
Apparently healthy (%)	$55.4^{a,b}$	71.1^{c}	79.3
Current smokers (%)	$12.0^{a,b}$	9.0^{c}	4.2
BMI (kg·m^{-2})	$27.3 \pm 6.7^{a,b}$	24.3 ± 4.9^{c}	22.1 ± 3.0
Nutrient data			
Energy (kCal)	1887.4 ± 607.5^{a}	1793.0 ± 508.2^{c}	1859.7 ± 514.7
kCal·kg^{-1}·d^{-1}	27.1 ± 9.4^{a}	28.1 ± 8.8^{c}	31.7 ± 9.8
Carbohydrate (% kCal)	47.7 ± 9.6^{b}	48.2 ± 9.0^{c}	51.1 ± 9.4
Protein (% kCal)	17.6 ± 3.7^{a}	18.1 ± 3.9	17.7 ± 3.9
Total fat (% kCal)	34.8 ± 7.6^{b}	33.7 ± 6.8^{c}	31.3 ± 7.5
SFA (% kCal)	11.1 ± 3.3^{b}	10.6 ± 3.2^{c}	9.6 ± 3.1
MUFA (% kCal)	$13.4 \pm 3.4^{a,b}$	12.8 ± 3.0^{c}	11.9 ± 3.2
PUFA (% kCal)	7.5 ± 2.2	7.5 ± 2.2	7.4 ± 2.4
Cholesterol (mg)	244.7 ± 132.8^{b}	224.6 ± 115.6^{c}	204.1 ± 103.6
Fiber (g)	$18.9 \pm 8.2^{a,b}$	20.0 ± 8.3^{c}	23.2 ± 10.7
Calcium (mg)	$765.2 \pm 361.8^{a,b}$	774.6 ± 342.8^{c}	828.3 ± 372.1
Sodium (mg)	3350.8 ± 980.8	3256.7 ± 927.7	3314.4 ± 952.7
Folate (μg)	$301.8 \pm 157.6^{a,b}$	319.7 ± 196.2	356.2 ± 232.5
Vitamin B6 (mg)	2.0 ± 0.8^{b}	2.0 ± 0.8^{c}	2.2 ± 0.9
Vitamin B12 (μg)	4.7 ± 4.2	4.9 ± 4.2	5.0 ± 4.2
Vitamin A (RE)	1421.9 ± 1135.3^{b}	1475.1 ± 1132.9^{c}	1699.0 ± 1346.9
Vitamin C (mg)	116.7 ± 7.5^{b}	131.5 ± 140.0	153.5 ± 161.1
Vitamin E (AE)	10.8 ± 7.5	10.3 ± 6.5^{c}	11.5 ± 8.1

From Brodney S, et al. Nutrient intake of physically fit and unfit men and women. Med Sci Sports Exerc 2001;33:459.

BMI, body mass index; SFA, saturated fatty acid; PUFA, polyunsaturated fatty acid; MUFA, monounsaturated fatty acid; RE, retinol equivalents; AE, α-tocopherol units.
[a]Significant difference between low and moderate fitness. P<.05. [b]Significant difference between low and high fitness. P<.05. [c]Significant difference between moderate and high fitness. P<.05.

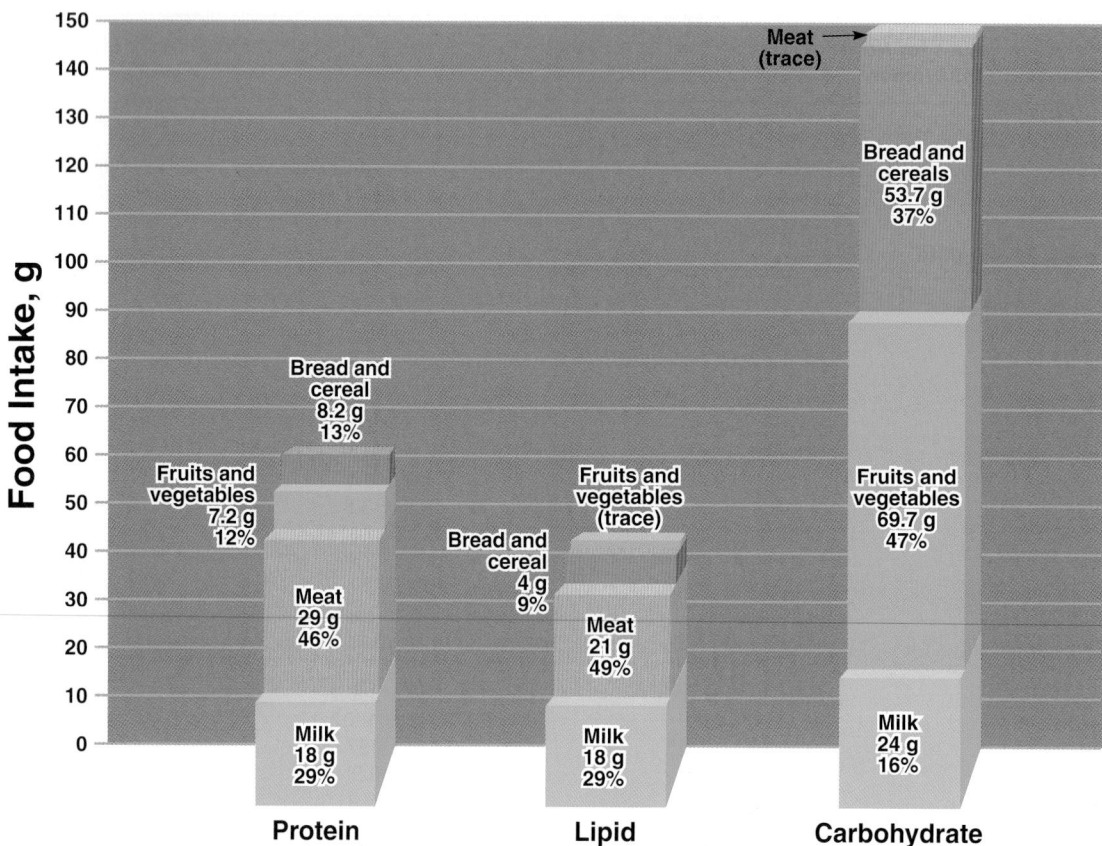

FIGURE 7.5 ■ Basic recommendations for carbohydrate, lipid, and protein components and the general categories of food sources in a balanced diet.

trients for active men and women. A daily energy requirement of 2000 kCal for women and 3000 kCal for men represents average values for typical young U.S. adults. *After meeting basic nutrient requirements (as recommended in* FIG. *7.5), a variety of food sources based on individual preference supply the extra energy needs for physical activity.*

Proteins

As discussed in Chapter 1, 0.8 g per kilogram of body mass $(0.35 \text{ g} \cdot \text{lb}^{-1})$ represents the RDA for protein intake. Thus, a person weighing 77 kg (170 lb) requires about 62 g or 2.2 oz of protein daily. Assuming that even during exercise relatively little protein loss occurs through energy metabolism (an assumption not entirely correct), this protein recommendation remains adequate for most active individuals. Also, the protein intake for the typical American exceeds the protein RDA; the competitive athlete's diet usually contains two to four times more protein than recommended values. One nutritional dilemma for the physically active vegetarian concerns obtaining an adequate balance of essential amino acids from a diet that obtains its protein from the plant kingdom. Chapter 1 discusses the use of complementary protein food sources to minimize this problem. It remains unclear if physically active children and adolescents require more protein for optimal growth and development than their sedentary counterparts.

Is the RDA Really Enough?

Studies of human protein needs in the mid-1800s postulated that muscular contraction destroyed a portion of the muscle's protein content to provide energy for biologic work. Based on this belief, prevailing wisdom recommended a high-protein diet for persons involved in heavy physical labor to provide for the structural content of skeletal muscle and its energy needs. In many ways, many modern-day athletes mimic these beliefs and practices. For men and women who devote considerable time and effort training with resistive equipment, dietary protein often represents their most important macronutrient. For one reason, many believe that resistance training in some way damages or "tears down" a muscle's inherent protein structure. This drain of muscle protein would require additional dietary protein above the RDA for subsequent tissue resynthesis to a new, larger, and more powerful state. Many endurance athletes also believe that training increases protein catabolism to sustain the energy requirements of exercise, particularly when glycogen reserves are low. They thus believe that consuming added dietary protein offsets the protein–energy drain and provides building blocks to resynthesize depleted muscle mass. To some extent, the reasoning of both groups of athletes has merit. The relevant question concerns whether the protein RDA provides a sufficient reserve should intense training increase demands for protein synthesis or catabolism.

SOME MODIFICATION REQUIRED FOR RECOMMENDED PROTEIN INTAKE? Much of current understanding of protein dynamics in exercise derives from studies that expanded the classic method to determine protein breakdown by measuring urea excretion. For example, the output of "labeled" carbon dioxide from amino acids either injected or ingested increases during exercise in proportion to metabolic rate. As exercise progresses, the concentration of plasma urea also increases, coupled with a dramatic rise in nitrogen excretion in sweat. This often occurs without any change in urinary nitrogen excretion. These observations run counter to prior conclusions concerning minimal protein breakdown during endurance exercise, because the early studies only measured nitrogen in urine. FIGURE 7.6 illustrates that the sweat mechanism serves an important role in excreting the nitrogen from protein breakdown during exercise. Urea production does not reflect all aspects of protein breakdown because the oxidation of both plasma and intracellular leucine (a branched-chain essential amino acid) increases during moderate exercise, independent of changes in urea production.[162]

FIGURE 7.6 also shows that protein use for energy reaches its highest level during exercise in a glycogen-depleted state (indicated *low CHO*). This emphasizes the important role carbohydrate plays as a protein sparer. It further indicates that carbohydrate availability inhibits protein catabolism in exercise.[156] Protein breakdown for energy and its role in gluconeogenesis undoubtedly serve important needs in endurance exercise (or in frequent intense training) when glycogen reserves diminish.

Eating a high-carbohydrate diet with adequate energy intake conserves muscle protein in individuals who engage in protracted intense training. The potential for increased protein use

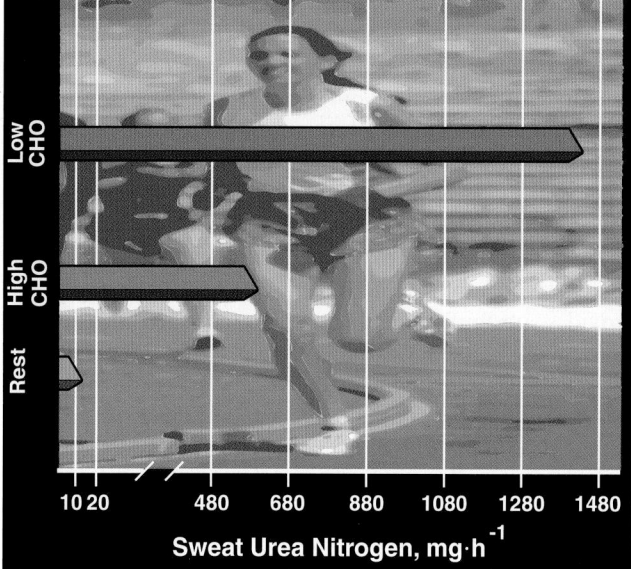

FIGURE 7.6 ■ Excretion of urea in sweat at rest, and during exercise after carbohydrate loading *(High CHO)* and carbohydrate depletion *(Low CHO)*. The largest use of protein (as reflected by sweat urea) occurs with low glycogen reserves. (From Lemon PWR, Nagel F. Effects of exercise on protein and amino acid metabolism. *Med Sci Sports Exerc* 1981;13:141.)

Sweat Urea Nitrogen, mg·h^{-1}

10 20 480 680 880 1080 1280 1480

Low CHO / High CHO / Rest

Prolonged Exercise and Starvation: A Similar Metabolic Mixture

Increased protein catabolism during endurance exercise and intense training often mirrors the metabolic mixture during short-term starvation. With depleted glycogen reserves, gluconeogenesis from amino acid-derived carbon skeletons largely sustains the liver's glucose output. More than likely, augmented protein breakdown reflects the body's attempt to maintain blood glucose concentration for central nervous system functioning.

for energy (and the depression of protein synthesis) during strenuous exercise helps to explain why individuals who resistance-train to augment muscle size generally refrain from glycogen-depleting, endurance-type exercise.

The beginning phase of an exercise training regimen also places a transient but increased demand on body protein, perhaps resulting from both muscle injury and associated increased energy requirements. A continuing area of controversy concerns whether initial increased protein demand contributes to a true long-term increase in protein requirement *above* the RDA. *Although a definitive answer remains elusive, protein breakdown above the resting level occurs during endurance exercise (and with resistance training) to a degree greater than previously believed.* Protein catabolism becomes most apparent when exercising with low carbohydrate reserves or low energy intake. Protein use may increase from a need to repair exercise-induced damaged tissue and from extra protein required for gains in lean tissue mass. Unfortunately, research has yet to pinpoint the protein requirements for individuals who train 4 to 6 hours daily by resistance-type exercise.

One hopes that future research will target protein intake recommendations for individuals who typically use resistance exercise to increase muscle size, strength, and power and individuals involved in prolonged endurance competitions and heavy training. *At this point (and without convincing evidence to the contrary), it seems prudent that those in endurance training should consume between 1.2 and 1.4 g of high-quality protein per kg of body mass daily; those who resistance train may benefit from 1.8 g per kilogram of body mass.* This level of protein intake falls within the range typically consumed by physically active men and women, thus obviating the need to consume supplementary protein.

Vegetarians May Require a Bit More Protein

Increase recommended protein intake values by 10% for vegetarians, to adjust for less-efficient digestion of plant protein. If protein intake remains adequate, consuming animal sources of protein does not facilitate muscle strength or size gains with resistance training compared with a similar protein intake from plant sources.[49]

Preparations of Simple Amino Acids

The usual reasons for using protein and amino supplements include stimulation of muscle growth and strength, enhanced energy capacity, and increased growth hormone output (see Chapter 12).[161] Supplement manufacturers often advertise that *only* simple amino acids are absorbed from the gut into the blood at a rate fast enough to stimulate muscle growth during resistance training. Male and female weightlifters, body builders, and other power athletes consume up to four times the RDA for protein.[74] This level of excess takes the form of liquids, powders, or pills of "purified" protein at a cost often in excess of $50 per pound of actual protein. Such preparations often contain proteins "predigested" to simple amino acids through chemical action in the laboratory. Advocates believe the body absorbs the simple amino acid molecule more readily (increased bioavailability) to optimize the expected muscle growth induced by training or to improve strength, power, and "vigor" in the short term for a strenuous workout. This does not occur. The healthy intestine absorbs amino acids rapidly when they exist in more complex di- and tripeptide molecules, not just in simple amino acid form (see Chapter 3). The intestinal tract handles protein quite efficiently in its more complex form. A concentrated amino acid solution creates an osmotic effect that draws water into the intestine, often precipitating irritation, cramping, and diarrhea. In addition, carbohydrate remains the preferred energy source to power the anaerobic energy system primarily relied on in resistance training. Multiple sets of single exercises can reduce a muscle's glycogen content by 40%. *Simply stated, adequate research design and methodology has not shown that protein (amino acid) supplementation in any form above the RDA increases muscle mass or improves muscular strength, power, or endurance.* Most individuals obtain adequate protein to sustain muscle growth with resistance training by consuming ordinary foods in a well-balanced diet. Provided caloric intake balances energy output by consuming a wide variety of foods, no need exists to consume supplements of protein or simple amino acids.

Lipids

No firm standards exist for optimal lipid intake. The amount of dietary lipid varies widely according to personal taste, money spent on food, and availability of lipid-rich foods. For example, lipid furnishes only about 10% of the energy in the average diet of people living in Asia, whereas in many Western countries lipid accounts for 40 to 45% of the energy intake. *To promote good health, lipid intake should probably not exceed 30% of the diet's energy content. Of this, at least 70% should come from unsaturated fatty acids.* For those who consume a Mediterranean-type diet, rich in monounsaturated fatty acids, a somewhat higher total fat percentage (35–40%) becomes tolerable.

No exercise performance benefit occurs by reducing the percentage lipid intake below the 30% value. In fact, significant reductions in dietary lipid compromise exercise performance. A diet of 20% lipid produced poorer endurance performance scores than a diet of identical caloric value containing about 40% lipid.[115] Such findings further fuel the controversy concerning the importance of dietary lipid for individuals involved in intense training and endurance competition (see "High-Fat Versus Low-Fat Diets for Endurance Training and Exercise Performance" in Chapter 8). Consuming low-fat diets during strenuous training also creates difficulty in increasing carbohydrate and protein intake enough to furnish energy to maintain body weight and muscle mass. In addition, essential fatty acids and fat-soluble vitamins enter the body in dietary lipids; thus, sustaining a low-fat or "fat-free" diet could create a relative state of malnutrition. A low-fat diet (20% total calories as lipid; see Chapter 12) also blunts the normal rise in plasma testosterone following a short-term bout of resistance exercise.[155] If additional research verifies these findings and if changes in hormonal milieu actually diminish training responsiveness and tissue synthesis, a low-fat intake may be contraindicated for intense training.

Carbohydrates

The negative end of the nutrition continuum includes low-calorie "semistarvation" diets and other potentially harmful practices such as high-fat, low-carbohydrate diets, "liquid-protein" diets, and single food-centered diets. These extremes counter good health, exercise performance, and optimum body composition. *A low-carbohydrate diet rapidly compromises energy reserves for vigorous physical activity or regular training.* Excluding sufficient carbohydrate energy from the diet causes an individual to train in a state of relative glycogen depletion; this may eventually produce "staleness" that hinders exercise performance.[12,89]

The prominence of dietary carbohydrates varies widely throughout the world, depending on availability and relative cost of lipid-rich and protein-rich foods. Complex carbohydrate-rich foods (unrefined grains, starchy roots, and dried peas and beans) usually are cheapest compared with their energy value. In the Far East, carbohydrates (rice) contribute 80% of the total energy intake; in contrast, in the United States, carbohydrate supplies only about 40 to 50% of the energy intake. *No hazard to health exists when subsisting chiefly on a variety of fiber-rich complex unrefined carbohydrates, with adequate intake of essential amino acids, fatty acids, minerals, and vitamins.*

Stored muscle glycogen and blood-borne glucose become prime energy contributors in maximal exercise with inadequate oxygen supply to active muscles. Stored glycogen also provides substantial energy during intense aerobic exercise. Consequently, dietary carbohydrate plays an important role for individuals who maintain a physically active lifestyle. *Their diet should contain at least 55 to 60% of calories as carbohydrates, predominantly starches from fiber-rich, unprocessed grains, fruits, and vegetables.* For competitive swimmers, rowers, and speed skaters, the importance of maintaining a relatively high daily carbohydrate intake relates more to the considerable and prolonged energy demands of their training than to the short-term demands of actual competition.

More Specific Carbohydrate Recommendations

General recommendations for carbohydrate range between 6 and 10 g per kg of body mass per day. This amount will vary with an individual's daily energy expenditure and type of ex-

Absolute Carbohydrate Amount Counts

Carbohydrate intake recommendations for physically active individuals assume that daily energy intake balances energy expenditure. Unless this condition exists, even consuming a relatively large *percentage* of carbohydrate calories will not adequately replenish this important energy macronutrient.

ercise performed. *Individuals undergoing endurance training should consume on a daily basis 10 g of carbohydrate per kg of body mass.* Thus, the daily carbohydrate intake for a small 46-kg (100-lb) person who expends about 2800 kCal each day should be approximately 450 g, or 1800 kCal. In contrast, the person weighing 68 kg (150 lb) should consume 675 g of carbohydrate (2700 kCal) daily to sustain an energy requirement of 4200 kCal. In both examples, carbohydrates represent 65% of total energy intake. Chapter 12 presents specific diet-exercise techniques to facilitate glycogen storage in the days before endurance competition.

Carbohydrate and the "Overtraining Syndrome"

Endurance runners, swimmers, cross-country skiers, and cyclists frequently experience chronic fatigue in which successive days of hard training become progressively more difficult. Normal exercise performance usually deteriorates because the individual undergoes increasing difficulty recovering from exercise training. The overtrained condition, commonly termed the **overtraining syndrome,** represents more than just a short-term inability to train as usual or a slight dip in competition-level performance. Rather, it reflects chronic fatigue experienced during workouts and in subsequent recovery periods. It also relates to increased incidence of infections, persistent muscle soreness, and general malaise and loss of interest in sustaining high-level training. Injuries occur more frequently in the overtrained state.[151] Specific symptoms of overtraining are highly individualized. The symptoms outlined in TABLE 7.8 generally represent the most common consequences of overtraining; they usually persist until the person rests. Complete recovery requires weeks or even months.

TABLE 7.8 The Overtraining Syndrome: Six Symptoms of Staleness

1. Unexplained, persistently poor performance

2. Disturbed mood states characterized by general fatigue, depression, and irritability

3. Elevated resting pulse, painful muscles, and increased susceptibility to upper respiratory infections and gastrointestinal disturbances

4. Insomnia

5. Weight loss

6. Overuse injuries

It Takes Time to Replenish Glycogen

Even with a diet high in carbohydrates, muscle glycogen does not rapidly replenish to pre-exercise levels. It takes at least 24 hours to replenish muscle glycogen levels following prolonged exhaustive exercise; liver glycogen restores at a faster rate. *One to 2 days of rest (or lighter exercise) combined with a high-carbohydrate intake re-establishes pre-exercise muscle glycogen levels after exhaustive training or competition.* Chapter 8 discusses in detail how to facilitate carbohydrate replenishment following exhaustive exercise.

Unmistakably, if a person performs unduly intense exercise on a regular basis, carbohydrate allowance must be adjusted to permit optimal glycogen resynthesis to maintain optimal training. This certainly provides a nutritional justification for the recommendation of many coaches and trainers to gradually reduce or *taper* the intensity of workouts several days before competition, while still maintaining a high-quality, carbohydrate-rich diet. TABLE 7.9 outlines practical nutritional guidelines to diminish the likelihood of chronic athletic fatigue or **staleness.** These guidelines were prepared for competitive swimmers, but the recommendations apply to all individuals in intense training.

VITAMINS AND EXERCISE PERFORMANCE: THE ATHLETE'S DILEMMA

Vitamin–mineral pills represent the most common form of nutritional supplement used by the general public—they account for 70 to 90% of all supplements marketed. Particularly susceptible marketing targets include the exercise enthusiast, the competitive athlete, and those who assist athletes to achieve peak performance. The following excerpts (including the letterwriter's emphasis in italics) come from a letter to a college athletic trainer from a physician extolling his concoction of micronutrients (with dosages as high as 15–25 times recommended levels) developed for the "unique" needs of the physically active individual. Such pseudoscientific promotional pitches from so-called experts continually bombard coaches, athletic trainers, and all individuals involved in regular exercise:

Dear:

I'm a physician with an interest in *biochemistry* and nutrition and the effects of both on *athletes.*

Today, *good nutrition requires supplementation.*

The product I developed is an "*all-natural* nutritional foundation for building strong, healthy bodies that perform at peak levels *without harmful side effects.* Using this formula, athletes notice increased energy and improved performance."

This product "is an alternative to steroids and other quick fixes."

This product "is the *only complete supplement* of its kind that combines 23 *essential vitamins, minerals*

TABLE 7.9　Practical Nutritional Guidelines for Prevention of Chronic Athletic Fatigue Among Athletes[a]

1. Consume easily digested high-carbohydrate drinks or solid foods 1–4 h before training and/or competition. Roughly 1 g of carbohydrate/kg body weight is the recommended intake 1 h before exercise, and up to 5 g of carbohydrate/kg body weight/h is suggested if the feeding occurs 4 h prior to exercise. For example, a 70-kg swimmer could drink 350 mL (12 oz) of a 20% carbohydrate beverage 1 h before exercise or eat 14 "energy bars," each containing 25 g carbohydrate, 4 h before exercise.

2. Consume an easily digested, high-carbohydrate, liquid or solid food containing at least 0.35–1.5 g of carbohydrate/kg body weight/h immediately after exercise for the first 4 h after exercise. Thus, a 70-kg swimmer could drink 100–450 mL (3.6–16 oz) of a 25% carbohydrate beverage or 1–4.5 energy bars, each containing 25 g of carbohydrate, immediately after exercise and every hour thereafter for 4 h.

3. Consume a 15–25% carbohydrate drink or a solid high-carbohydrate supplement with each meal. For example, reduce consumption of normal foods by 250 kCal and consume a high-carbohydrate beverage or solid food containing 250 kCal of carbohydrate with each meal.

4. Maintain a stable body weight during all phases of training by matching energy consumption to the energy demands of training. This will also help maintain body carbohydrate reserves.

From Sherman WJ, Maglischo EW. Minimizing chronic athletic fatigue among swimmers: special emphasis on nutrition. Sports Sci Exchange, Gatorade Sports Sci Inst 1991;35(4).)

[a]*In cooperation with a nutritionist or dietitian, athletes should maintain a record of foods consumed so that an accurate assessment can be made of total energy and total carbohydrate intake. Based on this assessment, dietary adjustments can be made to ensure that during intense training seasons, the athlete consumes roughly 10 g of carbohydrate/kg body weight daily.*

---

and antioxidants in the proper amounts needed for powerful performance. (You may be startled to see how dramatically my formulation *exceeds* the RDAs.) The amounts shown on the back of this letter are based on the latest research in nutrition . . . NOT outdated government information."

While developing this product, "I consulted with world famous biochemists . . . collaborated with leading nutritionists (the same ones physicians have ignored for years) . . . walked miles and miles in health food stores . . . *completed a comprehensive search of current medical literature.*"

This letter applies the typical psychological "tools" of advertising: *respect for authority* (I'm a physician, of course I am correct), *safety* (try it, it can't hurt you and it might help); *disdain for the conventional wisdom of science and governmental agencies* (the new scientists have the answers but the "old club" will not publish them), *prestige by association* (I've checked with experts [unnamed biochemists and nutritionists] and gone to the library), and *if a little is good, more must be better* (you'll get a dose dramatically above recommended values). One of the few items missing is a testimonial from a renowned athlete, perhaps wearing a nostril-dilating adhesive strip!

More than 50% of athletes in certain sports regularly consume vitamin–mineral supplements. They undertake such practices either to ensure adequate micronutrient intake or to achieve excess in hopes of enhancing exercise performance and training responsiveness.[19–21,102] If vitamin–mineral deficiencies become apparent in active people, they often occur among (1) vegetarians or groups with low energy intake (dancers, gymnasts, and weight-class sport athletes who continually strive to maintain or reduce body weight), (2) those

who eliminate one or more food groups from their diet, or (3) individuals who consume large amounts of processed foods and simple sugars with low micronutrient density (endurance athletes). Under these adverse situations, a multivitamin–mineral supplement at recommended dosages can upgrade the micronutrient density of the daily diet.

VITAMIN SUPPLEMENTS: THE COMPETITIVE EDGE?

Over 50 years of research fails to support the use of vitamin supplements to improve aerobic and anaerobic exercise performance or ability to train arduously in nutritionally adequate healthy people.[37,122,147,148,158] When vitamin intake achieves recommended levels, supplements neither improve exercise performance nor increase the blood levels of these micronutrients. The facts, however, remain clouded by "testimonials" from coaches and elite athletes who attribute their success to a particular dietary modification or specific vitamin supplements.

As noted in Chapter 2, many vitamins serve as coenzyme components or precursors of coenzymes to help regulate energy metabolism. FIGURE 7.7 illustrates that B complex vitamins play a key role as coenzymes in important energy-yielding reactions during carbohydrate, fat, and protein catabolism. They also contribute to hemoglobin synthesis and red blood cell production. The belief that "if a little is good, more must be better" has led many coaches, athletes, fitness enthusiasts, and even some "expert" scientists to advocate supplementing with vitamins above recommended levels.

Supplementing with vitamin B₆ (pyridoxine), an essential cofactor in glycogen and amino acid metabolism, did not ben-

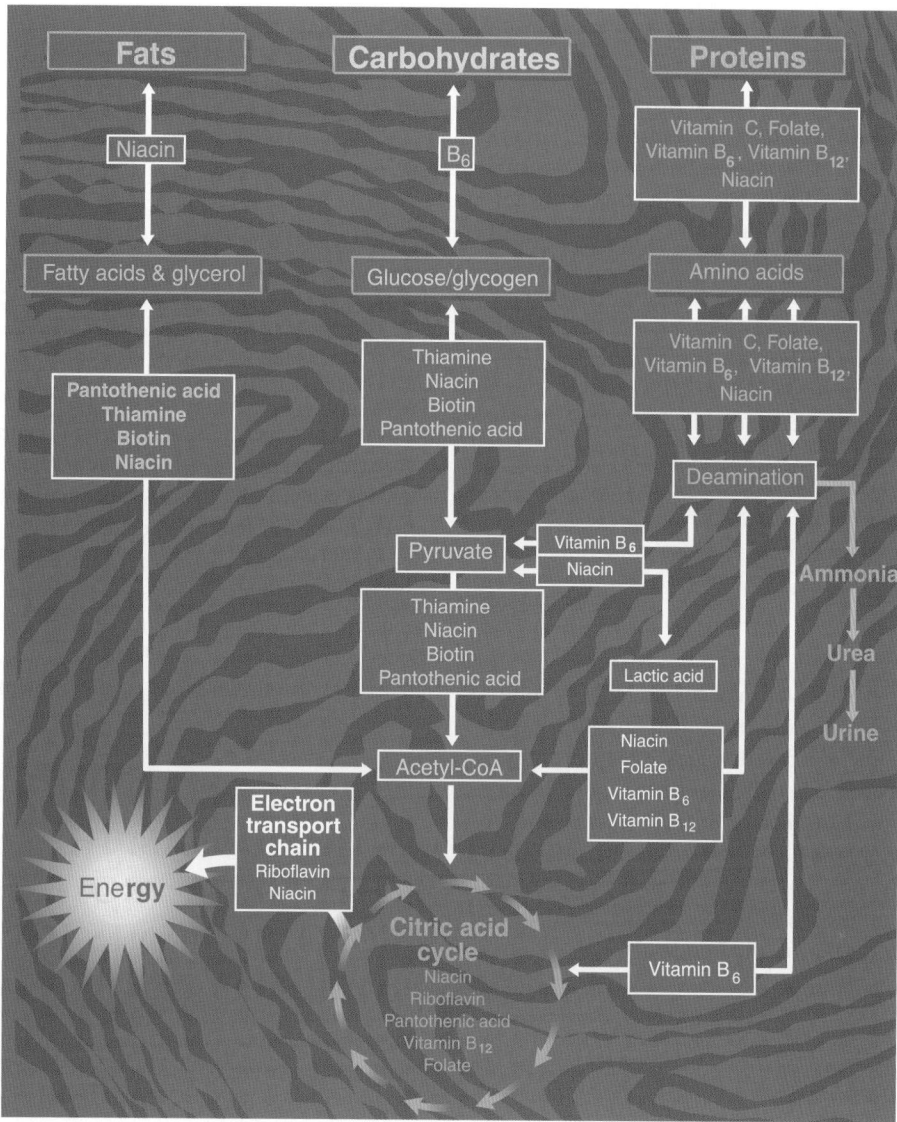

FIGURE 7.7 ■ General schema for the role of water-soluble vitamins in the metabolism of carbohydrates, fats, and proteins.

efit the metabolic mixture metabolized by women during high-intensity aerobic exercise.[93] In fact, the status of athletes for this vitamin normally equals reference standards for the population[91]; it does not decrease with strenuous exercise to levels warranting supplementation.[127] Supplementing for 4 days with a highly absorbable derivative of thiamin—a component of the five-enzyme complex pyruvate dehydrogenase that catalyzes movement of pyruvate into the citric acid cycle—offered no advantage over a placebo on measures of oxygen uptake, lactate accumulation, and cycling performance during exhaustive exercise.[158] The loss of water-soluble vitamins in sweat, even during extreme physical activity, is probably negligible.[50]

No exercise benefit exists for vitamins C and E with intakes above recommended values. Vitamin C, for example, serves as a factor to synthesize collagen and the adrenal hormone norepinephrine. Supplementing with vitamin C has negligible effects on endurance performance and does not alter the rate, severity, and duration of injuries, com-

pared with placebo treatment. Vitamin C status, assessed by serum concentration and urinary ascorbate levels, in diverse groups of highly trained athletes does not differ from that of untrained subjects, despite large differences in daily physical activity level.[130] Other investigators report similar findings for this and other vitamins.[34,46,129] Furthermore, the energy intake of active persons usually increases to match the increased energy requirement of physical activity; thus a proportionate increase also occurs in micronutrient intake, often in amounts greatly exceeding recommended levels.

Vitamin E deficiencies may impair muscular function,[23] yet no scientific data have established that vitamin E consumed in excess of the RDA benefits stamina, circulatory function, or energy metabolism. Chronic high-potency multivitamin–mineral supplementation for well-nourished healthy, individuals does not benefit aerobic fitness, muscular strength, or neuromuscular performance following prolonged runnings or athletic performance.[39,140]

A Unique Case for Vitamin C

Consuming vitamin C above recommended daily levels (75 mg for women and 90 mg for men) does not protect the general population against upper respiratory tract infection (URTI). Daily supplements of 500 to 1500 mg of vitamin C per day may confer some benefit to individuals engaged in strenuous exercise who experience frequent viral infections.[52,116,118]

Moderate exercise heightens immune function, whereas a prolonged period of intense physical activity (marathon running or an exceedingly intense training session) transiently suppresses and stresses the body's first line of defense against infectious agents. This increases risk of URTI within 1 or 2 weeks of exercise stress. For these individuals, additional vitamin C and E and perhaps carbohydrate ingestion before, during, and after a workout may boost the normal immune mechanisms for combating infection.[63,101,107] Page 218 presents a more complete discussion of exercise, nutritional supplementation, and URTI.

Megavitamins

Most nutritionists believe little harm occurs in taking a multivitamin capsule containing the recommended quantity of each vitamin. For some people, the psychological effects of supplementation may even confer a benefit. Of concern are those individuals who take **megavitamins,** or doses at least *10* and up to 1000 times the RDA, hoping that "supercharging" with vitamins improves exercise performance and training responsiveness. Such practices can be harmful, except for serious medical illness that requires above-normal vitamin intake.

More and "Natural" Not Necessarily Better

Vitamins synthesized in the laboratory are no less effective for bodily functions than vitamins from natural sources. Compared with the deficient state, vitamin supplements reverse the symptoms of vitamin deficiency and improve exercise performance. Once a person is cured of a deficiency, taking supplements does not further improve normal nutritional status.

Vitamins Behave as Chemicals

Once the enzyme systems catalyzed by specific vitamins become saturated, any excess taken in megadose function as chemicals or drugs in the body. For example, a megadose of water-soluble vitamin C raises serum uric acid levels and precipitates gout in people predisposed to this disease. At intakes above 1000 mg daily, urinary excretion of oxalate (a breakdown product of vitamin C) increases, accelerating kidney stone formation in susceptible individuals. Also, some American blacks, Asians, and Sephardic Jews have a genetic metabolic deficiency that becomes activated to hemolytic anemia with excessive vitamin C intake. For iron-deficient individuals, megadoses of vitamin C may destroy significant amounts of vitamin B_{12}. In healthy persons, vitamin C supplements frequently irritate the bowel and cause diarrhea.

Excess vitamin B_6 can induce liver disease and nerve damage. Excessive riboflavin (B_2) can impair vision, whereas a megadose of nicotinic acid (niacin) acts as a potent vasodilator and inhibitor of fatty acid mobilization during exercise. A blunted fatty acid metabolism could cause a more rapid than normal depletion of muscle glycogen during exercise. Folate in concentrated supplement form can trigger an allergic response producing hives, light-headedness, and breathing difficulties. Possible side effects of a vitamin E megadose include headache, fatigue, blurred vision, gastrointestinal disturbances, muscular weakness, and low blood sugar. Because unsaturated fatty acids usually contain vitamin E, it is difficult to "construct" a vitamin E-deficient diet. The toxicity to the nervous system of megadoses of vitamin A and the damaging effects to the kidneys of excess vitamin D are well known.

If vitamin supplementation does offer benefits to physically active individuals, benefits only apply to those with marginal vitamin stores or who restrict energy intake or make poor dietary choices.[92] Well-controlled research must fully determine if and under what circumstances such supplementation confers benefits.

EXERCISE, FREE RADICALS, AND ANTIOXIDANTS: THE POTENTIALLY PROTECTIVE MICRONUTRIENTS FOR PHYSICALLY ACTIVE PEOPLE

The benefits of physical activity are well known, but the possibility for negative effects remain controversial. Potentially negative effects occur because elevated aerobic exercise metabolism increases the production of free radicals (see Chapter 2).[3,15,72,84,111,152] Free-radical production in humans and subsequent tissue damage are not directly measured, but rather inferred from markers of free radical by-products. Increased free radicals could possibly overwhelm the body's natural defenses and pose a health risk from an elevated ox-

Green Tea and Health Benefits

The belief that drinking green tea confers health benefits has increased in popularity in recent years. However, Federal regulators have rejected a petition to allow green tea labels to claim that drinking at least 5 oz of green tea a day (or green tea extract) reduces heart disease risk. The FDA's review of 105 articles and other publications submitted with the petition concluded that no credible evidence exists to support claims of health benefits. A health claim characterizes a relationship between consuming a particular substance and a reduced risk of contracting a particular disease.

idative stress level.[65,131] Free radicals also play a role in muscle injury from exercise, particularly eccentric muscle actions and unaccustomed exercise. Muscle damage of this nature releases muscle enzymes and initiates inflammatory cell infiltration into the damaged tissue.

The opposing position maintains that although free radical production increases during exercise, the body's normal antioxidant defenses remain either adequate or improve as natural enzymatic defenses become "upregulated" through exercise training adaptations.[51,60,138] Upregulation of antioxidant defenses accompanies a reduced exercise-induced lipid peroxidation in red blood cell membranes, which increases their resistance to subsequent oxidative stress.[99] *Convincing epidemiologic evidence supports the beneficial effects of regular aerobic exercise on cancer and heart disease incidence, the occurrences of which link to oxidative stress.*[36]

Increased Metabolism and Free Radical Production

Exercise produces reactive oxygen (free radicals) in at least two ways. The first occurs via a mitochondrial electron leak, probably at the cytochrome level, that produces superoxide radicals. The second happens during alterations in blood flow and oxygen supply—underperfusion during intense exercise followed by reperfusion in recovery, which triggers excessive free radical generation. Some argue that the potential for free radical damage increases during trauma, stress, and contraction-induced muscle damage from exercise and can result from environmental pollutants including smog. With exercise, the risk depends on intensity and the participant's state of training, because exhaustive exercise by the untrained often produces oxidative damage in active muscles. FIGURE 7.8 illustrates how regular exercise affects oxidative response and potential for tissue damage, including protective adaptive responses.

Important Questions

Two questions arise concerning physical activity and free-radical production:

1. Are physically active individuals more prone to free-radical damage?
2. Are nutritional agents with antioxidant properties required in increased quantities by the physically active person?

In answer to the first question, research suggests that for well-nourished individuals, the body's natural defenses respond adequately to increased physical activity. A single bout of exercise increases oxidant formation, but the natural antioxidant defenses cope effectively in both healthy individuals and trained heart transplant recipients.[66] Even repeating multiple exercise bouts on consecutive days, various indices of oxidative stress indicated no depletion of antioxidant defenses. The second question requires an equivocal answer. Some evidence indicates that exogenous antioxidant compounds either slow exercise-induced free-radical formation or augment the

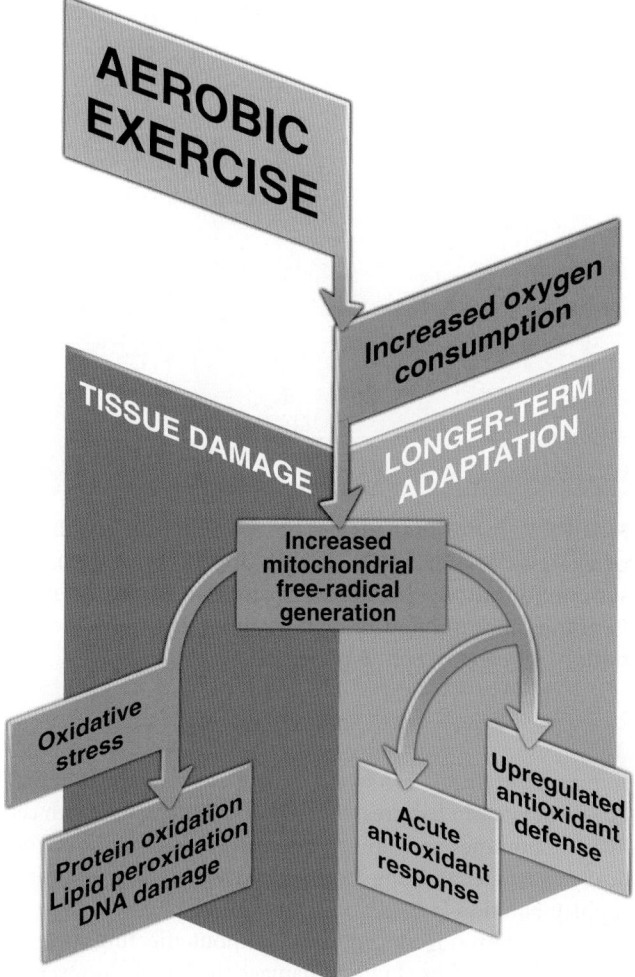

FIGURE 7.8 ■ Cascade of events and adaptations produced by regular aerobic exercise that lessen the likelihood of tissue damage.

body's natural antioxidant defense system. This would limit the extent and progression of muscle damage following and acute exercise bout.

If supplementation proves beneficial, vitamin E may be the most important antioxidant related to exercise.[22,42,61,128,131] In one study, vitamin E-deficient animals began exercise with plasma membrane function compromised from oxidative damage. These animals reached exhaustion earlier than animals with normal vitamin E levels. For animals fed a normal diet, vitamin E supplements diminished exercise-induced oxidative damage to skeletal muscle fibers[41] and myocardial tissue.[43] FIGURE 7.9 shows the effects of 3 weeks of a daily 200-mg vitamin E supplement on pentane elimination (pentane serves as a primary marker of free radical production). The vitamin E-supplemented trials dramatically reduced free radical production. Humans fed a daily antioxidant vitamin mixture of β-carotene, ascorbic acid, and vitamin E had lower serum and breath markers of lipid peroxidation at rest and following exercise than subjects not receiving supplements.[73] Five months of vitamin E supplementation in racing cyclists produced a protective effect on markers of oxidative stress induced by extreme

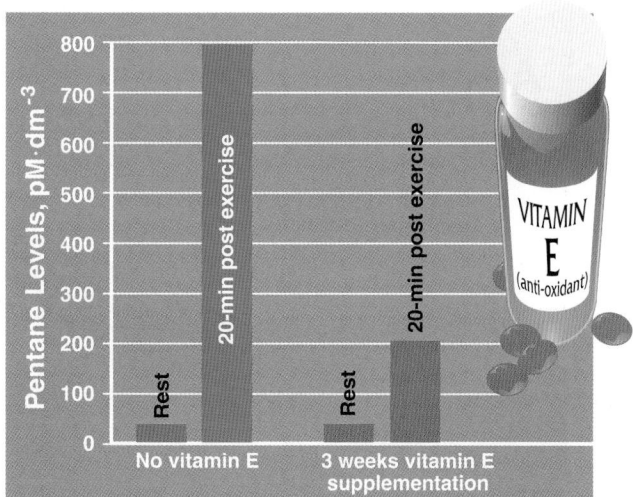

FIGURE 7.9 ■ Pentane levels before and after 20 minutes of exercise at 100% $\dot{V}O_{2max}$ with and without vitamin E supplementation. (Adapted from Pincemail J, et al. Pentane measurement in man as an index of lipid peroxidation. *Bioelectrochem Bioenerg* 1987;18:117.)

endurance exercise. Two weeks of daily supplementation with 120 IU of vitamin E decreased free-radical interaction with cellular membranes and slowed muscle tissue disruption from heavy resistance training.[97] In contrast, 30 days of vitamin E supplementation (1200 IU · d^{-1}) produced a 2.8-fold increase in serum vitamin E concentration without affecting contraction-induced indices of muscle damage (including postexercise force decrement) or inflammation caused by eccentric muscle actions.[9] Similarly, a 4-week daily vitamin E supplement of 1000 IU produced no effect on biochemical or ultrastructural indices of muscle damage in experienced runners after a half marathon.[27] No evidence emerged that vitamin E supplements effectively reduced oxidative damage induced by resistance training exercises.[154] Differences in exercise severity and oxidative stress could account for discrepancies in research findings.

Get Vitamin E from Dietary Sources, Not from Supplements

Rich sources of vitamin E in the diet include almonds, sunflower seeds, safflower and corn oils, hazelnuts, tomato sauce, peanuts, mangos, kidney beans, spinach, kiwi, and broccoli.

Selenium and some trace minerals such as copper, manganese, and zinc possess antioxidant properties owing to their incorporation within the structure of glutathione peroxidase and other enzymes that protect plasma membranes from free radical damage. In a double-blind, placebo-controlled cancer prevention trial, individuals received a selenium supplement of 200 μg daily or about 3 to 4 times the recommended value.[18] Supplementation reduced incidence of, and mortality from, prostate (71%), esophageal (67%), colorectal (62%), and lung (46%) cancers.

Proposed mechanisms for selenium's protection include its function as an essential component of antioxidant enzymes, how it alters carcinogen metabolism and inhibits tumor growth, its effects on the endocrine and immune systems, and its action through molecular mechanisms to regulate the programmed death (*apoptosis*) of damaged precancerous cells. The recommended daily selenium intake is 70 μg for adult men and 55 μg for women; intakes in excess of 1000 μg can produce toxicity—hair and fingernail loss and gastrointestinal dysfunction. Selenium-rich foods include cereals and other grains, Brazil nuts, seafood, meat, mushrooms, and asparagus.

Coenzyme Q$_{10}$ probably acts as an antioxidant either singularly within the respiratory chain or as a recycler of vitamin E. Little evidence exists that coenzyme Q$_{10}$ exerts the same direct antioxidant effect as vitamin E.

A PRUDENT RECOMMENDATION. Supplementing with various antioxidant compounds slows exercise-induced free radical formation and may augment the body's natural defense system. A prudent recommendation includes consuming a well-balanced diet of fruits, grains, and vegetables. Nutrient antioxidants are best obtained from diverse food sources, not from supplements. We endorse this position because of uncertainty whether health protection derives from the antioxidant per se or its interaction with the broad array of active compounds within the food source (e.g., the numerous "chemoprotectant" phytochemicals contained in plants). Three potential mechanisms for antioxidant health benefits include:

1. Influencing molecular mechanisms and gene expression
2. Providing enzyme-inducing substances that detoxify carcinogens
3. Blocking uncontrolled growth of cells

Three Rich Dietary Sources of Vitamin Antioxidants

1. β-Carotene: pigmented compounds or carotenoids that give color to yellow, orange, and green leafy vegetables and fruits; examples include carrots, dark-green leafy vegetables such as spinach, broccoli, turnips, beet and collard greens; sweet potatoes; winter squash; apricots, cantaloupe, mangos, and papaya
2. Vitamin C: citrus fruits and juices; cabbage, broccoli, turnip greens; cantaloupe; green and red sweet peppers, and berries
3. Vitamin E: poultry, seafood, vegetable oils, wheat germ, fish liver oils, whole-grain breads and fortified cereals, nuts and seeds, dried beans, green leafy vegetables, and eggs

According to the director of the division of cancer prevention and control at the National Cancer Institute (NCI; www.cancer.gov/), "More than 150 studies have clearly shown that groups of people who eat plenty of fruits and vegetables get less cancer at a number of cancer sites." The NCI encourages consumption of five or more servings (nine recommended for men) of fruits and vegetables daily, while the USDA's *Dietary Guidelines* recommend two to four servings of fruits and three to five servings of vegetables daily.

EXERCISE, INFECTIOUS ILLNESS, CANCER, AND THE IMMUNE RESPONSE

"Don't exercise until you're fatigued or you'll get sick," is a common perception held by many parents, athletes, and coaches that too much strenuous exercise increases susceptibility to certain illnesses. In contrast, the belief also exists that regular, more moderate exercise improves health and reduces susceptibility to infectious illness such as the common cold.

Studies as early as 1918 reported that most cases of pneumonia among boys in boarding school occurred among athletes. Respiratory infections seemed to progress toward pneumonia after intense sports training. Anecdotal reports also related the severity of poliomyelitis to participation in heavy physical activity at a critical time of infection. Current epidemiologic and clinical findings from the flourishing field of **exercise immunology**—the study of the interactions of physical, environmental, and psychologic factors on immune function—support the contention that unusually strenuous physical activity affects immune function to increase susceptibility to illness, particularly URTI.

The immune system comprises a highly complex and self-regulating grouping of cells, hormones, and interactive modulators that defend the body from invasion from outside microbes (bacterial, viral, and fungal), foreign macromolecules, and abnormal cancerous cell growth. This system has two functional divisions: (1) **innate immunity** and (2) **acquired immunity.** The innate immune system includes anatomic and physiologic components (skin, mucous membranes, body temperature, and specialized defenses such as natural killer [NK] cells, diverse phagocytes, and inflammatory barriers). The acquired immune system consists of specialized B- and T-lymphocyte cells. These cells when activated regulate a highly effective immune response to a specific infectious agent. If infection does occur, an optimal immune system blunts the severity of illness and speeds recovery.

FIGURE 7.10 proposes a model for interactions among exercise, stress, illness, and the immune system. Within this framework, exercise, stress, and illness interact, each with its own effect on immunity. For example, exercise affects susceptibility to illness, and certain illnesses clearly affect exercise capacity. Likewise, psychologic factors (via links between the hypothalamus and immune function) and other forms of stress, including nutritional deficiencies and acute alterations

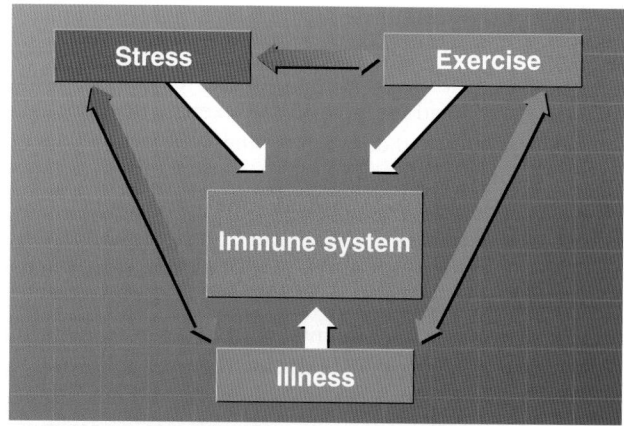

FIGURE 7.10 ■ Theoretical model of the interrelationships among stress, exercise, illness, and the immune system. (From MacKinnon LT. Current challenges and future expectations in exercise immunology: back to the future. *Med Sci Sports Exerc* 1994;26:191.)

in normal sleep schedule, influence resistance to illness. Concurrently, exercise either positively or negatively moderates the body's response to stress. Each factor—stress, illness, and short- and long-term exercise—exerts an independent effect on immune status, immune function, and resistance to disease.

Upper Respiratory Tract Infections

FIGURE 7.11 displays the general J-shaped curve to describe the relationship between short-term exercise (and unusually intense training) and susceptibility to URTI. The figure also indicates that markers of immune function follow an inverted J-shaped curve.[110,163] Although one may draw overly simplis-

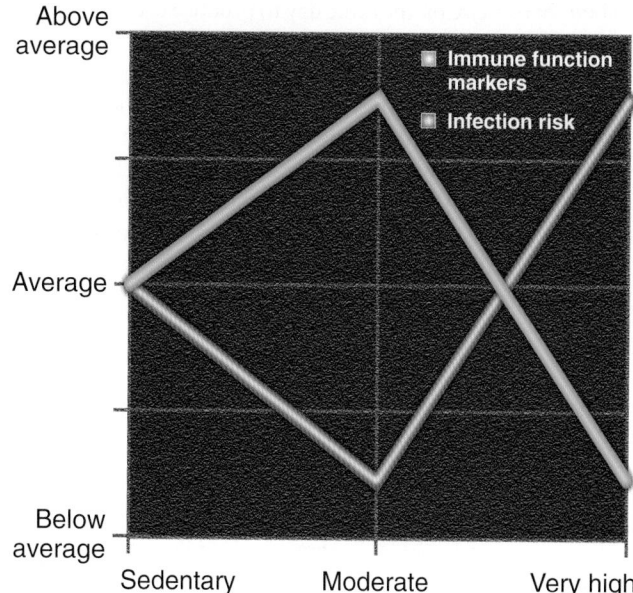

FIGURE 7.11 ■ Exercise intensity affects immune function and risk of infection.

tic implications from these relationships, light-to-moderate physical activity does appear to offer more protection against URTI and possibly diverse cancers than a sedentary lifestyle.[68,90,96] In addition, moderate exercise does not exacerbate the severity and duration of illness if infection does occur.[159] In contrast, strenuous physical activity (marathon run or intense training session) provides an "open window" (3–72 hours) that decreases antiviral and antibacterial resistance and increases risk of UTRI (by two to six times) that manifests itself within 1 or 2 weeks.[26,57] For example, approximately 13% of the participants in a Los Angeles marathon reported an episode of URTI during the week following the race. For runners of comparable ability who did not compete for reasons other than illness, the infection rate approximated 2%.[103]

Two Acute Exercise Effects

1. **Moderate exercise:** *A bout of moderate exercise boosts natural immune functions and host defenses for up to several hours.*[76,95] Noteworthy effects include the increase in NK cell activity. These phagocytic lymphocyte subpopulations enhance the disease-fighting capacity of the blood. They also provide the body's first line of defense against diverse pathogens. The NK cell does not require prior or specific sensitization to foreign bodies or neoplastic cells. Rather, these cells demonstrate spontaneous cytolytic activity that ultimately ruptures and/or inactivates viruses and the metastatic potential of tumor cells.

2. **Exhaustive exercise:** *A prolonged period of exhaustive exercise (and other forms of extreme stress or increased training) severely impairs the body's first line of defense against infection.*[75,80,113,160] Repeated cycles of unusually intense exercise further compound the risk. For example, impaired immune function from strenuous exercise "carries over" to a second bout of exercise on the same day to produce even more pronounced changes in neutrophils, lymphocytes, and select CD cells.[132] Elevated temperature, cytokines, and various stress-related hormones (epinephrine, growth hormone [GH], cortisol, β-endorphins) with exhaustive exercise may mediate depression of the body's innate (NK cell and neutrophil activity) and adaptive (T- and B-cell function) immune defenses.[7,104,146] The transient but diminished immunity after strenuous exercise remains apparent in the mucosal immune system of the upper respiratory tract.[95,100]

A Healthful Way to Reduce Cold Risk

For overweight, sedentary, postmenopausal women who participated in a program of moderate-intensity exercise 5 days per week for 12 months, the risk of colds decreased by more than threefold compared to a control group of women who attended once-weekly stretching sessions[16]

Some Prudent Advice

The negative effect of strenuous exercise on immune response clearly supports the wisdom of individuals with URTI symptoms to refrain from physical activity (or at least "go easy") to optimize normal immune mechanisms that combat infection.

Chronic Exercise Effects

Aerobic training positively affects natural immune functions and resistance to stress in young and older individuals and in the obese during periods of weight loss.[32,33,135] Areas of improvement include (1) enhanced functional capacity of natural cytotoxic immune mechanisms (e.g., antitumor actions of NK cell activity), and (2) slowing of the age-related decrease in T-cell function and associated cytokine production. The cytotoxic T cells defend directly against viral and fungal infections and contribute to regulating other immune mechanisms.

If exercise training enhances immune function, one might question why trained individuals show increased susceptibility to URTI after intense competition. The **open window hypothesis** maintains that an inordinate increase in training or actual competition exposes even the highly conditioned person to "nonnormal" stress that transiently but severely depresses NK cell function. This period of immunodepression ("open window") decreases natural resistance to infection. The inhibitory effect of strenuous exercise on adrenocorticotropic hormone output and cortisol's maintenance of optimal blood glucose concentrations may negatively affect the immune process. For individuals who exercise regularly but only at moderate levels, the window of opportunity for infection remains "closed," thus preserving the protective benefits of regular exercise on immune function.

RESISTANCE TRAINING. Nine years of prior resistance exercise training did not affect resting NK cell number or activity level when compared with sedentary controls.[106] Comparisons indicated that resistance training activated monocytes more than typically observed for regular aerobic exercise. Monocyte activation releases prostaglandins that downregulate NK cells following exercise; this inhibits the long-term positive effect of exercise on NK cells. These investigators had previously shown that NK cells increase a substantial 225% following an acute bout of resistance exercise, a response similar to the immediate effect of moderate aerobic exercise.[112,113]

Perhaps a Role for Nutritional Supplements

Nutritional factors influence immune function (and possibly susceptibility to infection) in response to strenuous exercise and training.[2,40,53,136,137] For example, consuming a fat-rich diet (62% energy from lipids) negatively affected the immune system compared with a carbohydrate-rich diet (65% energy from carbohydrates).[114] Supplementing with a 6% carbohydrate beverage (0.7l L before; 0.25 L every 15 minute during; 500 mL every hour throughout a 4.5-hour recovery) beneficially lowered cytokine levels in the inflammatory cascade after 2.5 hours of endurance running.[101] Subsequent research by the same laboratory showed that ingesting carbohydrates (4 mL per kg body mass) every 15 minutes during 2.5 hours of high-intensity running or cycling maintained higher plasma glucose levels in 10 triathletes during exercise than a placebo.[108] A 6% carbohydrate solution ingested during exercise by young adult male competitive cyclists and triathletes attenuated the exercise-induced immune response and stress, particularly by phagocytizing cells by the reduced release of cortisol, as effectively as a 12% beverage.[136] Similar beneficial results with carbohydrate ingestion for cortisol and select antiinflammatory cytokines have been observed following competition, regardless of age or gender.[109] A blunted cortisol response and diminished pro- and antiinflammatory cytokine response accompanied the higher plasma glucose levels with carbohydrate supplementation in exercise. *This suggests a carbohydrate-induced reduction in overall physiologic stress in prolonged high-intensity exercise.*

Combined supplementation with the antioxidant vitamins C and E produces more prominent immunopotentiating effects (enhanced cytokine production) in young, healthy adults than supplementation with either vitamin alone.[63] Also, a 200-mg daily vitamin E supplement enhanced clinically relevant indices of T-cell-mediated function for healthy elderly subjects.[98] However, long-term daily supplementation with a physiologic dose of vitamins and minerals or with 200 mg of vitamin E did not lower the incidence and severity of acute respiratory tract infections in noninstitutionalized persons aged 60 and older. Among individuals experiencing an infection, those receiving vitamin E had longer total illness duration and restriction of activity.[45]

Additional research must determine whether intake of vitamins C and E (and other antioxidants such as β-carotene) above recommended levels upgrades immune function to protect the general population against URTI. Daily supplementation with vitamin C does appear to benefit individuals engaged in strenuous physical activity exercise, particularly those predisposed to frequent viral URTI.[52,119] Runners who received a 600-mg daily vitamin C supplement before, and for 3 weeks after, a 90-km ultramarathon competition experienced significantly fewer symptoms of URTI—running nose, sneezing, sore throat, coughing, fever—than runners receiving a placebo.[116] Interestingly, infection risk inversely related to race performance; those with the fastest times suffered more symptoms. URTI also appeared most frequently in runners with strenuous training regimens. For these individuals, additional vitamin C and E and perhaps carbohydrate ingestion before, during, and after prolonged stressful exercise may boost normal immune mechanisms to combat infection.[104,107] More than likely, the presence of other stressors—lack of sleep, mental stress, poor nutrition, or weight loss—magnify the stress on the immune system from a single bout (or repeated bouts) of exhaustive exercise.

Glutamine and the Immune Response

The nonessential amino acid glutamine plays an important role in normal immune function. One protective aspect of glutamine concerns its use as an energy fuel for nucleotide synthesis by disease-fighting cells, particularly the lymphocytes and macrophages that defend against infection.[6,139] Sepsis, injury, burns, surgery, and endurance exercise lower glutamine levels in plasma and skeletal muscle. Lowered plasma glutamine most likely occurs because glutamine demand by the liver, kidneys, gut, and immune system exceeds its supply from the diet and skeletal muscle. A lowered plasma glutamine concentration contributes, at least in part, to the immunosuppression that accompanies extreme physical stress.[10,54,133,143] Thus, glutamine supplementation might reduce susceptibility to URTI following strenuous physical exertion.

Marathoners who ingested a glutamine drink (5 g of L-glutamine in 330 mL of mineral water) at the end of a race and then 2 hours later reported fewer URTI than unsupplemented runners.[13] Subsequent studies by the same researchers to determine a possible mechanism for glutamine's protective effect on postexercise infection risk reported no effect of supplementation on changes in blood lymphocyte distribution.[14] Appearance of URTI in athletes during intense training does not fluctuate with changes in plasma glutamine concentration. Pre-exercise glutamine supplementation does not affect the immune response following a single bout of sustained high-intensity exercise or repeated bouts of intense exercise.[79,126,157] Glutamine supplements taken 0, 30, 60, and 90 minutes following a marathon race prevented the drop in glutamine concentrations following the race but did not influence three factors: (1) lymphokine-activated killer cell activity, (2) the proliferative responses, or (3) exercise-induced changes in leukocyte subpopulations.[125] *Currently, insufficient data exist to recommend glutamine supplements to reliably blunt immunosuppression from exhaustive exercise.*

A General Recommendation

Optimum immune function generally occurs with a lifestyle that emphasizes regular physical activity, maintenance of a well-balanced diet, reducing stress to a minimum, and obtaining adequate sleep. For prudent weight loss, use a gradual approach, because more rapid weight loss with accompanying severe caloric restriction suppresses immune function.[105] With prolonged, high-intensity exercise, carbohydrate ingestion (about $1 L \cdot h^{-1}$ of a typical sports drink) lessens the negative changes in immunity brought about by physiologic stress and carbohydrate depletion. In general, endurance athletes who ingest carbohydrate during a race experience much lower disruption in hormonal and immune measures than do athletes not consuming carbohydrate. These responses indicate a diminished level of physiologic stress.

MINERALS AND EXERCISE PERFORMANCE

The use of single-mineral supplements is ill advised unless prescribed by a physician or registered dietitian because of potential adverse consequences. Excess magnesium supplementation, for example can cause gastrointestinal disturbances, including diarrhea. Magnesium intake can impair iron and zinc nutrition, while a15-mg zinc excess per day inhibits copper absorption and adversely affects HDL cholesterol concentrations. Concern also exists about the long-term effects of chromium supplementation on tissue chromium accumulation and toxic side effects. *Short- and long-term mineral supplementation above recommended levels does not benefit exercise performance or enhance training responsiveness.*

Mineral Losses in Sweat

Loss of water and accompanying mineral salts, primarily sodium chloride and some potassium chloride in sweat, poses an important challenge during prolonged exercise, especially in hot weather. Excessive water and electrolyte loss impairs heat tolerance and exercise performance and can cause severe dysfunction in the form of heat cramps, heat exhaustion, or heat stroke. The yearly number of heat-related deaths during spring and summer football practice tragically illustrates the importance of fluid and electrolyte replacement. During practice or a game, an athlete may lose up to 5 kg of water from sweating. This corresponds to about 8.0 g of salt depletion because each kg (1 L) of sweat contains about 1.5 g of salt (40% of NaCl represents sodium). *Replacement of water lost through sweating, however, becomes the crucial and immediate need.* As indicated in Chapter 10, some salt added to the ingested fluid facilitates this process.

Defense Against Mineral Loss

Vigorous exercise triggers a rapid and coordinated release of the hormones **vasopressin** and **aldosterone** and the enzyme **renin** to minimize sodium and water loss through the kidneys. Sodium conservation by the kidneys occurs even under extreme conditions such as running a marathon in warm, humid weather when sweat output often reaches 2 L per hour. Electrolytes lost in sweat are usually replenished by adding a slight amount of salt to fluid or food ingested. Runners in a 20-day road race in Hawaii maintained plasma minerals at normal levels by consuming an unrestricted diet without mineral supplements.[29] Ingesting "athletic drinks" offers no special benefit in replacing the minerals lost through sweating compared with consuming the same minerals in a well-balanced diet. Salt supplements may be necessary for prolonged exercise in the heat when fluid loss exceeds 4 or 5 kg. One can achieve proper supplementation by drinking a 0.1 to 0.2% salt solution (adding 0.3 tsp of table salt per liter of water). Chapter 10 presents more specific recommendations for electrolyte replacement via the rehydration beverage.

A mild potassium deficiency occurs with intense exercise during heat stress, but a diet with the recommended amount of potassium generally ensures adequate levels. Drinking an 8-oz glass of orange or tomato juice replaces the calcium, potassium, and magnesium lost in 3 L (7 lb) of sweat, a sweat loss not likely to occur with less than 60 minutes of vigorous exercise.

Trace Minerals and Exercise

Many athletes believe that supplementing with certain trace minerals enhances exercise performance and counteracts the demands of heavy training. Strenuous exercise may increase excretion of the following four trace elements:

1. *Chromium:* necessary for carbohydrate and lipid catabolism and proper insulin function and protein synthesis
2. *Copper:* required for red blood cell formation; influences specific gene expression, and serves as a cofactor or prosthetic group for several enzymes
3. *Manganese:* component of superoxide dismutase in the antioxidant defense system
4. *Zinc:* component of lactate dehydrogenase, carbonic anhydrase, superoxide dismutase, and enzymes related to energy metabolism, cell growth and differentiation, and tissue repair

Urinary losses of zinc and chromium were 1.5- and 2.0-fold higher on the day of a 6-mile run than on a rest day.[4] A relatively large loss of copper and zinc occurs in sweat during exercise.[25,81] However, the normal plasma volume expansion with aerobic training combined with zinc redistribution from the plasma to other body tissues (e.g., liver and skeletal muscles) dilutes plasma zinc concentrations to indicate an *apparent* zinc inadequacy.

Trace mineral losses with exercise do not necessarily mean that physically active individuals should supplement with these micronutrients. No benefit occurred, for example, from short-term 25 mg daily zinc supplementation on metabolic and endocrine responses and performance during strenuous exercise in eumenorrheic women.[141] Collegiate football players who supplemented with 200 μg of chromium (as chromium picolinate) daily for 9 weeks showed no beneficial changes in body composition or muscular strength during intense weightlifting compared with a control group that received a placebo.[17] Power and endurance athletes had higher, not lower, plasma levels of copper and zinc than nontraining controls.[124] However, men and women who train strenuously (with large sweat production) and show marginal nutrition and low body weight (e.g., weight-class wrestlers, endurance runners, ballet dancers, female gymnasts) should carefully monitor trace mineral intake to prevent overt deficiency.[88] For most physically active men and women, only transient, trace mineral losses occur with exercise, without impairing exercise performance, training responsiveness, and overall health.

Iron, zinc, and copper interact and compete for the same carrier during intestinal absorption. Thus, excessive intake of one mineral often causes deficiency in the other.[87] For example, consuming excess iron reduces zinc absorption, while excess zinc blunts copper absorption. In addition, supplementing with zinc above recommended levels can lower HDL cholesterol, diminishing the beneficial effect of aerobic exercise on this cardioprotective plasma lipoprotein. Chapter 12 discusses the possible ergogenic effects of chromium supplements and other trace minerals such as boron and vanadium. TABLE 7.10 outlines exercise-related functions and food sources of four

TABLE 7.10	Exercise-Related Functions and Food Sources of Selected Trace Minerals	
	Function	**Prominent Food Sources**
Zinc	Component of several enzymes involved in energy metabolism; cofactor to carbonic anhydrase	Oysters, wheat germ, beef, dark poultry meat, whole grains, liver
Copper	Required to synthesize cytochrome oxidase and for use of iron; constituent of ceruloplasmin; constituent of superoxide dismutase	Liver, kidney, shellfish, whole grains, legumes, nuts, eggs
Chromium	Enhances action of insulin	Mushrooms, prunes, nuts, whole grain bread and cereal, Brewer's yeast
Selenium	Functions as an antioxidant with glutathione peroxidase; complements vitamin E function	Seafood, kidney, liver

minerals—zinc, copper, chromium, and selenium—associated with exercise and training.

EXERCISE AND FOOD INTAKE

Balancing energy intake with energy expenditure represents a primary goal for the physically active individual of normal body weight. Energy balance not only optimizes physical performance, it also helps to maintain lean body mass, training responsiveness, and immune and reproductive function. Physical activity represents the most important factor affecting daily energy expenditure (see Chapter 14). A person can estimate daily energy requirements from tabled energy cost values for diverse activities (considering frequency, intensity, and duration) such as those presented in Appendix B.

FIGURE 7.12 illustrates age-related average daily energy intakes for males and females in the U.S. population. Energy intakes peak between ages 16 and 29 years and then decline for succeeding age-groups. A similar pattern occurs for males and females, although males achieve higher energy intakes than females at all ages. Between ages 20 and 29 years, women consume on average 35% fewer kCal than men on a daily basis (3025 kCal [12,657 kJ] vs 1957 kCal [8188 kJ]). Thereafter, the sex-related difference in energy intake becomes smaller; at age 70, women consume about 25% fewer kCal than their male counterparts.

Physical Activity Makes a Difference

Individuals who engage regularly in moderate-to-intense physical activity eventually increase daily energy intake to match their higher level of energy expenditure. Lumber workers, who expend approximately 4500 kCal each day, unconsciously adjust energy intake to balance energy output. Consequently, body mass remains stable despite a relatively large food intake. The body requires several days to attain energy equilibrium when balancing food intake to meet a new level of energy output. *Sedentary persons often do not maintain a fine energy balance, thereby allowing energy intake to exceed daily energy expenditure.* The lack of precision in regulating food intake at the low end of the physical activity spectrum undoubtedly contributes to the "creeping

obesity" in highly mechanized and technically advanced sedentary societies.

Daily food intake of athletes in the 1936 Olympics reportedly averaged more than 7000 kCal, or roughly three times the average intake.[1] These often-quoted energy values justify what many believe to be an enormous food requirement of athletes in training. These figures represent estimates because objective dietary data did not appear in the original report. In all likelihood, they are inflated estimates of the energy expended (and required) by the athletes. For example, distance runners who train upward to 100 miles per week (6 minutes per mile pace at about 15 kCal per minute) do not expend more than 800 to

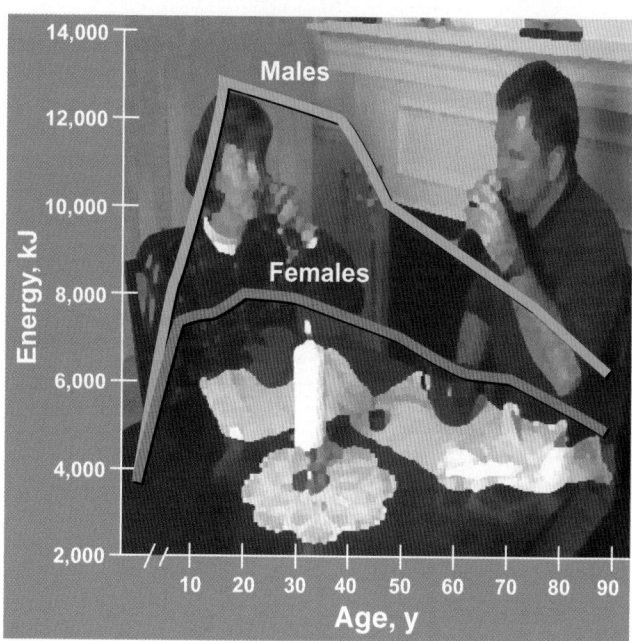

FIGURE 7.12 ■ Average daily energy intake for males and females by age in the U.S. population during the years 1988 to 1991. Multiply by 0.239 to convert kJ to kCal. (From Briefel RR, et al. Total energy intake of the US population: The third National Health and Nutrition Examination Survey, 1988–1991. *Am J Clin Nutr* 1995; 62(suppl):1072S.)

1300 "extra" calories daily. For these endurance athletes, about 4000 kCal from daily food intake should balance the increased exercise energy expenditure.

Potential for Negative Energy Balance with High-Volume Training

Many athletes, particularly females, do not meet energy intake recommendations. Research with elite female swimmers, using the doubly labeled water technique described in Chapter 6, noted that total daily energy expenditure increased to 5593 kCal daily during high-volume training. This value represents the highest level of sustained daily energy expenditure reported for female athletes.[149] Daily energy intake did not increase enough to match training demands and averaged only 3136 kCal, implying a negative energy imbalance. The possibility of a negative energy balance in the transition from moderate to intense training may ultimately compromise a person's full potential to train efficiently and compete.

FIGURE 7.13 presents energy intakes from a large sample of elite male and female endurance, strength, and team sport ath-

letes in the Netherlands. For the men, daily energy intake ranged between 2900 and 5900 kCal, whereas the intakes of women competitors ranged between 1600 and 3200 kCal. With the exception of the large energy intakes of athletes at extremes of performance and training, daily energy intake generally did not exceed 4000 kCal for the men and 3000 kCal for the women. TABLE 7.11 lists additional energy and macronutrient intakes for elite male and female athletes. The data, presented as daily caloric intake, include the percentage of total energy as carbohydrate, protein, and lipid. For men, daily energy intake ranges from 3034 to 5222 kCal; for women, it ranges between 1931 and 3573 kCal. Averaging values across studies for percentage of total calories for each macronutrient results in values of 14.8% protein, 35.0% lipid, and 49.8% carbohydrate for men and 14.4% protein, 31.8% lipid, and 54.0% carbohydrate for women.

Tour de France

Some physical activities require extreme energy output (in excess of 1000 kCal per hour in elite marathoners and professional cyclists) and a correspondingly large energy intake during competition or periods of high-intensity training. For example, the daily energy requirements of elite cross-country skiers during 1 week of training averaged 3740 to 4860 kCal for women and 6120 to 8570 kCal for men.[142] These values for women agree with recent evaluations of daily energy expenditure of seven elite lightweight female rowers, which averaged 3957 kCal over a 14-day training period.[56] FIGURE 7.14 outlines variation in daily energy expenditure for a male competitor during the most grueling event in sports, the Tour de France professional cycling race. Daily energy expenditure averaged 6500 kCal for nearly 3 weeks. Large variation occurred, depending on the level of activity for a particular day; energy expenditure decreased to 3000 kCal on a "rest" day and increased to 9000 kCal cycling over a mountain pass. By combining liquid nutrition with normal meals, this cyclist nearly matched daily energy expenditure with energy intake.

Ultraendurance Running Competition

Energy balance has been studied during a 1000-km (approximately 600-mile) race from Sidney to Melbourne, Australia. The Greek ultramarathon champion Kouros completed the race in 5 days, 5 hours, and 7 minutes, finishing 24 hours and 40 minutes ahead of the next competitor. Kouros did not sleep during the first 2 days of competition. He covered 463 km (287.8 miles) at an average speed of 11.4 km $\cdot$ h^{-1} during day 1 and 8.3 km $\cdot$ h^{-1} on day 2. During the remaining days, he took frequent rest periods, including periodic breaks for short "naps." Weather ranged from spring to winter conditions (30–8°C), and terrain varied. TABLE 7.12 lists the pertinent details of distance covered, energy expenditure, and food and water intake.

The near equivalence between Kouros' estimated total energy intake (55,970 kCal) and energy expenditure (59,079 kCal) represents a remarkable aspect of energy homeostasis during extremes of physical exertion. Of the total energy intake from food, carbohydrates represented 95.3%, lipids 3%,

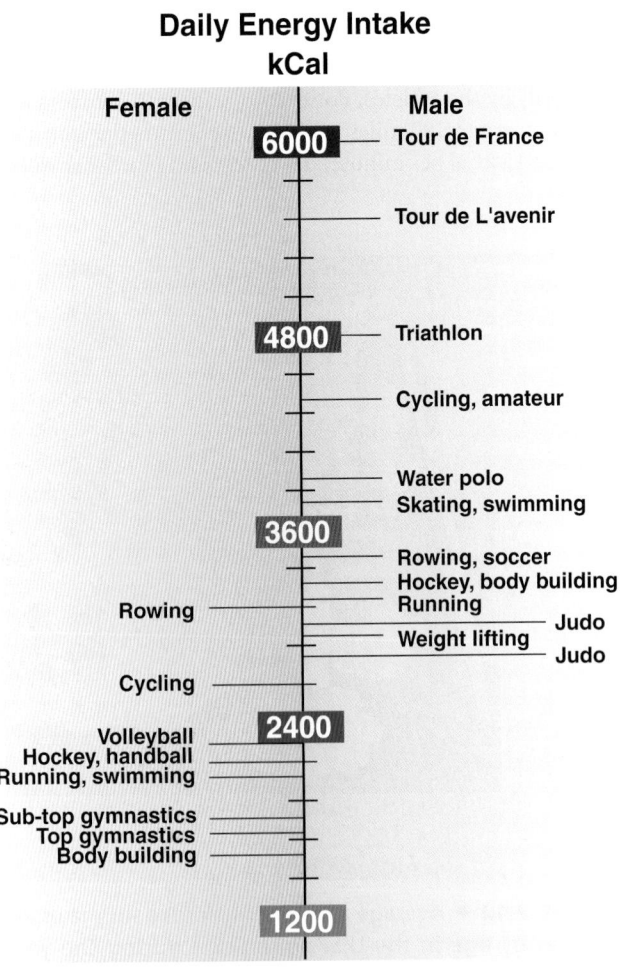

Daily Energy Intake
kCal

Female		Male
	6000	Tour de France
		Tour de L'avenir
	4800	Triathlon
		Cycling, amateur
		Water polo
		Skating, swimming
	3600	
		Rowing, soccer
		Hockey, body building
Rowing		Running
		Judo
		Weight lifting
		Judo
Cycling		
Volleyball	**2400**	
Hockey, handball		
Running, swimming		
Sub-top gymnastics		
Top gymnastics		
Body building		
	1200	

FIGURE 7.13 ■ Daily energy intake (in kCal) of elite male and female endurance, strength, and team sport athletes. (Modified from van Erp-Baart AMJ, et al. Nationwide Survey on Nutritional Habits in Elite Athletes. *Int J Sports Med* 1989;10:53.)

TABLE 7.11   Examples of Daily Intakes of Energy, Protein, Lipid, and Carbohydrate (CHO) of Well-Trained Male and Female Athletes

Group	Energy Intake (kCal)	Protein (g)	Protein (%)	Lipid (g)	Lipid (%)	CHO (g)	CHO (%)	Research Study
Well-Trained Males								
Distance runners (n=50)	3170	114	14	116	33	417	52	7
Distance runners (n=10)	3034	128	17	115	34	396	49	4
Triathletes (n=25)	4095	134	13	127	27	627	60	2
Marathon runners (n=19)	3570	128	15	128	32	487	52	2
Football players (n=56)	3395	126	15	141	38	373	44	2
Weight lifters (n=19)	3640	156	18	155	39	399	43	2
Soccer players (n=8)	4952	170	14	217	39	596	47	6
Swimmers (n=22)	5222	166	12	248	43	596	45	1
Swimmers (n=9)	3072	108	15	102	30	404	55	5
Well-Trained Females								
Distance runners (n=44)	1931	70	19	60	28	290	53	7
Distance runners, eumenorrheic (n=33)	2489	81	12	97	35	352	53	3
Distance runners, amenorrheic (n=12)	2151	74	13	67	27	344	60	3
Swimmers (n=21)	3573	107	12	164	41	428	48	1
Swimmers (n=11)	2130	79	16	63	28	292	55	5

From Williams C. Carbohydrate needs of elite athletes. In: Simopoulos AP, Parlou KN, eds. Nutrition and fitness for athletes. Basel: Karger, 1993.

[1] Berning JR, et al. The nutritional habits of adolescent swimmers. Int J Sports Nutr 1991;1:240.

[2] Burke LM, et al. Dietary intakes and food use of groups of elite Australian male athletes. Int J Sports Nutr 1991;1:278.

[3] Deuster PA, et al. Nutritional intakes and status of highly trained amenorrheic and eumenorrheic women runners. Fertil Steril 1986;46:636.

[4] Grandjean AC. Macro-nutrient intake of US athletes compared with the general population and recommendations for athletes. Am J Clin Nutr 1989;49:1070.

[5] Hawley JA, Williams MM. Dietary intakes of age-group swimmers. Br J Sports Med 1991;25:154.

[6] Jacobs I, et al. Muscle glycogen concentration and elite soccer players. Eur J Appl Physiol 1982;48:297.

[7] Courtesy of V. Katch (Unpublished).

with the remaining 1.7% proteins. Protein intake from food averaged considerably below the RDA level (although protein supplements were taken in tablet form). The unusually large daily energy intake (8600–13,770 kCal) came from Greek sweets (baklava, cookies, and donuts), some chocolate, dried fruit and nuts, various fruit juices, and fresh fruits. Every 30 minutes after the first 6 hours of running, Kouros replaced sweets and fruit with a small biscuit soaked in honey or jam. He consumed a small amount of roasted chicken on day 4, and drank coffee every morning. He took a 500-mg vitamin C supplement every 12 hours and a protein tablet twice daily.

The remarkable achievement by this champion exemplifies a highly conditioned athlete's exquisite regulatory control for energy balance during strenuous exercise. Kouros performed at a pace requiring a continuous energy supply averaging 49% of aerobic capacity during the first 2 days of competition (and 38% for days 3–5). He finished the competition without compromising overall health, with no muscular injuries or thermoregulatory problems, and his body mass remained unchanged. Reported difficulties included a severe bout of constipation during the competition and frequent urination that persisted for several days after the race.

Another case study of a 37-year-old male ultramarathoner further demonstrates the tremendous capacity for

prolonged, high daily energy expenditure. The doubly labeled water technique evaluated energy expenditure during a 2-week period of a 14,500-km run around Australia in 6.5 months (average 7–90 km · d[-1]) with no days for rest.[55] Daily energy expenditure over the measurement period averaged 6321 kCal; daily water turnover equaled 6.083 L. The subject ran about the same distance each day over the study period as in the entire race period. As such, these data likely represent energy dynamics for the entire run.

High-Risk Sports for Marginal Nutrition

Gymnasts, ballet dancers, ice dancers, and weight-class athletes in boxing, wrestling, and judo engage in arduous training. Yet due to the nature of their sport, these men and women continually strive to maintain a lean, light body mass (TABLE 7.13). As a result, energy intake often intentionally falls short of energy expenditure and a relative state of malnutrition develops. The daily nutrient intake (% of RDA) of 97 competitive female gymnasts 11 to 14 years of age, indicate that nutritional supplementation could prove beneficial to these individuals (FIG. 7.15). Twenty-three percent of the girls consumed less than 1500 kCal daily, and more than 40% consumed less than two thirds of the RDA for

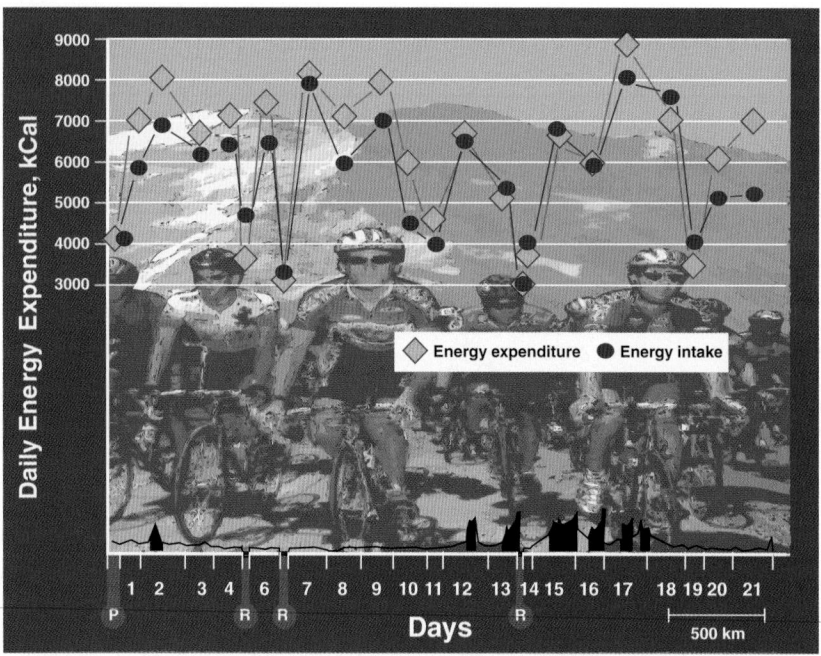

FIGURE 7.14 ■ Daily energy expenditure *(yellow squares)* and energy intake *(purple circles)* for a cyclist during the Tour de France competition. For 3 weeks in July, nearly 200 cyclists push themselves over and around the perimeter of France covering 2405 miles, more than 100 miles daily (only 1 day rest), at an average speed of 24.4 mph. Note the extremely high energy expenditure values and ability to achieve energy balance with liquid nutrition plus normal meals. *P*, stage; *R*, rest day. (Modified from Saris WHM, et al. Adequacy of vitamin supply under maximal sustained workloads; the Tour de France. In: Walter P, et al, eds. *Elevated Dosages of Vitamins.* Toronto: Huber Publishers, 1989.)

vitamin E, folate, iron, magnesium, calcium, and zinc. Clearly, a large number of these adolescent gymnasts needed to upgrade the nutritional quality of their diets or consider supplementation. For such athletes, carbohydrate intake fails to reach the level required by intense training. Consequently, they often train and perform in a carbohydrate-depleted state. Some protein supplementation to achieve a daily intake between 1.2 and 1.6 g per kg

of body mass also may be warranted to maintain nitrogen balance and reduce the potential for impaired training status.

EAT MORE, WEIGH LESS

The energy intakes of 61 middle-aged men and women who ran 60 km per week ranged between 40 and 60% more calories

TABLE 7.12   **Distance Covered and Daily and Total Energy Balance, Nutrient Distributions in Food, and Water Intake during an Elite Ultra Distance Running**

Day of the Race	Distance Covered (km)	Estimated Energy Expenditure (kCal)	Estimated Energy Intake (kCal)	Carbohydrates (g)	(%)	(kCal)	Lipids (g)	(%)	(kCal)	Proteins (g)	(%)	(kCal)	H₂O (L)
1	270	15,367	13,770	3375	98.0	13,502	20	1.3	180	22	0.7	88	22.0
2	193	10,741	8600	1981	92.2	7923	53	5.5	477	50	2.3	200	19.2
3	152	8919	12,700	3074	96.8	12,297	27	1.9	243	40	1.3	160	22.7
4	165	9780	7800	1758	90.1	7032	56	6.5	504	66	3.4	264	14.3
5	135	7736	12,500	3014	96.4	12,058	30	2.2	270	43	1.4	172	18.3
5 h	45	2536	550	138	100.0	550	—	—	—	—	—	—	3.2
Total	960	55,079	55,970	13,340		53,364	186		1674	221		734	99.7

Modified from Rontoyannis GP, et al. Energy balance in ultramarathon running. Am J Clin Nutr 1989;49:976.
The runner weighed 65 kg, was 171 cm tall, had a percentage body fat of 8%, and a $\dot{V}O_2$max of 62.5 mL·kg⁻¹·min⁻¹.

TABLE 7.13 High-Risk Sports for Marginal Nutrition

Criterion	Sports Discipline
Low weight—chronically low energy intakes to achieve low body fat	Gymnastics, jockeys, ballet, dancing, rhythmic gymnastics, ice dancing, aerobics
Competition weight—drastic weight loss regimens to achieve desired weight category	Weight class sports (e.g., judo, boxing, wrestling, rowing, ski jumping)
Low fat—drastic fat loss to achieve lowest possible fat	Body building
Vegetarian athletes	Endurance events

From Brouns F. Nutritional Needs of Athletes. New York: John Wiley & Sons, 1993.

per kg of body mass than intakes of sedentary controls. The extra energy required to run between 8 and 10 km daily accounted for the runners' larger caloric intake. Paradoxically, the most active runners who ate considerably more on a daily basis weighed considerably less than runners who exercised at a lower total caloric expenditure. These data agree with other studies of physically active people; they also support the argument that regular exercise provides an effective way to "eat more yet weigh less" while maintaining a lower percentage of body fat. Chapter 14 more fully explores the important role of regular exercise for weight control.

Eat More, Yet Stay Healthy

Physically active people maintain a lighter, leaner body and a more healthful disease risk profile, despite increased intake of the typical American diet.

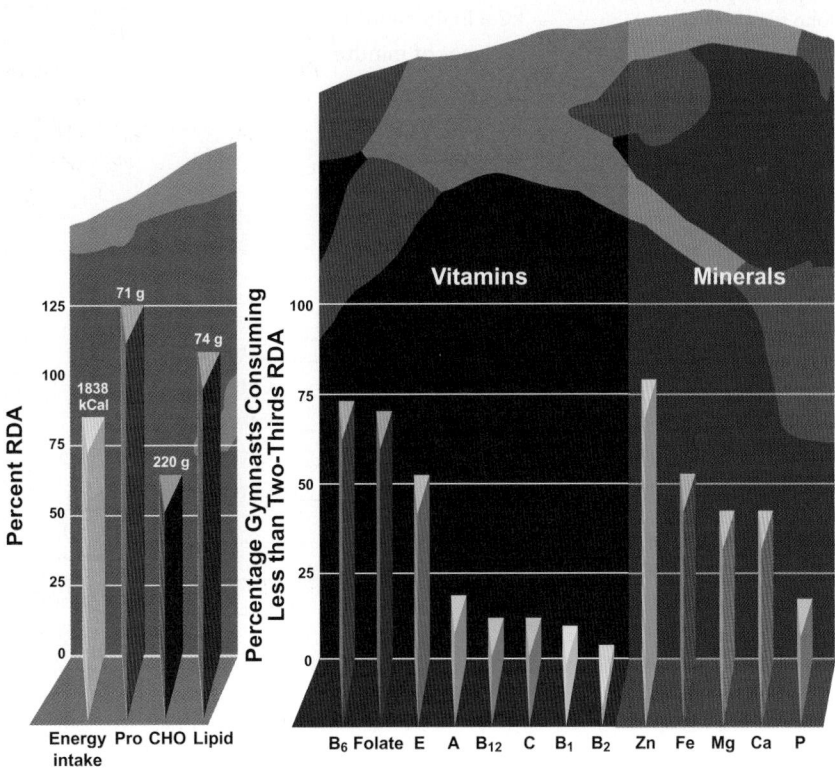

FIGURE 7.15 ■ Average daily nutrient intake of 97 adolescent female gymnasts (11–14 y) related to recommended values. The RDA on the *y* axis reflects only protein, while energy, CHO, and lipid reflect "recommended" values *(left)*. Percentage of gymnasts consuming less than two-thirds of the RDA *(right)*. Mean age, 13.1 years; mean stature, 152.4 cm (60 in.); mean body mass, 43.1 kg (94.8 lb). (Modified from Loosli AR, Benson J. Nutritional intake in adolescent athletes. *Sports Med* 1990;37:1143.)

Case Study

Personal Health and Exercise Nutrition 7–1

The ABCs of Good Nutrition: Applying the *Dietary Guidelines for Americans*

The *Dietary Guidelines for Americans* (www.usda.gov/cnpp), jointly developed by the U.S. Department of Agriculture and Department of Health and Human Services, represents medical and scientific consensus as a foundation for nutrition education for healthy Americans 2 years of age and older. When followed, the guidelines provide a prudent road map to reduce chronic disease risk and ensure nutritional adequacy.

One should learn the ABCs of the *Dietary Guidelines* and how to apply them to individual situations. After reviewing this information, you can evaluate your dietary habits, strengths, and shortcomings in comparison to the recommendations (TABLE 1).

TABLE 1   The ABCs of Your Dietary Habits

Part I. Aim for Fitness	Evaluation:
1. Determine your BMI.	BMI = ___kg/___cm² = +
2. Choose a physical activity that you do (e.g., jogging). Calculate the calories (kCal) you burn doing this activity for 10 and 45 minutes. How long would you have to do this activity to offset the calories in one small bag of M&Ms?	Activity: _____ kCal in 10 minutes _____ kCal in 45 minutes _____ Number of minutes _____
3. Determine your target heart rate (THR) for aerobic exercise training.	THR = Calories =
4. Determine how many calories you need to maintain your current level of body weight.	Calories =
5. Determine the number of calories in one pound of body fat.	

Aim for Fitness
- Aim for a health weight
- Be physically active every day

Build a Healthy Base
- Let MyPyramid guide your food choices
- Choose a variety of grains daily, especially whole grains
- Choose a variety of nuts and vegetables daily
- Keep food safe to eat

Part II. Build a Healthy Base	
1. Draw and label the Food Guide Pyramid.	Food _____ Category
2. List five foods you eat often and the corresponding Pyramid category.	Food _____ Category Food _____ Category Food _____ Category Food _____ Category

Identify one whole-grain cereal that you eat.
   Identify one whole-grain bread that you eat.
   Identify one whole-grain food that you eat.
	Whole grain cereal _____
	Whole grain bread _____
	Whole grain food _____

3. List the four principles of food safety and give an example of each from your experience	1. 2. 3. 4.
4. List one food as a potential source of harmful microorganisms. Have you ever eaten this food? Any consequences?	Food _____

Choose Sensibly
- Choose food low in saturated fat and cholesterol and moderate in total fat
- Choose beverages and foods to limit intake of sugar
- Choose and prepare foods with less salt
- If you drink alcoholic beverages, do so in moderation

Part III. Choose Sensibly

Go to the Interactive Healthy Eating Index at the USDA site [http://147.208.9.133/]. Enter the food you ate yesterday and compare your Healthy Eating Index score with the recommendations.

Case Study *continued*

Dietary Guidelines for Americans

The ABCs of the *Dietary Guidelines* consist of three components: (1) AIM FOR FITNESS, (2) BUILD A HEALTHY BASE, and (3) CHOOSE SENSIBLY. Refer to the following website for more specific up-to-date information: www. pueblo.gov/cictext/food/dietguide2000/toc.htm

Aim for Fitness

1. Aim for a healthy body weight as categorized by the body mass index (BMI). Maintain or improve body weight. See Chapter 13 for a discussion about BMI, and consult the following website for easy means of computation: www.keepkidshealthy.com/ welcome/bmicalculator.html

2. Become more physically active each day. Balance food intake with regular physical activity. The following website provides handy calculators to estimate calorie expenditure during exercise, determine target heart rates, and even compute how much exercise "burns off" your favorite desert: www.my.webmd.com/content/tools/ 1/calcdessert.htm?2–36288100000000704

Build a Healthy Base

1. Let MyPyramid guide your food choices. www.nal. usda.gov/fnic/Fpyr/pymid.gif

2. Choose diverse grains on a daily basis, particularly unrefined, whole grains. www.cspinet.org/nah/wwheat. html

3. Choose a variety of fruits and vegetables daily.

4. Keep food safe to eat. www.fightbac.org/main.cfm

Choose Sensibly

1. Choose a diet low in saturated fat and cholesterol and moderate in total fat. Eliminate *trans* fatty acids when possible.

2. Choose beverages and foods that lower intake of refined simple sugars. www.usda.gov/cnpp

3. Choose and prepare foods with less salt. www. pueblo.gsa.gov/cictext/food/dietguide2000/ lesssalt.htm

4. Drink alcoholic beverages in moderation. Some persons should not drink alcoholic beverages at all. www.pueblo.gsa.gov/cictext/food/dietguide2000/alcohol. htm

Applying the *Dietary Guidelines*

Once you understand the *Dietary Guidelines* you can assess your diet and fitness goals in relation to them. Assessment also helps you make wise decisions about changing current diet and exercise habits.

Summary

1. MyPyramid provides recommendations for healthful nutrition for physically active men and women. It emphasizes fruits, grains, and vegetables and deemphasizes foods high in animal protein, lipids, and dairy products.

2. The Diet Quality Index, a composite score based on eight food-and-nutrient recommendations of the National Academy of Sciences, provides a general indication of the "healthfulness" of one's diet.

3. Within rather broad limits, a balanced diet provides the nutrient requirements of athletes and other individuals who engage in exercise training programs. Well-planned menus of about 1200 kCal daily offer the vitamin, mineral, and protein requirements. Consuming additional food (depending on physical activity level) then meets daily energy needs.

4. The protein RDA of 0.8 g per kg of body mass represents a liberal requirement believed adequate for all people regardless of physical activity level.

5. A protein intake between 1.2 and 1.8 g per kg of body mass should adequately meet the possibility for added protein needs during strenuous training and prolonged exercise.

6. Physically active individuals readily achieve optimal protein values because they consume two to five times the protein RDA with their increased energy intake.

7. Precise recommendations do not exist for daily lipid and carbohydrate intake. A prudent recommendation suggests not to exceed 30 to 35% of daily calories from lipids; of this amount, most should be as unsaturated fatty acids.

Summary *continued*

8. For physically active people, carbohydrates should provide 60% or more of the daily calories (400 to 600 g), particularly as unrefined polysaccharides.

9. The American Heart Association (AHA) recommends lifestyle modifications that include increasing regular physical activity and eliminating use of all tobacco products.

10. A proper diet emphasizes fruits and vegetables, cereals and whole grains, nonfat and low-fat dairy products, legumes, nuts, fish, poultry, and lean meats.

11. To address the nation's obesity epidemic, the AHA urges men to maintain a waistline of 40 inches or less and for women, 35 inches or less.

12. Americans should devote at least 1 hour daily to moderately intense physical activity (brisk walking, swimming, or cycling) to maintain good health and a desirable body weight.

13. To meet daily energy and nutrient needs and minimize chronic disease risk, adults should consume between 45 and 65% of total calories from carbohydrates, with maximum intake of added sugars placed at 25% of total calories.

14. Acceptable lipid intake ranges between 20 and 35% of caloric intake, with protein intake between 10 to 35%.

15. Successive days of intense training gradually deplete carbohydrate reserves, even when maintaining the recommended carbohydrate intake. This could lead to "staleness," making continued training more difficult.

16. Vitamin supplementation above amounts in a well-balanced diet does not improve exercise performance or the potential for training. Serious illness can result from consuming a regular excess of fat-soluble and, in some instances, water-soluble vitamins.

17. Elevated metabolism in physical activity increases the production of potentially harmful free radicals. To reduce the possibility for oxidative stress and cellular damage, the daily diet should contain foods rich in antioxidant vitamins and minerals.

18. A J-shaped curve generally describes the relationship between short-term exercise intensity and susceptibility to upper respiratory tract infection (URTI).

19. Light-to-moderate physical activity offers greater protection against URTI and diverse cancers than a sedentary lifestyle. A bout of intense physical activity provides an "open window" that decreases antiviral and antibacterial resistance and increases UTRI risk.

20. Glutamine supplements are not recommended to reliably blunt immunosuppression from exhaustive exercise.

21. Excessive sweating during exercise causes loss of body water and related minerals. Mineral loss should be replaced following exercise through well-balanced meals.

22. Intensity of daily physical activity largely determines energy intake requirements. The daily caloric needs of athletes in strenuous sports probably do not exceed 4000 kCal unless (1) body mass is large, or (2) training level or competition is extreme.

Test Your Knowledge Answers

1. **False:** The human body functions in accord with the laws of thermodynamics. This also includes the dynamics of energy balance. In accord with the first law of thermodynamics, the energy balance equation dictates that body mass remains constant when caloric intake equals caloric expenditure. If the total food calories exceed daily energy expenditure, excess calories accumulate as fat in adipose tissue. Conversely, weight loss occurs when daily energy expenditure exceeds daily energy intake.

2. **True:** Thirty-five hundred "extra" kCal through either increased energy intake or decreased energy output approximates the energy contained in 1 pound (0.45 kg) of stored body fat.

3. **True:** Grouping of all fats and oils together (with sweets) does not distinguish differences between good fats (olive oil and canola oil, high in monounsaturated fats and omega-3 fatty acids) that fend off heart disease and fight inflammation and harmful fats such as saturated fats and *trans*-unsaturated fatty acids. Also, such a grouping does not clarify differences between refined carbohydrates (white rice, white bread) and the more healthful ones (whole grains, brown rice).

4. **False:** Guidelines from the U.S. government are similar to those advocated by other agencies (including the USDA); they place great emphasis on adopting healthy eating patterns and lifestyle behaviors rather than focusing on specific numeric goals such as for dietary fat intake.

5. **False:** Research in exercise nutrition, although far from complete, indicates that the large number of

Test Your Knowledge Answers   *continued*

teenagers and adults who exercise regularly to keep fit, including competitive athletes, do not require additional nutrients beyond those obtained through the regular intake of a nutritionally well-balanced diet. Endurance athletes and others who engage regularly in intense training must maintain adequate energy and protein intake and appropriate carbohydrate consumption to match this macronutrient's use for energy during exercise. However, attention to proper diet does not mean that a physically active person must join the ranks of the more than 40% of Americans who take supplements (spending about $6 billion yearly) to micromanage nutrient intake.

6. **False:** Adequate research design and methodology has not shown that amino acid supplementation in any form above the RDA significantly increases muscle mass or improves muscular strength, power, or endurance. Most individuals obtain adequate protein to sustain muscle growth with resistance training by consuming ordinary foods in a well-balanced diet. Provided caloric intake balances energy output (and one consumes a wide variety of foods), no need exists to consume protein supplements or simple amino acids.

7. **False:** Standards for optimal lipid intake are not firmly established, but to promote good health, lipid intake should probably not exceed 25 to 30%

of the diet's energy content. Of this, at least 70% should come from unsaturated fatty acids.

8. **False:** No hazard to health exists when subsisting chiefly on a variety of fiber-rich complex unrefined carbohydrates, with adequate intake of essential amino acids, fatty acids, minerals, and vitamins.

9. **False:** Over 50 years of research fails to support the use of vitamin supplements by nutritionally adequate healthy people to improve exercise performance or the ability to train arduously. When vitamin intake achieves recommended levels via diet, supplements neither improve performance nor increase the blood levels of these micronutrients.

10. **False:** The best sources of antioxidants are β-carotene found in pigmented compounds that give color to yellow and orange vegetables and fruits, including carrots; dark-green leafy vegetables such as spinach, broccoli, turnips, and beet and collard greens; sweet potatoes, winter squash, apricots, cantaloupe, mangos, and papaya; vitamin C found in citrus fruits and juices, cabbage, broccoli, turnip greens, cantaloupe, green and red sweet peppers, and berries; vitamin E found in poultry, seafood, vegetable oils, wheat germ, fish liver oils, whole-grain breads and fortified cereals, nuts and seeds, dried beans, green leafy vegetables, and eggs.

References

1. Abrahams A. The nutrition of athletes. *Br J Nutr* 1948;2:266.
2. Aguilo A, et al. Antioxidant diet supplementation influences blood iron status in endurance athletes. *Int J Sport Nutr Exerc Metab* 2004;14:147.
3. Aleisso HM, et al. Generation of reactive oxygen species after exhaustive aerobic and isometric exercise. *Med Sci Sports Exerc* 2000;32:1576.
4. Anderson RA, et al. Strenuous running: acute effects on chromium, copper, zinc, and selected variables in urine and serum of male runners. *Biol Trace Element Res* 1984;6:327.
5. Aoi W, et al. Exercise and functional foods. *Nutr J* 2006;5:15.
6. Ardawi MN, Newsholme EA. Metabolism in lymphocytes and its importance in the immune response. *Essays Biochem* 1985;21:1.
7. Baum M, et al. Moderate and exhaustive endurance exercise influences the interferon-levels in whole-blood culture supernatants. *Eur J Appl Physiol* 1997;76:165.
8. Bazzano LA, et al. Fruit and vegetable intake and risk of cardiovascular disease in US adults: the first National Health and Nutrition Examination Survey Epidemiologic Follow-up Study. *Am J Clin Nutr* 2002;76:93.
9. Beaton LJ, et al. Contraction-induced muscle damage is unaffected by vitamin E supplementation. *Med Sci Sports Exerc* 2002;34:798.
10. Blanchard MA, et al. The influence of diet and exercise on muscle and plasma glutamine concentrations. *Med Sci Sports Exerc* 2001;33:69.
11. Brooks GA, et al. Chronicle of the Institute of Medicine physical activity recommendation: how a physical activity recommendation came to be among dietary recommendations. *Am J Clin Nutr* 2004;79:921S.
12. Burke LM, et al. Energy and carbohydrate for training. *J Sport Sci* 2006;24:675.
13. Castell LM, et al. Does glutamine have a role in reducing infections in athletes? *Eur J Appl Physiol* 1996;73:488.
14. Castell LM, et al. Some aspects of the acute phase response after a marathon race, and the effects of glutamine supplementation. *Eur J Appl Physiol* 1997;75:47.
15. Cavas L, Tarhan L. Effects of vitamin-mineral supplementation on cardiac marker and radical scavenging enzymes, and MDA levels in young swimmers. *Int J Sport Nutr Exerc Metab* 2004;14:133.
16. Chubak J, et al. Moderate-intensity exercise reduces incidence of colds among postmenopausal women. *Am J Med* 2006;119:937.
17. Clancy SP, et al. Effects of chromium picolinate supplementation on body composition, strength, and urinary chromium loss in football players. *Int J Sport Nutr* 1994;4:142.
18. Clark LC, et al. Effects of selenium supplementation for cancer prevention in patients with carcinoma of the skin: a randomized trial. *JAMA* 1996;276:1957.
19. Clarkson PM. Minerals: exercise performance and supplementation in athletes. *J Sports Sci* 1991;9:91.
20. Clarkson PM, Haymes EM. Trace mineral requirements for athletes. *Int J Sports Nutr* 1994;4:104.
21. Clarkson PM, Haymes EM. Exercise and mineral status of athletes: calcium, magnesium, phosphorus, and iron. *Med Sci Sports Exerc* 1995;27:831.
22. Clarkson PM, Thompson HS. Antioxidants: what role do they play in physical activity and health? *Am J Clin Nutr* 2000;72:637.
23. Coombes JS, et al. Effect of vitamin E deficiency on fatigue and muscle contractile properties. *Eur J Appl Physiol* 2002;87:272.
24. Cordain L, et al. Origins and evolutions of the Western diet: health implications for the 21st century. *Am J Clin Nutr* 2005;81:341.

25. Couzy DL, et al. Zinc metabolism in the athlete: influence of training, nutrition and other factors. *Int J Sports Med* 1990;11:263.

26. Davis JM, et al. Exercise, alveolar macrophage function, and susceptibility to respiratory infection. *J Appl Physiol* 1997;83:1461.

27. Dawson B, et al. Effect of vitamin C and vitamin E supplementation on biochemical and ultrastructural indices of muscle damage after a 21 km run. *Int J Sports Med* 2002;23:10.

28. DeLorgeril M, et al. Mediterranean diet, traditional risk factors, and the rate of cardiovascular complications after myocardial infarction. *Circulation* 1999;99:779.

29. Dressendorfer RH, et al. Plasma mineral levels in marathon runners during a 20-day road race. *Phys Sportsmed* 1982;10:113.

30. Drewnowski A. Concept of a nutritious food: Toward a nutrient density score. *Am J Clin Nutr* 2005;82:721.

31. Eaton CB, et al. Cross-sectional relationship between diet and physical activity in two southeastern New England communities. *Am J Prev Med* 1995;11:238.

32. Fahlman M, et al. Effects of endurance training on selected parameters of immune function in elderly women. *Gerontology* 46:97, 2000.

33. Fleshner M. Exercise and neuroendocrine regulation of antibody production: protective effect of physical activity of stress-induced suppression of the specific antibody response. *Int J Sports Med* 2000;21(suppl 1):S214.

34. Fogelholm GM, et al. Dietary and biochemical indices of nutritional status in male athletes and controls. *J Am Coll Nutr* 1992;11:181.

35. Food and Nutrition Board, Institute of Medicine. Dietary reference intakes for energy, carbohydrates, fiber, fat, protein and amino acids. Washington, DC: National Academy Press, 2002.

36. Friedenreic CM. Physical activity and cancer: lessons learned from nutritional epidemiology. *Nutr Rev* 2001;59:349.

37. Fry AC, et al. Effect of a liquid multivitamin/mineral supplement on anaerobic exercise performance. *Res Sports Med* 2006;14:53.

38. Fung TT, et al. Whole-grain intake and risk of type-2 diabetes: a prospective study in men. *Am J Clin Nutr* 2002;76:535.

39. Gauche E, et al. Vitamin and mineral supplementation and neuromuscular recovery after a running race. *Med Sci Sports Exerc* 2006;38:2110.

40. Gleeson M, Bishop NC. Elite athlete immunology: importance of nutrition. *Int J Sports Nutr* 2000;21(suppl 1):S44.

41. Goldfarb AH, et al. Antioxidants: role of supplementation to prevent exercise-induced oxidative stress. *Med Sci Sports Exerc* 1993;25:232.

42. Goldfarb AH, et al. Vitamin E effects on indexes of lipid peroxidation in muscle from DHEA-treated and exercised rats. *J Appl Physiol* 1994;76:1630.

43. Goldfarb AH, et al. Vitamin E attenuates myocardial oxidative stress induced by DHEA in rested and exercised rats. *J Appl Physiol* 1996;80:486.

44. Grandjean AC. Macronutrient intakes of U.S. athletes compared with the general population and recommendations made for athletes. *Am J Clin Nutr* 1989;49:1070.

45. Gratt JM, et al. Effect of daily vitamin E and multivitamin-mineral supplementation on acute respiratory tract infections in elderly persons. *JAMA* 2002;288:715.

46. Guilland JC, et al. Vitamin status of young athletes including the effects of supplementation. *Med Sci Sports Exerc* 1989;4:441.

47. Hann CS, et al. Validation of the Healthy Eating Index with use of biomarkers in a clinical sample of healthy women. *Am J Clin Nutr* 2001;74:479.

48. Haraldsdottir J, Andersen LB. Dietary factors related to fitness in young men and women. *Prev Med* 1994;23:490.

49. Haub MD, et al. Effect of protein source on resistive-training-induced changes in body composition and muscle size in older men. *Am J Clin Nutr* 2002;76:511.

50. Haymes EM. Vitamin and mineral supplementation to athletes. *Int J Sport Nutr* 1991;1:146.

51. Hellsten Y, et al. Effect of sprint cycle training on activities of antioxidant enzymes in human skeletal muscle. *J Appl Physiol* 1996;81:1484.

52. Hemilüa H. Vitamin C and common cold incidence: a review of studies with subjects under heavy physical stress. *Int J Sports Med* 1996;17:379.

53. Henson DA, et al. Carbohydrate supplementation and lymphocyte proliferative response to long endurance running. *Int J Sports Med* 1998;19:574.

54. Hickson RC, et al. Glutamine prevents down-regulation of myosin heavy-chain synthesis and muscle atrophy from glucocorticoids. *Am J Physiol* 1995;31:E730.

55. Hill RJ, Davies PS. Energy expenditure during 2 wk of an ultra-endurance run around Australia. *Med Sci Sport Exerc* 2001;33:148.

56. Hill RJ, Davies PS. Energy intake and energy expenditure in elite light-weight female rowers. *Med Sci Sports Exerc* 2002;34:1823.

57. Hoffman-Goetz L, Pedersen BK. Exercise and the immune system: a model of the stress response? *Immunol Today* 1994;15:382.

58. Hu FB, Willett WC. Optimal diets for prevention of coronary heart disease. *JAMA* 2002;288:2569.

59. Hu FB, et al. Prospective study of major dietary patterns and risk of coronary heart disease in men. *Am J Clin Nutr* 2001;72:912.

60. Inal M, et al. Effect of aerobic and anaerobic metabolism on free radical generation in swimmers. *Med Sci Sports Exerc* 2001;33:564.

61. Itoh H, et al. Vitamin E supplementation attenuates leakage of enzymes following 6 successive days of running training. *Int J Sports Med* 2000;21:369.

62. Jeffery RW, et al. Physical activity and weight loss: does prescribing higher physical activity goals improve outcome? *Am J Clin Nutr* 2003;78:684.

63. Jeng KCG, et al. Supplementation with vitamins C and E enhances cytokine production by peripheral blood mononuclear cells in healthy adults. *Am J Clin Nutr* 1996;64:960.

64. Jensen MK, et al. Intakes of whole grains, bran, and germ and the risk of coronary heart disease in men. *Am J Clin Nutr* 2004;80:1492.

65. Ji LL. Exercise and oxidative stress: role of the cellular antioxidant systems. *Exerc Sport Sci Rev* 1995;23:135.

66. Jimenez K, et al. Exercise does not induce oxidative stress in trained heart transplant recipients. *Med Sci Sports Exerc* 2001;32:2018.

67. Johnston CS. Uncle Sam's diet sensation: MyPyramid—an overview and commentary. *Med Gen Med* 2005;7:78.

68. Jonsdottir IH, et al. Enhancement of natural immunity seen after voluntary exercise in rats: role of central opioid receptors. *Life Sci* 2000;66:1231.

69. Joshipura KJ, et al. Fruit and vegetable intake in relation to risk of ischemic stroke. *JAMA* 1999;282:1233.

70. Jula A, et al. Effects of a diet and simvastatin on serum lipids, insulin and antioxidants in hypercholesterolemic men: a randomized controlled trial. *JAMA* 2002;287:598.

71. Kant AK. Consumption of energy-dense, nutrient-poor foods by adult Americans: the third National Health and Nutrition Examination Survey, 1988–1994. *Am J Clin Nutr* 2000;72:929.

72. Kanter MM. Free radicals and exercise: effects of nutritional antioxidant supplementation. *Exerc Sport Sci Rev* 1995;23:375.

73. Kanter MM, et al. Effects of an antioxidant vitamin mixture on lipid peroxidation at rest and postexercise. *J Appl Physiol* 1993;74:965.

74. Kleiner SM, et al. Metabolic profiles, diet and health practices of championship male and female body builders. *J Am Diet Assoc* 1990;90:962.

75. Kohut ML, et al. Prolonged exercise suppresses antigen-specific cytokine response to upper respiratory infection. *J Appl Physiol* 2001;90:678.

76. Kosta T, et al. The symptomatology of upper respiratory tract infections and exercise in elderly. *Med Sci Sports Exerc* 2000;32:46.

77. Krauss RM, et al. AHA dietary guidelines revision 2000: a statement for health care professionals from the Nutrition Committee of the American Heart Association. *Circulation* 2000;102:2284.

78. Krester AJ. The new Dietary Reference Intakes in food labeling: the food industry's perspective, *Am J Clin Nutr* 2006;83:1231S.

79. Krzywkowski K, et al. Effect of glutamine and protein supplementation on exercise-induced decreases in salivary IgA. *J Appl Physiol* 2001;91:832.

80. Lambert CP, et al. Influence of acute submaximal exercise on T-lymphocyte suppressor cell function in healthy young men. *Eur J Appl Physiol* 2000;82:151.

81. Lane HW. Some trace elements related to physical activity: zinc, copper, selenium, chromium and iodine. In: Hickson JE, Wolinski I, eds. *Nutrition in Exercise and Sport.* Boca Raton, FL: CRC Press, 1989.

82. Lasheras C, et al. Mediterranean diet and age with respect to overall survival in institutionalized, nonsmoking elderly people. *Am J Clin Nutr* 2000;71:987.

83. Lauber RP, Sheard NF. The American Heart Association dietary guidelines for 2000: a summary report. *Nutr Rev* 2001;59:298.

84. Leaf DA, et al. The effect of exercise intensity on lipid peroxidation. *Med Sci Sports Exerc* 1997;29:1036.

85. Liu S, et al. A prospective study of dietary glycemic load, carbohydrate intake, and risk of coronary heart disease in US women. *Am J Clin Nutr* 2000;71:1455.

86. Liu S, et al. Fruit and vegetable intake and risk of cardiovascular disease: the Women's Health Study. *Am J Clin Nutr* 2000;72:922.

87. Lönnerdal B. Bioavailability of copper. *Am J Clin Nutr* 1996;63(suppl):821S.

88. Lukaski HC. Magnesium, zinc, and chromium nutriture and physical activity. *Am J Clin Nutr* 2000;72(suppl):585S.

89. Macdermid PW, Stannard SR. A whey-supplemented, high-protein diet versus a high-carbohydrate diet: effects on endurance cycling performance. *Int J Sport Nutr Exerc Metab* 2006;16:65.

90. Mackinnon LT. Future directions in exercise and immunology: regulation and integration. *Int J Sports Med* 1998;19:S205.

91. Manore MM. Vitamin B$_6$ and exercise. *Int J Sports Nutr* 1994;5:89.

92. Manore MM. Effects of physical activity on thiamine, riboflavin, and vitamin B$_6$ requirements. *Am J Clin Nutr* 2000;72(suppl):598S.

93. Manore MM, Leklem JE. Effect of carbohydrate and vitamin B$_6$ on fuel substrates during exercise in women. *Med Sci Sports Exerc* 1988;20:233.

94. Matthews CE, et al. Relationship between leisure-time physical activity and selected dietary variables in the Worcester Area Trial for Counseling in Hyperlipidemia. *Med Sci Sports Exerc* 1997;29:1199.

95. Matthews CE, et al. Physical activity and risk of upper-respiratory tract infection. *Med Sci Sports Exerc* 2000;32:S292.

96. Matthews CE, et al. Moderate to vigorous physical activity and risk of upper-respiratory tract infection. *Med Sci Sports Exerc* 2002;34:1242.

97. McBride JM, et al. Effect of resistance exercise on free radical production. *Med Sci Sports Exerc* 1998;30:67.

98. Meydani SN, et al. Vitamin E supplementation and in vivo immune response in healthy elderly subjects. *JAMA* 1997;277:1380.

99. Miyazaki H, et al. Strenuous endurance training in humans reduces oxidative stress following exhausting exercise. *Eur J Appl Physiol* 2001;84:1.

100. Müuns G, et al. Impaired nasal mucociliary clearance in long-distance runners. *Int J Sports Med* 1995;16:209.

101. Nehlsen-Cannarella S, et al. Carbohydrate and cytokine response to 2.5 hr of running. *J Appl Physiol* 1997;82:1662.

102. Nieman B, et al. Supplementation patterns in marathon runners. *J Am Diet Assoc* 1989;89:1615.

103. Nieman DC. Physical activity, fitness, and infection. In: Bouchard C, et al, eds. *Physical Activity, Fitness, and Health.* Champaign, IL: Human Kinetics, 1994.

104. Nieman DC. Immune response to heavy exertion. *J Appl Physiol* 1997;82:1385.

105. Nieman DC, Pedersen BK. *Nutrition and Exercise Immunology.* Boca Raton, FL: CRC Press, 2000.

106. Nieman D., et al. Natural killer cell cytotoxic activity in weight trainers and sedentary controls. *J Strength Condit Res* 1994;8:251.

107. Nieman DC, et al. Carbohydrate supplementation affects blood granulocyte and monocyte trafficking but not function following 2.5 hours of running. *Am J Clin Nutr* 1997;66:153.

108. Nieman DC, et al. Influence of mode and carbohydrate on the cytokine response to heavy exertion. *Med Sci Sports Exerc* 1998;30:671.

109. Nieman DC, et al. Cytokine changes after a marathon race. *J Appl Physiol* 2001;91:109.

110. Novas A, et al. Total daily energy expenditure and incidence of upper respiratory tract infection symptoms in young females. *Int J Sports Med* 2002;23:465.

111. Pattwell DM, Jackson MJ. Contraction-induced oxidants as mediators of adaptation and damage in skeletal muscle. *Exer Sport Sci Rev* 2004;32:14.

112. Pedersen BK. Influence of physical activity on the cellular immune system: mechanism of action. *Int J Sports Med* 1991;12:S23.

113. Pedersen BK, Hoffman-Goetz L. Exercise and the immune system: regulation, integration, and adaptation. *Physiol Rev* 2000;80:1055.

114. Pedersen BK, et al. Training and natural immunity: effects of diets rich in fat or carbohydrate. *Eur J Appl Physiol* 2000;82:98.

115. Pendergast DR, et al. The role of dietary fat on performance, metabolism and health. *Am J Sports Med* 1996;24:S53.

116. Peters EM, et al. Vitamin C supplementation reduces the incidence of postrace symptoms of upper-respiratory-tract infection in ultramarathon runners. *Am J Clin Nutr* 1993;57:170.

117. Peters EM, et al. Attenuation of the increase in circulating cortisol and enhancement of the acute phase response in vitamin C-supplemented ultramarathon runners. *Int J Sports Med* 2001;22:120.

118. Peters EM, et al. Vitamin C supplementation attenuates the increases in circulating cortisol, adrenaline and anti-inflammatory polypeptides following ultramarathon running. *Int J Sports Med* 2001;22:537.

119. Peters-Futre EM. Vitamin C, neutrophil function, and URTI risk in distance runners: the missing link. *Exerc Immunol Rev* 1997;3:32.

120. Pitsavos C, et al. Adherence to the Mediterranean diet is associated with total antioxidant capacity in healthy adults: the ATTICA study. *Am J Clin Nutr* 2005;82:694.

121. Popkin BM, et al. A comparison of dietary trends among racial and socioeconomic groups in the United States. *N Engl J Med* 1996;335:716.

122. Position of the American Dietetic Association. Nutrition for physical fitness and athletic performance for adults. *ADA Reports* 1987;87:933.

123 Quindry JC, et al. the effects of acute exercise on neutrophils and plasma oxidative stress. *Med Sci Sports Exerc* 2003;35:1139.

124. Rodriguez Tuya I, et al. Evaluation of the influence of physical activity on plasma concentrations of several trace metals. *Eur J Appl Physiol* 1996;23:299.

125. Rohde T, et al. Competitive sustained exercise in humans, lymphokine activated killer cell activity, and glutamine: an intervention study. *Eur J Appl Physiol* 1998;78:448.

126. Rohde T, et al. Effect of glutamine supplementation on changes in the immune system induced by repeated exercise. *Med Sci Sports Exerc* 1998;30:856.

127. Rokitzke L, et al. Acute changes in vitamin B$_6$ status in endurance athletes before and after a marathon. *Int J Sports Nutr* 1994;4:154.

128. Rokitzki L, et al. α-Tocopherol supplementation in racing cyclists during extreme endurance training. *Int J Sports Nutr* 1994;4:255.

129. Rokitzki L, et al. Assessment of vitamin B$_2$ status in performance athletes of various types of sports. *J Nutr Sci Vitaminol* 1994;40:11.

130. Rokitzki L, et al. Dietary, serum and urine ascorbic acid status in male athletes. *Int J Sports Med* 1994;15:435.

131. Rokitzki L, et al. Lipid peroxidation and antioxidative vitamins under extreme endurance stress. *Acta Physiol Scand* 1994;151:149.

132. Rosen O, et al. Leukocyte counts and lymphocyte responsiveness associated with repeated bouts of strenuous endurance exercise. *J Appl Physiol* 2001;91:425.

133. Rowbottom DG, et al. The emerging role of glutamine as an indicator of exercise stress and overtraining. *Sports Med* 1996;21:80.

134. Sarris WWM, et al. How much physical activity is enough to prevent unhealthy weight gain? Outcome of the IASO 1st Stock Conference and consensus statement. *Obesity Reviews* 2003;4:1201.

135. Scanga CB, et al. Effects of weight loss and exercise training on natural killer cell activity in obese women. *Med Sci Sports Exerc* 1998;30:1668.

136. Scharhag J, et al. Mobilization and oxidative burst of neutrophils are influenced by carbohydrate supplementation during prolonged cycling in humans. *Eur J Appl Physiol* 2002;87:584.

137. Scharhag J, et al. Effects of graded carbohydrate supplementation on the immune response in cycling. *Med Sci Sports Exerc* 2006;38:286.

138. Senturk UK, et al. Exercise-induced oxidative stress affects erythrocytes in sedentary rats but not exercise-trained rats. *J Appl Physiol* 2001;91:1999.

139. Shewchuk LD, et al. Dietary L-glutamine does not improve lymphocyte metabolism or function in exercise-trained rats. *Med Sci Sports Exerc* 1997;29:474.

140. Singh A, et al. Chronic multivitamin-mineral supplementation does not enhance physical performance. *Med Sci Sports Exerc* 1992;24:726.

141. Singh A, et al. Neuroendocrine response to running in women after zinc and vitamin E supplementation. *Med Sci Sports Exerc* 1999;31:536.

142. Sjödin AM, et al. Energy balance in cross-country skiers: a study using doubly labeled water. *Med Sci Sports Exerc* 1994;26:720.

143. Smith DJ, Norris SR. Changes in glutamine and glutamate concentrations for tracking training tolerance. *Med Sci Sports Exerc* 32:684, 2000.

144. Solfrizzi V, et al. High monounsaturated fatty acid intake protects against age-related cognitive decline. *Neurology* 1999;52:1563.

145. Stark AH, Madar Z. Olive oil as a functional food: epidemiology and nutritional approaches. *Nutr Rev* 2002;60:170.

146. Steensberg A, et al. Strenuous exercise decreases the percentage of type 1 T cells in the *circulation. J Appl Physiol* 2001;91:1708.

147. Telford R, et al. The effect of 7 to 8 months of vitamin/mineral supplementation on athletic performance. *Int J Sports Nutr* 1992;2:135.

148. Tiidus PM, Houston ME. Vitamin E status and response to exercise training. *Sports Med* 1995;26:12.

149. Trappe TA, et al. Energy expenditure of swimmers during high volume training. *Med Sci Sports Exerc* 1997;29:950.

150. Trichopoulou A, et al. Adherence to a Mediterranean diet and survival in a Greek population. *N Engl J Med* 2003;348:2599.

151. Uusitalo AL, et al. Overtraining: making a difficult diagnosis and implementing targeted treatment. *Phys Sportsmed* 2001;29(5):35.

152. Van Remmen H, et al. Oxidative damage to DNA and aging. *Exerc Sport Sci Rev* 2003;31;149.

153. Variyam JN, et al. USDA's Healthy Eating Index and nutrition information. Washington, DC: USDA, 1998.

154. Viitala PE, et al. The effects of antioxidant vitamin supplementation on resistance exercise induced lipid peroxidation in trained and untrained participants. *Lipids Health Dis* 2004;3:14.

155. Volek JS, et al. Testosterone and cortisol in relationship to dietary nutrients and resistance exercise. *J Appl Physiol* 1997;82:49.

156. Wagenmakers A, et al. Carbohydrate supplementation, glycogen depletion, and amino acid metabolism. *Am J Physiol* 1991;260:E883.

157. Walsh NP, Blannin AK. Effect of oral glutamine supplementation on human neutrophil lipopolysaccharide-stimulated degranulation following prolonged exercise. *Int J Sport Nutr Exerc Metab* 2000;1:39.

158. Webster MJ, et al. The effect of a thiamin derivative on exercise performance. *Eur J Appl Physiol* 1997;75:520.

159. Weidner TG, et al. The effect of exercise training on the severity and duration of viral upper respiratory illness. *Med Sci Sports Exerc* 1998;30:1578.

160. Weinstock C, et al. Effect of exhaustive exercise stress on the cytokine response. *Med Sci Sports Exerc* 1997;29:345.

161. Wolfe RR. Protein supplements and exercise. *Am J Clin Nutr* 2000;72(suppl):551S.

162. Wolfe RR, et al. Isotopic analysis of leucine and urea metabolism in exercising humans. *J Appl Physiol* 1982;52:458.

163. Woods JA, et al. Exercise and cellular innate immune function. *Med Sci Sports Exerc* 1999;31:57.

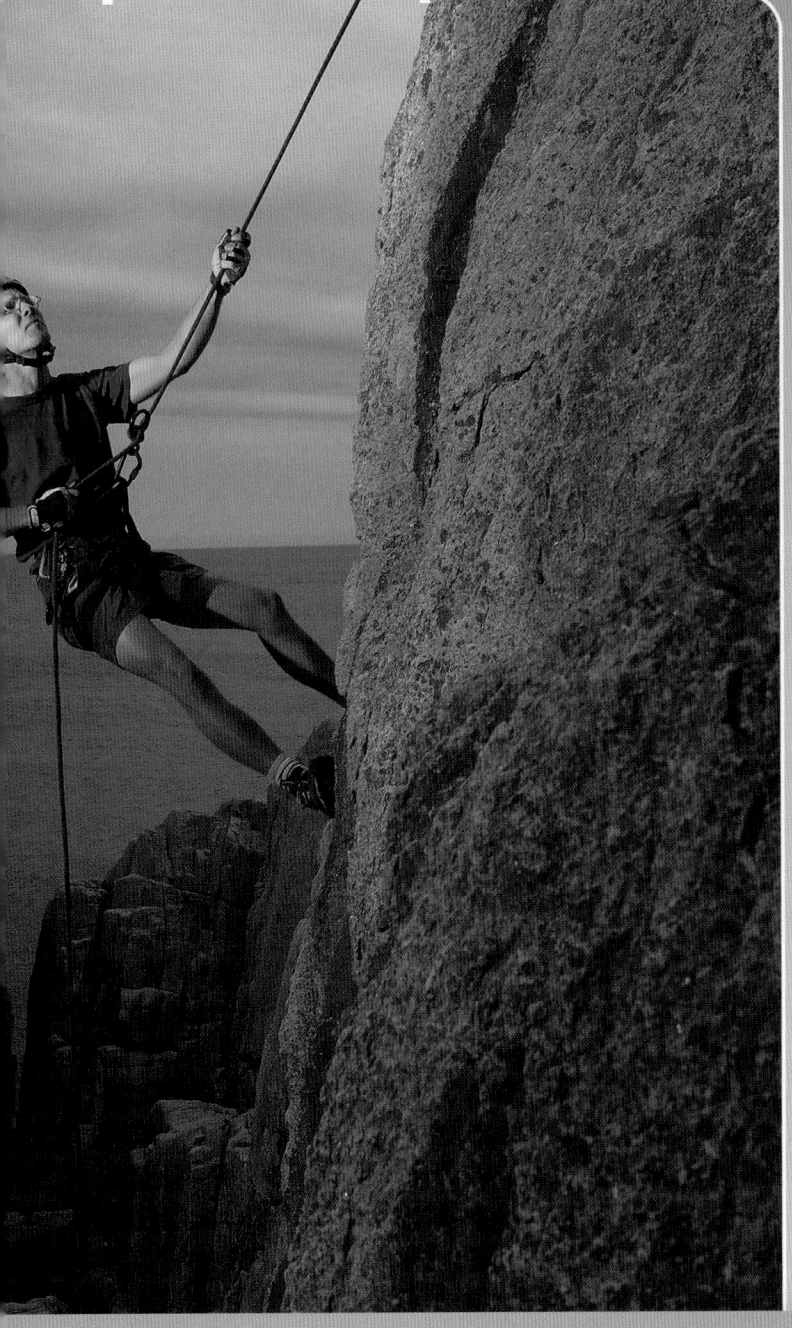

Chapter 8

Nutritional Considerations for Intense Training and Sports Competition

Test Your Knowledge

Answer these 10 statements about intense training and sports competition. Use the scoring key at the end of the chapter to check your results. Repeat this test after you have read the chapter and compare your results.

1. **T F** One should fast for 24 hours before sports competition or intense training to avoid an upset stomach caused by undigested food.

2. **T F** The ideal precompetition meal consists of high-protein foods to ensure elevated levels of muscle protein during competition.

3. **T F** It is unwise to eat during high-intensity aerobic exercise.

4. **T F** The glycemic index indicates the number of calories in different forms of carbohydrate.

5. **T F** Consuming high-glycemic carbohydrates provides the most effective means to rapidly replenish depleted glycogen following intense endurance exercise.

6. **T F** Glycogen reserves in muscle and liver usually replenish within 12 hours when consuming high-glycemic carbohydrates in the immediate postexercise period.

7. **T F** Avoid drinking liquids immediately before vigorous exercise to minimize intestinal disturbance and impaired exercise performance.

8. **T F** Plain cold water serves as the optimal oral rehydration beverage for consumption during exercise.

9. **T F** Sound research supports the wisdom of adding some sodium to an oral rehydration solution, particularly during prolonged exercise in the heat.

10. **T F** Drinking a concentrated sugar drink before and during exercise facilitates rehydration and enhances exercise performance.

The need to maintain optimal nutrient intake to sustain energy and tissue-building requirements of regular physical activity also requires unique dietary modifications to facilitate intense training and competition.

THE PRECOMPETITION MEAL

Athletes often compete in the morning following an overnight fast. As noted out in Chapter 1, considerable depletion occurs in carbohydrate reserves over an 8- to 12-hour period without eating, even if the person normally follows appropriate dietary recommendations. Consequently, precompetition nutrition takes on considerable importance. *The precompetition meal should provide adequate carbohydrate energy and ensure optimal hydration.* Within this framework, fasting before competition or intense training makes no sense physiologically because it rapidly depletes liver and muscle glycogen, which subsequently impairs exercise performance. If a person trains or competes in the afternoon, breakfast becomes the important meal to optimize glycogen reserves. For late afternoon training or competition, lunch becomes the important source for topping off glycogen

stores. Consider the following three factors when individualizing the precompetition meal plan:

1. Food preferences
2. Psychological set
3. Food digestibility

As a general rule, eliminate foods high in lipid and protein content on the day of competition because these foods digest slowly and remain in the digestive tract longer than carbohydrate foods of similar energy content. Timing of the precompetition meal also deserves consideration. The increased stress and tension that usually accompany competition decrease blood flow to the digestive tract, depressing intestinal absorption. *It takes 3 to 4 hours to digest, absorb, and store as muscle and liver glycogen a carbohydrate-rich, precompetition meal.*

Protein or Carbohydrate?

Many athletes become psychologically accustomed to, and even depend on, the classic "steak and eggs" precompetition meal. Such a meal may satisfy the athlete, coach, and restaurateur, but it provides no benefit to exercise performance. This type of meal, with its low carbohydrate content, can hinder optimal exercise performance.

There are five reasons for modifying or even abolishing the high-protein precompetition meal in favor of one high in carbohydrates:

1. Dietary carbohydrates replenish liver and muscle glycogen depletion from the overnight fast.
2. Carbohydrates digest and absorb more rapidly than either proteins or lipids. They provide energy faster and reduce the feeling of fullness following a meal.
3. A high-protein meal elevates resting metabolism considerably more than a high-carbohydrate meal owing to greater energy requirements for digestion, absorption, and assimilation. This additional metabolic heat potentially strains the body's heat-dissipating mechanisms and impairs hot weather exercise performance.
4. Protein breakdown for energy facilitates dehydration during exercise because the by-products of amino acid breakdown require water for urinary excretion. For example, approximately 50 mL of water "accompanies" excretion of each gram of urea in the urine.
5. Carbohydrate serves as the primary energy nutrient for short-term anaerobic activity and for prolonged, high-intensity aerobic exercise.

Make It Carbohydrate Rich

The ideal precompetition meal maximizes muscle and liver glycogen storage and provides glucose for intestinal absorption during exercise. The meal should:

1. Contain 150 to 300 g of carbohydrate (3 to 5 g per kg of body mass in either solid or liquid form)
2. Be consumed 3 to 4 hours before exercising
3. Contain relatively little fat and fiber to facilitate gastric emptying and minimize gastrointestinal distress

The importance of precompetition feeding occurs only if the person maintains a nutritionally sound diet throughout training. Pre-exercise feedings cannot correct existing nutritional deficiencies or inadequate nutrient intake in the weeks before competition. Chapter 11 discusses how endurance athletes can augment precompetition glycogen storage with the specific exercise/diet modifications of carbohydrate loading.

LIQUID AND PREPACKAGED BARS, POWDERS, AND MEALS

Commercially prepared nutrition bars, powders, and liquid meals offer an alternative approach to precompetition feeding or supplemental feedings during periods of competition.[57] These nutrient supplements also effectively enhance energy and nutrient intake in training, particularly if energy output exceeds energy intake from lack of interest or mismanagement of feedings.

Liquid Meals

Liquid meals provide a high-carbohydrate content but contain enough lipid and protein to contribute to satiety. They also can supply the person with fluid because they exist in liquid form. A liquid meal digests rapidly, leaving essentially no residue in the intestinal tract. Liquid meals prove particularly effective during day-long swimming and track meets or during tennis, soccer, and basketball tournaments. In these situations, the person usually has little time for (or interest in) food. Liquid meals offer a practical approach to supplementing caloric intake during the high-energy output phase of training. Athletes can also use liquid nutrition if they have difficulty maintaining body weight and as a ready source of calories to gain weight.

Nutrition Bars

Nutrition bars (called "energy bars," "protein bars," and "diet bars") contain a relatively high protein content that ranges between 10 and 30 g per bar. The typical 60-g bar contains 25 g (100 kCal) of carbohydrate (equal amounts of starch and sugar), 15 g (60 kCal) of protein, and 5 g (45 kCal) of lipid (3 g or 27 kCal of saturated fat), with the remaining weight as water. This represents about 49% of the bar's total 205 calories from carbohydrates, 29% from protein, and 22% from lipid. The bars often include vitamins and minerals (30–50% of recommended values), and some contain dietary supplements such as β-hydroxy-β-methylbutyrate (HMB). These bars must be labeled as dietary supplements, rather than foods.

While nutrition bars provide a relatively easy way to obtain important nutrients, they should not totally substitute for normal food intake because they lack the broad array of plant fibers and phytochemicals found in food and contain a relatively high level of saturated fatty acids. As an added warning, these bars are generally sold as dietary supplements; no independent assessment by the Food and Drug Administration (FDA) or other federal or state agency exists to validate the labeling claims for macronutrient content and composition.

Nutrient Composition of Nutrition Bars Varies with Purpose

So-called energy bars contain a greater proportion of carbohydrates while "diet" or "weight loss" bars are lower in carbohydrate content and higher in protein. "Meal-replacement bars" have the largest energy content (240–310 kCal), with proportionately more of the three macronutrients. "Protein bars" simply contain a larger amount of protein.

Nutrition Powders and Drinks

A high protein content, between 10 and 50 g per serving, represents a unique aspect of nutrition powders and drinks. They also contain added vitamins, minerals, and other dietary supplement ingredients. The powders come in canisters or packets that readily mix with water (or other liquid); the drinks come premixed in cans. These products often serve as an alternative to nutrition bars; they are marketed as meal replacements, dieting aids, energy boosters, or concentrated protein sources.

Nutrient composition of powders and drinks varies considerably from nutrition bars. For one thing, nutrition bars contain at least 15 g of carbohydrates to provide texture and taste, whereas powders and drinks do not. This accounts for the relatively high protein content of powders and drinks. Nutrition powders and drinks generally contain fewer calories per serving than do bars, but this can vary for a powder, depending on the liquid used for mixing.

> ## Supplement Use Among Elite Athletes
>
> A recent survey of high-performance Canadian athletes indicated that 88.4% reported taking one or more dietary supplements during the previous 6 months. Of the supplements used, sport drinks (22.4%), sport bars (14.0%), multivitamins and minerals (13.5%), protein supplements (9.0%), and vitamin C (6.4%) were the most frequently reported.[24]

The recommended serving of a powder averages about 45 g, the same amount as a nutrition bar (minus its water content), but wide variation exists in this recommendation. A typical serving of a high-protein powder mix contains about 10 g of carbohydrate (two thirds as sugar), 30 g of protein, and 2 g of lipid. This amounts to a total of 178 kCal or 23% of calories from carbohydrate, 67% from protein, and 10% from lipid. Thus, when mixed in water, these powdered nutrient supplements far exceed the recommended protein intake percentage and fall below recommended lipid and carbohydrate percentages. A drink typically contains slightly more carbohydrate and less protein than does a powder.

As with nutrition bars, the FDA or other federal or state agency makes no independent assessment of the validity of labeling claims for macronutrient content and composition.

TABLE 8.1 provides the macronutrient composition for commercially packaged liquid food supplements (rapid stomach emptying with low residue and gastrointestinal distress), high-carbohydrate drinks, and "high-energy" bars typically advocated for physically active individuals. Prudent use of some of these supplements can replenish glycogen reserves before and after high-intensity exercise and competition, especially because an athlete's appetite for "normal" food wanes.

CARBOHYDRATE FEEDING BEFORE, DURING, AND FOLLOWING INTENSE EXERCISE

The "vulnerability" of the body's glycogen stores during intense, prolonged exercise has focused considerable research on potential benefits of carbohydrate feedings immediately before and during exercise. This has also included ways to op-

timize carbohydrate replenishment in the postexercise recovery period.

Carbohydrate Feedings Before Exercise

Confusion exists about potential endurance benefits of pre-exercise ingestion of simple sugars. Some in exercise nutrition argue that consuming high-glycemic, rapidly absorbed carbohydrates (see Fig. 8.3) within 1 hour before exercising negatively affects endurance performance in one of two ways:

1. Inducing an overshoot in insulin from the rapid rise in blood sugar. Insulin excess causes a relative hypoglycemia (**rebound hypoglycemia**). Blood sugar reduction impairs central nervous system function during exercise to produce a fatiguing effect.
2. Facilitating glucose influx into muscle (through large insulin release) to increase carbohydrate catabolism for energy in exercise. At the same time, high insulin levels inhibit lipolysis, which reduces free fatty acid mobilization from adipose tissue. Both augmented carbohydrate breakdown and depressed fat mobilization contribute to premature glycogen depletion and early fatigue.

Research in the late 1970s indicated that drinking a highly concentrated sugar solution 30 minutes before exercise precipitated early fatigue in endurance activities. For example, endurance on a bicycle ergometer declined 19% when subjects consumed a 300-mL solution containing 75 g of glucose 30 minutes before exercise compared with riding time preceded by the same volume of plain water or a liquid meal of protein, lipid, and carbohydrate.[27] Paradoxically, consuming the concentrated pre-event sugar drink (in contrast to drinking plain water) prematurely depleted muscle glycogen reserves. This occurred because the dramatic rise in blood sugar within 5 to 10 minutes after ingestion produced an overshoot in insulin release from the pancreas (accentuated hyperinsulinemia) followed by a rapid decline in blood sugar (rebound hypoglycemia) as glucose moved rapidly into muscle.[35,108] At the same time, insulin inhibited fat mobilization for energy, an effect that can last for several hours after consuming a concentrated sugar solution. During exercise, therefore, intramuscular carbohydrate catabolized to a greater degree than under normal conditions. This increased the rate of glycogen depletion.

These negative research findings seem impressive and their explanation reasonable, yet subsequent investigations have *not* been replicated in healthy subjects[1,19,26,32] or patients with type 1 diabetes.[70] In fact, pre-exercise glucose ingestion *increased* muscle glucose uptake but *reduced* liver glucose output during exercise, to conserve liver glycogen.[52] The discrepancy among studies has no clear explanation. One way to eliminate any potential for negative effects of pre-exercise simple sugars is to consume them at least 60 minutes before exercising. This provides sufficient time to re-establish hormonal balance before exercise begins. In all likelihood, individual differences exist in the response to specific carbohydrate ingestion before exercise and the subsequent insulin release. The

---

TABLE 8.1 Composition of Commercial Carbohydrate Supplements in Liquid and Solid Form

Sports Nutrition and "Metabolic Optimizer"

Beverage	kCal per 8-oz Serving	Carbohydrate, g	Lipid, g	Protein, g
GatorPro Sports Nutrition	360	58 (65%)	7 (17%)	16 (18%)
Nutrament	240	34 (57%)	6.5 (25%)	11 (18%)
SportShake	310	45 (58%)	10 (29%)	11 (13%)
SegoVery	180	30 (67%)	2.5 (13%)	9 (20%)
Go	190	27 (56%)	3 (13%)	15 (31%)
Sustacal	240	33 (55%)	5.5 (21%)	14.5 (24%)
Ensure	254	35 (54%)	9 (32%)	9 (14%)
Endura Optimizer	279	57 (82%)	<1 (2%)	11 (16%)
Metabolol II	258	40 (62%)	2 (7%)	20 (31%)
ProOptibol	266	44 (66%)	2 (7%)	18 (27%)
Muscle Pep	261	45 (69%)	1 (3%)	18 (28%)
Protein Repair Formula	200	26 (52%)	1.5 (8%)	20 (40%)

High Carbohydrate Beverages

Beverage	Carbohydrate, type	Serving Size, oz	Carbohydrate, g per oz	% Carbohydrate
GatorLode	Maltodextrin & glucose	12	5.9	20
Carboplex	Maltodextrin		7.1	24
Exceed	Maltodextrin & sucrose	32	7.1	24
Carbo Fire	Glucose, polymers, fructose		7.1	24
Ultra Fuel	Maltodextrin	16	6.25	23
Carbo Power	Maltodextrin, high-fructose corn syrup		7.9	18

Sports Energy Bars

Bar	Size, oz	Total kCal	Carbohydrate, g	Protein, g	Lipid, g
Power Bar	2.25	225	42 (75%)	10 (17%)	2 (8%)
Exceed Sports Bar	2.9	280	53 (76%)	12 (17%)	2 (7%)
Edgebar	2.5	234	44 (75%)	10 (17%)	2 (8%)
K-Trainer	2.25	220	40 (73%)	10 (18%)	2 (9%)
Tiger Sport	2.3	230	40 (70%)	11 (19%)	3 (11%)
Thunder Bar	2.25	220	41 (74%)	10 (18%)	2 (8%)
Ultra Fuel	4.87	290	100 (82%)	15 (12%)	3 (6%)
Clif Bar	2.4	252	52 (80%)	5 (8%)	3 (12%)
Gator Bar	2.25	220	48 (87%)	3 (5%)	2 (8%)
Forza	2.5	231	45 (78%)	10 (18%)	1 (4%)
BTU Stoker	2.6	252	46 (73%)	10 (16%)	3 (11%)
PR Bar	1.6	190	19 (40%)	14 (30%)	6 (30%)

Carbohydrate content of common foods: 4 chocolate chip cookies = 28 g; 1 cup Wheaties (1 oz) = 23 g; 1 apple = 21 g; 1 cup apple juice = 29 g; 1 banana = 27 g

Protein content of common foods: 1 cup milk = 8 g; 3 oz baked salmon = 21 g; 1 cup cooked peas = 16 g; 3 oz steak = 22 g; 1 large egg = 6 g.

---

individual's pre-exercise glucose or glycogen status plays a role including the glycemic index of food ingested (see page 239).

Pre-exercise Fructose: Not a Good Alternative

Fructose absorbs more slowly from the gut than either glucose or sucrose. This causes only minimal insulin response with essentially no decline in blood glucose. These observations have stimulated debate about the possible benefits of fructose as an immediate pre-exercise exogenous carbohydrate fuel source for prolonged exercise. The theoretical rationale for fructose use appears plausible, but its exercise benefits remain inconclusive. From a practical standpoint, consuming a high-fructose beverage often produces gastrointestinal distress (vomiting and diarrhea); this negatively affects exercise performance. Once absorbed by the small intestine, fructose must first enter the liver for conversion to glucose. This further limits how quickly fructose becomes available as an energy source.

Carbohydrate Feedings During Exercise

High-intensity aerobic exercise for 1 hour decreases liver glycogen by about 55%, whereas a 2-hour strenuous workout almost totally depletes the glycogen content of the liver and exercised muscles (muscle fibers). Even maximal, repetitive 1- to 5-minute bouts of exercise interspersed with periods of lower intensity exercise—as occurs in soccer, ice hockey, field hockey, European handball, and tennis—dramatically lower liver and muscle glycogen reserves.[37,83] Physical and mental performance improves with carbohydrate supplementation during exercise.[2,99,103,106] The addition of protein to the car-bohydrate-containing beverage (4:1 ratio of carbohydrate to protein) may augment time to fatigue and reduce muscle damage compared to supplementation during exercise with carbohydrate only.[78] Carbohydrate feedings during prolonged exercise also allow individuals to exercise at greater intensity, although their perception of physical effort remains no different than for a placebo group.[92]

No Abnormal Insulin Response During Exercise

Consuming high-glycemic sugars *during* exercise does *not* augment the insulin response (and possible resulting hypoglycemia) that could occur with sugar consumption in the pre-exercise condition. This occurs because sympathetic nervous system hormones in exercise inhibit insulin release. Concurrently, exercise augments glucose uptake by muscle so the exogenous glucose moves into these cells with a lower insulin requirement.

Consuming about 60 g of liquid or solid carbohydrates each hour benefits high-intensity, long-duration ($\geq$1 h) aerobic exercise and repetitive short bouts of near-maximal effort.[3,15,44,58] As discussed in Chapter 5, sustained exercise at or below 50% of maximum intensity relies primarily on energy from fat oxidation, with relatively little demand on carbohydrate breakdown. This level of exercise does not tax glycogen reserves to a degree that would limit endurance. On the other hand, glucose feedings provide supplementary carbohydrate during intense exercise when glycogen demand for energy increases greatly. In fact, mixtures of glucose, fructose, and sucrose ingested simultaneously at a high rate (between 1.8 and 2.4 g · min^{-1}) result in a 20 to 55% higher exogenous carbohydrate oxidation rate peak as high as 1.7 g · min^{-1} (with reduced oxidation of endogenous carbohydrate) compared with ingestion of an isocaloric amount of glucose.[12,43,76,77] Exogenous carbohydrate intake during exercise provides the following two benefits:

1. Spares muscle glycogen, particularly in the type I, slow-twitch muscle fibers, because the ingested glucose powers exercise.[89–91]
2. Maintains a more optimal level of blood glucose. This elevates plasma insulin levels and lowers cortisol and growth hormone levels and prevents headache, lightheadedness, nausea, and other symptoms of central nervous system distress.[10,63,109] Blood glucose maintenance also supplies muscles with glucose when glycogen reserves deplete in the later stages of prolonged exercise.[18,34]

FIGURE 8.1 shows that training status does not alter the ability to oxidize glucose during exercise when the trained and untrained exercise at the same relative intensity. Seven trained cyclists and seven untrained subjects exercised for 2 hours at 60% of aerobic capacity. At the onset of exercise, each subject consumed 8 mL · kg^{-1} of an 8% naturally labeled [^{13}C]-glucose solution with 2 mL · kg^{-1} of the fluid ingested every 20 minutes thereafter. Total exogenous [^{13}C]-glucose use (3.2 kCal · min^{-1}) was similar in both groups despite a 24% higher absolute oxygen uptake in the trained subjects (36 vs. 29 mL O$_2$ · kg^{-1} · min^{-1}; FIG. 8.1A) and higher total fat oxidation. (About 1.5–1.7

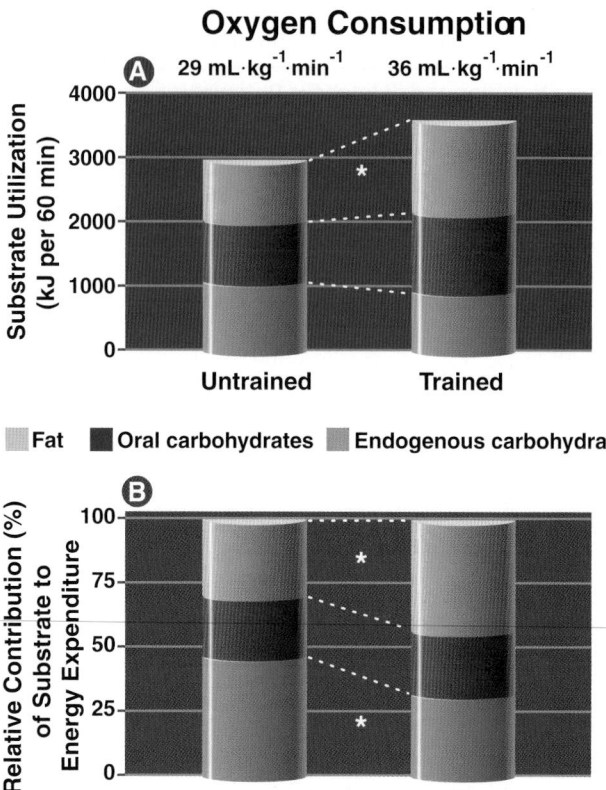

FIGURE 8.1 ■ **A,** Absolute (kJ per 60-min of exercise) and **B,** relative (%) contributions of substrates to energy expenditure in endurance trained and untrained men. (*) indicates statistically significant difference between trained and untrained. Multiply by 0.239 to convert kilojoules to kilocalories. (From Jeukendrup AE, et al. Exogenous glucose oxidation during exercise in endurance-trained and untrained subjects. *J Appl Physiol* 1997;83:835.)

g [6.0–to 6.8 kCal] per minute represents the upper limit for oxidizing exogenous carbohydrate.[43,45,100,101]) Equivalence in exogenous glucose use between trained and untrained subjects occurred even with a relatively smaller contribution of exogenous and endogenous carbohydrate to the higher total energy expenditure of the trained subjects (Fig. 8.1 B). This suggests that carbohydrate absorption from the gastrointestinal tract into the circulation limits ingested carbohydrate's catabolism rate during exercise independent of training state.

Keep It Glucose

Do not substitute exogenous fructose for glucose during prolonged exercise, because less fructose oxidizes when consuming equivalent amounts of both sugars.[53]

A Distinct Ergogenic Advantage in Intense Aerobic Exercise

Carbohydrate feeding during exercise at 60 to 80% of aerobic capacity postpones fatigue by 15 to 30 minutes, with performance improvement generally ranging between 15 and 35%. This effect, potentially important in marathon running, occurs because fatigue in well-nourished individuals usually becomes noticeable within 2 hours of intense exercise. A person can ward off fatigue and extend endurance with a single concentrated carbohydrate feeding approximately 30 minutes before anticipated fatigue. FIGURE 8.2 shows that this feeding restores the level of blood glucose, which then sustains the energy needs of active muscles.

Endurance benefits from carbohydrate feedings become apparent at about 75% of aerobic capacity. When exercise initially exceeds this intensity, an individual must reduce intensity to the 75% level during the final stages to maintain the benefits from carbohydrate intake.[18] Repeated feedings of solid carbohydrate (43 g sucrose with 400 mL water) at the beginning and at 1, 2, and 3 hours during exercise maintain blood glucose and slows glycogen depletion during 4 hours of cycling. Maintaining blood glucose and glycogen reserves also enhances high-intensity exercise performance to exhaustion at the end of the activity.[3,5,73,85] The winner of a marathon run is usually the athlete who sustains high-intensity aerobic effort and sprints to the finish.

REPLENISHING GLYCOGEN RESERVES: REFUELING FOR THE NEXT BOUT OF INTENSE TRAINING OR COMPETITION

All carbohydrates do not digest and absorb at the same rate. Plant starch composed primarily of amylose represents a resistant carbohydrate because of its relatively slow hydrolysis rate. Conversely, starch with relatively high amylopectin content digests and absorbs more rapidly.

The Glycemic Index

*The **glycemic index** serves as a relative (qualitative) indicator of how carbohydrate-containing food affects blood glucose levels.* The rise in blood sugar—termed the *glycemic response*—is determined after ingesting a food containing 50 g of a digestible carbohydrate (total carbohydrate minus fiber) and comparing it over a 2-hour period with a "standard" for carbohydrate (usually white bread or glucose) with an assigned value of 100.[7,107] The glycemic index expresses the percentage of total area under the blood glucose response curve for a specific food compared with glucose (FIG. 8.3). Thus, a food with a glycemic index of 45 indicates that ingesting 50 g of the food raises blood glucose concentrations to levels that reach 45% of that reached with 50 g of glucose. The glycemic index provides a more useful physiologic concept than simply classifying a carbohydrate on the basis of its chemical configuration as simple or complex, sugar or starch, or available or unavail-

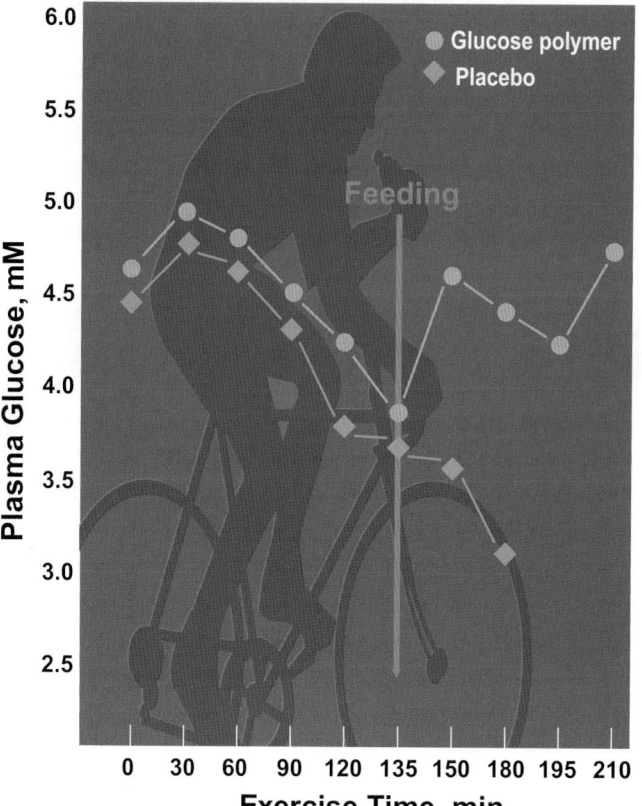

FIGURE 8.2 ■ Average plasma glucose concentration during prolonged high-intensity aerobic exercise when subjects consumed either a placebo or glucose polymer (3 g per kg body mass in a 50% solution). (Modified from Coggan AR, Coyle EF. Metabolism and performance following carbohydrate ingestion late in exercise. *Med Sci Sports Exerc* 1989;21:59.)

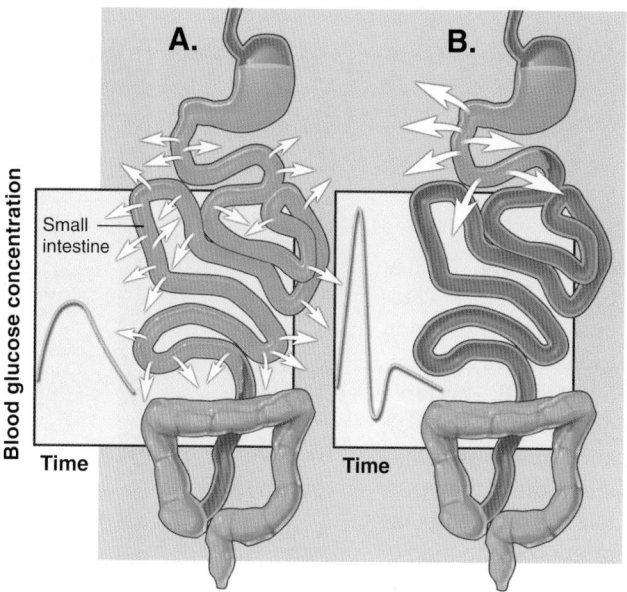

FIGURE 8.3 ■ General response of intestinal glucose absorption following feeding of foods with either **(A)** low glycemic index or **(B)** high glycemic index such as glucose. The low glycemic food absorbs at a slower rate throughout the full length of the small intestine to produce a more gradual rise in blood glucose.

Not Simply the Carbohydrate Form

The glycemic index is a function of glucose appearance in the systemic circulation and its uptake by peripheral tissues, which is influenced by the properties of the carbohydrate-containing food. For example, the food's amylose to amylopectin ratio and its fiber and fat content influence intestinal glucose absorption, whereas the protein content of the food may augment insulin release to facilitate tissue glucose uptake.[79]

able. One international listing of glycemic index values contains nearly 1300 entries that represent values of more than 750 different food types.[28] Differences in values exist within the literature, depending on the laboratory and exact food type evaluated (e.g., slight variations in type of white bread, rice, and potatoes used as the standard of comparison). Do not view the glycemic index as an unwavering standard because considerable variability exists among individuals consuming a specific carbohydrate-containing food. A high glycemic index rating does not necessarily indicate poor nutritional quality.[68] For example, carrots, brown rice, and corn, with their rich quantities of health-protective micronutrients, phytochemicals, and dietary fiber, have relatively high indices.

Individual differences in response to how food is digested and its preparation and ripeness affect the glycemic index. For example, a ripe banana has a higher glycemic index than a "greener" banana. Once foods are combined (i.e., a ripe banana eaten with three flavors of ice cream topped with nuts and chocolate fudge), the meal's glycemic index for that com-

bination of foods differs from the glycemic index for the separate items.

The revised glycemic index listing also includes the **glycemic load** associated with the specified serving sizes of different foods. Whereas the glycemic index compares equal quantities of a carbohydrate-containing food, the glycemic load quantifies the overall glycemic effect of a typical *portion* of food. This represents the product of the amount of available carbohydrate in that serving and the glycemic index of the food. A high glycemic load reflects a greater expected elevation in blood glucose and a greater insulin release. An increased risk for type 2 diabetes and coronary heart disease coincides with the chronic consumption of a diet with a high glycemic load.[41,50]

Not All Carbohydrates Are Equal

FIGURE 8.4A lists the glycemic index for common items in various food groupings. Inset table (B) gives examples of high- and low-glycemic index meals of similar calorie and macronutrient composition. For easy identification, we have placed foods into high, medium, and low categories for glycemic index. Interestingly, a food's index rating does not depend simply on its classification as a "simple" (mono- and disaccharides) or "complex" (starch and fiber) carbohydrate. This is because the plant starch in white rice and potatoes has a higher glycemic index than the simple sugars (particularly fructose) in apples and peaches. A food's fiber content slows digestion rate; thus, many vegetables (e.g., peas, beans, and other legumes) have a low glycemic index. Ingesting lipids and proteins tends to slow the passage of food into the small intestine, thus reducing the glycemic index of the meal's accompanying carbohydrate content. *Clearly, the most rapid method to replenish glycogen after exercise is to consume foods*

FIGURE 8.4 ■ **A.** Glycemic index categorization of common food sources of carbohydrates. **B.** This table gives examples of high and low glycemic-index diets that contain the same amounts of energy and macronutrients and derive 50% of energy from carbohydrate (CHO) and 30% of energy from lipid. (Diets from Brand-Miller J, Foster-Powell K. *Nutr Today* 1999;34:64.)

A High glycemic	
Glucose	100
Carrots	92
Honey	87
Corn flakes	80
Whole meal bread	72
White rice	72
New potatoes	70
White bread	69
Shredded wheat	67
Brown rice	66
Beets	64
Raisins	64
Bananas	62

Moderate glycemic	
Corn	59
Sucrose	59
All-bran	51
Potato-chips	51
Peas	51
White pasta	50
Oatmeal	49
Sweet potatoes	48
Whole wheat pasta	42
Oranges	40

Low glycemic	
Apples	39
Fish sticks	38
Butter beans	36
Navy beans	31
Kidney beans	29
Lentils	29
Sausage	28
Fructose	20
Peanuts	13

B	High GI Diet			Low GI Diet		
		CHO (g)	Contribution to Total GI		CHO (g)	Contribution to Total GI
	Breakfast			**Breakfast**		
	30 g Corn Flakes	25	9.9	30 g All-Bran	24	4.7
	1 banana	30	7.8	1 diced peach	8	1.1
	1 slice whole meal bread	12	3.8	1 slice grain bread	14	2.2
	1 tsp margarine			1 tsp margarine		
				1 tsp jelly		
	Snack			**Snack**		
	1 crumpet	20	6.4	1 slice grain fruit loaf	20	4.1
	1 tsp margarine			1 tsp margarine		
	Lunch			**Lunch**		
	2 slices whole-meal bread	23.5	7.6	2 slices grain bread	28	4.5
	2 tsp margarine			2 tsp margarine		
	25 g cheese			25 g cheese		
	1 cup diced cantaloupe	8	10.4	1 apple	20	3.6
	Snack			**Snack**		
	4 plain sweet biscuits	28	10.4	200 g low-fat fruit yogurt	26	4.1
	Dinner			**Dinner**		
	120 g lean steak			120 g lean minced beef		
	1 cup of mashed potatoes	32	12.1	1 cup boiled pasta	34	6.4
	1/2 cup of carrots	4	1.7	1 cup of tomato and onion sauce	8	2.5
	1/2 cup of green beans	2	0.6	Green salad with vinaigrette	1	0.6
	50 g broccoli					
	Snack			**Snack**		
	290 g watermelon	15	5.1	1 orange	10	2.1
	1 cup of reduced-fat milk throughout day	14	1.9	1 cup of reduced-fat milk throughout day	14	1.9
	Total	212	69.8	**Total**	212	39.0

For each diet, the carbohydrate choices are maximized for differences between the two diets.

with moderate-to-high glycemic indices rather than foods rated low,[11,19,20,84,102] *even if the replenishment meal contains a small amount of lipid and protein.*[12] In fact, the addition of liquid protein to the carbohydrate supplement may even enhance the magnitude of glycogen resynthesis.[6] During the first 2 hours of recovery, when muscle glycogen content is at its lowest level, consuming a glucose polymer solution (low osmolality) restores glycogen more rapidly than an energy-equivalent solution of monomers with high osmolality.[67] This beneficial effect of low-osmolality solutions on glycogen replenishment probably results from two factors: (1) more rapid gastric emptying and glucose delivery to the small intestine and (2) augmented postexercise-stimulated non–insulin-dependent glucose uptake by the muscles. The addition of L-arginine to a carbohydrate-containing beverage offers no additional benefit to carbohydrate replenishment.[74]

The need for glycogen in previously active muscle augments glycogen resynthesis in the postexercise period.[65] When food becomes available after exercise, the following four factors facilitate cellular uptake of glucose:

1. Hormonal milieu reflected by elevated insulin
2. Increased tissue sensitivity to insulin and other transporter proteins (e.g., GLUT 1 and GLUT 4, members of a family of facilitative monosaccharide transporters that mediate much of glucose transport activity)
3. Low catecholamine levels
4. Increased activity of a specific form of the glycogen-storing enzyme glycogen synthase

To speed glycogen replenishment after intense training or competition, one should consume high-glycemic carbohydrate-rich foods as soon as possible. Follow this practical advice to rapidly restore depleted glycogen reserves: Within 15 minutes after stopping exercise, consume 50 to 75 g (2–3 oz, or 1.0–1.5 g per kg body mass) of high- to moderate-glycemic carbohydrates. Continue eating 50 to 75 g of carbohydrate every 2 hours until achieving 500 to 700 g (7–10 g per kg of body mass) or until eating a large high-carbohydrate meal. If immediately ingesting carbohydrate after exercise proves impractical, an alternative strategy involves eating meals containing 2.5 g of high-glycemic carbohydrate per kg body mass at 2, 4, 6, 8, and 22 hours postexercise. This replenishes glycogen to levels similar to those achieved with the same protocol begun immediately postexercise.[64]

Insulin-Stimulating Effect of Protein Ingestion in Recovery: Does It Augment Glycogen Replenishment?

Consuming an amino acid-protein mixture of wheat protein hydrolysate with free leucine and phenylalanine ($0.4 \text{ g} \cdot \text{kg}^{-1} \cdot \text{h}^{-1}$) in a carbohydrate-containing beverage ($0.8 \text{ g} \cdot \text{kg}^{-1} \cdot \text{h}^{-1}$) facilitates more muscle glycogen storage without gastrointestinal discomfort than ingesting a carbohydrate-only beverage of the same concentration.[94] This advantage appears to relate to the insulinotropic effect of a higher level of plasma amino acids.[93,110] The benefit of added protein and/or amino acids (and the associated increased insulin release) on glyco-

gen replenishment, however, is no greater than achieved by simply adding additional carbohydrate to the recovery supplement.[75] For example, trained athletes attained glycogen synthesis rates equivalent to those with a glucose plus protein supplement with a carbohydrate-only intake of $1.2 \text{ g} \cdot \text{kg}^{-1} \cdot \text{h}^{-1}$.[94] Supplements were given at 30-minute intervals over a 5-hour recovery period. This replenishment protocol produced maximal glycogen resynthesis. Additional intake of protein or amino acids, while increasing the insulin response, does not increase the rate of glycogen synthesis.

What Is the Optimal Approach?

Research has addressed the following question: Is it better to consume large meals or more frequent snacks of high-glycemic carbohydrates to optimize glycogen replenishment? One study compared 24-hour carbohydrate replenishment with two patterns of consuming an energy-equivalent meal of high-glycemic carbohydrates: (1) "gorging" on a single large meal, with its greater incremental glucose and insulin response or (2) "nibbling" on frequent smaller snacks, which produces a more stable glucose and insulin response.[13] The two styles of eating produced *no difference* in final glycogen levels. These findings indicate that individuals should eat high-glycemic carbohydrates following intense exercise; the frequency of the meals and snacks should dovetail with a person's appetite and the availability of food after exercising.

Glycogen Replenishment Takes Time

Avoid legumes, fructose, and milk products when rapidly replenishing glycogen reserves because of their slow rates of intestinal absorption. More-rapid glycogen resynthesis takes place if the person remains inactive during recovery.[17] *With optimal carbohydrate intake, glycogen stores replenish at about 5 to 7% per hour. Thus, even under the best of circumstances, it takes at least 20 hours to re-establish glycogen stores following a glycogen-depleting exercise bout.*

Optimal glycogen replenishment benefits individuals involved in (1) regular intense training, (2) tournament competition with qualifying rounds, or (3) competitive events scheduled with only 1 or 2 days for recuperation. Before current methods for establishing a wrestler's minimal wrestling weight (see Chapter 14), wrestlers who lost considerable glycogen (and water) using food and fluid restriction before the weigh-in to "make weight" also benefited from a proper glycogen replenishment strategy.[40] For collegiate wrestlers, short-term weight loss through energy restriction without dehydration also impaired anaerobic exercise capacity.[71] Anaerobic performance recovered to near-baseline values when these athletes then consumed meals containing 75% carbohydrate (21 kCal per kg body mass) over the next 5 hours. No improvement occurred if the refeeding diet contained only 45% carbohydrate. Even without full glycogen replenishment, some replenishment in recovery benefits endurance in the next exercise bout. For example, replenishing carbohydrate after only a 4-hour recovery period from glycogen-depleting exercise yields better endurance in subsequent exercise than a similar scenario with no carbohydrate eaten in recovery.

Choose the Right Form of Carbohydrate

To evaluate the influence of a carbohydrate's structure on glycogen replenishment, eight male cyclists decreased the glycogen content of the vastus lateralis muscle with 60-minutes of cycling at 75% $\dot{V}O_{2max}$ followed by six 1-minute sprints at 125% $\dot{V}O_{2max}$.[46] Twelve hours after the glycogen-depleting exercise, they consumed a 3000-kCal meal (ratio of 65%:20%:15% carbohydrate to lipid to protein). A solution of glucose, maltodextrin (glucose polymer), waxy starch (100% amylopectin), or resistant starch (100% amylose) provided all of the recovery meal's carbohydrate. Muscle biopsies 24 hours into recovery (FIG. 8.5) revealed a lower glycogen repletion level from the resistant starch meal (high amylose

content, low glycemic index) than from meals with the other, more rapidly hydrolyzed carbohydrates. Keeping to the prescribed carbohydrate intake in the immediate recovery period produces more desirable glycogen replenishment than letting athletes eat the amount they wish.

THE GLYCEMIC INDEX AND PRE-EXERCISE FEEDINGS

Use the glycemic index to formulate the immediate pre-exercise feeding. The ideal meal immediately before exercising should provide a source of glucose to maintain blood sugar and sustain muscle metabolism; it also should not trigger a spike in insulin release. A relatively normal plasma insulin level theoretically preserves blood glucose availability and optimizes fat mobilization and catabolism while sparing glycogen reserves. As mentioned previously, consuming simple sugars (concentrated high-glycemic carbohydrates) immediately before exercising causes blood sugar to rise rapidly (**glycemic response**), often triggering excessive insulin release (**insulinemic response**). The resulting rebound hypoglycemia, depressed fat catabolism, and possible early depletion of glycogen reserves negatively affect endurance exercise performance.

In contrast, consuming low-glycemic index foods (starch with high amylose content) immediately before exercise provides a relatively slow rate of glucose absorption into the blood. This eliminates any possible insulin surge, while a steady supply of "slow-release" glucose becomes available from the digestive tract as exercise progresses. This effect theoretically proves beneficial during long-term, intense exercise, particularly in unusual events such as ocean swimming where the practicality of consuming carbohydrate during exercise remains a challenge.[105]

Several studies support the wisdom of consuming low-glycemic carbohydrates (starch with high amylose content or moderate-glycemic carbohydrate with high dietary fiber content) in the immediate 45- to 60-minute period before exercise, which allows for a slower rate of glucose absorption; this reduces the potential rebound glycemic response. For trained cyclists who performed high-intensity aerobic exercise, a pre-exercise low-glycemic meal of lentils significantly extended endurance over that with feedings of either glucose or a high-glycemic meal of potatoes of equivalent carbohydrate content.[11] Higher blood glucose levels near the end stages of exercise accompanied the low-glycemic, pre-exercise feeding.[22,33] Despite inducing potentially favorable alterations in blood glucose and fat catabolism, all research has not observed ergogenic benefits from low-glycemic pre-exercise carbohydrates.[26,32,88] Further study of the topic seems warranted.

GLUCOSE, ELECTROLYTES, AND WATER UPTAKE

As we discuss in Chapter 10, fluid ingestion before and during exercise minimizes the detrimental effects of dehydration on cardiovascular dynamics, temperature regulation, and exercise

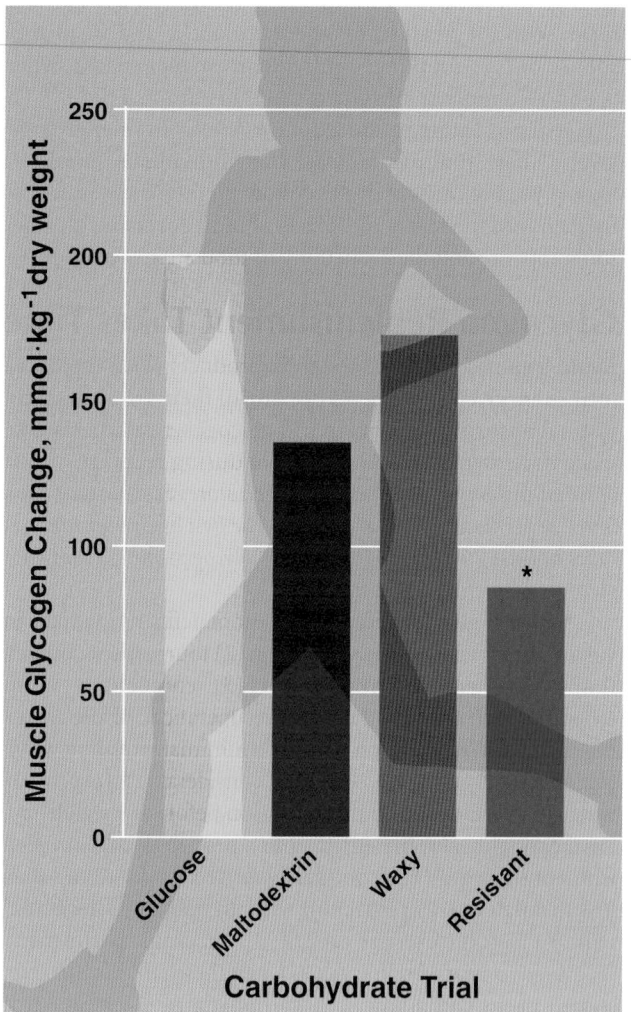

FIGURE 8.5 ■ Changes in muscle glycogen with various carbohydrate feedings of similar energy content in the 24-hour period following glycogen-depleting exercise. (*) Denotes significantly lower value than glucose, maltodextrin, and waxy starch. (From Jozsi AC, et al. The influence of starch structure on glycogen resynthesis and subsequent cycling performance. *Int J Sports Med* 1996;17:373.)

performance. *Adding carbohydrate to the **oral rehydration beverage** provides additional glucose energy for exercise as glycogen reserves deplete. Adding electrolytes to the rehydration beverage maintains the thirst mechanism and reduces the risk of hyponatremia* (see Chapter 10). The coach and athletes should work together to determine the optimal fluid/carbohydrate mixture and volume to minimize fatigue and prevent dehydration. Concern focuses on the dual observations that a large fluid volume intake impairs carbohydrate uptake, while a concentrated sugar/electrolyte solution impairs fluid replacement.

Important Considerations

Stomach emptying rate greatly affects fluid and nutrient absorption by the small intestine. FIGURE 8.6 illustrates important factors that influence gastric emptying. Little negative effect of exercise on gastric emptying occurs until an intensity of about 75% of maximum, after which, emptying rate slows.[49] Gastric volume, however, greatly influences gastric emptying because emptying rate declines exponentially as fluid volume decreases. *A major factor to speed gastric emptying and compensate for any inhibitory effects of the beverage's carbohydrate content involves maintaining a relatively large stomach fluid volume.*

Practical Recommendations

Consuming 400 to 600 mL of fluid 20 minutes before exercise optimizes the beneficial effect of increased stomach volume on fluid and nutrient passage into the small intestine. Regularly ingesting 150 to 250 mL of fluid (at 15-minute intervals) throughout exercise continually replenishes fluid passed into the intestine; this maintains a relatively large and constant gastric volume.[4,23,47,62] This protocol delivers about 1 L of fluid per hour to the small intestine, a volume that meets the needs of most endurance athletes. Prior research indicated that colder fluid emptied from the stomach more rapidly than fluid at room temperature, yet fluid temperature does *not* exert a major influence during exercise. Beverages containing alcohol or caffeine induce a diuretic effect (alcohol most pronounced), which facilitates water loss. Both beverages are contraindicated for fluid replacement.

Consider Fluid Concentration

Concern exists about the potential negative effect of sugar drinks on water absorption from the digestive tract. Gastric emptying slows when ingested fluids either contain increased concentrations of particles in solution (osmolality) or possess high caloric content.[8,72] Rehydration beverages hypertonic to plasma (>280 mOsm $\cdot$ kg^{-1}) retard net fluid uptake by the intestine. This negatively affects prolonged exercise in hot weather, when adequate fluid intake *and* absorption play prime roles in the participant's health and safety. The negative effect of concentrated sugar molecules on gastric emptying is diminished (and plasma volume maintained) if the drink contains a short-chain glucose polymer (**maltodextrin**) rather than simple sugars. Short-chain polymers (3–20 glucose units) derived from cornstarch breakdown reduce the number of particles in solution. Fewer particles facilitate water movement from the stomach for intestinal absorption.

Adding a small amount of glucose and sodium (glucose being the more important factor) to the oral rehydration solution does not negatively affect gastric emptying. It also facilitates fluid uptake by the intestinal lumen because rapid cotransport of glucose–sodium across the intestinal mucosa stimulates water's passive uptake by osmotic action.[29,30,81] Water replenishes effectively, and the additional glucose uptake contributes to blood glucose maintenance. This glucose then spares muscle and liver glycogen, and/or provides blood glucose should glycogen reserves fall during the later stage of exercise.

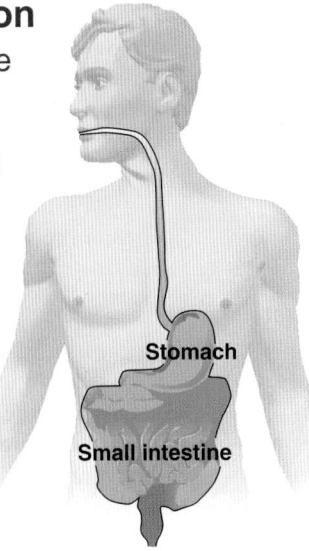

Intestinal Fluid Absorption
- Carbohydrate: low to moderate level of glucose + sodium *increases* fluid absorption
- Sodium: low to moderate level *increases* fluid absorption
- Osmolality: hypotonic to isotonic fluids containing NaCl and glucose *increase* fluid absorption

Stomach

Small intestine

Gastric Emptying
- Volume: *increased* volume *increases* emptying rate
- Caloric content: *increased* energy content *decreases* emptying rate
- Osmality: *increased* solute concentration *decreases* emptying rate
- Exercise: intensity exceeding rate of 75% of maximum *decreases* empting rate
- pH: marked deviations from 7.0 *decrease* emptying rate
- Hydration level: dehydration *decreases* gastric emptying and *increases* risk of gastrointestinal distress

FIGURE 8.6 ■ Major factors that affect gastric emptying (stomach) and fluid absorption (small intestine).

Rehydration solutions that combine two different transportable carbohydrate substrates (glucose, fructose, sucrose, or maltodextrins) produce greater water uptake at a particular intestinal lumen osmolality than solutions containing only one substrate from enhanced solute flux (and thus water flux) from the intestine (FIG. 8.7). The second substrate stimulates more intestinal transport mechanisms, thus facilitating net water absorption by osmosis.

POTENTIAL BENEFIT OF SODIUM. Adding moderate amounts of sodium (the most abundant ion in the extracellular space) to the ingested fluid minimally affects glucose absorption and does not

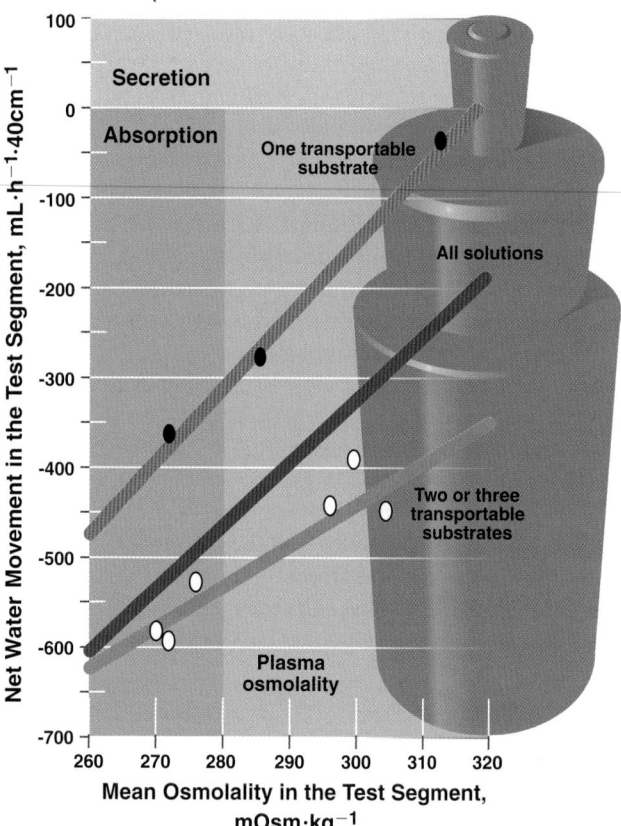

FIGURE 8.7 ■ Net water movement related to mean osmolality in the intestinal test segment. Water absorption from the intestine shows as a negative value (high negative values indicate greater absorption) while secretion into the intestinal lumen would show as a positive value. The *purple line* shows the relationship among the three test solutions containing one transportable substrate, while the *orange line* refers to six solutions containing two or three transportable substrates. The middle line *(red)* represents the relationship among all test solutions. For each test solution, net water absorption increases as osmolality decreases. However, for any osmolality value, greater net water absorption occurs from the gut into the body with solutions containing more than one transportable substrate. (From Shi X, et al. Effects of carbohydrate type and concentration and solution osmolality on water absorption. *Med Sci Sports Exerc* 1996;27:1607.)

Replace Fluid and Energy During Exercise

To optimize water and carbohydrate absorption, consume a 6% carbohydrate-electrolyte solution that combines fructose and sucrose, each transported by separate noncompetitive pathways.

---

alter the contribution of ingested glucose to the total energy yield in prolonged exercise.[31,36,54] The extra sodium (0.5–0.7 g per L) does, however, help to maintain plasma sodium concentrations. This effect benefits ultraendurance athletes at risk for hyponatremia. Hyponatremia occurs from a large sweat–sodium loss coupled with drinking copious amounts of plain water. Maintaining plasma osmolality with added sodium in the rehydration beverage also reduces urine output and sustains the sodium-dependent osmotic drive to drink. These factors promote continued fluid intake *and* fluid retention during recovery.[55,56,104] Chapter 10 discusses the optimal characteristics of a rehydration beverage following exercise-induced dehydration.

RECOMMENDED ORAL REHYDRATION BEVERAGE: EVALUATING THE SPORTS DRINKS

A 5 to 8% carbohydrate–electrolyte beverage consumed while exercising in the heat helps to regulate temperature and fluid balance as effectively as plain water. As an added bonus, this drink maintains glucose metabolism (provides an intestinal delivery rate of 5.0 kCal · min⁻¹) and preserves glycogen during prolonged exercise.[56,57,82] Consuming this solution in recovery from prolonged exercise in a warm environment also improves endurance capacity for subsequent exercise.

The Ideal Oral Rehydration Beverage

1. Tastes good
2. Abosrbs rapidly
3. Causes little or no gastrointestinal distress
4. Maintains extracellular fluid volume and osmolality
5. Offers the potential to enhance exercise performance

To determine the percentage carbohydrate in a drink, divide carbohydrate content (in grams) by fluid volume (in milliliters) and multiply by 100. For example, 80 g of carbohydrate in 1 L (1000 mL) of water provides an 8% solution. Environmental and exercise conditions interact to influence the optimal composition of the rehydration solution. Fluid replenishment becomes of utmost importance to health and safety when intense aerobic effort in hot, humid weather lasts between 30 and 60 minutes. Under these conditions, we recommend a more dilute carbohydrate–electrolyte solution containing less than 5% carbohydrate. In cooler weather, when dehydration is not a major factor, a more concentrated beverage of 15% carbohydrate suffices. Little difference exists among liquid glucose, sucrose, or starch as the preferred ingested carbohydrate fuel source during exercise.

Optimal carbohydrate replenishment ranges between 30 and 60 g (about 1–2 oz) per hour. TABLE 8.2 compares the carbohydrate and mineral content and osmolality of popular fluid replacement beverages. FIGURE 8.8 presents a general guideline for fluid intake each hour during exercise for a given amount of carbohydrate replenishment. Although a tradeoff exists between carbohydrate ingestion and gastric emptying, the stomach empties up to 1700 mL of water per hour, even when drinking an 8% carbohydrate solution. However, 1000 mL (about 1 quart) of fluid consumed per hour probably represents the optimal volume to offset dehydration, because larger fluid intakes can cause gastrointestinal discomfort.

TABLE 8.2   Comparison of Various Beverages Used by Athletes to Replace Fluid Lost in Exercise

Beverages	Flavors	CHO Source	CHO conc (%)	Sodium (mg)	Potassium (mg)	Other Minerals and Vitamins	Osmolality (mOsm · L⁻¹)
GATORADE[a] Thirst Quencher Stokely-Van Camp, Inc., a subsidiary of the Quaker Oats Company	Lemon-lime, lemonade, fruit punch, orange, citrus cooler	S/G (powder) S/G syrup solids (liquid)	6	110	25	Chloride, phosphorus	280–360
Exceed[a] Ross Laboratories	Lemon-lime, orange	G polymers/F	7.2	50	45		
Quickick[a] Cramer Products, Inc.	Lemon-lime, fruit punch, orange, grape, lemonade	F/S	4.7	116	23	Chloride, calcium, magnesium, phosphorus	250
Sqwincher, the Activity Drink Universal Products, Inc	Lemon-lime, fruit punch, lemonade, orange, grape, strawberry, grapefruit	G/F	6.8	60	36	Calcium, chloride, phosphorus	305
10-K Beverage Products, Inc.	Lemon-lime, orange, fruit punch, lemonade, iced tea	S/G/F	6.3	52	26	Chloride, phosphorus, calcium, magnesium, vitamin C	470
USA Wet Texas Wet, Inc	Lemon-lime, orange, fruit punch	S	6.8	62	44	Vitamin C, chloride, phosphorus	350
Coca-Cola Coca-Cola, USA	Regular, Classic, Cherry	HFCS/S	10.7–11.3	9.2	trace		
Sprite Coca-Cola, USA	Lemon-lime	HFCS/S	10.2	28	trace	Chloride, phosphorus	450
Cranberry juice cocktail		HFCS/S	15	10	61		
Orange juice		F/S/G	11.8	2.7	510	Phosphorus	600–715
Water				low[b]	low[b]		
PowerAde		HFCS/M	8	73	33		695
All-Sport		HFCS	8–9	55	55	Phosphorus, vitamin C	890
10 K		S/G/F	6.3	54	25	Phosphorus, calcium, iron, vitamins C and A, niacin, riboflavin, thiamine	690
Cytomax		FCS/S	7–11	10	150		
Breakthrough		M/F	8.5	60	45		
Everlast		S/F	6	100	20		
Hydra Charge		M/F	8	—	trace		
SportaLYTE		M/F/G	7.5	100	60		

[a]Serving size, 8 fluid oz.

[b]Depends on water source.

S = sucrose; F = fructose; G = glucose; HFCS= high fructose corn syrup; M = maltodextrin

Practical Recommendations for Fluid and Carbohydrate Replacement During Exercise

1. Monitor dehydration rate from changes in body weight. Require urination before postexercise body weight determination. Each pound of weight loss corresponds to 450 mL (15 fl oz) of dehydration.
2. Drink fluids at the same or somewhat greater rate as their estimated depletion (or at least at a rate close to 80% of the sweating rate) during prolonged exercise with accompanying cardiovascular stress, high metabolic heat, and dehydration.
3. Endurance athletes can meet both carbohydrate (30–60 g per hour) and fluid requirements by drinking during each hour 625 to 1250 mL (average about 250 mL every 15 minutes) of a beverage that contains 4 to 8% carbohydrate.

HIGH-FAT VERSUS LOW-FAT DIETS FOR ENDURANCE TRAINING AND EXERCISE PERFORMANCE

Debate concerns the wisdom of maintaining a high-fat diet (or even fasting) during training or before endurance competition.[21,25,61,96,97] Adaptations to high-fat diets consistently show a shift in substrate use toward higher fat oxidation in exercise.[14,38,39,87,111] Proponents of high-fat diets argue that a long-term increase in dietary fat stimulates fat burning by augmenting the capacity to mobilize and catabolize this energy nutrient. Any fat-burning enhancement should conserve glycogen reserves and/or contribute to improved endurance capacity under low-glycogen conditions. To investigate possible benefits, research compared endurance ca-

pacity in two groups of 10 young men matched for aerobic capacity who consumed either a high-carbohydrate diet (65% kCal from carbohydrate) or high-fat diet (62% kCal from lipid) for 7 weeks. Each group trained for 60 to 70 minutes at 50 to 85% of aerobic capacity, 3 days per week during weeks 1 to 3 and 4 days per week during weeks 4 to 7. Following 7 weeks of training, the group consuming the high-fat diet switched to the high-carbohydrate diet. FIGURE 8.9 displays the exercise performance for both groups. Endurance results were clear: the group consuming the high-carbohydrate diet performed significantly better after 7 weeks of training than the group consuming the high-fat diet (102.4 vs. 65.2 minutes). When the high-fat diet group switched to the high-carbohydrate diet during week 8, only a small additional improvement in endurance of 11.5 minutes occurred. Consequently, total overall endurance improvement over the 8-week period reached 115% for the high-fat diet group, whereas endurance for the group on the high-carbohydrate diet improved by 194%. The inset table shows daily energy and nutrient intakes before the experimental treatment (habitual diet) and during the 7-week experimental diet. The high-fat diet produced suboptimal adaptations in endurance performance, which were not fully remedied by switching to a high-carbohydrate diet.

Subsequent research from the same laboratory failed to demonstrate any endurance-enhancing effect of a high-fat diet containing only moderate carbohydrate (15% total kCal) in rats, regardless of their training status. For sedentary humans, maintaining either a low or high dietary fat intake for 4 weeks did not affect maximal or submaximal aerobic exercise performance.[69] A 6-day exposure to a high-fat, low-carbohydrate diet, followed by 1 day of carbohydrate restoration with a high-carbohydrate diet increased fat oxidation during prolonged submaximal exercise. This carbohydrate-sparing effect did not enhance 1-hour time trial performance following 4 hours of continuous cycling.[16]

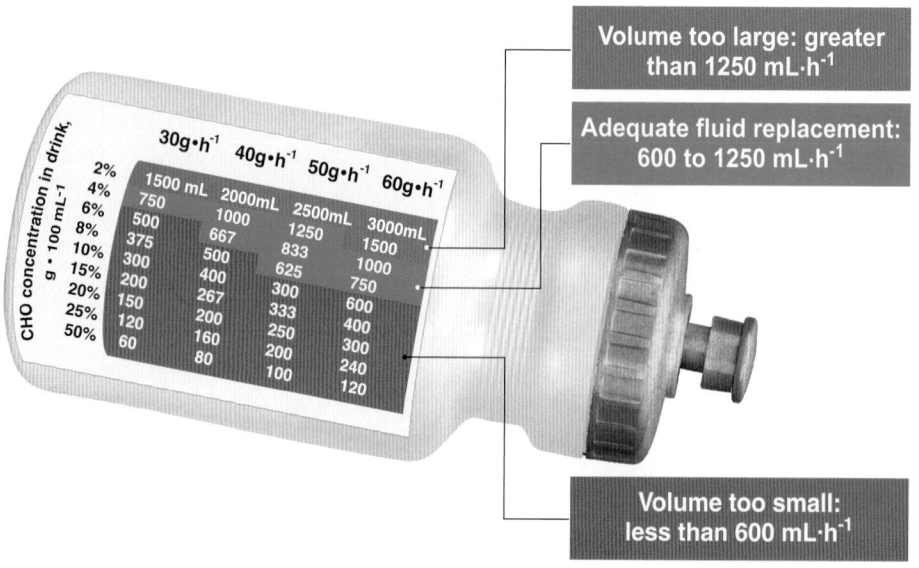

FIGURE 8.8 ■ Fluid volume to ingest each hour to obtain the noted amount of carbohydrate (CHO). (Modified from Coyle EF, Montain SJ. Benefits of fluid replacement. *Med Sci Sports Exerc* 1992;24: S324.)

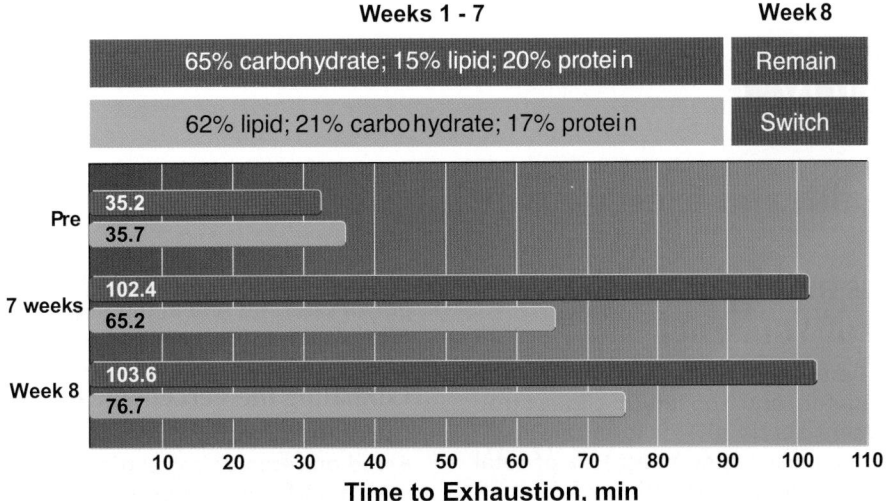

Daily intake of energy and nutrients in the subjects' habitual diet and during 7 weeks on an experimental diet

	Units	Habitual diet		Experimental diet	
		CHO	Lipid	CHO	Lipid
Energy, E	MJ	13.6	11.9	14.3	13.7*†
Protein	E%	13.2	14.3	14.6	16.5*†
	g	105.0	101.0	123.0	133.0*†
Carbohydrate	E%	48.2	53.4	65.0	22.0*†
	g	386.0	373.0	546.0	177.0*†
	g · kg body wt^{-1}	4.7	5.0	6.8	2.4*†
Simple sugars	E%	11.0	10.0	7.0	2.2*†
Dietary fiber	g · MJ^{-1}	2.3	2.6	4.3	2.2 †
Lipid	E%	34.3	39.0	20.4	62.0*†
	g	118.0	94.0	75.0	217.0*†
Cholesterol	mg · MJ^{-1}	31.0	29.0	26.0	44.0*†
Essential FA	E%	4.4	4.3	4.0	11.2*†
P/S ratio		0.39	0.43	0.53	0.62*†

Values are means; *significantly different between the habitual and the experimental diet; †significantly different between the two experimental diets; MJ, megajoule; E%, percent of total energy

FIGURE 8.9 ■ Effects of a high-carbohydrate (CHO) versus a high-fat diet on endurance performance. The group consuming the high-fat diet for 7 weeks switched to the high-CHO diet during week 8. The endurance test consisted of pedaling a bicycle ergometer at the desired rate. The inset table compares the average daily energy and nutrient intakes during the habitual and experimental diets. P/S ratio, polyunsaturated-to-saturated fatty acid ratio. (From Helge JW, et al. Interaction of training and diet on metabolism and endurance during exercise in man. *J Physiol* 1996;492:293.)

A high-fat diet stimulates adaptive responses that augment fat catabolism, yet reliable research has not demonstrated consistent exercise or training benefits from this dietary modification. Compromised training capacity and symptoms of lethargy, increased fatigue, and higher ratings of perceived exertion usually accompany exercise when subsisting on a high-fat diet[14,38,86] One must carefully consider the potential detrimental health risks when recommending a diet with 60% of total calories from lipid. This concern may prove unwarranted for athletes with high levels of daily energy ex-

penditure. Increasing the diet's percentage of lipid calories to 50% for physically active individuals who maintain a stable body weight does not adversely affect heart disease risk factors, including plasma lipoprotein profiles.[9,48] Overall, available research does not support the popular notion that reducing carbohydrate while increasing fat intake above a 30% level optimizes the metabolic "zone" for endurance performance.[80,95] Conversely, significant restriction of dietary fat intake below recommended levels also impairs endurance exercise performance.[38,94,95]

Case Study

Personal Health and Exercise Nutrition 8–1

How to Assess and Upgrade the Lipid Quality of Your Diet

The typical Western diet contains too much total lipid, too much saturated fat, and too much cholesterol. Dietary lipids represent about 36% of total caloric intake, with the average person consuming 15% of total calories as saturated fatty acids. Health professionals recommend that lipid intake should not exceed 30% of the diet's total energy content, and consuming less (about 20%) may confer even greater health benefits. Unsaturated fatty acids should account for at least 70%

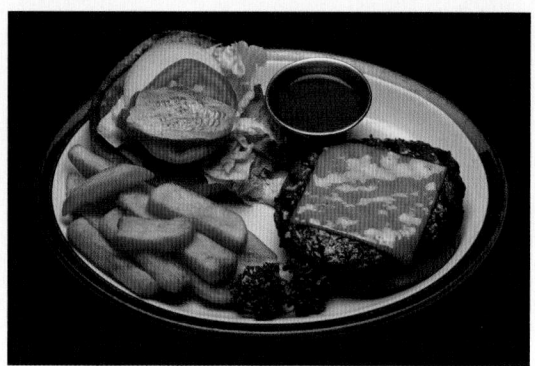

of the total lipid intake, equally distributed between polyunsaturates and monounsaturates, with cholesterol intake below 300 mg per day.

Estimating the Percentage of Total Calories Consumed from Fat

Based on research correlating food intake from a diary with data from a simple questionnaire it is possible to estimate the percentage of total calories from fat.

Choosing Among the Different Fats in Your Diet

Lipids (fats) not only provide fuel for energy but also aid in the absorption of fat-soluble vitamins, are an integral part of the plasma membrane, provide for hormone synthesis (steroids), and aid in insulation and protection of vital organs. Most lipids store in adipose tissue for subsequent release into the bloodstream as free fatty acids (FFAs), which broadly classify as monounsaturated, polyunsaturated, and saturated. Each exerts different effects on cholesterol and lipoprotein deposition in arteries and subsequent coronary heart disease risk.

Choosing the Proper Dietary Fat

Table 1 shows the available food choices for different types of lipids based on how they affect total cholesterol and the different lipoprotein fractions.

TABLE 1 Choose the Right Fat for Your Diet

Best Choice **Monounsaturated Fatty Acids**	Good Choice **Polyunsaturated Fatty Acids**	Occasional Choice **Saturated/Hydrogenated Fatty Acids**
Effects on Cholesterol and Lipoproteins		
• Decreases total cholesterol • Decreases LDL-cholesterol • No effect on HDL-cholesterol	• Decreases total cholesterol • Decreases LDL-cholesterol • Decreases HDL-cholesterol	• Increases total cholesterol • Increases LDL-cholesterol • Decreases HDL-cholesterol
	Food Examples	
Vegetable oils: avocado, canola, olive, peanut	**Vegetable oils:** corn, safflower, sesame, soybean, sunflower, trans-fat-free margarine, mayonnaise, Miracle Whip	**Tropical vegetable oils:** coconut, palm, palm kernel, cocoa butter **Hydrogenated oils:** margarine, shortening
Nuts: acorns, almonds, beechnuts, cashews, chestnuts, hazelnuts, hickory, macadamia, natural peanut butter, peanuts, pecans, pistachios	**Nuts:** Brazil, butternuts, pine, walnuts	**Animal fats:** bacon, beef fat, chicken fat, egg yolk, fatty meats, lamb fat, lard, pepperoni, pork fat, salt pork, sausage, kielbasa
Other: fish fat (omega-3 fatty acids)	**Seeds:** sesame, pumpkin, sunflower	**Dairy products:** butter, cheese (regular, light, low fat), cream cheese, half & half, ice cream, sour cream, whole milk, 2% milk

Hutchinson Cancer Research Center, Seattle, WA. www.shcrc.org

Case Study *continued*

Questionnaire

How Much Fat Do You Consume? Think of Your Diet Over the Past 3 Months and Answer the Following Questions.

Choices: 1 = Usually/always; 2 = Often; 3 = Sometimes; 4 = Rarely/never

1. _____ When I eat bread, rolls, muffins, or crackers, I eat them without butter or margarine.
2. _____ When I eat cooked vegetables, I eat them without butter, margarine, salt pork, or bacon fat.
3. _____ When I eat cooked vegetables, they are cooked by a method other than frying.
4. _____ When I eat potatoes, they are cooked by a method other than frying.
5. _____ When I eat boiled or baked potatoes I eat them without butter, margarine, or sour cream.
6. _____ When I eat green salads, I eat them without dressing.
7. _____ When I eat dessert, I eat it without cream or whipped-cream topping.
8. _____ When I eat spaghetti or noodles, I eat it plain or use a meatless sauce.
9. _____ My main meal for the day is usually meatless.
10. _____ When I eat fish, it is broiled, baked, or poached.
11. _____ When I eat chicken, it is broiled or baked.
12. _____ When I eat chicken, I remove the skin.
13. _____ When I eat red meat, I trim off all visible fat.
14. _____ When I eat ground beef, I choose extra lean.
15. _____ When I drink milk I choose skim or 1% fat milk instead of 2% fat or whole milk.
16. _____ When I eat cheese, it is the reduced fat variety.
17. _____ When I eat a frozen dessert, it is sherbet, ice milk, or nonfat versions of ice cream or yogurt.
18. _____ When I eat green salads with dressing, I use a low-fat or nonfat dressing.
19. _____ When I sauté or pan fry food I use a nonstick spray instead of oil, margarine, or butter.
20. _____ When I use mayonnaise or a mayonnaise-type dressing, I usually use a low-fat or nonfat variety.
21. _____ When I eat dessert, I usually eat fruit.
22. _____ When I eat snacks, I usually eat raw vegetables.
23. _____ When I eat snacks, I usually eat fresh fruit.

Scoring
Total your score and divide by 23.

Your average	Percentage kCal from fat
1.0 to 1.5	Less than 25%
1.5 to 2.0	25 to 29%
2.0 to 2.5	30 to 34%
2.5 to 3.0	35 to 39%
3.0 to 3.5	40 to 44%
3.5 to 4.0	45+%

Summary

1. The precompetition meal should include readily digestible foods and contribute to the energy and fluid requirements of exercise. Meals high in carbohydrates and relatively low in lipids and proteins serve this purpose. Three hours should provide sufficient time to digest and absorb the precompetition meal.

2. Commercially prepared liquid meals offer a practical approach to precompetition nutrition and energy supplementation. These "meals" (1) provide balance in nutritive value, (2) contribute to fluid needs, and (3) absorb rapidly, leaving practically no residue in the digestive tract.

3. High-intensity aerobic exercise for 1 hour decreases liver glycogen by about 55%, whereas a 2-hour strenuous workout nearly depletes the glycogen content of the liver and specifically exercised muscles

4. Carbohydrate-containing rehydration beverages consumed during exercise enhance endurance performance by maintaining blood sugar concentration. Glucose supplied in the blood can (1) spare existing glycogen in active muscles or (2) serve as "reserve" blood glucose for later use should muscle glycogen become depleted.

5. All carbohydrates do not digest and absorb at the same rate. The glycemic index provides a relative measure of blood glucose increase after consuming a food containing 50 g of a digestible carbohydrate (total carbohydrate minus fiber) and compares it over a 2-hour period to a "standard" for carbohydrate (usually white bread or glucose) with an assigned value of 100. The glycemic load quantifies the overall glycemic effect of a typical portion of food.

6. For rapid carbohydrate replenishment after exercise, begin immediately to consume moderate-to-high glycemic index carbohydrate-containing foods (50–75 g of carbohydrate each hour). With optimal carbohydrate intake, glycogen stores replenish at a rate of about 5 to 7% per hour.

7. Use the glycemic index to formulate the immediate pre-exercise feeding. Foods with a low glycemic index digest and absorb at a relatively slow rate. Ingesting these carbohydrates in the immediate pre-exercise period provides a steady supply of "slow- release" glucose from the intestinal tract during exercise.

8. Maintaining a relatively large stomach fluid volume throughout exercise enhances gastric emptying. Optimal gastric volume occurs by consuming 400 to 600 mL of fluid immediately before exercise, followed by regular fluid ingestion of 250 mL every 15 minutes thereafter.

9. Drinking concentrated sugar-containing beverages slows the gastric emptying rate. This could negatively upset fluid balance during exercise and heat stress.

10. The ideal oral rehydration beverage contains between 5 and 8% carbohydrates. This formulation permits carbohydrate replenishment without adversely affecting fluid balance and thermoregulation.

11. Adding moderate amounts of sodium to the ingested fluid helps to maintain plasma sodium concentration. This benefits the ultraendurance athlete at risk for hyponatremia.

12. Maintaining plasma osmolality with added sodium in the rehydration beverage reduces urine output and sustains the sodium-dependent osmotic drive to drink.

13. A high-fat diet stimulates adaptive responses that augment fat use—but reliable research has not yet demonstrated consistent exercise or training benefits from this dietary modification approach.

Test Your Knowledge Answers

1. **False:** Significant depletion occurs in carbohydrate reserves over an 8- to 12-hour period without eating, even if the person normally follows appropriate dietary recommendations. Thus, fasting before competition or intense training makes no sense physiologically because it rapidly depletes liver and muscle glycogen, which subsequently impairs exercise performance. In individualizing the precompetition meal plan, consider the following factors (1) food preference, (2) "psychological set" of the competitor, and (3) digestibility of the foods.

2. **False:** The ideal precompetition meal maximizes muscle and liver glycogen storage and provides glucose for intestinal absorption during exercise. The meal should contain 150 to 300 g of carbohydrate (3–5 g per kg of body mass in either solid or liquid form), be consumed 3 to 4 hours before exercising, and contain relatively little fat and fiber to facilitate gastric emptying and minimize gastrointestinal distress.

3. **False:** High-intensity aerobic exercise for 1 hour decreases liver glycogen by about 55%, whereas a 2-hour strenuous workout almost totally depletes the glycogen content of the liver and the exercised muscle fibers. Also, maximal, repetitive 1- to 5-minute bouts of exercise interspersed with periods of lower intensity exercise—as occurs in soccer, ice hockey, field hockey, European handball, and tennis—dramatically lower liver and muscle glycogen reserves. Research shows that physical and mental

Test Your Knowledge Answers   *continued*

performance under such conditions improves with carbohydrate supplementation during exercise. Carbohydrate feedings during high-intensity, prolonged exercise also enables individuals to exercise at greater intensity of effort.

4. **False:** The glycemic index serves as an indicator of a carbohydrate's ability to raise blood glucose levels. This index expresses the percentage of total area under the blood glucose response curve for a specific food, compared with glucose. Blood sugar increase—termed the *glycemic response*—is determined after ingesting a food containing 50 g of a carbohydrate and comparing it over a 2-hour period with a "standard" for carbohydrate (usually white bread or glucose) with an assigned value of 100.

5. **True:** The most rapid method of replenishing carbohydrate after exercise requires consuming foods with moderate-to-high glycemic indices rather than foods rated low, even if the replenishment meal contains a small amount of lipid and protein. Furthermore, ingesting lipids and proteins slows the passage of food into the small intestine, reducing the glycemic index of the meal's accompanying carbohydrate content.

6. **False:** More-rapid glycogen resynthesis takes place if the person remains inactive during recovery. With optimal carbohydrate intake (high glycemic foods), glycogen stores replenish at a rate of about 5 to 7% per hour. Thus, even under the best of circumstances, it takes at least 20 hours to re-establish glycogen stores following a glycogen-depleting exercise bout.

7. **False:** Consuming 400 to 600 mL of fluid 20 minutes before exercise optimizes the beneficial effect of an increased stomach volume on fluid and nutrient passage into the small intestine. Then, regularly ingesting 150 to 250 mL of fluid (at 15-minute intervals) throughout exercise continually replenishes fluid in the stomach; this maintains a relatively large and constant gastric volume. Such a protocol delivers about 1 L of fluid per hour to the small intestine, a volume that meets the needs of most endurance athletes.

8. **False:** A 5 to 8% carbohydrate–electrolyte beverage consumed during exercise in the heat contributes to temperature regulation and fluid balance as effectively as plain water. As an added bonus, this drink aids in maintaining glucose metabolism (providing an intestinal delivery rate of 5.0 kCal · min^{-1}) and glycogen reserves in prolonged exercise.

9. **True:** Adding moderate amounts of sodium to ingested fluids exerts a minimal effect on glucose absorption or the contribution of ingested glucose to the total energy yield in prolonged exercise. The extra sodium (0.5–0.7 g per L) does, however, contribute to maintaining plasma sodium concentrations and benefits the ultraendurance athlete at risk for hyponatremia. Hyponatremia occurs from large sweat–sodium loss coupled with drinking large amounts of plain water. Maintaining plasma osmolality with added sodium in the rehydration beverage also reduces urine output and sustains the sodium-dependent osmotic drive to drink.

10. **False:** Drinking concentrated sugar-containing beverages slows gastric emptying rate, which could ultimately upset fluid balance during exercise and heat stress. The ideal oral rehydration solution contains between 5 and 8% carbohydrates. This beverage formulation permits carbohydrate replenishment without adversely affecting fluid balance and thermoregulation.

References

1. Anantaraman R, et al. Effects of carbohydrate supplementation on performance during 1 hour of high-intensity exercise. I*nt J Sports Med* 1995;16:461.
2. Backhouse SH, et al. Effect of carbohydrate and prolonged exercise on affect and perceived exertion. *Med Sci Sports Exerc* 2005;37:1768.
3. Ball TC, et al. Periodic carbohydrate replacement during 50 min of high-intensity cycling improves subsequent sprint performance. *Int J Sports Nutr* 1995;5:151.
4. Beckers EJ, et al. Comparison of aspiration and scintigraphic techniques for the measurement of gastric emptying rates in man. *Gut* 1992;33:115.
5. Below PR, et al. Fluid and carbohydrate ingestion independently improve performance during 1 h of intense exercise. *Med Sci Sports Exerc* 1995;27:200.
6. Berardi JM, et al. Postexercise muscle glycogen recovery enhanced with a carbohydrate-protein supplement. *Med Sci Sports Exerc* 2006;38:1106.
7. Brand-Miller J, et al. The G.I. factor: the Glycaemic Index Solution. Sydney, Australia: Hodder & Stoughton, 1996.
8. Brouns F, Beckers E. Is the gut an athletic organ? *Sports Med* 1993;15:242.
9. Brown R, Cox CM. Effects of high fat versus high carbohydrate diets on plasma lipids and lipoproteins in endurance athletes. *Med Sci Sports Exerc* 1998;30:1677.
10. Burelle Y, et al. Oxidation of an oral [^{13}C] glucose load at rest and prolonged exercise in trained and sedentary subjects. *J Appl Physiol* 1999;86:52.
11. Burke LM, et al. Muscle glycogen storage after prolonged exercise: effect of the glycemic index on carbohydrate feedings. *J Appl Physiol* 1993;74:1019.
12. Burke LM, et al. Effect of coingestion of fat and protein with carbohydrate feedings on muscle glycogen storage. *J Appl Physiol* 1995;78:2187.
13. Burke LM, et al. Muscle glycogen storage after prolonged exercise: effect of the frequency of carbohydrate feeding. *Am J Clin Nutr* 1996;64:115.

14. Burke LM, et al. Effect of fat adaptation and carbohydrate restoration on metabolism and performance during prolonged cycling. *J Appl Physiol* 2000;89:2413.

15. Burke LM, et al. Energy and carbohydrate for training and recovery. J *Sports Sci* 2006;24:675.

16. Carey AL, et al. Effects of fat adaptation and carbohydrate restoration on prolonged endurance exercise. *J Appl Physiol* 2001;91:225.

17. Choi D, et al. Effect of passive and active recovery on the resynthesis of muscle glycogen. *Med Sci Sports Exerc* 1994;26:992.

18. Coggan AR, Coyle EF. Metabolism and performance following carbohydrate ingestion late in exercise. *Med Sci Sports Exerc* 1989;21:59.

19. Coyle EF. Timing and method of increased carbohydrate intake to cope with heavy training, competition and recovery. *J Sports Sci* 1991;9:29.

20. Coyle EF. Substrate utilization during exercise in active people. *Am J Clin Nutr* 1995;61(suppl):968S.

21. Cox CM, et al. The effects of high-carbohydrate versus high-fat dietary advice on plasma lipids, lipoproteins, apolipoproteins, and performance in endurance trained cyclists. *Nutr Metab Cardiovasc Dis* 1996;6:227.

22. DeMarco HD, et al. Pre-exercise carbohydrate meals: application of the glycemic index. *Med Sci Sports Exerc* 1999;31:164.

23. Duchman SM, et al. Upper limit for intestinal absorption of a dilute glucose solution in men at rest. *Med Sci Sports Exerc* 1997;29:482.

24. Erdman KA, et al. Influence of performance level on dietary supplementation in elite Canadian athletes. *Med Sci Sports Exerc* 2006;38:349.

25. Erlenbusch M, et al. Effect of high-fat or high-carbohydrate diets on endurance exercise: a meta-analysis. *Int J Sport Nutr Exerc Metabol* 2005;15:1.

26. Febbraio MA, Stewart, KL. CHO feeding before prolonged exercise: effect of glycemic index on muscle glycogenolysis and exercise performance. *J Appl Physiol* 1996;81:1115.

27. Foster C, et al. Effects of pre-exercise feedings on endurance performance. *Med Sci Sports* 1979;11:1.

28. Foster-Powell K, et al. International table of glycemic index and glycemic load values: 2002. *Am J Clin Nutr* 2002;76:5.

29. Gisolfi CV, et al. Human intestinal water absorption: direct vs indirect measurements. *Am J Physiol* 1990;258:G216.

30. Gisolfi CV, et al. Intestinal water absorption from select carbohydrate solutions in humans. *J Appl Physiol* 1992;7:2142.

31. Gisolfi CV, et al. Effect of sodium concentration in a carbohydrate-electrolyte solution on intestinal absorption. *Med Sci Sports Exerc* 1995;27:1414.

32. Goodpaster BH, et al. The effects of pre-exercise starch ingestion on endurance performance. *Int J Sports Med* 1996;17:366.

33. Guezennec CY, et al. The role of type and structure of complex carbohydrates on response to physical exercise. *Int J Sports Nutr* 1993;14:224.

34. Hargreaves M, Briggs CA. Effect of carbohydrate ingestion on exercise metabolism. *J Appl Physiol* 1988;65:1553.

35. Hargreaves M, et al. Effect of fructose ingestion on muscle glycogen usage during exercise. *Med Sci Sports Exerc* 1985;17:360.

36. Hargreaves M, et al. Influence of sodium on glucose bioavailability during exercise. *Med Sci Sports Exerc* 1994;26:365.

37. Hawley JA, et al. Carbohydrate, fluid, and electrolyte requirements of the soccer player: a review. *Int J Sports Med* 1994;4:221.

38. Helge JW, et al. Interaction of training and diet on metabolism and endurance during exercise in man. *J Physiol* 1996;492:293.

39. Helge JW, et al. Impact of a fat-rich diet on endurance in man: role of the dietary period. *Med Sci Sports Exerc* 1998;30:456.

40. Horswill CA. Weight loss and weight cycling in amateur wrestlers: implications for performance and resting metabolic rate. *Int J Sports Nutr* 1993;3:245.

41. Jenkins DJ, et al. Glycemic index: an overview of implications in health and disease. *Am J Clin Nutr* 2002;76(suppl):266S.

42. Jentiens RL, et al. Oxidation of combined ingestion of glucose and fructose during exercise. *J Appl Physiol* 2004;96:1277.

43. Jentjens RL, et al. High oxidation rates from combined carbohydrates ingested during exercise. *Med Sci Sports Exerc* 2004;36:1551.

44. Jeukendrup AE, et al. Carbohydrate-electrolyte feedings improve 1 h time trial cycling performance. *Int J Sports Med* 1997;18:125.

45. Jeukendrup AE, et al. Exogenous glucose oxidation during exercise in endurance-trained and untrained subjects. *J Appl Physiol* 1997;83:835.

46. Jozsi AC, et al. The influence of starch structure on glycogen resynthesis and subsequent cycling performance. *Int J Sports Med* 1996;17:373.

47. Lambert GP, et al. Simultaneous determination of gastric emptying and intestinal absorption during cycle exercise in humans. *Int J Sports Med* 1996;17:48.

48. Leddy J, et al. Effect of a high or a low fat diet on cardiovascular risk factors in male and female runners. *Med Sci Sports Exerc* 1997;29:17.

49. Leiper JB, et al. Effect of intermittent high-intensity exercise on gastric emptying in man. *Med Sci Sports Exerc* 2001;33:1270.

50. Liu S, et al. A prospective study of dietary glycemic load, carbohydrate intake, and risk of coronary heart disease in US women. *Am J Clin Nutr* 2000;71:1455.

51. Macdermid PW, Stannard SR. A whey-supplemented, high-protein diet versus a high-carbohydrate diet: effects on endurance cycling performance. *Int J Sport Nutr Exerc Metab* 2006;16:65.

52. Marmy-Conus N, et al. Preexercise glucose ingestion and glucose kinetics during exercise. *J Appl Physiol* 1996;81:853.

53. Massicotte D, et al. Effect of metabolic rate on the oxidation of ingested glucose and fructose during exercise. *Int J Sports Med* 1994;15:177.

54. Massicotte D, et al. Lack of effect of NaCl and/or metoclopramide on exogenous (^{13}C)-glucose oxidation during exercise. *Int J Sports Med* 1996;17:165.

55. Maughan RJ, Lieper JB. Sodium intake and post-exercise rehydration in man. *Eur J Appl Physiol* 1995;71:311.

56. Maughan RJ, et al. Restoration of fluid balance after exercise-induced dehydration: effect of food and fluid intake. *Int J Appl Physiol* 1996;73:317.

57. Maugham RJ, et al. Dietary supplements. *J Sports Sci* 2004;22:2004

58. McConell G, et al. Effect of timing of carbohydrate ingestion on endurance exercise performance. *Med Sci Sports Exerc* 1996;28:1300.

59. Millard-Stafford ML, et al. Carbohydrate-electrolyte replacement improves distance running performance in the heat. *Med Sci Sports Exerc* 1992;24:934.

60. Millard-Stafford ML, et al. Should carbohydrate concentration of a sports drink be less than 8% during exercise in the heat? *Int J Sports Nutr Exerc Metab* 2005;15:117.

61. Mudio DM. Effect of dietary fat on metabolic adjustments to maximal $\dot{V}O_2$ and endurance in runners. *Med Sci Sports Exerc* 1994;26:81.

62. Noakes TD, et al. The importance of volume in regulating gastric emptying. *Med Sci Sports Exerc* 1991;23:307.

63. Nybo L. CNS fatigue and prolonged exercise: effect of glucose supplementation. *Med Sci Sports Exerc* 2003;35:589.

64. Pabkin JAM, et al. Muscle glycogen storage following prolonged exercise: effect of timing of ingestion of high glycemic index food. *Med Sci Sports Exerc* 1997;29:220.

65. Pencek RR, et al. Mobilization of glucose from the liver during exercise and replenishment afterward. *Can J Appl Physiol* 2005;30:292.

66. Pendergast DR, et al. The role of dietary fat on performance, metabolism and health. *Am J Sports Med* 1996;24:s53

67. Piehl Aulin K, et al. Muscle glycogen resynthesis rate in humans after supplementation of drinks containing carbohydrates with low and high molecular masses. *Eur J Appl Physiol* 2000;81:347.

68. Pi-Sunyer X. Glycemic index and disease. *Am J Clin Nutr* 2002;76(suppl): 290S.

69. Pogliaghi S, Veicsteinas A. Influence of low and high dietary fat on physical performance in untrained males. *Med Sci Sports Exerc* 1999;31:149.

70. Ramires PR, et al. Oral glucose ingestion increases endurance capacity in normal and diabetic (type I) humans. *J Appl Physiol* 1997;83:608.

71. Rankin JW, et al. Effect of weight loss and refeeding diet composition on anaerobic performance in wrestlers. *Med Sci Sports Exerc* 1996;28:1292.

72. Rehrer NJ. The maintenance of fluid balance during exercise. *Int J Sports Med* 1994;15:122.

73. Riddell MC, et al. Substrate utilization during exercise with glucose and glucose plus fructose ingestion in boys ages 10–14 yr. *J Appl Physiol* 2001;90:903.

74. Robinson TM, et al. L-Arginine ingestion after rest and exercise: effects on glucose disposal. *Med Sci Sports Exerc* 2003;35:1309.

75. Roy LP, et al. Addition of protein and amino acids to carbohydrates does not enhance postexercise muscle glycogen synthesis. *J Appl Physiol* 2001;91:839.

76. Roy LP, et al. High oxidation rates from combined carbohydrates ingested during exercise. *Med Sci Sports Exerc* 2004;36:1551.

77. Roy LB, et al. Oxidation of exogenous glucose, sucrose, and maltose during prolonged cycling exercise. *J Appl Physiol* 2004;96:1285.

78. Saunders MJ, et al. Effects of a carbohydrate-protein beverage on cycling endurance and muscle damage. *Med Sci Sports Exerc* 2004;36:1233.

79. Schenk S, et al. Different glycemic indexes of breakfast cereals are not due to glucose entry into blood but to glucose removal by tissues. *Am J Clin Nutr* 2003;78:742.

80. Sears B, Lawren W. The zone. New York: Harper Collins, 1995.

81. Shirreffs SM, et al. Fluid and electrolyte needs for preparation and recovery from training and competition. *J Sports Sci* 2004;22:57.

82. Shi X, Gisolfi CV. Fluid and carbohydrate replacement during intermittent exercise. *Sports Med* 1998;25:157.

83. Simard C, et al. Effect of carbohydrate intake before and during and ice hockey match on blood and muscle energy substrates. *Res Q Exerc Sport* 1988;59:144.

84. Siu PM, Wong SH. Use of the glycemic index: effect on feeding patterns and exercise performance. *J Physiol Anthropol Appl Hum Sci* 2004; 22:57.

85. Spendiff O, Campbell IG. The effect of glucose ingestion on endurance upper-body exercise and performance. *Int J Sports Med* 2002;23:142.

86. Stepto NK, et al. Effect of short-term fat adaptation on high-intensity training. *Med Sci Sports Exerc* 2002;34:449.

87. Stellingwerff T, et al. Decreased PDH activation and glycogenolysis during exercise following fat adaptation with carbohydrate restoration. *Am J Physiol Endocrinol Metab* 2006;298:E380.

88. Thomas DE, et al. Plasma glucose levels after prolonged strenuous exercise correlate inversely with glycemic response to food consumed before exercise. *Int J Sports Nutr* 1994;4:361.

89. Tsintzas O-K, et al. Carbohydrate ingestion and glycogen utilization in different muscle fibre types in man. *J Physiol (Lond)* 1995;489:243.

90. Tsintzas O-K, et al. Carbohydrate ingestion and single muscle fiber glycogen metabolism during running in men. *J Appl Physiol* 1996;81:801.

91. Tsintzas O-K, et al. Influence of carbohydrate supplementation early in exercise on endurance running capacity. *Med Sci Sports Exerc* 1996;28:1373.

92. Utter AC, et al. Effect of carbohydrate ingestion on ratings of perceived exertion during a marathon. *Med Sci Sports Exerc* 2002;24:1779.

93. van Loon KJC. Plasma insulin responses after ingestion of different amino acid or protein mixtures with carbohydrate. *Am J Clin Nutr* 2000;72:2000.

94. van Loon KJC, et al. Maximizing postexercise muscle glycogen synthesis: carbohydrate supplementation and the application of amino acid or protein hydrolysate mixtures. *Am J Clin Nutr* 2000;72:106.

95. Venkatraman JT, Pendergast D. Effects of the level of dietary fat intake and endurance exercise on plasma cytokines in runners. *Med Sci Sports Exerc* 1998;30:1198.

96. Venkatraman JT, et al. Influence of the level of dietary lipid intake and maximal exercise on the immune status in runners. *Med Sci Sports Exerc* 1997;29:333.

97. Vogt M, et al. Effects of dietary fat on muscle substrates, metabolism, and performance in athletes. *Med Sci Sports Exerc* 2003;35:952.

98. Volek JS, et al. Testosterone and cortisol in relationship to dietary nutrients and resistance exercise. *J Appl Physiol* 1997;82:49.

99. Wagenmakers AJ. Carbohydrate feedings improve 1 h time trial cycling performance. *Med Sci Sports Exerc* 1996;28:S37.

100. Wagenmakers AJ, et al. Oxidation rates of orally ingested carbohydrates during prolonged exercise in men. *J Appl Physiol* 1993;75:2274.

101. Wallis GA, et al. Oxidation of combined ingestion of maltodextrins and fructose during exercise. *Med Sci Sports Exerc* 2005;37:426.

102. Walton P, Rhodes EC. Glycaemic index and optimal performance. *Sports Med* 1997;33:164.

103. Welsh RS, et al. Carbohydrates and physical/mental performance during intermittent exercise to fatigue. *Med Sci Sports Exerc* 2002;34;723.

104. Wilk B, Bar-Or O. Effect of drink flavor and NaCl on voluntary drinking and hydration in boys exercising in the heat. *J Appl Physiol* 1996;80:1112.

105. Williams C, Serratose L. Nutrition on match day. *J Sports Sci* 2006;24:687.

106. Winnick JJ, et al. Carbohydrate feeding during team sport exercise preserve physical and CNS function. *Med Sci Sports Exerc* 2005;37:306.

107. Wolever TMS, et al. Glycaemic index of 102 complex carbohydrate foods in patients with diabetes. *Nutr Res* 1994;14:651.

108. Yannick C, et al. Oxidation of corn starch, glucose, and fructose ingested before exercise. *Med Sci Sports Exerc* 1989;21:45.

109. Yaspelkis BB III, et al. Carbohydrate supplementation spares muscle glycogen during variable intensity exercise. *J Appl Physiol* 1993; 75:1477.

110. Zawadzki KM, et al. Carbohydrate-protein complex increases the rate of muscle glycogen storage after exercise. *J Appl Physiol* 1992;72:1584.

111. Zderic TW, et al. High-fat diet elevates resting intramuscular triglyceride concentration and whole body lipolysis during exercise. *Am J Physiol Endocrinol Metab* 2004;286:E217.

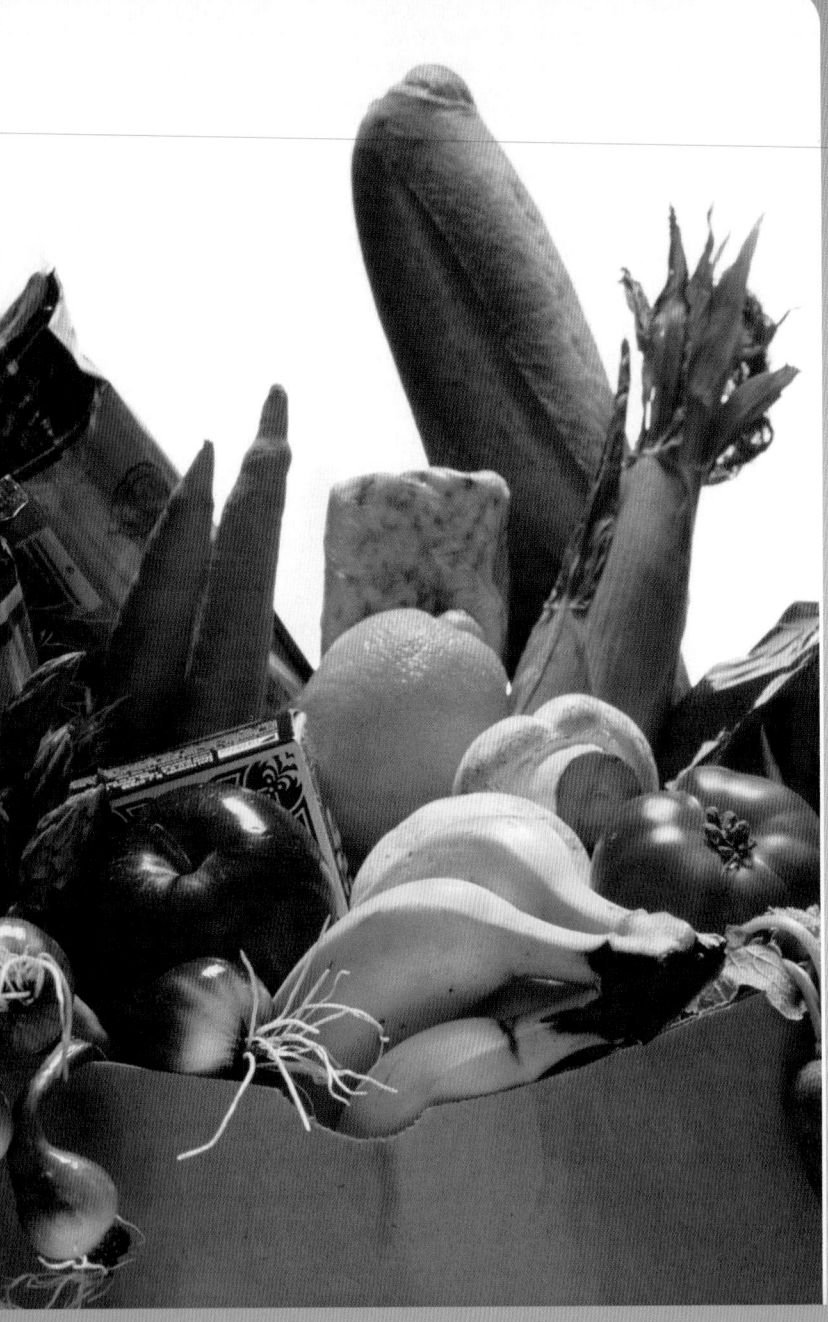

Chapter 9

Making Wise Choices in the Nutrition Marketplace

Test Your Knowledge

Answer these 10 statements about making wise choices in the nutrition marketplace. Use the scoring key at the end of the chapter to check your results. Repeat this test after you have read the chapter and compare your results.

1. **T F** The U.S. government oversees and guarantees that a nutritional supplement has been checked and rated safe to consume.
2. **T F** FTC stands for Federal Trade Commission; it regulates food-product advertising in different media.
3. **T F** FDA stands for the office of the Federal District Attorney; it prosecutes violators of food standards set by the Food and Drug Administration.
4. **T F** Federal law dictates that sellers of dietary supplements must guarantee their products as safe and effective.
5. **T F** Dietary supplements must provide precise information about their contents, clearly listed on the package.
6. **T F** The ATF stands for the Bureau of Alcohol, Tobacco and Firearms; it enforces laws related to alcohol, tobacco, and firearms.
7. **T F** The Daily Reference Values on food labels assume a 3000-kCal daily intake as representative of the average caloric intake for most adults.
8. **T F** The term "healthy" can be used on a food label without meeting any established criteria for making a claim for health benefits.
9. **T F** Computing a food's nutrient density provides a convenient way to compare the energy content of different foods.
10. **T F** Obesity continues to grow at an epidemic rate in the United States despite any significant change in eating patterns and behaviors.

D ramatic changes, both positive and negative, have affected the food and nutrition scene for the past 60 years. The most blatant example of negativism concerns how multinational companies focus on profit rather than consumer well-being. Companies allocate hundreds of millions of dollars annually to espouse supposed "health benefits" of micronutrient vitamins and minerals, specialty foods, and dietary supplements. Similarly, manufacturers of home exercise equipment use false and deceptive advertising to entice customers to purchase their products. Undoubtedly, big-budget advertising pays off. Almost 200 million Americans purchase billions of dollars of dietary supplements and over $3 billion worth of exercise equipment that includes abdominal "slimming" boards and gadgets, stationary bicycles, beltless treadmills, "gliders," face and neck "shapers," and exercise DVDs.

The Food and Drug Administration (FDA) is the government agency that regulates food, drugs (prescription, over-the-counter, generics), medical devices (pacemakers, contact lenses, hearing aids), biologics (vaccines), animal feed and drugs, cosmetics, radiation-emitting products (cell phones, lasers, microwaves), and combination products.

The FDA regulates dietary supplements under a different set of regulations than those covering "conventional" foods and drug products. Under the **Dietary Supplement Health and Education Act of 1994 (DSHEA)**, the dietary supplement

Case Study

Personal Health and Exercise Nutrition 9–1

What People Are Eating Around the World

Imagine eating for a week with 30 different families in 24 countries. Imagine shopping, cooking and eating with those families—taking note of every food purchased and consumed, every beverage poured, every package opened.[a] Well that's what photographer Peter Menzel and his writer-wife Faith D'Aluisio did for their book *Hungry Planet: What the World Eats* [*What the World Eats,* by Peter Menzel and Faith D'Aluisio. Photography: Peter Menzel. Copyright © 2005 Ten Speed Press, Berkeley, Calif.] The husband-and-wife team wanted to see how globalization, migration, and rising affluence are affecting the diets of communities around the globe.

Here is a sample of what they found from four different families of four to six people.

Family of six (2 adults and four young children) living in Refugee Camp, in eastern Chad, Africa	
Grains & Other Starchy Foods:**	Sorghum ration, unmilled, 39.3 lb; corn-soy blend ration (called CSB), 4.6 lb.
Dairy	Not available to them.
Meat, Fish, & Eggs: $0.58**	Goat meat, dried and on bone, 9 oz; fish, dried, 7 oz. (Note: Periodically, such as at the end of Ramadan, several families collectively purchase a live animal to slaughter and share. Some of its meat is eaten fresh in soup and the rest is dried.)
Fruits, Vegetables, & Nuts: $0.51**	Limes, small, 5; pulses ration, 4.6 lb, the seeds of legumes such as peas, beans, lentils, chickpeas, and fava beans. Red onions, 1 lb; garlic, 8 oz; okra, dried, 5 oz; red peppers, dried, 5 oz; tomatoes, dried, 5 oz.
Condiments: $0.13**	Sunflower oil ration, 2.1 qt; white sugar ration, 1.4 lb; dried pepper, 12 oz; salt ration, 7.4 oz; ginger, 4 oz.
Beverages:	Water, 77.7 gal, provided by Oxfam, and includes water for all purposes. Rations organized by the United Nations with the World Food Program.
Food Expenditure for One Week: 685 CFA francs/$1.23	
Market value of food rations, if purchased locally: $24.37	

Family of four (2 adults and 2 children age 10, 14 years) from Bavaria, Germany	
Grains & Other Starchy Foods: $31.98	Kölln muesli, 3.3 lb; Golden Toast whole grain bread, 3.3 lb; potatoes, 2.8 lb; brown bread, 2.2 lb; white bread (Italian style), 2.2 lb; bakery buns, 1.3 lb; Barilla linguini, 1.1 lb; Barilla rotini, 1.1 lb; Harry rye bread, 1.1 lb; wheat flour, 10.6 oz; croissants, with chocolate, 9 oz.
Dairy: $64.33	Milk, low fat, 3.2 gal; Onken yogurt, low fat, 9.9 oz; Velfrisk Danish fruit yogurt, 2.1 qt; Froop fruit yogurt, 3.6 lb; Langnese banana split ice cream, 2.2 lb; hard cheeses, assorted, 1.8 lb; Greek yogurt spreads, assorted, 1.1 lb; whipping cream, bio (organic), 14.1 oz; sour cream, 10.6 oz; Milsani butter, 8.8 oz.
Meat, Fish, & Eggs: $51.31	Beef, 2.6 lb; goulash beef, 2.5 lb; eggs, 12; cold cuts, 1.4 lb; beef, ground, 1.3 lb; Iglo fish sticks, frozen, 1.3 lb; pork, thinly sliced, 1.1 lb; Lloyd herring fillets, canned, 14.1 oz; bacon, 4.6 oz.
Fruits, Vegetables, & Nuts: $78.10	Oranges, 9 lb; apples, 3.9 lb, from family apple tree; yellow bananas, bio, 2.6 lb; red grapes, 10.6 oz; white cabbage, 1 large head, 11 lb; cherry tomatoes, 3.3 lb; green peas, frozen, 2.2 lb; yellow onions, 2.2 lb; cucumbers, 2.1 lb; kohlrabi (turnip-like vegetable), 2.1 lb; butter lettuce, 2 heads; iceberg lettuce, 2 heads; fennel root, 1.8 lb; sour pickles, 24.4 fl oz; arugula, 1.2 lb; carrots, 1.1 lb; leeks, 1.1 lb; mushrooms, 10.6 oz; radishes, 9.8 oz; red bell peppers, 8.6 oz; yellow bell peppers, 8.6 oz; pickled peppers, 7.2 oz; green onions, 6.4 oz; garlic, 0.2 oz.
Condiments: $31.83	Extra-virgin olive oil, 16.9 fl oz; Homann 1,000 Islands salad dressing, 10.6 oz; Kühne mustard, 8.8 oz; sugar, 8.8 oz; Heinz tomato ketchup, 8.5 fl oz; sea salt, 7.1 oz; lard, 4.4 oz, for frying; powdered sugar, 4.4 oz; LÄTTA margarine, low fat, 4.4 oz; paprika, 3.5 oz; black peppercorns, 1.8 oz; balsamic vinegar, 1.7 fl oz; oregano, 0.2 oz; Bourbon vanilla bean, 1.
Snacks & Desserts: $14.56	Chocolate, assorted, 1.1 lb; stollen (a buttery German cake), 1.1 lb; pistachios, 10.6 oz; bakery cinnamon rolls, 2.
Prepared Food: $66.78	Dr. Oetker pizza, frozen, 2.5 lb; Knorr tortelloni, frozen, 2 lb; vegetables in butter, frozen, 2 lb; Erbsen-Eintopf pea soup, canned, 27.1 fl oz; Bertolli tomato, garlic, and pecorino cheese pasta sauce, 13.5 fl oz; olives with almonds, 10 oz; dried tomatoes in olive oil, 8.6 oz; instant soup, 7.1 oz; vegetable stock, 6 tablespoons. Cafeteria meals, five days a week: Finn at school, pizza or spaghetti; Kjell eats lunch at home (already listed); Jörg at work, green salad, meat salad, rouladen with potatoes and vegetables, spinach with potatoes and sausage, chili con carne. Susanne eats yogurt at work.
Beverages: $70.17	Jakobus soda water, 12 25.4-fl -oz bottles; Erdinger beer, alcohol free, 10 16.9-fl-oz bottles; Frucht-Oase multivitamin fruit juice, 4 1.1-qt cartons; Einbecker Ur-Bock beer, 10 11.1-fl-oz bottles; Quinta Hinojal red wine, 4 25.4-fl-oz bottles; Flensburger malt beer, 8 11.2-fl-oz bottles; Frucht-Oase multivitamin orange juice, 2 1.1-qt cartons; cocoa powder, 14.1 oz; Lavazza espresso, 8.8 oz; fruit tea, 7.1 oz; black tea, 25 teabags; tap water, for cooking and drinking.
Miscellaneous: $91.01	Centrum vitamins, 7 pills, taken by Susanne daily. Vitamins and supplements taken by Susanne and children: Herbalife products: Formula 1, powder, 7.3 oz; AloeMAX, 2 fl oz; Formula 2, 45 pills; vitamin B, 45 pills; Formula 3, 23 pills; Formula 4, 23 pills; Herba-Lifeline, 23 pills; Coenzyme Q10 Plus, 8 pills.
Food Expenditure for One Week: Approximately 375.39 euros/$500.07	

Family of four (2 adults and 2 teenage children) from Raleigh, NC	
Grains & Other Starchy Foods: $17.92	Red potatoes, 2.3 lb; Natures Own bread, sliced, 1 loaf; Trix cereal, 1.5 lb; Mueller fettuccini, 1 lb; Mueller spaghetti, 1 lb; Uncle Ben's Original white rice, 1 lb; Flatout flatbread wraps, 14 oz; New York Original Texas garlic toast, 11.3 oz; Harris Teeter (store brand) Flaky Brown-n-Serve dinner rolls, 11 oz.
Dairy: $14.51	Harris Teeter milk, 1 gal; Kraft cheese, 8 oz; Kraft sharp cheddar, 8 oz; Kraft swiss cheese, 8 oz; Kraft cheese singles, 6 oz; parmesan cheese, grated, 3 oz; butter, 2 oz.
Meat, Fish, & Eggs: $54.92	Harris Teeter chicken wings, 1.5 lb; Armour Italian-style meat balls, 1 lb; Gwaltney bacon, Virginia-cured with brown sugar, 1 lb; Harris Teeter ground turkey, 1 lb; shrimp,‡ 1 lb; Star-Kist tuna, canned, 12 oz; honey-baked ham, sliced, 9 oz; smoked turkey, sliced, 7.8 oz.
Fruits, Vegetables, & Nuts: $41.07	Dole yellow bananas, 2.9 lb; red seedless grapes, 2.4 lb; green seedless grapes, 2.2 lb; Birds Eye baby broccoli, frozen, 4 lb; yellow onions, 3 lb; Green Giant corn, canned, 1.9 lb; Green Giant green beans, canned, 1.8 lb; Bush's vegetarian baked beans, canned, 1.8 lb; cucumbers, 1.4 lb; Harris Teeter tomatoes, vine-ripened, 1.2 lb; Del Monte whole leaf spinach, canned, 13.5 oz; garden salad, packaged, 10 oz; Italian salad mix, packaged, 8.8 oz; pickled mushrooms, 7.3 oz; Harris Teeter peanuts, 1 lb.
Condiments: $12.51	White sugar, 1.6 lb; Ruffles ranch dip, 11 oz; Crisco vegetable oil, 6 fl oz; Nestle Coffee-Mate, French vanilla, nonfat, 6 fl oz; Food Lion garlic salt, 5.3 oz; Hellmann's mayonnaise, 4 oz; Newman's Own salad dressing, 4 oz; Jiffy peanut butter,‡ 3 oz; black pepper, 2 oz; Harris Teeter Original yellow mustard, 2 oz; Heinz ketchup, 2 oz; salt, 2 oz; Colonial Kitchen meat tenderizer, 1 oz; Durkee celery seed, 1 oz; Encore garlic powder, 1 oz.
Snacks & Desserts: $21.27	Mott's apple sauce, 1.5 lb; Munchies Classic mix, 15.5 oz; Kellogg's yogurt-flavored pop tarts,‡ 14.7 oz; Orville Redenbacher's popcorn, 9 oz; Harris Teeter sunflower seeds, 7.3 oz; Lays Classic potato chips, 5.5 oz; Lays Wavy potato chips, 5.5 oz; Del Monte fruit in cherry gel, 4.5 oz; Extra chewing gum, 3 pks; Snickers candy bar, 2.1 oz; M&M's peanut candy, 1.7 oz.
Prepared Food: $24.27	Bertolli portobello alfredo sauce, 1 lb; Ragu spaghetti sauce, chunky mushroom and bell peppers, 1 lb; Maruchan shrimp flavored ramen, 15 oz; California sushi rolls, 14 oz; Campbell's cream of celery soup, 10.8 oz; Hot Pockets, jalapeño, steak & cheese, 9 oz; shrimp sushi rolls, 7 oz.
Fast Food: $71.61	McDonald's: 10-pc chicken McNuggets, large fries, large Coca-Cola, Filet-o-Fish meal; Taco Bell: 4 nachos Bell Grande, 2 soft tacos, taco supreme, taco pizza, taco, bean burrito, large lemonade; Burger King: double cheeseburger, onion rings, large Coca-Cola; KFC: 2-pc chicken with mashed potatoes, large Coca-Cola; Subway: 6-inch wheat veggie sub, 6-inch wheat seafood crab sub; Milano's Pizzeria: large sausage pizza, large pepperoni pizza; I Love NY Pizza: 4 pizza slices.
Restaurants: $6.15	China Market: shrimp fried rice, 2 orders; large fruit punch.
Beverages: $77.75	Budweiser, 24 12-fl -oz cans; bottled water, 2 gal; Harris Teeter cranberry-apple juice cocktail, 4 2-qt bottles; diet Coca-Cola, 12 12-fl-oz cans; A&W cream soda, 2 2.1-qt bottles; 7UP, 6 16.9- fl-oz bottles; Harris Teeter cranberry-raspberry juice cocktail, 2 2-qt bottles; Harris Teeter ruby grapefruit juice cocktail, 2 2-qt bottles; Capri Sun, 10 6.8-fl-oz pkgs; soda,‡ 5 12-fl-oz cans, purchased daily by Brandon at school; Arbor Mist strawberry wine blenders, 1.1 qt; Gatorade,‡ 16 fl oz; Powerade,‡ 16 fl oz; Snapple, Go Bananas juice drink, 16 fl oz; Maxwell House instant coffee, 1.5 oz; Kool-Aid, black cherry, 0.5 oz; breakfast tea, 5 teabags; tap water for drinking and cooking.
Food Expenditure for One Week: $341.98	

Family of four (2 adults and 2 teenage) children from Beijing, China	
Grains & Other Starchy Foods: $6.52	Xiaozhan rice (a type of rice grown in China), 11 lb; white bread, 2 loaves; French bread, 2 baguettes.
Dairy: $26.29	Bright yogurt, plain, 2.1 qt; Bright milk, whole, 1.1 qt; Häagen-Dazs ice cream, assorted flavors, 11.4 oz; butter, unsalted, 7.1 oz; Häagen-Dazs vanilla ice cream, 5.5 oz; Häagen-Dazs vanilla almond ice cream, 3 oz.
Meat, Fish, & Eggs: $26.97	Flatfish, 3 lb; beef flank, 2.4 lb; pigs feet, 1.8 lb; beef shank, 1.3 lb; chicken wings, 1.3 lb; eggs, 9; beef, marinated in soy sauce, 1 lb; salmon, fresh, 9.8 oz; pigs elbows, 8.6 oz; sausage links, 7 oz; sirloin steak, 5.3 oz
Fruits, Vegetables, & Nuts: $16.45	Cantaloupe, 6 lb; oranges, 4.2 lb; firedrake fruit (sweet flavored cactus fruit), 2.3 lb; lemons, 1.5 lb; plums, 1.1 lb; tomatoes, 2.4 lb; cucumbers, 2.3 lb; cauliflower, 1 head; celery, 1.4 lb; carrots, 1 lb; taro, 13.8 oz; cherry tomatoes, 13.4 oz; long beans, 10.6 oz; white onions, 10.6 oz; shiitake mushrooms, dried, 8.8 oz; shiitake mushrooms, fresh, 5.6 oz; black fungus (agaric), 3.5 oz.
Condiments: $17.26	Luhua peanut oil, 1.1 qt; Hijoblanca olive oil, 16.9 fl oz; soy bean juice, 16.9 fl oz; orange jam, 12 oz; hot pepper sauce, 9.7 oz; salad dressing, 7.1 oz; white sugar, 7.1 oz; Maxwell House coffee creamer, 6.7 oz; sesame oil, 6.8 fl oz; BB sweet hot sauce, 5.6 oz; citron day lily, 5.3 oz, dried flower bud is used for flavoring; honey, 5.3 oz; vinegar, 5.3 fl oz, eaten with boiled dumplings; pepper paste, 3.5 oz; sour cowpea (blackeyed peas), preserved, 3.5 oz; seafood sauce, 3.4 fl oz; Knorr chicken-flavored MSG, 1.8 oz; MSG, 1.8 oz; salt, 1.8 oz; curry powder, 0.4 oz.
Snacks & Desserts: $17.70	Snack chips, 7 bags; Ferrero Rocher chocolates, 14.1 oz; Xylitol gum, 1 bottle; Dove chocolate, 8.5 oz; Xylitol blueberry gum, 3 pk; Xylitol gum, 3 pk.
Prepared Food: $6.12	Sushi rolls, packaged, 1.1 lb; eel strips, baked, 8.2 oz; Knorr chicken bouillon, 0.7 oz.
Fast Food: $9.17	KFC: 2 chicken hamburgers, 2 chicken burritos; 4 Coca-Cola; 2 pkgs french fries.
Beverages: $27.95	Grapefruit juice, 2.1 gal; Asahi beer, 6 12-fl -oz cans; Bright orange juice, 2.1 qt; Tongyi orange juice drink, 2.1 qt; Coca- Cola, 3 12-fl-oz cans; Great Wall dry red wine, 25.4 oz; diet Coca-Cola, 12 fl oz; Jinliufu rice wine, 8.5 fl oz; Nescafe instant coffee, 3.5 oz; tap water, boiled for drinking and cooking.
Miscellaneous: $0.63	Zhongnanhai cigarettes, 1 pk.
Food Expenditure for One Week: 1,233.76 yuan/$155.06 USD	

[a]Menzel P, D'Aluiso F. *Hungry planet: what the world eats;* Berkeley, CA: Ten Speed Press, 2005.

manufacturer is responsible for ensuring that a dietary supplement is safe before marketing it. The FDA is responsible for taking action against any unsafe dietary supplement product after it reaches the market. Generally, manufacturers do not need to register their products with the FDA or get FDA approval before producing or selling dietary supplements. Manufacturers must make sure that product label information is truthful and not misleading.

The FDA's postmarketing responsibilities include monitoring safety such as voluntary dietary supplement adverse event reporting, and product information such as labeling, claims, package inserts, and accompanying literature. The Federal Trade Commission regulates dietary supplement advertising.

The Nutrition Labeling and Education Act of 1990 (**NLEA**) defines commonly consumed dietary supplements in the marketplace in the form of capsules, tablets, liquids, or powders and includes vitamins; essential minerals; protein; amino acids; botanicals such as ginseng and yohimbe; extracts from animal glands; garlic extract; fish oils; fibers such as acacia guar gum; compounds not generally recognized as foods or nutrients such as bioflavonoids, enzymens, germanium, nucleic acids, para-aminobenzoic acid, and rutin; and mixtures of these ingredients.

FOOD ADVERTISING AND PACKAGING

In the late 1970s, renewed interest in nutrition and healthful eating sparked worldwide attention when the medical community linked cholesterol-rich diets to high blood cholesterol, a primary risk factor for heart disease. In addition, large-scale epidemiologic studies linked many forms of cancer to dietary practices. Coincidentally, the emerging physical fitness movement that swept North America became superimposed on the diet-heart disease and diet-cancer connections. Health clubs flourished, and articles in the lay press championed the latest tips on how to improve fitness and health by eating well and exercising regularly.

Advertising's Goal: To Shape Behavior

Advertising purposely attempts to create, shape, and alter perceptions about what we eat and how we exercise. The food industry, for example, spends more than $40 billion a year for advertising and promotion to sell its products and countless millions more for lobbying. In addition, food companies provide funds to academic departments and research institutes; they support conventions, meetings, and conferences and contribute to the production of "fact sheets" such as those produced by the American Dietetic Association. Companies like Coca-Cola, Monsanto, Procter & Gamble, and Slim-Fast often sponsor nutrition journals. Food and drug companies underwrite the cost of publishing journal supplements of papers presented at conferences they frequently support. In some instances, corporate funding underwrites entire departments at universities.

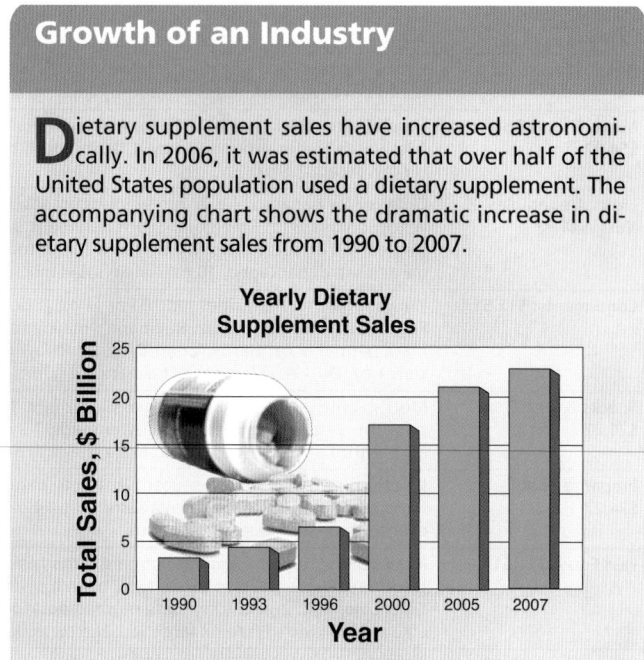

Growth of an Industry

Dietary supplement sales have increased astronomically. In 2006, it was estimated that over half of the United States population used a dietary supplement. The accompanying chart shows the dramatic increase in dietary supplement sales from 1990 to 2007.

Yearly Dietary Supplement Sales

McDonald's spends more than any other company in the world to advertise its products. McDonald's is the largest purchaser in the United States of pork, beef, and potatoes—and the second largest purchaser of chicken. Contrast this with the less than $1 million the National Cancer Institute spends to promote good nutrition. Soft drink manufacturers commit about $1 billion or more each year to advertise products. Small wonder the average American drinks over 50 gallons of soft drinks yearly compared with less than half that amount of milk!

The food industry does not stand alone when it comes to advertising hype and success. In 2007, American Consumers purchased over $14 billion worth of exercise equipment and sports-related activities. Television infomercials, newspapers, catalogs, direct phone marketing, magazines, and print-ads target specific groups for sales, often using misleading and deceptive advertising, especially targeted toward minorities (www.ftc.gov/opa/2006/libermanbroadcastingsample.pdf).

Product imagery definitely affects consumer purchases. Food manufacturers, for example, often pay a premium to supermarkets to locate and display products for easy identification. Obviously, such payments from a large manufacturer can cripple a less wealthy competitor's attempts to make inroads in a particular market segment. The practice, generally unknown to the consumer, makes good business sense (although morally questionable) because increased sales with fewer competitors trigger larger profits.

Governmental agencies try to police the food industry by legislating how manufacturers advertise their products. Unfortunately, no state or federal guidelines require that all the facts about a product need be made known to support a particular claim. Manufacturers of many dietary supplements, for example, retain the luxury of interpreting the "facts" about their product's effectiveness. Consequently, the consumer must decipher what the advertising actually means as well as interpret the information provided on food labels. According to the Federal Trade Commission (FTC) in a report made public in 2002 (www.ftc.gov/opa/2002/09/weightlossrpt.htm), nearly 40% of ads that appeared in mainstream, national publications made at least one representation that is "almost certainly false," and 55% of the ads made at least one representation that is "very likely to be false."

As we discuss later, the current food labeling law puts "teeth" into what manufacturers can and cannot state on food labels and what they can promote about their products' health benefits.

GOVERNMENT "WATCHDOG" AGENCIES

TABLE 9.1 presents an overview of the different agencies to ensure food safety in the United States. The agencies listed in the table also work with other governmental agencies such as the Consumer Product Safety Commission (www.cpsc.gov/) to enforce the Poison Prevention Packaging Act (www.cpsc.gov/businfo/pppa.pdf); the FBI (www.fbi.gov) to enforce the Federal Anti-Tampering Act (www.fda.gov/opacom/laws/fedatact.htm); and the U.S. Postal Service (www.usps.com) to enforce laws against mail fraud.

Federal Trade Commission (FTC)

The FTC (www.ftc.gov) regulates food product advertising in various media (TV, radio, newsprint) and pursues legal action against manufacturers who advertise unsubstantiated claims or deceptive ads. For example, if a TV ad states, "Consuming this supplement reduces your chances of colon cancer," the FTC can require the manufacturer to substantiate the claim. The FTC has authority to remove a product from the marketplace if the product's claims lack verification. Manufacturers often cooperate with the FTC and take affirmative corrective action of violations.

The FTC describes its mission as follows: "To enforce a variety of federal antitrust and consumer protection laws. The commission seeks to ensure that the nation's markets function competitively, and are vigorous, efficient, and free of undue restrictions." The Commission also works to enhance the smooth operation of the marketplace by eliminating acts or practices that are unfair or deceptive. In general, the Commission's efforts are directed toward stopping actions that threaten consumers' opportunities to exercise informed choice. Finally, the Commission undertakes economic analysis to support its law enforcement efforts and to contribute to the policy deliberations of the congress, the executive branch, other independent agencies, and state and local governments when requested. Additional consumer information from the FTC exists concerning tips for buying exercise equipment (www.ftc.gov/bcp/conline/edcams/exercise/index.html) as part of *Project Workout,* the FTC consumer education campaign (www.ftc.gov/opa/9706/workout.htm).

Food and Drug Administration (FDA)[b]

The FDA, which celebrated its centennial In June, 2006, represents one of 13 agencies within the Department of Health and Human Services (DHHS). With the exception of poultry and meat products, the FDA regulates what manufacturers state on food labels; the safety of cosmetics, medicines, and medical devices; and feed and drugs for pets and farm animals. The FDA also decides what additives manufacturers can add to foods, including potential hazards with food additives (contaminants), food-borne infections, toxicants, artificially constituted foods, and pesticide residues.

One of six major FDA agencies (see Table 9.1), the **Center for Food Safety and Applied Nutrition (CFSAN)**[c] regulates billions of dollars of imported food and cosmetic products sold across state lines. The CFSAN employs about 800 people

---

[b]FDA Internet site: (www.fda.gov). The FDA, a large public health agency, has the responsibility for protecting American consumers by enforcing the Federal Food, Drug, and Cosmetic Act and several related public health laws. The FDA employs 1100 investigators located in district and local offices in 157 cities who cover approximately 95,000 FDA-regulated businesses. Investigators and inspectors visit more than 15,000 facilities a year to oversee production and labeling. The FDA examines about 80,000 domestic and imported product samples for label checks. If a company violates any of the laws that the FDA enforces, the FDA encourages the firm to voluntarily correct the problem or to recall a faulty product from the market. The FDA can ask the courts to force a company to stop selling a product and to have items already produced seized and destroyed. Criminal penalties—including prison sentences—can be sought against manufacturers and distributors. About 3000 products a year are declared unfit for consumers and withdrawn from the marketplace (voluntarily or by court-ordered seizure). The FDA detains about 30,000 import shipments a year at the port of entry because the goods appear unacceptable. The FDA employs 2100 scientists who work in 40 laboratories around the country. These facilities provide evaluation of products seeking agency approval such as drugs, vaccines, food additives, coloring agents, and medical devices. The FDA also monitors the safety of the nation's blood supply and routinely examines blood bank operations, from record keeping to testing for contaminants. The FDA ensures the purity and effectiveness of biologics (medical preparations made from living organisms and their products) such as insulin and vaccines. The FDA collects and analyzes tens of thousands of reports each year on drugs and devices for any unexpected adverse reactions after they become commercially available.

[c]Kurtzwell P. Center for food safety and applied nutrition. FDA Consumer April 27, 1997. Internet site for CFSAN: http://vm.cfsan.fda.gov/list.html

TABLE 9.1   U.S. Food Safety Team. The United States Maintains a Monitoring System to Watch Over Food Production and Distribution at Every Level (Local, State, and National). Monitoring Proceeds by Food Inspectors, Microbiologists, Epidemiologists, and Other Food Scientists Working for City and County Health Departments, State Public Health Agencies, and Different Federal Departments and Agencies.

Agency	Functions
U.S. Department of Health and Human Services	
Food and Drug Administration www.cfsan.fda.gov/list.html; http://www.fda.gov/cvm/	Oversees all domestic and imported food sold in interstate commerce, including shell eggs, but not meat and poultry
Centers for Disease Control and Prevention www.cdc.gov	Oversees all foods; investigates with local, state, and other federal officials sources of food-borne disease outbreaks; develops and advocates public health policies to prevent food-borne diseases; conducts research to help prevent food-borne illness
U.S. Department of Agriculture	
Food Safety and Inspection Service www.fsis.usda.gov	Oversees domestic and imported meat and poultry and related products, such as meat- or poultry-containing stews, pizzas and frozen foods, processed egg products (generally liquid, frozen and dried pasteurized egg products)
Cooperative State Research, Education, and Extension Service www.reeusda.gov	Oversees all domestic foods, some imported (with U.S. colleges and universities, develops research and education programs on food safety for farmers and consumers)
National Agricultural Library Usda/Fda Foodborne Illness Education Information Center www.nal.usda.gov/fnic/	Oversees all foods (maintains a database of computer software, audiovisuals, posters, games, teachers' guides and other educational materials on preventing food-borne illness)
U.S. Environmental Protection Agency www.epa.gov	Oversees drinking water (regulates toxic substances and wastes to prevent their entry into the environment and food chain, assists states in monitoring quality of drinking water and finding ways to prevent contamination of drinking water, determines safety of new pesticides, sets tolerance levels for pesticide residues in foods, and publishes directions on safe use of pesticides)
U.S. Department of Commerce	
National Oceanic And Atmospheric Administration http://seafood.nmfs.noaa.gov/	Oversees fish and seafood products (through its fee-for-service seafood inspection program; inspects and certifies fishing vessels, seafood processing plants, and retail facilities for federal sanitation standards)
U.S. Department of the Treasury	
Bureau of Alcohol, Tobacco and Firearms www.atf.treas.gov/alcohol/index.htm	Oversees alcoholic beverages except wine beverages containing less than 7% alcohol (enforces food safety laws governing production and distribution of alcoholic beverages; investigates cases of adulterated alcoholic products, sometimes with help from FDA)
U.S. Customs Service www.customs.ustreas.gov	Oversees imported foods (works with federal regulatory agencies to ensure that all goods entering and exiting the United States do so according to U.S. laws and regulations)
U.S. Department of Justice www.usdoj.gov.	Oversees all foods (prosecutes companies and individuals suspected of violating food safety laws; through U.S. marshals service, seizes unsafe food products not yet in the marketplace, as ordered by courts)
Federal Trade Commission www.ftc.gov	Oversees all foods (enforces a variety of laws that protect consumers from unfair, deceptive, or fraudulent practices, including deceptive and unsubstantiated advertising)
State and Local Governments	Oversee all foods within their jurisdictions (work with FDA and other federal agencies to implement food safety standards for fish, seafood, milk, and other foods produced within state borders; inspect restaurants, grocery stores, and other retail food establishments, as well as dairy farms and milk processing plants, grain mills, and food manufacturing plants within local jurisdictions; embargo [stop the sale of] unsafe food products made or distributed within state borders)

to carry out its mission that (1) the food supply remains safe, nutritious, and wholesome and (2) labels on foods and cosmetics maintain a high degree of accuracy. These two goals make sense when one considers that about one fifth of every consumer dollar in the United States goes for food and cosmetic products. Consumers spend 25 cents of every consumer dollar on products regulated by the FDA. Of this amount, approximately 75% is spent on food.

The CFSAN specialized support staff includes chemists, microbiologists, toxicologists, food technologists, pathologists, pharmacologists, nutritionists, epidemiologists, mathematicians, and sanitarians. Their areas of responsibility include

- Cosmetics and colors
- Food labeling
- Plant and diary foods and beverages
- Premarket approval
- Special nutritionals such as dietary supplements and infant formulas

The law defines a **"dietary supplement"** (typically sold in the form of tablets, capsules, soft gels, liquids, powders, and bars) as a product taken by mouth that contains a "dietary ingredient" intended to supplement the diet. "Dietary ingredients" may include vitamins, minerals, herbs or other botanicals, amino acids, and substances (e.g., enzymes, organ tissues, glandular material, and metabolites). Dietary supplements may also be extracts or concentrates from plants or foods. Products sold as dietary supplements must be clearly labeled dietary supplements.

In 1994, Congress passed the Dietary Supplement Health and Education Act (DSHEA). This reduced the FDA's control over vitamin, mineral, enzyme, hormone, botanical, amino acid, and herb supplements, which it reclassified as "foods" not drugs. Under the DSHEA, FDA approval stringently requires proof of purity, safety, and effectiveness (via clinical trials) for public consumption of over-the-counter and prescription pharmaceuticals. Marketing of dietary supplements does *not* require such approval because they are considered foods. In contrast to medicines, which must meet safety and efficacy requirements before they come to market, legislation places the burden on the FDA to prove that a supplement is harmful before it can remove it from the market. Marketing a supplement can progress with *only* the manufacturer's assurance of safety as long as the supplement does not claim disease-fighting benefits. Since DSHEA passage, dietary supplements in the United States have skyrocketed, jumping to nearly $10 billion in 1997 from about $5 billion in 1994. Of this total amount, consumers spend nearly $1 billion on dietary supplements related to "sports nutrition."

A manufacturer of an iron-containing supplement cannot make a specific unsubstantiated health claim about a product such as "This product cures anemia." However, more generalized "structure and function" claims are permissible, such as: "Iron is important in the synthesis of hemoglobin in red blood cells." The frightening aspect of lessened control over the supplement industry means that many supplements consumed in excess mimic the harmful effects of illegally obtained chemicals and drugs.

Rules for Dietary Supplements

To add strength to the 1994 DSHEA, the FDA approved a dietary supplement bill in September 1997. The FDA published final rules that provided consumers with somewhat more complete information in the labeling of dietary supplement products. These rules implement some of the major provisions of the DSHEA of 1994 designed to facilitate public access to "natural" medicines. The act requires the FDA to develop labeling requirements specifically designed for products containing ingredients such as vitamins, minerals, herbs, or amino acids intended to supplement the diet.

The new rules require these products to be labeled as dietary supplements (e.g., "Vitamin C Dietary Supplement") and to carry a "Supplement Facts" panel with information similar to the "Nutrition Facts" panel that appears on most processed foods (see page 264). The rules also set parameters for use of the terms "high potency" and "antioxidant" when used in the labeling of dietary supplements. *Despite this attempt by the government to upgrade standards in this industry, consumers must recognize that quality control does not exist for dietary supplements.*

The rules also require that the labels of products containing botanical ingredients identify the part of the plant used. In addition, the source of the dietary ingredient may either follow the name or be listed in the ingredient statement below the "Supplement Parts" panel.

The following guidelines apply for use of the terms "high potency" and "antioxidant" on food labels:

- **High potency** may be used to describe a nutrient in a food product including dietary supplements, at 100% or more of the Reference Daily Intake (RDI) established for that vitamin or mineral. High potency can be used with multi-ingredient products if two thirds of the product's nutrients occur at levels more than 100% of the RDI.
- **Antioxidant** may be used in conjunction with currently defined claims for "good source" and "high" to describe a nutrient for which scientific evidence shows that following absorption of a sufficient quantity, the nutrient (e.g., vitamin C) inactivates free radicals or prevents free radical-initiated chemical reactions.

Summary of Nutritional Labeling Rules for Dietary Supplements, 1999

In March 1999, the FDA mandated that all supplements contain consistent information on a "Supplement Facts" panel. The label must contain a title, a clear identity statement, and a complete list of all ingredients.

Specifically, the "Supplement Facts" panel must contain the following:

1. Title: "Supplement Facts" to allow for easy identification.
2. Information must be listed "per serving." Serving sizes are determined by manufacturer's recommendations for consumption at one occasion.
3. Nutrients required in nutrition labeling of conventional foods must be listed when present and omitted when not present.
4. "Other dietary ingredients" (e.g., botanicals, phytochemicals) that do not have recommendations for daily consumption are listed beneath a bar (see sample). The quantity

present must be stated and identified as having no recommendations for consumption.

5. The list of dietary ingredients in the nutrition label (nutrients and non-nutrients) may include the source ingredient. If so, the source need not be listed again in the ingredient list.
6. Botanicals must state the part of the plant present and be identified by their common usual name. In addition, the Latin binomial name is needed if the sommon or usual name is not listed in *Herbs of Commerce,* published by the American Herbal Products Association.
7. Proprietary blends may be listed with the weight given for the total blend only. When this is done, components of the blend must be listed in descending order of predominance by weight.

The table below shows an example of the DSHEA "Supplement Facts" label.

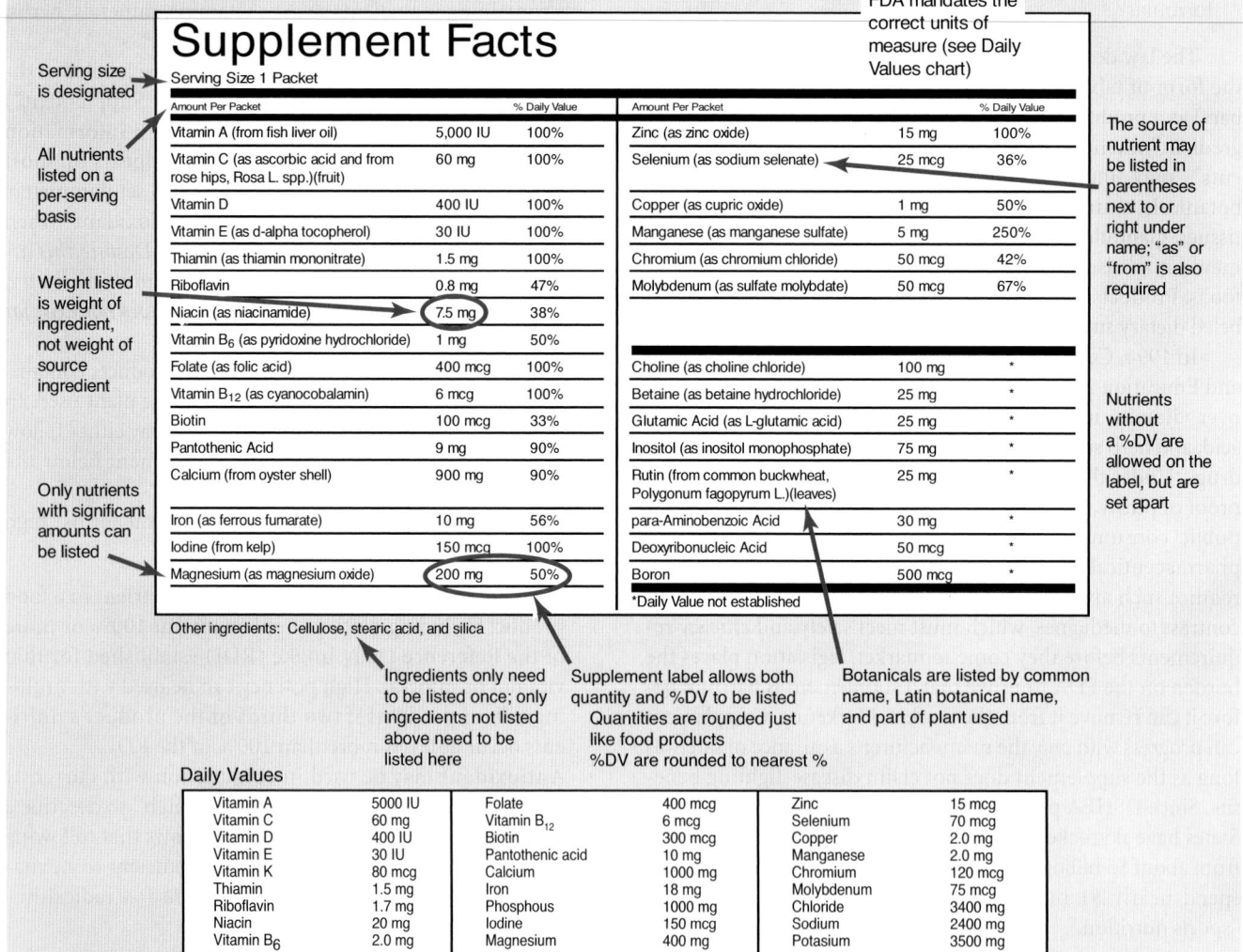

USER BEWARE. Because dietary supplements need not meet the same quality control for purity and potency as pharmaceuticals, considerable variation exists in the concentration of marker compounds.[8] So-called all natural pills and powders sold as dietary supplements have caused lead poisoning, impotence, lethargy and "unarousable" sleep, nausea, vomiting, diarrhea, and abnormal heart rhythms (from the presence of powerful pesticides, herbs, toxic contaminants, or potent prohibited drugs and hormones) in persons trying to self-treat diverse ailments or improve physical function.[1]

Advertisements for "health food" preparations containing natural herbs often promise weight loss, muscle growth, increased endurance capacity, and a drug-free "herbal high." As one government official said: "Some of these products are nothing more than street drugs masquerading as diet supplements." To compound matters, the preparations appear as dietary supplements and thus escape the FDA's rigid control over foods and pharmaceuticals. Many compounds fail to conform to labeling requirements of the DSHEA in terms of proper and correct identification of the strength of the product's ingredients.[3,4] Simply stated, supplement manufacturers need not guarantee that all ingredients are on its label. In this regard, independent organizations such as ConsumerLab (www.ConsumerLab.com) provide their "seal of approval" as to purity and quality control and the safety, effectiveness, and potential for adverse effects for numerous dietary and sport nutrition supplements. These include herbal, vitamin, and mineral supplements that affect health, wellness, and nutrition.

Bureau of Alcohol, Tobacco, and Firearms (ATF)[d]

The ATF, a law enforcement organization within the United States Department of Treasury, came into existence in 1972 after separating from the Internal Revenue Service (Alcohol, Tobacco and Firearms Division). The ATF has responsibilities dedicated to reducing violent crime, collecting revenue, and protecting the public. It enforces federal laws and regulations relating to alcohol, tobacco, firearms, explosives, and arson.

United States Department of Agriculture (USDA)[e]

The USDA deals with farm and foreign agricultural services, food, nutrition, and consumer services, food safety, marketing and regulatory programs, natural resources and environment, research, education, economics, marketing and regulatory

programs, and rural development. The Center for Nutrition Policy and Promotion coordinates nutrition policy in the USDA and provides overall leadership in nutrition education for consumers. The goals of the program include providing needy individuals with access to a more nutritious diet, improving the eating habits of American children, and helping America's farmers find an outlet for distributing food purchased under farmer assistance authorities. The Center serves as the link between basic science and the consumer. The Center coordinates with the DHHS the review, revision, and dissemination of the *Dietary Guidelines for Americans*. This represents the federal government's statement of nutrition policy, formed by a consensus of professionals in science and medicine. The USDA regulates food labels for poultry and meat products.

THE FOOD LABEL (NUTRITION PANEL)

The FDA and the Food Safety and Inspection Service (FSIS: www.fsis.gov) of the USDA issued new regulations concerning nutritional information about food labels to (1) help consumers choose more healthful diets and (2) offer an incentive to food companies to improve the nutritional qualities of their products. Also, the Nutrition Labeling and Education Act (NLEA) of 1990 (including 1993–1998 updates to the regulations) now requires food manufacturers to strictly adhere to regulations about what can and cannot be printed on food labels. The key provisions of food label reform include

- Nutrition labeling for almost all foods to assist consumers in making more healthful food choices
- Information on the amount per serving of saturated fat, cholesterol, dietary fiber, and other nutrients considered of major health concern to consumers
- The amount of *trans* fatty acids on nutrition labels in light of mounting evidence that *trans* fatty acids increase heart disease risk, food processors must also include, by the year 2006
- Nutrient reference values, expressed as % Daily Values, to help consumers determine how a food fits into an overall daily diet
- Uniform definitions for terms that describe a food's nutrient content, such as "light," "low-fat," and "high-fiber," to ensure that such terms have the same meaning for any product on which they appear
- Substantiating claims about the relationship between a nutrient or food and a disease or health-related condition, such as calcium and osteoporosis, and fat and cancer
- Standardized serving sizes to make nutritional comparisons among similar products easier
- Declaration of total percentage of juice in juice drinks so consumers can determine a product's juice content
- Voluntary nutrition information for many raw foods

---

[d]The ATF (www.atf.treas.gov) regulates the qualification and operation of distilleries, wineries, breweries, importers, and wholesalers. The ATF National Laboratory founded in 1886 tests new products coming onto the market and whether any products currently on the market pose a health risk to consumers. In 1996, the ATF laboratories analyzed 8400 alcohol and tobacco samples, processed over 3134 forensic cases, spent 342 days giving expert court testimony, 360 days at crime scenes, and 101 days training federal, state, and local investigators and examiners. To ensure that alcohol beverage labels do not contain misleading information and adhere to regulatory mandates, ATF examines all label applications for approval. The ATF maintains statistics about domestic alcohol and tobacco production.

[e]USDA Internet site: www.usda.gov. The Food and Nutrition Information Center, as part of the USDA, Agricultural Research Service, the National Agricultural Library, maintains an Internet presence (www.nal.usda.gov/fnic/) where users may read, download, or print information. The site links to other sites, including the Healthy School Meals Resource System (www.healthymeals.nal.usda.gov/nal_display/index.php?info_center=14&tax_level=1). Individuals can access full texts of the Food and Nutrition Information Center's (FNIC) bibliographies, resource lists, and fact sheets covering nutrition education, human nutrition, food service management, and others.

The food label must also list ingredients according to how much of the ingredient the food contains. In 2006, food makers were required to clearly state on food labels whether the product contained allergens such as milk, eggs, peanuts, wheat, soy, fish, shellfish, and tree nuts. The American Academy of Allergy Asthma & Immunology (www.aaaai.org/) estimates that food allergies affects up to 2 million or 8% of the children in the United States.

Nutrition Panel Title

The food label displayed in FIGURE 9.1, entitled "Nutrition Facts," differs from the previous title (Nutrition Information

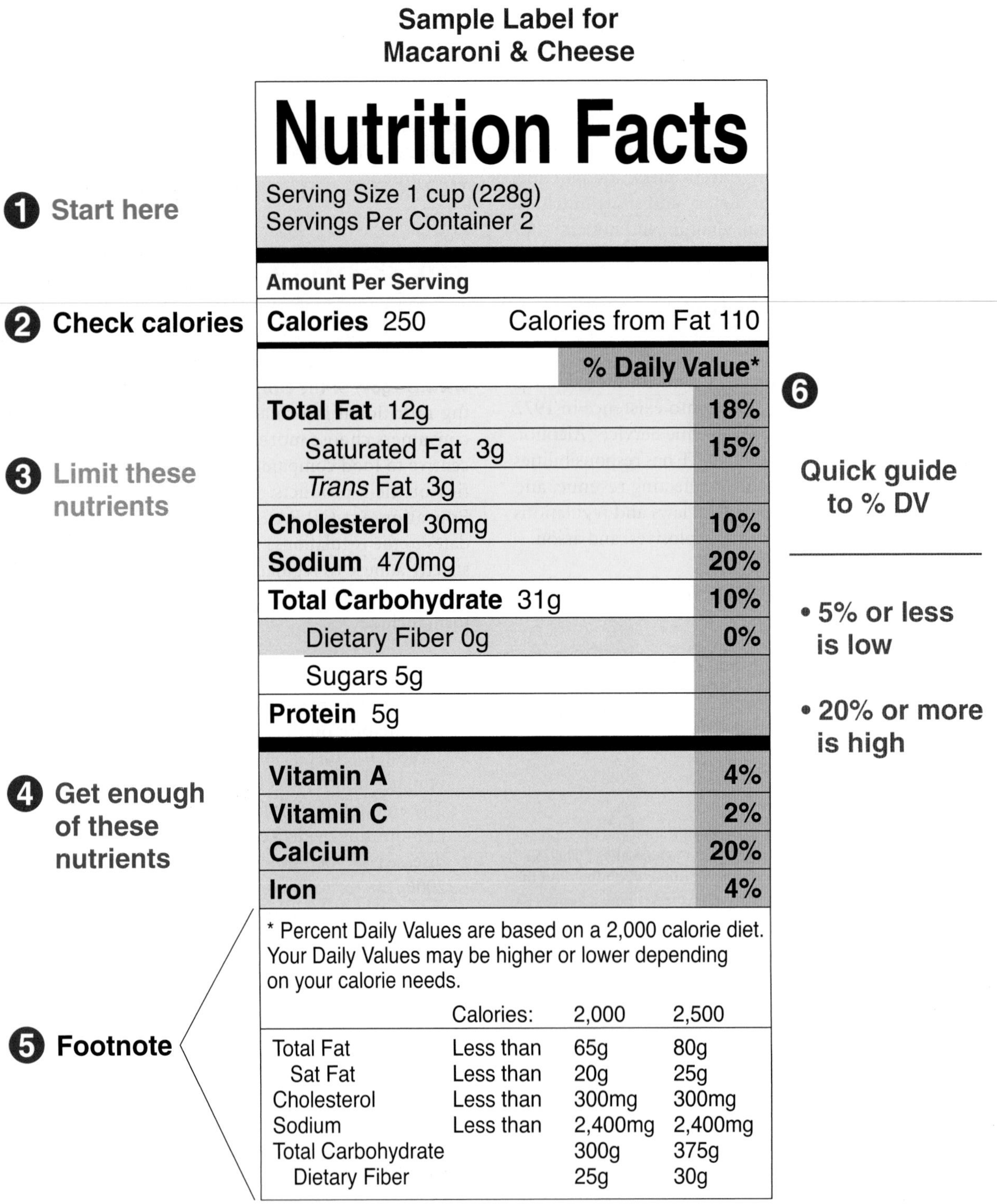

Sample Label for Macaroni & Cheese

Nutrition Facts

1 Start here

Serving Size 1 cup (228g)
Servings Per Container 2

Amount Per Serving

2 Check calories

Calories 250	Calories from Fat 110

	% Daily Value*
Total Fat 12g	**18%**
Saturated Fat 3g	**15%**
Trans Fat 3g	
Cholesterol 30mg	**10%**
Sodium 470mg	**20%**
Total Carbohydrate 31g	**10%**
Dietary Fiber 0g	**0%**
Sugars 5g	
Protein 5g	

Vitamin A	**4%**
Vitamin C	**2%**
Calcium	**20%**
Iron	**4%**

3 Limit these nutrients

4 Get enough of these nutrients

6 Quick guide to % DV

- 5% or less is low

- 20% or more is high

5 Footnote

* Percent Daily Values are based on a 2,000 calorie diet. Your Daily Values may be higher or lower depending on your calorie needs.

	Calories:	2,000	2,500
Total Fat	Less than	65g	80g
Sat Fat	Less than	20g	25g
Cholesterol	Less than	300mg	300mg
Sodium	Less than	2,400mg	2,400mg
Total Carbohydrate		300g	375g
Dietary Fiber		25g	30g

FIGURE 9.1 ■ Reading the nutrition facts panel. Food labels help one make informed choices. Foods that contain only a few of the nutrients required on the standard label have a shorter label format. What is on the label depends on what is in the food. Small- and medium-sized packages with limited label space also can use the short form.

Per Serving) and represents a more distinctive and easy to read label.

Nutrients Listed on Label

The following information must be listed on all food labels:

- Calories from fat/calories from saturated fat
- Total fat
- Saturated fat, stearic acid, polyunsaturated fat, monounsaturated fat, *trans* fat
- Cholesterol
- Sodium
- Potassium
- Total carbohydrate
- Dietary fiber (soluble and insoluble fiber)
- Sugars (sugar alcohols)
- Other carbohydrates
- Protein
- Vitamins and minerals (for which RDIs have been established)

Definitions

The definitions for each of the nutrients listed on the label are as follows:

- **Total fat:** total lipid fatty acids expressed as triglycerides
- **Saturated fat:** the sum of all fatty acids containing no double bonds
- **Polyunsaturated fat:** *cis, cis*-methylene interrupted polyunsaturated fatty acids
- **Monounsaturated fat:** *cis*-monounsaturated fatty acids
- **Total carbohydrate:** amount calculated by subtraction of the sum of crude protein, total fat, moisture, and ash from the total weight of food
- **Sugars:** the sum of all free mono- and disaccharides
- **Other carbohydrate:** the difference between total carbohydrate and the sum of dietary fiber, sugars, and, when declared, sugar alcohol

DAILY VALUES (DV)

The Nutrition Facts Panel must contain two sets of label references values (collectively termed Daily Values). These include daily reference values (DRVs) and reference daily intakes (RDIs).

Daily Reference Value (DRV)

The new label reference value, referred to as Daily Value, comprises two sets of dietary standards: Daily Reference Values (DRVs) and Reference Daily Intakes (RDIs). Only the DRV term appears on the label to make label reading less confusing. DRVs established for macronutrients include sources of energy (fat, carbohydrate [including fiber], and protein) and for non–calorie-contributing cholesterol, sodium, and potassium. A daily intake of 2000 kCal serves as the reference number of calories for determining the DRVs for the energy-producing nutrients. The 2000-kCal level was chosen, in part, because it approximates the caloric requirements for post-menopausal women, the group with the highest risk for excessive intake of calories and fat.

DRVs for the nutrients are calculated as follows based on a 2000-kCal diet:

- Total Fat: 65 g
- Saturated fat: 20 g
- Cholesterol: 300 mg
- Total carbohydrate: 300 g
- Dietary Fiber: 25 g
- Sodium: 2400 mg
- Protein: 50 g

Reference Daily Intake (RDI)

The RDI replaces the term "U.S. RDA," introduced in 1973 as a label reference value for vitamins, minerals, and protein in voluntary nutrition labeling. The name change was sought because of confusion over "U.S. RDA," the values determined by FDA and used on food labels, and "RDA" (Recommended Dietary Allowance), the values determined by the National Academy of Sciences for various population groups and used by the FDA to determine the U.S. RDAs. The values for the new RDIs remain the same as the old U.S. RDAs.

RDIs have been established for the following nutrients:

Vitamin A	Niacin	Magnesium
Vitamin C	Vitamin B_6	Zinc
Calcium	Folate	Selenium
Iron	Vitamin B_{12}	Copper
Vitamin D	Biotin	Manganese
Vitamin E	Pantothenic	Chromium
Vitamin K	acid	Molybdenum
Thiamin	Phosphorus	Chloride
Riboflavin	Iodine	

Nutrition Panel Format

The format for showing nutrient content per serving must be declared as percentages of the Daily Values—the new label reference values. The amount of nutrients (expressed in grams or milligrams) such as fat, cholesterol, sodium, carbohydrates, and protein must be listed to the immediate right of each named nutrient. A column headed "% Daily Value" also must appear on the label.

Declaring nutrients as a percentage of the Daily Values should prevent misinterpretations that arise with quantitative values. For example, one could mistake a food with 140 mg of sodium as a high-sodium food because the number 140 seems relatively large. In actuality, this amount represents less than 6% of the 2400-mg Daily Value for sodium. On the other hand, a food with 5 g of saturated fat could be construed as being low in that nutrient. However, that food provides one-fourth the total 20-g Daily Value for saturated fat based on a 2000-kCal diet. (The % Daily Value listing carries a footnote declaring that percentages are based on a 2000-kCal diet.)

NUTRIENT CONTENT DESCRIPTORS

TABLE 9.2 presents the guidelines about the claims and descriptions that manufacturers can use in food labeling to promote their products.

Additional Definitions

The labeling regulations also provide guidelines for additional definitions:

- **Percent fat free:** A product bearing this claim must be a low-fat or a fat-free product. In addition, the claim must accurately reflect the amount of fat present in 100 g of the food. Thus, if a food contains 2.5 g fat per 50 g, the claim must be "95% fat free."

- **Implied:** These types of claims are prohibited when they wrongfully imply that a food contains or does not contain a meaningful level of a nutrient. For example, a product claiming to be made with an ingredient known as a source of fiber (such as "made with oat bran") is prohibited unless the product contains enough of that ingredient (e.g., oat bran) to meet the definition for "good source" of fiber. As another example, a claim that a product contains "no tropical oils" is allowed, but only for foods that are "low" in saturated fat, because consumers have come to equate tropical oils with high saturated fat.

TABLE 9.2   Requirements for Manufacturers' Claims on Food Labels

Claim	Requirements That Must Be Met Before Using the Claim in Food Labeling
Fat-Free	Less than 0.5 g of fat per serving, with no added fat or oil
Low fat	3 g or less of fat per serving
Less fat	25% or less of fat than the comparison food
Saturated Fat Free	Less than 0.5 g of saturated fat and 0.5 g of *trans* fatty acids per serving
Cholesterol-Free	Less than 2 mg of cholesterol per serving, and 2 g or less of saturated fat per serving
Low Cholesterol	20 mg or less of cholesterol per serving and 2 g or less of saturated fat per serving
Reduced Calorie	At least 25% fewer calories per serving than the comparison food
Low Calorie	40 calories or less per serving
Extra Lean	Less than 5 g of fat, 2 g of saturated fat, and 95 mg of cholesterol per (100 g) serving of meat, poultry, or seafood
Lean	Less than 10 g of fat, 4.5 g of saturated fat, and 95 mg of cholesterol per (100 g) serving of meat, poultry, or seafood
Light (fat)	50% or less of the fat than in the comparison food (e.g., 50% less fat than a company's regular cheese)
Light (calories)	1/3 fewer calories than the comparison food
High-Fiber	5 g or more fiber per serving
Sugar-Free	Less than 0.5 g of sugar per serving
Sodium-Free or Salt-Free	Less than 5 mg of sodium per serving
Low Sodium	140 mg or less per serving
Very Low Sodium	35 mg or less per serving
Healthy	A food low in fat, saturated fat, cholesterol, and sodium, and contains at least 10% of the Daily Values for vitamin A, vitamin C, iron, calcium, protein, or fiber
"High," "Rich in," or "Excellent Source"	20% or more of the Daily Value for a given nutrient per serving
"Less," "Fewer" or "Reduced"	At least 25% less of a given nutrient or calories than the comparison food
"Low," "Little," "Few," or "Low Source of"	An amount that would allow frequent consumption of the food without exceeding the Daily Value for the nutrient; can only make the claim as it applies to all similar foods
"Good Source of," "More," or "Added"	The food provides 10% more of the Daily Value for a given nutrient than the comparison food

- **Meals and main dishes:** Claims that a meal or main dish is "free" of a nutrient, such as sodium or cholesterol, must meet the same requirements as those for individual foods. Other claims can be used under special circumstances. For example, "low-calorie" means the meal or main dish contains 120 kCal or less per 100 g. "Low-sodium" means the food has 140 mg or less per 100 g. "Low-cholesterol" means the food contains 20 mg of cholesterol or less per 100 g and no more than 2 g of saturated fat. "Light" means the meal or main dish is low fat or low calorie.
- **Standardized foods:** Any nutrient content claim, such as "reduced fat," "low calorie," and "light," may be used in conjunction with a standardized term if the new product has been specifically formulated to meet FDA's criteria for that claim, the product is not nutritionally inferior to the traditional standardized food, and the new product complies with certain compositional requirements set by the FDA. A new product bearing a claim also must have performance characteristics similar to those of the referenced traditional standardized food. If the product does not and the differences materially limit the product's use, its label must state the differences (e.g., not recommended for baking) to inform consumers.

What Does "Fresh" Mean?

Although not mandated by labeling regulations, the FDA has issued directions for use of the term "fresh." The agency took this step because of concern over possible misuse of this term on some food labels. The regulation defines "fresh" to suggest that a food is raw or unprocessed. In this context, "fresh" can describe a raw food, a food that has never been frozen or heated, and one that contains no preservatives (irradiation at low levels is allowed). "Fresh frozen," "frozen fresh," and "freshly frozen" can describe foods quickly frozen while still fresh. Blanching (brief scalding before freezing to prevent nutrient breakdown) is allowed. Other uses of the term "fresh," as in "fresh milk" or "freshly baked bread," are not affected.

How Sweetness Is Measured

Splenda (sucralose) is 600 times sweeter than sugar and three times sweeter than Equal (aspartame or Nutrasweet). How does one compare sweetness? Scientists measure the relative degree of sweetness with panels of trained participants who compare samples of plain water to those with progressively higher concentrations of sweetener until they notice a difference. The "threshold value" for a compound occurs when 50% of the testers detect a change from the taste of the nonsweetened water. Scientists measure relative sweetness by comparing the threshold values for various types of sugar and sugar substitutes. The average person can detect a solution of approximately 0.5% sucrose (1 tsp of table sugar dissolved in a glass of water). The compound neotame (FDA approved in 2002), is 7000 to 13,000 times sweeter than sucrose.

FOOD ADDITIVES

A manufacturer wishing to include an additive in a food must follow specific FDA guidelines. The manufacturer must test to ensure the additive meets its claims. The FDA also requires that the additive be detected and measured in the product and that it produces no undesirable health effects (e.g., cancer or birth defects) when given in large doses to animals. Strict guidelines exist once the FDA approves an additive.

Approximately 700 additives were initially included on a list of additives **generally recognized as safe (GRAS).** An expanded GRAS list currently includes about 2000 flavoring agents and 200 coloring agents. These substances do not receive permanent approval but face review periodically. Additives include emulsifiers, stabilizers, thickeners (to provide texture, smoothness, and consistency), nutrients such as vitamin C added to fruit juice or potassium iodide added to salt (to improve nutritive value), flavoring agents (to enhance taste), leavening agents (to make baked goods rise, or to control acidity or alkalinity), preservatives, antioxidants, sequestrants, and antimycotic agents (to prevent spoilage, rancidity of fats, and microbial growth), coloring agents (to increase attractiveness), bleaches (to whiten foods and speed up the maturing of cheese), and humectants and anticaking agents (to retain moisture and keep products such as salts and powders free flowing).

BABY FOODS

The FDA does not allow the broad use of nutrient claims on infant and toddler foods. The agency may propose later claims specifically for these foods. The terms "unsweetened" and "unsalted" can be used on these foods because they relate to taste and not nutrient content.

HEALTH CLAIMS

Current regulations now permit claims for relationships between intake of a nutrient or a food and the risk of disease or health-related condition. They can be made in several ways: through third-party references, such as the National Cancer Institute or the American Heart Association; statements; symbols, such as a heart; and vignettes or descriptions. Whatever the case, the claim must meet requirements for authorized health claims. For example, a claim cannot state the degree of risk reduction; it can only use "may" or "might" in discussing the nutrient–or food–disease relationship. In addition, claims must state that other factors play a role in that disease. Health claims also must be phrased so that consumers can understand the relationship between the nutrient and the disease and the nutrient's importance to a daily diet. The following exemplifies an appropriate health claim: "While many factors affect heart disease, diets low in saturated fat and cholesterol may reduce the risk of this disease."

Nutrient–disease relationship claims are as follows:

Approved health claims
- Soluble fiber and heart disease
- Dietary fat and cancer
- Saturated fat/cholesterol and heart disease
- Calcium and osteoporosis
- Fiber-containing grain products, fruits, and vegetables and cancer
- Folate and neural tube defects
- Dietary sugar alcohols and dental caries
- Whole oats, psyllium, and heart disease
- Soy protein and heart disease
- Calcium and hypertension
- Plant sterol and plant sterol esters and heart disease

Approved authoritative health claim statements
- Whole grains and heart disease and cancer (first health claim approved under the FDA Modernization Act of 1997)
- Potassium and high blood pressure

Qualified health claims (supportive but not conclusive research)
- Heart-healthy benefits of omega-3 fatty acids
- Eating 1.5 oz of walnuts a day may reduce coronary heart disease risk
- Eating 2 tbsp (23 g) of olive oil daily may reduce the risk of coronary heart disease due to the monounsaturated fat in olive oil

Health claims denied approval
- Dietary fiber and cancer (wheat bran and colon cancer)
- Dietary fiber and cardiovascular disease
- Antioxidant vitamins and cancer
- Zinc and immune function and the elderly

Possible future health claims (1–5 years)
- Folic acid/B_6/B_{12} and heart disease
- Low-fat dairy products and hypertension

TABLE 9.3 presents rules for the use of allowable health claims and an example of an accompanying label statement.

LABELING OF INGREDIENTS

The ingredient list on a food label is the listing of each ingredient in descending order of predominance. Descending order of predominance means that the ingredients are listed in order of predominance by weight, that is, the ingredient that weighs the most is listed first, and the ingredient that weighs the least is listed last.

> **Example:** INGREDIENTS: Pinto Beans, Water, and Salt

Water added in making a food is considered to be an ingredient. The added water must be identified in the list of ingredients and listed in its descending order of predominance by weight.

> **Example:** INGREDIENTS: Water, Navy Beans, and Salt

Always listed is the common or usual name for ingredients unless there is a regulation that provides for a different term. For instance, the term "sugar" is used instead of the scientific name "sucrose."

> **Example:** INGREDIENTS: Apples, Sugar, Water, and Spices

Listing trace ingredients depends on whether the trace ingredient is present in a significant amount and has a function in the finished food. If a substance is an incidental additive and has no function or technical effect in the finished product, then it need not be declared on the label. An incidental additive is usually present because it is an ingredient of another ingredient. Sulfites are considered to be incidental only if present at less than 10 ppm.

Listing alternative fat and oil ingredients ("and/or" labeling) is permitted only in the case of foods that contain relatively small quantities of added fat or oil ingredients (foods in which added fats or oils are not the predominant ingredient) and only if the manufacturer is unable to predict which fat or oil ingredient will be used.

> **Example:** INGREDIENTS: . . . Vegetable Oil (contains one or more of the following: Corn Oil, Soybean Oil, or Safflower Oil) . . . .

When an approved chemical preservative is added to a food, the ingredient list must include both the common or usual name of the preservative and the function of the preservative by including terms such as "preservative," "to retard spoilage," "a mold inhibitor," "to help protect flavor," or "to promote color retention."

> **Example:** INGREDIENTS: Dried Bananas, Sugar, Salt, and Ascorbic Acid to Promote Color Retention

Spices, natural flavors or artificial flavors may be declared in ingredient lists by using either specific common or usual names or by using the declarations "spices," "flavor" or "natural flavor," or "artificial flavor."

> **Example:** INGREDIENTS: Apple Slices, Water, Cane Syrup, Corn Syrup, Modified Corn Starch, Spices, Salt, Natural Flavor, and Artificial Flavor

Spices, such as paprika, turmeric, saffron, and others that are also colorings must be declared either by the term "spice and coloring" or by the actual (common or usual) names, such as "paprika."

Vegetable powders must be declared by common or usual name, such as "celery powder."

Artificial coloring agents must be listed if they are certified as coloring agents by the FD&C. They are listed by specific or abbreviated name such as "FD&C Red No. 40" or "Red 40."

Noncertified colors are listed as "artificial color," "artificial coloring," or by their specific common or usual names such as "caramel coloring" and "beet juice."

TABLE 9.3 Requirements for Approved Health Claims with an Example of Label Statement

Nutritional Requirements for Claims	Example of Label Statement
Dietary Fat and Cancer The food must meet the criteria for "low-fat."	Development of cancer depends on many factors. A diet low in total fat may reduce the risk of some cancers.
Saturated Fat/Cholesterol and Heart Disease The food must meet the criteria for "low-fat," "low saturated fat," and "low cholesterol."	Although many factors affect heart disease, diets low in saturated fat and cholesterol may reduce the risk of this disease.
Calcium and Osteoporosis The food must meet the criteria for "high in calcium." The calcium in the product must be bioavailable. The food shall not contain more phosphorus than calcium on a weight basis. *(For foods containing more than 40% recommended dietary intake of calcium, special requirements exist.)*	Regular exercise and a healthy diet with enough calcium helps teens and young adults and white and Asian women maintain good bone health and may reduce their high risk of osteoporosis later in life.
Fiber-Containing Grain Products, Fruits, Vegetables, and Cancer The claim is limited to foods that are or that contain a fruit, vegetable, or grain product. The food must meet the criteria for "low-fat" and "good source of fiber."	Low-fat diets rich in fiber-containing grain products, fruits, and vegetables may reduce the risk of some types of cancer, which is associated with many factors.
Fruit and Vegetables and Cancer The claim is limited to foods that are or that contain a fruit or vegetable. The food must meet the criteria for "low-fat." The food must meet the criteria for "good source" of vitamins A or C or dietary fiber (prior to fortification).	Low-fat diets rich in fruits and vegetables (foods that are low in fat and may contain dietary fiber, vitamins A and C) may reduce the risk of some types of cancer, which is associated with many factors.
Folate and Neural Tube Defects The food must meet the criteria for a "good source of folic acid."	Healthful diets with adequate folate may reduce a woman's risk of having a child with a brain or spinal cord birth defect.
Dietary Sugar and Dental Caries The food must meet the criteria for "sugar-free." Sugar alcohol in the food must be a xylitol, sorbitol, mannitol, maltitol, isomalt, lactitol, hydrogenated starch hydrolysates, hydrogenated glucose syrups, or a combination of these.	Frequent between-meal consumption of foods high in sugars and starches promotes tooth decay. The sugar alcohols in [name of food] do not promote tooth decay.
Oats and Psyllium and Heart Disease The food must meet the criteria for "low-fat," "saturated fat," and "low-cholesterol." The food must contain at least 0.75 g of soluble fiber from beta glucan or 7 g of soluble fiber from psyllium (prior to fortification)	[Number of] grams soluble fiber daily from [source of soluble fiber] such as [name of product] as part of a diet low in saturated fat and cholesterol, may reduce the risk of heart disease. [Name of product] provides [Number of] grams per [number of] cup.
Soy Protein and Heart Disease The food must meet the criteria for "low fat," "saturated fat," and "low-cholesterol." The food must contain at least 6.25 g of soy protein.	Diets low in saturated fat and cholesterol that include 25 g of soy protein may reduce the risk of heart disease. A serving of [name of food] provides [number of] grams soy protein.
Whole Grains and Heart Disease and Cancer Whole grain must contain all portions of the kernel: bran, germ, and endosperm. The food must contain at least 51% whole-grain ingredients by weight. The food must meet the criteria for "low-fat"	Low-fat diets rich in whole-grain foods and other plant foods may reduce the risk of heart disease and certain cancers.
Potassium and High Blood Pressure The food must meet criteria for "good source of potassium" and "low in sodium."	Diets containing foods that are good sources of potassium and low in sodium may reduce the risk of high blood pressure and stroke.
Plant Sterols and Plant Stanol Esters Among the foods that may qualify for claims based on plant sterol ester contents are spreads, salad dressings, snack bars, and dietary supplements in softgel form.	Foods containing at least 0.65 grams per serving of plant sterol esters, eaten twice per day with meals for a total daily intake of at least 1.3 grams, as part of a diet low in saturated fat and cholesterol, may reduce the risk of heart disease.

DETERMINING THE NUTRIENT PERCENTAGE IN A FOOD

Food labels must indicate the amount of a nutrient in packaged foods, yet no requirement exists to list nutrient composition in foods sold over-the-counter or in restaurants. Such information becomes quite revealing and often embarrassing to manufacturers who extol their "commitment to consumers" by providing "healthful" products.

Consider several popular franchise chains that tout their hamburgers for providing quality nutrition: McDonald's informs consumers that a "Big Mac" contains *only* 35 g of fat; Burger King lists the fat content of a "Whopper" at 42 g, and Roy Rogers' cheeseburger contains 37.3 g of fat. But these food retailers conceal important information about the food's fat content expressed as a percentage of total calories. For the Big Mac, 35 g of fat amounts to 315 kCal from fat (35 g × 9 kCal · g^{-1}). Because a Big Mac contains a total of 570 kCal, the percentage calories from fat ([315 ÷ 570] × 100) translates to 55.2% fat! Burger King's "Whopper" contains a whopping 57.7% fat, and the cheeseburger from Roy Rogers tops the list at 59.6% fat.

Not surprisingly, manufacturers downplay such information. TABLE 9.4 illustrates the importance of understanding the information in a product's label, particularly its lipid content. For example, most regular granola-type cereals contain a variety of nutritious whole grains; but they also contain considerable fat (Table 9.4A). Similarly, the number of fat grams in McDonald's french fries represents only 17.7% of the food's weight, but the percentage of total calories as fat jumps to 48.3% (Table 9.4B) Thus, fat contributes the largest percentage of this serving's 402 kCal. This occurs in spite of McDonald's commendable decision to replace the *trans* fatty acid component of the fries with a less harmful form of unsaturated fatty acid.

Learn to Read Food Labels

To illustrate the importance of understanding the components of a food label, TABLE 9.5 compares four popular products from the Hershey Foods company for protein, carbohydrate, and lipid content. The comparison includes the caloric value (kCal) and amount (g) of the nutrient, information provided by the manufacturer. Reading the table's footnote easily uncovers the percentage of a nutrient in relation to the product's total caloric content (not provided by the manufacturer). In Hershey's nutrition brochure widely distributed to consumers, a common question concerning their chocolate products states: "How many calories does a Hershey's Miniature Bar contain?" The manufacturer's answer: "There are 40 calories in a Hershey's Miniature Bar. This same calorie count applies for all the Hershey's Miniature Bars—Milk Chocolate, Special Dark, Mr. Goodbar, and Krackel." The brochure fails to reveal that the chocolate bars contain approximately 50% fat, whether they are small or large size! A consumer does not need the skills of Sherlock Holmes to revel in such discoveries. This applies to any food; just perform the same computations as done for the chocolate products listed in Table 9.5.

TABLE 9.4 **Reading Between the Lines: (A) Comparison of the Percentage of Total Calories from Lipid in Five Granola Cereals (one low-fat) with Wheaties and Cheerios and (B) Macronutrient Content as Weight and Percentage of Total Calories in One Large Serving of McDonald's French Fries**

A. Granola Cereals: Source of Hidden Fat

Type	Total kCal	Lipid (g)	kCal from Lipid (lipid, g^{-1})	% kCal from Lipid
Erewhon Honey Almond	130	6.0	54.0	41.5
Good Morning Pecan Splendor	130	6.0	54.0	41.5
Quaker 100% Natural	130	5.0	45.0	34.6
Homemade with nuts, raisins	138	7.7	69.0	50.0
Kellogg's Low-Fat	120	2.0	18.0	15.0
Wheaties	99	0.5	4.5	4.5
Cheerios	110	1.8	14.7	15.0

B. Food Weight versus Number of Calories (Food: McDonald's french fries, large; weight: 122.3 g [4.3 oz])

Nutrient	Weight (g)	kCal	% Weight	% kCal
Protein	6	24	4.9	6.0
Carbohydrate	45.9	183.6	37.5	45.7
Lipid	21.6	194.4	17.7	48.3
Ash	3.2	0	2.6	0
Water	45.6	0		0
Total	122.3	402	100	100

Conversion factors: protein and carbohydrate, 4 kCal per g; lipid, 9 kCal per g

Source of nutrient information: McDonald's Nutrition Information Center, McDonald's Corporation, Oak Brook, IL 60521

TABLE 9.5	Consumer Beware. Learn to Interpret the Nutritional Label to Determine the Percentage of a Particular Nutrient in Relation to a Food's Total Energy Content								
			Protein		**Carbohydrate**		**Lipid**		
Item	**Amount**	**Total kCal**	**(g)**	**% kCal[a]**	**(g)**	**% kCal[a]**	**(g)**	**% kCal[a]**	
Hershey's Chocolate milk (2% low fat)	1 cup (8 oz)	190	8	16.8	29	61.0	5	23.7	
Hershey's Chocolate Kisses	9 pieces (1.5 oz)	220	3	5.5	23	41.8	13	53.0	
Hershey's Reese's Peanut Butter Cup	2 cups (1.8 oz)	280	6	8.6	26	37.1	17	54.6	
Hershey's New Trail Granola Snack Bars, chocolate covered cocoa crème	1.3 oz	190	2	4.2	24	50.5	9	42.6	

Data from Nutrition Information for Consumers. Hershey Foods, Consumer Relations Department, P.O. Box 815, Hershey, PA 17033-0815. The percentage values were computed from the nutrient information listed in the table provided by Hershey's; data on percentages were not included as part of their table.

[a]This column, which represents the percentage of total calories for each of the macronutrients, was not provided by the manufacturer. To compute the percentage contribution of a particular nutrient, multiply the caloric value for the nutrient (protein and carbohydrate = 4 kCal·g⁻¹; lipid = 9 kCal·g⁻¹) times the number of grams. Express the value in relation to the total number of calories. For example, to compute the percentage of lipid in Hershey's Chocolate Kisses (last column), multiply 9 (kCal·g⁻¹) × 13 (number of grams) to obtain 117 kCal. Then (117 ÷ 220) × 100 = 53%, which is the percentage of total calories supplied by lipid!

NUTRIENT DENSITY

Determining a food's **nutrient density** or "healthfullness" provides useful information about its nutritional quality. One concept of nutrient density[2] refers to the quantity of a specific nutrient (protein, vitamins, and minerals) per 100 g of the food or per 1000 kCal of that food. In essence, comparing foods for nutrient density conveniently determines the better food source for a particular nutrient. Computing a food's **Index of Nutritional Quality (INQ)** makes this practical. Usually, the numerator of the INQ refers to the nutrient amount per 100 g of food divided by the RDA for that nutrient. The denominator represents the number of kCal per 100 g divided by the population average for energy intake (3000 kCal for men and 2000 kCal for women). An INQ greater than 1.0 means the food provides an adequate source of that nutrient; an INQ less than 1.0 indicates an inadequate nutritional source. For convenience in classification, a food considered "good" has an INQ between 2 and 6, while an INQ above 6 denotes an excellent source of the nutrient.

INQ = (Amount of nutrient per 100 g ÷ RDA for that nutrient) ÷ (kCal in 100 g ÷ Population average for energy intake)

Let's determine which food provides the best source of protein: whole milk, 1 and 2% low-fat milk, a raw egg, regular vanilla ice cream, chocolate chip cookies, or a McDonald's Big Mac hamburger. The calculations apply to an adult male (age 25–50) with an average daily energy intake of 3000 kCal.

First, refer to Appendix A for the protein content for 100 g (3.52 oz) of each of the six foods. The following example illustrates how to compute the INQ for protein in one raw egg:

Step 1. Compute the amount of protein in 100 g of egg. Appendix A presents the values in 1 oz, or 28.4 g. Because there is 3.52 g of protein per 28.4 g (0.124 per g of egg), 100 g of egg yields 12.4 g of protein.

Step 2. Divide the step 1 result by 63 g (protein RDA for adult males, age 25–50); 12.4 g ÷ 63 g = 0.197.

Step 3. Compute the number of Calories in 100 g of egg. Because 1 oz yields 40 (1.41 Calories per g of egg), then 100 g of egg yields 141 calories.

Step 4. Divide the step 3 result by 3000 (energy expenditure for average adult male): 141 calories ÷ 3000 kCal ÷ 0.047.

Step 5. Divide the step 2 result by the step 4 result to obtain the INQ for the protein in egg: 0.197 ÷ 0.047 = 4.2.

The other food items have the following protein INQ values: whole milk, 2.67; 2% milk, 3.24; 1% low-fat milk, 3.75; chocolate chip cookies, 0.61; Big Mac, 0.525. The inescapable conclusion: the egg ranks first and 1% low-fat milk second as best protein sources per quantity of food compared with the other food items.

A food's excellent INQ rating for a single nutrient does not reflect an equivalent rating for other nutrients. No single food ranks excellent for all of its nutrients. *In essence, no perfect food exists; some foods are just more nutritious than others per amount of a particular nutrient consumed.*

WHAT AMERICANS EAT

The panels A through E in FIGURE 9.2 display patterns of eating in the United States over a 20-year period for red meat, fish, and poultry; whole, low-fat, and nonfat milk; eggs; fats and oils from animal and vegetable sources; and refined sugars, corn sweeteners, honey, and low-calorie sweeteners.

For some classes of foods, the scorecard on a health basis rates as improved; most other items have a considerable way to go. For example, beef, mostly as hamburger, still maintains a prime position on the menus of American restaurants. Still, this popularity has failed to stem the decline in beef consumption. Twenty years ago, Americans consumed about 77 lb of beef per person and 51 lb of chicken, whereas in 2001 this figure changed to 66 lb of beef and 76 lb of chicken.

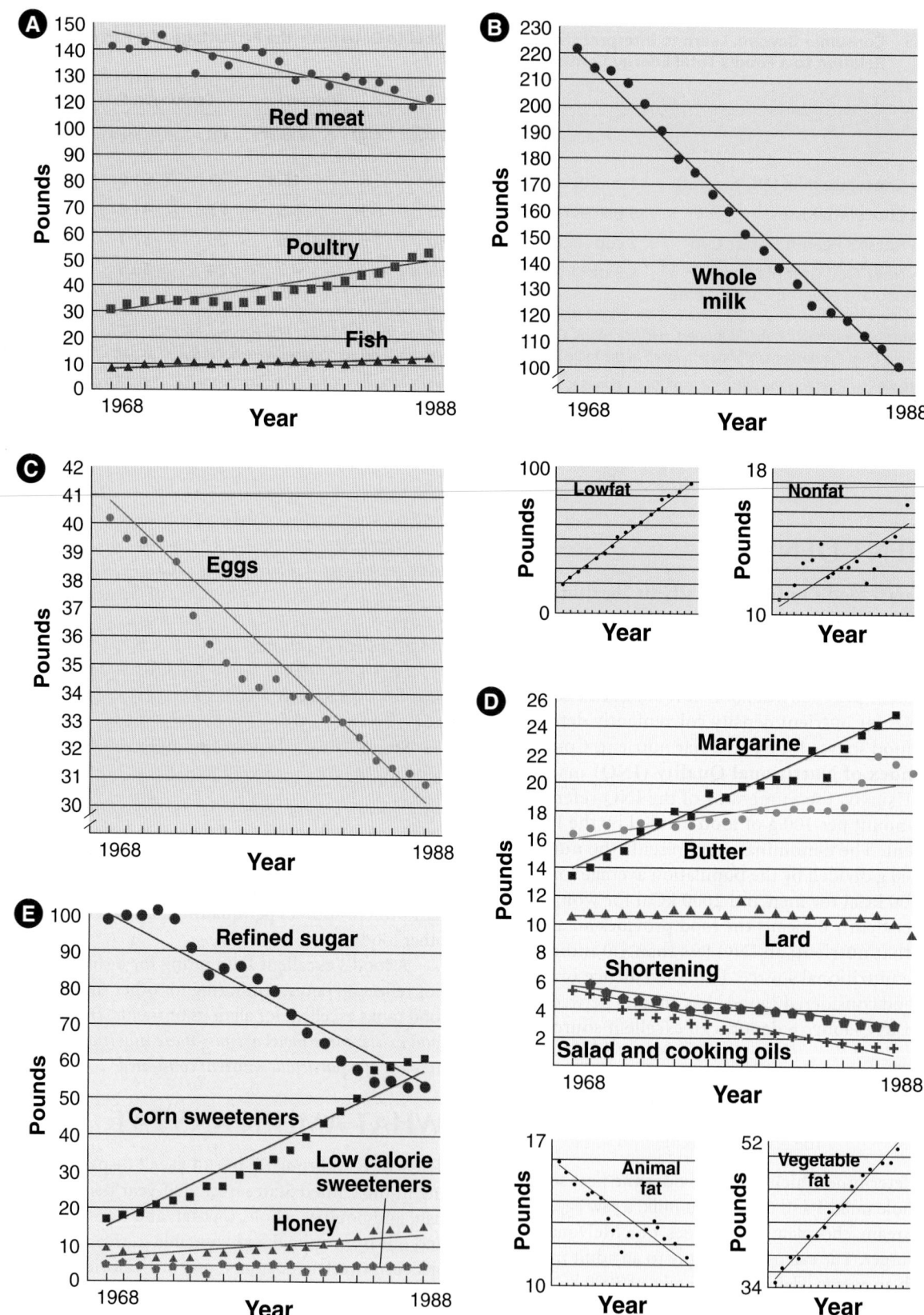

FIGURE 9.2 ■ Patterns of food consumption over a 20-year period. **A.** Red meat, fish, and poultry. **B.** Whole, lowfat, and nonfat milk. **C.** Eggs. **D.** Fats and oils from animal and vegetables. **E.** Refined sugars, corn sweeteners, honey, and low-calorie sweeteners. (Data from Putnam JJ. Food consumption, prices, and expenditures, 1967–1988. Unites States Department of Agriculture. Commodity Economics Division. Economic Research Service. statistical bulletin no. 804. Washington, DC, May 1990.)

The meaningful trends in the data summarize as follows:

- **Panel A:** An inverse relation exists between red meat consumption and consumption of poultry and fish. On a yearly per person basis over the 20-year period, Americans now consume 8.2 kg less red meat, 13.2 kg more poultry, and about 1 kg more fish and shellfish. The relatively small increase in fish consumption may relate to fear of contamination. Unlike red meat and poultry, seafood does not require federal inspection. The United States ranks twenty-seventh in fish and shellfish consumption among 45 other countries surveyed by the Food and Agricultural Organization of the United Nations. For example, the per capita yearly fish intake in Japan (86.2 kg) and Iceland (180.5 kg) far exceeded that in the United States (16.6 kg).
- **Panel B:** A marked increase occurred in drinking low-fat and nonfat milk compared with whole milk. This represents a 54% decline in consumption of whole milk and more than a 300% increase in low-fat and skim milk consumption (from 18.6 kg to 56.2 kg per person) over the study period.
- **Panel C:** Americans consume fewer eggs purchased in shells (285 per capita in 1968 vs. 184 in 1990), but eggs consumed in products such as pasta have correspondingly increased by 40.6% (14.5 kg in 1968 vs. 120.5 kg in 1989). The steady decline in shell egg consumption relates to media attention concerning dietary cholesterol and its link to coronary heart disease.
- **Panel D:** Since 1968, fat and oil consumption increased 19.5% from 23.1 kg to 27.6 kg per person yearly. The 4.77 ratio of vegetable to animal fats consumed in 1989 (22.9 kg ÷ 4.8 kg) averaged tenfold higher than the 0.475 ratio in 1968 (7.45 kg ÷ 15.7 kg). Animal fat accounted for 17% of total lipid intake in 1989, compared with 32% in 1968. Vegetable fat and oil represented 68% of total lipid consumption in 1968, compared with 83% in 1989. The shift from animal to vegetable sources of lipids reflects the consumer's health preference for reduced cholesterol and increased intake of unsaturated rather than saturated fatty acids. Of potential concern is the increase in total lipid consumption from (1) a greater intake of fried foods from various food outlets, particularly fast-food restaurants, and (2) the increased consumption of salad oils. Salad and cooking oil use has doubled, and shortening use has increased by one third, yet decreases occurred for whole-lard shortening, butter, and margarine. Of the total 6.6 billion kg of oils consumed in 1988, 4% (250 million kg) consisted of the highly saturated palm, palm kernel, and coconut tropical oils.
- **Panel E:** Per capita yearly consumption of sweeteners increased steadily from 56.8 kg in 1968 to 69.5 kg in 1988. Since 1968, intake of high-fructose corn syrup increased from 0.23 kg to 22.2 kg per person in 1990! The dramatic rise in low-calorie sweeteners reflects the 1981 introduction of aspartame, a sugar substitute almost 200 times sweeter than sucrose.

TABLE 9.6 shows the percentage change in dietary patterns over the study period between blacks and whites and the poor and affluent. Contrary to the conventional wisdom in 1965 (and perhaps presently), an apparent convergence exists between blacks and whites and across socioeconomic groups. The wealthier whites in 1965 had the lowest score for a healthful diet, while the poorer blacks consumed a diet rated more healthful, a difference attributed to inability of blacks to afford more "unhealthful" food choices of meat and other foods high in saturated fatty acids. In the 1991 analysis, affluent Americans ate more like their low-income counterparts. A higher percentage of both blacks and whites (the most dramatic gain among the wealthier whites) ate health-promoting diets; they reduced consumption of saturated fats and cholesterol and reduced total fat intake to 35% of total calories (down from 40%). An increase occurred in skim milk or low-fat milk consumption, yet negative trends persisted for both groups for increased intake of "hidden" fats in pizza, tacos, and pasta dishes. Intake of dietary fiber changed little.

Despite positive gains of all groups in nutrient intake, less than 25% of any group met four of the recommendations for dietary improvement. This resulted partly from the sharp increase in consuming packaged and restaurant food—foods high in lipid, saturated fatty acids, salt, and calories and low in fiber.

TABLE 9.6 Percentage Changes in High-Fat and Low-Fat Food Consumption among Americans of Different Races and Income Levels from 1965 to 1991

	Poorer Respondents		Wealthier Respondents[a]
	Whites	**Blacks**	**Whites**
High fat			
Milk	292	−66	−99
Cheese	+130	+271	+72
Egg items	−45	−24	−62
Red meat	−71	−89	−89
Low fat			
Milk	+607	+92	+256
Poultry	+77	−26	+157
Noncitrus fruits	24	−24	−25
Dark green or orange vegetables	+21	13	+44
Soy products and legumes	0	−24	+156

From Popkin BM, et al. A comparison of dietary trends among the racial and socioeconomic groups in the United States. N Engl J Med 1996;335:716.

[a]Blacks of high socioeconomic status are not listed because of the small number of respondents in the 1965 survey.

Popular Fast-Food Chains Offer "Healthier" Food Options

The table lists traditional fast-food items first (in red), followed by new alternatives (in blue).

Food	Calories	Total fat (grams)	Trans fat (grams)	Saturated fat (grams)	Sodium (mg)
BURGER KING					
Whopper with Cheese	760	47	1.5	16	1450
Tendergrill Chicken Sandwich	450	10	0	2	1210
BK Veggie Burger	420	16	0	2.5	1100
Tendergrill Chicken Caesar Salad					
• Light Italian Dressing	360	20	0	4	1160
• No dressing	240	9	0	2.5	720
McDonald's					
Quarter Pounder with Cheese	510	25	1.5	12	1150
Grilled Chicken Classic Sandwich	420	9	0	2	1240
Grilled Chicken Cobb Salad					
• Cobb Dressing	400	20	0	6.5	1560
• Low-Fat Balsamic Vinaigrette	320	14	0	5	1850
WENDY'S					
Big Bacon Classic Hamburger	580	29	1.5	12	1400
Classic Single Hamburger (no mayo)	400	16	1	6.5	840
Crispy Chicken Sandwich (no mayo)	350	12	2	3	760
Baked Potato with broccoli and cheese (no butter)	340	3.5	0	1	430

Thirty-Year Increase in Calorie Intake: More Food and More of It As Sugar

A 30-year study by the Centers for Disease Control and Prevention of Americas' eating habits shows that the amount of fat people eat has remained relatively steady while total energy intake has increased, particularly energy derived from increased simple sugar intake. FIGURE 9.3 indicates that from 1971 to 2000, women increased caloric intake by 22% and men increased intake by 7%. While the percentages of calories from fat has remained deceivingly stable over the 30-year period, the amount of fat eaten has actually gone up, because of the steadily rising increase in caloric intake. In 1971, women consumed 1542 kCal on average compared with the year 2000 value of 1887 kCal (+22%), while men increased from 2450 kCal to 2618 kCal (+7%).

Portion Size Distortion

Changing trends in eating behaviors coincide with the current classification by the Centers for Disease Control and Preven-

tion of about two thirds of U.S. adults 20 to 70 years of age are either overweight or overfat. Part of this upswing in the body weight relates to the nearly 350% increase between 1965 and 2005 in the proportion of foods that children consume from restaurants and fast-food outlets. Supersized servings of french fries and sodas are often two to five times larger than when they were first introduced. In 1954 a regular size hamburger at Burger King averaged 2.9 ounces and contained 202 kCal while the 2004 version weighs 4.3 ounces and contains 325 kCal. Likewise, the 1955 McDonald's French fries weighed 2.4 ounces (only a small size was available) with 210 kCals while in 2006 McDonald's offered a supersize version weighing in at 7 oz with 610 kCal! The 1950s 3-cup version of movie popcorn contained 174 kCal while the contemporary 21-cup buttered version contains 1700 kCal. Americans do not just supersize their portions in fast-food restaurants but they are doing it in their own kitchens. FIGURE 9.4 shows the progressive increase in portion size of such foods as hamburgers, burritos, tacos, French fries, sodas, ice cream, pie, cookies, and salty snacks between 1970s and the 1990s, regardless of whether people ate out or at home.[6] The size of hamburgers made at home increased from 5.7 oz in 1977 to

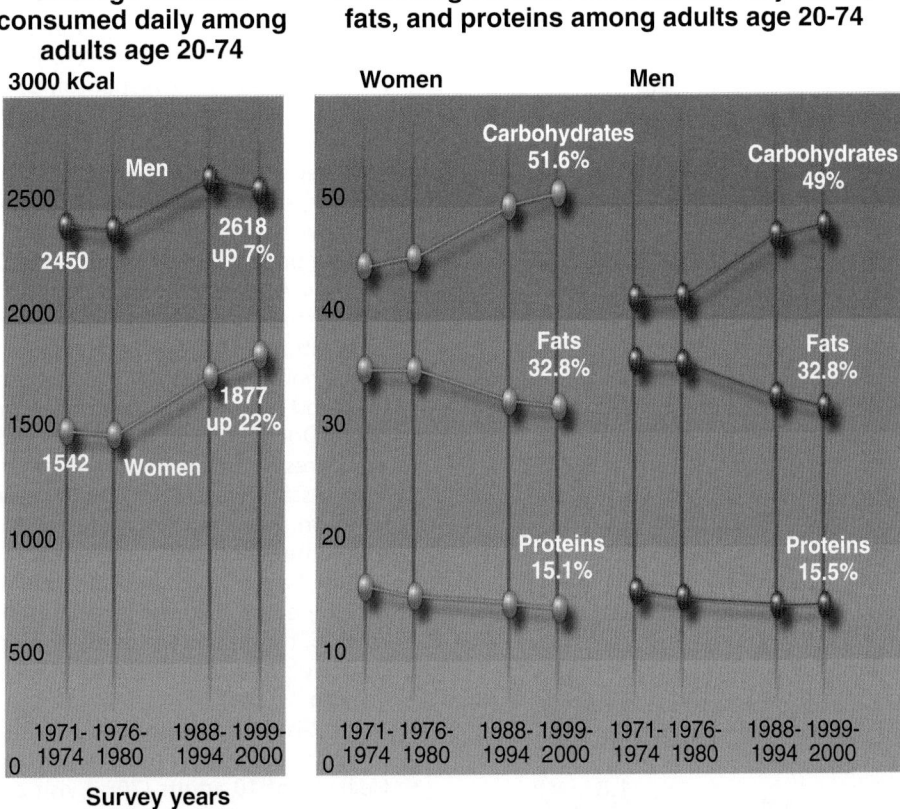

FIGURE 9.3 ■ Patterns of macronutrient and energy intake of men and women over a 30-year period (Centers for Disease Control and Prevention).

8.4 oz in 1996. Over the same time, fast food hamburgers increased from 6.1 to 7.2 oz. For Mexican food, a person consumed an average of 408 calories in one sitting in 1977 compared with 541 calories in 1996. Entrée size increase has also affected eating behaviors of preschool children. The large, fixed size of these portions may constitute an "obesigenic" environmental influence that contributes to excessive caloric intake at meals.[3] The USDA considers 2 to 3 oz of cooked lean meat a serving and suggests consuming between 1600 and 2800 kCal per day, depending on a person's age, gender, and physical activity level. These findings point to the need to evaluate not just what we eat but also the size of the portions we eat when assessing and modifying energy intake.

Increases in portion size and fat content of typical dietary items have not been limited to the United States. For example, on June 9, 2003, the British Medical Association proposed a 17.5% "fat-tax" on high-fat foods (e.g., biscuits and processed meats) to combat obesity-related problems, which cost the National Health Service approximately 500 million pounds ($825 million in U.S. currency) a year. Excess weight has reached epidemic proportions in Britain, where one in five men and one in four women classify as obese. The Australian Medical Association is also considering such a fat tax as one of several fat-fighting ideas for consideration by the country's health ministers.

SUPERSIZING: AN AMERICAN TREND

The increasing size of American food portions links to the U.S. food industry's growing reliance on "value" marketing, a technique used to increase food companies' profits. This process encourages customers to spend a little extra money to purchase larger portion sizes, which supposedly leaves the customer with the feeling that they have "gotten a deal."

The nutritional and caloric costs of getting "deals" at fast-food restaurants, convenience stores, and other retail food establishments is enormous. Upgrading to larger serving sizes often increases price only modestly, but substantially increases calorie and fat content (contributing to overeating and obesity.)

For food companies, the actual monetary costs of larger portions are small, because the cost of food itself is small (on average about 20% of retail costs) relative to labor, packaging, transportation, marketing, and other costs.[9] Thus, even the relatively small amounts of extra money consumers spend when "upgrading" to larger portion sizes means larger corporate profits.

In addition to using price to encourage the purchase of larger portion sizes, fast-food restaurants, in particular, actively encourage consumers to "upgrade" to larger sizes with

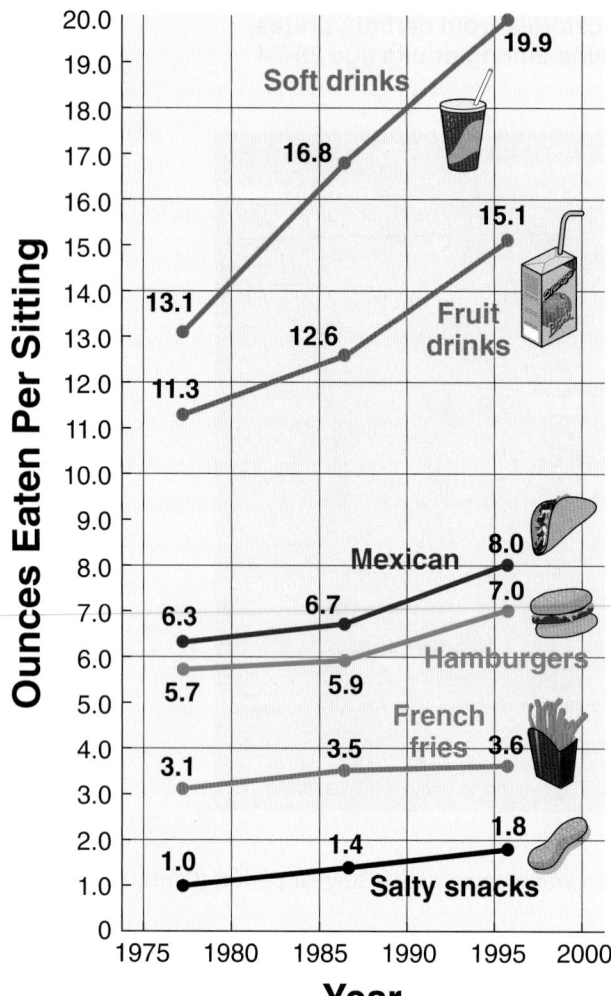

FIGURE 9.4 ▪ Portion size distortion. Trends in the portion size, shown as ounces consumed per sitting, of some common foods that Americans eat.

point-of-purchase displays and verbal sales prompts from employees. They also encourage consumers to combine their entrée with high-profit-margin, high-calorie soft drinks and side dishes like french fries ("Value Meal," "Combo Meal," etc.)—a technique known in the food industry as "bundling."

Some Fast-Food Sobering Facts

- Ninety-six percent of American schoolchildren can identify Ronald McDonald. The only fictional character with a higher degree of recognition is Santa Claus. The impact of McDonald's on the nation's culture, economy, and diet is hard to overstate. Its corporate symbol—the Golden Arches—is more widely recognized than the Christian cross. McDonald's represents the largest restaurant chain in the world with about 34,000 establishments. It is

one of a handful of companies showing substantial growth every year of its existance.
- Americans now spend more on fast food than on higher education, personal computers, software, or new cars. More is spent on fast food than on movies, books, magazines, newspapers, videos, and recorded music combined.
- The restaurant industry is now the largest private employer in the United States. In Colorado Springs (with a population of about 4,417,000), the restaurant industry (and particularly fast-food establishments) has grown at a faster rate than the city's population. In 1969, the city had a total of 20 fast-food chain restaurants. Today, there are 178 "fast-food and carry out" restaurants in the city's directory (33 McDonald's, 10 Burger King's and Wendy's, and 9 Arby's restaurants). This amounts to about one fast-food restaurant for every 24,800 residents.
- Houston, Texas, with a population of 1,953,631 has more than 772 fast-food restaurants listed in its Yellow Pages. This amounts to 1 fast-food restaurant for every 2530 residents!
- In 2006, the restaurant industry posted its 16th consecutive year of inflation-adjusted (real) sales growth.
- August is the most popular month to eat out, and Saturday is the most popular day of the week.
- Nearly 7 of 10 adults (70%) visit a restaurant for a birthday occasion, making this the most popular reason to dine out, followed by Mother's Day (38%) and Valentine's Day (28%).

The Economic and Caloric Costs of Supersizing

For small increases in price, people can purchase larger portions and, as a result, end up with substantially more calories and saturated fat (TABLE 9.7). Consider the following two examples:

- A Minibon (at Cinnabon) costs an average of $2.01 (in 2007) and provides 300 calories and 5 grams of saturated fat. For 48 cents more (a 24% increase in price), you can buy a Classic Cinnabon, which has 370 more calories (123% more) and almost three times as much saturated fat.
- At movie theaters, upgrading from a small ($3.13) to a medium-sized bag of popcorn without "butter" costs about 71 more cents. However, it also costs an additional 500 calories (i.e., a 23% increase in price buys 125% more calories). If you shell out another 60 cents, you can get a large, which brings the total to 1160 calories and almost three days' worth of saturated fat. (Getting "butter" topping adds even more calories and fat, and many movie theaters provide free refills with a large popcorn.)

Tips To Avoid Portion Distortion

Portion sizes served in restaurants have gotten larger in the last few years. The trend has also spilled over into grocery stores and vending machines, where a bagel has become a

TABLE 9.7   Economic Cost of Supersizing

Location	Item	Size	Ounces Cups	kCal	Total Fat (g)	Saturated Fat (g)	Average Price ($)
McDonald's	French Fries	Small	2.4 oz	210	10	2	1.03
		Medium	5.2 oz	450	22	4	1.50
		Large	6.2 oz	540	26	5	1.67
		Super Size	7 oz	610	29	5	1.90
	Coca-Cola Classic	Small	16 oz	150	0	0	1.04
		Medium	21 oz	210	0	0	1.20
		Large	32 oz	310	0	0	1.44
		Super Size	42 oz	410	0	0	1.64
	Chocolate Shake	Small	12 oz	350	11	7	1.53
		Medium	16 oz	510	15	10	1.90
		Large	21 oz	770	23	15	2.31
	Quarter Pounder w/Cheese		7 oz	530	30	13	2.33
	Quarter Pounder w/Cheese Extra Value Meal	Medium[f]		1190	52	17	3.74
		Large[g]		1380	56	18	4.32
		Super Size[h]		1550	59	18	4.47
	Chicken McNuggets	6 piece	3.8 oz	290	17	4	2.10
		9 piece	5.7 oz	430	25	5	2.82
Wendy's	Classic Double w/Cheese		11 oz	760	45	19	3.32
	Classic Double w/Cheese Old Fashioned Combo Meal 2	Regular[i]		1360	68	26	4.89
		Biggie Size[j]		1540	72	27	5.28
Cinnabon[a]	Minibon		3 oz	300	11	5	2.01
	Cinnabon		8 oz	670	34	14	2.49
"TCBY"	Frozen Yogurt, 96% Fat Free	Small Cup	7 oz	265	6	4	1.80
		Reg. Cup	9 oz	340	8	5	2.37
		Large Cup	11 oz	420	10	6.5	2.77
Baskin Robbins	Chocolate Chip Ice Cream	Kids Scoop	2.5 oz	150	10	6	1.26
		Single Scoop	4 oz	270	17	11	1.65
		Dbl Scoop	8 oz	540	34	22	2.88
Starbucks	Caffe Latte with Whole Milk	Tall	12 oz	210	11	7	2.44
		Grande	16 oz	260	14	9	2.99
		Venti	20 oz	350	18	12	3.29
Movie Theater	Popcorn without "Butter"	Small	7 cups	400	27	19	3.13
		Medium	16 cups	900	60	43	3.84
		Large	20 cups	1160	77	55	4.44
Subway	Tuna Sub	6-inch	8.8 oz	420	21	5	3.29
		12-inch	17.6 oz	840	42	10	4.82
Taco Bell	Nachos	Supreme	7 oz	440	24	7	1.60
		BellGrande	11 oz	760	39	11	2.74
		Mucho Grande	18 oz	1320	82	25	3.71
	Burrito	Bean	7 oz	370	12	4	0.90
		Beef Supreme	8.75 oz	430	18	7	2.01
		Beef Double	10.25 oz	510	23	9	2.47
		Supreme	10 oz	680	39	13	2.24
Burger King[a]	Whopper						
	Whopper Value Meal	Medium[c]		1270	57	23	3.93
		Large[d]		1510	64	26	4.39
		King[e]		1710	69	29	4.80

[a]Saturated fat numbers include trans fat; [b]Includes Big Grab Lay's Classic Potato Chips and Medium Coca-Cola Classic; [c]Includes medium French fries and medium Coca-Cola Classic; [d]Includes large French fries and large Coca-Cola Classic; [e]Includes king French fries and king Coca-Cola Classic; [f]Includes medium French fries and medium Coca-Cola Classic; [g]Includes large French fries and large Coca-Cola Classic; [h]Includes supersized French fries and supersized Coca-Cola Classic; [i]Includes biggie French fries and medium cola; [j]Includes great biggie French fries and biggie cola; [k]Includes ice.

BAGEL and an "individual" bag of chips can easily feed more than one. Here are some tips to help in avoiding some common portion-size pitfalls.

Practice Portion Control When Eating Out

- Eat a portion of low-calorie raw vegetables before going out; it's OK to try and "spoil" your dinner.
- Split an entrée with a friend.
- Ask the wait-person for a "to-go" box and wrap up half your meal as soon as it's brought to the table.
- Ask if the appetizer of choice can be "upgraded" in size to substitute for a full meal (it still would be smaller than a full-size portion).

Practice Portion Control When Eating at Home

- Replace the candy dish with a fruit bowl.
- To minimize temptations of second and third helpings, serve food on individual plates, instead of using serving dishes on the table.
- Keep excess food out of reach to discourage overeating.
- Eat a portion of low-calorie raw vegetables; it's OK to try and "spoil" your dinner.
- Drink a glass of water before eating.

Practice Portion Control in Front of the TV and When Snacking

- If possible, try to never eat in front of the TV.
- Put the amount that you plan to eat into a bowl or container instead of eating straight from the package.
- Prepare low-calorie snacks like raw vegetables to eat if you know your going to watch TV during dinner.
- Be aware of large packages; the larger the package, the more food consumed.
- Divide up the contents of one large package into a smaller container and put away the extra to.
- Replace the candy dish with a fruit bowl.
- Store especially tempting foods, like cookies, chips, or ice cream, out of immediate eyesight, such as on a high shelf or at the back of the freezer. Move the healthier food to the front at eye level.
- Add popcorn (of course, without the butter) to your diet.
- Snack on whole grain cereals or popcorn instead of chips and candy.

Related Web Resources

1. The Portion Distortion Quiz from the National Heart Lung and Blood Institute (NHLBI):
   http://hp2010.nhlbihin.net/portion/
2. Understanding food labels can help with portion size control:
   www.cfsan.fda.gov/~dms/foodlab.html
3. Test Your Food Label Knowledge (quiz), FDA, Center for Food Safety and Applied Nutrition:
   www.cfsan.fda.gov/~dms/flquiz1.html

ACTIVE PEOPLE ON THE GO: EATING AT FAST-FOOD RESTAURANTS

Athletes and other physically active men and women who follow prudent guidelines for food consumption still must choose from a plethora of foods. Like the typical person, these individuals endure a continual stream of advertising to lure them to consume a particular brand of food, or to "take a break" and eat at a favorite restaurant. Many athletes eat their meals at sport-specific "training tables" during the competitive season. However, the off season and summer months provide a unique challenge to maintain an optimal food intake that minimizes total fat intake and emphasizes unrefined complex carbohydrates, while ensuring adequate vitamins and minerals from the main food groups.

An occasional trip to a fast-food eatery may temporarily disrupt the recommended intake of higher complex-carbohydrate, lower fat foods. On the other hand, regular visits to franchise establishments can wreak havoc on consuming the recommended nutrients from the major food groups. Many physically active individuals often stray from planned nutritional regimens. Attending parties, going out to dinner with friends, and "hanging out" often include eating foods that provide nonnutritious or "empty" calories, high in saturated fatty acids.

Ethnic Sources for Poor Nutrition

The nongovernmental Center for Science in the Public Interest (CSPI; www.cspinet.org), publishes information about a variety of food–health related topics, including analyses of menu items from different ethnic eateries. Consider the nutritional consequences of eating at Chinese and Mexican restaurants. For the analysis of typical foods from Chinese restaurants, CSPI bought dinner-size takeout portions of 15 popular dishes from 20 midpriced Chinese restaurants in Washington, D.C., Chicago, and San Francisco. For the Mexican dishes, they purchased takeout portions of 15 popular appetizers and main dishes at 19 midpriced Mexican restaurants (including large and medium-sized chains, e.g., Chi-Chi's, El Torito, Chevys, El Chico) in Chicago, Dallas, San Francisco, and Washington, D.C. The CSPI constructed a "composite" from nine samples of each dish (e.g., equal portions of nine restaurants' chicken tacos were mixed together). An independent laboratory analyzed the food for total calories, lipid, saturated fat, cholesterol, and sodium. TABLE 9.8 provides examples of the lipid content of typical Chinese and Italian food, including appetizers, entrees, and side dishes from noted theme restaurants (Chili's, T.G.I. Friday's, Bennigan's, Hard Rock Cafe, and Planet Hollywood). The high fat content of such popular food items should serve as a beacon that the nutritional quality of many foods at popular ethnic and chain restaurants remains a nutritional quagmire. Consult Appendix A to compare the lipid content of foods in Table 9.8 with the lipid content of foods at 11 popular fast-food restaurants.

TABLE 9.8 Lipid Content of Foods from Chinese and Italian Eateries and Appetizers, Main Dishes, and Side Dishes at Popular "Theme" (Chain) Restaurants

Food	Total Calories	Lipid (g)	Lipid (kCal)	Lipid (%)
Chinese[a]				
Kung pao chicken	1275	75	675	53
Egg roll	190	75	99	52
Moo shu pork	1220	64	576	47
Sweet & sour pork	1635	71	639	39
Beef with broccoli	1180	46	414	35
General Tso's chicken	1607	59	531	33
Orange (crispy) beef	1798	66	594	33
Hot and sour soup	109	4	36	32
House lo mein	1048	36	324	31
House fried rice	1498	50	450	30
Chicken chow mein	1067	32	288	28
Hunan tofu	931	28	252	27
Shrimp with garlic sauce	972	27	243	25
Stir fried vegetables	778	19	171	22
Szechwan shrimp	949	19	171	18
Italian				
Fettucini Alfredo	1505	97	873	58
Lasagna	954	53	477	50
Cheese manicotti	697	38	342	49
Eggplant parmigiana	1212	62	558	46
Cheese ravioli	615	26	234	38
Veal parmigiana	1070	44	396	37
Spaghetti with sausage	1025	39	351	34
Chicken marsala with side of spaghetti	1155	39	351	30
Spaghetti with meatballs	1170	39	351	30
Spaghetti with meat sauce	900	25	225	25
Linguini with red clam sauce	899	23	207	23
Spaghetti with tomato sauce	850	17	153	18
Olive Garden (Italian chain restaurant)				
Garlic bread, 8 oz	818	40	360	44
Fried calamari	1032	70	630	61
Antipasto (assorted meats, cheeses, marinated vegetables, dressings, tomato, lettuce)	631	47	423	67
Hot artichoke spinach dip with garlic crisps	266	15	135	51
Bread sticks & dipping sauce, 1 stick	116	2.6	23	20
Chicken giardino	484	11	99	20
Capellini primavera	281	4.7	42	15
Appetizers				
Chili, 1 cup	350	16	144	41
Buffalo wings, 12 pieces (13 oz)	700	48	432	62
Fried mozzarella sticks, 9 pieces (8 oz)	830	51	459	55
Stuffed potato skins, 8 pieces (12 oz)	1120	79	711	64
Entrée & side dishes				
Grilled chicken, 6 oz	270	8	72	27
with baked potato + 1 Tbsp sour cream + 1 cup vegetable	640	14	126	20
with loaded potato + 1 cup vegetable	950	42	378	40
Sirloin steak, 7 oz	410	20	180	44
with baked potato + 1 Tbsp sour cream + 1 cup vegetable	780	26	234	30
with 2 cups french fries + 1 cup vegetable	1060	54	486	46
with loaded baked potato + 1 cup vegetable	1090	54	486	45
Chicken Caesar salad with dressing	660	46	414	63
Bacon & cheese grilled chicken sandwich	650	30	270	42
with 2 cups French fries	1230	61	549	45
with 11 onion rings	1550	94	846	55

(continues)

TABLE 9.8   Lipid Content of Foods from Chinese and Italian Eateries and Appetizers, Main Dishes, nd Side Dishes at Popular "Theme" (Chain) Restaurants *(continued)*

Food	Total Calories	Lipid (g)	Lipid (kCal)	Lipid (%)
Steak fajitas with 4 tortillas	860	31	279	32
with guacamole, sour cream, pico de gallo, diced cheese	1190	63	567	48
Chicken fajitas with 4 tortillas	840	24	216	26
Oriental chicken salad with dressing	750	49	441	59
Chicken fingers, 5 pieces (9 oz)	620	34	306	49
with 2 cups French fries + 1 cup cole slaw + 4 Tbsp dressing	1640	106	954	58
Hamburger with trimmings	660	36	324	49
with 2 cups French fries	1240	67	603	49
with 11 onion rings	1550	101	909	59
BBQ baby back ribs, 14 ribs (16 oz)	770	54	486	63
Fudge brownie sundae (10 oz)	1130	57	513	45
Philly cheese steak sandwich (6 inch)	680	35	315	46
with 2 cups French fries	1270	66	594	47
Chicken pot pie	680	37	333	49
Turkey club sandwich (13 oz)	740	34	306	41
Subway steak & cheese sub (6 inch)	370	13	117	32
Lobster, shrimp, scallop pasta	536	23	207	39

[a] *Food portions without rice.*

The following conclusions from the CSPI food analyses illustrate that "eating out" regularly at ethnic restaurants does not qualify as more healthful eating than eating at popular fast-food restaurants such as Arby's, Burger King, Kentucky Fried Chicken, McDonald's, Taco Bell, Roy Rogers, or Wendy's.

- The average Chinese dinner contains more sodium than the daily requirement. It also has 70% of a day's lipid, 80% of a day's cholesterol, and almost one-half day's saturated fatty acid recommendation.
- An order of lo mein contains as much salt as a whole Pizza Hut cheese pizza.
- An order of kung pao chicken (52% lipid) contains as much lipid as four McDonald's Quarter Pounders.
- An order of beef and cheese nachos contains the lipid in 10 glazed doughnuts from Dunkin' Donuts.
- A chicken burrito dinner yields one day's worth of sodium.
- A chile relleno dinner contains as much saturated fatty acid as 27 slices of bacon.
- An oriental chicken salad contains more fat than a footlong Subway cold-cut sub washed down with a Dunkin' Donuts Bavarian Kreme donut.
- Nine fried mozzarella sticks contain as much lipid as one-half stick of butter (1/4 cup or 4 tablespoons).

BEWARE OF THEATER POPCORN. In addition to revelations about the high lipid content of popular foods at ethnic restaurants, the

CSPI in 1994 evaluated the lipid content of movie theater popcorn. Popcorn samples came from 12 theaters from six chains in San Francisco, Chicago, and Washington, D.C. The CSPI combined the popcorn into three "composites" (coconut oil, coconut oil with topping, and canola shortening) for analysis by an independent laboratory for total calories from lipid, including artery-clogging saturated fatty acids. The results for popcorn's lipid content were as revealing as for Chinese and Mexican foods and in some cases worse.

Without adding butter, a large popcorn contained 80 g of lipid (720 kCal from using hydrogenated soybean oil, canola oil, or coconut oil-based fats during popping). More than 450 kCal (50 g) of these calories came from saturated fatty acids—the equivalent saturated fatty acid content of six McDonald's Big Macs! Buttering the popcorn boosted the total lipid content 50 more grams to 130 g or a whopping 1170 lipid kCal, equivalent to the saturated fatty acid content in eight McDonald's Big Macs (or the 4-day limit for the recommended amount of saturated fatty acids in the diet).

What can one do to avoid such high-fat "treats?" Become an activist consumer. Let theater managers know you want them to do the following: (1) Substitute liquid corn oil (it contains minimal saturated fatty acids and no harmful *trans* fatty acids) for hydrogenated and partially hydrogenated oils and shortenings. (2) Switch to air-popped popcorn, which eliminates any oil in the preparation and reduces total lipid content by over 95%! Also, making popcorn without salt spares an additional 300 to 700 mg of salt per bag.

Popcorn Buyers Beware!

Aware that popcorn, popped in coconut oil (as typically found in most theaters), with butter and salt does not represent a "healthy" snack, people have turned to other popcorn preparation methods to make it healthier. Below is nutritional breakdown of the contents of different types of popcorn. The quantity represents a typical serving of that product.

Contents	Popcorn Products					
	Air-popped 1 cup (0.3 oz)	Microwave, Butter, 94% Fat-Free, Unpopped 2 tablespoons (1.2 oz)	Microwave, Butter, Naturally Flavored, Unpopped 2 tablespoons (1.2 oz)	Oil-popped, unsalted 1 serving; (3.5 oz)	Caramel-coated w. peanuts 2/3 cup (1 oz)	Movie Theater w. butter, large (20 cups)
kCal	31	120	160	521	113	1500
Total fat	0.4 g	2 g	9 g	28.1	2.2 g	116 g
Saturated fat	0.1 g	–	2 g	4.9	0.3	–
Trans fat	–	–	3.5 g	–	–	–
Cholesterol	–		–	–	–	–
Sodium	1 mg	300 mg	400 mg	3 mg	84 mg	–
Carbohydrates	6.2 g	23 g	17 g	58.1 g	22.9 g	90 g
Dietary fiber	1.2 g	5 g	4 g	10 g	1.1 g	24 g
Sugars	Sugars	–	–	0.5 g	12.9 g	–
Calcium	0.6 mg	–	–	10 mg	18.7 mg	–
Potassium	26.3 mg	–	–	225 mg	100.6 mg	–
Protein	1.0 g	–	3 g	9 g	1.8 g	26.5 g

Source: http://www.calorieking.com/foods/calories-in-popcorn_c-Y2lkPTQxMDQ2JnBhcj0.html.

ICE CREAM IS ALSO IN THE CROSSHAIR. Even the most cherished of American staples, ice cream, has not escaped the close scrutiny of CSPI's calorie sleuths (www.cspinet.org/new/200307231.html). Some of CSPI's findings—published in the July/August 2003 issue of its *Nutrition Action Healthletter*—include

- **Ben & Jerry's** *empty Waffle Cone Dipped in Chocolate* has 320 kCal and a half-day's worth of saturated fat—the equivalent of a half-pound rack of BBQ baby back ribs. Fill it with a regular scoop of Chunky Monkey Ice Cream and the cone becomes worse (820 kCal and 30 g of saturated fat) than a full 1-lb rack of ribs.
- **Cold Stone Creamery's** *regular Mud Pie Mojo*—a mixture of coffee ice cream, roasted almonds, fudge, Oreos, peanut butter, and whipped topping—is the equivalent of two Pizza Hut Personal Pan Pepperoni Pizzas (1180 kCal and 26 g saturated fat).
- **Häagen-Dazs'** *Mint Chip Dazzler* is a portable sundae with three scoops of mint chip ice cream, hot fudge, Oreos, chocolate sprinkles, and whipped cream. Nutritionally, it's like eating a T-bone steak, Caesar salad, and a baked potato with sour cream (1270 kCal and 38 g saturated fat).

WHAT DOES FOOD MEAN TO YOU?

While our bodies have changed little from our ancient ancestors, the world we live in has changed dramatically over the last century. The technologic era has allowed industrialized countries to create an abundant low-cost food supply, massive transportation and communication networks to distribute it, and the luxuries of convenience foods and high-speed cooking equipment to support it. Individuals now have the freedom to choose foods from a far greater variety in local markets than ever before. Consequently, many factors act and interact to influence a person's food behaviors.

Factors Affecting Food Choices

About one fourth of the population consumes inordinately large quantities of food that often exceeds daily energy requirements. Besides hunger, food satisfies deep personal and social needs. Understanding the factors that compel us to eat certain foods helps to make wise decisions regarding food choices.

Age-Old Tradition

Seeking food and the pleasures of eating often intertwine with other human drives deeply imbedded in our culture. Food, for example, has become a central part of sharing. We offer food and drink to visitors in our homes; most of us also accept food and drink when we visit another's home, even if we are not hungry or dislike the food. Athletes learn what foods to eat (steak and eggs, special drinks) from coaches, many of whom have never taken a sport and exercise nutrition class or read a reputable book in the area. These early experiences persist well into adulthood and pass on as part of one's "eating tradition."

Early Experiences: Emotion and Family

Early food experiences became entangled with strong emotional forces, particularly from the main caregivers' influence of our parents. For many, food equates with security and love and associates with feelings of comfort and "good" (family gatherings, holidays, desserts, special occasions) and "bad" (punishment, lack of money, lack of food availability). As adults, we may reject some of these earlier food choices, but we still crave them because they remind us of positive childhood experiences.

Positive and Negative Associations

Specific memories of forgotten events influence food choices. In early childhood, sweets and snacks were often rewards for good behavior or were denied as punishment; thus, they become a necessity as a personal reward for doing something good or to make us feel good. This learned response plays a signigicant role in our current food choices and may help to explain why many adults overeat.

A noxious experience paired in time with the eating of a particular food imprints an aversion to that food. The food aversion persists, although the specific experience may be forgotten. Many athletes who experience a change in performance often associate this change with a particular food or meal. This sets the stage for some bizarre practices before athletic events. Many athletes, for example, insist that they eat precisely the same meal (at the same time) before every performance.

Fear of Foods

Children often resist eating newer or strange foods and only eat the familiar foods provided by their caregiver. Unfortunately, as we age we often classify foods that we eat as "normal," and different foods consumed by others as "odd" or "weird." This dictates certain food preferences creating a fear of some foods that persists from one generation to the next. Athletes who travel to other countries often cringe at foods they never considered eating (e.g., boiled dragonflies, grilled dog or cat meat, fried ants, monkey brains, raw snails) and perform poorly because they avoid the available yet unaccustomed foods. Developing a varied palate at an early age expands an individual's eating pleasures later in life.

Availability

Although food habits develop slowly over time, food availability can play a big role in the development of these habits. For example, fastfood chains are now within reach of most individuals in North American and Europe, offering cheap, calorie-laden alternatives to home-cooked meals. Busy parents often rely on these nutrient-poor foods to feed their children, totally neglecting fruits and vegetables, which are frequently absent from most fast food menus. Vending machines in schools and the workplace have replaced homemade meals. Indeed, the rush to find and eat cheap, high-fat, high-sugar meals has replaced the traditional family dinner consisting of grains, fruits, and vegetables. We have become a "fast-food nation," fixated on food that does not promote good eating habits or good health.

Choosing Food Based on Nutritional Value: A Tough Decision

The reasons for making food choices normally lie outside our conscious awareness. Choosing foods for nutritional value seldom dictates food choices. Learning to make wise choices in the marketplace enhances health and promotes longevity; choosing foods based on nutritional value, unlike the other reasons for choosing foods, is a consciously learned behavior. Choosing nutritious foods can be consistent with other gratifications such as physical pleasure, emotional satisfaction, economy, and convenience. Learing to eat nutritiously takes motivation, knowledge, and commitment, but once learned, it can become a lifelong "habit."

Try This

To learn to choose nutritious foods, one must first analyze food choices, beyond just recording the foods consumed (see Appendix C). As an exercise, record all of the food eaten for one day, indicating the reason for selecting the food from the following choices:

- Personal preference (I like it)
- Social pressure (it was offered; I couldn't refuse)
- Familiarity (it was familiar)
- Economy (it was the only choce I could afford)
- Convenience (it was readily available: I was too rushed to do anything else)
- Nutritional value (I know it is good for me)
- Other (explain your reason)

Case Study

Personal Health and Exercise Nutrition 9–2

Can We Trust the Organic Food Label?

The latest statistics indicate that approximately 75% of U.S. consumers buy organic products. They spend extra money for organics hoping to avoid chemicals, eat healthy, and support the environment. Though a small part of the overall food market, "organic" is growing at 20% a year since 1999, while overall food sales have risen only about 3%. This trend is likely to continue as big grocers, most recently Wal-Mart, Costco, and other "big-box" retailers, expand their organic offerings.

Organic foods are supposed to be free of most chemical pesticides, fertilizers, antibiotics, hormones, and genetic engineering. Organic farmers and ranchers must enrich the soil and be kind to their animals. But, can we really trust the USDA Organic Label to be what it is supposed to be?

Recent evidence suggests substantial cheating by farmers, growers, and others involved in the organic food industry. Even the USDA does not know how often organic rules are broken, and it has not consistently taken action when potential violations are exposed. In fact, since the organic standards were enacted in 2002, there has not been one prosecution of violations of the organic law.

The USDA organic program monitors at least 20,000 organic growers, ranchers, processing plants, and others worldwide. It has proven an impossible task to try and control the growing organics market throughout the United States and abroad. At least three reasons explain why organic shoppers may not be getting what they think:

- A review of 216 internal USDA audits show examples of violations at organic farms and production plants. Reports about problems that are supposed to filter up to the agency from on-the-ground monitors are incomplete.

- Much organic food is produced overseas, where there is less oversight. Inspectors in China, for example, describe obvious violations that are not well-tracked or known by the USDA or importers.

- Vague rules leave much to interpretation, particularly concerning animal treatment and feeding.

Organic Cheaters

Most organic farmers and food processors are "true believers" and go above and beyond what is required. But among 268 complaints released by the USDA in 2006, about 50 were products erroneously claiming to be organic or falsely using the organic label. The USDA ordered them to stop but had no way to enforce their order. Clearly, the USDA is under funded relative to the increase in sales of organic products (see accompanying figure).

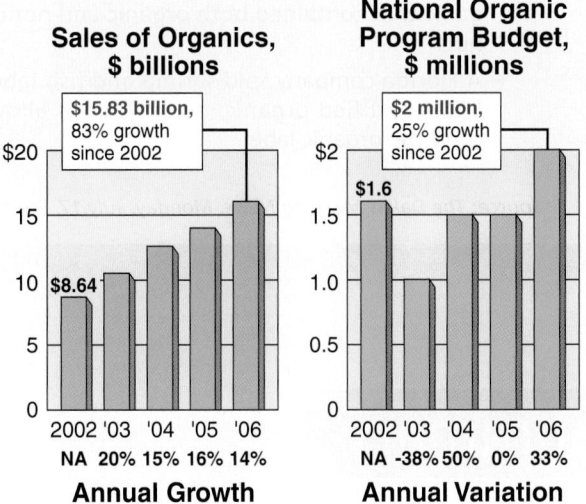

GROWING NATURALLY

U.S. sales of organic foods and drinks have risen by 83% since 2002. The budget for the government program established to watch over the industry has not grown at the same pace.

Sales of Organics, $ billions

$15.83 billion, 83% growth since 2002

$8.64

| 2002 | '03 | '04 | '05 | '06 |
| NA | 20% | 15% | 16% | 14% |

Annual Growth

National Organic Program Budget, $ millions

$2 million, 25% growth since 2002

$1.6

| 2002 | '03 | '04 | '05 | '06 |
| NA | -38% | 50% | 0% | 33% |

Annual Variation

Moreover, the USDA does not know how many violations occur because it often does not receive information from those who are supposed to police the industry at the base level.

The agency collects information from 56 certifiers in the United States and 40 certifiers in foreign countries, usually from in-state-run agencies or private companies. Farms and processing plants can choose any USDA-approved certifier. Certifiers hire inspectors to walk through fields, interview plant workers, and evaluate records. The certifiers are then supposed to notify the USDA when problems exist, but this rarely occurs.

Case Study *continued*

Potential Violators*
The following examples illustrate violations taken from hundreds of certifier audits and complaints provided by the USDA. However, the agency has not provided records of confirmed violations.

- A company in Italy produced butter and cheese from dairy cows described as eating organic feed not USDA certified
- A certifier in Idaho sent inspectors with little or no experience to certify farms, where they overlooked potential violations
- A California seed company listed synthetic fungicide—not allowed under USDA rules—to process seeds
- A brewery in Berkeley, CA distributed organic beer without using organically grown hops
- A Michigan farm sold beef as organic, although it was processed at a nonorganic facility
- A Georgia company sold boxes of pecans labeled organic that contained both organic and nonorganic nuts
- A Florida company sold shrimp and fish labeled as USDA-certified organic; no seafood is allowed to carry the organic label

*Source: The Dallas Morning News, Monday, July 17, 2006

- A noncertified organic Michigan farm advertised beef and buffalo meat as organic

When Can the USDA Organic Seal Be Used?
The label is allowed on raw food and packaged products that are "100% organic" or "organic" from certified producers. Organic products allow for up to 5% nonorganic ingredients. This mainly involves materials used in processing packaged foods.

If the product is at least 70% organic, it cannot use the USDA seal, but can use the phrase "made with organic ingredients." If it is less than 70%, but still has some organic content, it can only use the word "organic" to identify individual ingredients.

What Is Organic?
Organic food is grown without most conventional pesticides, fertilizers made with synthetic ingredients, sewage sludge, or bioengineering or ionizing radiation. Animals do not receive antibiotics or growth-stimulating hormones. The animals are supposed to have access to the outdoors so that they can exhibit more of their natural feeding behavior. The complete rules are lengthy and vary depending on the type of operation.

Who Says It's Organic?
A USDA-accredited certifier, whose name should be on the product label or package, makes declarations.

Summary

1. The past 55 years have witnessed a tremendous increase in public awareness of the health benefits of good nutrition. Concurrently, advertisers have linked many food products to health maintenance and enhancement. However, new regulations from the Food and Drug Administration (FDA) under the aegis of the United States Department of Agriculture's (USDA) Food Safety and Inspection Service now require manufacturers to adhere to guidelines when linking a nutrient(s) to medical or health benefits.

2. Four governmental agencies create the rules, regulations, and legal requirements concerning advertising, packaging, and labeling of foods and alcoholic beverages.

3. The Federal Trade Commission (FTC) regulates food product advertising in various media (TV, radio, and newsprint) and pursues legal action against manufacturers who advertise unsubstantiated claims or deceptive ads.

4. The FDA regulates (1) what manufacturers state on food labels, (2) safety of cosmetics, medicines, medical devices, feed and drugs for pets and farm animals, and (3) what additives manufacturers can add to foods, including potential hazards with food additives (contaminants), foodborne infections, toxicants, artificially constituted foods, and pesticide residues.

5. The USDA deals with farm and foreign agricultural services, food, nutrition and consumer services, food safety,

Summary   *continued*

marketing and regulatory programs, natural resources and environment, research, education, economics, marketing and regulatory programs, and rural development.

6. The Bureau of Alcohol, Tobacco and Firearms (ATF) enforces federal laws and regulations relating to alcohol, tobacco, firearms, explosives, and arson.

7. Before 1990, the law did not require manufactures (and their advertising agencies) to adhere to rules and regulations to describe foods. The Nutrition Labeling and Education Act (NLEA) of 1990 (including 1993–1998 updates to the regulations) now requires food manufacturers to strictly comply to regulations about what can and cannot be printed on food labels.

8. The format for the nutrition panel on foods must declare the nutrient content per serving as percentages of the Daily Values—the new label reference values.

9. The new "% Daily Value" comprises two sets of dietary standards: Daily Reference Values (DRVs) and Reference Daily Intakes (RDIs).

10. DRVs established for macronutrients include sources of energy (lipid, carbohydrate [including fiber], and protein) and noncalorie contributors (cholesterol, sodium, and potassium).

11. The RDI replaces the term "U.S. RDA." The new RDIs remain the same as the old U.S. RDAs.

12. Food labels must indicate the amount of a particular nutrient, but no requirement exists to list its relative percentage in a food. Consequently, a food may be advertised as "low fat" (absolute quantity) when, in reality, its percentage of fat might exceed 50%! The NLEA requires manufacturers to list on the food label the percentage of fat in relation to the DRV for total calorie intake for most food items.

13. A manufacturer wishing to include an additive in a food must follow specific FDA guidelines to ensure the additive's effectiveness (i.e., it meet its claims). A list of additives that are generally recognized as safe (GRAS) currently includes about 2000 flavoring agents and 200 coloring agents.

14. Many factors influence the amount, type, and quality of food consumed by a particular group or individual in the group. These include level of income and education, racial and ethnic background, and geographic locale and personal interests.

15. Significant changes have occurred in patterns of food consumption over the past 35 years. Partly this reflects heightened public awareness of the relationship between diet and health. Unfortunately, increased reliance on "eating out" at restaurants has a negative impact on nutrition quality.

16. People who often eat at fast-food restaurants usually double their kCal intake compared with eating at home.

17. The nongovernmental watchdog organization, Center for Science in the Public Interest, raises public awareness about the nutritional content of favorite foods and meals, often with alarming results about high fat content (particularly saturated fat) and excessive calorie content.

18. Many factors affect food choices: traditions, early food experiences, emotions, food fears, and availability.

Test Your Knowledge Answers

1. **False:** The Food and Drug Administration (FDA) is not required to provide adequate scientific data to support claims for food or chemicals classified as dietary supplements. They only intervene when a supplement causes documented injury or illness. Consequently, consumers must remain continually aware of advertising hype in the various media that promote the health and fitness benefits of products. Far too few "watchdog" organizations and adequately staffed and funded governmental agencies exist to patrol overzealous promoters whose products often pledge longer life, improved bodily functions, and instant cure for every possible ailment and misfortune.

2. **True:** The Federal Trade Commission (FTC) regulates food product advertising in various media (TV, radio, newsprint) and pursues legal action against manufacturers who advertise unsubstantiated claims or deceptive ads. The FTC has authority to remove a product from the marketplace if the product's claims cannot be verified.

3. **False:** FDA stands for Food and Drug Administration. This federal agency represents one of 13 agencies within the Department of Health and Human Services (DHHS). With the exception of poultry and meat products, the FDA regulates what manufacturers state on food labels and the safety of cosmetics, medicines, medical devices, and feed and drugs for

Test Your Knowledge Answers   *continued*

pets and farm animals. The FDA also decides what additives manufacturers can add to foods, including potential hazards with food additives (contaminants), food-borne infections, toxicants, artificially constituted foods, and pesticide residues.

4. **False:** The marketing of dietary supplements requires no government approval because supplements are considered foods and not drugs. In contrast to medicine, which must meet many safety and efficacy requirements before coming to market, legislation places the burden on the FDA to prove that a supplement is harmful before it can be removed from the market. Supplement marketing can progress with only the manufacturer's assurance of safety as long as the supplement does not claim disease-fighting benefits.

5. **True:** New rules in 1997 require supplements to be labeled as dietary supplements (e.g., "Vitamin C Dietary Supplement") and to carry a "Supplement Facts" panel with information similar to the "Nutrition Facts" panel that appears on most processed foods. Included on the facts panel must be an appropriate serving size; information on 14 nutrients, including sodium, vitamin A, vitamin C, calcium, and iron, when present at significant levels; other vitamins and minerals if added or part of a nutritional claim on the label; dietary ingredients with no established Reference Daily Intakes; if the product contains a proprietary blend of ingredients, the total amount of the blend and the identity of each dietary ingredient in the blend (although amounts of individual ingredients in the blend are not required). The rules also require that the labels of products containing botanical ingredients identify the part of the plant used.

6. **True:** The Bureau of Alcohol, Tobacco and Firearms (ATF) is a law enforcement organization within the United States Department of Treasury. It came into existence in 1972 after separating from the Internal Revenue Service (Alcohol, Tobacco and Firearms Division). The ATF has responsibilities dedicated to reducing violent crime, collecting revenue, and protecting the public. It enforces the federal laws and regulations relating to alcohol, tobacco, firearms, explosives, and arson.

7. **False:** A daily intake of 2000 kCal serves as the reference number of calories for determining Daily Reference Values for the energy-producing nutri-

ents. The 2000-kCal level was chosen, in part, because it approximates the caloric requirements for postmenopausal women, the group with the highest risk for excessive intake of calories and fat.

8. **False:** A "healthy" food must be low in fat and saturated fat and contain limited amounts of cholesterol and sodium. In addition, a single-item food must provide at least 10% of one or more of vitamins A or C, iron, calcium, protein, or fiber. A meal-type product, such as frozen entrees and multicourse frozen dinners, must provide 10% of two or three of these vitamins or minerals or of protein or fiber in addition to meeting the other criteria. Sodium content must be less than 360 mg per serving for individual foods and 480 mg per serving for meal-type products that carry the "healthy" claim.

9. **False:** Nutrient density refers to the quantity of a specific nutrient (protein, vitamins, and minerals) per 100 g of the food or per 1000 kCal of that food. In essence, comparing foods for nutrient density conveniently determines the better food source for a particular nutrient. Computing a food's Index of Nutritional Quality (INQ) makes this practical. Usually, the numerator of the INQ refers to the nutrient amount per 100 g of food divided by the RDA for that nutrient. The denominator represents the number of kCal per 100 g divided by the population average for energy intake (3000 kCal for men and 2000 kCal for women). For convenience in classification, a food considered "good" has an INQ between 2 and 6, while an INQ above 6 denotes an excellent source of the nutrient.

10. **False:** Significant trends have taken place in eating behaviors. For example, Americans are supersizing their portions not just in fast-food restaurants but also in their own kitchens. A progressive increase has occurred in portion size of hamburgers, burritos, tacos, French fries, sodas, ice cream, pie, cookies, and salty snacks between 1970s and the 1990s, regardless of whether people ate out or at home. The size of hamburgers made at home increased from 5.7 oz in 1977 to 8.4 oz in 1996. Over the same time, fast-food hamburgers increased from 6.1 oz to 7.2 oz. Entrée size increase also has affected the eating behaviors of preschool children. The large, fixed size of these portions may constitute an "obesigenic" environmental influence that contributes to excessive caloric intake at meals.

References

1. Angell M, Kassirer JP. Alternative medicine: the risks of untested and unregulated remedies. *N Engl J Med* 1998;339:831.
2. Drewnowski A. Concept of a nutritious food: toward a nutrient density score. *Am J Clin Nutr* 2005;82:721.
3. Fisher JO, et al. Children's bite size and intake of an entrée are greater with large portions than with age-appropriate or self-selected portions. *Am J Clin Nutr* 2003;77:1164.
4. Green GA, et al. Analysis of over-the-counter dietary supplements. *Clin J Sports Med* 2001;11:254.

5. Kamber M, et al. Nutritional supplements as a source for positive doping cases? *Int J Sport Nutr Exerc Metab* 2001;11:258.

6. Nielsen SJ, Popkin BM. Patterns and trends in food portion sizes, 1977-1998. *JAMA* 2003;289:450.

7. Nielsen SJ. Popkin BM. Changes in beverage intake between 1977 and 2001. *Am J Prev Med* 2004;27:205.

8. Sarubin A. Government regulation of dietary supplements. In: *The Health Professional's Guide to Dietary Supplements.* Chicago: The American Dietetic Association, 1999.

9. Young LR, Nestle M. The contribution of expanding portion sizes to the U.S. obesity epidemic." *Am J Public Health* 2002;92:246.

Additional Readings

American Institute for Cancer Research (AICR). As restaurant portions grow, vast majority of Americans still belong to clean plate club, new survey finds. Washington, DC: AICR News Release, January 15, 2001.

Conway JM, et al. Commercial portion-controlled foods in research studies: how accurate are label weights? *J Am Diet Assoc* 2004;104:1420.

Duffey KJ, Popkin BM. Adults with healthier dietary patterns have healthier beverage patterns. *J Nutr* 2006;136:2901.

Jacobson MF. High-fructose corn syrup and the obesity epidemic. *Am J Clin Nutr* 2004;80:1081.

Leary TB. The ongoing dialogue between the Food and Drug Administration and the Federal Trade Commission. *Food Drug Law J* 2004;59:209.

Lin CT, et al. Do dietary intakes affect search for nutrient information on food labels? *Soc Sci Med* 2004;59:1955.

Macon JF, et al. Food label use by older Americans: Data from the Continuing Survey of Food Intakes by Individuals and the Diet and Health Knowledge Survey 1994-1996. *J Nutr Elder* 2004;24:35.

Nestle M. *Food Politics: How the Food Industry Influences Nutrition and Health.* Berkeley, CA: University of California Press, 2002.

Popkin BM, et. al. A new proposed guidance system for beverage consumption in the United States. *Am J Clin Nutr* 2006;83:529.

Sitzman K. Expanding food portions contribute to overweight and obesity. *AAOHN J* 2004;52:356.

Wansink B. Can package size accelerate usage volume? *J Market* 1996;60:1.

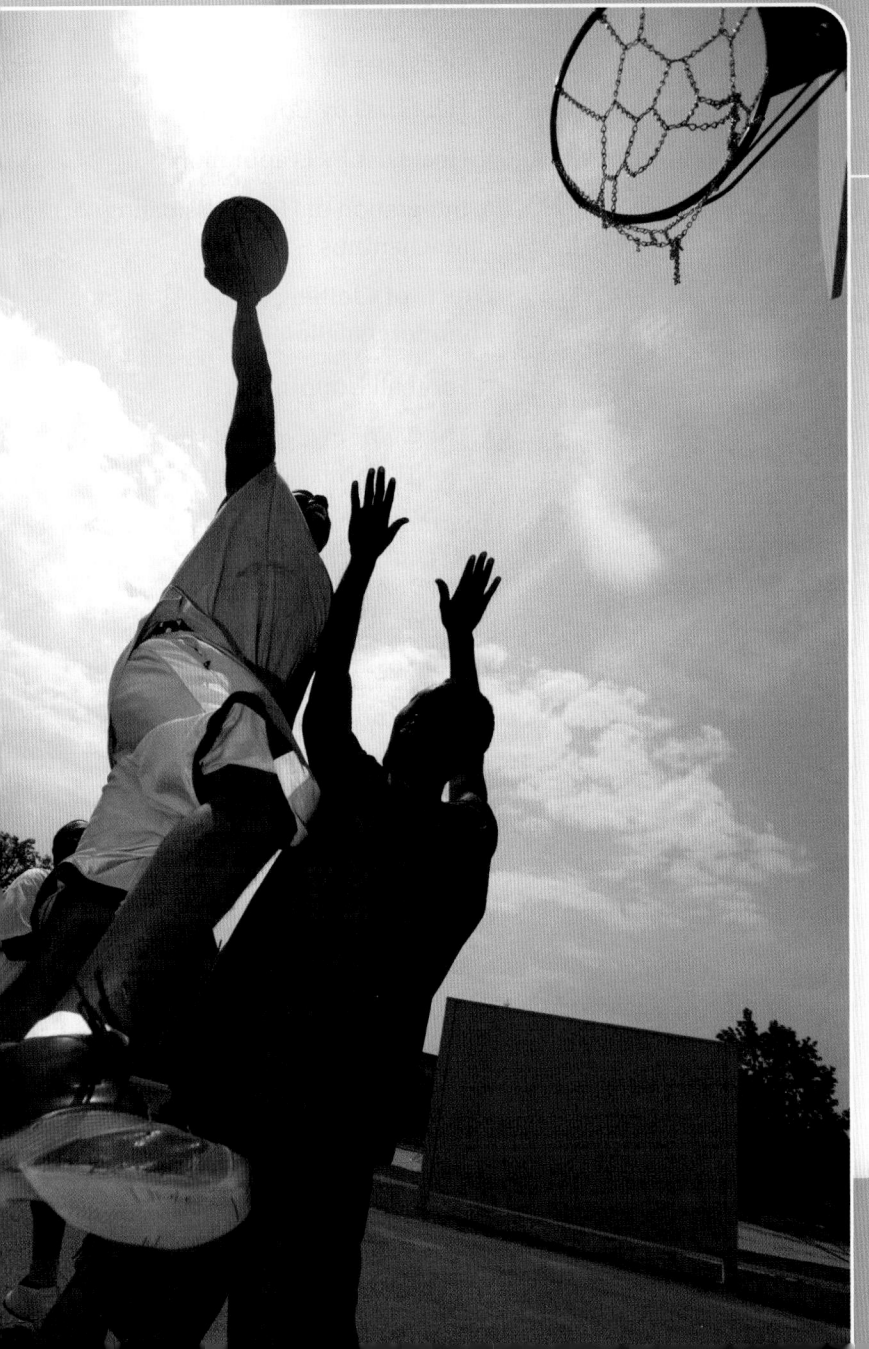

Part 4

Thermoregulation and Fluid Balance During Heat Stress

Chapter 10

Exercise Thermoregulation, Fluid Balance, and Rehydration

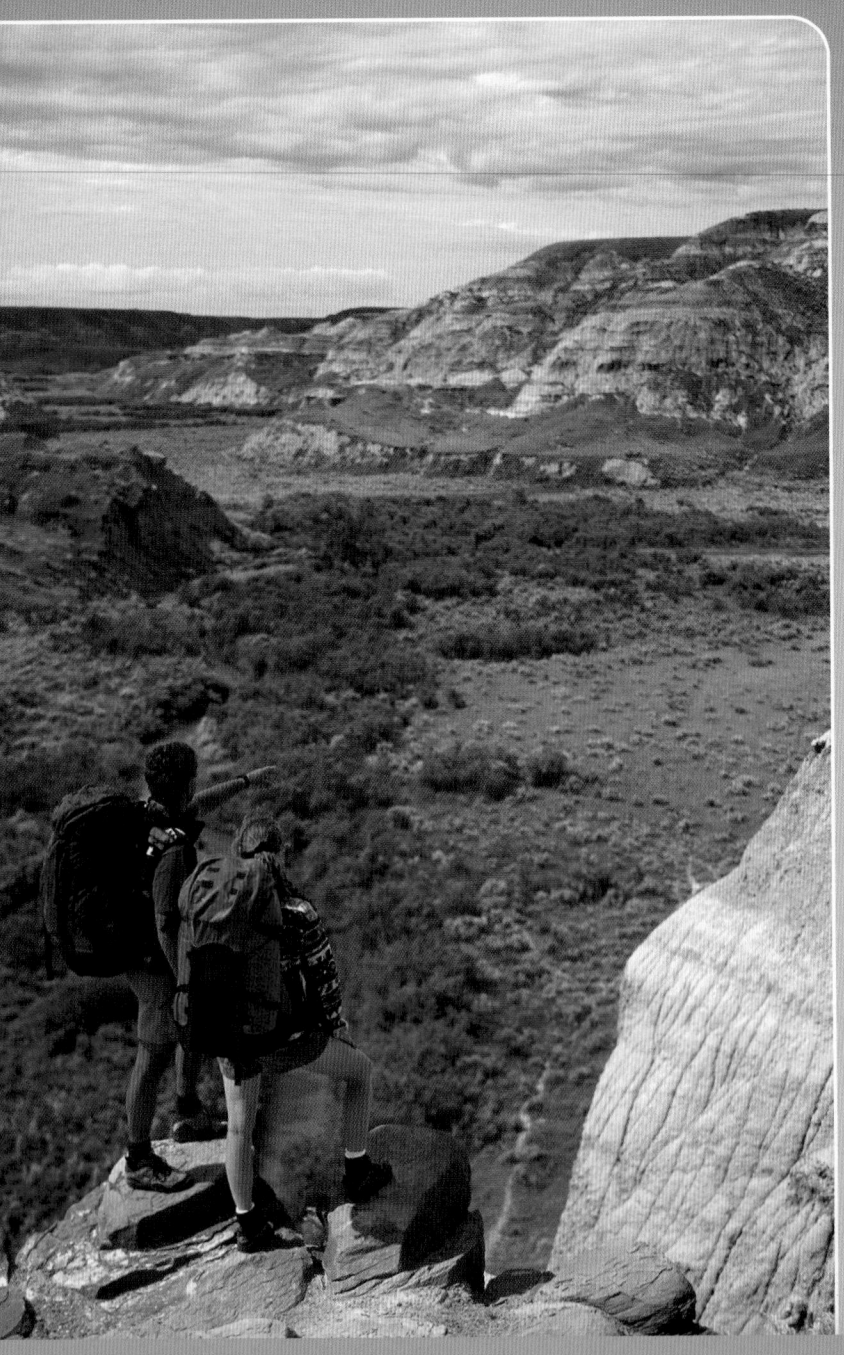

Factors That Improve Heat Tolerance

- Acclimatization
- Children
- Male/Female Differences
- Level of Body Fat

Evaluating Environmental Heat Stress

Heat Illness: Complications from Excessive Heat Stress

- Heat Cramps
- Heat Exhaustion
- Exertional Heat Stroke

Test Your Knowledge

Answer these 10 statements about exercise thermoregulation, fluid balance, and rehydration during heat stress. Use the scoring key at the end of the chapter to check your results. Repeat this test after you have read the chapter and compare your results.

1. **T F** Core body temperature remains stable despite significant changes in environmental temperature.
2. **T F** The hypothalamus contains the central coordinating center for temperature regulation.
3. **T F** The body loses heat primarily via the physical mechanism of radiation.
4. **T F** Relative humidity refers to how dry the environment becomes in the warm weather.
5. **T F** ADH is a major water conserving hormone.
6. **T F** Exercising while dehydrated greatly increases the risk for heat injury.
7. **T F** The thirst mechanism provides a precise gauge to replenish water lost during exercise.
8. **T F** You can never consume too much water.
9. **T F** Air temperature primarily determines the potential physiologic strain produced by environmental heat.
10. **T F** Oral temperature provides the most rapid and reliable estimate of core temperature after strenuous exercise.

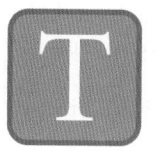

he requirements for thermoregulation are considerable—the price of failure is death. A person can tolerate a drop in deep body temperature of 10°C but an increase of only 5°C. The latter condition of **hyperthermia** occurred more than 100 times over the past 30 years in football players who died from excessive heat stress during practice or competition. Hyperthermia and dehydration were linked to the deaths of three collegiate wrestlers in the latter part of 1997. Heat injury also commonly occurs during military operations and longer duration athletic events. Athletes who illegally use erythropoietin, a hormone that boosts production of red blood cells, experience an even greater risk of heat injury. Their increased blood viscosity from increased hematocrit magnifies as dehydration progresses while exercising in the heat.

The decision to hold the 1996 Summer Olympics in Atlanta (average summer temperature between 21 and 31°C, relative humidity between 50 and 90%) refocused interest on temperature regulation during exercise. Particular emphasis was placed on understanding (1) the challenges from environmental heat and humidity on the exercising individual and (2) the appropriate means of diminishing the adverse effects of heat

stress on participants and spectators. Knowledge of thermoregulation and the most effective ways to support its mechanisms significantly reduces heat-related tragedies. Coaches, athletes, race and event organizers, and those who provide overall nutritional advice must use strategies based on factors that contribute to heat gain and dehydration during exercise in a hot environment. Concern also must focus on the most effective behavioral approaches (e.g., prudent scheduling of events, acclimatization, proper clothing, and fluid and electrolyte replacement before, during, and after exercise) to blunt the potential for negative effects on performance and safety.

An Ergogenic Aid in Its Own Right

Water becomes the most important performance-enhancing nutrient when exercise and heat stress combine. The exercise nutritionist must apply knowledge of the basic physics and physiology of thermoregulation to defend effectively against the potentially lethal challenge of heat stress.

Mechanisms of Thermoregulation

THERMAL BALANCE

FIGURE 10.1 shows body temperature (more specifically, the temperature of the deeper tissues or **core**) in dynamic equilibrium between factors that add and subtract body heat. This balance results from integrating mechanisms that:

- Alter heat transfer to the periphery (**shell**)
- Regulate evaporative cooling
- Vary the rate of heat production

Core temperature rises quickly when heat gain exceeds heat loss during vigorous exercise in a warm environment.

TABLE 10.1 presents thermal data for heat production (oxygen consumption) and heat loss from sweating at rest and during maximal exercise. The body gains considerable heat from the reactions of energy metabolism, particularly from ac-

tive muscle. From shivering alone, the total metabolic rate increases threefold to fivefold. During sustained exercise by aerobically fit men and women, metabolic rate often increases 20 to 25 times above the resting level to 20 kCal $\cdot$ min^{-1}; heat production of this magnitude could theoretically increase core temperature 1°C (1.8°F) every 5 to 7 minutes! The body also absorbs heat from the environment by solar radiation and from objects warmer than the body. Heat loss occurs by the physical mechanisms of radiation, conduction, and convection. However, water vaporization (evaporation) from the skin and respiratory passages provides the most important avenue for heat loss. Evaporative cooling under optimal conditions accounts for a heat loss of about 18 kCal $\cdot$ min^{-1}.

Circulatory adjustments provide "fine tuning" for temperature regulation. Heat conservation occurs by rapidly shunting blood deep to the cranial, thoracic, and abdominal cavities and portions of the muscle mass. This optimizes insulation from subcutaneous fat and other areas of the body's shell. Conversely, excessive internal heat buildup dilates peripheral vessels that channel warm blood to the cooler periphery. During exercise in the heat, the strong drive for thermal balance can increase sweat rate to as high as 3.5 L $\cdot$ h^{-1}.

HYPOTHALAMIC REGULATION OF CORE TEMPERATURE

*The **hypothalamus** contains the central coordinating center for temperature regulation.* This group of specialized neurons at the floor of the brain serves as a "thermostat" (usually set and carefully regulated at 37°C $\pm$ 1°C) that makes thermoregulatory adjustments to deviations from a temperature norm. Unlike a thermostat in a building, however, the hypothalamus cannot "turn off" the heat; it only initiates responses to protect the body from heat gain or heat loss.

Heat-regulating mechanisms become activated in two ways:

1. Temperature changes in blood perfusing the hypothalamus directly stimulate this thermoregulatory control center.
2. Thermal receptors in the skin provide input to modulate hypothalamic activity.

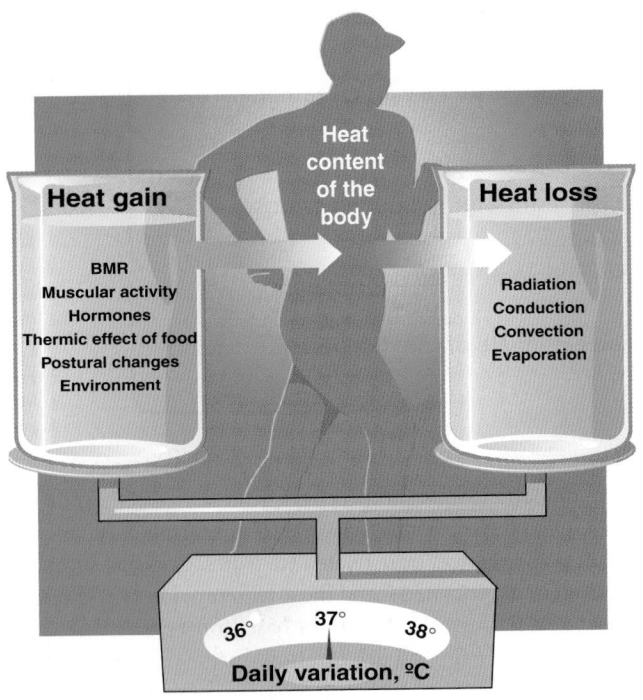

FIGURE 10.1 ■ Factors that contribute to heat gain and heat loss to regulate core temperature at about 37°C.

TABLE 10.1	**Thermodynamics at Rest and during Exercise**		
Body's heat production (1 L O$_2$ uptake = ~4.82 kCal); mixed diet	**Rest** ~0.25 L O$_2$·min^{-1} ~1.2 kCal·min^{-1}	**Maximal exercise** ~4.0 L O$_2$·min^{-1} ~20.0 kCal·min^{-1}	
Body's capacity for evaporative cooling (Each 1 mL sweat evaporation = ~0.6 kCal body heat loss)		**Maximal sweating** 30 mL·min^{-1} = ~18 kCal · min^{-1}	
Core temperature increase	No increase	~1°C every 5–7 min	

FIGURE 10.2 displays the diverse structures embedded within the skin and subcutaneous tissues. The inset on the right depicts the dynamics of sweat evaporation from the skin surface. Peripheral thermal receptors responsive to rapid changes in heat and cold exist predominantly as free nerve endings in the skin. The more numerous cutaneous cold receptors generally exist near the skin surface; they play an important role in initiating regulatory responses to cold environments. The cutaneous thermal receptors act as an "early warning system" that relays sensory information to the hypothalamus and cerebral cortex. This direct communication link evokes appropriate heat-conserving or heat-dissipating physiologic adjustments as the individual consciously seeks relief from the thermal challenge.

THERMOREGULATION IN HEAT STRESS: HEAT LOSS

The body's thermoregulatory mechanisms primarily protect against overheating. Defense against a rise in core temperature becomes particularly crucial during exercise in hot weather. Here, competition exists between mechanisms that maintain a large muscle blood flow to deliver oxygen and nutrients and remove waste products and mechanisms that provide for ade-

quate regulation of body temperature. FIGURE 10.3 illustrates the potential avenues for heat exchange in an exercising human. Body heat loss occurs in four ways: (1) **radiation**, (2) **conduction**, (3) **convection**, and (4) **evaporation**.

Heat Loss by Radiation

Objects continually emit electromagnetic heat waves. Because our bodies are usually warmer than the environment, the net exchange of radiant heat energy occurs from the body through the air to solid, cooler objects around us. This form of heat transfer, similar to how the sun's rays warm the earth, does not require molecular contact between objects. Despite subfreezing temperatures, a person can remain warm by absorbing sufficient radiant heat energy from direct sunlight (or reflected from the snow, sand, or water). The body absorbs radiant heat energy when the temperature of objects in the environment exceeds skin temperature.

Heat Loss by Conduction

Heat loss by conduction transfers heat directly through a liquid, solid, or gas from one molecule to another. The circulation transports most of the body heat to the shell, but a small amount continually moves by conduction directly through the deep tissues to the cooler surface. Conductive heat loss in-

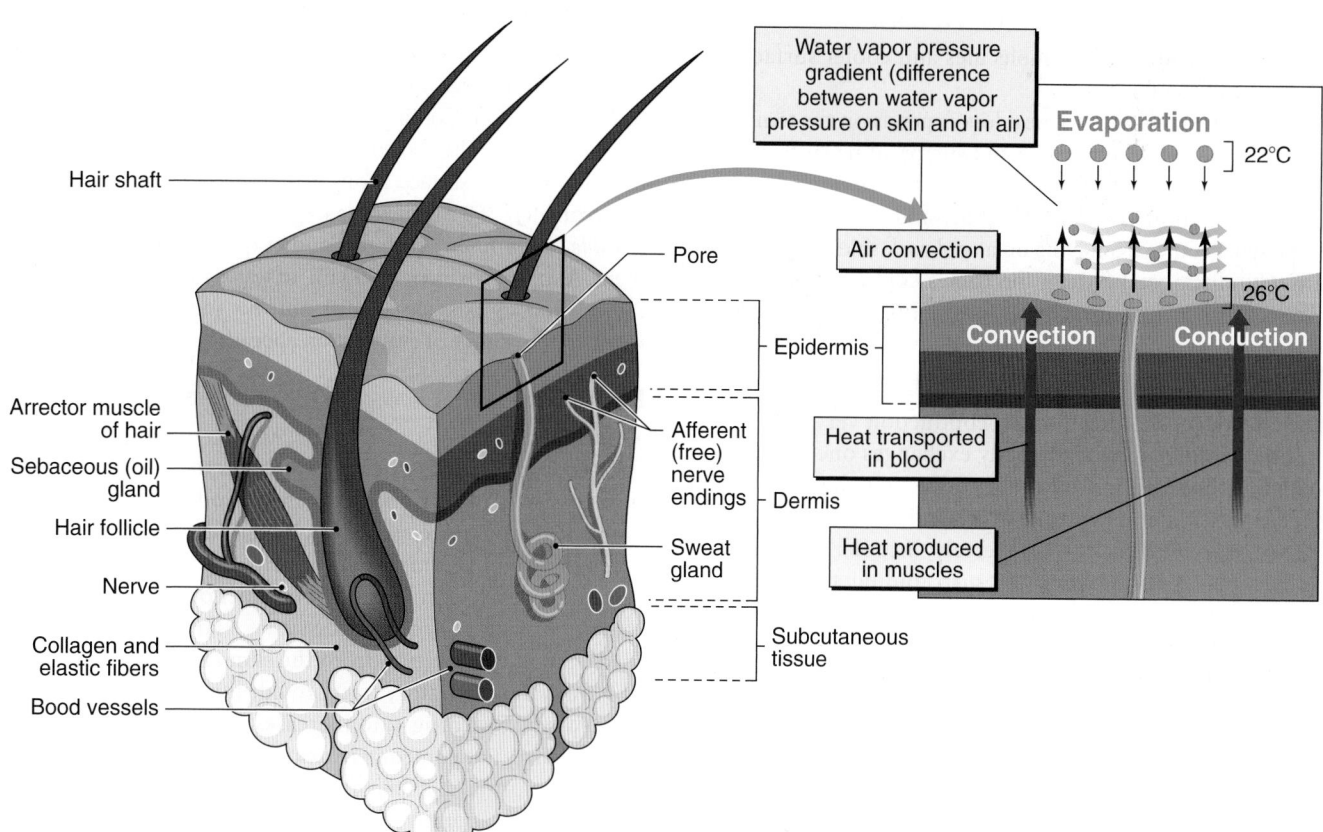

FIGURE 10.2 ■ *Left,* Schematic illustration of the skin and underlying structures. The enlargement of the skin surface at *right* shows the dynamics of conduction, convection, and sweat evaporation for heat dissipation from the body. Each 1 L of water evaporated from the skin transfers 580 kCal of heat energy to the environment.

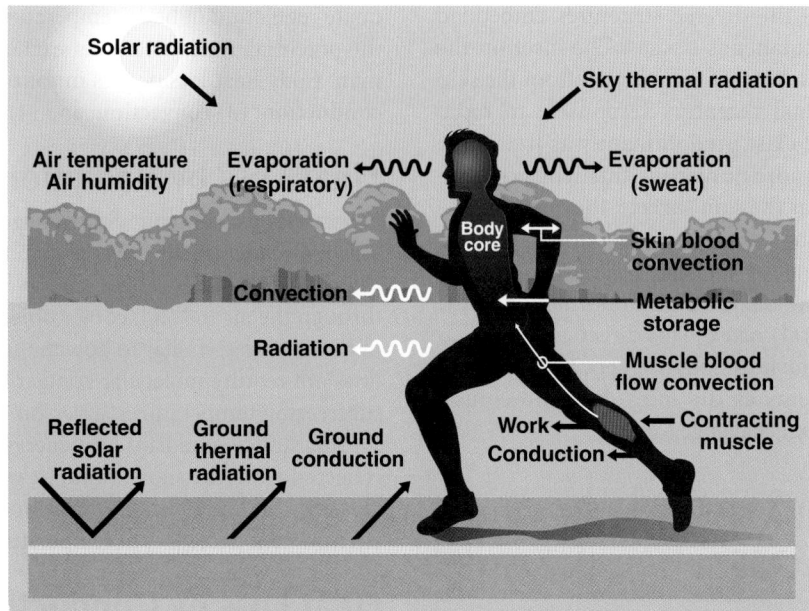

FIGURE 10.3 ▪ Heat production within active muscle and its subsequent transfer from the core to the skin. Under appropriate environmental conditions, excess body heat dissipates to the environment and core temperature stabilizes within a narrow range. (From Gisolfi CV, Wenger CB. Temperature regulation during exercise: old concepts, new ideas. *Exerc Sport Sci Rev* 1984;12:339.)

volves the warming of air molecules and cooler surfaces in contact with the skin.

The rate of conductive heat loss depends on the temperature gradient between the skin and surrounding surfaces and their thermal qualities. Warm-weather hikers gain considerable heat from their physical activity and the environment. Some relief comes from lying on a cool rock shielded from the sun. Conductance between the rock's cold surface and the hiker's warmer surface facilitates favorable loss of body heat.

Heat Loss by Convection

The effectiveness of heat loss by conduction via air depends on how rapidly air near the body exchanges once it warms. With little or no air movement or convection, the warmed air next to the skin acts as a zone of insulation, minimizing further conductive heat loss. Conversely, if cooler air continuously replaces the warmer air surrounding the body (as occurs on a breezy day, in a room with a fan, or during running), heat loss increases because convective currents carry the heat away. For example, air currents at 4 miles per hour cool twice as effectively as air moving at 1 mile per hour.

Heat Loss by Evaporation

Evaporation of sweat provides the major physiologic defense against overheating. Water vaporization from the respiratory passages and skin surface continually transfers heat to the environment. Each liter of water that vaporizes transfers 580 kCal of heat energy from the body to the environment.

In response to heat stress, 2 to 4 million sweat (eccrine) glands secrete large quantities of hypotonic saline solution (0.2–0.4% NaCl). Cooling occurs when sweat evaporates from the skin surface. The cooled skin then cools blood shunted from the interior to the surface. Along with heat loss through sweating, approximately 350 mL of water seeps through the skin (called *insensible perspiration*) each day and evaporates to the environment. Also, approximately 300 mL of water vaporizes daily from the respiratory passages' moist mucous membranes. In cold weather, this source of evaporation appears as "foggy breath."

Evaporative Heat Loss at High Ambient Temperatures

Increased ambient temperature reduces the effectiveness of heat loss by conduction, convection, and radiation. When ambient temperature exceeds body temperature, these three mechanisms of thermal transfer actually contribute to heat gain. When this occurs (or when conduction, convection, and radiation cannot adequately dissipate a large metabolic heat load), sweat evaporation from the skin and water vaporization from the respiratory tract provide the only avenue to dissipate heat. Sweating rate increases directly with ambient temperature. For someone relaxing in a hot, humid environment, the normal 2-L daily fluid requirement doubles or even triples from evaporative fluid loss.

Heat Loss in High Humidity

FIGURE 10.4 illustrates the influence of exercise intensity and environmental conditions on sweating rate. Sweat evapora-

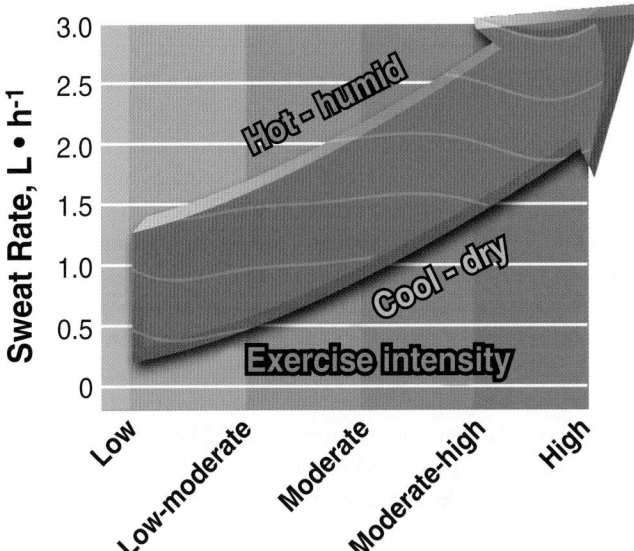

FIGURE 10.4 ■ Approximate hourly sweating rates related to environmental conditions and exercise intensity.

tion from the skin depends on three factors: (1) surface exposed to the environment, (2) temperature and relative humidity of ambient air, and (3) convective air currents around the body. *By far, relative humidity exerts the greatest impact on the effectiveness of evaporative heat loss.*

Relative humidity refers to the percentage of water in ambient air at a particular temperature compared with the total quantity of moisture that the air could carry. For example, 40% relative humidity means that ambient air contains only 40% of the air's moisture-carrying capacity at that specific temperature. With high humidity, ambient air's vapor pressure approaches that of moist skin (approximately 40 mm Hg). Consequently, evaporative heat loss becomes thwarted, even though a large quantity of sweat beads on the skin and eventually rolls off. This represents a useless water loss that can lead to dehydration and overheating.

Continually drying the skin with a towel before sweat evaporates also thwarts evaporative cooling. *Sweat does not cool the skin; rather, skin cooling occurs only when sweat evaporates.* One can tolerate relatively high environmental temperatures as long as humidity remains low. For this reason, people prefer the comfort of hot, dry desert climates to "cooler" but more humid tropical climates.

Integration of Heat-Dissipating Mechanisms

Circulation

The circulatory system serves as the "workhorse" to maintain thermal balance. At rest in hot weather, heart rate and blood flow from the heart (cardiac output) increase while superficial arterial and venous blood vessels dilate to divert warm blood to the body's shell. This manifests as a flushed or reddened face on a hot day or during vigorous exercise. With extreme heat stress, 15 to 25% of the cardiac output passes through the skin, greatly increasing the thermal conductance of peripheral tissues. Increased peripheral blood flow favors radiative heat loss, particularly from the hands, forehead, forearms, ears, and tibial area of the lower legs.

Evaporation

Sweating begins within several seconds of the start of vigorous exercise and, after about 30 minutes, reaches equilibrium directly related to exercise load. A large cutaneous blood flow coupled with evaporative cooling generally produces an effective thermal defense. The cooled peripheral blood then returns to the deeper tissues and picks up additional heat as it returns to the heart.

Hormonal Adjustments

Heat stress initiates hormonal adjustments to conserve the loss of salts and fluid in sweat. During heat exposure, the pituitary gland releases **antidiuretic hormone (ADH).** ADH increases water reabsorption from the kidney tubules, causing urine to become more concentrated. Concurrently, during a single bout of exercise or with repeated days of exercise in hot weather, the adrenal cortex releases the sodium-conserving hormone **aldosterone,** which increases the renal tubules' reabsorption of sodium. Aldosterone also decreases sodium concentration in sweat (i.e., reduces sweat osmolality); this aids in additional electrolyte conservation.

EFFECTS OF CLOTHING ON THERMOREGULATION IN THE HEAT

Different materials absorb water at different rates. Cottons and linens readily absorb moisture. In contrast, heavy "sweatshirts" and rubber or plastic garments produce high relative humidity close to the skin and retard the vaporization of moisture. This inhibits or even prevents evaporative cooling. Color also plays an important role; dark colors absorb light rays and add to radiant heat gain, whereas clothing of lighter color reflects heat rays away from the body.

Some Fabrics Are Better Than Others

Moisture-wicking fabrics (e.g., polypropylene, Coolmax, Drylite) that adhere close to the skin provide optimal transfer of heat and moisture from the skin to the environment, particularly during high-intensity exercise in hot weather. These fabrics wick moisture *away* from the skin. They also offer benefits during exercise in cold environments because dry clothing (in contrast to sweat-drenched clothing) greatly reduces the risk for hypothermia.

Football Uniforms

Football uniforms and equipment present a considerable barrier to heat dissipation during environmental heat exposure.[37] Even with loose-fitting porous jerseys, the wrappings, padding (with plastic covering), helmet, and other objects of "armor" effectively seal off 50% of the body's surface from the benefits of evaporative cooling. Just wearing the 6 to 7 kg of football equipment increases the metabolic load, not to mention the thermal challenge from a hot artificial playing surface and the body heat-retaining qualities of the equipment. The large body size of these athletes further magnifies the heat load, particularly for offensive and defensive linemen. They possess a relatively small body surface area-to-body mass ratio and a higher percentage of body fat than players at other positions.

The Modern Cycling Helmet Does Not Thwart Heat Dissipation

Wearing a commercial cycling helmet provides considerable protection against possible head injury, but does the helmet impede thermoregulatory processes in a hot–dry or hot–humid environment? Because the head provides an important avenue for heat loss during exercise,[49] many competitive cyclists believe that not wearing a helmet reduces thermal strain and physical discomfort. This belief persists even though the design of current commercial helmets remains aerodynamic and lightweight, with ventilation ports for convective and evaporative cooling. To evaluate the physiologic and perceptual responses to wearing a helmet, male and female competitive cyclists pedaled for 90 minutes at 60% peak oxygen uptake in both hot–dry (35°C, 20% relative humidity) and hot–humid (35°C, 70% relative humidity) environments with and without a protective helmet.[57] Measurements included oxygen uptake; heart rate; core, skin, and head skin temperatures; rating of perceived exertion; and perceived thermal sensations of the head and body. Results showed that exercising in a hot–humid environment produced significantly greater thermal stress, yet wearing the helmet during exercise did *not* increase the riders' level of heat strain or perceived heat sensation of the head or body.

Summary

1. Humans tolerate relatively small variations in internal (core) temperature. Consequently, exposure to heat or cold initiates thermoregulatory mechanisms that generate and conserve heat at low ambient temperatures and dissipate heat at high temperatures.

2. The hypothalamus serves as the "thermostat" for temperature regulation. This coordination center initiates adjustments from thermal receptors in the skin and changes in hypothalamic blood temperature.

3. Warm blood diverts from the body's core to the shell in response to heat stress. Heat loss occurs by radiation, conduction, convection, and evaporation. Evaporation provides the major physiologic defense against overheating at high ambient temperatures and during exercise.

4. Warm, humid environments dramatically decrease the effectiveness of evaporative heat loss. This increases one's vulnerability to a dangerous state of dehydration and spiraling core temperature.

5. The ideal warm-weather clothing consists of lightweight, loose-fitting, and light-color clothes. Moisture-wicking fabrics against the skin optimize heat and moisture transfer from the skin to the environment.

6. Football uniforms impose a significant barrier to heat dissipation because they effectively seal off about 50% of the body's surface from the benefits of evaporative cooling. They also add to the metabolic load imposed by exercise.

7. During exercise in hot–humid environments, the modern cycling helmet does not increase the level of heat strain or perceived heat sensation of the head or body above that with the no-helmet condition.

Thermoregulation During Exercise in the Heat

Cardiovascular adjustments and evaporative cooling dissipate metabolic heat during exercise, particularly in hot weather. A tradeoff occurs, because the fluid lost in thermoregulation often creates a relative state of dehydration. Excessive sweating leads to more serious fluid loss with accompanying reductions in plasma volume. This end result produces circulatory failure, and core temperature rises to lethal levels. During near-maximal exercise in the heat, with accompanying dehydration, relatively less blood diverts to peripheral areas for heat dissipation. Reduced peripheral blood flow reflects the body's attempt to maintain cardiac output despite a diminishing plasma volume caused by sweating.

CORE TEMPERATURE DURING EXERCISE

Heat generated by active muscles can raise core temperature to fever levels that incapacitate a person if caused by external heat stress alone. However, distance runners show no ill effects from rectal temperatures as high as 41°C (105.8°F) recorded at the end of a race.[8,27] Within limits, an increased core temperature with exercise does not reflect a failure of heat-dissipating mechanisms. To the contrary, a well-regulated rise in core temperature occurs even during exercise in the cold. *More than likely, a modest rise in core temperature reflects a favorable internal adjustment that creates an optimal thermal environment for physiologic and metabolic functions.*

WATER LOSS IN THE HEAT: DEHYDRATION

Dehydration refers to an imbalance in fluid dynamics when fluid intake does not replenish water loss from either hyperhydrated or normally hydrated states. A moderate exercise workout generally produces a 0.5- to 1.5-L sweat loss over a 1-hour period. Considerable water loss occurs during several hours of intense exercise in a hot environment. Even with exercise performed in less challenging thermal environments (e.g., swimming and cross-country skiing), sweating occurs.[30] For the swimmer, immersion in water per se also stimulates body water loss through cold-induced increased urine production. Non–exercise-induced water loss occurs when power athletes (boxers, weightlifters, and rowers) aggressively attempt to "make weight" through rapid weight loss induced by common dehydration techniques (e.g., heat exposure via sauna, steam room, hot whirlpool or shower; fluid and food restriction; diuretic and laxative drugs; or vomiting). These individuals often combine techniques, hoping to achieve even faster weight loss.

Intracellular and extracellular compartments contribute to the fluid deficit (dehydration), which can rapidly reach levels that impede heat dissipation, reduce heat tolerance, and severely compromise cardiovascular function and exercise capacity. *The risk of heat illness greatly increases when a person begins exercising in a dehydrated state.* Dehydration associated with a 3% decrease in body weight also slows gastric emptying rate, thus increasing epigastric cramps and feelings of nausea.[69] Avoiding dehydration not only optimizes exercise performance but also reduces the feelings of gastrointestinal discomfort associated with body fluid loss. Because sweat is hypotonic with other body fluids, the reduced plasma volume caused by sweating correspondingly increases blood plasma osmolality.

Magnitude of Fluid Loss

Water loss by sweating in an acclimatized person peaks at about 3 L per hour during intense exercise in the heat and averages nearly 12 L (26 lb) on a daily basis. Several hours of intense sweating can cause sweat-gland fatigue, which

ultimately impairs core temperature regulation. Elite marathon runners frequently experience fluid losses in excess of 5 L during competition; this represents between 6 and 10% of body mass. For slower paced marathons or ultramarathons, average fluid loss rarely exceeds 500 mL per hour. Even in a temperate climate, an average fluid loss of 2 L takes place in soccer players during a 90-minute game played at about 10°C (50°F).[32] A large sweat output and subsequent fluid loss occurs in sports other than distance running; football, basketball, and hockey players also lose large quantities of fluid during a contest.

Physiologic and Performance Consequences

Just about any degree of dehydration impairs the capacity of circulatory and temperature-regulating mechanisms to adjust to exercise demands. As dehydration progresses and plasma volume decreases, peripheral blood flow and sweating rate diminish and thermoregulation becomes progressively more difficult. Cumulatively, this contributes to larger increases in heart rate, perception of effort, and core temperature and premature fatigue than under normal hydration. A fluid loss of only 1% of body mass increases rectal temperature above that with the same exercise performed when fully hydrated.

Reduced peripheral blood flow and increased core temperature in exercise relate closely to dehydration level. Dehydration of as little as 2% body mass impairs physical work capacity and physiologic function and predisposes to heat injury when exercising in a hot environment.[7,11,12,19,34,59] For each liter of sweat-loss dehydration, exercise heart rate increases 8 beats $\cdot$ min^{-1} with a corresponding 1.0 L $\cdot$ min^{-1} decrease in cardiac output.[13] A large portion of water lost through sweating comes from blood plasma, so circulatory capacity progressively decreases as sweat loss progresses. Body fluid loss coincides with the following: (1) decreased plasma volume, (2) reduced skin blood flow for a given core temperature, (3) reduced stroke volume, (4) increased heart rate, and (5) general deterioration in circulatory and thermoregulatory efficiency in exercise. For exercise performance, dehydration equal to 4.3% of body mass reduced walking endurance by 18%; concurrently, $\dot{V}O_{2max}$ decreased by 22%. These same experiments showed decreased endurance performance (−22%) and $\dot{V}O_{2max}$ (−10%) when dehydration averaged only 1.9% of body mass. Clearly, even modest dehydration imposes adverse thermoregulatory and exercise performance effects during exercise. A moderate degree of hypohydration or hyperthermia exerts no effect on anaerobic exercise performance.[11]

CONSIDERABLE FLUID LOSS IN WINTER ENVIRONMENTS. The risk for dehydration increases during vigorous cold-weather exercise. For one thing, colder air contains less moisture than air at warmer temperature, particularly at higher altitudes. Consequently, greater fluid volumes leave the respiratory passages as the incoming cold, dry air becomes fully humidified and warmed to body temperature. This air-conditioning process can create a 1-L daily fluid loss. Cold stress also increases urine production, which adds to total body fluid loss. Furthermore, many people overdress for outdoor winter activities. As exercise progresses and body heat production increases, heat gain exceeds body heat loss, which initiates sweating. All of these factors become magnified, in that many individuals consider it unimportant to consume fluids before, during, and in recovery from prolonged exercise in cold weather. FIGURE 10.5 illustrates a back-mounted hydration system to provide ready access to water *during* such prolonged winter activities as Nordic or alpine skiing, serious outdoor winter trekking including ice and mountain climbing at high altitudes, or distance cycling or running. In the military, back-mounted hydration systems are often attached to load-bearing equipment. Many different styles and configurations of hydration systems are available at sporting goods or cycling shops and through sports equipment mail-order catalogues.

Diuretic Use

Athletes who use diuretics to lose body water to rapidly "make weight" place themselves at a distinct performance disadvantage because a disproportionate reduction in plasma volume occurs, which negatively affects thermoregulation and cardiovascular function. Diuretic drugs also can markedly impair neuromuscular function not noted when comparable fluid loss occurs by exercise. Athletes who use vomiting and diarrhea to lose weight not only produce dehydration but also cause excessive mineral loss with accompanying muscle weakness and impaired neuromuscular function. This clearly gives a competitive "edge" to the opponent—a result entirely opposite that anticipated.

WATER REPLACEMENT: REHYDRATION

Adequate fluid replacement sustains the exceptional potential for evaporative cooling of acclimatized humans. Properly scheduling fluid replacement maintains plasma volume so circulation and sweating progress optimally. Strictly following an adequate water replacement schedule prevents dehydration and its consequences, particularly hyperthermia. This replenishment is often "easier said than done" because some coaches and athletes still believe water consumption hinders performance. Left on their own, most individuals voluntarily replace only about half of the water lost (less than $500 \text{ mL} \cdot \text{h}^{-1}$) during exercise.[44] The enlightened exercise nutritionist must remain vigilant about the key role of hydration in thermoregulation and its impact on exercise performance and safety.

> ## There Are Risks and Then There Are Serious Risks
>
> Glycogen depletion during exercise impairs high-intensity endurance performance, yet failure to replenish this energy reserve does not impose a risk to health and safety. In contrast, inadequate water replenishment not only impairs exercise capacity but also creates life-threatening disturbances in fluid balance and core temperature.

"Cold treatments"—periodic application of cold towels to the forehead and abdomen during exercise, or taking a cold shower before exercising in a hot environment—do not facilitate heat transfer at the body's surface compared with the same exercise without skin wetting. Adequate hydration provides the most effective defense against heat stress by balancing water loss with water intake, not by pouring water over the head or body. Ingesting fluid at 4°C during exercise enhances fluid consumption and improves endurance by attenuating the rise in body temperature and thus reducing the effects of heat stress.[42] No evidence exists that restricting fluid intake during training prepares a person to perform better in the heat. *A well-hydrated individual always functions at a higher physiologic and performance level than a dehydrated one.*

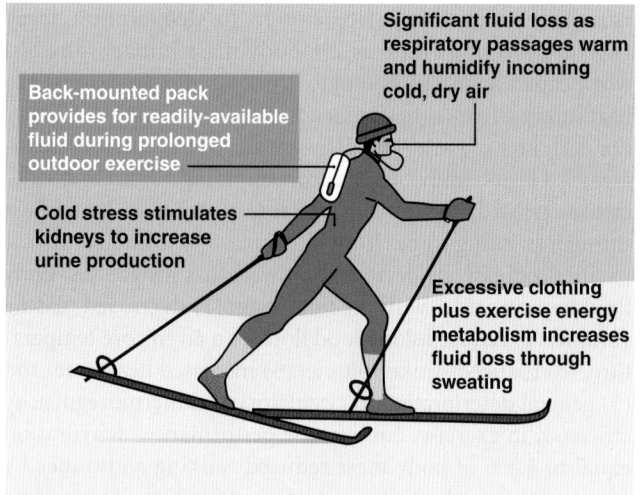

Back-mounted pack provides for readily-available fluid during prolonged outdoor exercise

Cold stress stimulates kidneys to increase urine production

Significant fluid loss as respiratory passages warm and humidify incoming cold, dry air

Excessive clothing plus exercise energy metabolism increases fluid loss through sweating

FIGURE 10.5 ■ Factors that increase the potential for dehydration during cold-weather exercise. The illustration depicts a back-mounted hydration system to provide ready access to fluid during continuous exercise in the outdoor environment.

Pre-exercise Hydration

Ingesting "extra" water (**hyperhydration**) before exercising in a hot environment protects to some extent against heat stress because it delays dehydration, increases sweating during exercise, and diminishes the rise in core temperature. These outcomes contribute to enhanced exercise performance and the participant's overall safety. In addition to increasing fluid intake 24 hours before strenuous exercise in the heat, we recommend consuming 400 to 600 mL (13–20 oz) of cool water about 20 minutes before such exercise. Pre-exercise fluid intake increases the stomach's volume, a major factor that optimizes gastric emptying (see Chapter 8). A systematic regimen of hyperhydration (4.5 L fluid per day) 1 week before soccer competition by acclimated elite young players in Puerto Rico increased body water reserves (despite greater urine output) and improved temperature regulation during the soccer match in warm weather.[52] This structured sequence of pre-exercise hyperhydration produced a body fluid volume 1.1 L greater than that produced when the players consumed their normal daily fluid volume of 2.5 L. In Chapter 12, we discuss the role of glycerol supplementation to augment pre-exercise hyperhydration.

Pre-exercise hyperhydration does not replace the need to continually replace fluid during exercise. In intense endurance activities in the heat, matching fluid loss with fluid intake often becomes impossible, because only about 1000 mL of fluid each hour empties from the stomach. This volume does not match a sweat loss that averages nearly 2000 mL per hour. Even individuals with unlimited access to water should be carefully monitored during exercise in the heat.

Adequacy of Rehydration

Body weight changes indicate the extent of water loss from exercise and adequacy of rehydration during and after exercise or athletic competition. Voiding small volumes of dark yellow urine with a strong odor provides a qualitative indication of inadequate hydration. Well-hydrated individuals typically produce urine in large volumes, light in color, and without a strong smell. For team athletes, assign each player a squeeze bottle for fluids to emphasize the importance of fluid replacement and monitor the fluid consumed. TABLE 10.2 recommends fluid intake with weight loss during exercise. Although these standards were developed for a 90-minute football practice, they easily adapt to most exercise situations. Menstrual cycle variations do not adversely affect rehydration.[35]

Coaches often require athletes to weigh-in before and after practice (following urination) to monitor fluid balance; each 1-lb weight loss represents 450 mL (15 fl oz) of dehydration. FIGURE 10.6 gives a practical illustration to determine quantity and rate of fluid loss from exercise. To properly match fluid loss with intake, partition the estimated hourly fluid loss from a workout or competition into 10- or 15-minute periods and ingest that amount of fluid at those intervals. For example, we recommend fluid intake every 15 minutes for hourly losses up to 1000 mL, whereas fluid ingestion at 10-minute intervals optimizes replenishing a fluid loss

Fluid Replacement with and without the Calories: The Added Cost of Replacing Fluid with Some Products

Beverage	Calories
Diet Pepsi (20 oz)	0
Water or club soda	0
Tea, with 2 sugar packets (8 oz)	20
Coffee, with 1 liquid creamer and 1 sugar packet (8 oz)	30
V-8 or tomato juice (8 oz)	70
Milk, fat-free (8 oz)	80
Beer, light (12 oz)	110
Orange juice (8 oz)	110
Starbucks Coffee Frappuccino Light, tall (12 oz)	110
with whipped cream	210
Gatorade (20 oz)	130
Wine, red (5 oz)	130
Cranberry juice cocktail (8 oz)	140
Grape juice (8 oz)	150
Milk, whole (8 oz)	150
Beer, regular (12 oz)	160
Dunkin' Donuts Coffee Coolatta (16 oz)	170
Gin and tonic, on the rocks (7 oz)	190
Yoplait Strawberry Smoothie (8 oz)	190
Snapple Lemonade (16 oz)	220
Coca-Cola or 7-Up (20 oz)	250
Dannon Strawberry Blend Frusion (10 oz)	260
Starbucks Caffe Latte, venti (prepared with whole milk) (20 oz)	340
Dunkin' Donuts Coffee Coolatta with cream (16 oz)	350
Nestle Nesquik Chocolate Milk (16 oz)	400
7-Eleven Super Big Gulp, Coca-Cola (44 oz)	410
Burger King Vanilla Shake, large (32 oz)	820
McDonald's Chocolate Triple Thick Shake, large (32 oz)	1160

Sources: Company web sites and U.S. Department of Agriculture.

in excess of 1000 mL per hour. Make water available (and ensure it is consumed) during practice and competition. Urge individuals to rehydrate themselves, because the thirst mechanism imprecisely indicates water needs, particularly in children and the elderly. The elderly generally require longer time to achieve rehydration after dehydration.[28] If rehydration were left entirely to a person's thirst, it could take several days after severe dehydration to re-establish fluid balance. *Drink at least 125 to150% of the existing fluid loss (body weight loss) as soon as possible after exercising. The 25 to 50% "extra" water accounts for that portion of ingested water lost in urine.*[60,61]

Flavored Drinks Help

Consuming highly palatable flavored beverages with added salt facilitates voluntary rehydration in children and young and older adults.[5,28,31,47] After exercise, dehydration, and

TABLE 10.2   Recommended Fluid Availability and Intake for a Strenuous 90-Minute Athletic Practice[a]

Weight Loss		Minutes Between Water Breaks	Fluid per Break		Fluid Availability for an 11-Member Squad	
lb	kg		oz	mL	gal	L
8	3.6	No practice recommended	–	–		
7.5	3.4		–	–		
7	3.2	10	8–10	266	6.5–8	27.4
6.5	3.0	10	8–9	251	6.5–7	25.5
6	2.7	10	8–9	251	6.5–7	25.5
5.5	2.5	15	10–12	325	5.5–6.5	22.7
5	2.3	15	10–11	311	5.5–6	21.8
4.5	2.1	15	9–10	281	5–5.5	19.9
4	1.8	15	8–9	251	4.5–5	18.0
3.5	1.6	20	10–11	311	4–4.5	16.1
3	1.4	20	9–10	281	3.5–4	14.2
2.5	1.1	20	7–8	222	3	11.4
2	0.9	30	8	237	2.5	9.5
1.5	0.7	30	6	177	1.5	5.7
1	0.5	45	6	177	1	3.8
0.5	0.2	60	6	177	0.5	1.9

[a]Based on 80% replacement of weight loss.

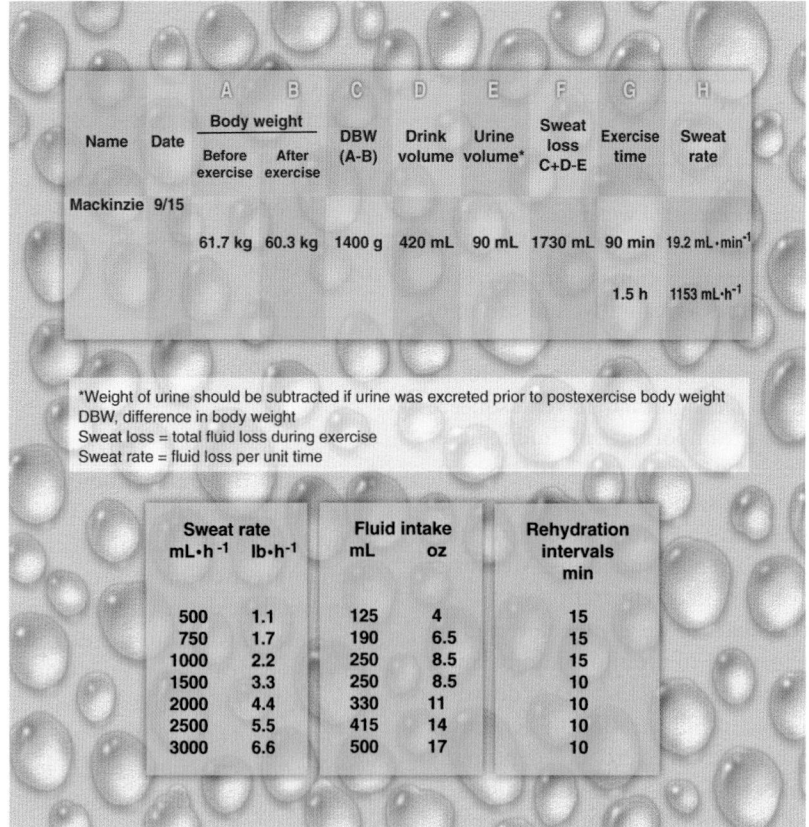

FIGURE 10.6 ■ Computing the magnitude of sweat loss and rate of sweating in exercise. In this example, Mackinzie should drink about 1000 mL (32 oz) of fluid during each hour of activity (250 mL every 15 minutes) to remain well hydrated. (Modified from Gatorade Sports Science Institute, 1996;9:4[suppl]:63.)

heat exposure, boys voluntarily consumed one of three beverages: (1) plain water, (2) grape-flavored water, or (3) grape-flavored water containing 6% carbohydrate (14 g per 8 oz) and 18 mmol · L^{-1} NaCl (110 mg per 8 oz).[76] The flavored carbohydrate–electrolyte drink elicited the largest total voluntary fluid intake (1157 mL), followed by the flavored drink (1112 mL), with the smallest volume recorded for plain water (610 mL).

Aging Affects Rehydration

Older men and women require particular attention when evaluating rehydration following exercise in the heat. These individuals do not recover from dehydration as effectively as younger adults, probably from a depressed thirst drive. This increases susceptibility to chronic hypohydration, which creates a suboptimal plasma volume and diminished thermoregulatory capacity. However, when palatable fluid (e.g., carbohydrate–electrolyte solution) is readily available, older adults drink enough to maintain fluid balance following exercise; the carbohydrate–electrolyte solution promotes greater voluntary fluid intake and restores plasma volume losses faster than water.[5]

Sodium Facilitates Rehydration

In Chapter 8, we pointed out that a moderate amount of sodium added to a rehydration beverage provides more complete rehydration after exercise and thermal induced dehydration than plain water.[50,56,58] Restoring water and electrolyte balance in recovery occurs most effectively by (1) adding moderate to high amounts of sodium (100 mmol · L^{-1}, an amount exceeding that in commercial beverages) to the rehydration drink or (2) combining solid food (with appropriate sodium content) with plain water.[31,33,36] In addition, a small amount of potassium (2–5 mmol · L^{-1}) enhances water retention in the intracellular space and may diminish any extra potassium loss that results from sodium retention by the kidneys.[14]

The kidneys continually form urine, so the volume of ingested fluid following exercise should exceed exercise sweat loss by 25 to 50% to restore fluid balance. Unless the beverage has a sufficiently high sodium content, excess fluid intake merely increases urine output with *no benefit* to rehydration.[62,63]

FIGURE 10.7 illustrates the effect of adding sodium to a rehydration beverage on retention of ingested fluid in recovery. Six healthy men exercised in a warm, humid environment until sweating produced a 1.9% loss of body mass. They then ingested 2045 mL of one of four test drinks containing sodium in a concentration of either 2, 26, 52, or 100 mmol · L^{-1} over a 30-minute period beginning 30 minutes after exercise stopped. (Typical "sports drinks" contain between 10 and 25 mmol of sodium · L^{-1}; normal plasma sodium concentration ranges between 138 and 142 mmol · L^{-1}.) From the 1.5-hour urine sample onward, urine volume inversely related to the rehydration beverage's sodium content. At the end of the study period, a difference in total body water content of 787 mL existed between trials using drinks with the lowest and highest sodium content. The drink containing sodium at a

Adding Salt Facilitates Rehydration

Pure water absorbed from the gut rapidly dilutes plasma sodium concentration. A decrease in plasma osmolality, in turn, stimulates urine production and blunts the normal sodium-dependent stimulation of the thirst mechanism. Maintaining a relatively high plasma concentration of sodium (by adding a pinch of sodium to ingested fluid) achieves three objectives:

1. Sustains the thirst drive
2. Promotes retention of ingested fluids (less urine output)
3. More rapidly restores lost plasma volume during rehydration

concentration of 100 mmol · L^{-1} contributed to the greatest fluid retention.

With prolonged exercise in the heat, sweat loss can deplete the body of 13 to 17 g of salt (2.3–3.4 g per L of sweat), about 8 g more than typically consumed daily in the diet. It seems prudent in this situation to replace the lost sodium by adding about one-third teaspoon of table salt to 1 L of water.

The American College of Sports Medicine (ACSM) recommends that sports drinks contain 0.5 to 0.7 g of sodium per liter of fluid consumed during exercise lasting more than 1 hour. Moderate exercise produces negligible losses of potassium in sweat. Even at intense physical activity levels, potassium lost in sweat ranges between 5 and 18 mEq, which poses no immediate danger. One can replace potassium lost with heavy sweating by increasing intake of potassium-rich foods (citrus fruits and bananas). A glass of orange juice or tomato juice replaces almost all the potassium, calcium, and magnesium excreted in 3 L of sweat. Except in unusual cases, minor adjustments in food intake and electrolyte conservation by the kidneys compensate adequately for mineral loss through sweating. TABLE 10.3 gives examples of drinks from five major sports-beverage categories including their carbohydrate and calorie content per 8-oz serving. Beverages in the recovery drink and energy drink categories most effectively facilitate glycogen replenishment because of their high carbohydrate content.

HYPONATREMIA: REDUCED SODIUM CONCENTRATION IN BODY FLUIDS

Major concerns in hot-weather exercise include the following:

- Dehydration
- Decreased plasma volume and resulting hemoconcentration
- Impaired physical performance and thermoregulatory capacity
- Increased risk of heat injury (especially heat stroke)

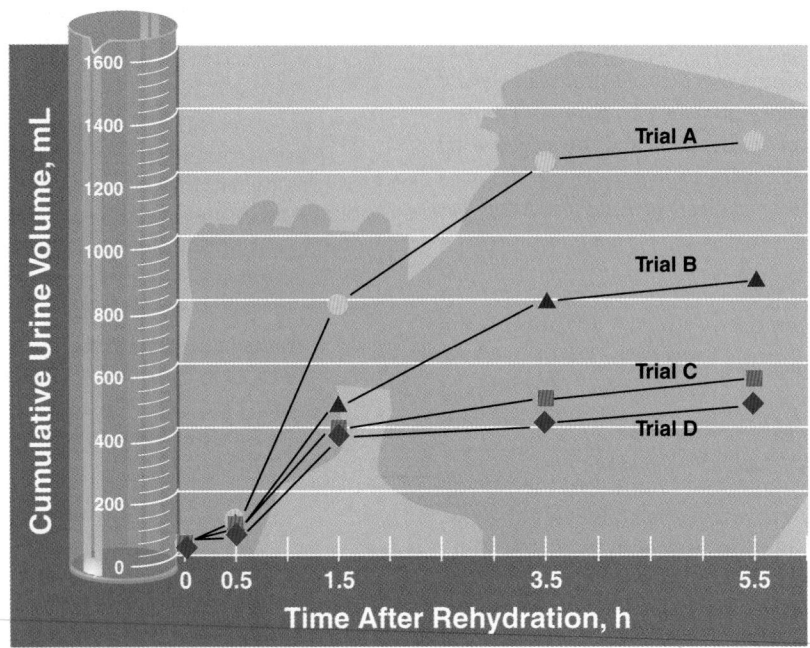

FIGURE 10.7 ■ Cumulative urine output during recovery from exercise-induced dehydration. The oral rehydration beverages consisted of four test drinks (equivalent to 1.5 times the body weight loss, or approximately 2045 mL) containing sodium (and matching anion) in a concentration of either 2 (trial A), 26 (trial B), 52 (trial C), or 100 (trial D) mmol · L^{-1}. (From Maughan J, Leiper JB. Sodium intake and post-exercise rehydration in man. *Eur J Appl Physiol* 1995;71:311.)

TABLE 10.3   How the Drinks Stack Up. Five Major Sports Drink Categories Including Their Calorie and Carbohydrate Content Plus Nutritional "Extras" per 8-oz Serving

	Calories	Carbohydrate (g)	Extras
Waters			
Tap water	0	0	Minerals—vary by source
Dasani	0	0	Spring source
Fiji	0	0	Artesian source
Penta	0	0	Purified
Fitness waters			
ChampionLyte	0	0	Electrolytes
Life O$_2$	0	0	10 times O$_2$ of tap water
Propel	10	3	Electrolytes, vitamins
Reebok	12	3	Electrolytes, vitamins, trace minerals
Sports drinks			
All Sport	70	20	No longer carbonated, vitamins B and C
G-Push (G^2)	70	18	Electrolytes, vitamins
Gatorade	50	14	Electrolytes
GU$_2$O	50	14	Electrolytes
Powerade	72	19	Electrolytes, vitamins
Simple Sports Drink	80	21	Electrolytes, vitamin C
Recovery drinks			
Endurox R^4	180	35	Electrolytes, vitamins
G-Push (G^4)	110	27	Electrolytes, vitamins, trace minerals
Gatorade Energy Drink	207	41	Vitamins
Energy drinks			
Red Bull	109	27	Taurine, caffeine, vitamins
SoBe Adrenaline Rush	135	35	Taurine, ribose, caffeine

The exercise physiology literature contains more than ample information about the need to consume fluid before, during, and after exercise. In many instances the recommended beverage remains plain, hypotonic water. However, we now know that excessive water intake under certain exercise conditions can produce potentially serious medical complications from the syndrome termed **hyponatremia** or "water intoxication." Hyponatremia exists when serum sodium concentration falls below 135 mEq $\cdot$ L^{-1}; a serum sodium concentration below 125 mEq $\cdot$ L^{-1} triggers severe symptoms. A sustained low plasma sodium concentration creates an osmotic imbalance across the blood–brain barrier that causes rapid water influx into the brain. The resulting swelling of brain tissue produces a cascade of symptoms that range from mild (headache, confusion malaise, nausea, cramping) to severe (seizures, coma, pulmonary edema, cardiac arrest, and death).[3,21,22]

More Prevalent Than Previously Thought

The exercise scenario conducive to the development of hyponatremia involves water overload during continuous high-intensity, ultramarathon-type exercise of 6- to 8-hours duration, particularly in hot weather.[4,24,25,39,40,45] It can also occur in events lasting less than 4 hours, such as standard marathons.[67] In a large study of more than 18,000 ultraendurance runners (including triathletes), approximately 9% of collapsed individuals presented with symptoms of hyponatremia.[46] The athletes, on average, drank fluids with low sodium chloride content (less than 6.8 mmol $\cdot$ L^{-1}). The runner with the most severe hyponatremia (serum sodium level of 112 mmol $\cdot$ L^{-1}) excreted more than 7.5 L of dilute urine during the first 17 hours of hospitalization.

Researchers monitored changes in body mass and blood sodium concentration in 95 competitors receiving medical care and 169 competitors not requiring care in the 1996 New Zealand Ironman Triathlon (swim 3.8 km, cycle 180 km, run 42 km).[66] For individuals with clinical evidence of fluid or electrolyte disturbance, body mass declined 2.5 kg (–2.9 kg in competitors without medical care). Hyponatremia accounted for 9% of medical abnormalities (identical to that reported earlier[46]). One person with hyponatremia (Na = 130 mEq $\cdot$ L^{-1}) drank 16 L of fluid over the course of the race, with a weight gain of 2.5 kg (consistent with the hypothesis that fluid overload causes hyponatremia). An inverse relationship existed between postrace sodium concentration and percentage change in body mass; individuals who lost less weight tended to have a higher serum sodium concentration.

Level of acclimatization affects sodium loss. For example, sodium concentration in sweat ranges from 5 to 30 mmol $\cdot$ L^{-1} (115–690 mg $\cdot$ L^{-1}) in individuals fully acclimatized to the heat to 40 to 100 mmol $\cdot$ L^{-1} (920–2300 mg $\cdot$ L^{-1}) in the unacclimatized. In addition, some individuals produce relatively highly concentrated sweat regardless of their degree of acclimatization. *Development of hyponatremia requires extreme sodium loss through prolonged sweating coupled with dilution of existing ex-*

Some Important Influencing Factors

Data obtained from the finishers of the 2002 Boston Marathon indicate that 13% had hyponatremia.[1] Most prevalent factors associated with this disorder that occurs in many nonelite marathoners include:

1. Substantial pre-post race weight gain
2. Consumption of more than 3 L of fluid during race
3. Race time greater than 4:00 hours
4. Low body mass index

tracellular sodium (and accompanying reduced osmolality) from consuming large fluid volumes containing low or no sodium (FIG. 10.8A). A reduced extracellular solute concentration promotes movement of water into the cells (Fig. 10.8B). Water movement of sufficient magnitude congests the lungs, swells brain tissue, and adversely affects central nervous system function. Hyponatremia has not been reported from participation in a marathon under only mild environmental stress and where aggressive hydration practices were not promoted.[51]

Predisposing Factors to Hyponatremia

1. Prolonged intense exercise in hot weather
2. Large sodium loss associated with sweat containing high sodium concentration; particularly prevalent in relatively unfit individuals
3. Beginning physical activity in a sodium-depleted state owing to "salt-free" or "low-sodium" diet
4. Use of diuretic medication for hypertension
5. Frequent intake of large quantities of sodium-free fluid before, during, and after prolonged exercise

Several hours of exercise in the heat can cause considerable sodium loss. Exercise in hot, humid weather produces a sweat rate of more than 1 L per hour, with a sweat-sodium concentration ranging between 20 and 100 mEq $\cdot$ L^{-1}. Also, frequently ingesting large volumes of plain water draws sodium from the extracellular fluid compartment into the unabsorbed intestinal water, further diluting serum sodium concentration. Exercise compounds the problem because urine production decreases during exercise owing to a significantly reduced renal blood flow. This reduces the body's ability to excrete excess water.

Competitive athletes, recreational participants, and occupational workers should be aware of the dangers of excessive hydration and that fluid intake should not exceed fluid loss. To reduce risk of overhydration and hyponatremia in prolonged exercise, we recommend the following five steps:

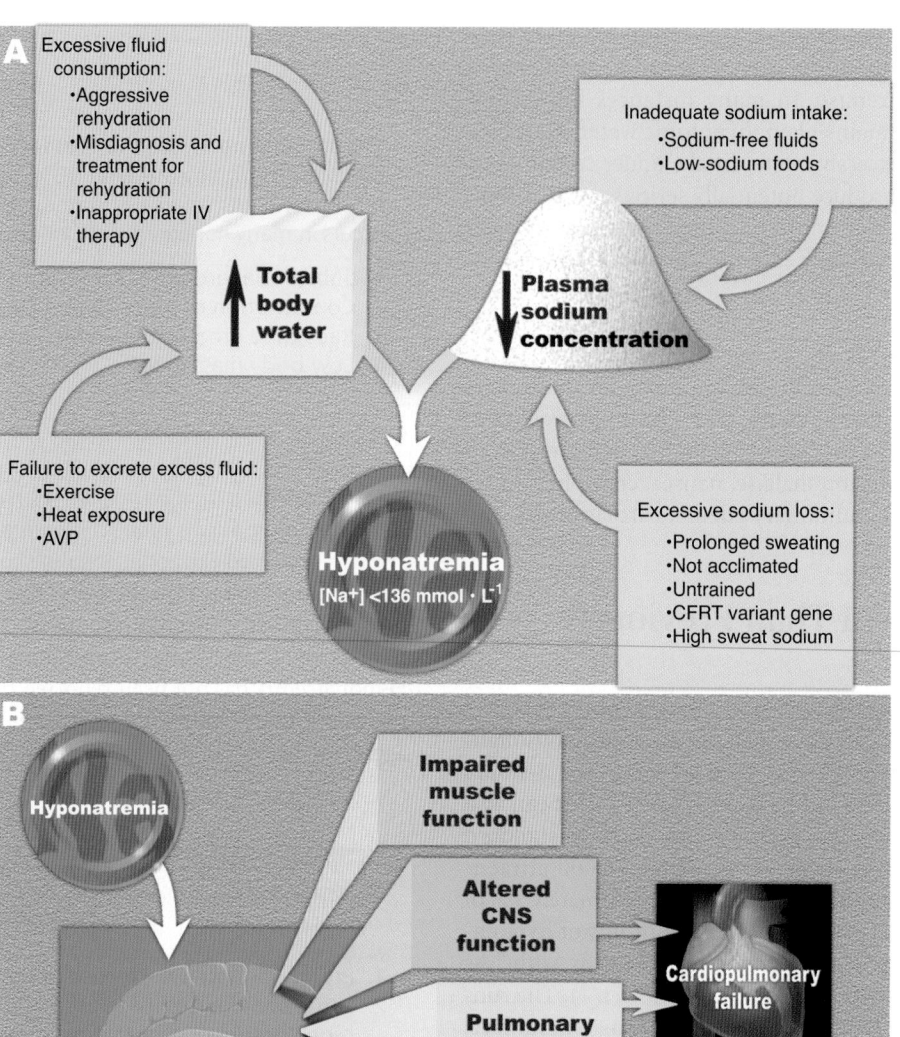

FIGURE 10.8 ■ **A.** Factors that contribute to the development of hyponatremia. AVP, arginine vasopressin; CFTR, cystic fibrosis transmembrane regulatory gene. **B.** Physiologic consequences of hyponatremia. CNS, central nervous system. (Modified from Montain SJ, et al. Hyponatremia associated with exercise: risk factors and pathogenesis. *Exerc Sport Sci Rev* 2001;2:113.)

1. Two to three hours before exercise drink 400 to 600 mL (14–22 oz) of fluid.
2. Drink 150 to 300 mL (5–10 oz) of fluid about 30 minutes before exercise.
3. Drink no more than 1000 mL · h⁻¹ (32 oz) of plain water spread over 15-minute intervals during or after exercise.
4. Add a small amount of sodium (approximately ¼ to ½ tsp

of salt per 32 oz) to the ingested fluid. Commercial sports drinks are also effective in providing water, carbohydrate fuel, and electrolytes.
5. Do not restrict dietary salt.

Including some glucose in the rehydration drink facilitates intestinal water uptake via the glucose–sodium transport mechanism (see Chapters 3 and 8).

FACTORS THAT IMPROVE HEAT TOLERANCE

Relatively moderate exercise performed in cool weather becomes taxing if attempted on the first hot day of spring. The early stages of spring training can present a hazard for heat injury because thermoregulatory mechanisms have not adjusted to the dual challenge of exercise and environmental heat. *Repeated exposure to hot environments, particularly when combined with physical activity, improves capacity for exercise with less discomfort upon heat exposure.*

Acclimatization

Heat acclimatization refers to the physiologic adaptations that improve heat tolerance. FIGURE 10.9 shows that the major acclimatization to heat stress occurs during the first week of heat exposure (2–4 hours each day) with essentially complete acclimatization after 10 days. In practical terms, use 15 to 20 minutes of light-intensity exercise during the first several exercise sessions in a hot environment. Thereafter, exercise sessions can increase systematically to reach the normal duration and intensity for training.

Increased Production of a More Dilute Sweat

TABLE 10.4 summarizes eight physiologic adjustments during heat acclimatization. As acclimatization progresses, larger quantities of blood shunt to cutaneous vessels to facilitate heat transfer from the core to the periphery during exercise. More effective cardiac output distribution maintains blood pressure during exercise; a lowered threshold (earlier onset) for sweating complements this cardiovascular acclimatization. An earlier onset of sweating initiates cooling before internal temperature increases too markedly. After 10 days of heat exposure, sweating capacity nearly doubles and sweat becomes dilute (less salt lost) and more evenly distributed on the skin surface. Increased sweat loss in an acclimatized individual creates a greater need to rehydrate during and following exercise. Adjustments in circulatory function and evaporative cooling enable a heat-acclimatized person to exercise with lower skin and core temperatures and heart rate than an unacclimatized individual. Optimal acclimatization necessitates adequate hydration. Also, one loses the major benefits of heat acclimatization within 2 to 3 weeks upon return to a more temperate climate.

Full Acclimatization Requires Hot-Weather Training

As one might expect, exercise "heat conditioning" in cool weather produces less effective results than acclimatization from similar exercise training in the heat. *Full heat acclimatization cannot take place without exposure to environmental heat stress.* Individuals who train and compete in hot weather show a distinct thermoregulatory advantage over those who train in cooler climates and only periodically compete in hot weather.[26]

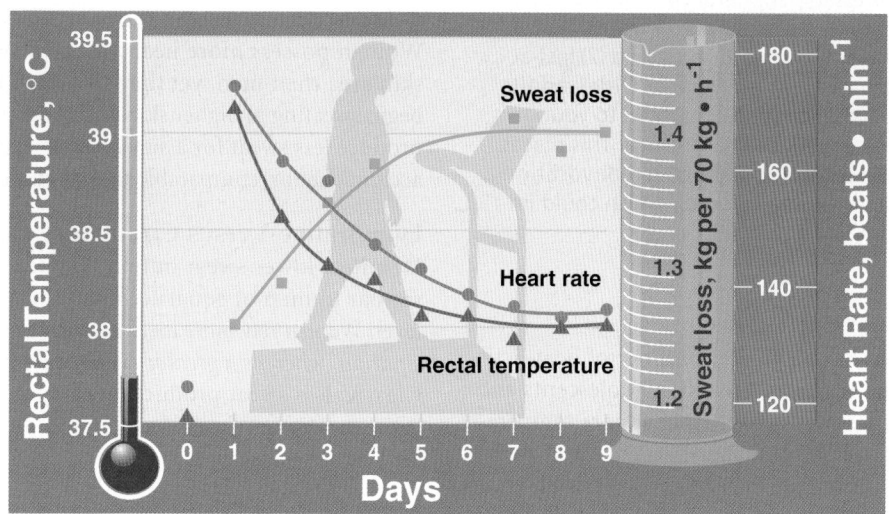

FIGURE 10.9 ■ Average rectal temperature (▲), heart rate (●), and sweat loss (■) during 100 minutes of daily heat-exercise exposure for 9 consecutive days. On day 0, the men walked on a treadmill at an exercise intensity of 300 kCal · h⁻¹ in a cool climate. Thereafter, the same daily exercise took place in the heat at 48.9°C (26.7°F wet bulb). (From Lind R, Bass DE. Optimal exposure time for development of acclimatization to heat. *Fed Proc* 1963;22:704.)

TABLE 10.4 Physiologic Adjustments during Heat Acclimatization	
Acclimatization Response	**Effect**
1. Improved cutaneous blood flow	• Transports metabolic heat from deep tissues to the body's shell
2. Effective distribution of cardiac output	• Appropriate circulation to skin and muscles to meet demands of metabolism and thermoregulation; greater stability of blood pressure during exercise
3. Lowered threshold for start of sweating	• Evaporative cooling begins early during exercise
4. More effective distribution of sweat over skin surface	• Optimum use of effective surface for evaporative cooling
5. Increased sweat output	• Maximizes evaporative cooling
6. Lowered salt concentration in sweat	• Dilute sweat preserves electrolytes in extracellular fluid
7. Lower skin and core temperature and heart rate for standard exercise	• Frees greater portion of cardiac output for distribution to active muscles
8. Less reliance on carbohydrate catabolism during exercise	• Carbohydrate-sparing effect

An Age-Related Difference

Age-related factors affect thermoregulatory dynamics despite equivalence between young and older adults in capacity to regulate core temperature during heat stress. Aging delays the onset of sweating and blunts the magnitude of the sweating response in possibly three ways: (1) modified sensitivity of thermoreceptors, (2) limited sweat gland output per se, or (3) dehydration-limited sweat output with insufficient fluid replacement. Aging also alters the intrinsic structure and function of the skin itself and its vasculature. Vascular changes include depressed peripheral vascular sensitivity that impairs local cutaneous vasodilation from two factors: (1) smaller release of vasomotor tone and (2) less-active vasodilation once sweating begins. Older adults recover less well from dehydration compared to younger counterparts because of reduced thirst drive. This places elderly individuals in a chronic state of hypohydration (with less than optimal plasma volume), which could impair thermoregulatory dynamics.[28,29]

Children

Prepubescent children have a greater number of heat-activated sweat glands per unit skin area than adolescents and adults, yet they sweat less and achieve higher core temperatures during heat stress.[6,18] These thermoregulatory differences probably last through puberty but only limit exercise capacity during extreme environmental heat stress.[17] Sweat composition differs between children and adults; adults have higher concentrations of sodium and chloride, but lower lactate, H^+, and potassium concentrations.[18,38] Children also take longer to acclimatize to heat than adolescents and young adults. *From a practical standpoint, children exposed to environmental heat stress should exercise at reduced intensity and receive more time to acclimatize than more mature competitors.*

Male/Female Differences

Early comparisons between men and women showed that men had greater tolerance to environmental heat stress during exercise. However, the research was flawed because women consistently exercised at higher intensities relative to their aerobic capacity. When comparing men and women of equal fitness, the sex differences in thermoregulation became much less pronounced.[23] *Generally, women tolerate the physiologic and thermal stress of exercise as well as men of comparable fitness and level of acclimatization; both sexes acclimatize to a similar degree.*[2,53,68]

Sweating

A distinct sex difference in thermoregulation exists for sweating. Women possess more heat-activated sweat glands per unit skin area than men, yet they sweat *less* prolifically. Women begin sweating at higher skin and core temperatures; they also produce less sweat for a similar heat–exercise load, even with acclimatization comparable to that of men.

Evaporative Versus Circulatory Cooling

Despite a lower sweat output, women show heat tolerance similar to men of equal aerobic fitness at the same exercise level. *Women rely more on circulatory mechanisms for heat dissipation, whereas a greater evaporative cooling occurs in men.* Clearly, less sweat production to maintain thermal balance protects women from dehydration during exercise at high ambient temperatures.

Ratio of Body Surface Area to Body Mass

Women possess a relatively large body surface area-to-body mass ratio, a favorable dimensional characteristic for heat dissipation. Stated differently, the smaller woman has a larger external surface per unit of body mass exposed to the environment. Consequently, under identical conditions of heat exposure, women cool at a faster rate than men through a smaller body mass across a relatively large surface area. In this regard, children also possess a "geometric" advantage during heat stress, because boys and girls have larger surface areas per unit body mass than adults.

Level of Body Fat

Excess body fat negatively affects exercise performance in hot environments. Because body fat's specific heat exceeds that of muscle tissue, fat increases the insulatory quality of the shell to retard heat conduction to the periphery. The relatively large, obese person also possesses a relatively small body surface area-to-body mass ratio for sweat evaporation compared to a leaner, smaller person.

Excess body fat directly adds to the metabolic cost of weight-bearing activities in addition to retarding effective heat exchange. The additional demands of equipment weight (such as football gear), intense competition, and a hot, humid environment compound these effects. Thus, a fat person experiences considerable difficulty in temperature regulation and exercise performance.[20] Fatal heat stroke occurs 3.5 times more frequently in obese young adults than in individuals whose body mass falls within reasonable limits.

EVALUATING ENVIRONMENTAL HEAT STRESS

Factors other than air temperature that determine the physiologic strain imposed by heat include (1) body size and fatness, (2) level of training, (3) acclimatization, (4) adequacy of hydration, and (5) external factors (convective air currents; radiant heat gain; intensity of exercise; amount, type, and color of clothing; and, most importantly, relative humidity). Several football deaths from hyperthermia occurred when air temperature dipped below 75°F (23.9°C) but relative humidity exceeded 95%.

Prevention represents the most effective way to control heat-stress injuries. Acclimatization greatly reduces the chance for heat injury. Another defense involves use of the **wet bulb-globe temperature** (WB-GT) to evaluate the environment for its potential thermal challenge. This index of environmental heat stress, developed by the United States military, incorporates ambient temperature, relative humidity, and radiant heat in its calculations as follows:

$$\text{WB-GT} = 0.1 \times \text{DBT} + 0.7 \times \text{WBT} + 0.2 \times \text{GT}$$

where

DBT = dry-bulb (air) temperature in the shade recorded by an ordinary mercury thermometer that measures air temperature.

WBT (accounts for 70% of the index) = temperature recorded by an ordinary mercury thermometer and a thermometer with a wet wick that surrounds the mercury bulb (wet bulb) exposed to rapid air movement in direct sunlight. With high relative humidity, little evaporative cooling occurs from the wetted bulb, so the temperature of this thermometer remains similar to that of the dry-bulb. On a dry day, evapora-

tion occurs from the wetted bulb. This maximizes the difference between the two thermometer readings. A small difference between readings indicates high relative humidity, whereas a large difference indicates little air moisture and a high rate of evaporation.

GT = globe temperature in direct sunlight recorded by a thermometer with a black metal sphere surrounding the bulb. The black globe absorbs radiant energy from the surroundings to provide a measure of radiant heat gain.

FIGURE 10.10 illustrates the apparatus to measure WB-GT. The top portion of the inset table presents WB-GT guidelines for athletic activities to reduce the chance of heat injury. These standards apply to lightly clothed humans; they do not consider the specific heat load imposed by football uniforms or other types of equipment. For football, the lower end of each temperature range serves as a more prudent guide.

American College of Sports Medicine WB-GT Recommendations for Continuous Activities Such as Endurance Running and Cycling

- **Very high risk:** Above 28°C (82°F)—postpone race
- **High risk:** 23 to 28°C (73–82°F)—heat-sensitive individuals (e.g., obese, low physical fitness, unacclimatized, dehydrated, previous history of heat injury) should not compete
- **Moderate risk:** 18 to 23°C (65–73°F)
- **Low risk:** Below 18°C (65°F)

An indication of ambient heat load also comes from the wet-bulb thermometer because this reading reflects both air temperature and relative humidity. An inexpensive wet-bulb thermometer can be purchased at most industrial supply companies. The bottom portion of the inset table of Figure 10.10 presents heat stress recommendations based on the wet-bulb temperature. Without the WBT, but knowing relative humidity via local meteorologic stations' media reports and the Internet (www.weather.com), the **Heat Index** (FIG. 10.11) devised by the U.S. National Weather Service also evaluates the relative heat stress. Sometimes referred to as the "apparent temperature," the index provides an accurate measure of how hot it feels when the relative humidity combines with the air temperature. The heat index values were determined for shady, light wind conditions, so exposure to full sunshine increases values by up to 15°F. In addition, strong winds (particularly with hot, dry air) present an extreme hazard. Determine the index close to the race site to eliminate potential error from using meteorologic data some distance from the event. Data collected for the 24-hour trend of ambient temperature and relative humidity justified changing the race time for the 1996 Olympic Marathon run in Atlanta from 6:30 PM to 7:00 AM to reduce heat injury risk.

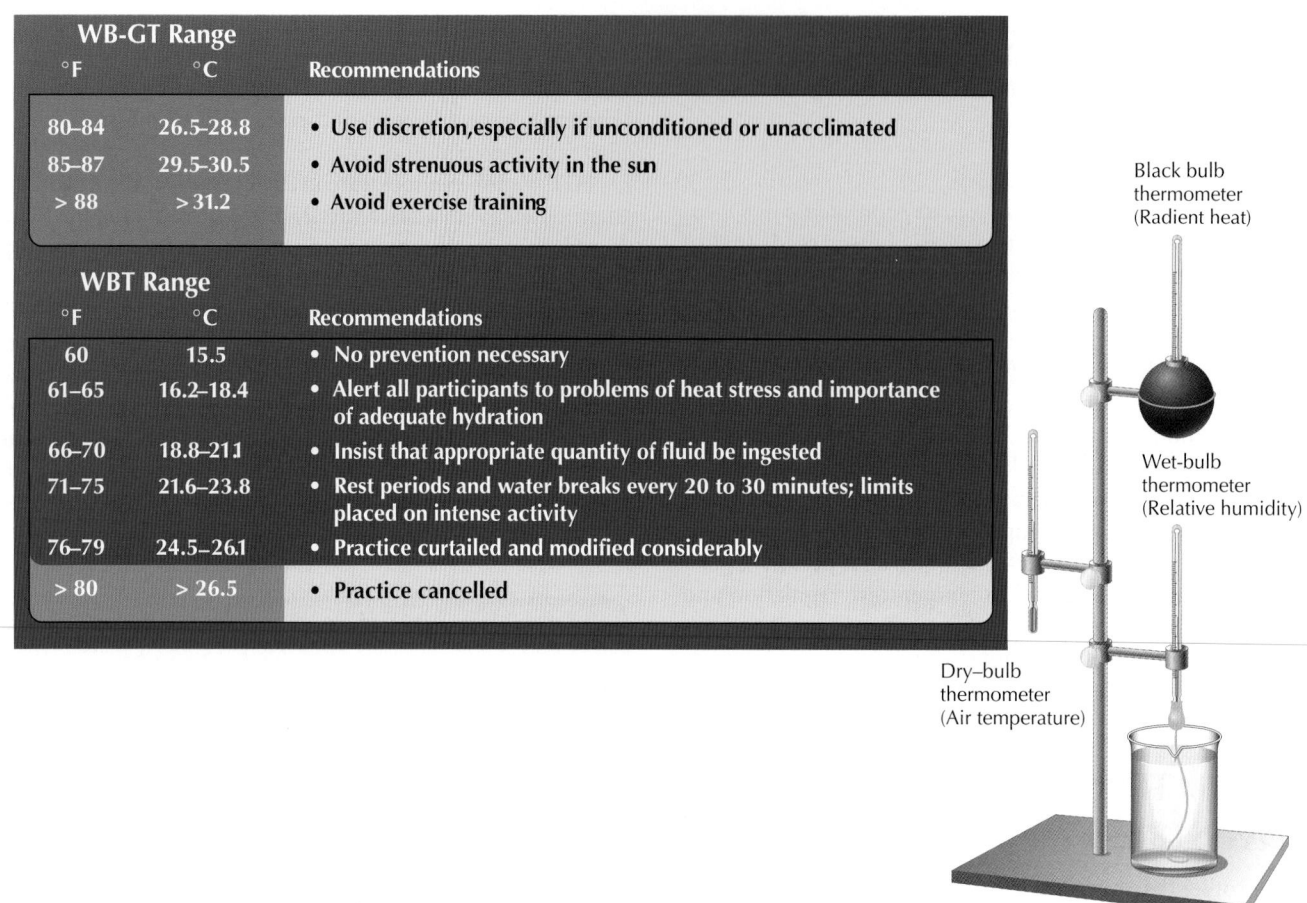

WB-GT Range		
°F	°C	Recommendations
80–84	26.5–28.8	• Use discretion, especially if unconditioned or unacclimated
85–87	29.5–30.5	• Avoid strenuous activity in the sun
> 88	> 31.2	• Avoid exercise training

WBT Range		
°F	°C	Recommendations
60	15.5	• No prevention necessary
61–65	16.2–18.4	• Alert all participants to problems of heat stress and importance of adequate hydration
66–70	18.8–21.1	• Insist that appropriate quantity of fluid be ingested
71–75	21.6–23.8	• Rest periods and water breaks every 20 to 30 minutes; limits placed on intense activity
76–79	24.5–26.1	• Practice curtailed and modified considerably
> 80	> 26.5	• Practice cancelled

Black bulb thermometer (Radient heat)

Wet-bulb thermometer (Relative humidity)

Dry–bulb thermometer (Air temperature)

FIGURE 10.10 ■ Wet bulb-globe temperature (WB-GT) for outdoor activities and wet-bulb temperature (WBT) guide. (Modified from Murphy RJ, Ashe WF. Prevention of heat illness in football players. *JAMA* 1965;194:650.)

HEAT ILLNESS: COMPLICATIONS FROM EXCESSIVE HEAT STRESS

From the perspective of health and safety, it is far easier to prevent heat injury than remedy it. However, if one fails to heed the normal signs of heat stress—thirst, tiredness, grogginess, and visual disturbances—cardiovascular decompensation triggers a series of disabling complications termed **heat illness.** Heat-related disabilities become more apparent among overweight and poorly conditioned individuals, those with prior heat intolerance, and those who exercise when dehydrated.[15,19,48] Heat illness, in order of increasing severity, includes heat cramps, heat exhaustion, and exertional heat stroke. No clear-cut demarcation exists between these maladies because symptoms usually overlap: the cumulative effects of multiple adverse interacting stimuli can produce exercise-induced heat injury.[64] When serious heat illness occurs, only immediate corrective action can reduce heat stress using rehydration until medical help arrives.[16]

Heat Cramps

Heat cramps (involuntary muscle spasms) occur during or after intense physical activity, usually in the specific muscles exercised. Cramping most likely occurs from an imbalance in hydration level and electrolyte concentrations. During heat exposure, sweating augments salt loss. If electrolytes are not replenished, this increases the chance for muscle pain and spasm (most commonly in the muscles of the abdomen and extremities). Crampers tend to have high sweat rates and/or high sweat sodium concentrations. With heat cramps, body temperature does not necessarily increase. Prevention involves two factors: (1) providing copious amounts of water that contains salt (e.g., Gatorade or GatorLytes) and (2) increasing daily salt intake (e.g., adding salt to foods at mealtime) several days before heat stress.

Heat Exhaustion

Heat exhaustion, the most common heat illness among the physically active, usually develops in dehydrated, untrained, and

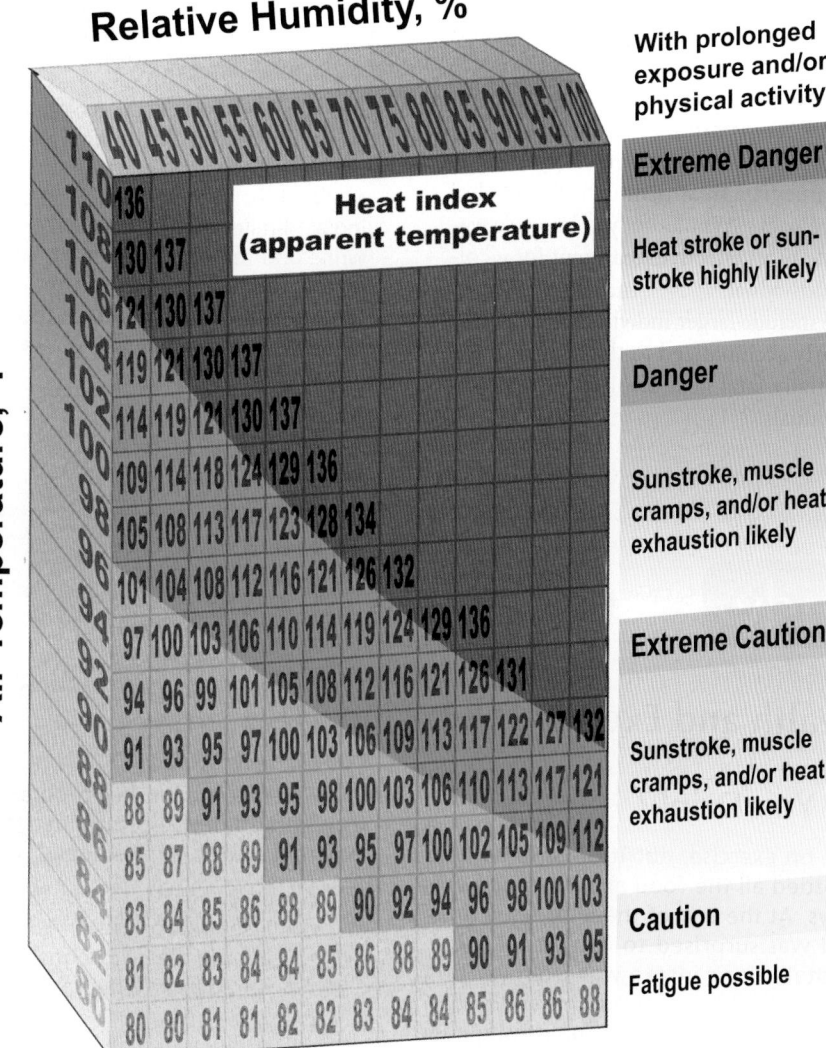

FIGURE 10.11 ■ How hot is too hot? The Heat Index.

unacclimatized people; it mainly occurs during the first summer heat wave or first hard training session on a hot day. Exercise-induced heat exhaustion occurs because of ineffective circulatory adjustments compounded by depletion of extracellular fluid (plasma volume) from excessive sweating. Blood pools in the dilated peripheral vessels. This drastically reduces the central blood volume required to maintain cardiac output. Characteristics of heat exhaustion include weak, rapid pulse; low blood pressure in the upright position; headache; nausea; dizziness; "goose bumps"; and general weakness. Sweating may decrease somewhat, but body temperature does not rise to dangerous levels (i.e., above 104°F or 40°C). A person experiencing heat exhaustion symptoms should stop exercising and move to a cooler environment; administer fluids orally or via intravenous therapy with 5% dextrose sugar in either 0.45% NaCl or 0.9% NaCl.[2]

Exertional Heat Stroke

Exertional heat stroke, the most serious and complex heat-stress malady, requires immediate medical attention. Heat stroke syndrome reflects a failure of the heat-regulating mechanisms induced by excessively high body temperature. With thermoregulatory failure, sweating usually ceases, the skin becomes dry and hot, body temperature rises to 41.5°C or higher, and the circulatory system becomes excessively strained.

Subtle symptoms often confound the complexity of exertional hyperthermia. Sweating can occur during intense exercise (e.g., 10-km running race) in young, hydrated, and highly motivated individuals. However, the body's heat gain greatly exceeds avenues for heat loss because of the high metabolic heat production. If left untreated, the disability becomes fatal from circulatory collapse, oxidative damage, systemic inflamatory response, and damage to the central nervous system and other organs.[9,55,73] Heat stroke represents a medical emergency! *While awaiting medical care, only aggressive treatment to rapidly lower elevated core temperature can avert death; the magnitude and duration of hyperthermia determine organ damage and mortality risk.* Immediate treatment includes alcohol rubs and application of ice packs. Whole-body cold or ice water immersion remains the most effective treatment for a collapsed hyperthermic individual.[41,43,65] Individuals most susceptible to heat stroke include larger individuals, especially those who are unfit, poorly acclimatized to the heat, and excessively fat. This potentially fatal heat disorder also affects physically fit young individuals.[55,71]

Don't Rely on Oral Temperature

Oral temperature taken following strenuous exercise does not accurately measure deep body (core) temperature. Large and consistent differences exist between oral and rectal temperatures; rectal temperature following a 14-mile race in a tropical climate averaged 103.5°F, while oral temperature remained normal at 98°F.[54] Part of this discrepancy lies in the lowering effect on oral temperature of evaporative cooling in the mouth and airways during high levels of exercise and recovery pulmonary ventilation.

Case Study

Personal Health and Exercise Nutrition 10–1

Think Before You Drink?

As part of a course on exercise, nutrition, and weight control, Leslie recorded all the food and beverage she consumed for 5 days. At the end of the 5 days she analyzed her diet and was surprised to learn that more than 25% of her total caloric intake was from various beverages she consumed. This was troubling and might be an explanation for her recent weight gain—she had gained about 10 lb toward the end of her freshman year.

Leslie went to her nutrition instructor to ask for advice. During their discussion, Leslie was surprised to find that she was not alone. Beverage and snack overconsumption is a big problem for many college students. Leslie's professor pointed out the following facts regarding beverage (including snack) consumption among college-age individuals:

- The portion sizes of actual meals consumed have increased over the last 5 years.

- There has been an increasing trend toward greater consumption of calorically sweetened beverages (in 2006, 23% of total kCal intake came from beverages).

- Snacks are consistently more energy dense and less nutrient dense (calcium, fiber, folate) than meals.

- Beverage intake does not affect food intake (drinking more fluid does not reduce total food intake).

- Calorically sweetened beverages sold is higher than at any time in history.

After reviewing her food and beverage intake history, Leslie's professor outlined the pros and cons of the different available beverages.

1. Water
   - Essential for life
   - People need to consume a minimum amount for adequate hydration

2. Tea and Coffee
   - No adverse health effects in terms of obesity and chronic diseases; the only issue is added cream and sugar
   - Animal research suggests a protective role against selected cancers (data are unclear for humans; the potential health benefits of flavonoids in tea are unclear)
   - Coffee acts as a mild antidepressant and may lower risk of type 2 diabetes

3. Low-Fat and Skim Milk and Soy Beverage
   - Skim milk: unclear benefits on weight and bone density
   - Major provider of calcium and vitamin D
   - Adult milk intake may adversely affect several chronic diseases (e.g., prostate cancer, ovarian cancer)

4. Noncalorically Sweetened Beverages
   - May condition a preference for sweetness leading to overfatness and type 2 diabetes

5. Caloric Beverages with Some Nutrients
   - Fruit juices are high in energy content yet contribute limited nutrients
   - Vegetable juices have fewer calories but contain significant amounts of sodium

Case Study *continued*

- Whole milk contains saturated fat, not needed beyond infancy
- Sport drinks have reduced energy density compared to soft drinks and are helpful for rehydration
- Alcohol: only the ethanol benefits are known (1 drink daily for women, 2 for men) and linked with reduced mortality, coronary heart disease, and type 2 diabetes.

6. Calorically Sweetened Beverages
- Associated with increased dental caries, type 2 diabetes, and weight gain

Leslie was now ready to make an informed decision regarding her beverage consumption. She planned to try and adhere to the following guidelines, assuming she maintained her 2200-kCal diet (see figure).

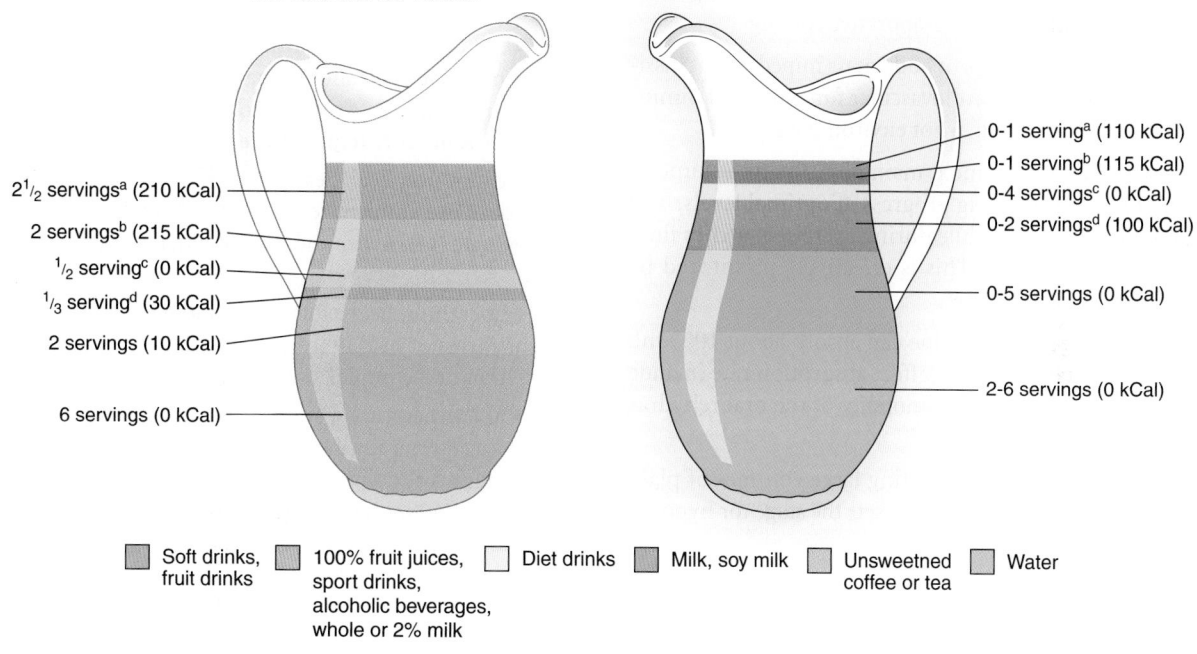

UNDESIRABLE
What the average American adult currently drinks. Most of the non-water fluids consumed contains calories from beverages with essentially no nutritional value.

$2^1/_2$ servings[a] (210 kCal)
2 servings[b] (215 kCal)
$^1/_2$ serving[c] (0 kCal)
$^1/_3$ serving[d] (30 kCal)
2 servings (10 kCal)
6 servings (0 kCal)

DESIRABLE
A more desirable fluid intake for someone who consumes 2200 kCal a day.

0-1 serving[a] (110 kCal)
0-1 serving[b] (115 kCal)
0-4 servings[c] (0 kCal)
0-2 servings[d] (100 kCal)
0-5 servings (0 kCal)
2-6 servings (0 kCal)

■ Soft drinks, fruit drinks   ■ 100% fruit juices, sport drinks, alcoholic beverages, whole or 2% milk   ■ Diet drinks   ■ Milk, soy milk   ■ Unsweetned coffee or tea   ■ Water

[a]1 serving = 8 fluid oz.;
[b]0-2 servings of alcohol are okay for men;
[c]Includes diet soft drinks and tea or coffee with sugar substitutes;
[d]Includes fat-free or 1% milk and unsweetened fortified soy milk.

- Water: 20 to 50 fl oz/d
- Tea and Coffee: (unsweetened) 0 to 40 fl oz/d (can replace water; caffeine a limiting factor—up to 400 mg/d or about 32 fl oz/d of coffee)
- Low-Fat and Skim Milk and Soy Beverages: 0 to 16 fl oz/d
- Noncalorically Sweetened Beverages: 0 to 32 fl oz/d (could substitute for tea and coffee with the same limitations regarding caffeine)

- Caloric Beverages with Some Nutrients: 100% fruit juices 0 to 8 fl oz/d, alcoholic beverages 0 to 1 drink per day for women and 0 to 2 drinks per day for men (one drink = 12 fl oz of beer, 5 fl oz of wine, or 1.5 fl oz of distilled spirits), whole milk 0 fl oz/d
- Calorically Sweetened Beverages: 0 to 8 fl oz/d

Reference: Nielsen SJ. Popkin BM. Changes in beverage intake between 1977 and 2001. Am J Prev Med 2004;27:205.

Summary

1. Cutaneous and muscle blood flow increase during exercise in the heat, whereas other tissues temporality compromise their blood supply.

2. Core temperature normally increases in exercise; the relative stress of exercise determines the magnitude of the increase. A well-regulated temperature increase creates a more favorable environment for physiologic and metabolic functions.

3. Increased sweating strains fluid reserves, creating a relative state of dehydration. Excessive sweating without fluid replacement decreases plasma volume and core temperature rises precipitously.

4. Exercise in a hot, humid environment poses a thermoregulatory challenge because a large sweat loss in high humidity contributes little to evaporative cooling.

5. Fluid loss in excess of 2% of body mass impedes heat dissipation, compromises cardiovascular function, and diminishes exercise capacity in a hot environment.

6. Adequate fluid replacement maintains plasma volume so circulation and sweating progress at optimal levels. The ideal replacement schedule during exercise matches fluid intake with fluid loss. This is effectively monitored by changes in body weight.

7. Each hour, the small intestine can absorb about 1000 mL of water. Prime factors that affect absorption rate include stomach volume and the osmolality of the oral rehydration beverage.

8. Excessive sweating plus ingesting large volumes of plain water during prolonged exercise sets the stage for hyponatremia (water intoxication). A decrease in extracellular sodium concentration causes this potentially dangerous malady.

9. A small amount of electrolytes in the rehydration beverage facilitates fluid replenishment more than drinking plain water.

10. Repeated heat stress initiates thermoregulatory adjustments that improve exercise capacity and reduce discomfort on subsequent heat exposure. Heat acclimatization triggers favorable redistribution of cardiac output and increases sweating capacity. Full acclimatization generally occurs in about 10 days of heat exposure.

11. Aging affects thermoregulatory function, yet acclimatization to moderate heat stress does not appreciably deteriorate with age.

12. When controlling for fitness and acclimatization levels, women and men show equal thermoregulatory efficiency during exercise. Women produce less sweat than men do at the same core temperature.

13. Various practical heat-stress indices (e.g., Heat Stress Index) use ambient temperature and relative humidity to evaluate the environment's potential thermal challenge to an exercising person.

14. Heat cramps, heat exhaustion, and heat stroke are the major forms of heat illness. Heat stroke represents the most serious and complex of these maladies

15. Oral temperature underestimates core temperature following strenuous exercise. This discrepancy results from evaporative cooling of the mouth and airways during high levels of pulmonary ventilation.

Test Your Knowledge Answers

1. **False:** Core temperature (the temperature of deep tissues) remains in dynamic equilibrium between factors that add and subtract body heat. This balance results from integrating mechanisms that alter heat transfer to the periphery (shell), regulate evaporative cooling, and vary the rate of heat production

2. **True:** The hypothalamus contains the central coordinating center for temperature regulation. This group of specialized neurons at the floor of the brain serves as a "thermostat" (usually set and carefully regulated at 37°C ± 1°C) for making thermoregulatory adjustments to deviations from a temperature norm. Unlike a thermostat in a building, the hypothalamus cannot "turn off" the heat; it only initiates responses to protect the body from heat gain or heat loss.

3. **False:** Body heat loss occurs in four ways: radiation, conduction, convection, and evaporation. Evaporation of sweat provides the major physiologic defense against overheating. Water vaporization from the respiratory passages and skin surface continually transfers heat to the environment. For each liter of water that vaporizes, 580 kCal of heat energy transfers from the body to the environment.

4. **False:** Sweat evaporation from the skin depends on three factors: (1) surface exposed to the environ-

Test Your Knowledge Answers   *continued*

ment, (2) temperature and relative humidity of ambient air, and (3) convective air currents around the body. By far, relative humidity exerts the greatest impact on the effectiveness of evaporative heat loss. Relative humidity refers to the percentage of water in ambient air at a particular temperature compared with the total quantity of moisture that the air could carry. For example, 40% relative humidity means that ambient air contains only 40% of the air's moisture-carrying capacity at that specific temperature.

5. **True:** During heat stress, the pituitary gland releases antidiuretic hormone (ADH). ADH increases water reabsorption from the kidney tubules, causing urine to become more concentrated during heat stress. This action of ADH helps to protect against dehydration during heat stress.

6. **True:** Dehydration refers to an imbalance in fluid dynamics when fluid intake does not replenish water loss from either hyperhydrated or normally hydrated states. A moderate exercise workout generally produces a moderate 0.5- to 1.5-L sweat loss over a 1-hour period. Significant water loss occurs during several hours of intense exercise in a hot environment. The risk of heat illness greatly increases when a person begins exercising in a dehydrated state. Dehydration associated with a 3% decrease in body weight also slows the rate of gastric emptying, thus increasing epigastric cramps and feelings of nausea.

7. **False:** Urge individuals to rehydrate themselves, because the thirst mechanism imprecisely indicates water needs, particularly in children and the elderly. If left to depend on thirst, most individuals

voluntarily replace only about half of the water lost during exercise. It could take several days after severe dehydration to re-establish fluid balance. Drink at least 125 to 150% of the existing fluid loss (body weight loss) as soon as possible after exercising. The 25 to 50% "extra" water accounts for that portion of ingested water lost in urine.

8. **False:** Excessive water intake under certain exercise conditions produces potentially serious medical complications from the syndrome termed *hyponatremia* (water intoxication). Hyponatremia exists when serum sodium concentration falls below 136 mEq · L^{-1} and serum sodium concentrations below 130 mEq · L^{-1}. A sustained low plasma sodium concentration creates an osmotic imbalance across the blood–brain barrier, which causes rapid water influx into the brain. The resulting swelling of brain tissue produces a cascade of symptoms that range from mild (headache, confusion malaise, nausea, cramping) to severe (seizures, coma, pulmonary edema, cardiac arrest, and death).

9. **False:** Factors other than air temperature determine the physiologic strain imposed by heat. These include (1) body size and fatness, (2) level of training, (3) acclimatization, (4) adequacy of hydration, and (5) external factors (convective air currents; radiant heat gain; intensity of exercise; amount, type, and color of clothing; and, most importantly, the relative humidity of ambient air).

10. **False:** Oral temperature underestimates core temperature after strenuous exercise. This discrepancy largely results from evaporative cooling of the mouth and airways during high levels of pulmonary ventilation.

References

1. Almond CS, et al. Hyponatremia among runners in the Boston Marathon. *N Engl J Med* 2005;352:1550.
2. American College of Sports Medicine: American College of Sports Medicine position stand on heat and cold illnesses during distance running. *Med Sci Sports Exerc* 1996;28:1.
3. Androgué HJ, Madias NE. Hyponatremia. *N Engl J Med* 2000;342:1581.
4. Ayus JC, et al. Hyponatremia, cerebral edema, and noncardiogenic pulmonary edema in marathon runners. *Ann Intern Med* 2000;132:711.
5. Baker LB, et al. Sex differences in voluntary fluid intake by older adults during exercise. *Med Sci Sports Exerc* 2005;37:789.
6. Bar-Or O. Temperature regulation during exercise in children and adolescents. In: Gisolfi CV, Lamb DR, eds. *Perspectives in Exercise Science and Sports Medicine.* Vol. 2. Indianapolis, IN: Benchmark Press, 1989.
7. Burge CM, et al. Rowing performance, fluid balance, and metabolic function following dehydration and rehydration. *Med Sci Sports Exerc* 1993;25:1358.
8. Byrne C, et al. Continuous thermoregulatory responses to mass-participation distance running in heat. *Med Sci Sports Exerc* 2006;38:803.
9. Casa DJ, et al. Exertional heat stroke in competitive athletes. *Curr Sports Med Rep* 2005;4:309.
10. Cheuvront SN, et al. No effect of moderate hypohydration or hyperthermia on anaerobic exercise performance. *Med Sci Sports Exerc* 2006;38:1093.
11. Cheuvront SN, et al. Fluid balance and endurance exercise performance. *Curr Sports Med Rep* 2003;2:202.
12. Coyle EF. Fluid and fuel intake during exercise. *J Sports Sci* 2004;22:39.
13. Coyle EF, Montain SJ. Benefits of fluid replacement with carbohydrate during exercise. *Med Sci Sports Exerc* 1992;24:S324.
14. Cunningham JJ. Is potassium needed in sports drinks for fluid replacement during exercise? *Int J Sport Nutr* 1997;7:154.
15. Day TK, Grimshaw D. An observational study of the spectrum of heat-related illness, with a proposal on classification. *J R Army Med Corps* 2005;151:11.
16. Donaldson GC, et al. Cardiovascular responses to heat stress and their adverse consequences in healthy and vulnerable human populations. *Int J Hyperthermia* 2003;19:225.
17. Falk B. Exercise in the pediatric population: effects of thermal stress. In: Doubt T, ed. *Environmental and Exercise Physiology.* Champaign, IL: Human Kinetics, 1997.
18. Falk, et al. Longitudinal analysis of the sweating response of pre-, mid-, and late-pubertal boys during exercise in the heat. *Am J Hum Biol* 1992;4:527.

19. Frye AJ, Kamon E. Responses to dry heat of men and women with similar capacities. *J Appl Physiol* 1981;50:65.

20. Gardner JW, et al. Risk factors predicting exertional heat illness in male Marine Corps recruits. *Med Sci Sports Exerc* 1996;28:939.

21. Gardner JW. Death by water intoxication. *Milit Med* 2002;5:432.

22. Goudie AM, et al. Exercise-associated hyponatremia after a marathon: case series. *J R Soc Med* 2006;99:363.

23. Haymes EM. Physiological responses of female athletes to heat stress: a review. *Phys Sportsmed* 1984;12:45.

24. Hew TD, et al. The incidence, risk factors, and clinical manifestations of hyponatremia in marathon runners. *Clin J Sports Med* 2003;13:41.

25. Hsieh M, et al. Hyponatremia in runners requiring on-site medical treatment at a single marathon. *Med Sci Sports Exerc* 2002;34:185.

26. Hue O, et al. The effect of 8 days of training in tropical environment on performance in neutral climate in swimmers. *Int J Sports Med* 2007;28:48.

27. Irving RA, et al. Evaluation of renal function and fluid homeostasis during recovery from exercise induced hyponatremia. *J Appl Physiol* 1991;70:342.

28. Kenney WL, Chiu P. Influence of age on thirst and fluid intake. *Med Sci Sports Exerc* 2001;332:1524.

29. Kenney WL, Ho C-W. Age alters regional distribution of blood flow during moderate-intensity exercise. *J Appl Physiol* 1995;79:1112.

30. Leiper JB, Maughan RJ. Comparison of water turnover rates in young swimmers in training and age-matched non-training individuals. *Int J Sport Nutr Exerc Metab* 2004;14:347.

31. Maughan RJ, Leiper JB. Post-exercise rehydration in man: effects of voluntary intake of four different beverages. *Med Sci Sports Exerc* 1993;25(suppl):S2.

32. Maughan RJ, Leiper JB. Fluid replacement requirements in soccer. *J Sports Sci* 1994;12(special issue):S29.

33. Maughan RJ, Lieper JB. Sodium intake and post-exercise rehydration in man. *Eur J Appl Physiol* 1995;71:311.

34. Maughan RJ, Sherriffs S. Exercise in the heat; challenges and opportunites. *J Sports Sci* 2004;22:917.

35. Maughan RJ, et al. Influence of menstrual status on fluid replacement after exercise dehydration in healthy young women. *Br J Sports Med* 1996;30:41.

36. Maughan RJ, et al. Restoration of fluid balance after exercise-induced dehydration: effect of food and fluid intake. *Eur J Appl Physiol* 1996;73:317.

37. McCullough EA, Kenney WL. Thermal insulation and evaporative resistance of football uniforms. *Med Sci Sports Exerc* 2003;35:832.

38. Meyer F, et al. Sweat electrolyte loss during exercise in the heat: effects of gender and maturation. *Med Sci Sports Exerc* 1992;24:776.

39. Montain SJ, et al. Exercise associated hyponatraemia: quantative analysis to understanding etiology. *Br J Sports Med* 2006;40:98.

40. Montain SJ, et al. Hyponatremia associated with exercise: risk factors and pathogenesis. *Exerc Sport Sci Rev* 2001;2:113.

41. Muldoon S, et al. Is there a link between malignant hyperthermia and exertional heat illness. *Exerc Sport Sci Rev* 2004;32:174.

42. Mundel T, et al. Drink temperature influences fluid intake and endurance capacity during exercise in a hot, dry environment. *Exp Physiol* 2006;91:925.

43. Mustafa S, et al. Hyperthermia-induced vasoconstriction of the carotid artery: a possible causative factor in heatstroke. *J Appl Physiol* 2004;96:1875.

44. Noakes D. Fluid replacement during exercise. *Exerc Sports Sci Rev* 1993;21:297.

45. Noakes TD, Speedy DB. Case proven: exercise associated hyponatremia is due to over drinking. So why did it take 20 years before the original evidence was accepted? *Br J Sports Med* 2006;40:567.

46. Noakes TD, et al. The incidence of hyponatremia during prolonged ultraendurance exercise. *Med Sci Sports Exerc* 1990;22:165.

47. Passe DH, et al. Palatability and voluntary intake of sports beverages, diluted orange juice, and water during exercise. *Int J Sport Nutr Exerc Metab* 2004;14:272.

48. Porter AM. Collapse from exertional heat illness: implications and subsequent decisions. *Milit Med* 2003;168:76.

49. Rasch W, Cabanac M. Selective brain cooling is affected by wearing headgear during exercise. *J Appl Physiol* 1993;74:1229.

50. Rehrer NJ. The maintenance of fluid balance during exercise. *Int J Sports Nutr* 1996;15:122.

51. Reid SA, et al. Study of hematological and biochemical parameters in runners completing a standard marathon. *Clin J Sport Med* 2004;14:344.

52. Rico-Sanz J, et al. Effects of hyperhydration on total body water, temperature regulation and performance of elite young soccer players in a warm climate. *Int J Sports Med* 1996;17:85.

53. Rivera-Brown AM, et al. Exercise tolerance in a hot and humid climate in heat-acclimatized girls and women. Int J Sports Med 2006;27:943.

54. Rozycki TJ. Oral and rectal temperatures in runners. *Phys Sportsmed* 1984;12:105.

55. Ruell PA, et al. Plasma Hsp72 is higher in runners with more serious symptoms of exertional heat illness. *Eur J Appl Physiol* 2006;97:732.

56. Sharp RI. Role of sodium in fluid homeostasis with exercise. *J Am Coll Nutr* 2006;25(suppl 3):231S.

57. Sheffield-Moore M, et al. Thermoregulatory responses to cycling with and without a helmet. *Med Sci Sports Exerc* 1997;29:755.

58. Shi X, et al. Effects of carbohydrate type and concentration and solution osmolality on water absorption. *Med Sci Sports Exerc* 1995;27:1607.

59. Shibasaki M, et al. Non-thermoregulatory modulation of sweating in humans. *Exer Sport Sci Rev* 2003;31:34.

60. Shirreffs SM. The importance of good hydration for work and exercise performance. *Nutr Rev* 2005;63(6 Pt 2):S14.

61. Shirreffs SM, Maughan RJ. Rehydration and recovery of fluid balance after exercise. *Exerc Sport Sci Rev* 2000;28:27.

62. Shirreffs SM, et al. Post-exercise rehydration in man: effects of volume consumed and drink sodium content. *Med Sci Sports Exerc* 1996;28:1260.

63. Shirreffs SM, et al. Fluid and electrolyte needs for preparation and recovery from training and competition. *J Sports Sci* 2004;22:57.

64. Smith JE. Cooling methods used in treatment of exertional heat illness. *Br J Sports Med* 2005;39:503.

65. Sonna LA, et al. Exertional heat injury and gene expression changes: A DNA microarray analysis study. *J Appl Physiol* 2004;96:1943.

66. Speedy DB, et al. Hyponatremia and weight changes in an ultradistance triathlon. *Clin J Sport Med* 1997;7:180.

67. Speedy DB, et al. Hyponatremia in ultradistance triathletes. *Med Sci Sports Exerc* 1999;31:809.

68. Stephenson LA, Kolka MA. Thermoregulation in women. *Exerc Sport Sci Rev* 1993;21:231.

69. van Niewenhoven MA, et al. Effect of dehydration on gastrointestinal function at rest and during exercise in humans. *Eur J Appl Physiol* 2000;83:578.

70. Von Duvillard SP, et al. Fluids and hydration in prolonged endurance performance. *Nutrition* 2004;20:651.

71. Wallace RF, et al. Risk factors for exertional heat illness by gender and training period. *Avait Space Environ Med* 2006;77:415.

72. Wilk B, Bar-Or O. Effect of drink flavor and NaCl on voluntary drinking and hydration in boys exercising in the heat. *J Appl Physiol* 1996;80:1112.

73. Yan YE, et al. Pathophysiological factors underlying heatstroke. *Med Hypotheses* 2006;67:609.

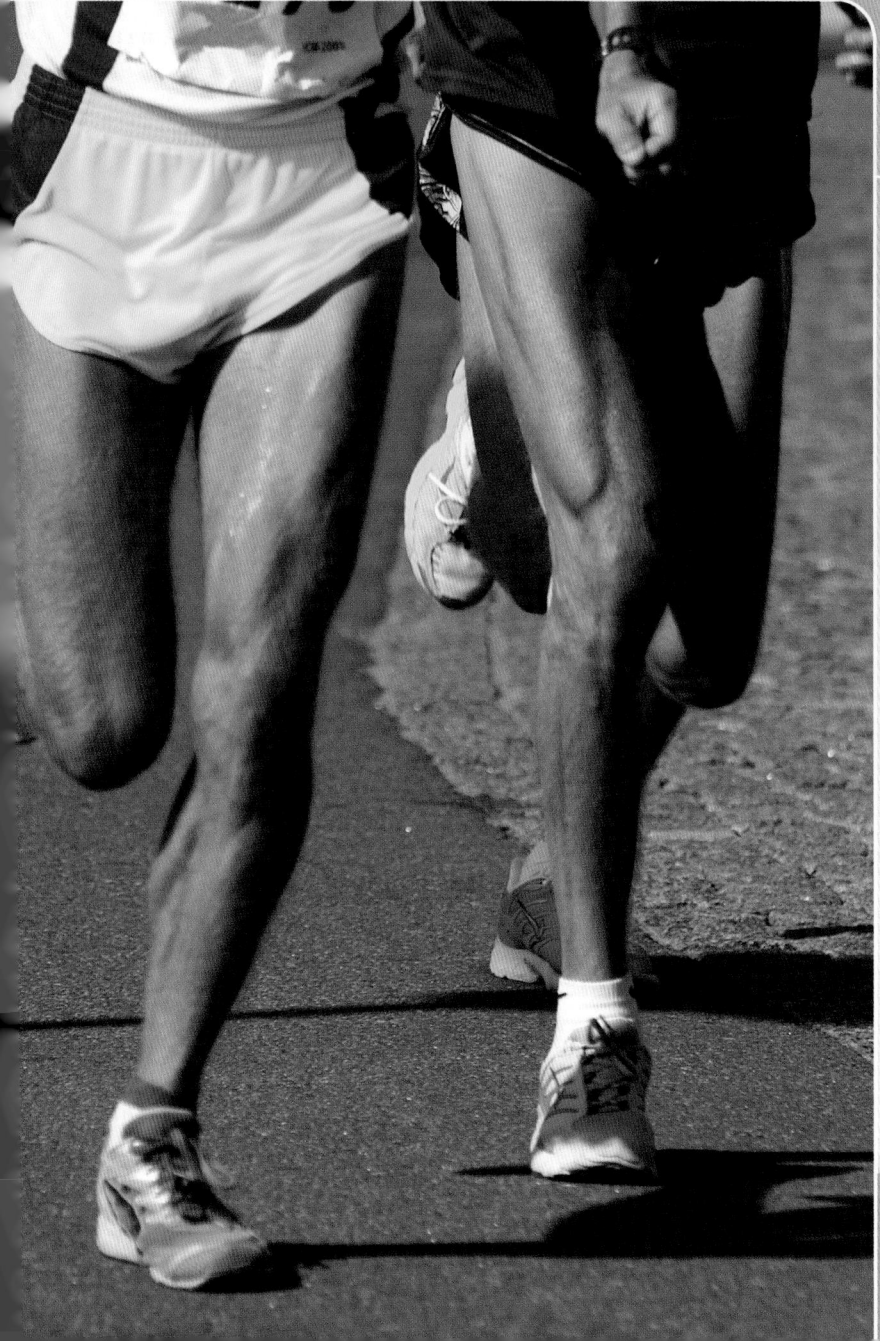

Part 5

Purported Ergogenic Aids

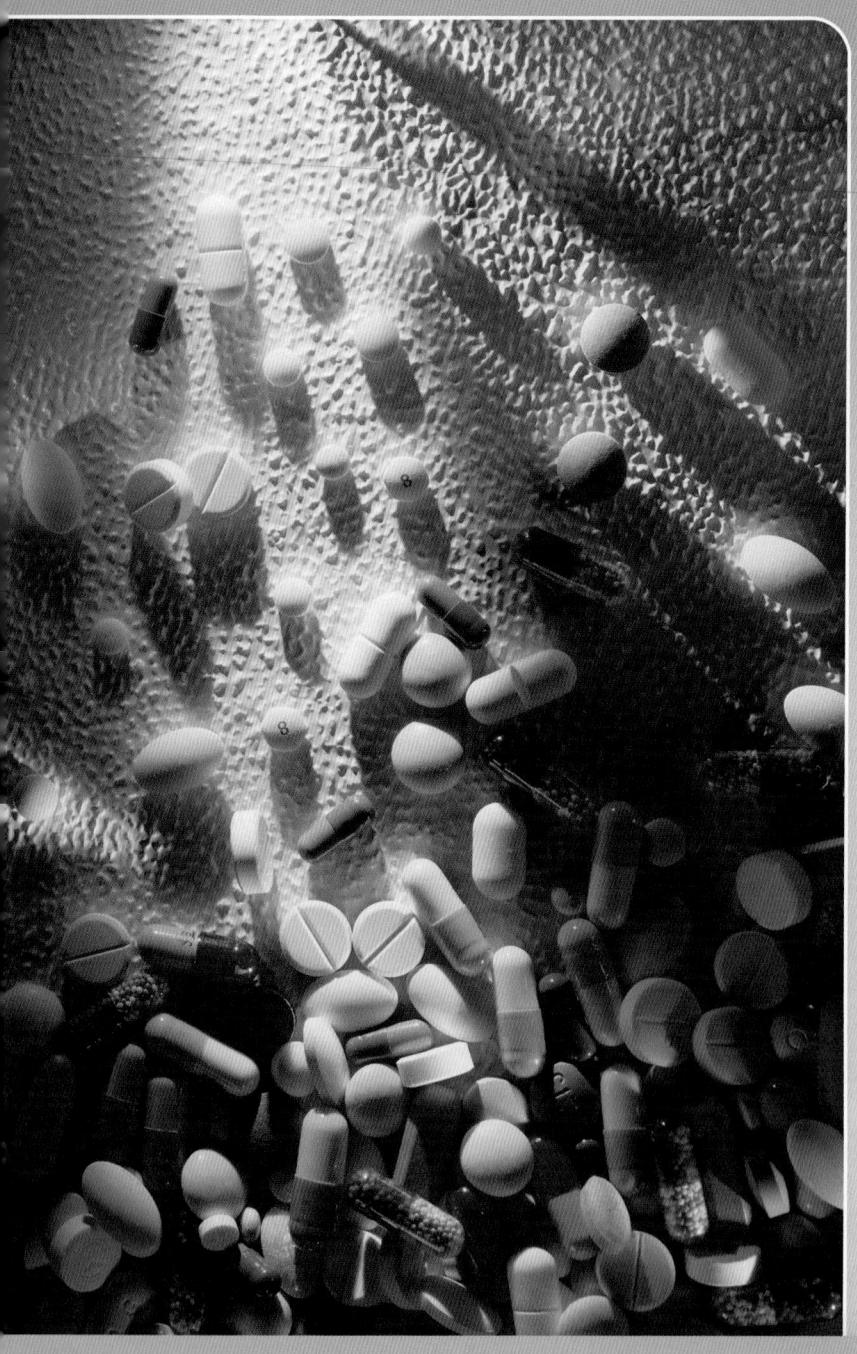

Chapter 11

Pharmacologic and Chemical Ergogenic Aids Evaluated

Androstenedione: Benign Prohormone Nutritional Supplement or Potentially Harmful Drug?

Amphetamines

- Dangers of Amphetamines
- Amphetamine Use and Athletic Performance

Caffeine

- Ergogenic Effects
- Proposed Mechanism for Ergogenic Action
- Effects on Muscle
- Warning About Caffeine

Ginseng and Ephedrine

- Ginseng
- Ephedrine

Alcohol

- Alcohol Use Among Athletes

- Alcohol's Action and Effect on Athletic Performance
- Alcohol and Fluid Replacement
- Perhaps of Some Benefit

Buffering Solutions

- Effects Related to Dosage and Degree of Exercise Anaerobiosis

Phosphate Loading

Anticortisol Compounds: Glutamine and Phosphatidylserine

- Glutamine
- Phosphatidylserine

β-Hydroxy-β-Methylbutyrate

A New Twist: Hormonal Blood Boosting

In the Future

Test Your Knowledge

Answer these 10 statements about pharmacologic and chemical ergogenic aids. Use the scoring key at the end of the chapter to check your results. Repeat this test after you have read the chapter and compare "before and after" results.

1. **T F** Use of ergogenic drugs by athletes reportedly began with the modern era (after 1900) and coincides with the ability to create "new" laboratory chemicals.
2. **T F** The term "placebo effect" in exercise research refers to the ability of a treatment or a compound to affect a person psychologically in a manner that improves physical performance independent of any real physiologic effect.
3. **T F** Anabolic steroids mimic the function of the hormone testosterone, so little chance exists for harmful side effects.
4. **T F** Androstenedione, an intermediate or precursor hormone between DHEA and testosterone, significantly increases endurance performance.
5. **T F** Amphetamines (pep pills) are dangerous and should not be taken by athletes.
6. **T F** Caffeine exerts no ergogenic effect other than to increase alertness in some persons.
7. **T F** The term *functional food* relates to the effects specific foods exert on muscular function and responsiveness to resistance training.
8. **T F** The herbal remedy ephedrine provides safe and positive effects for sports participants, particularly as a substance to facilitate fat loss.
9. **T F** Consuming a light-to-moderate amount of alcohol (e.g., a beer or two) after exercise speeds rehydration and replenishes depleted carbohydrate stores.
10. **T F** β-Hydroxy-β-methylbutyrate (HMB), a bioactive metabolite generated from the breakdown of the essential branched-chain amino acid leucine, decreases protein loss during stress by inhibiting protein catabolism.

Many men and women at all levels of physical prowess use pharmacologic and chemical agents, believing that a specific drug positively influences skill, strength, power, endurance, or responsiveness to training. In our drug-oriented, competitive culture, drug use for ergogenic[a] purposes continues to be on the upswing among high school and even junior high school athletes. Among older, more highly competitive athletes, illegal drug use is a cancer infecting the very foundation of sports competition. Before the 1996 Atlanta Olympic Games, only women's field hockey and gymnastics remained free from detection of anabolic steroids. When winning becomes all-important, cheating to win becomes pervasive.[192] Often, one can do little to prevent the use *and* abuse of drugs by athletes, despite scant "hard" scientific evidence indicating a performance-enhancing effect of many of these compounds. Ironically, athletes go to great lengths to promote all aspects of their health. They train hard, eat well-balanced meals, and receive medical attention even for minor injuries, yet they purposely ingest synthetic agents, many of which trigger negative health effects ranging from nausea, hair loss, itching, and nervous irritability to an array or potential life-threatening conditions.

Considerable information exists concerning possible ergogenic effects of nutritional and pharmacologic aids on exercise performance and training. These include testimonials and endorsements from sports professionals and organizations, media publicity, television infomercials, and Internet home pages for untested products. This also includes research studies that extol potential performance benefits from alcohol, amphetamines, hormones, carbohydrates, amino acids (either consumed singularly or in combination), fatty acids, caffeine, buffering compounds, wheat-germ oil, vitamins, minerals, catecholamine agonists, steroid hormone precursors and stimulants, and even marijuana and cocaine[b] TABLE 11.1 gives examples of ingredients and the frequently *unsubstantiated* (and largely incorrect) claims advertised by makers of nutritional supplements in the physical fitness marketplace. Active individuals routinely use many of these compounds, believing that they enhance the response to exercise. The general population considers supplementation a way to improve physical appearance; in this regard, products aggressively marketed to reduce fat and increase muscle mass become "best sellers."

---

[a]"Ergogenic ("work producing") refers to the application of a nutritional, physical, mechanical, psychologic, physiologic, or pharmacologic procedure or aid to improve exercise capacity, athletic performance, and responsiveness to training. Included are aids that prepare an individual to exercise, improve exercise efficiency, or facilitate the recovery process.

[b]Well-documented evidence exists about the addictive nature of cocaine and potential for significant health risks. Research has never shown that cocaine provides an ergogenic effect. Studies have been limited to animals (for obvious reasons), and results show that cocaine triggers an exaggerated catecholamine response during submaximal exercise, augments glycogen depletion in skeletal muscle, and causes lactate to rapidly accumulate in the blood.[12,26,27,52,136] These effects all impair exercise performance.

AN AREA OF INCREASING COMPLEXITY AND CONTROVERSY

Several explanations account for heightened interest in factors other than innate physical ability and commitment to training that might enhance capacity for exercise and training. First, more persons participate in high-level competitive amateur and professional athletics. Second, competitive success brings personal recognition and approval, but also more tangible rewards ranging from valuable college scholarships to lucrative professional contracts and commercial endorsements. Concurrently, exercise science continues to produce research about how pharmacologic agents and nutritional modification and supplementation affect energy supply, muscle metabolism, physiologic function, and growth and development.

In Use Since Antiquity

Ancient athletes of Greece reportedly used hallucinogenic mushrooms plant seeds and ground dog testicles for ergogenic purposes, while Roman gladiators ingested the equivalent of "speed" to enhance performance in the Circus Maximus. Athletes of the Victorian era routinely used caffeine, alcohol, nitroglycerine, heroin, cocaine, and the rat poison strychnine for a competitive edge. For today's exercise enthusiast, dietary supplements consist of nonprescription plant extracts, vitamins, minerals, enzymes, and hormonal products. To positively influence overall health and exercise performance, these supplements must provide a nutrient undersupplied in the diet or exert a druglike influence on cellular function.

In today's technologic society, little demarcation exists between diet, nutrient supplements (often at exposure levels greater than in foods), and chemical agents used to enhance training and gain a competitive edge. For example, vitamin intake in megadose quantities often exerts druglike effects once these chemicals saturate tissues, while the trace minerals chromium, vanadium, copper, and iron become harmful chemicals with potentially lethal side effects in excess. One could ask: "Does an inordinate intake of a particular amino acid, fatty acid, pyruvate salt, leucine metabolite, or other `natural' chemical simply reflect manipulation of one's normal diet or an abnormal pharmacologic intervention of a potentially harmful compound?"

Not Without Risk

The indiscriminate use of alleged ergogenic substances increases the likelihood of adverse side effects ranging from relatively benign physical discomfort to life-threatening episodes.[8] Many of these compounds fail to conform to labeling requirements to correctly identify the strength of the product's ingredients.[96,128] Results from a study at the Institute of Biochemistry at the German Sports University of Cologne (www.dopinginfo.de) and supported by the Medical Commission of the International Olympic Committee (IOC) indicate that up to 20% of the nutritional supplements sam-

---

TABLE 11.1 **Ingredients Commonly Advertised by Nutritional Supplement Manufacturers**

The definition/alleged attributes are verbatim from literature supplied by manufacturers, product labels, promotional material about the product on the Internet, and advertisements in muscle and body building magazines.

Supplement	Alleged Attribute	Supplement	Alleged Attribute
American ginseng	Restores energy after great fatigue. Reported to have invigorating and stimulating power. Acts as a general tonic. A booster.	Mexican wild yam	Increases physical well-being, enhances energy, and decreases body fat. Improves ability to deal with stressful situations. Clears the mind.
Barley Green	Used by athletes for energy. Extremely nutritious and loaded with vitamins, proteins, minerals, chlorophyll, and enzymes.	Muirapuama	Stimulant to enhance sports performance because of the rush it produces. Increases energy.
BCAAs	Branched-chain amino acids that assist the muscles in synthesizing other amino acids to aid muscle growth. Helps muscles absorb blood sugar for energy.	NAC	Reduces fatigue in muscles and improves liver metabolism. Aids the main antioxidant enzyme, glutathione peroxidase.
Chromium (picolinate)	Activates enzymes involved in glucose and protein for burning and increasing lean body mass. Builds stamina.	Nettle root	Rich in vitamins, lipids, and chlorophyll. Increases aerobic power and muscle strength. Mild antiinflammatory and diuretic.
Cinnamon	Promotes internal energy and strengthens the body. Strong tonic that promotes good circulation.	Orchic	Main source of natural testosterone production. Helps the body retain more protein and nitrogen to increase muscle mass and strength.
Codonopsis	Restores energy, balances metabolism, and stimulates the production of blood.	PAK	Significantly improves aerobic and anaerobic performance by increasing energy production. Reduces lactic acid.
Colostrum	Increases strength and lean body mass.		
CoQ$_{10}$	Plays a role in energy production. Powerful antioxidant. Enhances the body's total systems.	Peony	Nourishes the blood. Helps detoxify the liver and improve blood circulation.
Cordyceps	Renown as a supertonic. Builds physical power and mental energy.	Phosphatidyl serine	Stops exercise-induced increase in cortisol, which has an anticatabolic effect in muscles and tissues.
Creatine monohydrate	Enhances energy and athletic performance and significantly increases muscle mass and strength.	Plant sterols	Improves physical performance. Has general anabolic activity within muscle cells. Allows athletes to adapt to harder training loads.
Dendrobium	Quickly and effectively restores spent energy. A tonic and longevity herb.		
DHEA	Regulates metabolism and increases muscle mass while burning fat. Strengthens and maintains the immune system and enhances energy. Increases physical well-being. A wonder supplement.	Potassium chloride	Essential in maintaining fluid balance within the muscles. Aids in muscle contraction and transmission of glucose into glycogen for energy.
Digestive enzymes	Breaks down food particles for storage in the liver and muscles for energy. Helps to construct new muscle tissue.	Quebracho bark	Highly effective stimulant. Known to elevate mood and increase energy. Builds overall strength and power. Great for endurance.
Epemedium	A powerful tonic and stimulant. Helps strengthen bones and joints.	Radix angelicae	Used as a muscle building tonic. Nourishes the blood and activates blood circulation.
Eucommia	Superb energy tonic. Often used by athletes to strengthen the joints and the body.	Radix astragali	Strengthens muscle and improves metabolic function. Potent immune system tonic. Fabulous for fighting injuries.
Guarana extract	Increases energy and alertness. Increases fat-burning process.	RNA–DNA	Increases cell energy and protein synthesis. Helps rebuild cells to ensure postworkout repair and growth. A good protein.
Ho Shu Wu (FoTi)	Increases and builds essential energy and cleanses the blood. Oriental wonder.		
Kola nut	Increases energy and alertness. Increases fat-burning process.	Royal jelly	High concentration of nutrients, especially B-complex vitamins. High concentration of vitamins, minerals, enzymes, and amino acids.
L-Carnitine	Controls increases in body-fat stores by converting nutrients into energy. Burns body fat and improves athletic performance.	Saw palmetto	Contains plant sterols that improve physical performance and has profound effects on testosterone metabolism.
L-Glutamine	Promotes protein and glycogen synthesis in muscles and liver. Prevents muscle catabolism. Helps buffer lactic acid buildup while training. Alleviates fatigue. Promotes recovery.	Schizandra.	Increases endurance and strengthens the whole body. A powerful tonic that improves memory.
		Selenium	Boosts immunity and neutralizes many free radicals and carcinogens. Vital antioxidant.
Licorice root	Strengthens muscles. Regulates blood sugar levels. Strongest detoxifier known to man without side effects.	Siberian ginseng	Helps one adapt to all kinds of stresses. Improves the blood oxygen-carrying capacity. Promotes mental and physical vigor, metabolism, stamina, and endurance under stressful conditions. "Gets the body going."
Lipoic acid	Key compound for producing energy in muscles and normalizing blood sugar levels. Combats free radical formation.		
L-Lysine	Essential building block for all proteins. Uses fatty acids required in energy production. Important for recovery from sports injuries.	Silica	Excellent for building strong bones and connective tissue.
Lycii fructus	Nourishes the blood and liver. Excellent energy and blood tonic. Pain reliever.	Smilax	Increases muscle strength and size. Augments the body's natural production of its own testosterone.
Magnesium carbonate	Essential for vital enzymes. Aids in transmitting nerve and muscle impulses. Prevents muscle weakness.	Sumac	High in nutrients. Contains 19 different amino acids and electrolytes. Helps oxygenate the system and build and maintain lean muscle mass.

(continues)

TABLE 11.1	Ingredients Commonly Advertised by Nutritional Supplement Manufacturers *(continued)*		
Supplement	**Alleged Attribute**	**Supplement**	**Alleged Attribute**
Vanadyl sulfate	Helps increase muscle growth and development and reduces body fat stores.	**Yohimbe bark**	Male athletes use this herb because of its reputed muscle-building effects. Improves sports performance and increases energy.
Vitamin C	Powerful antioxidant required for tissue growth and repair. Protects against infection and enhances immunity.	**Zinc aspartate**	Helps protein synthesis and collagen formation. Essential to athletes for growth and development, and to increase performance.
Vitamin E	A powerful antioxidant. Improves oxygen use. Enhances immune response and improves athletic performance.		
Wild oats	Aids digestion and increases testosterone levels. Increases aerobic power and muscle strength. A great muscle builder.		
Yerba mate	Helps to relieve fatigue and stress. Cleanses the blood and stimulates the mind. A fat-burner in vital body areas.		

pled contain substances that produce a positive result for doping, including nandrolone, testosterone, and other steroids not declared on the label. The supplements analyzed included vitamins and minerals, protein, and creatine. These findings, plus those of other researchers, raise the real possibility that cross contamination occurs in laboratories that produce both prohormone products and nutrient supplements.[13] Use of a dietary supplement contaminated with the prohibited anabolic substance 19-norandrosterone was the explanation offered by a member of the United States Olympic bobsled team for his disqualification just before the start of the Salt Lake City Winter Games. This was particularly ironic because the Unites States Olympic Committee[c] and Salt Lake City Olympic organizers signed a $20 million deal with Nu Skin, a Utah-based company, to supply Olympic training centers with dietary supplements.

ON THE HORIZON

The day may not be far off when individuals born lacking certain "lucky" genes that augment growth and development and exercise performance will simply add them, doping undetectably with DNA, not drugs. In these instances, the use of "gene doping" misappropriates the medical applications of gene therapy that treats atherosclerosis, cystic fibrosis, and other diseases and uses them to increase the size, speed, and strength of healthy humans. For example, genes that cause muscles to enlarge would be ideal for sprinters, weightlifters, and other power athletes. On the other hand, endurance athletes would benefit from genes that boost the production of red blood cells (e.g., gene for erythropoietin) or stimulate the development of blood vessels (e.g., gene for vascular endothelial growth factor).

An increasing belief in the potential for selected foods to promote health has led to coining of the term **functional food** (see Case Study 6.1). Beyond meeting three basic nutrition needs for survival, hunger satisfaction, and preventing adverse

effects, functional foods comprise those foods and their bioactive components (e.g., olive oil, soy products, n-3 fatty acids) that promote well-being, health, and optimal body function or reduce disease risk (FIG. 11.1).[164,174,213,235] Examples include many polyphenolic substances (simple phenols and flavinoids found in fruits, vegetables, and nuts), carotinoids, soy isoflavones, fish oils, and components of nuts that possess antioxidant and other properties that decrease risk of vascular diseases and cancers. Primary targets for this expanding branch of food science include gastrointestinal functions, antioxidant systems, and macronutrient metabolism. Clearly, enormous implications exist for society from a greater understanding of nutrition's role in optimizing an individual's genetic potential, resistance to disease, and overall performance. Unfortunately, the science base generated by research in this

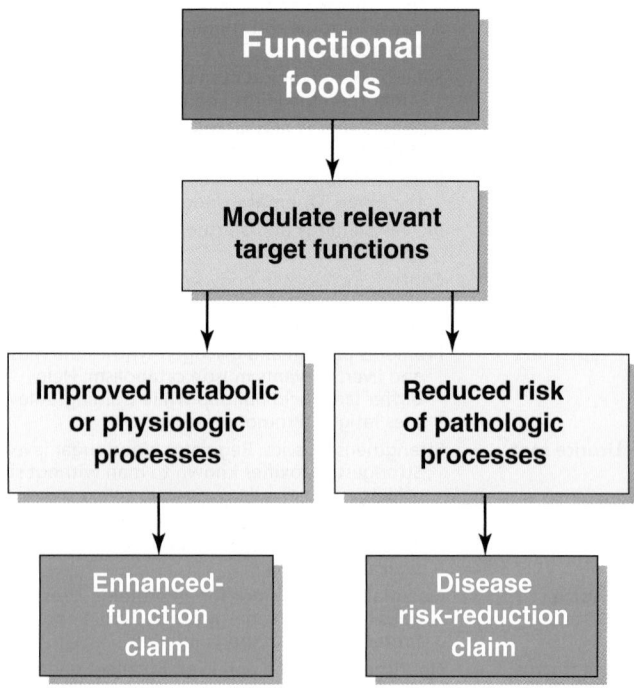

FIGURE 11.1 ■ Strategy of functional food science. Basis for enhanced structure–function or disease risk-reduction claims. (From Roberfroid MB. Concepts and strategy of functional food science: the European perspective. *Am J Clin Nutr* 2000;71[suppl]:1163S.)

---

[c]The United States Olympic Committee (USOC) provides background information about prohibited substances and methods on their web site (http://test.olympic-usa.org/insiide/in_1_1_4_6_5.html#TOC) with links to different sport organization web sites (NGB) and International Federations (IF). Contact the USOC Drug Control Program in Colorado Springs to obtain the most recent "*Guide to Prohibited Substances and Methods.*"

valid field of human nutrition often falls prey to nutritional hucksters and scam artists.

Biotechnology also has created the emerging field of **transgenic nutraceuticals**—modifying a biochemical pathway by use of genes introduced into a host plant or animal. This produces a new class of "natural" bioactive components of food in a nonfood matrix with physiologic and therapeutic functions (e.g., pharmaceutical proteins such as vaccines and monoclonal antibodies) to promote disease prevention and treatment. Nutraceuticals differ from functional foods that deliver their active ingredients within the food matrix. By definition, nutraceutical compounds fall along the continuum from food to food supplements to drugs. Examples of such genetic engineering of nutrients include remodeling of mammary gland milk of cows (adding or deleting specific milk proteins or adding oligosaccharides) to provide medical benefits and development of novel food oils that do not require chemical hydrogenation (and thus no harmful *trans* fatty acids). Through genetic tinkering, scientists can dramatically augment the vitamin C levels in the leaves and seeds of crop plants by increasing expression of a gene that causes recycling of vitamin C within the plant. Undoubtedly, some of these biotechnology products will make their way into the exercise enthusiast's nutritional armamentarium to form the next wave of alleged performance enhancers.

A NEED TO CRITICALLY EVALUATE

Companies expend considerable money and effort, often illegally, to show a beneficial effect of an "aid." Often, however, a **"placebo effect,"** not the "aid," improves performance because of psychological factors—the individual performs at a higher level because of the suggestive power of believing that a substance or procedure should work. Sports nutritionists must evaluate the scientific merit of articles and advertisements about nutrition products. To separate marketing "hype" from scientific fact, we pose five areas for questioning the validity of research claims concerning the efficacy of chemical, pharmacologic, and nutritional ergogenic aids:

I. Justification
Scientific rationale: Does the study represent a "fishing expedition" or is there a sound rationale that the specific treatment should produce an effect? For example, a theoretical basis exists to believe that ingesting creatine elevates intramuscular creatine and phosphocreatine to possibly improve short-term power output capacity. In contrast, no rationale exists to hypothesize that hyperhydration, breathing hyperoxic gas, or ingesting medium-chain triglycerides should enhance 100-m dash performance.

II. Subjects
Animals or humans: Many diverse mammals exhibit similar physiologic and metabolic dynamics, yet significant species differences exist, which often limit generalizations to humans. For example, the models for disease processes, nutrient requirements, hormone dynamics, and growth

and development often differ markedly between humans and different animal groups.

Sex: Sex-specific responses to the interactions between exercise, training, and nutrient requirements and supplementation limit generalizability of findings to the sex studied.

Age: Age often interacts to influence the outcome of an experimental treatment. Effective interventions for the elderly may not apply to growing children or young and middle-aged adults.

Training status: Fitness status and training level can influence the effectiveness (or ineffectiveness) of a particular diet or supplement intervention. Treatments that benefit the untrained (e.g., chemicals or procedures that enhance neurologic disinhibition) often have little effect on elite athletes who practice and compete routinely at maximal arousal levels.

Baseline level of nutrition: The research should establish the subjects' nutritional status before experimental treatment. Clearly, a nutrient supplement administered to a malnourished group typically improves exercise performance and training responsiveness. Such nutritional interventions fail to demonstrate whether the same effects occur if subjects received the supplement with their baseline nutrient intake at recommended levels. It should occasion little surprise, for example, that supplemental iron enhances aerobic fitness in a group with iron-deficiency anemia. One cannot infer, however, that iron supplements provide such benefits to all individuals.

Health status: Nutritional, hormonal, and pharmacologic interventions profoundly affect the diseased and infirmed yet offer no benefit to those in good health. Research findings from diseased groups should not be generalized to healthy populations.

III. Research sample, subjects, and design
Random assignment or self-selection: Apply research findings only to groups similar to the sample studied. If subject volunteers "self-select" into an experimental group, does the experimental treatment produce the results or did a change occur from the individual's motivation to take part in the study? For example, desire to enter a weight loss study may elicit behaviors that produce weight loss independent of the experimental treatment per se. Great difficulty exists in assigning truly random samples of subjects into an experimental group and a control group. When subjects volunteer to take part in an experiment they must be randomly assigned to a control or experimental condition, a process termed **randomization.** When all subjects receive the experimental supplement and the placebo treatment (see below), supplement administration is counterbalanced, and half the subjects receive the supplement first, while the other half takes the placebo first.

Double-blind, placebo-controlled: The ideal experiment to evaluate performance-enhancing effects of an exogenous supplement requires that experimental and control subjects remain unaware or "blinded" to the substance administered. To achieve this goal, subjects should receive a similar quantity and/or form of the proposed aid. In contrast, control group subjects receive an inert compound or placebo. The placebo treatment evaluates the possibility of subjects performing well or responding better simply because they receive a substance they believe should benefit them (psychological or placebo effect). To further reduce experimental bias from influencing the outcome, those administering the treatment and recording the response must not know which subjects receive the treatment or placebo. In such a **double-blinded** experiment, both investigator and subjects remain unaware of the treatment condition.

Control of extraneous factors: Under ideal conditions, experiences should be similar for both experimental and control groups, except for the treatment variable. Random assignment of subjects to control or experimental groups goes a long way to equalize factors that could influence the study's outcome.

Appropriateness of measurements: Reproducible, objective, and valid measurement tools must evaluate research outcomes. For example, a step test to predict aerobic capacity, or infrared interactance to evaluate components of body composition represent imprecise tools to answer meaningful questions about the efficacy of a proposed ergogenic aid.

IV. Conclusions

Findings should dictate conclusions: The conclusions of a research study must logically follow from the research findings. Frequently, investigators who study ergogenic aids extrapolate conclusions beyond the scope of their data. The implications and generalizations of research findings must remain within the context of the measurements made, the subjects studied, and the magnitude of the response. For example, increases in anabolic hormone levels in response to a dietary supplement reflect just that; they do not necessarily indicate an augmented training responsiveness or an improved level of muscular function. Similarly, improvement in brief anaerobic power output capacity with creatine supplementation does not justify the conclusion that exogenous creatine improves overall "physical fitness."

Appropriate statistical analysis: Appropriate inferential statistical analysis must be applied to quantify the potential that chance caused the research outcome. Other statistics must objectify averages, variability, and degree of association between variables.

Statistical versus practical significance: The finding of statistical significance of a particular experimental treatment only means a high probability exists that the result did not occur by chance. One must also evaluate the magnitude of an effect for its real impact on physiology and/or performance. A reduced heart rate of 3 beats per minute during submaximal exercise may reach statistical significance, yet have little practical effect on aerobic fitness or cardiovascular function.

V. Dissemination of findings

Published in peer-reviewed journal: High-quality research withstands the rigors of critical review and evalua-

tion by colleagues with expertise in the specific area of investigation. **Peer review** provides a measure of quality control over scholarship and interpretation of research findings. Publications in popular magazines or quasi-professional journals do not undergo the same rigor of evaluation as peer review. In fact, self-appointed "experts" in sports nutrition and physical fitness pay eager publishers for magazine space to promote their particular viewpoint. In some cases, the expert owns the magazine!

Findings reproduced by other investigators: Findings from one study do not necessarily establish scientific fact. Conclusions become stronger and more generalizable when support emerges from the laboratories of other independent investigators. Consensus reduces the influence of chance, flaws in experimental design, and investigator bias.

TABLE 11.2 summarizes recommendations for future research on performance-enhancing products put forth at the Conference on the Science and Policy of Performance-Enhancing Products held in January 2002.

SUPPLEMENT USE AND ABUSE AMONG ELITE ATHLETES

A survey of college student athletes by the National Collegiate Athletic Association (NCAA) indicated 29% of the respondents used nutritional supplements during the previous year.[97] The most popular supplement was creatine (26%), followed by amino acids (10%), with androstenedione, chromium, and ephedra each used by about 4% of the athletes. Prevalence for doping occurs among athletes in sports that emphasize speed and power.[3] The IOC initiated drug testing for stimulants in Olympic competition in the 1968 Mexico City games following the death of a famed Tour de France British cyclist from amphetamine overdose a year earlier. Testing has consistently expanded, with the initiation of random unannounced drug testing in track and field in 1989 to the administration of 3500 tests before the opening ceremonies of the 2002 Winter Games in Salt Lake City. The following broad categories encompass substances and methods banned by the IOC as of 2006 (no change in 2007).

- Stimulants
- Narcotic analgesics
- Androgenic anabolic steroids
- β-Blockers and alcohol
- β$_2$-Agonists
- Diuretics and other masking agents
- Agents with antiestrogenic activity
- Peptide hormones and analogues
- Substances that alter the integrity of urine samples
- Enhancers of oxygen transport, chemical and physical manipulation, and gene doping
- Cannabinoids
- Glucocorticosteroids

TABLE 11.2   Research-Based Recommendations for Investigating the Optimal Dosing, Health Risks, and Efficacy of Alleged Performance-Enhancing Products

- Evaluation of the risks and benefits of performance-enhancing supplements among subpopulations with diverse dietary patterns and nutrient intakes, such as adolescents, body builders, military personnel, and the elderly
- Monitoring and surveillance of the effects of chronic, prolonged use of performance-enhancing supplements, particularly androstenedione, ephedrine, and creatine
- Identification and characterization of mechanism(s) of action of performance-enhancing ingredients
- Characterization of the patterns of use (e.g., type of product, frequency) and psychosocial behavioral aspects of use among various subpopulations in the United States
- Characterization of dose-response curves for performance-enhancing supplements, particularly those containing ephedrine, alkaloids, and steroid hormone precursors such as androstenedione
- Characterization of the endocrine effects of performance-enhancing supplements, especially those containing hormonal ingredients such as androstenedione and dehydroepiandrosterone (DHEA), according to age, gender, and physiological life stage (e.g., female athletes with amenorrhea or disordered eating or at high risk for osteoporosis)
- Comparative studies of analytical grade dietary supplement ingredients (particularly caffeine and ephedrine) with formulations currently in the marketplace
- Evaluation of the effects of combining performance-enhancing ingredients as in "stacking formulas" or the simultaneous use of multiple sports supplements
- Comparative studies that examine the effect of frequency and timing of supplementation on physical performance
- Determining targeted approaches to communicate the risks and benefits of performance-enhancing products to various segments of the U.S. population (professional and lay audiences)
- Determining whether other stimulant and thermogenic ingredients might serve as substitutes for ephedrine alkaloids

From Fomous CM, et al. Symposium: conference on the science and policy of performance-enhancing products. Med Sci Sports Exerc 2002;34:1685.

In the next sections, we discuss common pharmacologic and chemical agents purported to enhance exercise performance, increase the quality and quantity of training, and augment the body's adaptation to regular exercise. Chapter 12 discusses the role of nutritional supplementation for ergogenic purposes. The following presents five mechanisms by which such foods, food components, and pharmacologic agents might enhance exercise performance:[117]

Five Mechanisms for How Purported Ergogenic Aids Might Work

1. Act as a central or peripheral nervous system stimulant (e.g., caffeine, choline, amphetamines, alcohol)
2. Increase storage or availability of a limiting substrate (e.g., carbohydrate, creatine, carnitine, chromium)
3. Act as supplemental fuel source (e.g., glucose, medium-chain triacylglycerols)
4. Reduce or neutralize performance-inhibiting metabolic by-products (e.g., sodium bicarbonate or sodium citrate, pangamic acid, phosphate)
5. Facilitate recovery (e.g., high-glycemic carbohydrates, water)

ANABOLIC STEROIDS

Anabolic steroids for medical use became prominent in the early 1950s to treat patients deficient in natural androgens or with muscle-wasting diseases (muscular dystrophies). Other legitimate steroid uses include treatment for osteoporosis and severe breast cancer in women and to counter the excessive decline in lean body mass and increase in body fat often observed among elderly men, patients infected with human immunodeficiency virus (HIV), and individuals undergoing kidney dialysis.

Anabolic steroids have become an integral part of the high-technology scene of competitive American sports, beginning with the U.S. weightlifting team (1955), who used Dianabol (modified, synthetic testosterone molecule, methandrostenolone). From the early 1960s until the fall of the Berlin Wall, a new era ushered in the systematic "drugging" of East German competitive athletes with formulation of other anabolic steroids.[81,246]

Up to 4 million athletes (90% of male and 80% of female professional bodybuilders) currently use androgens, often combined with stimulants, hormones, and diuretics, believing their use augments training effectiveness. Even in the sport of baseball, *estimates* based on interviews of strength trainers and current players indicate that up to 30% of professionals use anabolic steroids in their quest to enhance performance.

Interestingly, a recent survey of 500 steroid users reported that nearly 80% are nonathletes who take these drugs for cosmetic purposes. The majority self-administer with intramuscular injections, with nearly 1 in 10 reporting hazardous injection techniques.[200]

Method of Detection

Testing of urine samples provides the primary method for drug detection. The standard testing procedure adds chemicals to the dried urine, vaporizes it with heat, and then blows the vapor through an absorbent column and an electric or magnetic field (gas chromatography-mass spectrometry). The pattern made by the molecules deflected by the field is compared with patterns of known chemicals. Drug testing by use of gas chromatography coupled to high-resolution mass spectrometry introduced in the 1996 Atlanta Olympic Games detects most anabolic steroid use for the prior 18 months.

Structure and Action

Anabolic steroids function in a manner similar to the chief male hormone testosterone. By binding with special receptor sites on muscle and other tissues, testosterone contributes to male secondary sex characteristics. These include sex differences in muscle mass and strength that develop at the onset of puberty. Testosterone production takes place mainly in the testes (95%), with the remainder produced by the adrenal glands. One can minimize the hormone's androgenic or masculinizing effects by synthetically manipulating the steroid's chemical structure to increase muscle growth from nitrogen retention and anabolic tissue building. Nevertheless, the masculinizing effect of synthetically derived steroids still occurs despite chemical alteration, particularly in females.

Athletes who take these drugs typically do so during the active years of their athletic careers. They combine supraphysiologic dosages of multiple steroid preparations in oral and injectable form (combined because they believe the various androgens differ in physiologic action)—a practice called **"stacking"**—progressively increasing drug dosage (**"pyramiding"**), usually during 4- to 18-week cycles. A drug-free period is included between cycles. The drug quantities far exceed the recommended medical dose, often up to 200 times or more the therapeutic amounts. The athlete then progressively reduces the dosage in the months before competition to reduce risk of detection during drug testing. The difference between dosages in research studies and the excess typically abused by athletes has largely contributed to credibility gap between scientific findings (often, no effect of steroids) and what most in the athletic community "know" to be true.

Designer Drug Unmasked

Researchers in the Department of Molecular and Medical Pharmacology at the University of California–Los Angeles' (UCLA's) IOC-accredited Olympic Analytical Laboratory have unmasked a potentially illegal "designer" compound that mimics the chemical structure similar to the prohibited steroids gestrinome and trenbolone. The researchers called the discovery a new stand-alone steroid chemical entity, not a "pro-steroid"

or "precursor steroid" like many performance-boosting substances on the market—a drug with no prior record of manufacture or existence. The U.S. Anti-Doping Agency (USADA: www.usantidoping.org), which oversees drug testing for all sports federations under the U.S. Olympic umbrella, said an anonymous tipster provided a syringe sample of a steroid identified as tetrahydrogestrinone, or THG. Athletes who test positive face 2-year suspensions that would prohibit participation in international meets. As of October 17, 2003, the National Football League began testing players for THG to avoid the scandal that has embarrassed track and field.

In subsequent events, scientists with the World Anti-Doping Agency announced on February 1, 2005 the discovery of a designer steroid, one of considerable more complexity than THG. The drug was uncovered after an anonymous e-mail directed the agency to investigate a substance seized by Canadian customs officials in June 2004. The drug, desoxymethyltestosterone, dubbed DMT, is a clear, oily substance modified from methylestosterone. Although no evidence exists as yet of use of the drug by athletes, scientists with the anti-doping agency, Canadian customs, and the University of Laval in Quebec are working to uncover the structure of the compound and its metabolic pathways. This will eventually lead to a means to test for it in urine.

On October 23, 2003, the **American College of Sports Medicine (ACSM)**, the largest sports medicine and exercise science organization in the world (www. acsm-msse.org), issued a statement that called for increased vigilance in identifying and eradicating steroid use. They condemned the development and use of new "designer" steroids such as THG that are cloaked to avoid detection by doping tests. ACSM considers use of these chemicals "serious threats to the health and safety of athletes, as well as detriments to the principle of fair play in sports. Any effort to veil or disguise steroid use in sports through stealth, designer, or precursor means, puts elite, amateur and even recreational athletes at risk."

A Drug with a Considerable Following

Anabolic steroid use usually combines with resistance training and augmented protein intake to improve strength, speed, and power. The image of the steroid abuser often pictures massively developed body builders; abuse also occurs frequently among athletes in road cycling, tennis, track and field, baseball, American collegiate and professional football, and swimming. Federal authorities conservatively estimate that the business of illegal trafficking in steroids exceeds $100 million yearly.

Increasingly Prevalent Among Young Athletes and Nonathletes

Because many competitive and recreational athletes obtain steroids on the "black market" or the legal equivalent, androstenedione, from mall nutrition stores, misinformed individuals take massive and prolonged dosages without medical monitoring for possible harmful alterations in physiologic function. Particularly worrisome is steroid abuse among boys and girls as young as 10 and high school students who do not play team sports.[5,72,89] Accompanying risks including extreme virilization and irreversible premature cessation of bone growth in children who would otherwise continue to develop. Those teenagers who use steroids cite improved athletic performance as the most common reason for taking them, although 25% acknowledged enhanced appearance—simply wanting to look good—as the main reason.[34] In this struggle for self-image, a disturbance in body image (dissatisfaction/unhappiness with upper and lower body parts, facial features) and with marked symptoms of muscle dysmorphia (see Chapter 15)[36,129] contributes to anabolic steroid abuse among teenagers and young men.[268] A Blue Cross/Blue Shield national survey noted a 25% increase in steroid and similar drug use from 1999 to 2000 among boys ages 12 to 17 (FIG. 11.2). Twenty percent of these teenagers took steroids to improve their looks, not to enhance sports performance.

Effectiveness Questioned

For more than five decades, researchers and athletes have debated the true effect of anabolic steroids on human body composition and exercise performance. Much of the confusion about anabolic steroids' ergogenic effectiveness stems from variations in experimental design: poor selection of controls; differences in specific drugs, dosages, treatment duration, accompanying nutritional supplementation, training intensity, evaluation techniques; and individual variation in response.[39,105,106] The relatively small residual androgenic effect of the steroid also may augment central nervous system function to make the athlete more aggressive (so-called "roid" rage), competitive, and fatigue resistant. Such facilitory effects allow the athlete to train harder for a longer time or to believe that training improvement actually occurred. Abnormal alterations in mood and psychiatric dysfunction also are associated with androgen use.[46,240]

Research with animals suggests that anabolic steroid treatment, when combined with exercise and adequate protein intake, stimulates protein synthesis and increases a muscle's protein content (myosin, myofibrillar, and sarcoplasmic factors).[215] In contrast, other data show no benefit from steroid treatment on the leg muscle weight of rats subjected to functional overload by surgically removing the

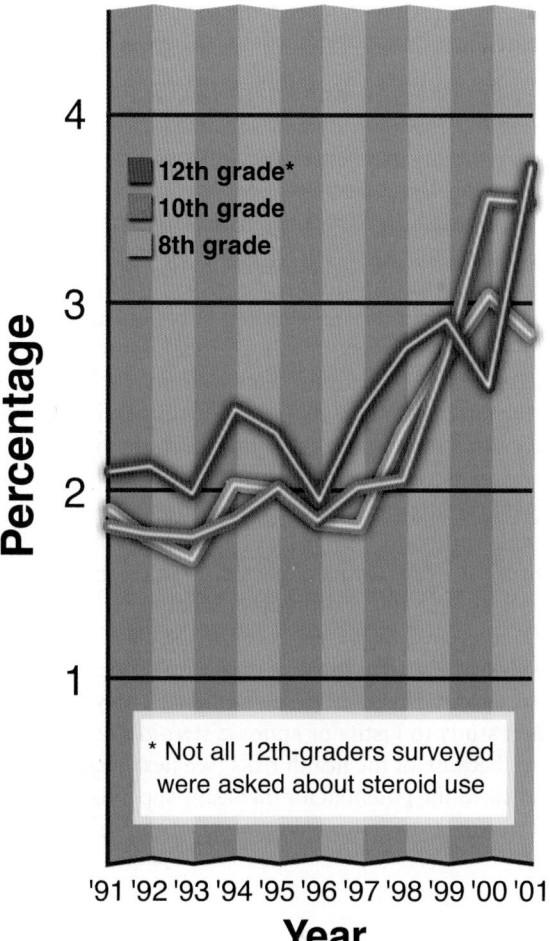

FIGURE 11.2 ■ On the upswing: percentage of adolescent students claiming to have used anabolic steroids at least once. (Source: Blue Cross/Blue Shield. University of Michigan.)

synergistic muscle.[167] In this study, treatment with anabolic steroids did not complement functional overload to stimulate muscle development.

The response of humans is often difficult to interpret. Some studies show augmented body weight gains and reduced body fat with steroid use in men who train, whereas other studies show no effects on strength and power or body composition, even with sufficient energy and protein intake to support an anabolic effect.[76,104] When steroid use produced body weight gains, the compositional nature of these gains (water, muscle, fat) remains unclear.

Patients receiving dialysis and those infected with the HIV commonly experience malnutrition, reduced muscle mass, and chronic fatigue. For dialysis patients, a 6-month supplement with the anabolic steroid nandrolone decanoate increased lean body mass and the level of daily function.[123] Similarly, a moderate supraphysiologic androgen regimen that included the anabolic steroid oxandrolone substantially facilitated lean tissue accrual and muscle strength gains from resistance training in men with HIV compared with testosterone replacement alone.[238]

Dosage Becomes an Important Factor

Variations in drug quantity may account for confusion (and create a credibility gap between scientist and steroid abuser) about the true ergogenic effectiveness of anabolic steroids.[103] Research focused on 43 healthy men with some resistance training experience. Diet (energy and protein intake) and exercise (standard weight-lifting, three times weekly) were controlled, and steroid dosage (600 mg testosterone enanthate injected weekly or placebo) exceeded that in previous human studies. FIGURE 11.3 illustrates changes from baseline average values for fat-free body mass (FFM), triceps and quadriceps cross-sectional muscle areas, and muscle strength (1-RM) after 10 weeks of treatment. The men who received the hormone while continuing to train gained about 0.5 kg (1 lb) of lean tissue weekly, with no increase in body fat over the relatively brief 10-week treatment period. Even the group receiving the drug and not training increased muscle mass and strength compared with men receiving the placebo, but their increases were less than those of men who trained while taking testosterone. The researchers emphasized they did not design their study to justify or endorse steroid use for athletic purposes because of the health risks (see next section). Their data indicated the potential for medically supervised anabolic steroid treatment to restore muscle mass from tissue-wasting diseases.

Do Risks Exist?

Debate exists about the health risks of anabolic steroids used by the athletic population because much of the research on steroid risk comes from medical observations. Prolonged high dosages of steroids often impair normal testosterone endocrine function. Twenty-six weeks of steroid administration to male power athletes reduced serum testosterone to less than half the level when the study began; this effect lasted throughout a 12- to 16-week steroid-free follow-up.[76] Infertility, reduced sperm concentrations (azoospermia), and decreased testicular volume pose additional problems for the steroid abuser.[87] Gonadal function usually returns to normal after several months of steroid cessation.

Other hormonal alterations that accompany steroid use in men include a sevenfold increase in estradiol concentration, the major female hormone. The higher estradiol level represents the average value for normal women and possibly explains the **gynecomastia** (excessive development of the male mammary glands, sometimes secreting milk) noted in men who take anabolic steroids. Steroid use with exercise training also causes connective tissue damage that decreases the tensile strength and elastic compliance of tendons.[148,186] Furthermore, steroids use causes the following five worrisome responses: (1) chronic stimulation of the prostate gland (may increase prostate size), (2) possible kidney malfunction, (3) injury and alterations in cardiovascular function and myocardial cell cultures, (4) possible pathologic ventricular growth and dysfunction when combined

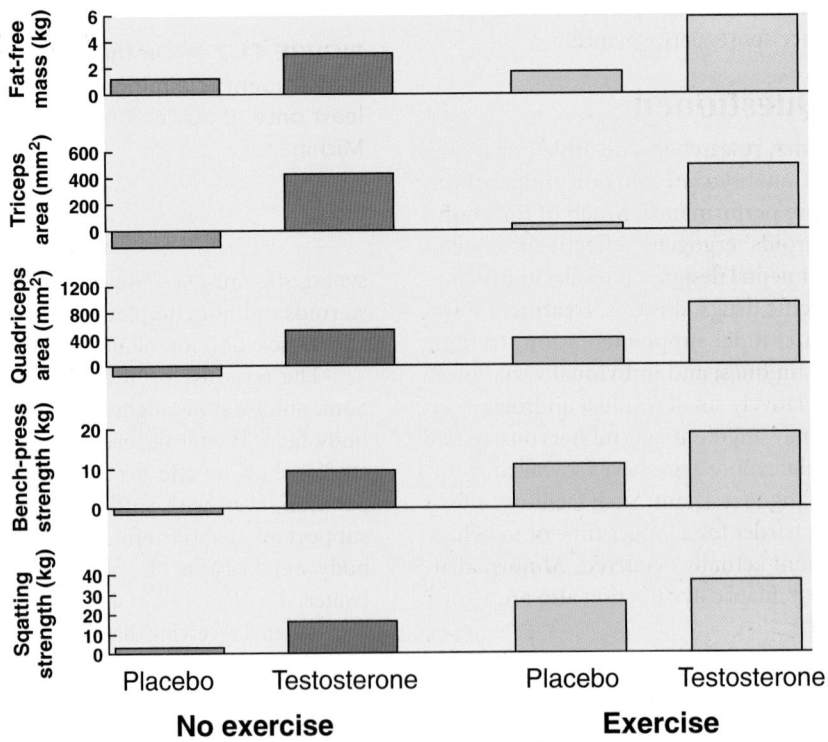

FIGURE 11.3 ■ Changes from baseline in mean fat-free body mass, triceps and quadriceps cross-sectional areas, and muscle strength in bench press and squatting exercises over 10 weeks of testosterone treatment. (From Bhasin S, et al. The effects of supraphysiological doses of testosterone on muscle size and strength in normal men. *N Engl J Med* 1996;335:1.)

with resistance training, and (5) impaired cardiac microvascular adaptation to exercise training and increased blood platelet aggregation.[2,61,105,114,131,160,173,175,243] Increased blood platelet aggregation and impaired myocardial blood supply could increase risk of stroke and acute myocardial infarction. For rats, anabolic steroids exerted a direct action on the thyroid gland and peripheral metabolism of thyroid hormones in a manner that could precipitate thyroid gland dysfunction.[79]

Steroid Use and Life-Threatening Disease

Dramatic life-shortening effects of steroids occurred in adult rats exposed to the type and relative levels of steroids taken by physically active humans. One year after terminating the 6-month steroid exposure, 52% of the mice given the high dosage had died compared with 35% of the mice given the low dosage and only 12% of the control animals not given the exogenous hormone (FIG. 11.4). Autopsy of steroid-treated mice revealed a broad array of pathologic effects that did not appear until long after cessation of steroid use. Most prevalent pathologies included liver and kidney tumors, lymphosarcomas, and heart damage, frequently in combinations. A 6-month exposure period represents about one-fifth of a male mouse's life expectancy, a relative duration considerably longer than exposures of most humans to steroid use. However, several of the pathologies, particularly liver damage, are typically seen in humans on steroids. These findings, if applicable to humans, indicate that it may require several decades before the true negative effects of anabolic steroid use emerge.

TABLE 11.3 lists the undesirable side effects and medical risks of anabolic steroid use. Concern centers on evidence about possible links between androgen abuse and abnormal liver function.[233] Because the liver almost exclusively metabolizes androgens, it becomes susceptible to damage from long-term steroid use and toxic excess. One of the serious effects of androgens on the liver occurs when it (and at times splenic tissue) develops localized blood-filled lesions, a condition called **peliosis hepatis.** In the extreme, the liver eventually fails and the patient dies. We present these data to emphasize the potentially serious side effects, even when a physician prescribes the drug in the recommended dosage. Although patients often take steroids for a longer duration than athletes, some athletes take steroids on and off for years, with daily doses exceeding typical therapeutic levels (5–20 mg vs. 50–200 mg used by athletes).

Steroid Use and Plasma Lipoproteins

Anabolic steroid use, particularly the orally active 17-alkylated androgens, in healthy men and women rapidly reduces high-density lipoprotein cholesterol (HDL-C), elevates both low-density lipoprotein cholesterol (LDL-C) and total cholesterol,[115,264] and reduces the HDL-C to LDL-C ratio.[49] The HDL-C of weightlifters who used anabolic steroids averaged 26 mg · dL^{-1} compared with 50 mg · dL^{-1} for weightlifters not taking the drug.[130] Reduced HDL-C at this level increases a steroid user's coronary artery disease risk. HDL-C remained low among weightlifters, even after abstaining from steroid use for at least 8 weeks between consecutive steroid cycles.[220] The long-term effects of steroid use on cardiovascular morbidity and mortality remain undetermined.

Position Statement on Anabolic Steroids

As part of their long-range educational program, the ACSM has taken a stand on the use and abuse of anabolic–androgenic steroids.[7] We endorse their position, which follows:

American College of Sports Medicine Position Stand on Use of Anabolic Steroids

Based on a comprehensive survey of the world literature and a careful analysis of the claims made for and against the efficacy of anabolic–androgenic steroids in improving human physical performance, it is the position of the American College of Sports Medicine that:

1. Anabolic–androgenic steroids in the presence of an adequate diet and training can contribute to increases in body weight, often in the lean mass compartment.
2. The gains in muscular strength achieved through high-intensity exercise and proper diet can occur by the increased use of anabolic–androgenic steroids in some individuals.
3. Anabolic–androgenic steroids do not increase aerobic power or capacity for muscular exercise.
4. Anabolic–androgenic steroids have been associated with adverse effects on the liver, cardiovascular system, reproductive system, and psychologic status in therapeutic trials and in limited research on athletes. Until further research is completed, the potential hazards of the use of the

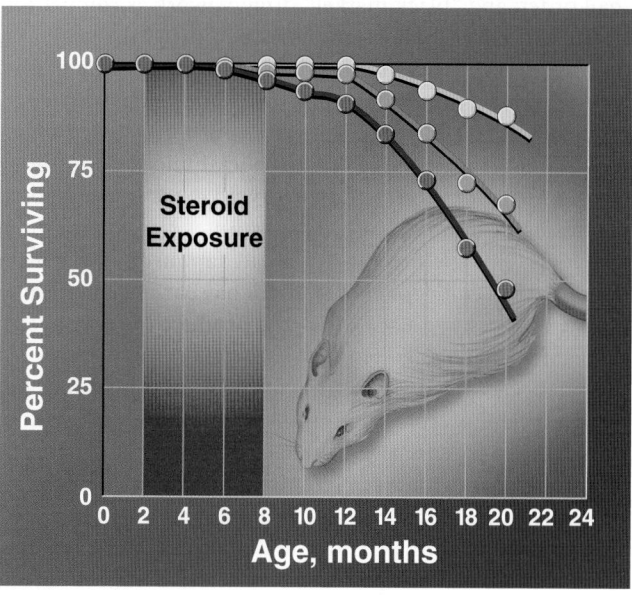

FIGURE 11.4 ■ Life-shortening effects of exogenous anabolic steroid use in mice. (Modified from Bronson FH, Matherne CM. Exposure to anabolic-androgenic steroids shortens life span of male mice. *Med Sci Sports Exerc* 1997;29:615.)

TABLE 11.3   Side Effects and Medical Risks of Anabolic Steroids

Males		Females	
Increase	**Decrease**	**Increase**	**Decrease**
Testicular atrophy	Sperm count	Voice change	Breast tissue
Gynecomastia	Testosterone levels	Facial hair	
		Menstrual irregularities	
		Clitoral enlargement	

Males and Females		
Increase	**Decrease**	**Possible**
LDL-C	HDL-C	Hypertension
LDL-C/HDL-C		Connective tissue damage
Potential for neoplastic disease of the liver		Myocardial damage
Aggressiveness, hyperactivity, irritability		Myocardial infarction
Withdrawal and depression upon stopping steroid use		Impaired thyroid function
Acne		Altered myocardial structure
Peliosis hepatitis		

LDL-C, low-density lipoprotein cholesterol; HDL-C, high-density lipoprotein cholesterol.

anabolic–androgenic steroids in athletes must include those found in therapeutic trials.

5. The use of anabolic–androgenic steroids by athletes is contrary to the rules and ethical principles of athletic competition as set forth by many of the sports governing bodies. The American College of Sports Medicine supports these ethical principles and deplores the use of anabolic–androgenic steroids by athletes.

Steroid Side Effects in Females

Besides the broad range of side effects from anabolic steroid use, females have additional concerns about their dangers. These include virilization (more apparent than in men), disruption of normal growth pattern by premature closure of the plates for bone growth (also for boys), deepened voice, altered menstrual function, dramatic increase in sebaceous gland size, acne, hirsutism (excessive body and facial hair), decreased breast size, and enlarged clitoris.

CLENBUTEROL AND OTHER β_2-ADRENERGIC AGONISTS: ANABOLIC STEROID SUBSTITUTES?

Extensive, random testing of competitive athletes for anabolic steroid use worldwide has ushered in a number of steroid "substitutes." These have appeared on the illicit health food, mail order, and "black market" drug network as competitors try to circumvent detection. One such drug, the sympathomimetic amine **clenbuterol** (brand names Clenasma, Monores, Novegan, Prontovent, and Spiropent) has become popular among athletes because of its purported tissue-building, fat-reducing benefits. When a body builder discontinues steroid use before competition to avoid detection and possible disqualification, the athlete substitutes clenbuterol to retard loss of muscle mass and facilitate fat burning to achieve the required "cut" look. Clenbuterol has particular appeal to female athletes because it does not produce the androgenic side effects of anabolic steroids.

Clenbuterol, one of a group of chemical compounds (albuterol, clenbuterol, salbutamol, salmeterol, terbutaline) classified as a β_2-adrenergic agonist, facilitates responsiveness of adrenergic receptors to circulating epinephrine, norepinephrine, and other adrenergic amines. A review of the available studies of animals (no human studies) indicates that when fed to sedentary, growing livestock in dosages in excess of those prescribed in Europe for human use for bronchial asthma, clenbuterol repartitions body composition by increasing skeletal and cardiac muscle protein deposition and slows fat gain (enhanced lipolysis). It also increases FFM and decreases fat mass when administered long term at therapeutic levels to thoroughbred racehorses partly owing to changes in plasma concentrations of adiponectin and leptin.[132,133]

Clenbuterol has been used experimentally in animals to counter the effects on muscle of aging, immobilization, malnutrition, and pathologic tissue-wasting conditions. In these situations, the β_2-agonists show specific growth-promoting actions on skeletal muscle.[68,269,274] In rats, clenbuterol altered muscle fiber type distribution, inducing enlargement and increased proportion of type II muscle fibers.[56] Decreased protein breakdown and increased protein synthesis accounted for the animals' increased muscle size from clenbuterol treatment.[1,21,161]

Potential Negative Effects on Muscle, Bone, and Cardiovascular Function

Female rats treated with clenbuterol injected subcutaneously or sham injected with the same volume of fluid carrier each day for 14 days increased (1) muscle mass, (2) absolute maximal force-generating capacity, and (3) hypertrophy of fast- and slow-twitch muscle fibers.[63] A negative finding showed hastened fatigue during short-term, intense muscle actions. Others have noted similar positive and negative effects. For example, regular exercise and regular exercise combined with clenbuterol decreased the progression of muscular dystrophy in *mdx* mice as reflected by increases in muscle force-generating capacity.[274] The group receiving clenbuterol also experienced increased muscle fatigability and cellular deformities not noted in the exercise-only group. This negative effect on muscle structure and function may explain findings that clenbuterol treatment negated the beneficial effects of exercise training on endurance performance of animals, despite increases in muscle protein content.[116] Clenbuterol treatment induced muscular hypertrophy in young male rats, but it concomitantly inhibited the longitudinal growth of bones.[141] This effect may relate to clenbuterol's acceleration of epiphyseal closure in the bones of growing animals and certainly would contraindicate its use for prepubescent and adolescent humans.

Echocardiographic evaluations from Standardbred mares indicate that chronic clenbuterol administration, even at low therapeutic levels, changes the heart's structural dimensions in a manner that negatively alters cardiac function.[232] Effects occurred whether the animals exercised or remained inactive. Furthermore, clenbuterol caused the aorta to enlarge after exercise to a degree indicating increased risk of aortic rupture and sudden death. Clenbuterol treatment when combined with aerobic training also blunts the normal training-induced increase in plasma volume in Standardbred mares; this related to a decrease in aerobic exercise performance and ability to recover.[132]

Clenbuterol, not approved for human use in the United States, is commonly prescribed abroad as an inhaled bronchodilator for treating obstructive pulmonary disorders. Reported short-term side effects in humans accidentally "overdosing" from eating clenbuterol-tainted meat include skeletal muscle tremor, agitation, palpitations, dizziness, nausea, muscle cramps, rapid heart rate, and headache. Despite such negative side effects, supervised use of clenbuterol may benefit humans in treating muscle wasting in disease, forced immobilization, and aging. Unfortunately, no data exist for potential toxicity level or its efficacy and safety in long-term use. Clearly, clenbuterol cannot be justified or recommended for use as an ergogenic aid.

Other β_2-Adrenergic Agonists

Research has focused on possible strength-enhancing effects of sympathomimetic β_2-adrenergic agonists other than clenbuterol. Men with cervical spinal-cord injuries took 80 mg of metaproterenol daily for 4 weeks in conjunction with physical therapy. Increases occurred in estimated muscle cross-sectional area and strength of the elbow flexors and wrist extensors compared with the placebo condition.[230] Albuterol administration (16 mg per day for 3 weeks) without exercise training improved muscular strength 10 to 15%.[162] Therapeutic doses of albuterol also facilitated isokinetic strength gains from slow-speed concentric/eccentric isokinetic training.[38] Recent studies indicate that salbutamol ingestion both over the short-term and with a single dose increased maximal anaerobic power output on the Wingate anaerobic exercise test.[51,152]

Training State Makes a Difference

Animals

Untrained skeletal muscle responds to the effects of β_2-adrenergic agonists. The increase in muscle mass with clenbuterol treatment plus exercise training becomes more pronounced in animals without prior training experience than in trained animals that continue training and then receive this β_2-adrenergic agonist.[184]

Humans

Some research shows augmented muscle power output with albuterol administration.[229] No ergogenic effect on short-term performance emerged from salbutamol administration in two 10-minute cycling trials.[50] Similarly, no effect on power output during a 30-second Wingate test occurred in nonasthmatic trained cyclists who received 360 μg (twice the normal dose administered by inhaler in four measured doses of 90 μg each) 20 minutes before testing.[151] In other research, twice the recommended dose of salbutamol (albuterol; 400 μg administered in four inhalations 20 minutes before exercising) did not enhance anaerobic power output, endurance performance, ventilatory threshold, or dynamic lung function of trained endurance cyclists.[193] In other research, no beneficial effect occurred in the pulmonary function and oxygen loading characteristics of the blood of trained male athletes who inhaled bronchodilators that contained β_2-adrenergic agonists before exercising.[111] Such findings support the argument that competitive athletes should not be prohibited from using these compounds because they provide no ergogenic benefit, yet they "normalize" individuals with obstructive pulmonary disorders. Differences in the groups' training status may explain discrepancies among studies concerning albuterol's effect on short-term power output.

A Blunted Response With Training

Albuterol's ergogenic benefit supposedly comes from its stimulating effects on skeletal muscle β_2-receptors to increase muscle force and power. With exercise training, the muscle β_2-receptors undergo down regulation (become less sensitive to a given stimulus) from long-term exposure to training-induced elevations in blood catecholamine levels. This makes the trained athlete less responsive to a sympathomimetic drug than an untrained counterpart.

GROWTH HORMONE: GENETIC ENGINEERING COMES TO SPORTS

Human growth hormone (**GH** or **hGH**), also known as *somatotropin,* now competes with anabolic steroids in the illicit market of alleged tissue-building, performance-enhancing drugs. The adenohypophysis of the pituitary gland produces GH, which serves as a potent anabolic and lipolytic agent for tissue building and growth and increasing fat catabolism. Specifically, GH stimulates bone and cartilage growth, enhances fatty acid oxidation, and slows glucose and amino acid breakdown. Reduced GH secretion (about 50% less at age 60 than age 30) accounts for some of the decreases in FFM and increases in fat mass that accompany aging. Exogenous recombinant GH supplements (whose use is difficult to detect) produced by genetically engineered bacteria can reverse these negative changes in body composition. Such results have led to a dramatic rise in the number of antiaging clinics throughout the country that provide GH to thousands of older persons looking to "turn back the clock," at a cost of $1000 or more a month.

Research has produced equivocal results concerning the true benefits of GH supplementation to counter the effects of aging—loss of muscle mass, thinning bones, increase in body fat, particularly abdominal fat, and a depressed energy level. For example, healthy men 70 to 85 years old who received GH supplements increased FFM by 4.3% and decreased fat mass by 13.1%.[194] Supplementation, however, did not reverse the negative effects of aging on functional measures of muscular strength and aerobic capacity. Furthermore, men receiving the supplement experienced hand stiffness, malaise, arthralgias, and lower extremity edema. One of the largest studies to date determined the effects of GH on changes in body composition and functional capacity of healthy men and women ranging in age from mid-60s to late 80s.[24] Men who took GH gained 7 lb of lean body mass and lost a similar amount of fat mass. Women gained about 3 lb of lean body mass and lost 5 lb of body fat compared with counterparts who received a placebo. The subjects remained sedentary and did not change their diet over the 6-month study period. Unfortunately, serious side effects afflicted between 24 and 46% of the subjects. These included swollen feet and ankles, joint pain, carpal tunnel

syndrome (swelling of tendon sheath over a nerve in the wrist), and development of diabetes or a prediabetic condition. As in previous research, no effects were noted for GH treatment on measures of muscular strength or endurance capacity despite increased lean body mass.

Excessive GH production during the growth period produces **gigantism,** an endocrine and metabolic disorder that triggers abnormal size or overgrowth of the entire body or any of its parts. Excessive GH production following cessation of growth produces the irreversible disorder **acromegaly.** Enlarged hands, feet, and facial features characterize this malady. Medically, children who suffer from kidney failure or GH deficiency receive thrice-weekly injections of this hormone until adolescence to help achieve near-normal size.[109] In young adults with hypopituitarism, GH replacement therapy improves muscle volume, isometric strength, and exercise capacity. It also increases endurance capacity in growth hormone-deficient patients.[47]

Disagreement Concerning Ergogenic Effects

At first glance, GH use seems appealing to the strength and power athlete because at physiologic levels this hormone stimulates amino acid uptake and muscle protein synthesis while enhancing lipid breakdown and conserving glycogen reserves. It also appears to enhance connective tissue protein synthesis.[64] However, few well-controlled studies have examined how GH supplements affect healthy subjects who undertake exercise training.[222] In one study, well-trained men maintained a high-protein diet while taking either biosynthetic GH or a placebo.[55] During 6 weeks of standard resistance training with GH, percentage body fat decreased and FFM increased. No changes in body composition occurred for the group training with the placebo. Subsequent investigations have not supported these findings.[60,272] Previously sedentary young men who participated in a 12-week resistance-training program received daily recombinant human GH supplements (40 $\mu g \cdot kg^{-1}$) or a placebo.[271] FFM, total body water, and whole body protein synthesis increased more in the GH recipients. No differences emerged between groups in fractional rate of protein synthesis in skeletal muscle and torso and limb circumferences. TABLE 11.4 shows equivalent effects of control and experimental treatments on muscle function in dynamic and static strength measures. The authors attributed the greater increase in whole body protein synthesis in the group receiving GH to a possible increase in nitrogen retention in lean tissue other than skeletal muscle (e.g., connective tissue, fluid, and noncontractile proteins).

Until fairly recently, healthy persons could obtain GH only on the black market and often in an adulterated form. Human cadaver-derived GH (used until 1985 by U.S. physicians to treat children of short stature) greatly increases the risk for contracting Creutzfeldt-Jakob disease, an infectious, incurable brain-deteriorating disorder. Currently, a synthetic form of GH (Protoropin and Humantrope) produced by genetic engineering is approved for treating GH-deficient chil-

TABLE 11.4	Maximal Force Production of Knee Extensor and Flexor Muscle Groups Before and After Training With or Without Growth Hormone (GH) Supplements					
	Exercise plus Placebo			Exercise plus GH		
Force	Initial[a]	Final[a]	% Change	Initial[a]	Final[a]	% Change
Concentric						
Knee extensors	212 ± 13	248 6 10	+17	191 ± 11	214 ± 9	+12
Knee flexors	137 ± 11	158 ± 7	+15	122 ± 12	143 ± 6	+17
Isometric						
Knee extensor	220 ± 13	252 ± 13	+14	198 ± 15	207 ± 7	+5
Knee flexors	131 ± 8	158 ± 8	+20	127 ± 13	140 ± 16	+10

From Yarasheski KF, et al. Effect of growth hormone and resistance exercise on muscle growth in young men. Am J Physiol 1992;262:E261.

[a]Values are mean ± SE. Maximum force (N) determined using a Cybex dynamometer. Concentric force measured at $60° \cdot s^{-1}$ angular velocity. Isometric force measured at 135° of knee extension. The maximum concentric force production of the knee flexor and extensor muscles increased significantly in both groups ($P < .05$), but these increments and the increments in maximum isometric force production were not greater in the exercise plus GH group.

dren. But once a drug reaches market, doctors can prescribe it at their discretion. For example, over a 4-year period from 1997 to 2001, prescriptions for GH have more than tripled from 6000 to 21,000. Men's fitness magazines currently advertise GH, providing telephone numbers of doctors who prescribe it.

Are The Benefits Worth The Risks?

Child athletes who take growth hormone (GH) believing they gain a competitive edge suffer increased incidence of gigantism, and adults develop acromegalic syndrome. Additional, less visual side effects include insulin resistance that leads to type 2 diabetes, water retention, and carpal tunnel compression.

DHEA: A WORRISOME TREND

Increased use of synthetic **dehydroepiandrosterone (DHEA)** by exercise enthusiasts and the general population has raised concerns about its safety and effectiveness among sports medicine personnel and the medical community in general. DHEA (and its sulfated ester, DHEA sulfate, or DHEAS), a relatively weak steroid hormone, is synthesized from cholesterol, primarily by the adrenal cortex. A small amount of DHEA (commonly referred to as "mother hormone") and other related **prohormone compounds** are naturally derived precursors to testosterone or other anabolic steroids. FIGURE 11.5 outlines the major pathways for synthesizing DHEA, androstenedione, and related compounds. The quantity of DHEA the body produces surpasses all other known steroids with its largest concentrations in the brain. Its chemical structure closely resembles that of the sex hormones testosterone and estrogen. News reports and advertisements tout DHEA as

a "superhormone," a "Holy Grail" that increases testosterone production, preserves youth, invigorates sex life, and counters the debilitating effects of aging. Home pages on the World Wide Web regularly extol its benefits.

Because DHEA occurs naturally, the Food and Drug Administration (FDA) has no control over its distribution or claims for its action and effectiveness. The lay press, mail order companies, and health food industry describe DHEA as a pill (even available as a chewing gum, each piece containing 25 mg) to cure just about any bodily ill. Advocates claim that it extends life; protects against cancer, heart disease, diabetes, and osteoporosis; enhances sexual drive; facilitates lean tissue gain and body fat loss; enhances mood and memory; improves muscular capacity; and boosts immunity against a variety of infectious diseases including acquired immune deficiency syndrome (AIDS). The hormone's detractors consider it "snake oil." The IOC and USOC have placed DHEA on their banned substance lists at zero tolerance levels.

FIGURE 11.6 illustrates the generalized trend for plasma DHEA levels during a lifetime. For boys and girls, DHEA levels are substantial at birth and then decline sharply. A steady increase in DHEA production occurs from age 6 to 10 years, an occurrence that some researchers feel contributes to the beginning of puberty and sexuality. Peak production occurs between ages 18 and 25 (higher in males than in females). In contrast to the glucocorticoid and mineralocorticoid adrenal steroids whose plasma levels remain relatively high with aging, a long, slow decline in DHEA begins after age 30. By age 75, the plasma level decreases to only about 20% of the value in young adulthood. This fact has fueled speculation that plasma DHEA levels might serve as a marker of biologic aging and disease susceptibility. Popular reasoning concludes that supplementing with DHEA blunts the negative effects of aging by raising plasma levels to more "youthful" concentrations.[202] Many persons supplement with this "natural" hormone just in case it proves beneficial, without considering the potential for harm.

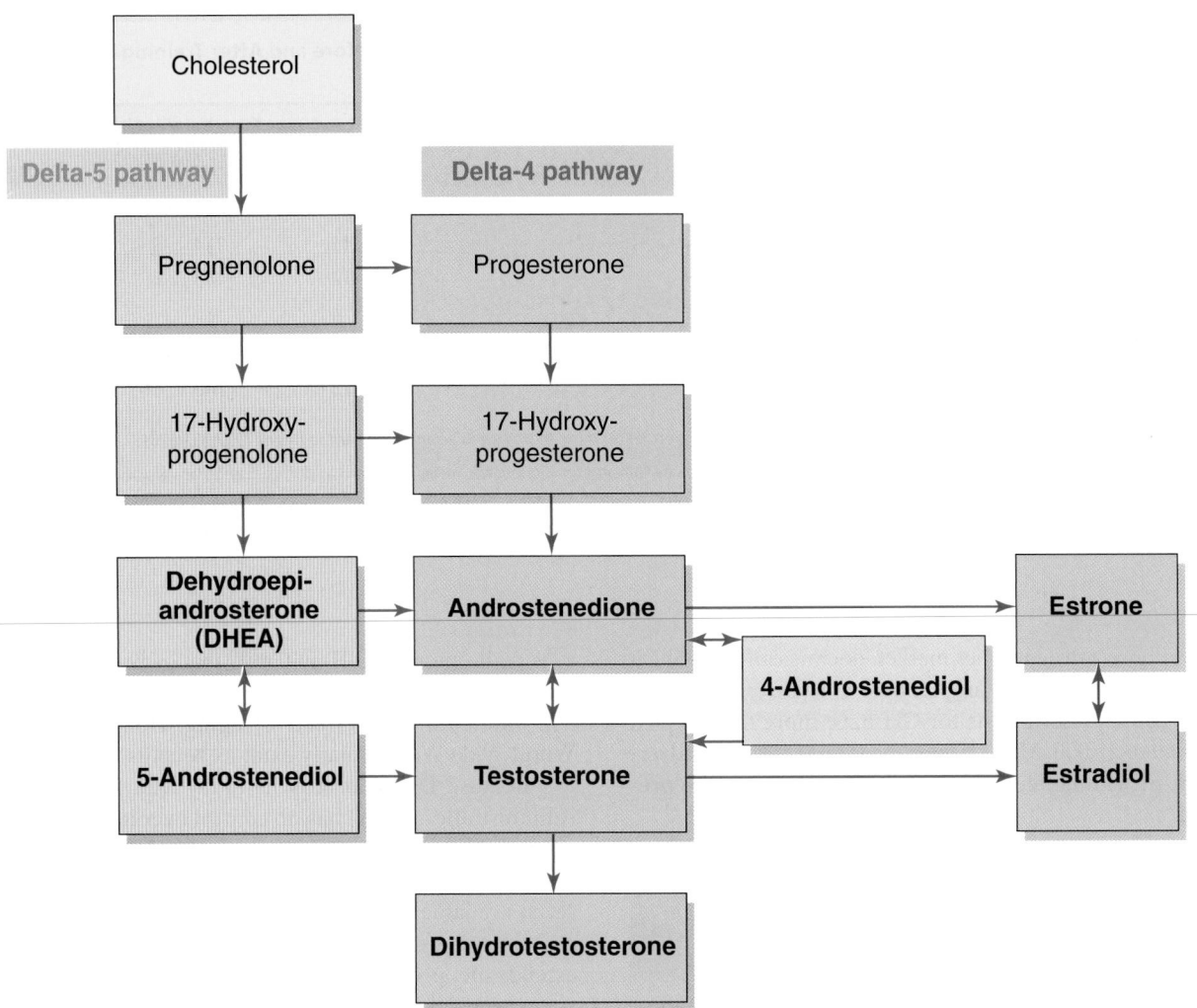

FIGURE 11.5 ■ Proposed metabolic pathways for dehydroepiandrosterone (DHEA), androstenedione, and related compounds. *Directional arrows* signify one-way and two-way conversions. Compounds in *bold print* are products currently available on the market.

An Unregulated Compound with Uncertain Safety

In 1994, the FDA reclassified DHEA (along with many other "natural" chemicals under the Dietary Supplement and Education Act) from the category of unapproved new drug (prescription required) to a dietary supplement for sale over the counter without a prescription. Pharmaceutical companies synthesize DHEA from chemicals found in soybeans and wild yams. In this process, other compounds such as androstenedione may be produced that contaminate the DHEA. Many consider the current unregulated and unmonitored use of DHEA by healthy men and women (daily dosage varies from 5 to 10 mg to as much as 2000 mg) a disaster waiting to happen.

Much Remains Unknown

Despite its quantitative significance as a hormone, researchers know little about DHEA, particularly with respect to the following four areas:

1. Health and aging
2. Cellular or molecular mechanism(s) of action
3. Possible receptor sites (although its sulfate interacts with brain receptors for the neurotransmitter γ-aminobutyric acid [GABA])
4. Potential for adverse effects from exogenous dosage, particularly among young adults with normal DHEA levels

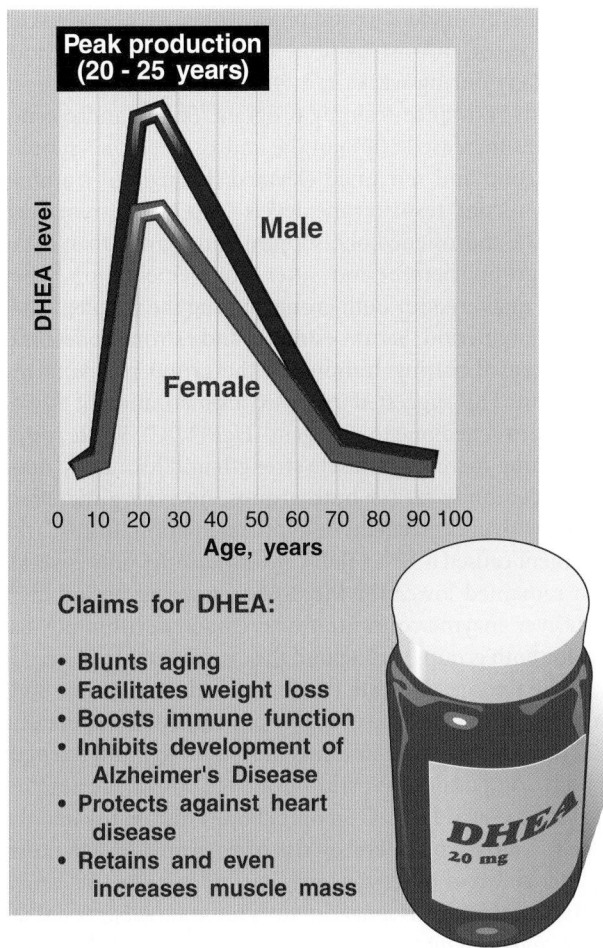

FIGURE 11.6 ■ Generalized trend for plasma levels of de-hydroepiandrosterone (DHEA) for men and women during a lifetime.

The appropriate DHEA dosage for humans has not been determined. Concern exists about possible harmful effects on blood lipids, glucose tolerance, and prostate gland health. The major reason is because medical problems associated with hormone supplementation often do not appear until years after initiation of use. A number of over-the-counter supplements contain DHEA (and other prohormones). One can readily purchase DHEA through mainstream grocery chains, drug and nutrition stores, health clubs, mail-order catalogues, and the Internet.

Early support for DHEA came from studies of rodents fed daily supplements of this hormone. Treatment indicated beneficial effects in preventing cancer, atherosclerosis, viral infections, obesity, and diabetes; enhancing immune function; and even extending life span. Scientists have argued that the findings from research on rats and mice—who produce little, if any, DHEA—do not necessarily apply to healthy humans. Cross-sectional observations relating levels of DHEA to risk of death from heart disease provided the early indirect evidence for a possible beneficial effect in humans. A high DHEA level conferred protection in men, while women with a high DHEA level increased their heart disease risk. Subsequent research showed only a

moderate protective association for men and no association for women. Studies also suggested that DHEA supplements might provide a cardioprotective effect with aging (more beneficial in men than in women),[121] boost immune function in disease,[215] and provide antioxidant protection during aging.[10]

In other research on humans, middle-aged men and women received either 100 mg of DHEA or a placebo daily for 3 months, and the other treatment for the next 3 months.[181] Both groups exhibited a slight increase of 1.2% in lean body mass during DHEA supplementation. Fat mass decreased in the men, but a small increase occurred for the women. Chemical markers also indicated improved immune function. An increase in muscle mass and strength induced by intense resistance training occurred with DHEA supplementation in elderly men and women.[257] These findings suggest some possible positive effects of exogenous DHEA on muscle mass and immune system function, and responsiveness to resistance training, in middle-aged and elderly adults.

Research in young men evaluated short-term ingestion of 50 mg of DHEA daily on serum steroid hormones and the effect of 8 weeks of supplementation (150 mg daily) on resistance-training adaptations.[29] Short-term DHEA supplementation rapidly increased serum androstenedione concentrations, although it exerted *no effect* on serum testosterone and estrogen concentrations. Furthermore, longer term DHEA supplementation raised serum androstenedione levels, but had *no effect* on anabolic hormones, serum lipids, liver enzymes, muscular strength, and lean body mass compared with a placebo given to men undergoing similar training. These and similar results of other investigators indicate that relatively low dosages of DHEA do not increase serum testosterone levels, enhance muscular strength or change muscle and fat cross-sectional areas, or facilitate adaptations to resistance training.[202,261]

Concern exists about the effect of unregulated long-term DHEA supplementation (particularly in doses >50 mg daily) on body function and overall health. Converting DHEA into potent androgens like testosterone in the body promotes facial hair growth in females and alters normal menstrual function. As with exogenous anabolic steroids, DHEA lowers HDL-C, which increases heart disease risk. Limited, conflicting data exist concerning its effects on breast cancer risk. Clinicians have expressed fear that elevated plasma DHEA through supplementation might stimulate growth of otherwise dormant prostate gland tumors or cause benign hypertrophy of the prostate gland itself. If cancer is present, DHEA may accelerate its growth. On a positive note, recent data show that supplements of DHEA for elderly men and women decreased abdominal (visceral) fat and improved the body's use of insulin.[256] Such findings indicate a potential for DHEA in treating components of the metabolic syndrome.

Despite its popularity among exercise enthusiasts, no data exist concerning ergogenic effects of DHEA supplements on young adult men and women. On a brighter side, DHEA supplementation may reduce the required dose of corticosteroid medication required by patients with the autoimmune disease lupus. This effect would certainly reduce side effects such as accelerated osteoporosis that accompany steroid therapy.

ANDROSTENEDIONE: BENIGN PROHORMONE NUTRITIONAL SUPPLEMENT OR POTENTIALLY HARMFUL DRUG?

Many physically active individuals use the legal over-the-counter "nutritional" supplement **androstenedione** (and androstenediol and norandrostenediol), believing that these steroid products (1) directly stimulate endogenous testosterone production or form androgen-like derivatives (as shown in Fig. 11.5) and (2) enable them to train harder, build muscle mass, and repair injury more rapidly. Androstenedione is found naturally in meat and extracts of some plants; the World Wide Web touts it as "a prohormone, a metabolite only one step away from the biosynthesis of testosterone."

Originally developed by East Germany in the 1970s to enhance performance of their elite athletes, androstenedione was first commercially manufactured and sold in the United States in 1996. By calling the substance a supplement and avoiding any claims of medical benefits, the 1994 FDA rules enable androstenedione to be marketed as a food. Because many countries consider androstenedione a controlled substance, individuals travel to the United States to purchase it, further contributing to the supplement industry's yearly sales. Currently available are an androstenedione-containing chewing gum and a steroid lozenge that dissolves under the tongue.

Androstenedione, an intermediate or precursor hormone between DHEA and testosterone, aids the liver in synthesizing other biologically active steroid hormones. Normally produced by the adrenal glands and gonads, it converts to testosterone enzymatically by 17β-hydroxysteroid dehydrogenase, found in diverse body tissues. Androstenedione also serves as an estrogen precursor.

Little scientific evidence supports claims about the ergogenic effectiveness or anabolic qualities of andro-type compounds.[15,58,80,208] One study showed that oral treatment with 200 mg of 4-androstene-3,17-dione or 200 mg of 4-androstene-3β,17β-diol increased peripheral plasma total and free testosterone concentrations compared with a placebo.[69] Androstenedione dosages as high as 300 mg per day have elevated testosterone levels by 34%.[149] However, chronic androstenedione administration also elevates serum estradiol and estrone in men and women. This response could offset any potential anabolic effect.

A two-phase investigation systematically evaluated whether short- or long-term androstenedione supplementation elevates blood testosterone concentrations or enhances muscle size and strength gains during resistance training.[138] In one phase, young-adult men received either a single 100-mg dose of androstenedione or a placebo containing 250 mg of rice flour. FIGURE 11.7A shows that serum androstenedione rose 175% during the first 60 minutes following ingestion and then increased further to 350% above baseline values between minutes 90 and 270. On the other hand, short-term supplementation did not affect serum concentrations of either free or total testosterone.

In the experiment's second phase, young men received either 300 mg of androstenedione or 250 mg of a rice flour placebo daily during weeks 1, 2, 4, 5, 7, and 8 of an 8-week whole-body resistance-training program. Serum androstenedione levels increased 100% in the androstenedione-supplemented group and remained elevated throughout training. Although serum testosterone levels (Fig.11.7B) remained higher in the androstenedione-supplemented group than in the placebo group before and after supplementation, they remained unaltered for both groups during the supplementation–training period. Serum estradiol and estrone concentrations increased during training in the group receiving the supplement. This suggested increased aromatization of the ingested androstenedione to estrogens (Fig. 11.7C). While resistance training increased muscle strength and lean body mass and reduced body fat for both groups, no synergistic effect emerged with androstenedione supplementation. Instead, the supplement caused a 12% HDL-C *reduction* after only 2 weeks, which remained lower for the 8-week training period.[30,138] Serum liver enzyme concentrations remained within normal limits for both groups throughout the experimental period.

These findings indicate *no effect* of androstenedione supplementation on (1) basal serum concentrations of testosterone or (2) training response in terms of muscle size and strength and body composition. Worrisome are the potentially negative effects of a lowered HDL-C on overall heart disease risk and the elevated serum estrogen level on risk of gynecomastia and possibly pancreatic and other cancers. *The findings must be viewed within the context of this specific study because test subjects took far smaller dosages of androstenedione (≤ 300 mg · d⁻¹) than those routinely taken by body builders and other athletes.*

> ### Eight Research Findings Concerning Androstenedione
>
> 1. Little or no elevation of plasma testosterone concentrations
> 2. No favorable effect on muscle mass
> 3. No favorable effect on muscular performance
> 4. No favorable alterations in body composition
> 5. Elevates a variety of estrogen subfractions
> 6. No favorable effects on muscle protein synthesis or tissue anabolism
> 7. Impairs the blood lipid profile in apparently healthy men
> 8. Increases likelihood of testing positive for steroid use

A MODIFIED VERSION. Norandrostenedione and norandrostenediol are norsteroid compounds available over-the-counter in the United States. They are chemically similar to androstenedione and androstenediol, respectively, with slight chemical modification that supposedly enhances anabolic properties without converting to testosterone but to the steroid nandrolone. These modifications should theoretically confer anabolic effects via the compounds' direct activation of the androgen receptors in skeletal muscle. To test this hypothesis, research evaluated 8 weeks of

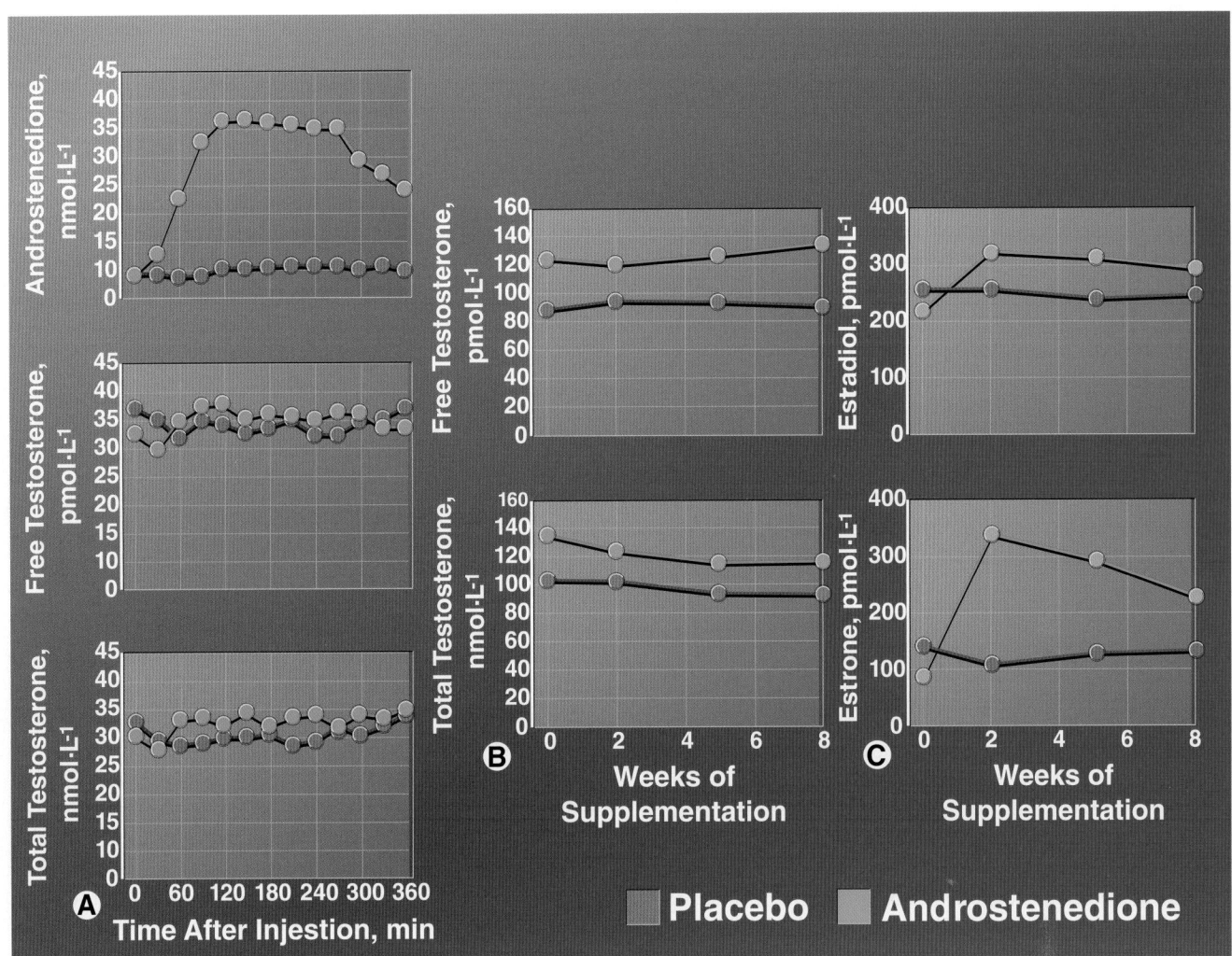

FIGURE 11.7 ▪ **A.** Effect of short-term (single dose) exogenous supplementation with 100 mg of androstenedione or placebo on serum concentrations of androstenedione and free and total testosterone. **B.** Serum free and total testosterone, and **(C)** serum estradiol and estrone with 300-mg daily supplementation and androstenedione (n = 9) during 8 weeks of resistance training. (From King DS, et al. Effect of oral androstenedione on serum testosterone and adaptations to resistance training in young men. *JAMA* 1999;281:2020.)

low-dose norsteroid supplementation on body composition, girth measures, muscular strength, and mood states of young adult, resistance-trained men.[248] The men received either 100 mg of 19-nor-4-androstene-3,17-dione plus 56 mg of 19-nor-4-androstene-3,17-diol (156 mg total norsteroid per day) or a multivitamin placebo. Each subject also resistance-trained 4 days a week for the duration of the study. Norsteroid supplementation provided *no additional effect* on any of the body composition or exercise performance variables measured.

AMPHETAMINES

Amphetamines, or *"pep pills,"* consist of pharmacologic compounds that exert a powerful stimulating effect on central nervous system function. Athletes most frequently use amphetamine (Benzedrine) and dextroamphetamine sulfate (Dexedrine).

Competitive Athletes Beware

Consuming trace amounts as low as 10 μg of 19-norandrostenedione daily (levels common in over-the-counter androstenedione supplements) often cause many users to test positive for 19-norandrosterone, the standard marker for the banned anabolic steroid nandrolone. Many nutritional supplements may be tainted with 19-norandrostenedione (and undisclosed by product labeling), so the caveat "buyer beware" is all too apropos. Ironically, while androgen prohormone supplements taken in large dosages may transiently increase serum testosterone, they exert no *ergogenic effects* on muscular strength, no favorable alterations in body composition, and no enhancement of overall health profile.

Amphetamines are sympathomimetic because their effects mimic actions of the sympathetic hormones epinephrine and norepinephrine. These hormones increase blood pressure, pulse rate, cardiac output, breathing rate, metabolism, and blood sugar. Taking 5 to 20 mg of amphetamine usually produces an effect for 30 to 90 minutes after ingestion, although the drug's influence persists for much longer. Besides arousing sympathetic function, amphetamines supposedly increase alertness and wakefulness and augment work capacity by depressing sensations of muscle fatigue. The deaths of two famed cyclists in the 1960s during competitive road racing were attributed to amphetamine use for just such purposes. In one of these deaths in 1967, British Tour de France rider Tom Simpson overheated and suffered a fatal heart attack during the ascent of Mont Ventoux. Soldiers in World War II commonly used amphetamines to increase alertness and reduce feelings of fatigue. Consequently, it should come as little surprise that athletes use amphetamines believing they gain an ergogenic edge; ironically, little or no performance advantage exists.

Dangers of Amphetamines

The following five facts argue against amphetamine use:

1. Chronic use leads to physiologic or emotional drug dependency. This often causes cyclical use of "uppers" (amphetamines) and "downers" (barbiturates)—the barbiturates reduce or tranquilize the "hyper" state brought on by amphetamines.
2. General side effects include headache, tremulousness, agitation, insomnia, nausea, dizziness, and confusion, all of which negatively affect sports performance requiring rapid reaction and judgment and a high level of steadiness and mental concentration.
3. Taking larger doses eventually requires more drug to achieve the same effect because drug tolerance increases with prolonged use; this may aggravate or even precipitate cardiovascular and mental disorders.
4. The drugs suppress normal mechanisms for perceiving and responding to pain, fatigue, or heat stress; this effect severely jeopardizes health and safety.
5. Prolonged intake of high doses produces weight loss, paranoia, psychosis, repetitive compulsive behavior, and nerve damage.

Amphetamine Use and Athletic Performance

TABLE 11.5 summarizes the results of seven experiments on amphetamine use and physical performance. In almost all instances, amphetamines produced little or no affect on exercise capacity or the performance of simple psychomotor skills.

Athletes take amphetamines to get "up" psychologically for competition. On the day or evening before a contest, competitors often seem nervous and irritable and have difficulty relaxing. Under these circumstances, they take a barbiturate to induce sleep. They then regain the "hyper" condition by popping an "upper." This cycle of depressant-to-stimulant becomes potentially dangerous because the stimulant acts abnormally following barbiturate intake. The IOC, American Medical Association, and most sport-governing groups have rules that disqualify athletes for amphetamine use. Ironically, most research indicates that amphetamines do *not* enhance exercise performance. Perhaps their greatest influence pertains to the psychologic realm, where naive athletes believe that taking any supplement contributes to a superior performance. A placebo containing an inert substance often produces identical results.

CAFFEINE

Caffeine represents a compound whose classification and prior regulatory status depends on its use as a drug (over-the-counter migraine products), food (in coffee and soft drinks), or dietary supplement (alertness products).[75] Caffeine is a possible exception to the general rule against taking stimulants.[119,135,143,161,273] The most widely consumed behaviorally active substance in the world, caffeine belongs to a group of lipid-soluble compounds called *purines* (chemical name, 1,3,7-trimethylxanthine) found naturally in coffee beans, tea leaves, chocolate, cocoa beans, and cola nuts and often added to carbonated beverages and nonprescription medicines. Sixty-three plant species contain caffeine in their leaves, seeds, or fruits. In the United States, 75% (14 million kg) of caffeine intake comes from coffee (3.5 kg per person per year), 15% from tea, and the remainder from the items listed in TABLE 11.6. Depending on preparation, one cup of brewed coffee contains 60 to 150 mg of caffeine, instant coffee about 100 mg, brewed tea between 20 and 50 mg, and caffeinated soft drinks about 50 mg. For comparison, 2.5 cups of percolated coffee contain 250 to 400 mg of caffeine or between 3 and 6 mg per kg of body mass. This produces urinary caffeine concentrations within the previously established IOC acceptable limit of 12 $\mu g \cdot mL^{-1}$ and NCAA limit of 15 $\mu g \cdot mL^{-1}$. *In January 2004, the IOC removed caffeine from its list of restricted substances.*

The intestinal tract absorbs caffeine rapidly. with peak plasma concentration reached within 1 hour. Caffeine clears from the body fairly rapidly, taking about 3 to 6 hours for blood caffeine concentrations to decrease by half. As a frame of reference, it requires about 10 hours for clearance of other stimulants like methamphetamine.

Typical Caffeine Sources

About 70% of caffeine is consumed in coffee, while soft drinks make up 15% and chocolate about 2%.

TABLE 11.5 Summary of Results on the Effects of Amphetamines on Athletic Performance

Study	Dose (mg)	Type of Experiment	Effect of Amphetamines
1.	10–20	Two all-out treadmill runs with 10-min rest between runs	None
		Consecutive 100-yd swims with 10-min rest intervals	None
		220- to 440-yd swims for time	None
		220-yd track runs for time	None
		100-yd to 2-mile track runs for time	None
2.	10	Bench stepping to fatigue carrying weights equal to 1/3 body mass, 3 times with 3-min rest intervals	None
3.	5	100-yd swim for speed	None
4.	10	All-out treadmill runs	None
5.	10	Stationary cycling at work rates of 275–2215 kg-m·min^{-1} for 25–35 min followed by treadmill run to exhaustion	None on submaximal or maximal oxygen uptake, heart rate, ventilation volume, or blood lactate; work time on the bicycle and treadmill increased
6.	20	Reaction and movement time to a visual stimulus	None; subjective feelings of alertness or lethargy unrelated to reaction or movement time
7.	5	Psychomotor performance during a simulated airplane flight	Enhanced performance and lessened fatigue, but if preceded by secobarbital (barbiturate), decreased performance

1. Karpovich PV. Effect of amphetamine sulfate on athletic performance. JAMA 1959;170:558.
2. Foltz EE, et al. The influence of amphetamine (Benzedrine) sulfate and caffeine on the performance of rapidly exhausting work by untrained subjects. J Lab Clin Med 1943;28:601.
3. Haldi J, Wynn W. Action of drugs on efficiency of swimmers. Res Q 1959;17:96.
4. Golding LA, Barnard RJ. The effects of d-amphetamine sulfate on physical performance. J Sports Phys Med Fitness 1963;3:221.
5. Wyndham CH, et al. Physiological effects of the amphetamines during exercise. S Afr Med J 1971;45:247.
6. Pierson WR, et al. Some psychological effects of the administration of amphetamine sulfate and meprobamate on speed of movement and reaction time. Med Sci Sports 1961;12:61.
7. McKenzie RE, Elliot LL. Effects of secobarbital and d-amphetamine on performance during a simulated air mission. Aerospace Med 1965;36:774.

Ergogenic Effects

Drinking 2.5 cups of regularly percolated coffee 1 hour before exercising extends endurance in strenuous aerobic exercise under laboratory and field conditions, as it also does in shorter duration maximal effort and repeated exercise bouts typical of high-intensity team sports.[28,32,65,66,239] An ergogenic effect even occurs with caffeine ingestion in the minutes just before exercising. Elite distance runners who consumed 10 mg of caffeine per kg of body mass immediately before a treadmill run to exhaustion improved performance time by 1.9% compared with placebo or control conditions.[83] Ergogenic effects during exhaustive exercise at 80% $\dot{V}O_{2max}$ that follows a 5-mg · kg^{-1} caffeine dose is maintained 5 hours later during a subsequent exercise challenge.[17] Thus, there is no need to ingest a smaller additional caffeine dose to preserve high blood caffeine levels to sustain the ergogenic effect during subsequent exercise within 5 hours.

Caffeine and Heart Attacks: Perhaps Risk Relates to Age and How Fast You Metabolize It

Research published in the *Journal of the American Medical Association* indicates that coffee intake may raise heart attack risk, but only if you are younger than age 50 and possess genes that produce the enzyme that metabolizes caffeine slowly (cytochrome P450 1A2). Those who metabolize caffeine rapidly have no increased risk, even if they drink four or more cups of regular coffee daily. The same holds true for slow metabolizers age 60 and older. In contrast, younger slow metabolizers had a 64% higher risk if they drank four cups a day compared to only one cup. If additional research confirms these findings, an easy, effective method must be devised to determine if individuals metabolize caffeine slowly or rapidly.

TABLE 11.6   Caffeine Content (mg) of Some Common Foods, Beverages, and Over-the-Counter and Prescription Medications

Substance	Caffeine content (mg)	Substance	Caffeine content (mg)
Beverages and Foods			
Coffee[a]		Pepsi Cola	38
Coffee, Starbucks, decaf, 12 oz	10	Diet Pepsi, Pepsi Light, Diet RC, RC Cola, Diet Rite	36
Coffee, Starbucks, grande, 16 oz	550		
Coffee, Starbucks, tall, 12 oz	375	Red Bull, 8 oz	80
Coffee, Starbucks, short, 8 oz	250	**Frozen Desserts**	
Caffe, Starbucks, Americano, grande, 16 oz	105	Ben and Jerry's no fat coffee fudge frozen yogurt, 1 cup	85
Caffe, Starbucks, Americano, tall, 12 oz	70	Starbucks coffee ice cream, assorted flavors, 1 cup	40–60
Caffe, Starbucks, Americano, short, 8 oz	35	Haagen-Dazs coffee ice cream, 1 cup	58
Caffe, Starbucks, latte or cappucinno, grande, 16 oz	70	Haagen-Dazs coffee frozen yogurt, fat-free, 1 cup	42
Caffe Mocha, Starbucks, short (8 oz) or tall (12 oz)	35	Haagen-Dazs coffee fudge ice cream, low-fat, 1 cup	30
Espresso, Starbucks, 8 oz	280		
Brewed, drip method	110–150	Starbucks frappuccino bar, 1 bar (2.5 oz)	15
Brewed, percolator	64–124		
Instant	40–108	Healthy Choice cappuccino, chocolate chunk, or cappuccino mocha fudge ice cream, 1 cup	8
Espresso	100		
Decaffeinated, brewed or instant; Sanka	2–5	**Over-the-counter Products**	
Coffe Frappuccino, Starbucks, grande, 16 oz	170	**Cold remedies**	
		Dristan, Coryban-D, Triaminicin, Sinarest	30–31
Tea, 5 oz cup[a]		Excedrin	65
Brewed, 1 min	9–33	Actifed, Contac, Comtrex, Sudafed	0
Brewed, 3 min	20–46	**Diuretics**	
Brewed, 5 min	20–50	Aqua-ban	200
Nestea Sweetened Lemon Ice Tea	20	Pre-Mens Forte	100
Iced tea, 12 oz; instant tea	12–36	Pain remedies	
Green tea, 8oz	30	Vanquish	33
Chocolate		Anacin; Midol	32
Baker's semi-sweet, 1 oz; Baker's chocolate chips, 1/4 cup	13	Aspirin, any brand; Bufferin, Tylenol, Excedrin P.M.	0
Cocoa, 5 oz cup, made from mix	6–10	**Stimulants**	
Milk chocolate candy, 1 oz	6	Vivarin tablet, NoDoz maximum strength caplet, Caffedrine	200
Sweet/dark chocolate, 1 oz	20		
Baking chocolate, 1 oz	35	NoDoz tablet	100
Chocolate bar, 3.5 oz	12–15	Enerjets lozenges	75
Jello chocolate fudge mousse	12	**Weight control aids**	
Ovaltine	0	Dexatrim, Dietac	200
Soft Drinks		Prolamine	140
7-Eleven Big Gulp Cola, 64 oz	190	**Pain drugs**[b]	
Jolt	100	Cafergot	100
Sugar Free Mr. Pibb	59	Migrol	50
Mellow Yellow, Mountain Dew	53–54	Fiorinal	40
Tab	47	Darvon	32
Coca Cola, Diet Coke, 7-Up Gold	46		
Shasta-Cola, Cherry Cola, Diet Cola	44		
Dr. Pepper, Mr. Pibb	40–41		
Dr. Pepper, sugar free	40		

Data from product labels and manufacturers, and National Soft Drink Association, 1997.
[a]*Brewing tea or coffee for longer periods slightly increases the caffeine content.*
[b]*Prescription, 1 oz ; 30 mL.*

Caffeinism

Refers to caffeine intoxication characterized by restlessness, tremulousness, nervousness, excitement, insomnia, flushed face, diuresis, gastrointestinal complaints, rambling flow of thought and speech, tachycardia or cardiac arrhythmia, periods of inexhaustibility, and/or psychomotor agitation.

FIGURE 11.8 shows that subjects exercised for 90.2 minutes with 330 mg of pre-exercise caffeine compared with 75.5 minutes without it. Despite similar heart rate and oxygen uptake values during the two trials, the caffeine made the work "feel easier." Consuming caffeine 60 minutes before exercise in-

creased exercise fat catabolism and reduced carbohydrate oxidation as assessed by plasma glycerol and free fatty acids levels and the respiratory quotient. The ergogenic effect of caffeine on endurance performance also applies to similar exercise performed at high ambient temperatures.[48]

Caffeine provides an ergogenic benefit during maximal swimming for durations less than 25 minutes. In a double-blind, crossover research design, competent male and female distance swimmers (<25 min for 1500-m swims) consumed caffeine (6 mg · kg body mass^{-1}) 2.5 hours before swimming 1500 m. FIGURE 11.9 illustrates that split times improved with caffeine for each 500-m of the swim. Total swim time averaged 1.9% faster with caffeine than without it (20:58.6 vs 21:21.8). Enhanced performance associated with lower plasma potassium concentration before exercise and higher blood glucose levels at the end of the trial. These responses

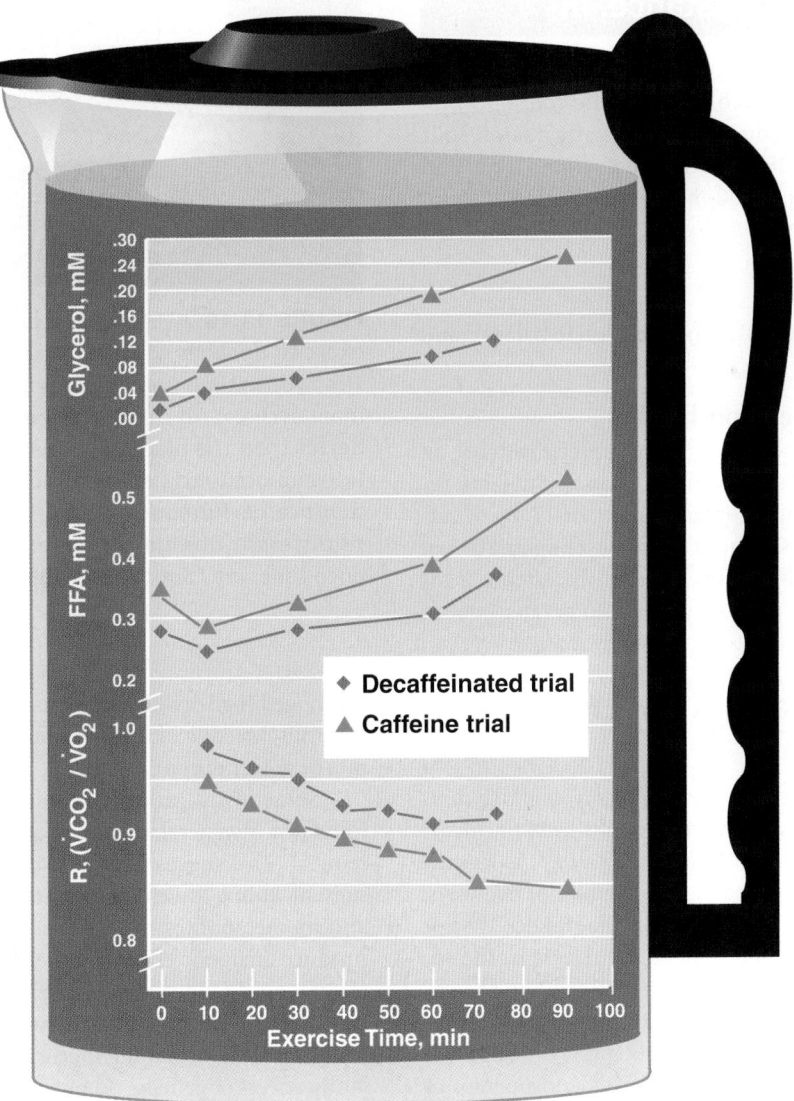

FIGURE 11.8 ■ Average values for plasma glycerol, free fatty acids *(FFA)*, and the respiratory exchange ratio *(R)* during endurance exercise trials after ingesting caffeine and decaffeinated liquids. (From Costill DL, et al. Effects of caffeine ingestion on metabolism and exercise performance. *Med Sci Sports* 1978;10:155.)

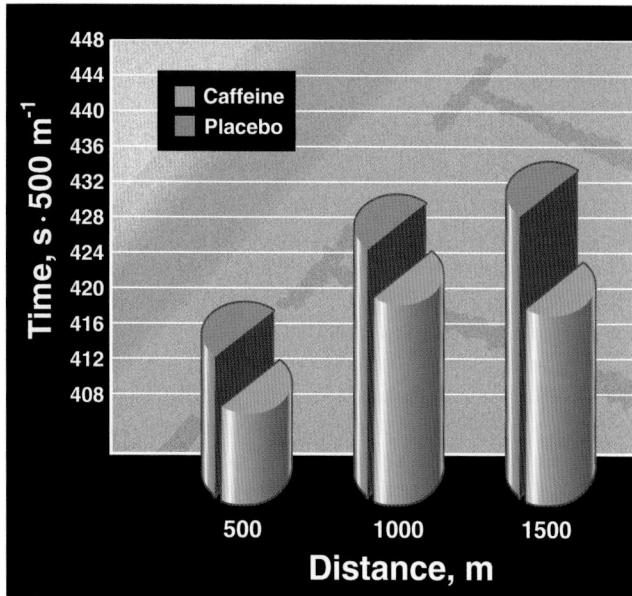

FIGURE 11.9 ■ Split times for each 500-m of a 1500-m swim for caffeine *(light purple)* and placebo *(dark purple)* time trials. Caffeine produced significantly faster split times. (From MacIntosh BR, Wright BM. Caffeine ingestion and performance of a 1,500-metre swim. *Can J Appl Physiol* 1995;20:168.)

suggest a possible caffeine effect on electrolyte balance and glucose availability.

No Dose-Response Relationship

FIGURE 11.10 illustrates the effects of pre-exercise caffeine on endurance time of well-trained male cyclists. Subjects received a placebo or a capsule containing 5, 9, or 13 mg of caffeine per kg of body mass 1 hour before cycling at 80% of maximal power output on a $\dot{V}O_{2max}$ test. All caffeine trials improved exercise performance by 24%. No greater benefit occurred for quantities above 5 mg · kg body mass^{-1}.

Proposed Mechanism for Ergogenic Action

The ergogenic effect of caffeine (or related methylxanthine compounds) in intense, endurance exercise results from the facilitated use of fat as an exercise fuel, thus sparing the limited glycogen reserves. Caffeine probably acts in either of two ways: (1) directly on adipose and peripheral vascular tissues,[93,252] or (2) indirectly from stimulating epinephrine release by the adrenal medulla; epinephrine then acts to inhibit adipocyte cell adenosine receptors that normally repress lipolysis.[190]

Caffeine's inhibition of adenosine receptors on adipocyte cells increases cellular levels of cyclic-3′,5′-adenosine monophosphate (cyclic-AMP). Cyclic-AMP, in turn, activates hormone-sensitive lipases to promote lipolysis, which releases free fatty acids into the plasma. Increased levels of free fatty acids contribute to increased fat oxidation, thus conserving liver and muscle glycogen. Sparing glycogen reserves benefits

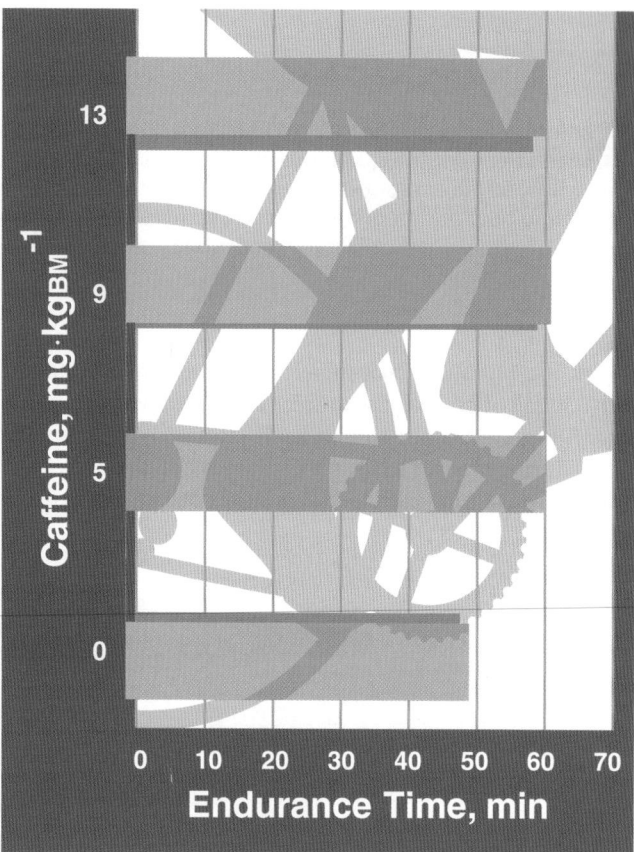

FIGURE 11.10 ■ Endurance performances following pre-exercise dosages of caffeine in different concentrations. The cycling time (min) represents the average for the nine male cyclists. All of the caffeine trials were significantly better than the placebo condition. No dose-response relationship occurred between caffeine concentration and endurance performance. (From Pasman WJ, et al. The effect of different dosages of caffeine on endurance performance time. *Int J Sports Med* 1995;16:225.)

prolonged high-intensity exercise; diminished glycogen in active muscles coincides with reduced capacity to sustain a high rate of power output.

Some investigators have found the ergogenic effect to be unrelated to general hormonal or metabolic changes with caffeine.[245] This suggests possible caffeine action on specific tissues, including those of the central nervous system.[127] Caffeine and its metabolites readily cross the blood–brain barrier to produce analgesic effects on the central nervous system. This effect would reduce the perception of effort and muscle pain during exercise.[182] Caffeine also enhances motoneuronal excitability, thus facilitating motor unit recruitment. The stimulating effects of caffeine do not result from its direct action on the central nervous system. Rather, caffeine indirectly stimulates the nervous system by blocking another chemical neuromodulator, adenosine, which calms brain and spinal cord neurons. Four factors likely interact to produce caffeine's facilitating effect on neuromuscular activity:

1. Lowered threshold for motor unit recruitment
2. Altered excitation/contraction coupling
3. Facilitated nerve transmission
4. Increased ion transport within the muscle itself

Conflicting evidence concerns the effect of pre-exercise caffeine on $\dot{V}O_{2max}$. Little effect has been noted for caffeine on repeated 20-m sprint running performance for team-sport female athletes.[201]

Effects Are Often Inconsistent

Prior nutrition partly accounts for the variation frequently observed among individuals in their exercise response after consuming caffeine. While caffeine generally elicits group improvements in endurance, individuals who normally consume a high-carbohydrate diet show little effect of caffeine on free fatty acid mobilization.[265] Individual differences in caffeine sensitivity, tolerance, and hormonal response from short- and long-term patterns of caffeine consumption also affect this drug's ergogenic qualities.[40,62] Interestingly, the ergogenic effects on endurance occur less for caffeine in coffee than for an equivalent dose from a caffeine capsule in water.[94] Apparently, components in coffee antagonize caffeine's actions. Beneficial effects do not consistently occur among habitual caffeine users[251,253]; thus, an athlete must consider "caffeine tolerance" before assuming it provides a consistent benefit to all persons.

Most Effective Way to Benefit

From a practical standpoint, individuals should omit caffeine-containing foods and beverages 4 to 6 days before competition to optimze caffeine's potential for ergogenic effects.

Effects on Muscle

Caffeine acts directly on muscle to enhance exercise capacity.[127,176,217,241] A double-blind research design study evaluated voluntary and electrically stimulated muscle actions under "caffeine-free" conditions and following oral administration of 500 mg of caffeine.[157] Electrically stimulating the motor nerve enabled the researchers to remove central nervous system control and quantify caffeine's direct effects on skeletal muscle. Caffeine produced no effect on maximal muscle force during voluntary or electrically stimulated muscle actions. For submaximal effort, however, caffeine increased force output for low-frequency electrical stimulation before and after muscle fatigue. In addition, caffeine extended time to exhaustion on short-term tests of anaerobic power.[19] Pre-exercise caffeine administration also increased by 17% repeated submaximum isometric muscular endurance.[203] Caffeine probably exerts a direct and specific effect on skeletal muscle and its sensory processes during repetitive stimulation. Perhaps caffeine increases the sarcoplasmic reticulum's permeability to Ca^{2+}, thus making this mineral readily available for contraction. Caffeine could also influence the myofibril's sensitivity to Ca^{2+} to augment excitation–contraction coupling. In Chapter 12, we discuss how caffeine diminishes the ergogenic effect of creatine supplementation on short-term muscular power.

Warning About Caffeine

Individuals who normally avoid caffeine can experience undesirable side effects when they consume it. Caffeine stimulates the central nervous system and in quantities greater than 1.5 g per day, can produce typical symptoms of caffeinism: restlessness, headaches, insomnia, and nervous irritability, muscle twitching, tremulousness, psychomotor agitation, and elevated heart rate and blood pressure and trigger premature left ventricular contractions. From the standpoint of temperature regulation, caffeine's effect as a potent diuretic could cause unnecessary pre-exercise loss of fluid that negatively affects thermal balance and exercise performance in a hot environment. This dehydrating effect is probably minimal when consumed in fluids during exercise because (1) an exercise-induced catecholamine release greatly reduces renal blood flow (and thus urine production) and (2) enhanced renal solute reabsorption in exercise facilitates water conservation (osmotic effect).[74,266]

Normal caffeine intake generally poses no significant health risk, yet death from caffeine overdose has occurred. The LD_{50} (lethal oral dose required to kill 50% of the population) for caffeine is estimated at 10 g (150 mg · kg body mass^{-1}). Thus, for a 50-kg woman, acute health risk occurs at a caffeine intake of 7.5 g. Moderate caffeine toxicity has been reported in small children consuming 35 mg · kg body mass^{-1}. Such observations provide clear indication of the *inverted U-shaped relationship* between certain exogenous chemicals and exercise performance (and health and safety). For caffeine, if ingesting small-to-moderate quantities produces desirable effects, consuming significant excess can wreak havoc.

GINSENG AND EPHEDRINE

Ginseng and ephedrine are botanical remedies commonly marketed as nutritional supplements to "reduce tension," "revitalize," "burn calories," and "optimize mental and physical performance," particularly during times of fatigue and stress. The herb ginseng also plays a role as an alternative therapy to treat diabetes, stimulate immune function, and counter male impotence. Clinically, 1 to 3 g of ginseng administered 40 minutes before an oral glucose challenge reduces postprandial glycemia in nondiabetic subjects.[260] As with caffeine, ephedrine and ginseng occur naturally and for years have been used in folk medicine to enhance "energy."

Ginseng

Currently used in Asian medicine to prolong life, strengthen and restore sexual functions, and invigorate the body, the **ginseng** root (*Panax ginseng* C.A., Meyer), often sold as Panax or Chinese or Korean ginseng, currently serves no recognized medical use in the United States except as a soothing agent in skin ointments. Commercial ginseng root preparations generally take the form of powder, liquid, tablets, or capsules; widely marketed foods and beverages also contain various types and amounts of ginsenosides.

No Guarantee As To Purity: What You See May Not Be What You Get

Dietary supplements need not meet the same quality control for purity and potency as pharmaceuticals; this allows for considerable variation in the concentrations of marker compounds for ginseng, including levels of potentially harmful impurities and toxins such as pesticide and heavy metal contamination.[102] Neither the FDA nor other state or federal agencies routinely test ginseng-containing products or other nutritional supplements for quality or purity.

A common claim for ginseng in the Western world is its ability to boost energy and diminish the negative effects of overall stress on the body. Reports of an ergogenic effect often appear in nontraditional journals.[33] Some peer-reviewed research has demonstrated a facilitating effect of ginseng on endurance performance and recovery from exercise.[137,153] However, a review of the majority of research on the topic provides little objective evidence to support the effectiveness of ginseng as an ergogenic aid.[4,15,91] For example, volunteers consumed either 200 or 400 mg of the standardized ginseng concentrate each day for 8 weeks in a double-blind research protocol.[71] Neither treatment affected submaximal or maximal exercise performance, ratings of perceived exertion, or physiologic parameters of heart rate, oxygen consumption, or blood lactate concentrations. Similarly, no ergogenic effects emerged on diverse physiologic and performance variables following a 1-week treatment with a ginseng saponin extract administered in two doses of either 8 or 16 mg per kg of body mass.[179] When effectiveness has been demonstrated, the research has failed to use adequate controls, placebos, or double-blind testing protocols.[77] At present, no compelling scientific evidence exists that ginseng supplementation offers any ergogenic benefit for physiologic function or exercise performance.[154,258]

Ephedrine

Based on an analysis of existing data, including commissioning a safety study by an independent research group (the Rand Corporation), the FDA announced in April, 2004 a ban on ephedra, the first time this federal agency has moved to ban a dietary supplement.

Unlike with ginseng, Western medicine recognizes the potent amphetamine-like alkaloid compound ephedrine (with sympathomimetic physiologic effects) found in several species of the plant ephedra (dried plant stem called ma huang [ma wong; *Ephedra sinica*]). The ephedra plant contains two major active components first isolated in 1928,

ephedrine and pseudoephedrine, which exert weaker effects than ephedrine. The medicinal role of this herb has included use to treat asthma, symptoms of the common cold, hypotension, and urinary incontinence and as a central stimulant to treat depression. Physicians in the United States discontinued using ephedrine as a decongestant and asthma treatment in the 1930s in favor of safer medications. The milder pseudoephedrine remains common in nonprescription cold and flu medications and has been clinically used to treat mucosal congestion that accompanies hay fever, allergic rhinitis, sinusitis, and other respiratory conditions. In January 2004, it was removed from the banned substances list by the IOC and placed on its monitoring program because of lack of evidence showing ergogenic effect. It is now banned.

Ephedrine exerts both central and peripheral effects, with the latter reflected in increased heart rate, cardiac output, and blood pressure. Owing to its β-adrenergic effect, ephedrine produces bronchodilation in the lungs. High ephedrine dosages can produce hypertension, insomnia, hyperthermia, and cardiac arrhythmias. Other possible side effects include dizziness, restlessness, anxiety, irritability, personality changes, gastrointestinal symptoms, and difficulty concentrating.

The potent physiologic effects of ephedrine have led researchers to investigate its potential as an ergogenic aid—sold commercially (before its ban by the FDA) as *Ripped Fuel, Metabolift, Xenadrine RFA-1, Hyrocut,* and *ThermoSpeed*. No effect of a 40-mg dose of ephedrine occurred on indirect indicators of exercise performance or ratings of perceived exertion (RPE).[59] The less concentrated pseudoephedrine also produced no effect on $\dot{V}O_{2max}$, RPE, aerobic cycling efficiency, anaerobic power output (Wingate test), time to exhaustion on a bicycle ergometer,[110,242] and a 40-km cycling trial,[88] or physiologic and performance measures during 20 minutes of running at 70% of $\dot{V}O_{2max}$ followed by a 5000-m time trial.[44] Conversely, a series of double-blind, placebo-controlled studies by the Canadian Defense and Civil Institute of Environmental Medicine using relatively high pre-exercise ephedrine dosage (0.8–1.0 mg $\cdot$ kg body mass^{-1}), either alone or combined with caffeine, produced small but statistically significant effects on endurance performance[16,18,20] and anaerobic power output during the early phase of the Wingate test.[19] Also, ephedrine supplementation increased muscular endurance during the first set of traditional resistance-training exercise.[120] Recent research has demonstrated improved 1500-m running performance with no reported side effects by male athletes who receive 2.5 mg of ephedrine per kg of body mass compared to a maltodextrin placebo 90 minutes before the all-out run trial.[112] Ergogenic effects were attributed to central nervous system effects rather than to altered metabolism.

Numerous anecdotal reports exist of adverse effects from ephedra-containing compounds, but a cause-and-effect relationship between use and untoward responses, including death, remains hotly debated. On February 28, 2003, the FDA (www.fda.gov) ordered that a prominent warning label be emblazoned on the front of all ephedra products, listing death, heart attack, or stroke as possible consequences of use.

The IOC and NCAA currently ban ephedrine use, and the National Football League (NFL; 2007–2008) represents the first professional sports league to do so. Professional baseball also bans ephedrine use. As of July 1, 2002, the NFL tested for this stimulant under the league's Policy on Anabolic Steroids and Related Substances. Any player who tests positive for ephedra is subject to a four-game suspension. Many players have acknowledged using the herbal stimulant seeking to lose weight or get a "quick burst of energy." The rationale for testing put forth by the NFL and the NFL Players Association was the growing evidence linking ephedrine-containing products to life-threatening strokes, seizures, thermoregulatory disorders that predispose to heat stroke, and heart arrhythmia.

ALCOHOL

Alcohol, more specifically ethyl alcohol or ethanol (a form of carbohydrate), classifies as a depressant drug. Alcohol provides 7 kCal of energy per gram (mL) of pure (100% or 200 proof) substance. Adolescents and adults, athletes and nonathletes, abuse alcohol more than any other drug in the United States.[100,101]

Alcohol Use Among Athletes

Statistics remain equivocal about alcohol use among athletes compared with the general population. In a study of athletes in Italy, 330 male high school nonathletes consumed more beer, wine, and hard liquor and had greater episodes of heavy drinking (including greater cigarette smoking rates) than 336 athletes.[67] Interestingly, the strongest predictor of the participants' alcohol consumption was their best friend and girlfriend's drinking habits. In other research, physically active men drank less alcohol than sedentary counterparts.[99] Some athletes possess a more negative attitude about drinking than the general population,[197] but collegiate athletes generally drink more heavily and are more likely to drive while intoxicated than their nonathletic peers.[185] In a sample of former world-class Finnish athletes who competed between 1920 and 1965, the current alcohol consumption of the endurance athletes (average age, 57.5 years) was less than that of an age-matched control group.[73] A study of the relationship between athletic participation and depression, suicidal ideation, and substance use among high school students in Kentucky reported no greater alcohol consumption for 823 athletes than for the school's general student body.[194] Athletes also reported less depression, thoughts about suicide, and cigarette smoking and marijuana use than nonathletes. Teenage male athletes also drank 25.5% less beer and 39.9% less wine and whiskey than nonathletes.[78]

Several studies indicate that athletes are more likely to engage in binge drinking.[142,150,186] A self-reported questionnaire assessed alcohol intake of randomly selected students in a representative national sample of 4-year colleges in the United States.[187] Compared with nonathletic students, athletes were at high risk for binge drinking (≥5 alcoholic drinks on at least one occasion in the past 2 weeks for men and ≥4 for women),

heavier alcohol use, and a greater number in drinking-related harm. Athletes were also more likely than nonathletes to surround themselves with (1) others who binge drink and (2) a social environment conducive to excessive alcohol consumption. These findings support the position that future alcohol prevention programs targeted to athletes should address the unique social and environmental influences that affect the current athletes' heavier alcohol use.

TABLE 11.7 compares serious male and female recreational runners and matched controls on responses to the Michigan Alcoholism Screening Test (MAST).[98] Male runners drank more (14.2 vs 5.4 drinks per week) and felt guiltier about their drinking behavior (26.6%) than nonexercising controls (3.8%). Male and female runners drank more frequently than controls (2.8 vs 2.3 times per week), while runners with MAST scores suggesting a history of problems with alcohol drank less than nonathletic controls with a similar score. Men also consumed more alcohol and drank more frequently (including binge drinking) than women. This study illustrates that problems associated with alcohol consumption do not exclude adult runners. However, running may serve as a healthy substitute for runners prone to alcoholic behavior.

Alcohol's Action and Effect on Athletic Performance

Levels of Alcohol in Beverages and in the Body

One alcoholic drink contains 1.0 oz (28 g or 28 mL) of 100 proof (50%) alcohol. This translates into 12 oz of regular beer (about 4% alcohol by volume) or 5 oz of wine (11–14% alcohol by volume). The stomach absorbs between 15 and 25% of the alcohol ingested. The small intestine rapidly takes up the remainder for distribution throughout the body's water compartments, particularly the water-rich tissues of the central nervous system. The absence of food in the digestive tract facilitates alcohol absorption. The liver, the major organ for alcohol metabolism, removes alcohol at a rate of about 10 g per hour, equivalent to the alcohol content of one drink. Consequently, consuming more than one drink per hour increases blood alcohol concentration, expressed in grams per deciliter $(g \cdot dL^{-1})$.

Consuming two alcoholic drinks in 1 hour produces a blood alcohol concentration between 0.04 and 0.05 $g \cdot dL^{-1}$. However, factors such as age, body mass, body fat content, and gender influence blood alcohol level. Depending on the state, the legal limit for alcohol intoxication generally ranges between a blood alcohol concentration of 0.11 and 0.16 $g \cdot dL^{-1}$. Blood alcohol concentration above 0.40 (≥19 drinks in 2 hours) leads to coma, respiratory depression, and eventual death.

Psychologic and Physiologic Effects

Athletes use alcohol to enhance performance because of its psychologic and physiologic effects. In the psychologic realm, some have argued that alcohol before competition reduces tension and anxiety (**anxiolytic effect**), enhances self-confidence, and promotes aggressiveness. It also facilitates neuro-

---

TABLE 11.7   Responses from Male and Female Recreational Runners and Matched Controls to the Shortened[a] and Brief[b] Versions of the Michigan Alcoholism Screening Test (MAST)

MAST Item	Men (N = 536)		Women (N = 262)	
	Runners, % (N)	Controls, % (N)	Runners, % (N)	Controls, % (N)
1. I am not a normal drinker.[a,b]	19.1 (75)	22.8 (31)	12.1 (17)	13.9 (16)
2. My friends and relatives think I'm not a normal drinker.[a,b]	14.5 (56)	22.8 (31)	10.1 (14)	13.0 (15)
3. Attended Alcoholics Anonymous for drinking.[a,b]	4.5 (18)	8.9 (12)	2.1 (3)	4.3 (5)
4. Lost friends because of drinking.[a]	6.1 (24)	7.9 (11)	1.4 (2)	4.3 (5)
5. Trouble at work because of drinking.[a,b]	3.8 (15)	5.0 (7)	0.7 (1)	3.4 (4)
6. Feel guilty about drinking.[b]	26.6 105)	13.8 (19)	16.7 (24)	15.5 (18)
7. Neglected obligations, family, work for 2 or more days in a row due to drinking.[a,b]	4.8 (19)	5.0 (7)	1.4 (2)	0.9 (1)
8. Experienced delirium tremens.[a]	4.3 (17)	2.9 (4)	0.7 (1)	3.4 (4)
9. Unable to stop drinking when desired.[b]	5.4 (21)	7.2 (10)	4.3 (6)	3.4 (4)
10. Sought help for drinking.[a,b]	5.3 (21)	7.2 (10)	2.1 (3)	6.0 (7)
11. Hospitalized for drinking.[a,b]	1.5 (6)	4.3 (6)	0.7 (1)	3.4 (4)
12. Drinking caused problems with spouse, parent, or other relative.[b]	20.6 (81)	21.0 (29)	2.8 (4)	8.5 (10)
13. Arrested for drunk driving.[a,b]	9.4 (37)	11.5 (16)	2.8 (4)	2.6 (3)
14. Arrested for drunken behavior.[b]	5.5 (22)	5.8 (8)	0.7 (1)	1.7 (2)

Adapted from Gutgesell M, et al. Reported alcohol use and behavior in long-distance runners. Med Sci Sports Exerc 1996;28:1063.

[a]*Shortened MAST; from Binokur A, VanRooijen I. A self-administered Short Michigan Alcoholism Screening Test (SMAST). J Stud Alcohol 1975;36:117.*

[b]*Brief MAST; from Pokorny AD, et al. The brief MAST: a shortened version of the Michigan Alcoholism Screening Test. Am J Psychiatry 1972;129:342.*

---

logic "disinhibition" because of its initial, though transitory, stimulatory effect. Thus, the athlete believes that alcohol facilitates physical performance at or close to physiologic capacity, particularly for activities requiring maximal strength and power. *Research does not substantiate any ergogenic effect of alcohol on muscular strength, short-term anaerobic power, or longer term aerobic activities.*

Initially acting as a stimulant, alcohol's ultimate effect produces generalized central neurologic depression (memory, visual perception, speech, motor coordination).[228] These effects relate directly to blood alcohol concentration. Damping of psychomotor function causes the antitremor effect of alcohol ingestion. Consequently, alcohol use has been particularly prevalent in rifle and pistol shooting and archery, which require steadiness and accuracy. Achieving an antitremor effect also provides the primary rationale for using drugs called β-blockers, such as propranolol, which diminish the arousal effect of sympathetic stimulation. Most research indicates that alcohol at best provides no ergogenic benefit; at worst, it precipitates undesirable side effects that impair performance (**ergolytic effect**). For example, alcohol's depression of nervous system function profoundly impairs all sports performances requiring balance, hand–eye coordination, reaction time, and overall need to process information rapidly. Although these effects vary considerably among individuals, they become apparent in a dose–response relationship at blood alcohol levels

above $0.05 \text{ g} \cdot \text{dL}^{-1}$. In the extreme, it seems unlikely that a legally intoxicated person or team could perform optimally in competitive sports such as ping pong, volleyball, baseball, tennis, gymnastics, diving, soccer, or figure skating.

Alcohol impairs cardiac function. Ingesting 1 g of alcohol per kg of body mass during 1 hour raised blood alcohol level to just over $0.10 \text{ g} \cdot \text{dL}^{-1}$.[147] This level, often observed among "social drinkers," acutely depresses myocardial contractility. In terms of metabolism, alcohol blunts the liver's capacity to synthesize glucose from noncarbohydrate sources via gluconeogenesis. Each of these effects impairs performance in high-intensity aerobic activities that rely heavily on cardiovascular capacity and energy from carbohydrate catabolism. Alcohol provides no benefit as an energy substrate and does not favorably alter the metabolic mixture in endurance exercise. In addition, substituting alcohol for high glycemic carbohydrates in the postexercise replenishment period decreases optimal glycogen storage in recovery.[35]

Alcohol and Fluid Replacement

Alcohol exaggerates the dehydrating effect of exercise in a warm environment; it acts as a potent diuretic by depressing antidiuretic hormone release from the posterior pituitary and blunting the arginine–vasopressin response.[221] Both of these effects impair thermoregulation during heat stress, thus placing the athlete at greater risk for heat injury during exercise.

Case Study

Personal Health and Exercise Nutrition 11–1

Alcohol Metabolism and Use: The Correct Approach

Background

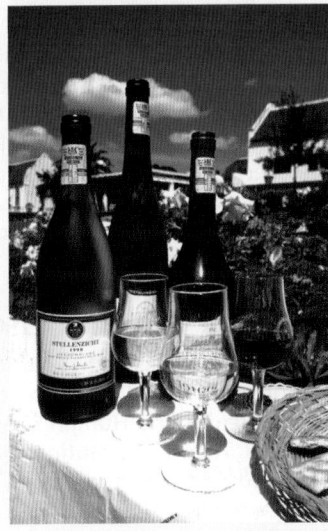

Abraham Lincoln, who enjoyed whiskey every now and then, once said, "It is true that many were injured by intoxicating drink, but none seemed to think the injury arose from the use of a bad thing, but from the abuse of a very good thing." President Lincoln most likely knew little about the medicinal benefits of "lighter drinking"; he simply enjoyed an occasional drink, like many persons in present-day society.

Alcohol abuse among college students, however, remains a persistent problem, representing the leading cause of death among individuals between ages 15 and 24. In America, more than 100,000 people die each year from alcohol-related deaths (mostly related to driving). Advertisers have touted the health benefits of "light" drinking. Many individuals have used this as justification to increase alcohol consumption.

Much confusion exists regarding (1) alcohols' metabolic effects, (2) defining levels of intake, (3) determining safe intake limits, and (4) the role of alcohol as a nutrient.

Alcohol Chemistry and Metabolism

Some alcohol metabolizes in the cells lining the stomach, while most breaks down in the liver. About 10% is directly eliminated by diffusion through the kidneys or the lungs. From a structural standpoint, ethanol contains a hydroxyl group (OH^-) and therefore resembles a carbohydrate. Because it converts directly to acetyl-CoA during catabolism, it does not proceed through glycolysis, in contrast to glucose and glycogen breakdown. Consequently, ethanol cannot provide substrate for glucose synthesis (gluconeogenesis). In metabolic terms, alcohol metabolizes more like a lipid than a sugar.

Alcohol concentration varies with the type of beverage. "Proof" value indicates its concentration, which equals two times the percentage concentration. For example, an 80-proof beverage contains 40% alcohol. When discussing alcohol consumption, "one drink" refers to a 12-oz bottle of beer, a 5-oz glass of table wine, or a cocktail with 1.5 oz of 80-proof liquor. Each of these drinks contains about 0.6 oz of alcohol by weight.

ALCOHOL METABOLISM WITH LOW BLOOD ALCOHOL LEVELS

At low consumption and correspondingly low blood levels, alcohol reacts with nicotinamide adenine dinucleotide (NAD) in the cell's cytosol to form acetaldehyde and NADH under the influence of the zinc-requiring enzyme alcohol dehydrogenase. Acetaldehyde then converts to acetyl-CoA (see Chapter 4) to yield more NADH. Acetyl-CoA enters the citric acid cycle; the NADH, $FADH_2$, and guanosine triphosphate molecules produced in acetaldehyde and acetyl-CoA formation and in the citric acid cycle provide energy to synthesize ATP (see figure below).

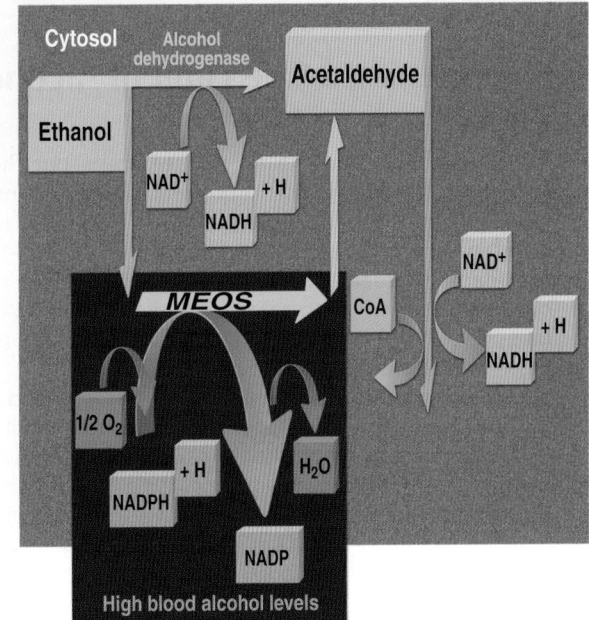

ALCOHOL METABOLISM WITH HIGH BLOOD ALCOHOL LEVELS

When blood alcohol levels increase with high alcohol intake, alcohol dehydrogenase cannot sustain the metabolism of all alcohol into acetaldehyde. In this situation, an alternative metabolic pathway, the microsomal ethanol-oxidizing system (MEOS), becomes activated. MEOS uses considerable energy to break down alcohol, in contrast to the simpler alcohol dehydrogenase pathway that readily produces useful energy as ATP. Normally, the MEOS metabolizes drugs and other "foreign" substances

Case Study

in the liver. Under the stress of excessive alcohol intake, the liver "registers" alcohol as a foreign substance for breakdown by MEOS. Chronic MEOS activation increases alcohol tolerance because high alcohol intake proportionally increases its rate of breakdown.

Rather than forming NADH by use of alcohol dehydrogenase (as occurs with moderate alcohol intake), the MEOS uses nicotinamide adenine dinucleotide phosphate (NADPH), a compound similar to NADH. However, instead of yielding potential ATP molecules via formation of NADH from the first step in alcohol breakdown, MEOS uses potential ATP energy (in the form of NADPH) as NADPH converts to NADP. The use of different pathways to catabolize alcohol, depending on intake level, helps to explain why alcoholics do not gain the weight expected based on the alcohol-derived energy consumed. High alcohol use damages liver function in a manner that hampers other metabolic pathways. This cascading effect also contributes to the reduced energy yield associated with high alcohol use. In addition, alcohol increases metabolic rate to further contribute to an alcoholic's increased weight loss.

Determining a Safe Limit of Alcohol Intake

Arbitrary limits define a "safe" alcohol intake, but "light," "moderate," and "heavy" represent the most common classifications. Historically, Anstie's rule (attributed to the British neurologist Sir Francis Edmund Anstie [1833–1874]) provided a frequently used operational definition, based on a person's ability to safely "handle" alcohol. At the time, the safe level for a typical male amounted to about three standard drinks daily (over 8 hours).

We now know that three factors—age, sex, and body weight (size)—determine a person's ability to "handle" alcohol. For a standard alcohol intake, blood alcohol levels inversely relate to body weight; the lower the weight, the greater is the effect. Blood alcohol levels below 0.01% almost never impair function; levels from 0.01 to 0.04% sometimes impair function; 0.05 to 0.07% usually impair function; and levels of 0.08% and above always impair function. For most individuals who weigh less than 170 lb, blood alcohol levels achieve the usually impaired level with only two drinks over 2 hours. For those who exceed 170 lb, three drinks in 2 hours impair function. Consequently, consuming no more than two drinks daily classifies as light-to-moderate drinking.

Benefits and Risks of Light-to-Moderate Drinking

For adults older than 18 years, light-to-moderate drinking associates with a lower risk of coronary heart dis-

ease, decreased incidence of ischemic stroke, and reduced occurrence of gallstones compared with alcohol abstinence. Moderate drinking is not risk free, however. Obviously, any level of drinking increases addiction risk, particularly for individuals with a family history of alcoholism. Links exist between light-to-moderate drinking and female breast cancer risk, harm to the fetus, and increased colon cancer risk in men and women.

Risks of Heavy Drinking

Heavy drinkers experience the highest overall risk of morbidity (contracting illness) and mortality, compared with nondrinkers or to those who drink moderately. Heavy drinking associates with diverse health problems including cirrhosis of the liver, inflammation of the pancreas and stomach, certain cancers, high blood pressure, diseases of the heart muscle, heart arrhythmias, hemorrhagic stroke, and increased accidents and suicide.

General Guidelines for Alcohol Use

Neither the Surgeon General's office, the National Academy of Science, nor the U.S. Department of Agriculture/ Department of Health and Human Services recommends drinking alcohol. All groups caution that if adults consume alcohol, it should be in moderation and with meals (no more than two drinks a day for men and one for women). Avoid drinking any alcohol before or while driving, operating machinery, taking medications, or engaging in other activity requiring sound judgment; no alcohol should be consumed while pregnant.

Do You Have a Problem?

Asking a person about the quantity and frequency of alcohol consumption provides an important means to detect abuse and dependence. The following CAGE questionnaire is popular for use in routine health care.

CAGE Questionnaire to Screen for Alcohol Abuse

C: Have you ever felt you ought to CUT down on drinking?

A: Have people ANNOYED you by criticizing your drinking?

G: Have you ever felt bad or GUILTY about your drinking?

E: Have you ever had a drink first thing in the morning to steady your nerves or get rid of a hangover (EYE-OPENER)?

More than one positive response to the CAGE questionnaire suggests an alcohol problem.

Marks DB, et al. Basic Medical Biochemistry. Baltimore: Williams & Wilkins, 1996.

Mayfield D, et al. The CAGE questionnaire: validation of a new alcoholism instrument. Am J Psychiatry 1974;131:1121.

Suter PM. Effects of alcohol on energy metabolism and body weight regulation: is alcohol a risk factor for obesity. Nutr Rev 1997;55:157

Because many athletes consume alcohol-containing beverages after exercising or sports competition, one question concerns the degree to which alcohol impairs rehydration in recovery. Alcohol's effect on rehydration has been studied following exercise-induced dehydration of about 2% of body mass.[227,228] Subjects consumed rehydration fluid volumes equivalent to 150% of fluid lost and containing 0, 1, 2, 3, or 4% alcohol. Urine volume produced during the 6-hour study period directly related to the beverage's alcohol concentration—greater alcohol consumption produced more urine. Increases in plasma volume in recovery compared with the dehydrated state averaged 8.1% when the rehydration fluid contained no alcohol, but only 5.3% for the beverage with 4% alcohol content. The bottom line: *Alcohol-containing beverages impede rehydration.*

Alcohol acts as a peripheral vasodilator, so it should not be consumed during cold exposure or to facilitate recovery from hypothermia. A good "stiff drink" just won't warm you up! Debate exists as to whether moderate alcohol intake exacerbates body cooling during mild cold exposure.[124]

No Ergogenic Benefit Whatsoever

The major conclusions of a position statement of the American College of Sports Medicine on alcohol use in sports remain as germane today as when first published in 1982.[6] Two main conclusions emerged:

1. Acute alcohol ingestion impairs psychomotor skill, including reaction time, balance, accuracy, hand–eye coordination, and complex coordination.
2. Alcohol does not improve and may even decrease strength, power, speed, local muscular endurance, and cardiovascular endurance.

Perhaps of Some Benefit

A moderate daily alcohol intake—2 oz or 30 mL of 90-proof alcohol, three 6-oz glasses of wine, or slightly less than three 12-oz beers—reduces a healthy person's risk of heart attack and stroke, independent of physical activity level,[14,70,220] and improves the likelihood of surviving a myocardial infarction.[183] The heart-protective benefit of moderate alcohol consumption also applies to individuals with type 2 diabetes.[247,263] The mechanism for benefit remains elusive, yet moderate alcohol intake increases HDL-C, particularly its subfractions HDL_2 and HDL_3.[86] In addition, certain components of red wine (e.g., polyphenols) may inhibit LDL-C oxidation, thus blunting a critical step in arterial plaque formation.[189,212] Moderate wine intake also associates with more "heart-healthy" dietary choices that positively affect plasma lipids.[244] For nondiabetic postmenopausal women, consuming 30 g (2 drinks) of alcohol each day benefited insulin and triacylglycerol concentrations and insulin sensitivity.[57] In contrast, excessive alcohol consumption offers no lipoprotein benefit and increases liver disease and cancer risk.

BUFFERING SOLUTIONS

Dramatic alterations occur in the acid–base balance of the intracellular and extracellular fluids during maximal exercise of between 30- and 120-seconds duration because the muscle fibers rely predominantly on anaerobic energy transfer. As a result, significant quantities of lactate accumulate, with a concurrent fall in intracellular pH. Increased acidity inhibits the energy transfer and contractile capabilities of active muscle fibers, thereby causing exercise performance to decline.

The **bicarbonate** aspect of the body's buffering system provides a major line of defense against increased intracellular H^+ concentration (see Chapter 3). Maintaining high levels of extracellular bicarbonate rapidly releases H^+ from the cells and delays the onset of intracellular acidosis. Increasing bicarbonate (alkaline) reserves might enhance anaerobic exercise performance because increased H^+ concentration in intense exercise reduces the calcium sensitivity of the contractile proteins, which impairs muscle function.[45,237] Research in this area has produced conflicting results, perhaps from variations in the pre-exercise sodium bicarbonate dose and the type of exercise to evaluate the effects of pre-exercise alkalosis.[95,171,236,249]

To improve experimental design, one early study evaluated the effects of acute induced alkalosis on short-term fatiguing exercise that greatly increased anaerobic metabolites. Trained middle-distance runners ran an 800-m race under normal (control) conditions or after ingesting either a sodium bicarbonate solution (300 mg $\cdot$ kg^{-1} body mass) or a similar quantity of calcium carbonate placebo. TABLE 11.8 shows that the alkaline drink raised pH and standard bicarbonate levels before exercise. Subjects ran an average of 2.9 seconds faster under alkalosis and achieved higher postexercise values for blood lactate, pH, and extracellular H^+ concentration than those under placebo or control conditions.

The ergogenic benefit of pre-exercise alkalosis also occurs in women (FIG. 11.11). Moderately trained women performed one bout of maximal cycle ergometer exercise for 60 seconds on separate days in a double-blind research design under the following conditions: (1) control, no treatment, (2) 300 mg $\cdot$ kg^{-1} body mass dose of sodium bicarbonate in 400 mL of low-calorie flavored water 90 minutes before testing, and (3) placebo of equimolar dose of sodium chloride (to maintain intravascular fluid status as in bicarbonate condition) 90 minutes before testing. Exercise capacity represented total work accomplished during the ride. The figure's inset box shows that total work performed and peak power output reached higher levels with pre-exercise bicarbonate treatment than with either control or placebo conditions. The bicarbonate treatment also produced a higher level of blood lactate in the immediate and 1-minute postexercise periods, which explained the greater anaerobic exercise capacity. Similar benefits of induced alkalosis occur in short-term anaerobic performance using exogenous **sodium citrate** as the alkalinizing agent.[107,169]

Augmented anaerobic energy transfer during exercise probably explains the ergogenic effect of pre-exercise alkalosis.[113,205,207,209] More than likely, increased extracellular

TABLE 11.8 **Performance Time and Acid–Base Profiles for Subjects Under Control (Placebo) and Induced Preexercise Alkalosis Conditions Immediately Before and After an 800-m Race**

Variable	Condition	Pretreatment	Preexercise	Postexercise
pH	Control	7.40	7.39[a]	7.07[b]
	Placebo	7.93	7.40[a]	7.09[b]
	Alkalosis	7.40	7.49[a]	7.18[b]
Lactate (mmol·L^{-1})	Control	1.21	1.15[a]	12.62[b]
	Placebo	1.38	1.23[a]	13.62[b]
	Alkalosis	1.29	1.31[a]	14.29[b]
Standard HCO$_3^-$ (mEq·L^{-1})	Control	25.8	24.5[a]	9.9[b]
	Placebo	25.6	26.2[a]	11.0[b]
	Alkalosis	25.2	33.5[a]	14.3[b]
	Control	**Placebo**	**Alkalosis**	
Performance Time (min)	2:05.8	2:05.1	2:02.9[c]	

From Wilkes D, et al. Effects of induced metabolic alkalosis on 800-m racing time. Med Sci Sports Exerc 1983;15:277.

[a] *Preexercise values significantly higher than pretreatment values.*

[b] *Alkalosis values significantly higher than placebo and control values after exercise.*

[c] *Alkalosis time significantly faster than control and placebo times.*

buffering from exogenous bicarbonate or citrate facilitates coupled transport of lactate and H$^+$ across the muscle cell membrane during anaerobic exercise.[23,126,237] This delays the fall in intracellular pH and its subsequent negative effects on muscle function. Nearly 3 seconds represents a dramatic improvement in 800-m race time; it transposes to a distance of about 19 m at race pace, bringing a last place finisher to first place!

Effects Related to Dosage and Degree of Exercise Anaerobiosis

The interaction between bicarbonate dosage and the cumulative anaerobic nature of the exercise influences the ergogenic effects of pre-exercise alkalosis. Doses of at least 0.3 g · kg^{-1} (ingested about 1–2 hours precompetition) facilitate H$^+$ efflux from the cell. This enhances a single maximal effort of 1 to 2 minutes duration,[90,163,170] including longer term arm or leg exercise that exhausts within 6 to 8 minutes.[214] Even long-term bicarbonate ingestion (0.5 g per kg body mass) for 5 days added to the normal diet raised plasma pH and increased performance in a 60-second maximal effort. No ergogenic effect emerges for typical resistance training exercises (e.g., squat, bench press), perhaps because of the generally lower absolute anaerobic metabolic load compared with continuous, maximal whole-body activities. Bicarbonate loading with all-out effort of less than 1 minute improves performance *only* with both short- and longer term repetitive exercise bouts that repeatedly produce high intracellular H$^+$ concentrations.[22,23,54]

Inconsistencies in the research literature cloud the issue concerning the effectiveness of pre-exercise alkalosis. For example, despite dose-dependent changes in pH, base excess, and HCO$_3^-$ after ingestion of sodium citrate, no effect occurred on measures of performance in a bicycling time trial, even when the simulated race contained a multiple-sprint component.[223]

High-Intensity Endurance Performance

Pre-exercise alkalosis does not benefit low-intensity, aerobic exercise (because pH and lactate remain near resting levels), but some research indicates benefits in prolonged aerobic exercise of higher intensity.[172] More specifically, race times of trained male cyclists were better after consuming sodium citrate (0.5 g per kg body mass) before a 30-km time trial than in placebo trials.[204] Despite the relatively small anaerobic component in high-intensity aerobic exercise (compared with short-term, all-out exercise), ingesting buffer before exercise facilitates lactate and hydrogen ion efflux. This maintains pH closer to normal resting levels to improve muscle function in prolonged effort.

More research must clarify the ergogenic benefits (and possible dangers) of short-term induced alkalosis. Individuals who bicarbonate-load often experience abdominal cramps and diarrhea about 1 hour after ingestion. This adverse effect would surely minimize any potential ergogenic benefit. Substituting the buffering agent sodium citrate (0.4–0.5 g · kg^{-1}) for sodium bicarbonate can reduce or eliminate adverse gastrointestinal effects.[155,168]

PHOSPHATE LOADING

The rationale concerning pre-exercise phosphate supplementation (**"phosphate loading"**) focuses on increasing the levels of extracellular and intracellular phosphate. This may in turn (1) increase the potential for adenosine triphosphate (ATP) phosphorylation, (2) increase aerobic exercise performance and myocardial functional capacity, and (3) augment peripheral oxygen extraction in muscle tissue by stimulating red blood cell glycolysis and subsequent elevation of erythrocyte

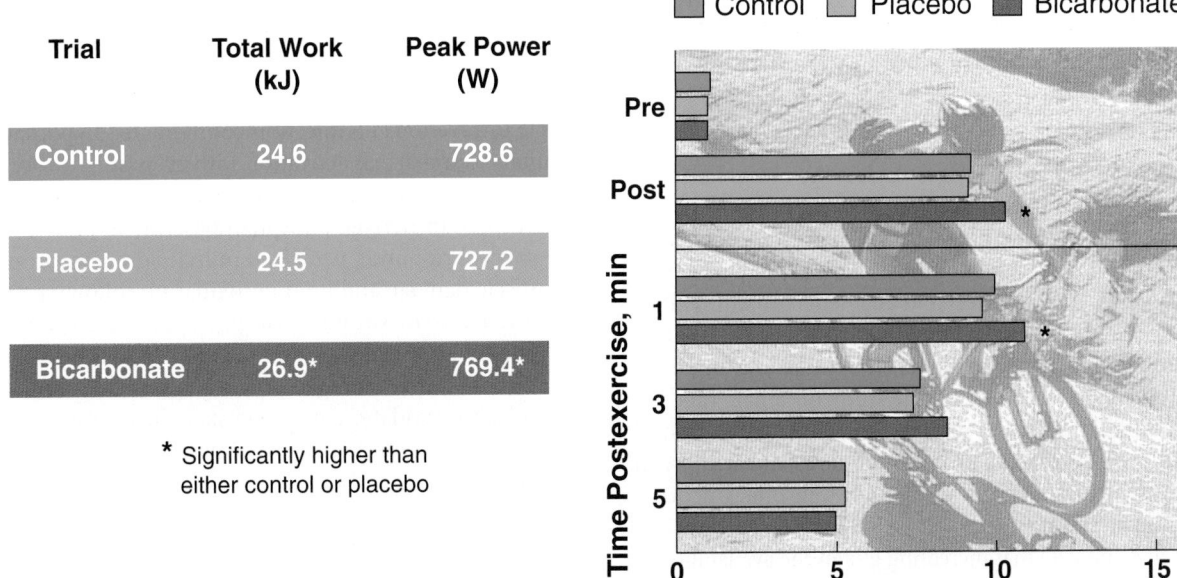

Trial	Total Work (kJ)	Peak Power (W)
Control	24.6	728.6
Placebo	24.5	727.2
Bicarbonate	26.9*	769.4*

* Significantly higher than
either control or placebo

FIGURE 11.11 ■ Bicarbonate loading and its effects on total work, peak power output, and postexercise blood lactate levels in moderately trained women. (From McNaughton LR, et al. Effect of sodium bicarbonate ingestion on high intensity exercise in moderately trained women. *J Strength Cond Res* 1997;11:98.)

2,3-diphosphoglycerate (2,3-DPG). The compound 2,3-DPG, produced within the red blood cell during the anaerobic reactions of glycolysis, binds loosely with subunits of hemoglobin, thus reducing its affinity for oxygen. Additional oxygen then releases to the tissues for a given decrease in the cellular oxygen pressure.

Despite the theoretical rationale for ergogenic effects with phosphate loading, benefits have not consistently emerged. Some studies show improvement in $\dot{V}O_{2max}$ and arteriovenous oxygen difference following phosphate loading, whereas others report no effects on aerobic metabolism and cardiovascular function.[159]

The major reasons for the inconsistencies in research findings include variations in exercise mode and intensity, dosage and duration of supplementation, standardization of pretest diets, and subjects' fitness level. In one study, subjects with low and high aerobic capacities consumed a drink containing either 22.2 g of dibasic calcium phosphate or a calcium carbonate placebo.[85] Each subject then pedaled a cycle ergometer for 20 minutes at an exercise intensity equivalent to 70% $\dot{V}O_{2max}$, followed by a 30-minute rest and then an incremental ride to exhaustion. For high- and low-fitness groups, no differences occurred for any of the variables measured, including erythrocyte 2,3-DPG, submaximal or maximal oxygen consumption exercise time to exhaustion, and plasma lactate in submaximal exercise.

Little reliable scientific evidence exists to recommended exogenous phosphate as an ergogenic aid. On the negative side, excess plasma phosphate stimulates secretion of **parathormone,** the parathyroid hormone. Excessive production of this hormone accelerates the kidneys' excretion of phosphate and facilitates reabsorption of calcium salts from

bones to cause loss of bone mass. Research has not yet determined whether short-term phosphate supplementation poses a risk to normal bone dynamics

ANTICORTISOL COMPOUNDS: GLUTAMINE AND PHOSPHATIDYLSERINE

The hypothalamus secretes corticotrophin-releasing factor as a normal response to emotional stress, trauma, infection, surgery, and physical exertion such as resistance training. This releasing factor, in turn, stimulates the anterior pituitary gland to secrete adrenocorticotropic hormone (ACTH), which induces the adrenal cortex to release the glucocorticoid hormone cortisol (hydrocortisone). Cortisol decreases amino acid transport into the cell; this depresses anabolism and stimulates protein breakdown to its building-block amino acids in all cells except liver cells. The circulation delivers these "liberated" amino acids to the liver for synthesis to glucose (gluconeogenesis). Cortisol also serves as an insulin antagonist by inhibiting glucose uptake and oxidation.

A prolonged, elevated serum concentration of cortisol (usually from therapeutic exogenous glucocorticoid intake in drug form) leads to excessive protein breakdown, tissue wasting, and negative nitrogen balance. The potential catabolic effect of cortisol has convinced many bodybuilders and other strength and power athletes to use supplements thought to inhibit the body's normal cortisol release. They believe that blunting cortisol's normal rise following exercise augments muscular development with resistance training by attenuating catabolism. In this way, muscle tissue synthesis progresses unimpeded in recovery. Glutamine and phosphatidylserine are two supplements used to produce an anticortisol effect.

Glutamine

Glutamine, a nonessential amino acid, is the most abundant amino acid in plasma and skeletal muscle. It accounts for more than half of the muscles' free amino acid pool. Glutamine exerts many regulatory functions, one of which provides an anticatabolic effect and augments protein synthesis.[122,166,267] Glutamine supplementation effectively counteracts the decline in protein synthesis and muscle wasting from repeated glucocorticoid use. In one study of female rats, infusing glutamine for 7 days inhibited the downregulation of myosin (muscle contractile protein) synthesis and atrophy in skeletal muscle that normally accompanies chronic glucocorticoid administration.[108]

Data also indicate that increasing glutamine availability by supplementation modulates glucose homeostasis during and after exercise in a direction that facilitates postexercise recovery.[118] It also promotes muscle glycogen accumulation in human muscle in recovery, perhaps by serving as a gluconeogenic substrate in the liver.[255] The practical application of these findings for promoting glycogen replenishment in recovery or enhancing glycogen accumulation in the pre-exercise period requires further research. The potential anticatabolic and glycogen-synthesizing effects of exogenous glutamine have promoted speculation that glutamine supplementation might benefit responses to resistance training.[9] However, daily glutamine supplementation (0.9 g per kg lean tissue mass) during 6 weeks of resistance training in healthy young adults did not affect muscle performance, body composition, or muscle protein degradation compared with a placebo.[37]

Immune Response

Glutamine plays an important role in normal immune function through its use as metabolic fuel by disease-fighting cells that defend against infection.[211,262] Glutamine plasma concentrations decrease following prolonged high-intensity exercise, so a glutamine deficiency has been linked to the immunosuppression caused by strenuous exercise.[25,188,210,216]

Chapter 7 discusses glutamine and the immune response in regard to supplementation and the incidence and severity of upper respiratory tract infections.

Phosphatidylserine

Phosphatidylserine (PS) is a glycerophospholipid typical of a class of natural lipids that constitute the structural components of biologic membranes, particularly the internal layer of the plasma membrane that surrounds all cells. Through its potential for modulating functional events in the plasma membrane (e.g., number and affinity of membrane receptor sites), PS might modify the neuroendocrine response to stress. In one study, healthy men consumed 800 mg of PS derived from bovine cerebral cortex daily for 10 days.[178] Three 6-minute intervals of cycle ergometer exercise of increasing

intensity induced physical stress. Compared with the placebo condition, the PS treatment diminished ACTH and cortisol release without affecting growth hormone release. These results confirmed earlier findings by the same researchers that a single intravenous PS injection counteracted hypothalamic–pituitary–adrenal axis activation with exercise.[177] More recent research observed that 10 days of supplementation with 750 mg of soybean-derived phosphatidylserine did not attenuate the cortisol response, perceived muscle soreness, or markers of muscle damage and lipid peroxidation following exhaustive intermittent running compared to a glucose polymer placebo.[139] Supplementation increased cycle time to exhaustion, but no effect emerged on oxygen kinetics, serum cortisol, substrate oxidation, or mood state during the exercise.[140] The physiologic mechanism for any ergogenic effect remains unknown.

Soybean lecithin provides most PS used for supplementation by athletes, yet research showing physiologic effects have used bovine-derived PS. Subtle differences in the chemical structure of these two forms of PS may create differences in physiologic action, including the potential for ergogenic effects.

Is Cortisol Release Really "Bad"?

Research must determine if the normal release and rise in serum cortisol with intense training counteracts muscular growth and development and recovery and repair. One could argue that cortisol release with exercise represents an appropriate and beneficial response to physiologic function and overall good health. It also remains unclear whether a supplement-induced decrease in cortisol output with resistance training translates into greater improvements in muscular strength and size.

β-HYDROXY-β-METHYLBUTYRATE

β-Hydroxy-β-methylbutyrate (HMB), a bioactive metabolite generated from the breakdown of the essential branched-chain amino acid leucine, may decrease protein loss during stress by inhibiting protein catabolism. A marked decrease in protein breakdown and a slight increase in protein synthesis occurred in muscle tissue of rats and chicks (*in vitro*) exposed to HMB.[195] Data also suggest an HMB-induced increase in fatty acid oxidation *in vitro* in mammalian muscle cells exposed to HMB.[43] Depending on the amount of HMB contained within foods—relatively rich sources include catfish, grapefruit, breast milk—the body synthesizes between 0.3 and 1.0 g daily, of which about 5% derives from dietary leucine catabolism. Because of its possible nitrogen-retaining effects, many resistance-trained athletes supplement directly with HMB to prevent or slow muscle damage and depress muscle breakdown (proteolysis) associated with intense physical effort.

Research has studied the effects of exogenous HMB on skeletal muscle's response to resistance training.[83,125,146,191,198,231] For example, young adult men participated in two randomized trials. In *study 1,* 41 subjects received 0, 1.5, or 3.0 g of HMB (calcium salt of HMB mixed with orange juice) daily at two protein levels, either 115 g or 175 g per day for 3 weeks. The men lifted weights during this time for 1.5 hours, 3 days per week for 3 weeks. In *study 2,* subjects consumed either 0 or 3.0 g of HMB per day and weight lifted for 2 to 3 hours, 6 days per week for 7 weeks. In the first study, HMB supplementation depressed the exercise-induced rise in muscle proteolysis as reflected by urine 3-methylhistidine and plasma creatine phosphokinase (CPK) levels during the first 2 weeks of training. These biochemical indices of muscle damage ranged between 20 and 60% lower in the HMB-supplemented group. In addition, this group lifted more total weight than the unsupplemented group during each training week (FIG. 11.12A), with the greatest effect in the group receiving the largest HMB supplement. Specifically, muscular strength increased 8% for the unsupplemented group, whereas it increased 13% for the 1.5-g HMB per day group and 18.4% for the 3.0-g HMB per day group. Additional protein (not indicated in graph) provided no augmenting effect on any of the measurements. The lack of effect with additional protein should be viewed in proper context because the group consuming the "lower" protein quantity (115 g per day) received the equivalent of about twice the protein RDA. Other investigators have replicated the finding of reduced signs and symptoms of exercise-induced muscle damage following resistance exercise with HMB supplementation.[250]

In *study 2,* subjects who received the HMB supplement had higher FFM than unsupplemented subjects at 2 and 4 to 6 weeks of training (Fig. 11.12B). However, at the last measurement during training the difference between groups decreased to the point at which no statistical significance between pre-training baseline values occurred.

The mechanism for HMB's action on muscle metabolism, strength improvement, and body composition remains unknown. Researchers speculate that this metabolite inhibits normal proteolytic processes that accompany intense muscular overload. While the results appear to demonstrate an ergogenic effect of HMB supplementation, it remains to be shown just what component of the FFM (protein, bone, water) HMB affects. Furthermore, the data in Figure 11.12B indicate potentially transient body-composition benefits of supplementation that tend to revert toward the unsupplemented state as training progresses. Additional studies must verify the present findings and assess the long-term effects of HMB supplements on body composition, training responsiveness, and overall health and safety.

Not all research shows beneficial effects of HMB supplementation with resistance training.[83,206,231] One study evaluated the effects of varied amounts of HMB (approximately 3 vs 6 g · d^{-1}) on muscular strength during 8 weeks of resistance training in untrained young men.[80] The study's primary finding indicated that HMB supplementation, regardless of

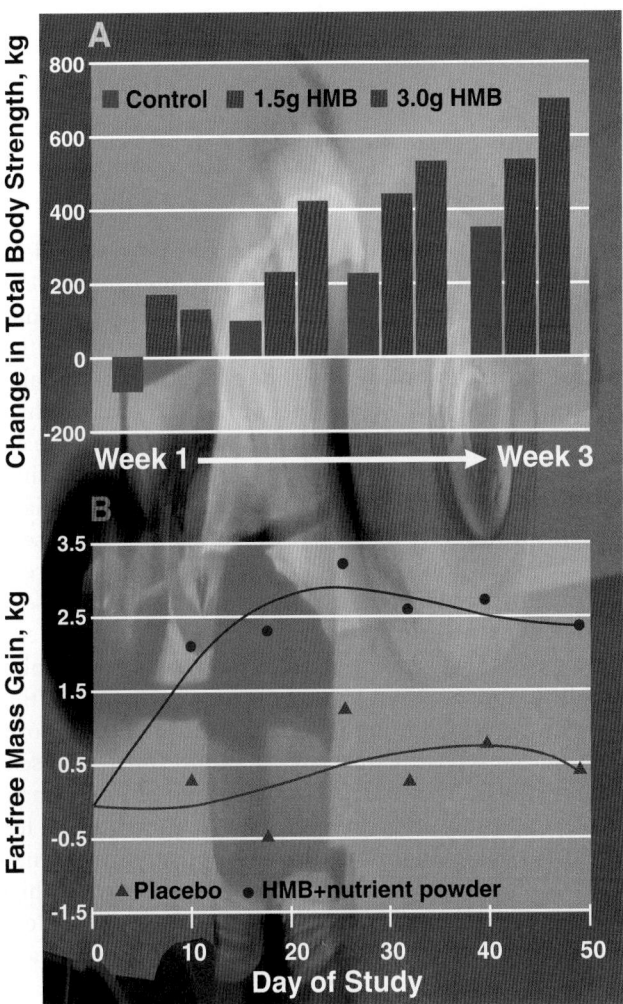

FIGURE 11.12 ■ **A.** Change in muscle strength (total of upper and lower body exercises) during *study 1* from week 1 to week 3 in subjects supplemented with HMB (β-hydroxy-β-methylbutyrate). Each grouping of bars represents one complete set of upper and lower body workouts. **B.** Total body electrical conductivity assessed change in fat-free body mass during *study 2* for a control group that received a carbohydrate drink *(placebo)* and an HMB group that received 3 g Ca-HMB per day mixed in a nutrient powder *(HMB 1 nutrient powder).* (From Nissen S, et al. Effect of leucine metabolite b-hydroxy-b-methylbutyrate on muscle metabolism during resistance-exercise training. *J Appl Physiol* 1996;81:2095.)

dosage, produced *no difference* in most of the strength data (including 1-RM strength) compared with placebo treatment. Increases in training volume remained similar among groups. Lower levels of CPK in both HMB-supplemented groups in recovery indicate some potential effect of HMB in inhibiting muscle breakdown with resistance training. HMB supplementation with a dosage as high as 6 g · d^{-1} during 8 weeks of resistance training does not appear to cause adverse effects on hepatic enzyme function, blood lipid profile, renal dynamics, or immune function.[84] Age does not affect responsiveness to HMB supplementation.[259]

A NEW TWIST: HORMONAL BLOOD BOOSTING

To eliminate the cumbersome and lengthy process of blood doping, endurance athletes now use recombinant **epoietin (EPO)**, a synthetic form of **erythropoietin.** This hormone, produced by the kidneys regulates red blood cell production within the marrow of the long bones. It also is essential in the resynthesis and proper functioning of several erythrocyte membrane proteins involved in facilitating lactate exchange.[53] Exogenous epoietin, commercially available since 1988, has proven clinically useful in combating anemia in patients with severe renal disease. Normally, a decrease in red blood cell concentration or decline in the pressure of oxygen in arterial blood—as in severe pulmonary disease or on ascent to high altitude—releases EPO to stimulate erythrocyte production. The 5 to12% increase in hemoglobin and hematocrit (% red blood cells in 100 mL blood) that typically occurs following a 6-week EPO treatment improves endurance-exercise performance.[218] Unfortunately, if self-administered in an unregulated and unmonitored manner—simply injecting the hormone requires much less sophistication than procedures for blood doping—hematocrit can increase by more than 60%. This dangerously high hemoconcentration (and corresponding increase in blood viscosity) increases the likelihood for stroke, heart attack, heart failure, and pulmonary edema.

EPO use has become prevalent in cycling competition and allegedly has contributed to at least 18 deaths (attributed to heart attacks) among competitive bicyclists. EPO cannot be detected in urine, so blood hematocrit level serves as a surrogate marker. During the 1997 and 1998 competitive seasons, Tour de France officials spot-checked the hematocrits of riders, suspending for 2 weeks any rider with an abnormally high value. This resulted in suspension of 12 riders during 1997 and 6 riders midway through the 1998 competitive season. The International Cycling Union has set a hematocrit threshold of 50% for males and 47% for females, while the International Skiing Federation uses a hemoglobin concentration of 18.5 g · dL^{-1} as the disqualification threshold. Hematocrit cutoff values of 52% for men and 48% for women (roughly 3 standard deviations above the mean normal value) represents "abnormally high" or extreme values in triathletes.[196] Of course, use of a hematocrit level cutoff raises the unanswered question concerning the number of disqualified "clean" cyclists. Estimates place this number at between 3 and 5%, due mainly to factors that affect normal variation in hematocrit such as genetics, posture, altitude training, and hydration level.[11,31]

The medical community's concern centers on an anomaly in iron metabolism frequently observed among elite international cyclists. Large numbers of these athletes typically show serum iron levels in excess of 500 ng · L^{-1} (normal iron level, 100 ng · L^{-1}) with some values as high as 1000 ng · L^{-1}. The elevated iron level results from regular injections of supplemental iron to support the increased synthesis of red blood cells induced by repeated EPO use. Chronic iron overload increases the risk of liver dysfunction among these athletes.

Other Means to Enhance Oxygen Transport

New classes of substances may emerge to enhance aerobic exercise performance.[224] These doping threats include perfluorocarbon emulsions and solutions formulated from either bovine or human hemoglobin that improve oxygen transport and delivery to muscle. Despite their potential benefits in clinical use, these substances exhibit potentially lethal side effects that include increased systemic and pulmonary blood pressure, renal toxicity, and impaired immune function.

IN THE FUTURE

As we envision the future, we see many physically active individuals, particularly athletes, with medicine chests containing an array of pharmaceutics that guarantee "even more fantastic" benefits than today's armamentarium of natural and synthetic "aids." As long as winning remains the priority, individuals will experiment with substances to improve exercise and sports performance and the response to training. Realistically, we see little hope for curbing this trend. We wish for optimism and decry presenting a negative perspective, but at this time we can offer little in constructive comment on how to stem the onslaught of commercial exploitation. The quest for an ergogenic boost in athletics had its roots 2500 years ago in the ancient Olympic Games. Perhaps the new generation of testing equipment can stay one step ahead of the abusers, but this seems doubtful. Increased legal statutes and penalties can curb the abuse, but drug enforcement remains difficult. Maintaining stricter laws at the local, state, and national levels may provide some relief, but thus far, additional vigilance by law enforcement has not curbed the problem. Perhaps a clearer identification of the characteristics of at-risk athletes and a vigorous education about drug abuse (coupled with a focus on improving the individual's decision-making skills and substituting more healthful alternatives) beginning in the early school years and continuing through college offers some limited hope for future generations. We certainly hope so.

Summary

1. Ergogenic aids consist of substances or procedures that improve physical work capacity, physiologic function, or athletic performance.

2. Anabolic steroids, pharmacologic agents commonly used as ergogenic aids, function similarly to the hormone testosterone. Research findings often are inconsistent, and the precise mechanism(s) of action unclear.

3. Negative side effects of anabolic steroid use in males include at least nine deleterious effects: infertility, reduced sperm concentrations, decreased testicular volume, gynecomastia, connective tissue damage that decreases the tensile strength and elastic compliance of tendons, chronic stimulation of the prostate gland, injury and functional alterations in cardiovascular function and myocardial cell cultures, possible pathologic ventricular growth and dysfunction, and increased blood platelet aggregation that can compromise cardiovascular system health and function and increase risk of stroke and acute myocardial infarction.

4. Unique negative side effects of anabolic steroid use in females include virilization (more apparent than in men), deepened voice, increased facial and body hair (hirsutism), altered menstrual function, dramatic increase in sebaceous gland size, acne, decreased breast size, and enlarged clitoris. The long-term effects of steroid use on reproductive function remain unknown.

5. The β_2-adrenergic agonists clenbuterol and albuterol increase skeletal muscle mass and slow fat gain in animals to counter the effects of aging, immobilization, malnutrition, and tissue-wasting pathology. A negative finding showed hastened fatigue during short-term, intense muscle actions.

6. Debate exists as to whether administration of exogenous growth hormone to normal, healthy people augments increases in muscle mass when combined with resistance training.

7. DHEA levels decrease steadily throughout adulthood, prompting many individuals (including large numbers of athletes) to supplement with this hormone in the hope of optimizing training and countering the effects of aging.

8. No data support ergogenic effect of DHEA supplements on young adult men and women.

9. Research findings generally indicate *no effect* of androstenedione supplementation on basal serum concentrations of testosterone or training response in terms of muscle size and strength and body composition. Worrisome are the potentially negative effects of a lowered HDL-C on overall heart disease risk and the elevated serum estrogen level on risk of gynecomastia and possibly pancreatic and other cancers

10. Little credible evidence exists that amphetamines ("pep pills") aid exercise performance or psychomotor skills any better than an inert placebo. Side effects of amphetamines include drug dependency, headache, dizziness, confusion, and upset stomach.

11. Caffeine can exert an ergogenic effect in extending aerobic exercise duration by increasing fat use for energy, thus conserving glycogen reserves. These effects become less apparent in individuals who (1) maintain a high-carbohydrate diet or (2) habitually use caffeine.

12. No compelling scientific evidence exists to conclude that ginseng supplementation offers positive benefit for physiologic function or performance during exercise. Accumulating evidence indicates significant health risk accompany ephedrine use.

13. Consuming ethyl alcohol produces an acute anxiolytic effect because it temporarily reduces tension and anxiety, enhances self-confidence, and promotes aggression. Other than the antitremor effect, alcohol conveys no ergogenic benefits and likely impairs overall athletic performance (ergolytic effect).

14. Increasing the body's alkaline reserve before anaerobic exercise by ingesting buffering solutions of sodium bicarbonate or sodium citrate improves performance. Buffer dosage and the cumulative anaerobic nature of the exercise interact to influence the ergogenic effect of bicarbonate (or citrate) loading.

15. Little scientific evidence exists to recommend exogenous phosphates as an ergogenic aid.

16. An objective decision about the potential benefits and risks of glutamine, phosphatidylserine, and β-hydroxyl-β-methyl butyrate to provide a "natural" anabolic boost with resistance training for healthy individuals awaits further research.

17. Erythropoietin (EPO), a hormone produced by the kidneys that regulates red blood cell production within the marrow of the long bones, increases hemoglobin and hematocrit to improve endurance performance. Significant risks accompany its unsupervised use.

Test Your Knowledge Answers

1. **False:** Ancient athletes of Greece reportedly used hallucinogenic mushrooms for ergogenic purposes, while Roman gladiators ingested the equivalent of "speed" to enhance performance in the Circus Maximus. Athletes of the Victorian era routinely used chemicals such as caffeine, alcohol, nitroglycerine, heroin, cocaine, and the rat poison strychnine for a competitive edge.

2. **True:** A "placebo effect" refers to improved performance due to psychologic factors in that the individual performs at a higher level simply because of the suggestive power of believing that a substance or procedure should work.

3. **False:** Anabolic steroids function in a manner similar to testosterone, the chief male hormone. Prolonged high dosages of anabolic steroids often impair normal testosterone endocrine function, cause infertility, reduce sperm concentrations (azoospermia), decrease testicular volume, induce connective tissue damage, increase prostate size, cause injury and alterations in cardiovascular function and myocardial cell cultures, produce possible pathologic ventricular growth and dysfunction when combined with resistance training, impair cardiac microvascular adaptations, and diminish myocardial blood supply, leading to stroke and acute myocardial infarction.

4. **False:** Little scientific evidence supports claims about the effectiveness or anabolic qualities of andro-type compounds. Research findings show that androstenedione (1) elevates plasma testosterone concentrations, (2) exerts no favorable effect on muscle mass, (3) does not favorably affect muscular performance, (4) does not favorably alter body composition, (5) provides no beneficial effects on muscle protein synthesis or tissue anabolism, and (6) impairs the blood lipid profile in apparently healthy men.

5. **True:** The following reasons argue against amphetamine use by athletes: it leads to physiologic or emotional drug dependency; induces headache, tremulousness, agitation, insomnia, nausea, dizziness, and confusion, all of which negatively affect sports performance requiring rapid reaction and judgment; taking larger doses eventually requires more of the drug to achieve the same effect because drug tolerance increases with prolonged use; aggravates or even precipitates cardiovascular and mental disorders; or suppresses normal mechanisms for perceiving and responding to pain, fatigue, or heat stress; and it can produce unwanted weight loss, paranoia, psychosis, repetitive compulsive behavior, and nerve damage.

6. **False:** Drinking 2.5 cups of regularly percolated coffee about 1 hour before exercising extends endurance in strenuous aerobic exercise under laboratory conditions, as it does in higher intensity, shorter duration effort. An ergogenic effect even occurs with caffeine ingestion in the minutes just before exercising. Elite distance runners who consume 10 mg of caffeine per kg of body mass immediately before a treadmill run to exhaustion improve performance time by 1.9% compared with placebo or control conditions.

7. **False:** An increasing belief in the potential for selected foods to promote health has led to coining the term *functional food*. Beyond meeting three basic nutrition needs (survival, hunger satisfaction, and preventing adverse effects), functional foods comprise those foods and their bioactive components (e.g., olive oil, soy products, n-3 fatty acids) that promote well-being, health, and optimal body function or reduce disease risk. Examples include many polyphenolic substances (simple phenols and flavinoids found in fruits and vegetables), carotinoids, soy isoflavones, fish oils, and components of nuts that possess antioxidant and other properties that decrease risk of vascular diseases and cancers. Primary targets for this expanding branch of food science include gastrointestinal functions, antioxidant systems, and macronutrient metabolism.

8. **False:** Many commercial weight-loss products have contained combinations of ephedra and caffeine, supposedly designed to accelerate metabolism. No evidence exists that the initial weight loss obtained with high doses of ephedrine plus caffeine lasts beyond 6 months. In 2003, the FDA ordered that a prominent warning label be emblazoned on the front of all ephedra products listing death, heart attack, or stroke as possible consequences of use. In addition, a recent evaluation of more than 16,000 adverse reactions showed "five deaths, five heart attacks, 11 cerebrovascular accidents, four seizures, and eight psychiatric cases as 'sentinel events' associated with prior consumption of ephedra or ephedrine." In December 2003 the FDA banned the use of ephedra as a dietary supplement.

9. **False:** Alcohol's effect on rehydration has been studied following exercise-induced dehydration of about 2% of body mass. Increases in plasma volume in recovery compared with the dehydrated state averaged 8.1% when the rehydration fluid contained no alcohol, but only 5.3% for the beverage with 4% alcohol content. The bottom line: Alcohol-containing beverages impede rehydration.

10. **True:** Many resistance-trained athletes supplement directly with HMB to prevent or slow muscle damage and depress muscle breakdown (proteolysis) associated with intense physical effort. Subjects who received an HMB supplement showed higher FFM mass than unsupplemented subjects. Not all research has shown beneficial effects of HMB supplementation with resistance training. Furthermore, available data indicate potentially transient body-composition benefits of supplementation that revert toward the unsupplemented state as training progresses. Additional studies must verify beneficial findings, and assess the long-term effects of HMB supplements on body composition, training responsiveness, and overall health and safety.

References

1. Agbenyega ET, Warham AC. Effect of clenbuterol on normal and denervated muscle growth and contractility. *Muscle Nerve* 1990;13:199.
2. Ajayi AAL, et al. Testosterone increases human platelet thromboxane A_2 receptor density and aggregation responses. *Circulation* 1995;91:2742.
3. Alaranta A, et al. Self-reported attitudes of elite athletes towards doping: Differences between types of sport. *Int J Sports Med* 2006;27:842.
4. Allen JD, et al. Ginseng supplementation does not enhance healthy young adults peak aerobic exercise performance. *J Am Coll Nutr* 1998;17:462.
5. American Academy of Pediatrics. Adolescents and anabolic steroids: a subject review. *Pediatrics* 1997;99:904.
6. American College of Sports Medicine. The use of alcohol in sports. *Med Sci Sports Exerc* 1982;14:481.
7. American College of Sports Medicine. The use of anabolic-androgenic steroids in sports. *Sports Med Bull* 1984;19:13.
8. Angell M, Kassirer JP. Alternative medicine: the risks of untested and unregulated remedies. *N Engl J Med* 1998;339:831.
9. Antonio J, Street C. Glutamine: a potentially useful supplement for athletes. *Can J Appl Physiol* 1999;24:1.
10. Araghiniknam M, et al. Antioxidant activity of dioscorea and dehydroepiandrosterone (DHEA) in older humans. *Life Sci* 1996; 59:11.
11. Audran M, et al. Effects of erythropoietin administration in training athletes and possible indirect detection in doping control. *Med Sci Sports Exerc* 1999;31:639.
12. Avois L, et al. Central nervous system stimulants and sport practice. *Br J Sports Med* 2006;40 Suppl 1:16.
13. Ayotte C. significance of 19-norandrosterone in athletes' urine samples. *Br J Sports Med* 2006;40(suppl 1):25.
14. Baer DJ, et al. Moderate alcohol consumption lowers risk factors for cardiovascular disease in postmenopausal women fed a controlled diet. *Am J Clin Nutr* 2002;75:593.
15. Bahrke M, Morgan WP. Evaluation of the ergogenic properties of ginseng. *Sports Med* 2000;29:113.
16. Bell DG, Jacobs I. Combined effects of caffeine and ephedrine ingestion improves run times of Canadian Forces Warrior Test. *Aviat Space Environ Med* 1999;70:325.
17. Bell DG, McLellan TM. Effect of repeated caffeine ingestion on repeated exhaustive exercise endurance. *Med Sci Sports Exerc* 2003;35:1348.
18. Bell DG, et al. Effects of caffeine, ephedrine and their combination on time to exhaustion during high-intensity exercise. *Eur J Appl Physiol* 1998;778:427.
19. Bell DG, et al. Effect of caffeine and ephedrine ingestion on anaerobic performance. *Med Sci Sports Exerc* 2001;33:1399.
20. Bell DG, et al. Effect of ingesting caffeine and ephedrine on 10-km run performance. *Med Sci Sports Exerc* 2002;34:344.
21. Benson DW, et al. Decreased myofibrillar protein breakdown following treatment with clenbuterol. *J Surg Res* 1991;50:1.
22. Bishop D, Claudius B. Effect of induced metabolic alkalosis on prolonged intermittent-sprint performance. *Med Sci Sports Exerc* 2005;37:759.
23. Bishop D, et al. Induced metabolic alkalosis affects muscle metabolism and repeated-sprint ability, *Med Sci Sports Exerc* 2004;36:807.
24. Blackman MR, et al. Growth hormone and sex steroid administration in healthy aged women and men: a randomized controlled trial. *JAMA* 2002;288:2282.
25. Blanchard MA, et al. The influence of diet and exercise on muscle and plasma glutamine concentrations. *Med Sci Sports Exerc* 2001;33:69.
26. Bracken ME, et al. The effect of cocaine on exercise endurance and glycogen use in rats. *J Appl Physiol* 1988;64:884.
27. Braiden RW, et al. Effects of cocaine on glycogen metabolism and endurance during high intensity exercise. *Med Sci Sports Exerc* 1994;26:695.
28. Bridge CA, Jones MA. The effects of caffeine ingestion on 8 km run performance in a field setting. *J Sports Sci* 2006;24:433.
29. Brown GA, et al. Effect of oral DHEA on serum testosterone and adaptations to resistance training in young men. *J Appl Physiol* 1999;87:2274.
30. Brown GA et al. Endocrine response to chronic androstenedione intake in 30- to 56-year-old men. *J Clin Endocrinol Metab* 2000;85:4074.
31. Browne A, et al. The ethics of blood testing as an element of doping control in sport. *Med Sci Sports Exerc* 1999;31:497.
32. Bruce CR, et al. Enhancement of 2000-m rowing performance after caffeine ingestion. *Med Sci Sports Exerc* 2000;32:1958.
33. Bucci LR. Selected herbals and human exercise performance. *Am J Clin Nutr* 2000;72(suppl):624S.
34. Buckley WE, et al. Estimated prevalence of anabolic steroid use among male high school seniors. *JAMA* 1988;260:3441.
35. Burke LM, et al. Effect of alcohol intake on muscle glycogen storage after prolonged exercise. *J Appl Physiol* 2003 95:983.
36. Cafri G, et al. Pursuit of muscularity in adolescent boys: relations among biopsychosocial variables and clinical outcomes. *J Clin Adolesc Psychol* 2006;35:282.
37. Candow DG, et al. Effect of glutamine supplementation combined with resistance training in young adults. *Eur J Appl Physiol* 2001;86:142.
38. Caruso JF, et al. The effects of albuterol and isokinetic exercise on the quadriceps muscle group. *Med Sci Sports Exerc* 1995;27:1471.
39. Casaburi R, et al. Androgen effects on body composition and muscle performance. In: Bhasin S, et al, eds. *Pharmacology, Biology, and Clinical Applications of Androgens: Current Status and Future Prospects.* New York: Wiley-Liss, 1996.
40. Casal DC, Leon AS. Failure of caffeine to affect substrate utilization during prolonged exercise. *Med Sci Sports Exerc* 1985;17:174.
41. Castell LM, et al. Some aspects of the acute phase response after a marathon race, and the effects of glutamine supplementation. *Eur J Appl Physiol* 1997;75:47.
42. Catlin DH, et al. Trace contamination of over-the-counter androstenedione and positive urine test results for nandrolone metabolite. *JAMA* 2000;285:2618.
43. Cheng W, et al. Beta-hydroxy-beta-methyl butyrate increases fatty acid oxidation by muscle cells. *FASEB J* 1997;11:A381.
44. Chester N, et al. Physiological, subjective and performance effects of pseudoephedrine and phenylpropanolamine during endurance running exercise. *Int J Sports Med* 2003;24:3.
45. Chin ER, Allen DG. The contribution of pH-dependent mechanisms to fatigue at different intensities in mammalian single muscle fibres. *J Physiol (Lond)* 1998;512:831.
46. Clark AS, Henderson LP. Behavioral and physiological responses to anabolic-androgenic steroids. *Neurosci Biobehav Rev* 2003;27:413.
47. Climent VE, et al. Growth hormone therapy and the heart. *Am J Cardiol* 2006;97:1097.
48. Cohen BS, et al. Effects of caffeine ingestion on endurance racing in heat and humidity. *Eur J Appl Physiol* 1996;73:358.
49. Cohen LI, et al. Lipoprotein (a) and cholesterol in body builders using anabolic androgenic steroids. *Med Sci Sports Exerc* 1996;28:176.
50. Collomp K, et al. Effects of salbutamol and caffeine ingestion on exercise metabolism and performance. *Int J Sports Med* 2002;23: 549.
51. Collomp K, et al. Effects of acute salbutamol intake during a Wingate test. *Int J Sports Med* 2005;26:513.
52. Conlee RK, et al. Effect of cocaine on plasma catecholamine and muscle glycogen concentrations during exercise in the rat. *J Appl Physiol* 1991;70:1323.
53. Connes P, et al. Injections of recombinant human erythropoietin increases lactate influx into erythrocytes. *J Appl Physiol* 2004;97:165.
54. Costill DL, et al. Acid-base balance during repeated bouts of exercise: influence of HCO_3. *Int J Sports Med* 1984;5:228.
55. Crist DM, et al. Body composition response to exogenous GH during training in highly conditioned adults. *J Appl Physiol* 1988;65:579.
56. Criswell DS, et al. Clenbuterol-induced fiber type transition in the soleus of adult rats. *Eur J Appl Physiol* 1996;74:391.
57. Davis MJ, et al. Effects of moderate alcohol intake on fasting insulin and glucose concentrations and insulin sensitivity in postmenopausal women: a randomized controlled trial. *JAMA* 2002;287:2559.
58. DeCree C. Androstenedione and dehydroepiandrosterone for athletes. *Lancet* 1999;354:779.

59. DeMeersman R, et al. Sympathomimetics and exercise enhancement: all in the mind? *Pharmacol Biochem Behav* 1987;28:361.

60. Deyssig R, et al. Effect of growth hormone treatment on hormonal parameters, body composition and strength in athletes. *Acta Endocrinol* 1993;128:313.

61. Dickerman RD, et al. Echocardiography in fraternal twin bodybuilders with one abusing anabolic steroids. *Cardiology* 1997;88:50.

62. Dodd SL, et al. The effects of caffeine on graded exercise performance in caffeine naive versus habituated subjects. *Eur J Appl Physiol* 1991;62:424.

63. Dodd SL, et al. Effects of clenbuterol on contractile and biochemical properties of skeletal muscle. *Med Sci Sports Exerc* 1996;28:669.

64. Doessing S, Kjaer M. Growth hormone and connective tissue in exercise. *Scand J Med Sci Sports* 2005;15:2002.

65. Doherty M, Smith PM. Effects of caffeine ingestion on exercise testing: a meta-analysis. *Int J Sport Nutr Exerc Metab* 2004;14:626.

66. Doherty M, et al. Caffeine is ergogenic after supplementation of oral creatine monohydrate. *Med Sci Sports Exerc* 2002;34:1785.

67. Donato T. Alcohol consumption among high school students and young athletes in north Italy. *Rev Epidemiol Sante Publique* 1994;42:198.

68. Dupont-Versteegdn EE. Exercise and clenbuterol as strategies to decrease progression of muscular dystrophy in mdx rats. *J Appl Physiol* 1995;80:734.

69. Earnst DP, et al. In vivo 4-androstene-3,17-dione and 4-androstene-3β,17β-diol supplementation in young men. *Eur J Appl Physiol* 2000;81:229.

70. ElSayed MS, et al. Interaction between alcohol and exercise: Physiological and haematological implications. *Sports Med* 2005;35:257.

71. Engels HJ, et al. No ergogenic effects of ginseng (Panax ginseng C.A. Meyer) during graded maximal aerobic exercise. *J Am Diet Assoc* 1997;97:1110.

72. Faigenbaum A, et al. Anabolic androgenic steroid use by 11- to 13-yearold boys and girls: knowledge, attitudes, and prevalence. *J Strength Cond Res* (abstr) 1996;10:285.

73. Fiala KA, et al. Rehydration with a caffeinated beverage during the nonexercise periods of 3 consecutive days of 2-a-day practices. *Int J Sport Nutr Exerc Metab* 2004;14:419.

74. Fogelholm M, et al. Healthy lifestyles of former Finnish world class athletes. *Med Sci Sports Exerc* 1994;26:224.

75. Fomous CM, et al. Symposium: conference on the science and policy of performance-enhancing products. *Med Sci Sports Exerc* 2002;34:1685.

76. Forbes GB, et al. Sequence of changes in body composition induced by testosterone and reversal of changes after drug is stopped. *JAMA* 1992;267:397.

77. Forgo I, Kirchdorfer AM. The effect of different ginsenoside concentrations on physical work capacity. *Notabene Medici* 1982;12:721.

78. Forman ES, et al. High-risk behaviors in teenage male athletes. *Clin J Sports Med* 1995;5:36.

79. Fortunato RS, et al. Chronic administration of anabolic androgenic steroid alters murine thyroid function. *Med Sci Sports Exerc* 2006;38:256.

80. Foster ZJ, Housner JA. Anabolic-androgenic steroids and testosterone precursors: ergogenic AIDS and sport. *Curr Sports Med Rep* 2004;3:234.

81. Franke WW, Berendonk B. Hormonal doping and androgenization of athletes: a secret program of the German Democratic Republic government. *Clin Chem* 1997;43:1262.

82. French C, et al. Caffeine ingestion during exercise to exhaustion in elite distance runners. *J Sports Med Phys Fitness* 1991;31:425.

83. Gallagher PM, et al. β-Hydroxy-β-methylbutyrate ingestion. Part I. Effects on strength and fat free mass. *Med Sci Sports Exerc* 2000; 32:2116.

84. Gallagher PM, et al. β-Hydroxy-β-methylbutyrate ingestion. Part II. Effects on hematology, hepatic and renal function. *Med Sci Sports Exerc* 2000;32:2116.

85. Galloway SDR, et al. The effects of acute phosphate supplementation in subjects of different aerobic fitness levels. *Eur J Appl Physiol* 1996;72:224.

86. Gaziano JM, et al. Moderate alcohol intake, increased levels of high-density lipoprotein and its subfractions, and decreased risk of myocardial infarction. *N Engl J Med* 1993;329:1829.

87. Gazvani M, et al. Conservative management of azoospermia following steroid abuse. *Hum Reprod* 1997;12:1706.

88. Gillies H, et al. Pseudoephedrine is without ergogenic effects during prolonged exercise. *J Appl Physiol* 1996;81:2611.

89. Goldberg L, et al. Effects of a multidimensional anabolic steroid prevention intervention: the Adolescents Training and Learning to Avoid Steroids (ATLAS) Program. *JAMA* 1996;276:1555.

90. Goldfinch J, et al. Induced metabolic alkalosis and its effects on 400-m racing time. *Eur J Appl Physiol* 1988;57:45.

91. Goulet ED, Dionne IJ. Assessment of the effects of eleutherococcus senticosus on endurance performance. *Int J Sport Nutr Exer Metab* 2005;15:75.

92. Grace F, et al. Blood pressure and rate pressure product response in males using high-dose anabolic androgenic steroids (AAS). *J Sci Med Sport* 2003;6:307.

93. Graham TE, Spriet LL. Metabolic, catecholamine and exercise performance responses to varying doses of caffeine. *J Appl Physiol* 1996;78:867.

94. Graham TE, et al. Metabolic and exercise endurance effects of coffee and caffeine ingestion. *J Appl Physiol* 1998;85:883.

95. Granier PL, et al. Effect of NaHCO₃ on lactate kinetics in forearm muscles during leg exercise in man. *Med Sci Sports Exerc* 1996;28:692.

96. Green GA, et al. Analysis of over-the-counter dietary supplements. *Clin J Sports Med* 2001;11:254.

97. Green GA, et al. NCAA study of substance use and abuse habits of college student-athletes. *Clin J Sports Med* 2001;11:56.

98. Gutgesell M, et al. Reported alcohol use and behavior in long-distance runners. *Med Sci Sports Exerc* 1996;28:1063.

99. Hallfrisch J, et al. Physical conditioning status and diet intake in active and sedentary older men. *Nutr Res* 1994;14:817.

100. Harburg E, et al. Using the Short Michigan Alcoholism Screening Test to study social drinkers: Tecumseh, Michigan. *J Stud Alcohol* 1988;49:522.

101. Harburg E, et al. Psychosocial factors, alcohol use and hangover signs among social drinkers: a reappraisal. *J Clin Epidemiol* 1993;46:413.

102. Harkey MR, et al. Variability in commercial ginseng products: an analysis of 25 preparations. *Am J Clin Nutr* 2001;73:1101.

103. Hartgens F, Kuipers H. Effects of androgenic-anabolic steroids in athletes. *Sports Med* 2004;3:513.

104. Hartgens F, et al. Body composition and anthropometry in bodybuilders: regional changes due to nandrolone deconate administration. *Int J Sports Med* 2001;22:235.

105. Hartgens F, et al. Prospective echocardiographic assessment of androgenic-anabolic steroid effects on cardiac structure and function in strength athletes. *Int J Sports Med* 2003;24:344.

106. Hartgens F, et al. Misuse of androgenic-anabolic steroids and human deltoid muscle fibers: differences between polydrug regimes and single drug administration. *Eur J Appl Physiol* 2002;86:233.

107. Hausswirth C, et al. Sodium citrate ingestion and muscle performance in acute hypobaric hypoxia. *Eur J Appl Physiol* 1995;71:362.

108. Hickson RC, et al. Glutamine prevents down-regulation of myosin heavy-chain synthesis and muscle atrophy from glucocorticoids. *Am J Physiol* 1995;31:E730.

109. Hintz RL, et al. Effect of growth hormone treatment on adult height of children with idiopathic short stature. *N Engl J Med* 1999;340:502.

110. Hodges AN, et al. Effects of pseudoephedrine on maximal cycling power and submaximal cycling efficiency. *Med Sci Sports Exerc* 2003;35:1316.

111. Hodges AN, et al. Effects of inhaled bronchodialtors and corticosteroids on exercise induced arterial hypoxaemia in trained male athletes. *Br J Sports Med* 2005;39:518.

112. Hodges K, et al. Pseudoephedrine enhances performance in 1500-m runners. *Med Sci Sports Exerc* 2006;38:329.

113. Hollidge-Horvat MG, et al. Effect of induced metabolic alkalosis on human skeletal muscle metabolism during exercise. *Am J Physiol* 2000;278:E316.

114. Huie MJ. An acute myocardial infarction occurring in an anabolic steroid user. *Med Sci Sport Exerc* 1994;26:408.

115. Hurley BF, et al. High density lipoprotein cholesterol in body builders vs. power-lifters. Negative effects of androgen use. *JAMA* 1984;252:4.

116. Ingalls CP, et al. Interaction between clenbuterol and run training: effects on exercise performance and MLC isoform control. *J Appl Physiol* 1996;80:795.

117. Ivy JL. Food components that may optimize physical performance: an overview. In: Marriott BM, ed. *Food Components to Enhance Performance.* Committee on Military Nutrition Research. Washington, DC: National Academy Press, 1994.

118. Iwashita S, et al. Impact of glutamine supplementation on glucose homeostasis during and after exercise. *J Appl Physiol* 2005;99:1858.

119. Jackman MP, et al. Metabolic, catecholamine and endurance responses to caffeine during intense exercise. *J Appl Physiol* 1996;81:1658.

120. Jacobs I, et al. Effects of ephedrine, caffeine, and their combination on muscular endurance. *Med Sci Sports Exerc* 2003;35:987.

121. Jakaubowicz D, et al. Effect of dehydroepiandrosterone on cyclic-guanosine monophosphate in men of advancing age. *Ann NY Acad Sci* 1995;774:312.

122. Jepson MM, et al. Relationship between glutamine concentration and protein synthesis in rat skeletal muscle. *Am J Physiol* 1988;255(Endocrinol Metab 18):E166.

123. Johansen KL, et al. Anabolic effects of nandrolone decanoate in patients receiving dialysis: a randomized controlled trial. *JAMA* 1999;281:1275.

124. Johnson CE, et al. Alcohol lowers the vasoconstriction threshold in humans without affecting core cooling rate during mild cold exposure. *Eur J Appl Physiol* 1996;74:293.

125. Jowko E, et al. Creatine and beta-hydroxy-beta-methylbutyrate (HMB) additively increase lean body mass and muscle strength during a weight training program. *Nutrition* 2001;17:558.

126. Juel C. Lactate-proton cotransport in skeletal muscle. *Physiol Rev* 1997;77:321.

127. Kalmar JM. The influence of caffeine on voluntary muscle activation. *Med Sci Sports Exerc* 2005;37:2113.

128. Kamber M, et al. Nutritional supplements as a source for positive doping cases? *Int J Sport Nutr Exerc Metab* 2001;11:258.

129. Kanayama G, et al. Body image attitudes toward male roles in anabolic-androgenic steroid users. *Am J Psychiatry* 2006;163:697.

130. Kantor MA, et al. Androgens reduce HDL$_2$-cholesterol and increase hepatic triglyceride lipase activity. *Med Sci Sports Exerc* 1985;17:462.

131. Karila TA, et al. Anabolic androgenic steroids produce dose-dependent increase in left ventricular mass in power athletes, and this effect is potentiated by concomitant use of growth hormone. *Int J Sports Med* 2003;24:337.

132. Kearns CF, McKeever J. Clenbuterol diminishes aerobic performance in horses. *Med Sci Sports Exerc* 2002;34:1976.

133. Kearns CF, et al. Chronic administration of therapeutic levels of clenbuterol acts as a repartitioning agent. *J Appl Physiol* 2001;91:2064.

134. Keisler BD, Armsey TD. Caffeine as an ergogenic aid. *Curr Sports Med Rep* 2006;5:215.

135. Keisler BD, Hosey RG. Ergogenic aids: an update on ephedra. *Curr Sports Med Rep* 2005;4:231.

136. Kelly KP, et al. Cocaine and exercise: physiological responses of cocaine-conditioned rats. *Med Sci Sports Exerc* 1995;27:65.

137. Kim SH, et al. Effects of Panex ginseng extract on exercise-induced oxidative stress. *J Sports Med Phys Fitness* 2005;45:178.

138. King DS, et al. Effect of oral androstenedione on serum testosterone and adaptations to resistance training in young men. *JAMA* 1999;281:2020.

139. Kingsley MI, et al. Effects of phosphatidylserine on oxidative stress following intermittent running. *Med Sci Sports Exerc* 2005;37:1300.

140. Kingsley MI, et al. Effects of phosphatidylserine on exercise capacity during cycling in active males. *Med Sci Sports Exerc* 2006;38:64.

141. Kitaura T, et al. Inhibited longitudinal growth of bones in young male rats by clenbuterol. *Med Sci Sports Exerc* 2002;34:267.

142. Kokotailo PK, et al. Substance use and other health risk behaviors in collegiate athletes. *Clin J Sport Med* 1996;6:183.

143. Kovacs EM, et al. The effect of ad libitum ingestion of caffeinated carbohydrate-electrolyte solution on urinary caffeine concentration after 4 hours of endurance exercise. *Int J Sports Med* 2002;23:237.

144. Kovacs EM, Mela DJ. Metabolically active functional food ingredients for weight control. *Obes Rev* 2006;7:58.

145. Kreider R.B, et al. Effects of phosphate loading on metabolic and myocardial responses to maximal and endurance exercise. *Int J Sports Nutr* 1992;2:20.

146. Kreider RB, et al. Effects of calcium beta-hydroxy-beta-methylbutyrate (HMB) supplementation during resistance training on markers of catabolism, body composition, and strength. *Int J Sports Med* 1999;20:503.

147. Lang RM, et al. Adverse cardiac effects of alcohol ingesting in young adults. *Ann Intern Med* 1985;102:742.

148. Laseter JT, Russell JA. Anabolic steroid-induced tendon pathology: a review of the literature. *Med Sci Sports Exerc* 1991;23:1.

149. Leder BZ, et al. Oral androstenedione administration and serum testosterone concentrations in young men. *JAMA* 2000;283:779.

150. Leichliter JS, et al. Alcohol use and related consequences among students with varying levels of involvement in college athletics. *J Am School Health* 1998;46:257.

151. Lemmer JT, et al. The effects of albuterol on power output in non-asthmatic athletes. *Int J Sports Med* 1995;16:243.

152. LePanse B, et al. Effects of short term salbutamol ingestion during a Wingate test. *Int J Sports Med* 2005;26:518.

153. Liang MT, et al. Panax notoginseng supplementation enhances physical performance during endurance exercise. *J Strength Cond Res* 2005;19:108.

154. Lieberman HR. The effects of ginseng, ephedrine, and caffeine on cognitive performance, mood and energy. *Nutr Rev* 2001;50:91.

155. Linossier M-T, et al. Effect of sodium citrate on performance and metabolism of human skeletal muscle during supramaximal cycling exercise. *Eur J Appl Physiol* 1998;76:48.

156. Liow RYL, Tavares S. Bilateral rupture of the quadriceps tendon associated with anabolic steroids. *Br J Sports Med* 1995;29:77.

157. Lopes JM, et al. Effect of caffeine on skeletal muscle function before and after fatigue. *J Appl Physiol* 1983;54:1303.

158. MacLennan PA, Edwards RHT. Effects of clenbuterol and propranol on muscle mass. *Biochem J* 1989;264:573.

159. Mannix ET, et al. Oxygen delivery and cardiac output during exercise following oral glucose phosphate. *Med Sci Sports Exerc* 1990;22:341.

160. Maravelias C, et al. Adverse effects of anabolic steroids in athletes: a constant threat. *Toxicol Lett* 2005;158:167.

161. Margos F, Kavouras SA. Caffeine use in sports, pharmolinetics in man, and cellular mechanisms of action. *Crit Rev Food Sci Nutr* 2005;45:535.

162. Martineau L, et al. Salbutamol, a β-agonist, increases skeletal muscle strength in young men. *Clin Sci* 1992;83:615.

163. Matson LG, Tran ZV. Effects of sodium bicarbonate ingestion on anaerobic performance: a meta-analytic review. *Int J Sports Nutr* 1993;3:2.

164. Matvienko OA, et al. A single dose of soybean phytosterols in ground beef decreases total serum cholesterol and LDL cholesterol in young, mildly hypercholesterolemic men. *Am J Clin Nutr* 2002;76:57.

165. Maughan RJ. Contamination of dietary supplements and positive drug tests in sport. *J Sport Sci* 2005;23:883.

166. Max SR. Glucocorticoid-mediated induction of glutamine synthetase in skeletal muscle. *Med Sci Sports Exerc* 1990;22:325.

167. Max SR, Rance NE. No effect of sex steroids on compensatory muscle hypertrophy. *J Appl Physiol* 1984;56:1589.

168. McNaughton LR. Sodium citrate and anaerobic performance: implications of dosage. *Eur J Appl Physiol* 1990;61:392.

169. McNaughton LR, Cedaro R. Sodium citrate ingestion and its effects on maximal anaerobic exercise of different durations. *Eur J Appl Physiol* 1992;64:36.

170. McNaughton LR, et al. Effect of sodium bicarbonate ingestion on high intensity exercise in moderately trained women. *J Strength Cond Res* 1997;11:98.

171. McNaughton L, et al. Effects of chronic bicarbonate ingestion on the performance of high-intensity work. *Eur J Appl Physiol* 1999;80:333.

172. McNaughton L, et al. Sodium bicarbonate can be used as an ergogenic aid in high-intensity, competitive cycle ergometry of 1 h duration. *Eur J Appl Physiol* 1999;80:64.

173. Melchert RB, Lelder AA. Cardiovascular effects of androgenic-anabolic steroids. *Med Sci Sports Exerc* 1995;27:1252.

174. Milner JA. Functional foods: the US perspective. *Am J Clin Nutr* 2000;71(suppl):1654S.

175. Modlinski R, Fields KB. The effect of anabolic steroids on the gastrointestinal system, kidneys, and adrenal glands. *Curr Sports Med* 2006;5:104.

176. Mohr T, et al. Caffeine ingestion and metabolic responses of tetraplegic humans during electrical cycling. *J Appl Physiol* 1998;85:979.

177. Monteleone P, et al. Effects of phosphatidylserine on the neuroendocrine response to physical stress in humans. *Neuroendocrinology* 1990;52:243.

178. Monteleone P, et al. Blunting by chronic phosphatidylserine administration of the stress-induced activation of the hypothalmo-pituitary-adrenal axis in healthy men. *Eur J Clin Pharmacol* 1992;41:385.

179. Morris AC, et al. No ergogenic effects of ginseng ingestion. *Int J Sport Nutr* 1996;6:263.

180. Morrison LJ, et al. Prevalent use of dietary supplements among people who exercise at a commercial gym. *Int J Sport Nutr Exerc Metab* 2004;4:481.

181. Mortola J, Yen SSC. The effects of oral dehydroepiandrosterone on endocrine-metabolic parameters in postmenopausal women. *J Clin Endocrinol Metab* 1990;71:696.

182. Motl TW, et al. Effect of caffeine on leg muscle pain during cycling exercise among females. *Med Sci Sports Exerc* 2006;38:598.

183. Mukamal KJ. Prior alcohol consumption and mortality following acute myocardial infarction. *JAMA* 2001;285:1965.

184. Murphy RJ, et al. Clenbuterol has a greater influence on untrained than previously trained skeletal muscle in rats. *Eur J Appl Physiol* 1996;73:304.

185. Nativ A, Puffer JC. Lifestyles and health risks of collegiate athletes. *J Fam Pract* 1991;33:585.

186. Nativ A, et al. Lifestyle and health risks of collegiate athletes: a multi-center study. *Clin J Sport Med* 1997;7:262.

187. Nelson TF, Wechsler H. Alcohol and college athletes. *Med Sci Sports Exerc* 2001;33:43.

188. Nieman DC, Bishop NC. Nutritional strategies to counter stress to the immune system in athletes, with special reference to football. *J Sports Sci* 2006;24:763.

189. Nigdikar SV, et al. Consumption of red wine polyphenols reduces susceptibility of low-density lipoproteins to oxidation in volunteers. *Am J Clin Nutr* 1998;68:258.

190. Nishijima Y, et al. Influence of caffeine ingestion on autonomic nervous system activity during endurance exercise in humans. *Eur J Appl Physiol* 2002;87:475.

191. Nissen S, et al. Effect of leucine metabolite β-hydroxy-β-methylbutyrate on muscle metabolism during resistance-exercise training. *J Appl Physiol* 1996;81:2095.

192. Noakes TD. Tainted glory-doping and athletic performance. *N Engl J Med* 2004;351:847–849.

193. Norris SR, et al. The effect of salbutamol on performance in endurance cyclists. *Eur J Appl Physiol* 1996;73:364.

194. Oler MJ, et al. Depression, suicidal ideation, and substance use among adolescents: are athletes at less risk? *Arch Fam Med* 1994;3:791.

195. Ostaszewksi P, et al. The effect of the leucine metabolite 3-hydroxy 3-methyl butyrate (HMB) on muscle protein synthesis and protein breakdown in chick and rat muscle. *J Anim Sci* 1996;74(suppl):138A.

196. O'Toole M., et al. Hematocrits of triathletes: is monitoring useful? *Med Sci Sports Exerc* 1999;31:372.

197. Overmann SJ, Terry T. Alcohol use and attitudes: a comparison of college athletes and non-athletes. *J Drug Educ* 1991;2:107.

198. Panton LB, et al. Nutritional supplementation of the leucine metabolite beta-hydroxy-beta-methylbutyrate (HMB) during resistance training. *Nutrition* 2000;16:734.

199. Papadakis MA, et al. Growth hormone replacement in healthy older men improves body composition but not functional ability. *Ann Inter Med* 1996;124:708.

200. Parkinson AM, Evans NA. Anabolic androgenic steroids: a survey of 500 users. *Med Sci Sports Exerc* 2006;38:644

201. Paton CD, et al. Little effect of caffeine ingestion on repeated sprints in team-sport athletes. *Med Sci Sports Exerc* 2001;33:822.

202. Percheron G, et al. Effect of 1-year oral administration of dehydroepiandrosterone to 60- to 80-year-old individuals on muscle function and cross-sectional area: a double-blind placebo-controlled trial. *Arch Intern Med* 2003;163:720.

203. Plaskett CJ, Cafarelli E. Caffeine increases endurance and attenuates force sensation during submaximal isometric contractions. *J Appl Physiol* 2001;91:1535.

204. Potteiger JA, et al. Sodium citrate ingestion enhances 30 km cycling performance. *Int J Sports Med* 1996;17:7.

205. Price M, et al. Effects of sodium bicarbonate ingestion on prolonged intermittent exercise. *Med Sci Sports Exerc* 2003;35:1303.

206. Ransone J, et al. The effect of beta-hydroxy beta-methylbutyrate on muscular strength and body composition in collegiate football players. *J Strength Cond Res* 2003; 17:34.

207. Raymer GH, et al. Metabolic effects of induced Alkaloids during progressive forearm exercise to fatigue. *J Appl Physiol* 2004;96: 2050.

208. Rasmussen BB, et al. Androstenedione does not stimulate muscle protein anabolism in young healthy men. *J Clin Endocrinol Metab* 2000;85:55.

209. Requena B, et al. Sodium bicarbonate and sodium citrate: ergogenic aids? *J Strength Cond Res* 2005;19:213.

210. Rhode T, et al. Competitive sustained exercise in humans, lymphokine activated killer cell activity, and glutamine: an intervention study. *Eur J Appl Physiol* 1998;78:448.

211. Rhode T, et al. Effect of glutamine supplementation on changes in the immune system induced by repeated exercise. *Med Sci Sports Exerc* 1998;30:856.

212. Rifici VA, et al. Red wine inhibits the cell-mediated oxidation of LDL and HDL. *J Am Coll Nutr* 1999;18:137.

213. Roberfroid MB. Concepts and strategy of functional food science: the European perspective. *Am J Clin Nutr* 2000;71(suppl):1660S.

214. Robertson RJ, et al. Effect of induced alkalosis on physical work capacity during arm and leg exercise. *Ergonomics* 1987;30:19.

215. Rogozkin V. Metabolic effects of anabolic steroids on skeletal muscle. *Med Sci Sports* 1979;11:160.

216. Rowbottom DG, et al. The emerging role of glutamine as an indicator of exercise stress and overtraining. *Sports Med* 1996;21:80.

217. Roy BD, et al. An acute oral dose of caffeine does not alter glucose kinetics during prolonged dynamic exercise in trained endurance athletes. *Eur J Appl Physiol* 2001;85:280.

218. Russell G, et al. Effects of prolonged low dosage of recombinant human erythropoietin during submaximal and maximal exercise. *Eur J Appl Physiol* 2002;86:442.

219. Sacco RL, et al. The protective effect of moderate alcohol consumption on ischemic stroke. *JAMA* 1999;28:913.

220. Sachtleben TR, et al. Serum lipoprotein patterns in long-term anabolic steroid users. *Res Q Exerc Sport* 1997;68:110.

221. Saini J, et al. Influence of alcohol on the hydromineral hormone responses to exercise in a warm environment. *Eur J Appl Physiol* 1995;72:32.

222. Saugy M, et al. Human growth hormone doping in sport. *Br J Sports Med* 2006;40(suppl 1):35.

223. Schabort EJ, et al. Dose-related evaluations in venous pH with citrate ingestion do not alter 40-km cycling time-trial performance. *Eur J Appl Physiol* 2000;83:320.

224. Schumacher YO, et al. Artificial oxygen carriers: the new doping threat in endurance sport? *Int J Sports Med* 2001;22:566.

225. Shekelle PG, et al. Efficacy and safety of ephedra and ephedrine for weight loss and athletic performance: a meta-analysis. *JAMA* 2003;289:1463.

226. Shirreffs SM, Maughan RJ. The effect on alcohol consumption on fluid retention following exercise-induced dehydration in man. *J Physiol* 1995;489:33P.

227. Shirreffs SM, Maughan RJ. The effect of alcohol consumption on the restoration of blood and plasma volume following exercise-induced dehydration in man. *J Physiol* 1996;491:64P.

228. Shirreffs SM. Maughan RJ. The effect of alcohol on athletic performance. *Curr Sports Med Rep* 2006;5:192.

229. Signorile JF, et al. Effects of acute inhalation of the bronchodilator, albuterol, on power output. *Med Sci Sports Exerc* 1992;24:638.

230. Signorile JF, et al. The effects of the chronic administration of metaproterenol on muscle size and function. *Arch Phys Med Rehab* 1995;76:55.

231. Slater B, et al. Beta-hydroxy-beta-methylbutyrate (HMB) supplementation does not affect changes in strength or body composition during resistance training in trained men. *Int J Sport Nutr Exerc Metab* 2001;11:384.

232. Sleeper MM, et al. Chronic clenbuterol, administration negatively alters cardiac function. *Med Sci Sports Exerc* 2002;34:643.

233. Soe LJ, et al. Liver pathology associated with the use of anabolic-androgenic steroids. *Liver* 1992;12:73.

234. Spriet LL, et al. Caffeine ingestion and muscle metabolism during prolonged exercise in humans. *Am J Physiol* 1992;262:E891.

235. Stark AH, Madar Z. Olive oil as a functional food: epidemiology and nutritional approaches. *Nutr Rev* 2002;60:170.

236. Stephens TJ, et al. Effect of sodium bicarbonate on muscle metabolism during intense endurance cycling. *Med Sci Sports Exerc* 2002;34:614.

237. Street C, et al. Metabolic alkalosis reduces exercise-induced acidosis and potassium accumulation in human skeletal muscle interstitium. *J Appl Physiol* 2005;566(Pt. 2):481.

238. Strawford A, et al. Resistance exercise and supraphysiologic androgen therapy and supraphysiologic androgen therapy in eugonadal men with HIV-related weight loss: a randomized controlled trial. *JAMA* 1999;281:1282.

239. Stuart GR, et al. Multiple effects of caffeine on simulated high-intensity team-sport performance. *Med Sci Sports Exerc* 2005;37:1998.

240. Su TP, et al. Neuropsychiatric effects of anabolic steroids in male normal volunteers. *JAMA* 1993;269:2760.

241. Supinski GS, et al. Caffeine effect on respiratory muscle endurance and sense of effort during loaded breathing. *J Appl Physiol* 1986;60:2040.

242. Swain RA, et al. Do pseudoephedrine or phenylpropanolamine improve maximum oxygen uptake and time to exhaustion? *Clin J Sports Med* 1997;7:168.

243. Tagarakis CV, et al. Anabolic steroids impair the exercise-induced growth of the cardiac capillary bed. *Int J Sports Med* 2000; 21:412.

244. Tjønneland A, et al. Wine intake and diet in a random sample of 48,763 Danish men and women. *Am J Clin Nutr* 1999;69:49.

245. Trice I, Haymes EM. Effects of caffeine ingestion on exercise-induced changes during high-intensity, intermittent exercise. *Int J Sports Nutr* 1995;5:37.

246. Ungerleider S. *Faust's Gold.* New York: St. Martin's Press, 2001.

247. Valmadrid CT, et al. Alcohol intake and risk of coronary heart disease mortality in persons with older-onset diabetes mellitus. *JAMA* 1999;282:239.

248. Van Gammeren D, et al. The effects of supplementation with 19-nor-4-androstene-3,17-dione and 19-nor-4-androstene-3,17-diol on body composition and athletic performance in previously weight-trained male athletes. *Eur J Appl Physiol* 2001;84:426.

249. Van Montfoort MC, et al. Effects of ingestion of bicarbonate, citrate, lactate, and chloride on sprint running. *Med Sci Sports Exerc* 2004;36:1239.

250. Van Simeren KA, et al. Supplementation with beta-hydroxy-beta-methylbutyrate (HMB) and alpha-ketoisocaproic acid (KIC) reduces signs and symptoms of exercise-induced muscle damage in man. *Int J Sport Nutr Exerc Metab* 2005;15:413.

251. Van Soeren MH, et al. Caffeine metabolism and epinephrine responses during exercise in users and nonusers. *J Appl Physiol* 1994;75:805.

252. Van Soeren MH, et al. Acute effects of caffeine ingestion at rest in humans with impaired epinephrine responses. *J Appl Physiol* 1996;80:999.

253. Van Soeren MH, Graham TE. Effect of caffeine on metabolism, exercise endurance, and catecholamine responses after withdrawal. *J Appl Physiol* 1998;85:1493.

254. Van Vollenhoven RF, et al. An open study of dehydroepiandrosterone in systemic lupus erythematosus. *Arthritis Rheum* 1994;37:1305.

255. Varnier M, et al. Stimulatory effect of glutamine on glycogen accumulation in human skeletal muscle. *Am J Physiol* 1995;269:E309.

256. Villareal DT, Holloszy JO. Effect of DHEA on abdominal fat and insulin action in elderly women and men. *JAMA* 2004;292:2243.

257. Villareal DT, Holloszy JO. DHEA enhances effects of weight training on muscle mass and strength in elderly women and men. *Am J Physiol Endocrinol Metab* 2006;291,1003.

258. Vogler BK, et al. The efficacy of ginseng: a systematic review of randomized clinical trials. *Eur J Clin Pharmacol* 1999;55:567.

259. Vukovich MD, et al. Body composition in 70-year-old adults responds to dietary beta-hydroxy-beta-methylbutyrate similarly to that of young adults. *J Nutr* 2001;131:2049.

260. Vuksan V, et al. American ginseng (*Panex quinquefolius* L.) attenuates postprandial glycemia in a time-dependent but not dose-dependent manner in healthy individuals. *Am J Clin Nutr* 2001;73:753.

261. Wallace MB, et al. Effects of dehydroepiandrosterone vs androstenedione supplementation in men. *Med Sci Sports Exerc* 1999;31:1788.

262. Walsh NP, Blannin AK. Effect of oral glutamine supplementation on human neutrophil lipopolysaccharide-stimulated degranulation following prolonged exercise. *Int J Sport Nutr Exerc Metab* 2000; 1:39.

263. Wannamethee SG, et al. Alcohol and diabetes risk. *Arch Intern Med* 2003;163:1329.

264. Webb OL, et al. Severe depression of high density lipoprotein cholesterol levels in weight lifters and body builders by self-administered exogenous testosterone and anabolic-androgenic steroids. *Metabolism* 1984;33:11.

265. Weir J, et al. A high carbohydrate diet negates the metabolic effects of caffeine during exercise. *Med Sci Sports Exerc* 1987;19:100.

266. Wemple R.D, et al. Caffeine vs caffeine-free sports drinks: effects on urine production at rest and during prolonged exercise. *Int J Sports Med* 1997;18:40.

267. Wernerman J, et al. Glutamine and ornithine-α-ketoglutarate but not branched-chain amino acids reduce the loss of muscle glutamine after surgical trauma. *Metabolism* 1989;38(supp 11):63.

268. Wroblewska A-M. Androgenic-anabolic steroids and body dysmorphia in young men. *J Psychosom Res* 1997;42:225.

269. Yang YT, McElligott MA. Multiple actions of β-adrenergic agonists on skeletal muscle and adipose tissue. *Biochem J* 1989;261:1.

270. Yanovski SZ, Yanovski JA. Drug therapy: Obesity. *N Engl J Med* 2002;346:591.

271. Yarasheski KE, et al. Effect of growth hormone and resistance exercise on muscle growth in young men. *Am J Physiol* 1992;262: E261.

272. Yarasheski KE, et al Short-term growth hormone treatment does not increase muscle protein synthesis in experienced weight lifters. *J Appl Physiol* 1993;74:3073.

273. Yeo SE, et al. Caffeine increases exogenous carbohydrate oxidation during exercise. *J Appl Physiol* 2005;99:844.

274. Zeman RJ, et al. Clenbuterol, a β_2-agonist, retards wasting and loss of contractility in irradiated dystrophic *mdx* muscle. *Am J Physiol* 1994;267:C865.

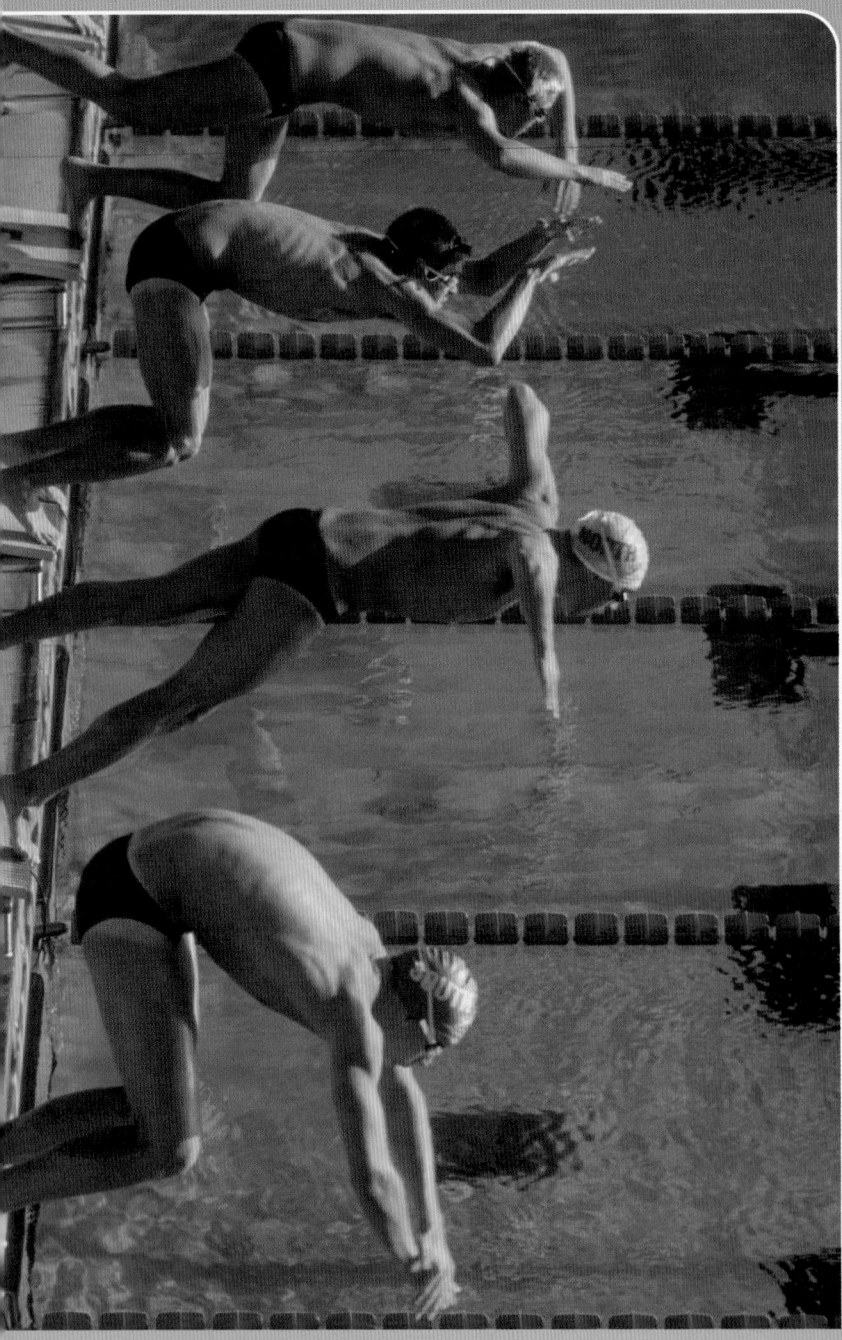

Chapter 12

Nutritional Ergogenic Aids Evaluated

- Creatine Loading

- Some Research Shows No Benefit

Ribose: The Next Creatine on the Supplement Scene?

Inosine and Choline

- Inosine

- Choline

Lipid Supplementation with Medium-Chain Triacylglycerols

- Exercise Benefits Inconclusive

(—)-Hydroxycitrate: A Potential Fat Burner?

Vanadium

Pyruvate

- Effects on Endurance Performance

Glycerol

Test Your Knowledge

Answer these 10 statements about nutritional ergogenic aids. Use the scoring key at the end of the chapter to check your results. Repeat this test after you have read the chapter and compare your results.

1. **T F** Reduced levels of muscle glycogen induce fatigue in intense aerobic exercise.

2. **T F** It is possible to modify nutrition to "superpack" muscle with glycogen and thereby delay the onset of fatigue in prolonged intense marathon running.

3. **T F** Amino acid supplements augment muscular strength and size with resistance training.

4. **T F** L-Carnitine supplementation aids endurance athletes by enhancing fat burning and sparing liver and muscle glycogen; it also promotes fat loss in body builders.

5. **T F** Chromium, the second largest selling mineral supplement in the United States is a well-documented "fat burner" and "muscle builder."

6. **T F** Creatine supplementation improves performance in short-duration, intense exercise.

7. **T F** Limited research indicates a potential for exogenous pyruvate as a partial replacement for dietary carbohydrate to augment endurance exercise performance and to promote fat loss.

8. **T F** The hyperhydration effect of glycerol supplementation reduces overall heat stress during exercise, lowers heart rate and core temperature, and enhances endurance performance under heat stress.

9. **T F** Because of its role in electron transport–oxidative phosphorylation, athletes supplementing with coenzyme Q_{10} (CoQ_{10}) improve aerobic capacity and cardiovascular dynamics in exercise.

10. **T F** Well-designed research clearly indicates that supplementation with (-)-hydroxycitrate or HCA facilitates the rate of fat oxidation at rest and during moderate-intensity exercise to effectively act as an antiobesity agent and ergogenic aid.

C hapter 11 highlighted that physically active individuals often resort to using banned pharmacologic and chemical agents to augment training and gain a competitive edge. They also focus on gaining a performance-enhancing advantage from specific foods and food components consumed in the diet.

MODIFICATION OF CARBOHYDRATE INTAKE

Exercise performance benefits from increased carbohydrate intake before and during high-intensity aerobic exercise and intense training. Vigilance and mood also improve with a carbohydrate beverage administered during a day of sustained aerobic activity interspersed with rest.[117] Carbohydrate loading represents one of the more popular nutritional modifications to increase glycogen reserves. Judicious adherence to this dietary technique improves specific exercise performance, yet some aspects of carbohydrate loading could prove detrimental.

Nutrient-Related Fatigue in Prolonged Exercise

Glycogen stored in the liver and active muscle supplies most of the energy for intense aerobic exercise. Prolonging such exercise reduces glycogen reserves and causes fat catabolism to supply a progressively greater percentage of energy from liver and adipose tissue fatty acid mobilization. Exercise that severely lowers muscle glycogen precipitates fatigue, even though active muscles have sufficient oxygen and unlimited potential energy from stored fat. Ingesting a glucose and water solution near the point of fatigue allows exercise to continue, but for all practical purposes the muscles' "fuel tank" reads empty. A corresponding decrease in exercise power output occurs from the slower rate of fat's mobilization and catabolism compared with carbohydrate.

A Unique Descriptive Term

Marathon runners use the term **"hitting the wall"** (endurance cyclists use *bonking*) to describe sensations of fatigue and discomfort in the active muscles associated with severe glycogen depletion.

In the late 1930s, Nordic scientists reported a startling discovery—athletes' endurance performance improved markedly when they consumed a carbohydrate-rich diet in the days before exercising. Conversely, switching to a high-fat diet markedly lowered glycogen reserves and reduced capacity in intense aerobic exercise (see Fig. 5.6 and Chapters 1 and 5). In a classic series of experiments, endurance capacity tripled for subjects fed a high-carbohydrate diet compared with a high-fat diet of similar energy content.[10] Because carbohydrate represents the important energy substrate during 1 to 2 hours of high-intensity exercise, researchers began to investigate additional relatively "simple" ways to elevate the body's glycogen reserves.

Enhanced Glycogen Storage: Carbohydrate Loading

Combining a specific dietary regimen with exercise produces significant "packing" of muscle glycogen, a procedure termed **carbohydrate loading,** or **glycogen supercompensation.** Endurance athletes often use carbohydrate loading before competition because it increases muscle glycogen even more than a high-carbohydrate diet. Normally, each 100-g of mus-

cle contains about 1.7 g of glycogen; carbohydrate loading packs up to 5 g of glycogen per 100 g of skeletal muscle.

Classic Loading Procedure

TABLE 12.1 indicates that the classic procedure for achieving the supercompensation effect first reduces the muscle's glycogen content with prolonged exercise about 6 days before competition. Because glycogen supercompensation occurs *only* in the specific muscles depleted by exercise, athletes must use the muscles involved in their sport in the depletion phase. Preparing for a marathon requires a 15- or 20-mile run, whereas for swimming and bicycling, approximately 90 minutes of moderately intense submaximal exercise in each activity takes place. The athlete then maintains a low-carbohydrate diet (about 60 to 100 g per day) for several days to further deplete glycogen stores. Glycogen depletion increases formation of intermediate forms of the glycogen-storing enzyme **glycogen synthetase** in the muscle fiber. Moderate training continues during this time. Then at least 3 days before competing, the athlete switches to a high-carbohydrate diet (400 to 700 g per day) and maintains this regimen up to the precompetition meal. The supercompensation diet should also contain adequate protein, minerals, and vitamins and abundant water. For athletes who follow the classic loading procedure, the supercompensated muscle glycogen levels remain stable in a resting, nonexercising individual for at least 3 days if the diet contains 60% of calories from carbohydrate.[61]

Exercise training facilitates both the rate and magnitude of glycogen replenishment. For sports competition and exercise training, a diet containing between 60 and 70% of calories as carbohydrates generally provides adequate muscle and liver glycogen reserves. This diet ensures about twice the level of muscle glycogen obtained with consumption of a typical diet. For well-nourished, physically active individuals, the supercompensation effect remains relatively small. During intense training, however, individuals who do not increase daily caloric and carbohydrate intakes to meet increased energy demands may experience chronic muscle fatigue and staleness.

Individuals should learn all they can about carbohydrate loading before trying to manipulate diet and exercise habits to achieve a supercompensation effect. If a person decides to supercompensate, after weighing the pros and cons (see page 363), the new food regimen should progress in stages during training, not for the first time before competition. For example, a runner should start with a long run followed by a high-carbohydrate diet. The runner should keep a detailed log of how the dietary manipulation affects performance and note subjective feelings during exercise depletion and replenishment phases. With positive results, he or she should then try the entire series of depletion, low-carbohydrate diet, and high-carbohydrate diet but maintain the low-carbohydrate diet for only 1 day. If no adverse effects appear, the low-carbohydrate diet should gradually extend to a maximum of 4 days.

SAMPLE DIETS TO ACHIEVE THE SUPERCOMPENSATION EFFECT. TABLE 12.2 gives meal plans for carbohydrate depletion (*stage 1*) and carbohydrate loading (*stage 2*) preceding an endurance event.

| TABLE 12.1 | Two-Stage Dietary Plan to Increase Muscle Glycogen Storage |

Stage 1—Depletion

Day 1: Exhausting exercise performed to deplete muscle glycogen in specific muscles

Days 2, 3, 4: Low-carbohydrate food intake (high percentage of protein and lipid in the daily diet)

Stage 2—Carbohydrate loading

Days 5, 6, 7: High-carbohydrate food intake (normal percentage of protein in the daily diet)

Competition day

Follow high-carbohydrate precompetition meal

Limited Applicability

Carbohydrate loading benefits only intense aerobic activities lasting more than 60 minutes, unless the person begins competing in a relative state of glycogen depletion. In contrast, less than 60 minutes of intense exercise requires only normal carbohydrate intake and glycogen reserves. For example, carbohydrate loading did not benefit trained runners in a 20.9-km (13-mile) run compared with a run following a low-carbohydrate diet. Similarly, no ergogenic effect emerged in time trial performance, heart rate, and rating of perceived exertion (RPE) for endurance-trained cyclists in a 100-km trial that simulated continuous changes in exercise intensity typical of competition.[21] In addition, ingesting 40 g of carbohydrate immediately before exercise did not benefit a 30-minute maximal cycling performance by trained cyclists.[135] Variations in the carbohydrate percentage between 40 and 70% for an isocaloric diet produced no effect on intense exercise of either 10 or 30 minutes duration.[138] Furthermore, anaerobic power output for 75 seconds or repetitive power performance did not improve when pre-exercise dietary manipulation increased muscle glycogen above normal levels.[71,75] A 2-day maintenance on a high-carbohydrate diet (61% carbohydrate) or a low–moderate carbohydrate diet (31% carbohydrate) produced no effect on intermittent anaerobic exercise consisting of five 20-second bouts interspersed with a 100-second recovery period followed by a sixth 30-second bout to exhaustion.[120] Ergogenic benefits did emerge for high-carbohydrate versus low-carbohydrate intakes when performing *multiple bouts* of short-term sprints.[6]

Negative Aspects of Carbohydrate Loading

The addition of 2.7 g of water with each gram of glycogen stored makes this a heavy fuel compared with equivalent energy stored as fat. The added body mass in the carbohydrate loaded state often makes the person feel "heavy" and uncomfortable; any extra load also directly adds to the energy cost of running, racewalking, or cross-country skiing, all weight-bearing activities. This effect of extra weight may negate any potential benefits from increased glycogen storage. On the

TABLE 12.2	Sample Meal Plan for Carbohydrate Depletion and Carbohydrate Loading Diets Preceding an Endurance Event	
Meal	**Stage 1—Depletion**	**Stage 2—Carbohydrate Loading**
Breakfast	0.5 cup fruit juice 2 eggs 1 slice whole-wheat toast 1 glass whole milk	1 cup fruit juice 1 bowl hot or cold cereal 1 to 2 muffins 1 Tbsp butter Coffee (cream/sugar)
Lunch	6 oz hamburger 2 slices bread Salad (normal size) 1 Tbsp mayonnaise and salad dressing 1 glass whole milk	2–3 oz hamburger with bun 1 cup juice 1 orange 1 Tbsp mayonnaise Pie or cake (8-inch slice)
Snack	1 cup yogurt	1 cup yogurt, fruit, or cookies
Dinner	2–3 pieces of chicken, fried 1 baked potato with sour cream 0.5 cup vegetables Iced tea (no sugar) 2 Tbsp butter	1–1.5 pieces of chicken, baked 1 baked potato with sour cream 1 cup vegetables 0.5 cup sweetened pineapple Iced tea (sugar) 1 Tbsp butter
Snack	1 glass whole milk	1 glass chocolate milk with 4 cookies

During stage 1, the intake of carbohydrate approaches approximately 100 g, 400 kCal; in stage 2, the carbohydrate intake increases to 400 to 625 g or about 1600 to 2500 kCal.

positive side, water liberated during glycogen breakdown aids in temperature regulation, which provides benefits during exercise in the heat.

The classic model for supercompensation poses a potential hazard for individuals with specific health problems. A severe, long-term carbohydrate overload, interspersed with periods of high lipid or high protein intake, can increase blood cholesterol and urea nitrogen levels. This could negatively affect individuals susceptible to type 2 diabetes and heart disease or those with muscle enzyme deficiencies (e.g., McArdle's disease) or renal disease. High lipid intake causes gastrointestinal distress, plus poor recovery from the exercise depletion sequence of the loading procedure. During the low-carbohydrate phase, marked ketosis can occur among individuals who exercise while carbohydrate-depleted. Failure to eat a balanced diet often produces mineral and vitamin deficiencies, particularly of the water-soluble vitamins, which then require supplementation. The glycogen-depleted state certainly reduces one's capability to train hard, possibly resulting in a detraining effect during the loading period. Adverse alterations in mood state also appear in individuals who train while consuming low-carbohydrate diets. Dramatically reducing dietary carbohydrate for 3 or 4 days sets the stage for lean tissue loss because muscle protein serves as gluconeogenic substrate to maintain blood-glucose levels in the glycogen-depleted state.

Modified Loading Procedure

Following the less stringent modified dietary protocol outlined in FIGURE 12.1 eliminates many of the negative outcomes of the classic glycogen-loading sequence. This 6-day protocol does not require prior exercise to exhaustion. The athlete exercises at about 75% of $\dot{V}O_{2max}$ (85% HR_{max}) for 1.5 hours and then on successive days, gradually reduces or tapers exercise duration. During the first 3 days, carbohydrates supply about 50% of total calories. Three days before competition, the diet's carbohydrate content then increases to 70% of total energy intake. This causes glycogen reserves to accumulate to about the *same level* as the classic protocol. The modified approach to carbohydrate loading increases the glycogen-storing enzyme (glycogen synthetase), without requiring the dramatic glycogen depletion with exercise and diet required by the classic loading procedure.[93,206]

Rapid Loading Procedure: A One-Day Requirement

The 2 to 6 days required to achieve supranormal muscle glycogen levels represent a limitation of typical carbohydrate loading procedures. Research has evaluated whether a shortened time period that combines a relatively brief bout of high-intensity exercise with only 1 day of high-carbohydrate intake achieves the desired loading effect. Endurance-trained athletes cycled for 150 seconds at 130% of $\dot{V}O_{2max}$ followed by 30 seconds of all-out cycling. In the recovery period, the men consumed 10.3 g · kg body mass^{-1} of high glycemic carbohydrate foods. Biopsy data presented in FIGURE 12.2 indicated that carbohydrate levels increased in all muscle fiber types of the vastus lateralis muscle from a 109.1 mmol · kg^{-1}

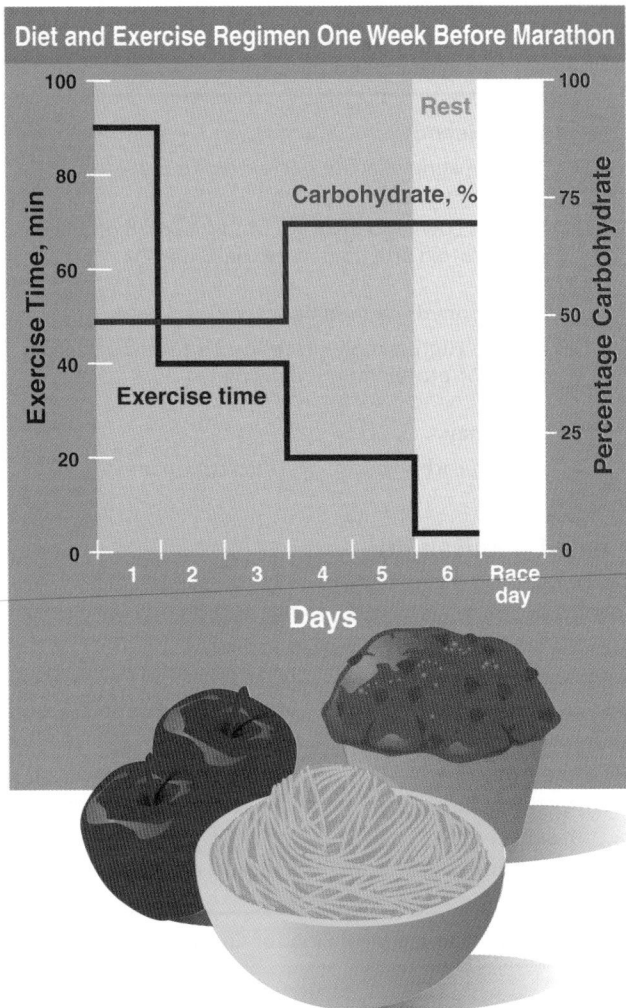

FIGURE 12.1 ■ The modified carbohydrate-loading approach. Recommended combination of diet and exercise for overloading muscle glycogen stores in the week before an endurance contest. Time devoted to exercise becomes gradually reduced during the week, while the diet's carbohydrate content increases for the last 3 days. (From Sherman WM, et al. Effect of exercise-diet manipulation on muscle glycogen and its subsequent utilization during performance. *Int J Sports Med* 1981;2:114.)

preloading average to 198.3 mmol · kg^{-1} after only 24 hours. This 82% increase in glycogen storage equaled or exceeded values reported by others using a 2- to 6-day regimen. The short-duration loading procedure benefits individuals who do not wish to disrupt normal training with the time required and potential negative aspects of other loading protocols.

Gender Differences in Glycogen Supercompensation and Glucose Catabolism in Exercise

Gender-related differences in muscle glycogen supercompensation remain controversial. One study reported a relatively small 13% increase in the muscle glycogen content of women

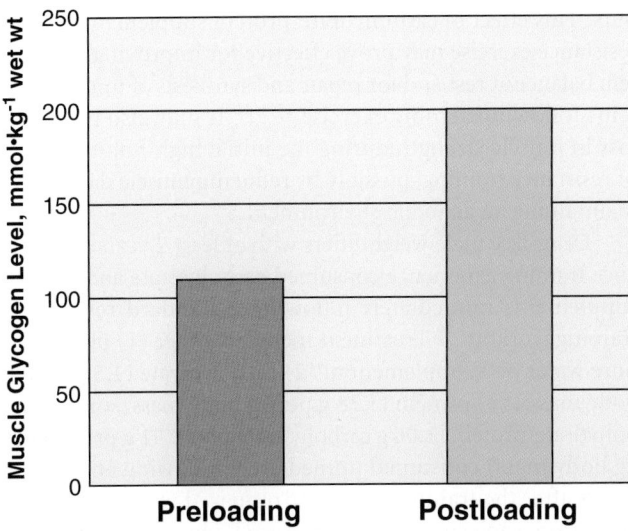

FIGURE 12.2 ■ Muscle glycogen concentration of the vastus lateralis before (preloading) and after 180 seconds of near-maximal intensity cycling exercise followed by 1 day of high carbohydrate intake (postloading). (From Fairchild TJ, et al. Rapid carbohydrate loading after short bout of near maximal-intensity exercise. *Med Sci Sports Exerc* 2002;34:980.)

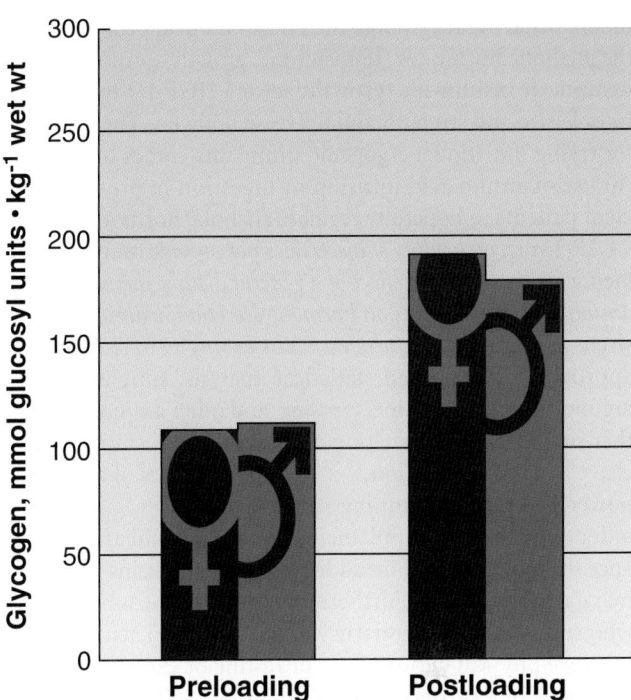

FIGURE 12.3 ■ Muscle glycogen concentrations pre- and post-carbohydrate loading in exercise-trained men and women. (From James AP, et al. Muscle glycogen supercompensation: absence of a gender-related difference. *Eur J Appl Physiol* 2001;85:533.)

when they switched from a mixed diet to a high-carbohydrate diet.[195] Other research also indicated that women stored less glycogen than men when dietary carbohydrate increased from 60 to 75% of total energy intake.[174] This increase in carbohydrate intake as a percentage of total calories represents *significantly less total carbohydrate intake* relative to lean body mass for women than for men. FIGURE 12.3 illustrates that equalizing daily carbohydrate intake for endurance-trained men and women at 12 g per kg of lean body mass for 3 consecutive days produced no gender differences in glycogen loading. These and other findings[175] support the notion that men and women possess an equal capacity to accumulate muscle glycogen when fed comparable amounts of carbohydrate relative to their lean body mass.

Gender differences exist in carbohydrate metabolism during exercise before and after endurance training. During submaximal exercise at equivalent percentages of $\dot{V}O_{2max}$ (same relative workload), women derive a smaller proportion of total energy from carbohydrate oxidation than men.[87] This gender difference in substrate oxidation does not persist into recovery.[81]

With similar endurance-training protocols, both women and men decrease glucose use during a given submaximal power output.[32,55] However, at the same relative workload after training, women show an exaggerated shift toward fat catabolism, whereas men do not.[87] This suggests that endurance training induces greater glycogen-sparing at a given percentage of maximal effort for women. Gender differences in exercise substrate metabolism may reflect sympathetic nervous system adaptation to training with a more-diminished catecholamine response for women. A glycogen-sparing metabolic adaptation could benefit a woman's performance during intense endurance competition.

Muscle Glycogen Supercompensation Enhanced by Prior Creatine Supplementation

A synergy exists between glycogen storage and creatine supplementation. For example, preceding a glycogen loading protocol with a 5-day creatine loading protocol (20 g per day) produced 10% more glycogen packing in the vastus lateralis muscle than achieved with glycogen loading alone.[155] More than likely, increases in creatine and cellular volume with creatine supplementation facilitate subsequent storage of muscle glycogen.

AMINO ACID SUPPLEMENTS AND OTHER DIETARY MODIFICATIONS FOR AN ANABOLIC EFFECT

Chapter 11 focused on anabolic–androgenic steroid use by an alarming number of male and female athletes in diverse sports. Coincidentally, an emerging trend involves using nutrition as a legal alternative for activating the body's normal anabolic mechanisms. Highly specific dietary changes supposedly create a hormonal milieu to facilitate protein synthesis in skeletal muscle. More than 100 companies in the United States market alleged ergogenic stimulants. Weightlifters, body builders, and fitness enthusiasts use amino acid supplements believing they boost the body's natural production of the anabolic hormones (testosterone, growth hormone [GH], insulin, or insulin-like growth factor I [IGF-I]) to increase muscle size and strength and decrease body fat. The rationale for trying nutritional ergogenic stimulants comes from clinical use of amino acid infusion or ingestion in protein-deficient patients to hopefully regulate anabolic hormones.

Research on healthy subjects does not provide convincing evidence for an ergogenic effect of a general dietary increase of oral amino acid supplements on hormone secretion, training responsiveness, or exercise performance. For example, in studies with appropriate design and statistical analysis, supplements of arginine, lysine, ornithine, tyrosine, and other amino acids, either singly or in combination, produced no effect on GH levels,[53,173] insulin secretion,[19,53] diverse measures of anaerobic power,[52] or all-out running performance at $\dot{V}O_{2max}$.[170] For older men, protein supplementation before and after resistance training provided no additional effect on gains in muscle mass and strength.[24] Furthermore, elite junior weightlifters who supplemented regularly with all 20 amino acids did not improve physical performance or resting or exercise-induced responses of testosterone, cortisol, or GH.[57] The indiscriminate use of amino acid supplements at dosages considered pharmacologic rather than nutritional increases risk of direct toxic effects or creation of an amino acid imbalance.[123]

Prudent Means to Possibly Augment an Anabolic Effect

Manipulation of exercise and nutritional variables in the immediate pre-exercise and postexercise periods can have an impact on the responsiveness to resistance training via mechanisms that alter nutrient availability, circulating metabolites and hormonal secretions and interactions with receptors on target tissues, and gene translation and transcription.[189] With resistance training, muscle enlargement (hypertrophy) occurs from a shift in the body's normal dynamic state of protein synthesis and degradation to greater tissue synthesis. The normal hormonal milieu (e.g., insulin and GH levels) in the period following resistance exercise stimulates the muscle fiber's anabolic processes while inhibiting muscle protein degradation. Specific dietary modifications that increase amino acid transport into muscle, raise energy availability, or increase anabolic hormone levels would theoretically augment the training effect by increasing the rate of anabolism and/or depressing catabolism. Either effect should create a positive body protein balance for improved muscular growth and strength.

Carbohydrate–Protein Supplementation Immediately in Recovery Augments Hormonal Response to Resistance Exercise

Studies of hormonal dynamics and muscle protein anabolism indicate a transient but potential ergogenic effect (up to four-fold increase in protein synthesis[146]) of carbohydrate and/or protein supplements consumed *before,*[178,204] or *immediately following,*[48,104,105,127,145,151,158,199] resistance exercise workouts. This effect of carbohydrate-protein supplementation in resistance exercise may prove effective for improving net protein balance at rest and for repair and synthesis of muscle proteins following aerobic exercise.[115,116] It may also blunt the loss in muscle strength during the initial high-volume stress of resistance training, possibly by reducing muscle damage by maintaining an anabolic environment.[108]

Drug-free male weightlifters with at least 2 years of resistance training experience consumed carbohydrate and protein supplements immediately following a standard resistance-training workout.[29] Treatment included either (1) placebo of pure water or a supplement of (2) carbohydrate (1.5 g per kg body mass), (3) protein (1.38 g per kg body mass), or (4) carbohydrate/protein (1.06 g carbohydrate plus 0.41 g protein per kg body mass) consumed immediately following and then 2 hours after the training session. Compared with the placebo condition, each supplement produced a hormonal environment in recovery conducive to protein synthesis and muscle tissue growth (elevated plasma concentrations of insulin and GH). Subsequent research from the same laboratory showed that protein–carbohydrate supplementation before and after resistance training favorably altered metabolic and hormonal responses to three consecutive days of intense resistance training.[107] Changes in the immediate recovery period included increased concentrations of glucose, insulin, GH, and IGF-I and decreased blood lactate concentration. Such data provide indirect evidence for a possible training benefit of increasing carbohydrate and/or protein intake immediately after a resistance-training workout.

POSTEXERCISE GLUCOSE AUGMENTS PROTEIN BALANCE AFTER RESISTANCE TRAINING. Research with postexercise glucose ingestion complements the previously described studies of carbohydrate/protein supplementation following resistance training.[157] Healthy men familiar with resistance training performed unilateral knee extensor exercise consisting of eight sets of 10 repetitions at 85% of maximum strength (1-RM) in a placebo-controlled, randomized, double-blind trial. Immediately following the exercise session and 1 hour later, subjects received either a carbohydrate supplement (1.0 g per kg body mass) or a placebo (NutraSweet). Measurements consisted of (1) urinary 3-methylhistidine excretion (3-MH) to indicate muscle protein degradation, (2) vastus lateralis muscle incorporation rate for the amino acid leucine (L-[l-^{13}C]) to indicate protein synthesis, and (3) urinary nitrogen excretion to reflect protein breakdown. FIGURE 12.4 shows that glucose supplementation reduced myofibrillar protein breakdown reflected by decreased excretion of both 3-MH and urinary urea. Glucose supplementation also increased leucine incorporation into the vastus lateralis over the 10-hour postexercise period (not statistically significant). These alterations indicated a more positive protein balance after exercise in the supplemented condition. The beneficial effect of glucose supplementation immediately following resistance exercise most likely resulted from increased insulin release. This hormone would enhance a positive muscle protein balance in recovery.

Although of possible significance as a "natural" means to stimulate anabolic processes and augment protein accre-

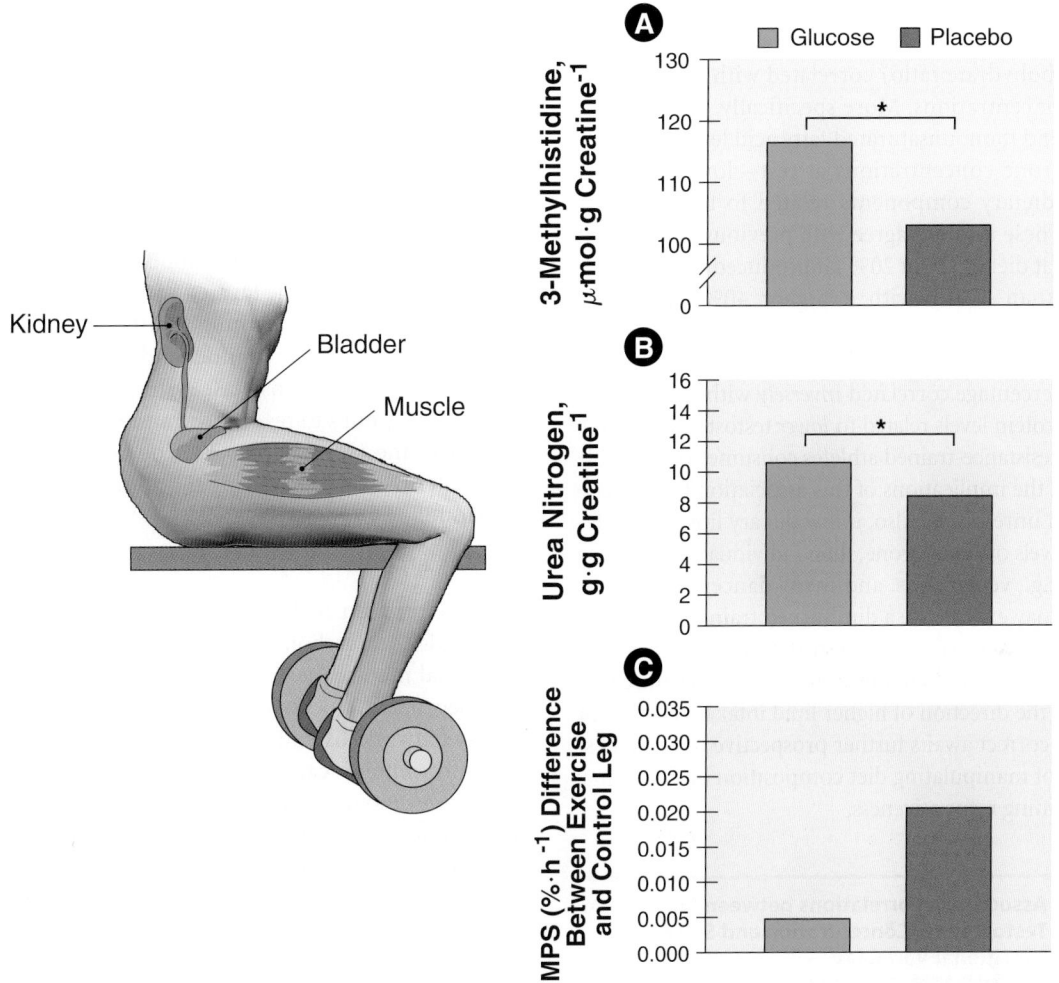

FIGURE 12.4 ■ The effects of glucose (1.0 g per kg body mass) versus NutraSweet placebo ingested immediately after exercise and 1 hour later on protein degradation reflected by 24-hour urinary output of **(A)** 3-methylhistidine and **(B)** urea nitrogen, and **(C)** the rate of muscle protein synthesis *(MPS)* measured by vastus lateralis muscle incorporation rate for the amino acid leucine (L-[l-^{13}C]). *Bars* for MPS indicate difference between exercise and control leg for glucose and placebo conditions. *Significantly different from placebo condition. (From Roy BD, et al. Effect of glucose supplement timing on protein metabolism after resistance training. *J Appl Physiol* 1997;82:1882.)

tion, the effects of immediate postexercise carbohydrate and/or protein supplementation must be viewed in perspective. The question awaiting an answer is the degree to which any transient (albeit positive) change in hormonal milieu favoring anabolism and net protein synthesis caused by postexercise dietary maneuvers contributes to *long-term* muscle growth and strength enhancement. In this regard, recent research failed to show any effect of immediate postexercise ingestion of an amino acid–carbohydrate mixture on muscular strength or size gains of older men undergoing 12 weeks of knee extensor resistance training.[59] Differences in study population, criterion variables, specific amino acid mixtures, diet composition, and subjects' age may account for future discrepancies in research findings.

Dietary Lipid Affects Hormonal Milieu

The diet's lipid content modulates resting neuroendocrine homeostasis in a direction that may modify tissue synthesis. Research evaluated the effects of an intense resistance exercise bout on postexercise plasma testosterone, an anabolic and anticatabolic hormone released by the Leydig cells of the testes.[191] In agreement with prior research, testosterone levels significantly increased 5 minutes postexercise. A more impressive finding revealed a close association between the individual's regular dietary nutrient composition and resting plasma testosterone levels. TABLE 12.3 shows that dietary macronutrient amount and composition (protein, lipid, saturated fatty acids, monounsaturated fatty acids, polyunsaturated unsaturated fatty acid/saturated fatty acid ratio, and protein-to-carbohydrate ratio) correlated with pre-exercise testosterone concentrations. More specifically, dietary lipid and saturated and monounsaturated fatty acid levels best predicted testosterone concentrations at rest—lower levels of each of these dietary components related to lower testosterone levels. These findings agree with previous studies that showed a low-fat diet of about 20% fat produced lower testosterone levels than a diet with a higher 40% lipid content.[144,150,176]

Interestingly, the data in TABLE 12.3 also show that the diet's protein percentage correlated *inversely* with testosterone levels (higher protein levels related to *lower* testosterone levels). Because many resistance-trained athletes consume considerable dietary protein, the implications of this association for exercise training remain unresolved. Also, if low dietary lipid levels decrease resting levels of testosterone, then individuals consuming low-fat diets (e.g., vegetarians, and many dancers, gymnasts, and wrestlers) may experience a diminished training response. Athletes who show reduced plasma testosterone with overtraining might benefit from changing their diet's macronutrient composition in the direction of higher lipid intake. Whether or not this proves correct awaits further prospective trials that assess the effects of manipulating diet composition on hormonal balance *and* training responsiveness.

TABLE 12.3 **Association Correlations between Preexercise Testosterone Concentration and Selected Nutritional Variables**

Nutrient	Correlation with testosterone[a]
Energy, kJ	−0.18
Protein, %[b]	−0.71*
CHO, %	−0.30
Lipid, %	0.72*
SFA, g·1000 kCal^{-1}·day^{-1}	0.77†
MUFA, g·1000 kCal^{-1}·day^{-1}	0.79†
PUFA, g·1000 kCal^{-1}·day^{-1}	0.25
Cholesterol, g·1000 kCal^{-1}·day^{-1}	0.53
PUFA/SFA	−0.63‡
Dietary fiber, g·1000 kCal^{-1}·day^{-1}	−0.19
Protein/CHO	−0.59‡
Protein/lipid	0.16
CHO/lipid	0.16

From Volek JS, et al.: Testosterone and cortisol in relationship to dietary nutrients and resistance exercise. J Appl Physiol 1997;82:49.

[a]*Correlation coefficients, Pearson product-moment correlations.*

[b]*Nutrient percentage values expressed as percentage of total energy per day.*

*P ≤ .01. †P ≤ .005. ‡P ≤ .05.

SFA, saturated fatty acids; MUFA, monounsaturated fatty acids; PUFA, polyunsaturated fatty acids; CHO, cholesterol.

L-CARNITINE

L-Carnitine (L-3-hydroxytrimethylamminobutanoate), a short-chain carboxylic acid containing nitrogen, is a vitamin-like compound with well-established functions in intermediary metabolism. It is found mostly in meat and dairy products. (*Note:* DL-carnitine is toxic and should never be consumed.) The liver and kidneys synthesize L-carnitine from methionine and lysine, with about 95% of the 20-g (120 mmol) total of carnitine located within muscle cells. Vital to normal metabolism, carnitine facilitates the influx of long-chain fatty acids into the mitochondrial matrix as part of the carnitine–acyl-CoA transferase system. The system causes activated acyl groups to reversibly transfer between coenzyme A and carnitine (see Chapter 4). The fatty acid components then enter β-oxidation during mitochondrial energy metabolism as follows:

$$\text{Carnitine} + \text{acyl-CoA} \leftrightarrow \text{acylcarnitine} + \text{CoA}$$

The reaction enables the acyl components of long-chain fatty acyl-CoA (carbon chain lengths ≥10) to cross the mitochondrial membrane as substrate for oxidation. This carnitine-dependent process is probably an important rate-limiting step in fatty acid oxidation.

Intracellular carnitine helps to maintain the acetyl-CoA/CoA ratio within the cell. Optimizing this ratio augments skeletal muscle energy metabolism by limiting inhibition of the pyruvate dehydrogenase enzyme; this effect facilitates conversion of pyruvate (and lactate) to acetyl-CoA, particularly in the type I, slow-twitch muscle fibers.[28,56] Theoretically, enhanced carnitine function could inhibit lactate accumulation and enhance exercise performance.[34,97] TABLE 12.4 outlines the potential mechanisms by which carnitine supplementation could enhance exercise performance.

TABLE 12.4 **Potential Mechanisms for a Beneficial Effect of Carnitine Supplementation on Exercise Performance in Healthy Humans**

- Enhance muscle fatty acid oxidation in exercise
- Decrease muscle glycogen depletion
- Shift substrate use in muscle from glucose to fatty acids
- Replace muscle carnitine redistributed into acylcarnitine
- Activate pyruvate dehydrogenase via lowering of acetyl-CoA content
- Improve muscle fatigue resistance
- Replace carnitine lost during training

From Brass EP. Supplemental carnitine and exercise. Am J Clin Nutr 2000;72(suppl):618S.

Rate of Fatty Acid Oxidation Affects Aerobic Exercise Intensity

During prolonged aerobic exercise, plasma free fatty acids (FFAs) often rise to a greater extent than required by the actual energy expenditure. The plasma lipid elevation could result from inadequate mitochondrial fatty acid uptake and oxidation because of insufficient L-carnitine concentration. Increasing intracellular L-carnitine levels through dietary supplementation should elevate aerobic energy transfer from fat breakdown while conserving limited glycogen reserves. Supplementation should prove most beneficial under conditions of glycogen depletion, which places the greatest demand on fatty acid oxidation.

A Compound for All

Marketers of L-carnitine target endurance athletes who believe this "metabolic stimulator" enhances fat burning and spares glycogen. Not surprisingly, the alleged fat-burning benefits of carnitine also appeal to body builders as a practical way to reduce body fat.

Although patients with progressive muscle weakness have benefited from carnitine administration, few data suggest that healthy adults require carnitine above levels in a well-balanced diet. *Research shows no ergogenic benefits, positive metabolic alterations (aerobic or anaerobic), enhanced recovery effect, or body fat-reducing effects from L-carnitine supplementation.*[1,18,33,159,171] For example, no difference exists in muscle carnitine levels between young and middle-aged men who consume a normal carnitine intake of about 100 to 200 mg daily. For these individuals, typical variations in carnitine levels do not reflect capacity for aerobic metabolism.[168] Furthermore, no L-carnitine deficit occurs during long-term exercise or intense training.[39,86,134] The low bioavailability and rapid renal excretion of oral carnitine make it highly unlikely that supplementation affects muscle carnitine stores in healthy subjects. Taking up to 2000 mg of L-carnitine, either orally or intravenously, during aerobic exercise does not affect the fuel mixture catabolized or endurance performance, aerobic capacity, or the exercise level for the onset of blood lactate accumulation (OBLA).[16,194]

Short-term administration of 2000 mg of L-carnitine to endurance athletes 2 hours before a marathon and after 20 km of the run increased plasma concentrations of all carnitine fractions.[33] The carnitine increases did not affect running performance, alter metabolic mixture during the run, or enhance recovery. Even with exercise prolonged and intense enough to deplete glycogen reserves, L-carnitine supplements did not alter substrate metabolism to indicate enhanced fat oxidation.[40] Carnitine supplementation also exerts no effect on repetitive short-term anaerobic exercise. Lactate accumulation, acid–base balance, or performance in five, 100-yard swims with 2-minute rest intervals did not differ between competitive swimmers who consumed 2000 mg of L-carnitine in a citrus drink twice daily for 7 days and swimmers who only consumed the citrus drink.[179]

Perhaps of Some Benefit

L-Carnitine acts as a vasodilator in peripheral tissues, thus possibly enhancing regional blood flow and oxygen delivery. In one study, subjects took either L-carnitine supplements (3000 mg per day for 3 weeks) or an inert placebo to evaluate the effectiveness of L-carnitine supplementation on delayed-onset muscle soreness (DOMS).[58] They then performed eccentric muscle actions to induce muscle soreness. Compared with placebo conditions, subjects receiving L-carnitine experienced less postexercise muscle pain and tissue damage as indicated by lower plasma levels of the muscle enzyme creatine kinase (CK). The vasodilation property of L-carnitine might improve oxygen supply to injured tissue and promote clearance of muscle damage by-products, thus reducing DOMS.

CHROMIUM

Chromium occurs widely in soil as chromite at a concentration that averages 250 μg per kg of soil. Its distribution in plants ranges between 100 and 500 μg per kg and in foodstuffs between 20 and 590 μg per kg. This trace mineral serves as a cofactor (as trivalent chromium) for a low-molecular-weight protein that potentiates insulin function, although chromium's precise mechanism of action remains unclear. Insulin promotes glucose transport into cells, augments fatty acid metabolism, and triggers cellular enzyme activity to facilitate protein synthesis.

Chronic chromium deficiency increases blood cholesterol and decreases sensitivity to insulin, thus increasing the chance for developing type 2 diabetes. Some adult Americans consume less than the 50 to 200 μg of chromium each day considered the estimated safe and adequate daily dietary intake (ESADDI). This occurs largely because chromium-rich foods—brewer's yeast, broccoli, wheat germ, nuts, liver, prunes, egg yolks, apples with skins, asparagus, mushrooms, wine, and cheese—do not usually form part of the regular diet. Processing also removes considerable chromium from foods, and strenuous exercise and associated high carbohydrate intake promote urinary chromium losses, thus increasing the potential for chromium deficiency.

For athletes with chromium-deficient diets, modifications to increase chromium intake or prudent use of chromium supplements seem appropriate. Touted as a "fat burner" and "muscle builder," chromium represents one of the largest selling mineral supplements in the United States (second only to calcium). Used by more than 10 million people, it commands annual sales of roughly $500 million. Poor intestinal absorption of chromium in its inorganic form (chromium chloride) provides a main hindrance to effective oral chromium supplementation. Supplement intake of chromium, usually as

chromium picolinate (picolinic acid, an organic compound in breast milk that helps transport minerals), often reaches 600 μg daily. This chelated picolinic acid combination supposedly improves chromium absorption. Millions of Americans believe the unsubstantiated claims of health food faddists, television infomercials, and exercise zealots that additional chromium promotes muscle growth, curbs appetite, fosters body fat loss, and lengthens life.

A Nutritional Link to Bigger Muscles?

Advertisers target chromium supplements to body builders and other resistance-trained individuals as a safe alternative to anabolic steroids to favorably modify body composition. Chromium supplements supposedly potentiate insulin's action, thus increasing skeletal muscle's amino acid anabolism. This belief persists despite sufficient scientific evidence that chromium supplements exert no effect on glucose or insulin concentrations in nondiabetic individuals.[2]

Generally, studies suggesting beneficial effects of chromium supplements on body fat and muscle mass inferred body composition modifications from changes in body weight (or unvalidated anthropometric measurements) instead of a more appropriate assessment by hydrostatic weighing or dual energy x-ray absorptiometry (DXA). One study observed that supplementing daily with 200 μg (3.85 μmol) of chromium picolinate for 40 days produced a small increase in fat-free body mass (FFM; estimated from skinfold thickness) and a decrease in body fat in young men undergoing 6 weeks of resistance training.[49] Another study reported increased body mass without changes in muscular strength or body composition in previously untrained female college students (no change in males) receiving daily chromium supplements of 200 μg during a 12-week resistance training program compared with unsupplemented controls.[74]

Other research evaluated the effects of a daily 200-μg chromium supplement on muscle strength, body composition, and chromium excretion in untrained men during 12 weeks of resistance training.[70] Muscular strength improved 24% for the supplemented group and 33% for the placebo group. No changes occurred in any of the body composition variables. The group receiving the supplement did show higher chromium excretion than the controls after 6 weeks of training. The researchers concluded that chromium supplements provided *no ergogenic effect* on any of the measured variables.

Daily supplementation of 400 μg of chromium picolinate for 9 weeks did not promote weight loss for sedentary obese women, but actually caused weight gain during the treatment period.[64] In support of chromium supplementation, greater body fat loss (no increase in FFM) occurred in subjects "recruited from a variety of fitness and athletic clubs" who consumed 400 μg daily over 90 days than in subjects receiving a placebo.[96] Hydrostatic weighing and DXA assessed body composition. The pretest versus posttest body composition data from hydrostatic weighing were not presented, and the DXA-derived analysis indicated average percentage body fat values of 42% for both control and experimental subjects, a seemingly extraordinary level of obesity for fitness club members.

Collegiate football players who received daily supplements of 200 μg of chromium picolinate for 9 weeks showed no changes in body composition and muscular strength from intense weight-lifting training compared with a control group who received a placebo.[31] Similar findings of no benefit on body composition and exercise performance variables emerged from a 14-week study of NCAA Division I wrestlers who combined chromium picolinate supplementation with a typical preseason training program, compared with identical training without supplementation.[196]

Muscle mass loss commonly affects older individuals, so any potential benefit on muscle from chromium supplementation should readily emerge in this group. This did not occur for older men involved in high-intensity resistance training. A daily high dose of 924 μg of chromium picolinate did not augment gains in muscle size, strength, or power or FFM compared with the no-supplement condition.[23] Among obese personnel enrolled in the U.S. Navy's mandatory remedial physical conditioning program, consuming additional 400 μg of chromium picolinate daily caused no greater loss in body weight and percentage body fat or increase in FFM than occurred in a group receiving a placebo.[180]

A comprehensive double-blind research design studied the effect of a daily chromium supplement (3.3–3.5 μmol either as chromium chloride or chromium picolinate) or a placebo for 8 weeks during resistance training in young men.[119] For each group, dietary intakes of protein, magnesium, zinc, copper, and iron equaled or exceeded recommended levels during training; subjects also maintained adequate baseline chromium intakes. Supplementation increased serum chromium concentration and urinary chromium excretion equally, regardless of its ingested form. TABLE 12.5 shows that compared with placebo treatment, chromium supplementation did not affect training-related changes in muscular strength, physique, FFM, or muscle mass. The Federal Trade Commission has ordered manufacturers of chromium supplements to cease promoting unsubstantiated weight loss and health claims (reduced body fat, increased muscle mass, increased energy level) for chromium picolinate. Companies can no longer claim benefits for this compound unless reliable research data substantiated such claims.

Not without a Potential Down Side

Chromium competes with iron for binding to transferrin, a plasma protein that transports iron from ingested food and damaged red blood cells and delivers it to tissues in need. The chromium picolinate supplements for the group whose data appear in TABLE 12.5 did reduce serum transferrin (a measure of current iron intake) compared with chromium chloride or placebo treatments. However, other researchers have ob-

---

TABLE 12.5   **Effects of Two Different Forms of Chromium Supplementation on Average Values for Anthropometric, Bone, and Soft Tissue Composition Measurements before and after Weight Training**

	Placebo		Chromium chloride		Chromium picolinate	
	Pre	Post	Pre	Post	Pre	Post
Age (y)	21.1	21.5	23.3	23.5	22.3	22.5
Stature (cm)	179.3	179.2	177.3	177.3	178.0	178.2
Weight (kg)	79.9	80.5[a]	79.3	81.1[a]	79.2	80.5
Σ4 skinfold thickness (mm)[b]	42.0	41.5	42.6	42.2	43.3	43.1
Upper arm (cm)	30.9	31.6[a]	31.3	32.0[a]	31.1	31.4[a]
Lower leg (cm)	38.2	37.9	37.4	37.5	37.1	37.0
Endomorphy	3.68	3.73	3.58	3.54	3.71	3.72
Mesomorphy	4.09	4.36[a]	4.25	4.42[a]	4.21	4.33[a]
Ectomorphy	2.09	1.94[a]	1.79	1.63[a]	2.00	1.88[a]
FFMFM (kg)[c]	62.9	64.3[a]	61.1	63.1[a]	61.3	62.7[a]
Bone mineral (g)	2952	2968	2860	2878	2918	2940
Fat-free mass (kg)	65.9	67.3[a]	64.0	65.9[a]	64.2	66.1[a]
Fat (kg)	13.4	13.1	14.7	15.1	14.7	14.5
Fatness (%)	16.4	15.7	18.4	18.2	18.4	17.9

From Lukaski HC, et al. Chromium supplementation and resistance training: effects on body composition, strength, and trace element status of men. Am J Clin Nutr 1996;63:954.

[a]*Significantly different from pretraining value*

[b]*Measured at biceps, triceps, subscapular, and suprailiac sites*

[c]*Fat-free, mineral-free mass*

---

served that giving middle-aged men 924 μg of supplemental chromium picolinate daily for 12 weeks did not affect hematologic measures or indices of iron metabolism or iron status.[22] Further research must determine whether chromium supplementation above recommended values adversely affects iron transport and distribution within the body. No studies have evaluated the safety of long-term supplementation with chromium picolinate or the ergogenic efficacy of supplementation in individuals with suboptimal chromium status. Concerning the bioavailability of trace minerals in the diet, excessive dietary chromium inhibits zinc and iron absorption. At the extreme, this could induce iron-deficiency anemia, blunt the ability to train intensely, and negatively affect exercise performance requiring a high level of aerobic metabolism.

Further potential bad news emerges from studies in which human tissue cultures that received extreme doses of chromium picolinate show eventual chromosomal damage. Critics contend that such high laboratory dosages do not occur with supplement use in humans. Nonetheless, one could argue that cells continually exposed to excessive chromium (e.g., long-term supplementation) accumulate this mineral and retain it for years.

COENZYME Q10 (UBIQUINONE)

Coenzyme Q_{10} (CoQ_{10}, *ubiquinone* in oxidized form and *ubiquinol* when reduced), found primarily in meats, peanuts,

and soybean oil, functions as an integral component of the mitochondrion's electron transport system of oxidative phosphorylation. This lipid-soluble natural component of all cells exists in high concentrations within myocardial tissue. CoQ_{10} has been used therapeutically to treat cardiovascular disease because of (1) its role in oxidative metabolism and (2) its antioxidant properties that promote scavenging of free radicals that damage cellular components.[88,187] Owing to its positive effect on oxygen uptake and exercise performance in cardiac patients, some consider CoQ_{10} a potential ergogenic nutrient for endurance performance. Based on the belief that supplementation could increase the flux of electrons through the respiratory chain and thus augment aerobic resynthesis of adenosine triphosphate (ATP), the popular literature touts CoQ_{10} supplements to improve "stamina" and enhance cardiovascular function.

Supplementation with CoQ_{10} increases serum CoQ_{10} levels, but it does not improve aerobic capacity, endurance performance, plasma glucose, or lactate levels at submaximal workloads, or cardiovascular dynamics compared with a placebo.[17,153,208] One study evaluated oral supplements of CoQ_{10} on the exercise tolerance and peripheral muscle function of healthy, middle-aged men. Measurements included $\dot{V}O_{2max}$, lactate threshold, heart rate response and upper-extremity exercise blood flow and metabolism.[141] For 2 months, subjects received either CoQ_{10} (150 mg per day) or a placebo. Blood levels of CoQ_{10} increased during the treatment period and remained unchanged in the controls. No differences occurred between groups for any of the physiologic or metabolic variables. Similarly, for trained young and older men, CoQ_{10} supplementation of 120 mg per day for 6 weeks did not benefit aerobic capacity or lipid peroxidation, a marker of oxidative stress.[113] More recent data also indicate that CoQ_{10} supplements (60 mg daily combined with vitamins E and C) did not affect lipid peroxidation during exercise in endurance athletes.[187] On the other hand, rats supplemented with CoQ_{10} (10 mg per day for 4 days), showed marked suppression of exercise-induced lipid peroxidation in liver, heart, and gastrocnemius muscle tissues.[50]

Future research must elucidate any potential benefits from exogenous CoQ_{10} supplementation. If benefits result, do they depend on the health status of one's cardiovascular system? On a negative note, CoQ_{10} supplementation may induce harmful effects. Increased cell damage (increased plasma CK) occurred during intense exercise in subjects receiving 60 mg of CoQ_{10} twice daily for 20 days.[124] Researchers speculate that under conditions of high proton concentrations as occur in intense aerobic exercise, CoQ_{10} supplementation augments free radical production.[42,124] If this proves true, supplementation could trigger plasma membrane lipid peroxidation and eventual cellular damage. This is indeed paradoxical in light of CoQ_{10}'s wide use as an oral antioxidant supplement.[76]

CREATINE

Meat, poultry, and fish provide rich sources of creatine; they contain approximately 4 to 5 g per kg of food weight. The body synthesizes only about 1 to 2 g of this nitrogen-containing organic compound daily, primarily in the kidneys, liver, and pancreas, from the amino acids arginine, glycine, and methionine. Thus, adequate dietary creatine usually becomes important for obtaining required amounts of this compound.[205] Because the animal kingdom contains the richest creatine-containing foods, vegetarians experience a distinct disadvantage in obtaining ready sources of exogenous creatine.

Creatine supplements, sold as **creatine monohydrate (CrH$_2$O),** come as a powder, tablet, capsule, and stabilized liquid. A person can purchase creatine over-the-counter or via mail order as a nutritional supplement (without guarantee of purity). Ingesting a liquid suspension of creatine monohydrate at the relatively high dosage of 20 to 30 g per day for up to 2 weeks increases intramuscular concentrations of free creatine and phosphocreatine by 10 to 30%. These levels remain high for weeks after only a few days of supplementation.[67,73,125] An athlete can supplement with creatine in international competition because governing bodies (including the IOC) do not consider creatine an illegal substance.

Important Component of High-Energy Phosphates

The precise physiologic mechanisms underlying the potential ergogenic effectiveness of supplemental creatine remain poorly understood. Creatine passes through the digestive tract unaltered for absorption into the bloodstream by the intestinal mucosa. Just about all ingested creatine incorporates

within skeletal muscle (120–150 g total with average concentration of 125 mM [range, 90–160 mM] per kg dry muscle) via insulin-mediated active transport. About 40% of the total exists as free creatine; the remainder combines readily with phosphate (in the CK reaction shown below) to form phosphocreatine (PCr). Type II, fast-twitch muscle fibers store about 4 to 6 times more PCr than ATP.[27] As emphasized in Chapter 4, PCr serves as the cells' "energy reservoir" to provide rapid phosphate-bond energy to resynthesize ATP (more rapid than ATP generated in glycogenolysis) in the reversible CK reaction:

$$PCr + ADP \xleftrightarrow{\text{creatine kinase}} Cr + ATP$$

PCr may also "shuttle" intramuscular high-energy phosphate between the mitochondria and the cross-bridge sites that initiate muscle action. Maintaining a high sarcoplasmic ATP/ADP ratio by energy transfer from PCr becomes important in all-out effort lasting up to 10 seconds. Such short-duration exercise places considerable demands on the rate of ATP resynthesis, the breakdown of which greatly exceeds energy transfer from the intracellular macronutrients.[13] Improved energy transfer capacity from PCr also lessens reliance on energy transfer from anaerobic glycolysis with its associated increase in intramuscular H^+ and decrease in pH from lactate accumulation. Owing to limited amounts of intramuscular PCr, it seems reasonable that any increase in PCr availability should have the following four effects:[13,26,68,184]

1. Accelerating ATP turnover rate to maintain power output during short-term muscular effort
2. Delaying PCr depletion
3. Diminishing dependence on anaerobic glycolysis with subsequent lactate formation
4. Facilitating muscle relaxation and recovery from repeated bouts of an intense, brief effort via increased rate of ATP and PCr resynthesis; rapid recovery allows continued high-level power output

---

Three Important Benefits to Strength/Power Athletes

Creatine supplementation at recommended levels exerts the following three effects in individuals involved in power-type physical activities:

1. Improves repetitive performance in muscular strength and short-term power activities
2. Augments short bursts of muscular endurance
3. Provides greater muscular overload to enhance training effectiveness.

Documented Benefits Under Certain Exercise Conditions

Creatine received notoriety as an ergogenic aid when used by British sprinters and hurdlers in the 1992 Barcelona Olympic Games. Creatine supplementation at the recommended level exerts ergogenic effects in short-duration, high-intensity exercise (5–10% improvement) without producing harmful side effects (TABLE 12.6). Anecdotes indicate a possible association between creatine supplementation and cramping in multiple muscle areas during competition or lengthy practice by football players. This effect may result from (1) altered intracellular dynamics from increased free creatine and PCr levels or (2) an osmotically induced enlarged muscle cell volume (greater cellular hydration) caused by the increased creatine content. Gastrointestinal tract disturbances such as nausea, indigestion, and difficulty absorbing food have also been linked to exogenous creatine ingestion.

FIGURE 12.5 clearly illustrates the positive ergogenic effects of creatine loading on total work accomplished during repetitive sprint cycling performance. Physically active but untrained males performed sets of maximal 6-second bicycle sprints interspersed with various recovery periods (24, 54, or 84 s) between sprints to simulate sport conditions. Performance evaluations took place under creatine-loaded (20 g per day for 5 days) or placebo conditions. Supplementation increased muscle creatine (48.9%) and PCr

(12.5%) over the placebo levels. Increased intramuscular creatine produced a 6% increase in total work accomplished (251.7 kJ presupplement vs 266.9 kJ creatine loaded) compared with the group that consumed the placebo (254.0 kJ presupplement vs 252.3 kJ placebo). Creatine supplements have benefited an on-court "ghosting" routine of simulated positional play of competitive squash players.[156] It augments repeated sprint cycle performance after 30 minutes of constant load, submaximal exercise in the heat, without adversely affecting thermoregulatory dynamics.[193] These benefits to muscular performance also occur in normally active older men.[62]

FIGURE 12.6 outlines mechanisms of how elevating intramuscular free creatine and PCr with creatine supplementation might enhance exercise performance and the training response. Improved immediate anaerobic power output capacity also aids sprint running, swimming, kayaking, and cycling, and in jumping, football, and volleyball. Increased intramuscular PCr concentrations should also enable individuals to increase training intensity.

TABLE 12.6   Selected Studies Showing Increase in Exercise Performance Following Creatine Monohydrate Supplementation

Reference	Exercise	Protocol	Exercise Performance
1.	Cycle ergometry (140 rev·min^{-1})	Ten 6-s bouts w/ 1-min rest periods	Better able to maintain pedal frequency during 4–6 s of each bout
2.	Cycle ergometry (80 rev·min^{-1})	Three 30-s bouts w/ 4-min rest periods	Increase in peak power during bout 1 and increase in mean power and total work during bouts 1 and 2
3.	Bench press	1-RM bench press and total reps at 70% of 1-RM	Increase in 1-RM; increase in reps at 70% of 1-RM
4.	Isokinetic, unilat. knee extensions (180°·s^{-1})	5 bouts of 30 ext. w/ 1-min rest periods	Reduction in decline of peak torque production during bouts 2, 3, and 4
5.	Running	Four 300 m w/ 4-min rest periods; four 1000 m w/ 3-min rest periods	Improved time for final 300- and 1000-m runs; improved total time for four 1000-m runs; reduction in best time for 300- and 1000-m runs
6.	Cycle ergometry (140 rev·min^{-1})	Five 6-s bouts w/ 30- s recovery followed by one 10-s bout	Better able to maintain pedal frequency near the end of 10-s bout
7.	Bench press	5 sets bench press w/ 2-min rest periods	Increase in reps completed during all 5 sets
	Jump squat	5 sets jump squat w/ 2-min rest periods	Increase in peak power during all 5 sets

From Volek JS, Kraemer WJ. Creatine supplementation: its effect on human muscular performance and body composition. J Strength Cond Res 1996;10:200.

1. Balsom PD, et al. Creatine supplementation and dynamic high-intensity intermittent exercise. Scand J Med Sci Sports 1993;3:143.

2. Birch R, et al. The influence of dietary creatine supplementation on performance during repeated bouts of maximal isokinetic cycling in man. Eur J Appl Physiol 1994; 69:268.

3. Earnest CP, et al. The effect of creatine monohydrate ingestion on anaerobic power indices, muscular strength and body composition. Acta Physiol Scand 1995;153:207.

4. Greenhaff PL, et al. Influence of oral creatine supplementation on muscle torque during repeated bouts on maximal voluntary exercise in man. Clin Sci 1993;84:565.

5. Harris RC, et al. The effect of oral creatine supplementation on running performance during maximal short-term exercise in man. J Physiol 1993;467:74P.

6. Soderlund K, et al. Creatine supplementation and high-intensity exercise: influence on performance and muscle metabolism. Clin Sci 1994;87(suppl.):120.

7. Volek JS, et al. Creatine supplementation enhances muscular performance during high-intensity resistance exercise. J Am Diet Assoc 1997;97:765.

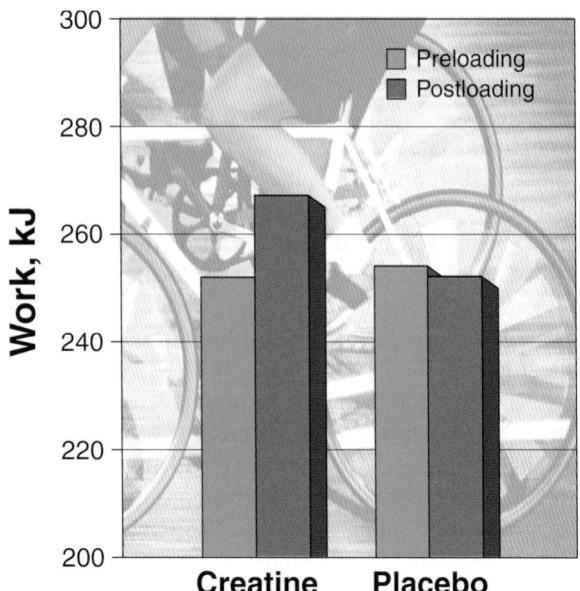

FIGURE 12.5 ▪ Effects of creatine loading versus placebo on total work accomplished during long-term (80-min) repetitive sprint-cycling performance. (From Preen CD, et al. Effect of creatine loading on long-term sprint exercise performance and metabolism. *Med Sci Sports Exerc* 2001;33:814.)

Creatine supplementation effects occur in animals. Specifically, supplementation combined with exercise training enhanced repetitive high-intensity running performance of rats to a greater extent than only training or only supplementing.[15] In addition, in vitro preparations of myogenic satellite cells obtained from young adult sheep showed increased proliferation or differentiation when exposed to creatine.[188] In humans, oral creatine supplementation combined with resistance training affected cellular functional processes in a manner that increased protein deposition within the muscle's contractile mechanism.[202] This response could possibly explain any increase in muscle size and strength associated with creatine supplementation in vivo. From a clinical perspective, exogenous creatine may reduce damage when administered after traumatic head injury. It also enhances neuromuscular functions in severe diseases, including muscular dystrophy.[137]

Oral supplements of creatine monohydrate (20–25 g per day) increase muscle creatine and performance of men and women in intense exercise, particularly repeated intense muscular effort.[14,35,46,131,142,183] The ergogenic effect does not vary between vegetarians and meat eaters.[161] Even daily doses as low as 6 g for 5 days promote improvements in repeated power performance.[47] Other research evaluated the effects of a 6-day creatine supplement of 30 g daily on the exercise performance of trained runners under two conditions: (1) four repeated 300-m runs with 4-minute recovery and (2) four 1000-m runs with 3-minute recovery.[72] Compared with placebo treatment, creatine supplementation improved performance in both running events. The most impressive improvements occurred in repeated 1000-m runs.

A Practical Finding

Creatine supplementation (0.3 g per kg of body weight) offered no benefit to endurance exercise performance in elderly women. Importantly, it did increase their ability to perform functional living tasks involving rapid movements of the lower body.[25]

For Division I football players, creatine supplementation with resistance training increased body mass, lean body mass, cellular hydration, and muscular strength and performance.[8] Similarly, supplementation augmented muscular strength and size increases during 12-weeks of resistance training.[201] The enhanced hypertrophic response with supplementation and resistance training possibly resulted from accelerated myosin heavy chain synthesis. For resistance-trained men classified as "responders" to creatine supplementation, (i.e., an increase of $\geq$32 mmol · kg dry wt muscle^{-1}), 5 days of supplementation increased body weight, FFM, peak force, and total force during repeated maximal isometric bench-presses.[101] For men classified as "nonresponders" to supplementation (i.e., increase of $\leq$21 mmol · kg dry wt muscle^{-1}), no ergogenic effect occurred.

Creatine supplementation does *not* improve exercise performance that requires a high level of aerobic energy transfer[4,5,47] or cardiovascular and metabolic responses during continuous incremental treadmill running.[65] It also exerts little effect on isometric muscular strength or dynamic muscle force measured during a brief *single* movement.[7,54,147,148]

Age Effects Uncertain

Whether or not creatine supplementation augments the training response in older individuals remains equivocal. For 70-year-old men, a creatine supplementation loading phase (0.3 g per kg body mass for 5days) followed by a daily maintenance phase (0.07 g per kg body mass) increased lean tissue mass, leg strength, muscular endurance, and average power of the legs during resistance training to a greater extent than a placebo.[30] Additional research shows no enhancement in resistance training response to creatine ingestion among sedentary and weight-trained older adults.[11] The investigators attributed their results to an age-related decline in creatine transport efficiency. Short-term creatine supplementation per se, without resistance training, does not increase muscle protein synthesis or FFM.[136]

Metabolic Reloading of High-Energy Phosphates

A large dose of creatine helps to replenish muscle creatine levels following intense exercise bouts.[27,68] Such metabolic "reloading" should facilitate recovery of muscle contractile capacity to enable athletes to sustain repeated bouts of exercise. Whether this potential to maintain "quality" workouts enhances the training response for strength athletes and power athletes awaits further research.

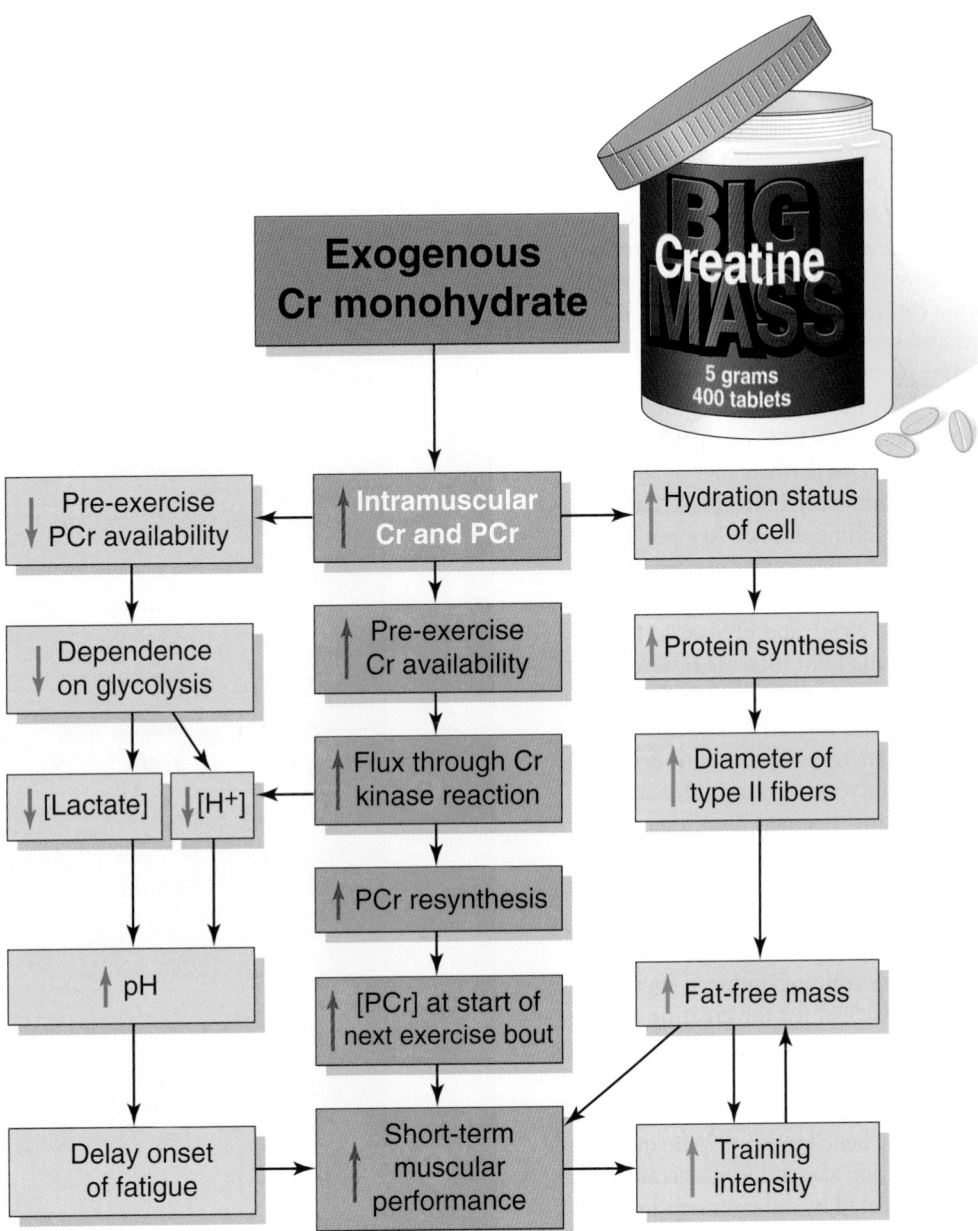

FIGURE 12.6 ■ Possible mechanisms of how elevating intracellular creatine *(Cr)* and phosphocreatine *(PCr)* enhance intense, short-term exercise performance and the exercise-training response. (Modified from Volek JS, Kraemer WJ. Creatine supplementation: its effect on human muscular performance and body composition. *J Strength Cond Res* 1996;10:200.)

Are There Risks?

Limited research exists about the potential dangers of creatine supplementation in healthy individuals, particularly the effects on cardiac muscle and kidney function (creatine degrades to creatinine before excretion in urine). Short-term use (e.g., 20 g per day for 5 consecutive days) in healthy men produced no detrimental effect on blood pressure, plasma creatine, plasma CK activity, or the renal response as measured by glomerular filtration rate and total protein and albumin excretion rates.[95,111,126,139] In addition, no differences emerged in healthy subjects in plasma contents and urine excretion rates for creatinine, urea, and albumin between control subjects and those who consumed creatine for between 10 months and 5 years.[140] Glomerular filtration rate, tubular reabsorption, and glomerular membrane permeability remained normal with chronic creatine use. Individuals with suspected renal malfunction should refrain from creatine supplementation because of the potential for exacerbating the disorder.[143] As a nutritional supplement, creatine requires less stringent regulations governing its manufacturing standards, purity, and reporting of adverse side effects than if classified as a drug. Clearly, more research needs to focus on the safety of long-term creatine supplementaion.[160]

Effects on Body Mass and Body Composition

Body mass increases of between 0.5 and 2.4 kg often accompany creatine supplementation,[45,68,84,94,128] *independent of short-term changes in testosterone or cortisol concentrations.*[190] In fact, short-term creatine supplementation exerts no effect on the hormonal responses to resistance training.[132] It remains unclear how much of the weight gain occurs from (1) the anabolic effect of creatine on muscle tissue synthesis, (2) osmotic retention of intracellular water from increased creatine stores, or (3) other factors.

Research has determined the effect of creatine supplementation plus resistance training on body composition, muscle fiber hypertrophy, and exercise performance adaptations. In one study of young adult women, creatine intake during resistance training (4 days pretraining dose of 20 g per day followed by 5 g per day during training) caused greater increases in muscle strength (20–25%), maximal intermittent exercise capacity of the arm flexors (10–25%), and FFM (6%) than the placebo condition.[182] Part of the FFM increase resulted from muscle water content. Data indicate that a 2.42-kg body mass gain with creatine supplementation plus resistance/agility training partly resulted from increases in fat/bone-free body mass that did not relate to an increase in total body water.[109]

In other research, resistance-trained men, matched on physical characteristics and maximal strength, randomly received either a placebo or a creatine supplement. Supplementation consisted of 25 g daily followed by maintenance with 5 g daily. Both groups engaged in resistance training for 12 weeks. FIGURE 12.7 shows the greater training-induced increase in body mass (6.3%) and FFM (6.3%) for the creatine-supplemented group than for controls (3.6% increase body mass and 3.1% increase FFM). Maximum bench press (+24%) and squat strength (+32%) increases were greater in the creatine group than in controls (+16% bench press; +24% squat; Fig. 12.7B). Creatine supplementation also induced a greater muscle fiber hypertrophy as indicated by enlargement in types I (35 vs 11%), IIA (36 vs 15%), and IIAB (35 vs 6%) muscle fiber cross-sectional areas (Fig. 12.7C). The larger average volume of weight lifted in the bench press during weeks 5 to 8 for the creatine supplement group suggests that a higher quality of training mediated more favorable adaptations in FFM, muscle morphology, and strength.

Creatine Loading

Many creatine users pursue a "loading" phase by ingesting 20 to 30 g of creatine daily (usually in tablet from or as powder added to liquid) for 5 to 7 days. A maintenance phase follows the loading phase where the person supplements daily with as little as 2 to 5 g of creatine. Individuals who consume vegetarian-type diets show the greatest increase in muscle creatine because of the already low creatine content of their diets. Large increases also characterize "responders," that is, individuals with normally low basal levels of intramuscular creatine.[67]

Practical questions for the person desiring to elevate intramuscular creatine with supplementation concern the following:

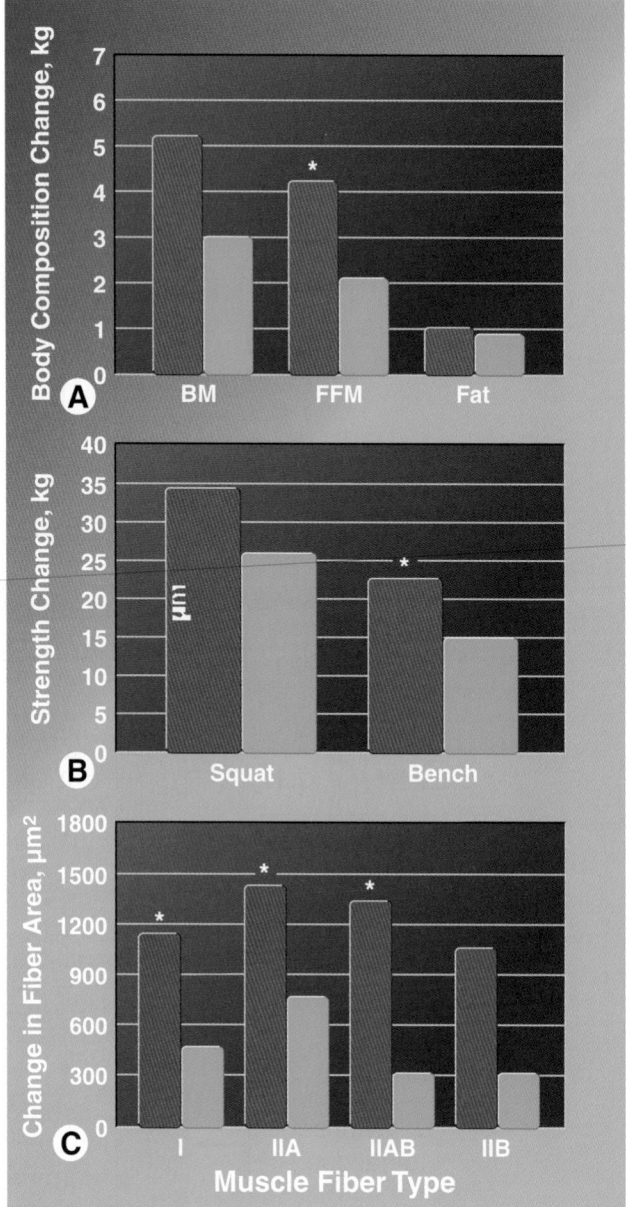

FIGURE 12.7 ▪ Effects of 12 weeks of creatine supplementation plus heavy resistance training on changes in **(A)** body mass *(BM)*, fat-free body mass *(FFM)*, and body fat, **(B)** muscular strength in the squat and bench press, and **(C)** cross-sectional areas of specific muscle fiber types. The placebo group underwent identical training and received an equivalent quantity of powdered cellulose in capsule form. *Change significantly greater than in placebo group. (From Volek JS, et al. Performance and muscle fiber adaptations to creatine supplementation and heavy resistance training. *Med Sci Sports Exerc* 1999;31:1147.)

1. The magnitude and time course of intramuscular creatine increase
2. The dosage necessary to maintain a creatine increase
3. The rate of creatine loss or "washout" following cessation of supplementation

To provide insight into these questions, researchers studied two groups of men. In one experiment, the men ingested 20 g of creatine monohydrate (approximately 0.3 g per kg of body mass) for 6 consecutive days, at which time supplementation ceased. Muscle biopsies were taken before supplement ingestion and at days 7, 21, and 35. Similarly, another group of men took 20 g of creatine monohydrate daily for 6 consecutive days. Instead of discontinuing supplementation, they reduced dosage to 2 g daily (approximately 0.03 g per kg body mass) for an additional 28 days. FIGURE 12.8A shows that after 6 days, muscle creatine concentration increased by approximately 20%. Without continued supplementation, muscle creatine content gradually declined to baseline in 35 days. The group that continued to supplement with reduced creatine intake for an additional 28 days maintained muscle creatine at the increased level (Fig. 12.8B).

For both groups, the increase in total muscle creatine content during the initial 6-day supplement period averaged 23 mmol per kg of dry muscle, which represented about 20 g (17%) of the total creatine ingested. Interestingly, a similar 20% increase in total muscle creatine concentration occurred with only a 3-g daily supplement. This increase progressed more gradually and required 28 days in contrast to only 6 days with the 6-g supplement.

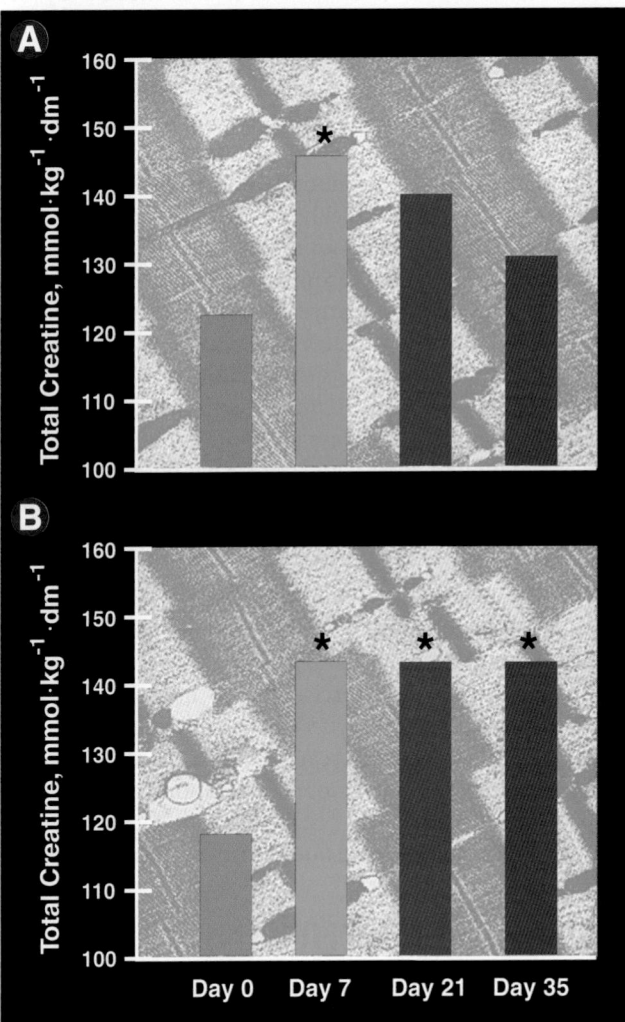

FIGURE 12.8 ■ Muscle total creatine concentration in six men who ingested 20 g of creatine for 6 consecutive days. Muscle biopsy samples were obtained before ingestion (day 0) and on days 7, 21, and 35. **B.** Muscle total creatine concentration in nine men who ingested 20 g of creatine for 6 consecutive days and thereafter ingested 2 g of creatine daily for the next 28 days. Muscle biopsy samples taken before ingestion (day 0) and on days 7, 21, and 35. Values refer to averages per dry mass (dm). *Significantly different from day 0. Dm, dry muscle. (From Hultman E, et al. Muscle creatine loading in men. *J Appl Physiol* 1996;81:232.)

To Load Quickly

To rapidly "creatine load" skeletal muscle, ingest 20 g of creatine monohydrate daily for 6 days; switch to a reduced dosage of 2 g per day to keep levels elevated for up to 28 days. If rapidity of "loading" is not a consideration, supplementing 3 g daily for 28 days achieves the same high levels.

Carbohydrate Ingestion Augments Creatine Loading

Research supports the common belief among athletes that consuming creatine with a sugar-containing drink increases creatine uptake and storage in skeletal muscle (FIG. 12.9).[66,162] For 5 days, subjects received either 5 g of creatine four times daily, or a 5-g supplement followed 30 minutes later by 93 g of a high glycemic simple sugar four times daily. For the creatine-only supplement group, increases occurred for muscle PCr (7.2%), free creatine (13.5%), and total creatine (20.7%). However, much larger increases took place for the creatine plus sugar-supplemented group (14.7% for muscle PCr, 18.1% in free creatine, and 33.0% in total creatine). Creatine supplementation alone did not affect insulin secretion, whereas adding sugar elevated plasma insulin. More than likely, augmented creatine storage with a creatine plus sugar supplement results from insulin-mediated glucose absorption by skeletal muscle, which also facilitates transport of creatine into muscle fibers.

Stop Caffeine When Using Creatine

Caffeine diminishes the ergogenic effect of creatine supplementation. To evaluate the effect of pre-exercise caffeine ingestion on intramuscular creatine stores and intense exercise performance, subjects consumed either a placebo, a daily creatine supplement (0.5 g per kg body mass), or the same daily creatine supplement plus caffeine (5 mg per kg body mass) for 6 days.[181] Under each condition, they performed maximal intermittent knee extension exercise to fatigue on an isokinetic dynamometer. Creatine supplementation, with or without caffeine, increased intramuscular PCr by between 4 and

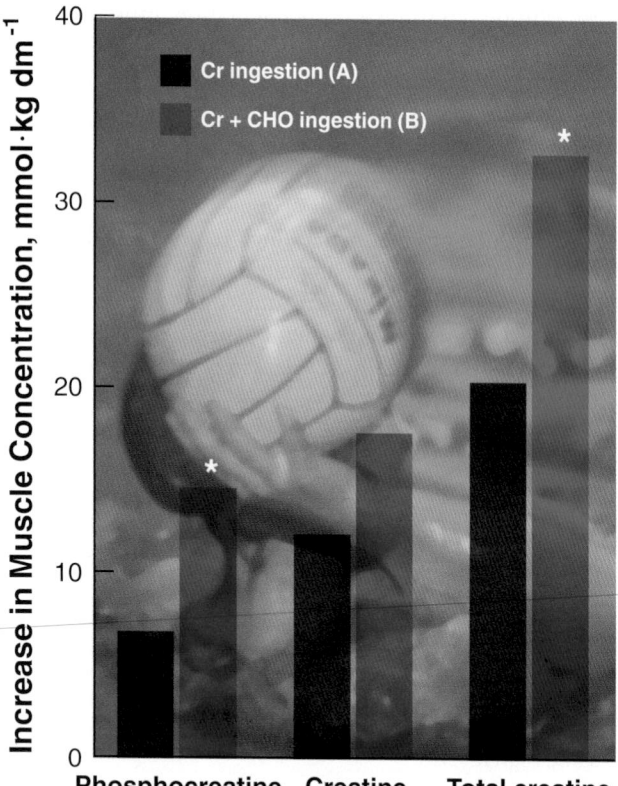

FIGURE 12.9 ■ Increases in dry muscle *(dm)* concentrations of phosphocreatine, creatine *(Cr)*, and total creatine in group A after 5 days of Cr supplementation and in group B after 5 days of Cr plus carbohydrate *(CHO)* supplementation. Values represent averages. *Significantly greater than creatine-only supplementation. (From Green AL, et al. Carbohydrate ingestion augments skeletal muscle creatine accumulation during creatine supplementation in humans. *Am J Physiol* 1996;E821.)

6%. Dynamic torque production also increased by 10 to 23% with creatine-only treatment compared with the placebo. Consuming caffeine *totally negated* creatine's ergogenic effect.

The researchers initially speculated that caffeine, through its action as a sympathomimetic agent, might facilitate the uptake and trapping of exogenous creatine by skeletal muscle. However, no enhanced retention occurred. From a practical standpoint, caffeine supplements totally counteracted any ergogenic effect of muscle creatine loading. *Athletes who load creatine should refrain from caffeine-containing foods and beverages for several days before competition.*

Some Research Shows No Benefit

Not all research reports ergogenic results from standard creatine supplementation. For example, no effects on exercise performance, fatigue resistance, and recovery appeared for untrained subjects performing a single 15-second bout of sprint cycling[35]; trained subjects performing sport-specific physical activities such as swimming, cycling, and running[20,51,128,149]; trained and untrained older adults[85,203] resist-

ance-trained individuals[172]; or trained rowers[43] or when short-term supplementation failed to significantly increase muscle PCr.[51,128] The reason for these discrepancies could include variations in subject population, length of exercise and recovery intervals, training methods, inadequate statistical power, inappropriate or unreliable performance measures, and the degree that supplementation increases intramuscular creatine and PCr concentrations.

RIBOSE: THE NEXT CREATINE ON THE SUPPLEMENT SCENE?

Ribose has emerged as a competitor to creatine as a supplement to increase power and replenish high-energy compounds after intense exercise. The body readily synthesizes ribose, and the diet provides small amounts through ripe fruits and vegetables. Metabolically, this 5-carbon sugar serves as an energy substrate for ATP resynthesis. Because of this role in energy metabolism, exogenous ribose ingestion has been touted as a means to quickly restore the body's limited amount ATP. To maintain optimal ATP levels and thus provide its ergogenic effect, recommended ribose doses range from 10 to 20 g per day. Clearly, any compound that either increases ATP levels or facilitates its resynthesis would benefit short-term, high-power physical activities. Only limited experimentation exists to assess this potential for ribose. A double-blind randomized study evaluated the effects of oral ribose supplementation (4 doses per day at 4 g per dose) on repeated bouts of maximal exercise and ATP replenishment after intermittent maximal muscle contractions.[133] No difference in any measure (e.g., intermittent isokinetic knee extension force, blood lactate, and plasma ammonia concentration) emerged between ribose and placebo trials. Although the exercise decreased intramuscular ATP and total adenine nucleotide content immediately after exercise and 24 hours later, ribose supplementation proved ineffective in facilitating recovery of these compounds. Other researchers have demonstrated no ergogenic effects of ribose supplementation in healthy untrained or trained groups,[9,44,100,110] yet it facilitated ATP resynthesis following intense intermittent exercise training.[78]

INOSINE AND CHOLINE

Inosine

Many popular articles and advertisements tout inosine as an amino acid, when in fact it is a nucleic acid derivative found naturally in brewer's yeast and organ meats. Inosine (and choline) are not considered essential nutrients. The body synthesizes inosine from precursor amino acids and glucose. Metabolically, inosine participates in forming purines such as adenine, one of the structural components of ATP. Strength and power athletes supplement with inosine believing that it increases ATP stores to improve training quality and competitive performance. Some also theorize that inosine supplementation augments synthesis of red blood cell 2,3-diphosphoglycerate, thus facilitating oxygen release from hemoglobin at the tissue level. Others suggest that inosine plays an ergogenic role by:

1. Stimulating insulin release to speed glucose delivery to the myocardium
2. Augmenting cardiac contractility
3. Acting as a vasodilating agent

These theoretical considerations, including anecdotal claims, provide the basis for popular marketing themes that extol inosine as a supplement to boost anaerobic and aerobic exercise performance.

Objective data do not support an ergogenic role for inosine supplementation. Highly trained young and older men and women who supplemented daily with 6000 mg of inosine for 2 days failed to improve 3-mile treadmill run time, peak oxygen uptake, blood lactate level, heart rate, or RPE.[200] Interestingly, subjects could not exercise as long on a test for aerobic capacity when supplemented with inosine as in the unsupplemented state. In another study, male competitive cyclists received either a placebo or a 5000-mg per day oral inosine supplement for 5 days.[169] They then performed a Wingate bicycle test, a 30-minute self-paced bicycle endurance test, and a constant load, supramaximal cycling sprint to fatigue. FIGURE 12.10 shows the results for maximal anaerobic power output

on the 30-second Wingate test (*A*) and heart rate (*B*), RPE (*C*), and total work accomplished (*D*) during segments of the 30-minute endurance ride. No significant differences occurred in any of the criterion variables between placebo and supplemented conditions. In agreement with the ergolytic effect of inosine noted previously,[200] cyclists fatigued nearly 10% faster on the supramaximal sprint test when they consumed inosine than without it. Additionally, serum uric acid levels increased nearly twofold following 5 days of inosine supplementation—a level normally associated with gout, an inherited metabolic disorder characterized by recurrent acute arthritis and deposition of crystalline urate in connective tissues and articular cartilage. *These findings alone contraindicate any use of inosine supplements for possible ergogenic effects.*

Choline

All animal tissues contain choline, an important compound for normal cellular functioning. Although humans synthesize choline, it (like inosine) also must be obtained in the diet. Lecithin, a structural component of the lipoproteins and the cells' phospholipid plasma membrane, and the neurotransmitter acetylcholine (which controls skeletal muscle activation at the myoneural junction) incorporate choline into their chemical structures. Choline functions as a lipotrophic agent

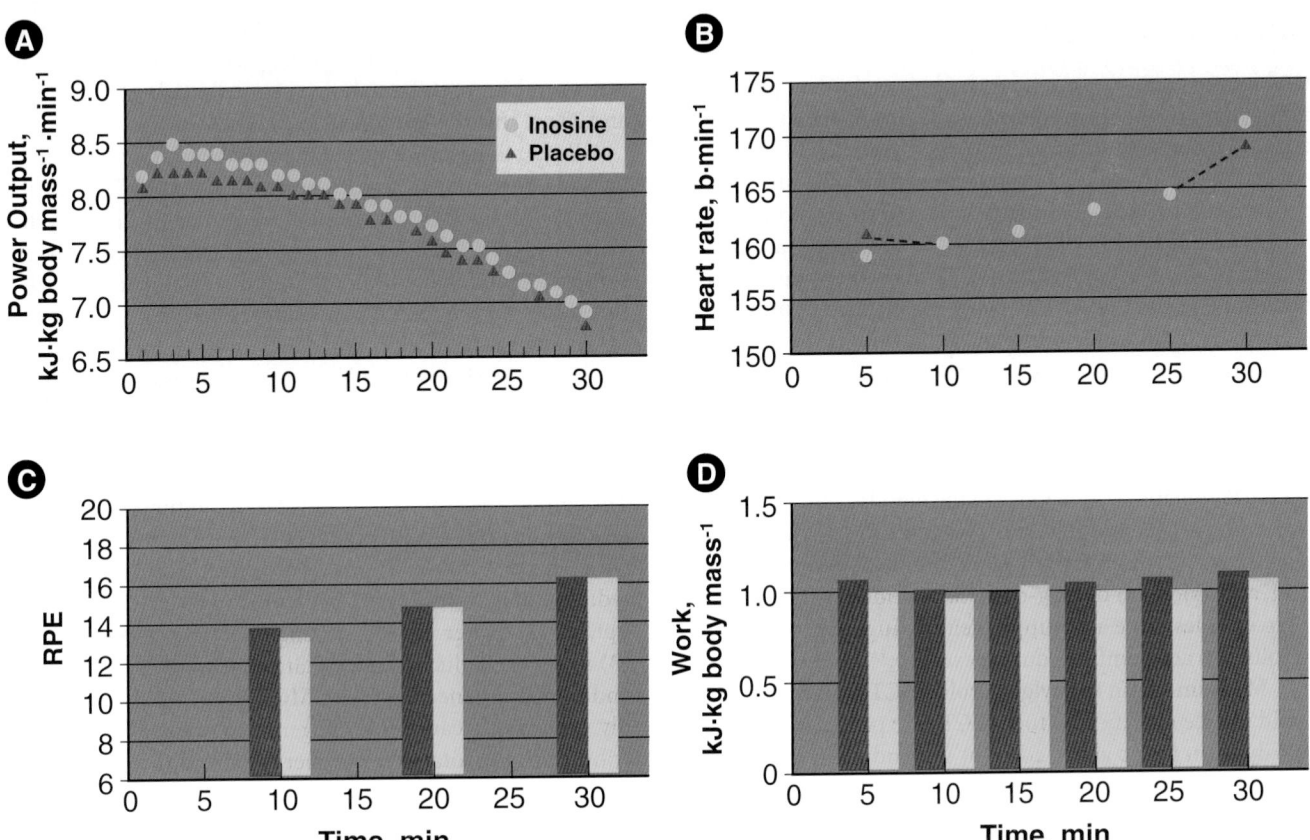

FIGURE 12.10 ■ Maximal anaerobic power output on the 30-second Wingate test **(A)** and for heart rate **(B)**, ratings of perceived exertion *(RPE)* **(C)**, and total work accomplished **(D)** during segments of the 30-minute endurance ride for inosine and placebo trials for 10 male competitive cyclists. (From Starling RD, et al. Effect of inosine supplementation on aerobic and anaerobic cycling performance. *Med Sci Sports Exerc* 1996;28:1193.)

as part of the lecithin molecule either to depress accumulation of fat in the liver or to increase fatty acid uptake by the liver. Very low density lipoproteins (the major transporting vehicle of triacylglycerols synthesized in the liver) also contain choline. A subpar choline intake increases the triacylglycerol content of the liver. Many foods contain ample choline; top food sources include eggs (yolk), brewer's yeast, liver (beef, pork, lamb), wheat germ, soybeans, dehydrated potatoes, oatmeal, and vegetables in the cabbage (cucurbrit) family.

Inositol and choline supplements depress fat accumulation in the liver when given to animals deficient in these compounds. Supplements did not affect percentage carcass fat of aerobically trained rats, although the supplemented animals gained less weight during the training period.[99] In addition, no depletion of plasma choline occurred with prolonged exhaustive exercise and no ergogenic effect was noted with supplementation in humans.[198] Body builders frequently take choline- and inositol-containing "metabolic optimizing powders" and "fat-burning tablets" before competition, hoping to increase their muscle mass/fat mass ratio to achieve the "cut" look. We are unaware of any research on humans that supports supplementation with inositol–choline products for such purposes.

LIPID SUPPLEMENTATION WITH MEDIUM-CHAIN TRIACYGLYCEROLS

Do high-fat foods or supplements elevate plasma lipid levels to make more energy available during prolonged aerobic exercise? One must consider several factors to achieve such an effect. For one thing, consuming triacylglycerols composed of predominantly long-chain fatty acids (12 to 18 carbons) *delays* gastric emptying. This negatively affects the rapidity of exogenous fat availability and also fluid and carbohydrate replenishment. Both are crucial factors in intense endurance exercise. In addition, following digestion and intestinal absorption (normally 3 to 4 hours), long-chain triacylglycerols reassemble with phospholipids, fatty acids, and a cholesterol shell to form fatty droplets called chylomicrons. Chylomicrons then travel slowly to the systemic circulation via the lymphatic system. Once in the bloodstream, the tissues remove the triacylglycerols bound to chylomicrons. Consequently, the relatively slow rate of digestion, absorption, and oxidation of long-chain fatty acids make this energy source undesirable as a supplement to augment energy metabolism in active muscle during exercise.[41,89]

Medium-chain triacylglycerols (MCTs) provide a more rapid source of fatty acid fuel. MCTs are processed oils (primarily from lauric acids, coconut oil, and palm kernal oils) frequently produced for patients with intestinal malabsorption and tissue-wasting diseases. Marketing for the sports enthusiast hypes MCT as a "fat burner," "energy source," "glycogen sparer," and "muscle builder." Unlike longer-chain triacylglycerols, MCTs contain saturated fatty acids with 8 to 10 carbon atoms along the fatty acid chain. During digestion (see Chapter 3), they hydrolyze by lipase action in the mouth, stomach, and intestinal duodenum to glycerol and medium-chain fatty acids (MCFAs). The water-solubility of MCFAs enables them to move across the intestinal mucosa directly into the bloodstream (portal vein) without the necessity of slow transport in chylomicrons by the lymphatic system as required for long-chain triacylglycerols. Once at the tissues, MCFAs readily move through the plasma membrane, where they diffuse across the inner mitochondrial membrane for oxidation. They pass into the mitochondria largely independent of the carnitine–acyl-CoA transferase system, which contrasts with the relatively slower transfer and mitochondrial oxidation rate of long-chain fatty acids. Owing to their relative ease of oxidation, MCTs do not usually store as body fat. Ingesting MCTs elevates plasma FFAs rapidly, so supplements of these lipids might spare liver and muscle glycogen during high-intensity aerobic exercise.

Exercise Benefits Inconclusive

Consuming MCTs does not inhibit gastric emptying, as does conusing common fat, but conflicting research exists about their use in exercise.[3,92] In early studies, subjects consumed 380 mg of MCT oil per kg of body mass per hour before exercising 1 hour at between 60 and 70% of aerobic capacity.[38] Plasma ketone levels generally increased with MCT ingestion, but the exercise metabolic mixture did not change compared with a placebo trial or a trial after subjects consumed a glucose polymer. By consuming 30 g of MCTs (an estimated maximal amount tolerated in the gastrointestinal tract) before exercising, MCT catabolism contributed only between 3 and 7% of the total exercise energy cost.[90]

Research has investigated the metabolic and ergogenic effects of consuming a large quantity of 86 g of MCTs (surprisingly well tolerated by subjects). Endurance-trained cyclists rode for 2 hours at 60% $\dot{V}O_{2peak}$; they then immediately performed a simulated 40-km cycling time trial. During each of three rides they drank 2 L containing either 10% glucose, 4.3% MCT emulsion, or 10% glucose plus 4.3% MCT emulsion. FIGURE 12.11 shows the effects of the beverages on average speed in the 40-km trials. Replacing the carbohydrate beverage with only the MCT emulsion impaired exercise performance by approximately 8% (in agreement with another study[92]). The combined carbohydrate plus MCT solution consumed repeatedly during exercise produced a 2.5% improvement in cycling speed. This small ergogenic effect occurred with (1) reduced total carbohydrate oxidation at a given level of oxygen uptake, (2) higher final circulating FFA and ketone levels, and (3) lower final glucose and lactate concentrations. The small endurance enhancement with MCT supplementation probably occurred because this exogenous fatty acid source contributed to the total exercise energy expenditure and total fat oxidation.[91]

Consuming MCT does not stimulate the release of bile, the fat-emulsifying agent from the gallbladder. Thus, cramping and diarrhea often accompany excess intake of this lipid form.[60,89] Additional research must validate the ergogenic claims for MCT, including the tolerance level for these lipids during exercise. In general, relatively small alterations in sub-

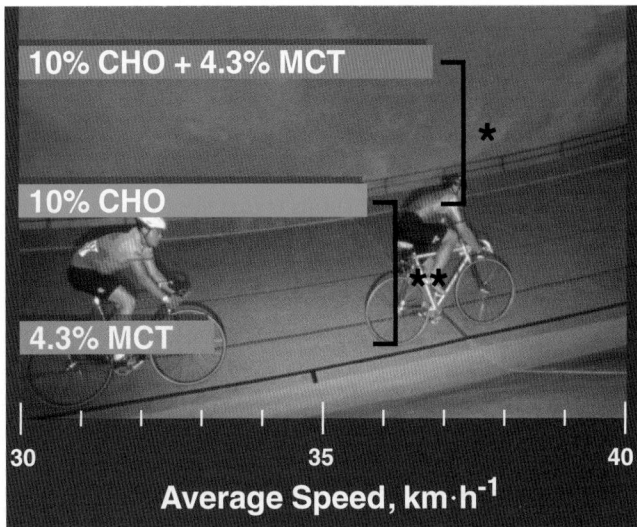

FIGURE 12.11 ■ Effects of carbohydrate (*CHO*; 10% solution), medium-chain triglyceride (*MCT*; 4.3% emulsion), and carbohydrate + MCT ingestion during exercise on simulated 40-km time-trial cycling speeds after 2 hours of exercise at 60% of peak oxygen uptake. *Significantly faster than 10% CHO trials; **significantly faster than 4.3% MCT trials. (From Van Zyl CG, et al. Effects of medium-chain triglyceride ingestion on fuel metabolism and cycling performance. *J Appl Physiol* 1996;80:2217.)

strate oxidation occur by increasing the availability of FFAs during exercise at 65 to 90% of aerobic capacity; this likely accounts for its small effect on exercise capacity.[77]

(—)-HYDROXYCITRATE: A POTENTIAL FAT BURNER?

(—)-Hydroxycitrate (HCA), a principal constituent of the rind of the fruit of *Garcinia cambogia* used in Asian cuisine, is promoted as a "natural fat burner" to facilitate weight loss and enhance endurance performance. Metabolically, HCA operates as a competitive inhibitor of citrate lyase, which catalyzes the breakdown of citrate to oxaloacetate and acetyl-CoA in the cytosol. Inhibition of this enzyme limits the pool of 2-carbon acetyl compounds and thus reduces cellular ability to synthesize fat. Inhibition of citrate catabolism also slows carbohydrate breakdown, so HCA supplementation should provide a means to conserve glycogen and increase lipolysis during exercise.[106,118]

Research has evaluated short-term effects of HCA ingestion on (1) HCA availability in the plasma, and (2) fat oxidation rates at rest and during moderate-intensity exercise.[185] Endurance-trained cyclists received either a 3.1 mL per kg of body mass HCA solution (19 g · L^{-1}; 6 to 30 times the dosage in weight-loss studies) or a placebo at 45 and 15 minutes before starting exercise (resting measure) and 30 and 60 minutes after a 2-hour exercise bout at 50% maximal working capacity. Plasma concentrations of HCA increased at rest and during exercise after supplementation, but no difference occurred be-

tween trials in energy expenditure or in fat and carbohydrate oxidation. These findings indicate that increasing plasma HCA availability with supplementation exerts no effect on skeletal muscle fat oxidation during rest or exercise, at least in endurance-trained humans. In addition, no effects of HCA supplementation occurred for resting or postexercise energy expenditure and markers of lipolysis in healthy men[112] or weight or fat loss in obese subjects.[79] Taken together, these findings cast serious doubt on the usefulness of large quantities of HCA as an antiobesity agent or ergogenic aid—claims frequently made by supplement purveyors.

VANADIUM

Vanadium, a trace element widely distributed in nature, comes from the bluish salt of vanadium acid and was named in 1831 for the Norse goddess of beauty (Vanadis) because of how it forms multicolored compounds. This important element (without an Recommended Dietary Allowance [RDA]) exhibits insulin-like properties by facilitating glucose transport and use in skeletal muscle, stimulating glycogen synthesis, and activating glycolytic reactions. In animals, vanadium supplements attenuated the effects of diabetes, perhaps by augmenting the action of available insulin.[12,130,177] In humans, administering 50 mg of vanadium twice daily for 3 weeks improved hepatic and skeletal muscle insulin sensitivity in patients with type 2 diabetes, partly by enhancing insulin's inhibitory effect on fat breakdown. No altered insulin sensitivity occurred in nondiabetic subjects.[69] Optimal iodine metabolism and thyroid function may also require adequate vanadium intake. The best "natural" sources of vanadium include cereal and grain products and dietary oils, although meat, fish, and poultry also contain moderate amounts of this element.

Body builders ingest vanadium supplements, usually in its oxidized form as vanadyl sulfate, often combined with additional minerals or coatings, or as bis-maltolato-oxovanadium (BMOV).[207] Enthusiasts believe that vanadium provides the "pumped look" to give the appearance of muscular hypertrophy (hardness, density, and size) because of enhanced muscle glycogen storage and amino acid uptake. Research does not support an ergogenic role for vanadium supplements. Individuals should not supplement with this element because an extreme excess of vanadium becomes toxic (particularly to the liver) in mammals.

PYRUVATE

Ergogenic effects have been extolled for pyruvate, the 3-carbon end product of the cytoplasmic breakdown of glucose in glycolysis. Exogenous pyruvate, as a partial replacement for dietary carbohydrate, allegedly augments endurance exercise performance and promotes fat loss. Pyruvic acid, a relatively unstable chemical, causes intestinal distress. Consequently, various forms of the salt of this acid (sodium, potassium, calcium, or magnesium pyruvate) are provided in capsule, tablet, or powder form. Supplement manufacturers recommend taking 2 to 4 capsules daily. One capsule usually contains 600 mg of pyruvate. The calcium form of pyruvate contains approximately 80 mg of calcium with 600 mg of pyruvate. Some advertisements recommend a dose of one capsule per 20 lb of body weight. Manufacturers also combine creatine monohydrate and pyruvate; 1 g of creatine pyruvate provides about 80 mg of creatine and 400 mg of pyruvate. Recommended pyruvate dosages range from 5 to 20 g per day. Pyruvate content in the normal diet ranges from 100 mg to 2000 mg daily. The largest dietary amounts occur in fruits and vegetables, particularly red apples (500 mg each), with smaller quantities in dark beer (80 mg per 12 oz) and red wine (75 mg per 6 oz).

Effects on Endurance Performance

Several reports indicate beneficial effects of exogenous pyruvate on endurance performance. Two double-blind, crossover studies by the same laboratory showed that 7 days of daily supplementation of a 100-g mixture of pyruvate (25 g) plus 75 g of dihydroxyacetone (DHA; another 3-carbon compound of glycolysis) increased upper- and lower-body aerobic endurance by 20% compared with exercise with a 100-g supplement of an isocaloric glucose polymer.[164,165] The pyruvate–DHA mixture increased cycle ergometer time to exhaustion of the legs (lower body) by 13 minutes (66 vs 79 minutes), while upper-body arm-cranking exercise time increased by 27 minutes (133 vs 160 minutes). Local muscle and overall body ratings of perceived exertion were also lower when subjects exercised with the pyruvate–DHA mixture than with the placebo condition.[154] Dosage recommendations range between a total of 2 and 5 g of pyruvate spread throughout the day and taken with meals.

Proponents of pyruvate supplementation maintain that elevations in extracellular pyruvate augment glucose transport into active muscle. Enhanced "glucose extraction" from blood provides the important carbohydrate energy source to sustain intense aerobic exercise while at the same time conserving intramuscular glycogen stores.[83] When the individual's diet contains a normal level of carbohydrate (approximately 55% of total energy), pyruvate supplementation also increases pre-exercise muscle glycogen levels.[165] Both of these effects—higher pre-exercise glycogen levels and facilitated glucose uptake and oxidation by active muscle—benefit endurance exercise in much the same way as pre-exercise carbohydrate loading and glucose feedings during exercise exert their ergogenic effects. The question awaiting research concerns whether pyruvate ingestion provides any greater ergogenic benefit than carbohydrate loading and/or carbohydrate consumption during exercise.

Body Fat Loss

Subsequent research by the same investigators who showed ergogenic effects of pyruvate supplementation indicates that pyruvate intake also augments body fat loss when accompanied by a low-energy diet. Obese women in a metabolic ward maintained a liquid 1000-kCal daily energy intake (68% car-

bohydrate, 22% protein, 10% lipid). Adding 20 g of sodium pyruvate plus 16 g of calcium pyruvate (13% of energy intake) daily for 3 weeks induced greater weight loss (13.0 vs 9.5 lb) and fat loss (8.8 vs 5.9 lb) than in a control group on the same diet who received an equivalent amount of extra energy as glucose.[166] These findings complement the researchers' previous study with obese subjects that showed that adding DHA and pyruvate (substituted as equivalent energy for glucose) to a severely restricted low-energy diet facilitated weight and fat loss (without increased nitrogen loss).[167] The inhibition of weight and fat gain through dietary substitution with 3-carbon compounds, originally observed in growing animals, indicated that pyruvate might cause a greater effect than DHA.[36,163] The precise role of pyruvate in facilitating weight loss remains unknown. Taking pyruvate may stimulate small increases in futile metabolic activity (metabolism not coupled to ATP production) with a subsequent wasting of energy.

Adverse side effects of a 30- to 100-g daily pyruvate intake include diarrhea as well as gastrointestinal gurgling and discomfort. *Until additional studies from independent laboratories reproduce existing findings for exercise performance and body fat loss, one should view the effectiveness of pyruvate supplementation with caution.* To complicate matters, recent research indicates *no beneficial effect* of pyruvate supplementation on measures of body composition, the metabolic response to exercise, or exercise performance.[102,186]

GLYCEROL

Glycerol is a component of the triacylglycerol molecule, a gluconeogenic substrate, an important constituent of the cells' phospholipid plasma membrane, and an osmotically active natural metabolite. The 2-carbon glycerol molecule achieved clinical notoriety (along with mannitol, sorbitol, and urea) for helping to produce an osmotic diuresis. The capacity for influencing water movement within the body makes glycerol effective in reducing excess accumulation of fluid (edema) in the brain and eye. Glycerol's effect on water movement occurs because extracellular glycerol enters the tissues of the brain, cerebrospinal fluid, and eye's aqueous humor at a relatively slow rate; this creates an osmotic effect that draws fluid from these tissues.

Ingesting a concentrated mixture of glycerol plus water increases the body's fluid volume and glycerol concentrations in plasma and interstitial fluid compartments. This sets the stage for fluid excretion from increased renal filtrate and urine flow. The proximal and distal tubules reabsorb much of this glycerol, so a large fluid portion of renal filtrate also becomes reabsorbed, which averts a marked diuresis. Renal reabsorption does not occur with tissue dehydrators such as mannitol and sorbitol, which produce a true osmotic diuresis.

The kidneys generally reabsorb from the renal filtrate almost all of the glycerol from food and metabolism. Normal plasma glycerol concentration at rest averages 0.05 mmol · L^{-1}; it often rises to 0.5 mmol · L^{1} during prolonged exercise with accompanying carbohydrate depletion and elevated fat catabolism. Exaggerated increases in urine glycerol concentration most likely indicate the use of exogenous glycerol, usually ingested at quantities of 1.2 g per kg of body mass.

When consumed with 1 to 2 L of water, glycerol facilitates water absorption from the intestine and causes extracellular fluid retention, mainly in the plasma fluid compartment.[103,152,197] The hyperhydration effect of glycerol supplementation reduces overall heat stress during exercise as reflected by increased sweating rate; this lowers heart rate and body temperature during exercise and enhances endurance performance under heat stress.[80,121] Reducing heat stress with hyperhydration using glycerol plus water supplementation before exercise increases safety for the exercise participant. The typically recommended pre-exercise glycerol dosage of 1.0 g of glycerol per kg of body mass in 1 to 2 L of water lasts up to 6 hours.

Not all research demonstrates meaningful thermoregulatory, cardiovascular, or exercise performance benefits of glycerol hyperhydration over pre-exercise hyperhydration with plain water.[63,98,114,122] For example, exogenous glycerol diluted in 500 mL of water consumed 4 hours before exercise failed to promote fluid retention or ergogenic effects.[82] Also, no cardiovascular or thermoregulatory advantages occurred when consuming glycerol with small volumes of water during exercise.[129] Side effects of exogenous glycerol ingestion include nausea, dizziness, bloating, and light-headedness. Proponents of glycerol supplementation argue that any ban on glycerol use only increases the risk of elite athletes to heat injury, including potentially fatal heat stroke. This area clearly requires further research.

Case Study

Personal Health and Exercise Nutrition 12–1

How to Identify the Metabolic Syndrome

Modification of risk factors greatly reduce the likelihood of coronary heart disease (CHD). Specifically, a major target of therapy includes a constellation of lipid and non-lipid risk factors of metabolic origin known as the *metabolic syndrome*. This syndrome closely links to the generalized metabolic disorder of *insulin resistance*, in which the normal actions of insulin are impaired. Excess body fat (particularly abdominal obesity) and physical inactivity promote the development of insulin resistance. Some individuals are genetically predisposed to this condition.

The risk factors for the metabolic syndrome are highly concordant; in aggregate they enhance risk for CHD at any given low density lipoprotein (LDL) cholesterol level. Diagnosis of the metabolic syndrome is made when three or more of the risk determinants shown in Table 1 are present. These determinants include a combination of categorical and borderline risk factors that can be readily measured.

Management of Underlying Causes of the Metabolic Syndrome

Weight reduction and increased physical activity represent the first-line therapy for the metabolic syndrome. Weight reduction facilitates the lowering of LDL cholesterol and reduces all of the risk factors of the syndrome. Regular physical activity reduces very low density lipoprotein (VLDL) levels, raises high density lipoprotein

Table 1 Clinical Identification of the Metabolic Syndrome

Risk Factor	Defining Level
Abdominal obesity[a]	**Waist girth**[b]
Men	>102 cm (>40 in.)
Women	>88 cm (>35 in.)
Triacylglycerols	$\geq$150 mg $\cdot$ dL^{-1}
HDL-cholesterol	
Men	<40 mg $\cdot$ dL^{-1}
Women	<50 mg $\cdot$ dL^{-1}
Blood pressure	$\geq$130/$\geq$85 mm Hg
Fasting glucose	$\geq$110 mg $\cdot$ dL^{-1}

From Third Report of the National Cholesterol Education Program (NCEP) Expert Panel on Detection, evaluation, and treatment of high blood cholesterol in adults (Adult Treatment Panel III). National Heart, Lung, and Blood Institute. NIH publ. no. 01-3670, May 2001.
[a] *Overweight and obesity are associated with insulin resistance and the metabolic syndrome. However, the presence of abdominal obesity is more highly correlated with the metabolic risk factors than is an elevated body mass index (BMI). Therefore, the simple measure of waist girth is recommended to identify the body weight component of the metabolic syndrome.*
[b] *Some males can develop multiple metabolic risk factors when the waist girth is only marginally increased, e.g., 94 to 102 cm (37–39 in.). Such patients may have a strong genetic contribution to insulin resistance. They would benefit from changes in life habits, similar to men with larger increases in waist girth.*

(HDL) cholesterol, and in some persons lowers LDL cholesterol. It also can lower blood pressure, reduce insulin resistance, and favorably influence overall cardiovascular function.

Summary

1. Carbohydrate loading generally increases endurance in prolonged submaximal exercise. A modification of the classic loading procedure provides for the same high level of glycogen storage without dramatic alterations in one's diet and exercise routine. A 1-day rapid loading procedure produces nearly as high glycogen storage as the more prolonged loading techniques.

2. Men and women achieve equal supramaximal muscle glycogen levels when fed comparable amounts of carbohydrate in relation to their lean body mass.

3. Many resistance-trained athletes supplement their diets with amino acids, either singly or in combination to create a hormonal milieu to facilitate protein synthesis in skeletal muscle. Research shows no benefit of such general supplementation on levels of anabolic hormones or measures of body composition, muscle size, or exercise performance.

4. Carbohydrate–protein supplementation immediately in recovery from resistance training produces a hormonal environment conducive to protein synthesis and muscle tissue growth (elevated plasma concentrations of insulin and growth hormone).

5. Long-term exercise or intense training does not adversely affect intracellular carnitine levels. This explains why most research with carnitine supplementation fails to show an ergogenic effect, positive metabolic alterations, or body fat reductions.

6. Many tout chromium supplements (usually as chromium picolinate) for their fat- burning and muscle-building properties. For individuals with adequate dietary chromium intakes, research fails to show any beneficial effect of chromium supplements on training-related changes in muscular strength, physique, fat-free body mass, or muscle mass.

7. Excess chromium can adversely affect iron transport and distribution in the body. Prolonged excess may even contribute to chromosomal damage.

8. Because of its role in electron transport-oxidative phosphorylation, athletes supplement with coenzyme Q_{10} (CoQ_{10}) to improve aerobic capacity and cardiovascular dynamics. CoQ_{10} supplements in healthy individuals provide no ergogenic effect on aerobic capacity, endurance, submaximal exercise lactate levels, or cardiovascular dynamics.

9. In supplement form, creatine increases intramuscular creatine and phosphocreatine, enhances short-term anaerobic power output capacity and facilitates recovery from repeated bouts of intense effort. Creatine loading occurs by ingesting 20 g of creatine monohydrate for 6 consecutive days. Reducing intake to 2 g daily then maintains elevated intramuscular levels.

10. Consuming creatine with a glucose-containing drink increases creatine uptake and storage in skeletal muscle. More than likely, this results from insulin-mediated glucose uptake by skeletal muscle, which facilitates creatine uptake.

11. Limited research indicates no effect of inosine supplements on physiologic or performance measures during aerobic or anaerobic exercise. A decidedly negative effect includes an increase in serum uric acid levels after only 5 days of supplementation.

12. Choline forms part of the cells' phospholipid plasma membrane; it is also a constituent of the neurotransmitter acetylcholine. Body builders frequently supplement with choline to enhance fat metabolism and achieve the "cut look." Research does not support such effects.

13. Some believe that consuming medium-chain triacylglycerols (MCTs) enhances fat metabolism and conserves glycogen during endurance exercise. Ingesting about 86 g of MCT enhances performance by an additional 2.5%.

14. Increasing plasma (—)-hydroxycitrate (HCA) availability via supplementation exerts no effect on skeletal muscle fat oxidation at rest or during exercise. These findings cast doubt on the usefulness of HCA, even when provided in large quantities as an antiobesity agent or ergogenic aid.

15. Vanadium exerts insulin-like properties in humans. No research documents an ergogenic effect, and extreme intake produces toxic effects.

16. Pyruvate supplementation purportedly augments endurance performance and promotes fat loss. A definitive conclusion concerning pyruvate's effectiveness requires verification by other investigators.

17. Pre-exercise glycerol ingestion promotes hyperhydration, which supposedly protects the individual from heat stress and heat injury during high-intensity exercise.

Test Your Knowledge Answers

1. **True:** Glycogen stored in the liver and active muscle supplies most of the energy for intense aerobic exercise. Reduced glycogen reserves allow fat catabolism to supply a progressively greater percentage of energy from fatty acid mobilization from the liver and adipose tissue. Exercise that severely lowers muscle glycogen precipitates fatigue, even though the active muscles have sufficient oxygen and unlimited use of potential energy from stored fat. This occurs because the aerobic breakdown of FFAs progresses at about 50% the rate of glycogen breakdown. Ingesting a glucose and water solution near the point of fatigue allows exercise to continue, but for all practical purposes, the muscles' "fuel tank" reads empty.

2. **True:** A particular combination of diet plus exercise significantly "packs" muscle glycogen, a procedure termed *carbohydrate loading* or *glycogen supercompensation*. Endurance athletes often use carbohydrate loading for competition because it increases muscle glycogen even more than a high-carbohydrate diet. Normally, each 100 g of muscle contains about 1.7 g of glycogen; carbohydrate loading packs up to 5 g of glycogen.

3. **False:** Research on healthy subjects does not provide convincing evidence for an ergogenic effect of oral amino acid supplements on hormone secretion, training responsiveness, or exercise performance. For example, in studies with appropriate design and statistical analysis, supplements of arginine, lysine, ornithine, tyrosine, and other amino acids, either singly or in combination, produced no effect on GH levels, insulin secretion, diverse measures of anaerobic power, or all-out running performance at $\dot{V}O_{2max}$.

4. **False:** Vital to normal metabolism, carnitine facilitates the influx of long-chain fatty acids into the mitochondrial matrix as part of the carnitine–acyl-CoA transferase system. Theoretically, enhanced carnitine function could inhibit lactate accumulation and enhance exercise performance. Increasing intracellular L-carnitine levels through dietary supplementation should elevate aerobic energy transfer from fat breakdown while conserving limited glycogen reserves. Research shows no ergogenic benefits, positive metabolic alterations (aerobic or anaerobic), or body fat-reducing effects from L-carnitine supplementation.

5. **False:** For individuals with adequate dietary chromium intakes, research fails to show any beneficial effect of chromium supplements on training-related changes in muscular strength, physique, fat-free body mass, or muscle mass. Excess chromium can possibly adversely affect iron transport and distribution in the body. Prolonged excess may damage chromosomes.

6. **True:** Creatine monohydrate supplementation at the recommended level (20–25 g per day) exerts ergogenic effects in short-duration, high-intensity exercise (5–10% improvement) without producing harmful side effects. Anecdotes indicate a possible association between creatine supplementation and cramping in multiple muscle areas during competition or lengthy practice by football players.

7. **True:** Several reports indicate beneficial effects of exogenous pyruvate on endurance performance. Two double-blind crossover studies by the same laboratory showed that 7 days of daily supplementation of a 100-g mixture of pyruvate (25 g) plus 75 g of dihydroxyacetone (DHA; another 3-carbon compound of glycolysis) increased upper- and lower-body aerobic endurance by 20% compared with exercise with a 100-g supplement of an isocaloric glucose polymer. Proponents of pyruvate supplementation maintain that elevations in extracellular pyruvate augment glucose transport into active muscle. Enhanced "glucose extraction" from blood provides the important carbohydrate energy source to sustain high-intensity aerobic exercise while at the same time conserving intramuscular glycogen stores. Subsequent research by the same investigators also indicates that exogenous pyruvate intake augments body fat loss when accompanied by a low-energy diet. Until additional studies from independent laboratories reproduce existing findings for exercise performance and body fat loss, one should view with caution conclusions about the effectiveness of pyruvate supplementation.

8. **False:** Not all research demonstrates meaningful thermoregulatory or exercise performance benefits of glycerol hyperhydration over preexercise hyperhydration with plain water. Side effects of exogenous glycerol ingestion include nausea, dizziness, bloating, and light-headedness.

9. **False:** CoQ_{10} functions as an integral component of the mitochondrion's electron transport system of oxidative phosphorylation. The popular literature touts CoQ_{10} supplements to improve "stamina" and enhance cardiovascular function based on the belief that supplementation could increase the flux of electrons through the respiratory chain and thus augment aerobic resynthesis of adenosine triphosphate. Although positive benefits have been reported for cardiac patients, CoQ_{10} supplements in healthy individuals provide no ergogenic effect on aerobic capacity, endurance, submaximal exercise lactate levels, or cardiovascular dynamics. On the negative side, supplementation could trigger plasma membrane lipid peroxidation and eventual cellular damage.

10. **False:** Plasma concentrations of HCA increase at rest and during exercise after supplementation, but no effect emerges in energy expenditure or in fat and carbohydrate oxidation. Consequently, increasing plasma HCA availability with supplementation does not influence skeletal muscle fat oxidation during rest or exercise. In addition, no effects of HCA supplementation occurred for resting or postexercise energy expenditure and markers of lipolysis in healthy men, or weight or fat loss in obese subjects. Taken together, these findings cast serious doubt on the usefulness of large quantities of HCA as an antiobesity agent or ergogenic aid—claims frequently made by supplement purveyors.

References

1. Abromowicz WN, Galloway SD. Effects of acute versus chronic L-carnitine L-tartrate supplementation on metabolic responses to steady state exercise in males and females. *Int J Sports Nutr Exerc Metab* 2005;15:386.

2. Althuis MD, et al. Glucose and insulin responses to dietary chromium supplements: a meta-analysis. *Am J Clin Nutr* 2002;76:148.

3. Auclair E, et al. Metabolic effects of glucose, medium chain triglyceride and long chain triglyceride feeding before prolonged exercise in rats. *Eur J Appl Physiol* 1988;57:126.

4. Balsom PD, et al. Creatine supplementation and dynamic high-intensity intermittent exercise. *Scand J Med Sci Sports* 1993;3:143.

5. Balsom PD, et al. Creatine supplementation per se does not enhance endurance exercise performance. *Acta Physiol Scand* 1993;149:521.

6. Balsom PD, et al. High-intensity exercise and muscle glycogen availability in humans. *Acta Physiol Scand* 1999;168:357.

7. Bemben MG. Effects of creatine supplementation on isometric force-time curve characteristics. *Med Sci Sports Exerc* 2001;33:1876.

8. Bemben MG, et al. Creatine supplementation during resistance training in college football athletes. *Med Sci Sports Exerc* 2001;33:1667.

9. Berardi JM, Ziegenfuss TN. Effects of ribose supplementation on repeated sprint performance in men. *J Strength Cond Res* 2003;17:47.

10. Bergstrom J, et al. Diet, muscle glycogen and physical performance. *Acta Physiol Scand* 1967;71:140.

11. Bermon S, et al. Effects of creatine monohydrate ingestion in sedentary and weight-trained older adults. *Acta Physiol Scand* 1998;164:147.

12. Bhanot S, McNeil JH. Vanadyl sulfate lowers plasma insulin and blood pressure in spontaneously hypertensive rats. *Hypertension* 1994;24:625.

13. Bogandis GC, et al. Contribution of phosphocreatine and aerobic metabolism to energy supply during repeated sprint exercise. *J Appl Physiol* 1996;80:876.

14. Branch JD. Effect of creatine supplementation on body composition and performance: a meta-analysis. *Int J Sport Nutr Exerc Metab* 2003;13:198.

15. Brannon TA, et al. Effects of creatine loading and training on running performance and biochemical properties of rat skeletal muscle. *Med Sci Sports Exerc* 1997;29:489.

16. Brass EP, et al. Effect of intravenous L-carnitine on carnitine homeostasis and fuel metabolism during exercise in humans. *Clin Pharmacol Ther* 1994;55:681.

17. Braun B, et al. The effect of coenzyme Q_{10} supplementation on exercise performance, $\dot{V}O_2$ max, and lipid peroxidation in trained cyclists. *Int J Sport Nutr* 1991;1:353.

18. Broad EM, et al. Effects of four weeks L-carnitine L-tartrate ingestion on substrate utilization during prolonged exercise. *Int J Sport Nutr Exerc Metab* 2005;15:665.

19. Bucci L, et al. Ornithine supplementation and insulin release in bodybuilders. *Int J Sports Nutr* 1992;2:287.

20. Burke LM, et al. Oral creatine supplementation does not improve sprint performance in elite swimmers. *Med Sci Sports Exerc* 1995;27:S146.

21. Burke LM, et al. Carbohydrate loading failed to improve 100-km cycling performance in a placebo-controlled trial. *J Appl Physiol* 2000;88:1284.

22. Campbell WW, et al. Chromium picolinate supplementation and resistive training by older men: effects on iron-status and hematologic indexes. *Am J Clin Nutr* 1997;66:944.

23. Campbell WW, et al. Effects of resistance training and chromium picolinate on body composition and skeletal muscle in older men. *J Appl Physiol* 1999;86:29.

24. Candon DG, et al. Protein supplementation before and after resistance training in older men. *Eur J Appl Physiol* 2006;97:548.

25. Canete S, et al. Does creatine supplementation improve functional capacity in elderly women? *J Strength Cond Res* 2006;20:22.

26. Casey A, et al. Creatine ingestion favorably affects performance and muscle metabolism during maximal exercise in humans. *Am J Physiol* 1996;271:E31.

27. Casey A, et al. Metabolic response of type I and II muscle fibers during repeated bouts of maximal exercise in humans. *Am J Physiol* 1996;271:E38.

28. Cerretelli P, Marconi C. L-Carnitine supplementation in humans: the effects on physical performance. *Int J Sports Med* 1990;11:1.

29. Chandler RM, et al. Dietary supplements affect the anabolic hormones after weight-training exercise. *J Appl Physiol* 1994;76:839.

30. Chrsuch MJ, et al. Creatine supplementation combined with resistance training in older men. *Med Sci Sports Exerc* 2001;33:2111.

31. Clancy S, et al. Effects of chromium picolinate supplementation on body composition, strength, and urinary chromium loss in football players. *Int J Sports Nutr* 1994;4:142.

32. Coggan AR, et al. Endurance training increases plasma glucose turnover and oxidation during moderate-intensity exercise in men. *J Appl Physiol* 1990;68:990.

33. Colombani P, et al. Effects of L-carnitine supplementation on physical performance and energy metabolism of endurance-trained athletes: a double-blind crossover field study. *Eur J Appl Physiol* 1996;73:434.

34. Constantin-Teodosiu D, et al. Carnitine metabolism in human muscle fiber types during submaximal dynamic exercise. *J Appl Physiol* 1996;80:1061.

35. Cooke WH, et al. Effect of oral creatine supplementation on power output and fatigue during bicycle ergometry. *J Appl Physiol* 1995;78:670.

36. Cortez MY, et al. Effects of pyruvate and dihydroxyacetone consumption on the growth and metabolic state of obese Zucker rats. *Am J Clin Nutr* 1991;53:847.

37. Costill DL, et al. Effects of repeated days of intensified training on muscle glycogen and swimming performance. *Med Sci Sports Exerc* 1988;20:249.

38. Décombaz J, et al. Energy metabolism of medium-chained triglycerides versus carbohydrates during exercise. *Eur J Appl Physiol* 1983;52:9.

39. Décombaz J, et al. Muscle carnitine after strenuous endurance exercise. *J Appl Physiol* 1992;72:423.

40. Décombaz J, et al. Effect of L-carnitine on submaximal exercise metabolism after depletion of muscle glycogen. *Med Sci Sports Exerc* 1993;25:773.

41. DeLany JP, et al. Differential oxidation of dietary fatty acids in humans. *Am J Clin Nutr* 2000;72:905.

42. Demopoulous H, et al. Free radical pathology: rationale and toxicology of antioxidants and other supplements in sports medicine and exercise science. In: Katch FI, ed. *Sport, Health, and Nutrition.* Champaign, IL: Human Kinetics, 1996.

43. Deutekom M, et al. No acute effects of short-term creatine supplementation on muscle properties and sprint performance. *Eur J Appl Physiol* 2000;82:223.

44. Dunne L, et al. Ribose versus dextrose supplementation, association with rowing performance: a double-blind study. *Clin Sport Med* 2006;16:68.

45. Earnest CP, et al. The effect of creatine monohydrate ingestion on anaerobic power indices, muscular strength and body composition. *Acta Physiol Scand* 1995;153:207.

46. Eckerson JM, et al. Effect of two and five days of creatine loading on anaerobic working capacity in women. *J Strength Cond Res* 2004;18:168.

47. Engelhardt M, et al. Creatine supplementation in endurance sports. *Med Sci Sports Exerc* 1998;30:1123.

48. Esmarck B, et al. Timing of postexercise protein intake is important for muscle hypertrophy with resistance training in elderly humans. *J Physiol* 2001;535:301.

49. Evans GW. The effect of chromium picolinate on insulin controlled parameters in humans. *Int J Biosoc Med Res* 1969;11:163.

50. Faff J, Frankiewicz-Józko A. Effect of ubiquinone on exercise-induced lipid peroxidation in rat tissues. *Eur J Appl Physiol* 1997;75:413.

51. Finn JP, et al. Effect of creatine supplementation on metabolism and performance in humans during intermittent sprint cycling. *Eur J Appl Physiol* 2001;84:238.

52. Fleck SJ, et al. Anaerobic power effects of an amino acid supplement containing no branched amino acids in elite competitive athletes. *J Strength Cond Res* 1995;9:132.

53. Fogelholm GM, et al. Low-dose amino acid supplementation: no effects on serum human growth hormone and insulin in male weight lifters. *Int J Sports Nutr* 1993;3:290.

54. Francaux M, Poortmans JR. Effects of training and creatine supplement on muscle strength and body mass. *Eur J Appl Physiol* 1999;80:165.

55. Friedlander AL, et al. Training induced alterations of carbohydrate metabolism in women: women respond differently than men. *J Appl Physiol* 1998;85:1175.

56. Friolet R, et al. Relationship between the coenzyme A and the carnitine pools in human skeletal muscle at rest and after exhaustive exercise under normoxic and acutely hypoxic conditions. *J Clin Invest* 1994; 94:1490.

57. Fry A, et al. Endocrine and performance responses to high volume training and amino acid supplementation in elite junior weightlifters. *Int J Sports Nutr* 1993;3:306.

58. Giamberardino MA, et al. Effect of prolonged L-carnitine administration on delayed muscle pain and CK release after eccentric effort. *Int J Sports Med* 1996;17:320.

59. Godard MP, et al. Oral amino-acid provision does not affect muscle strength or size gains in older men. *Med Sci Sports Exerc* 2002;34:1126.

60. Goedecke JH, et al. The effects of medium-chain triacylglycerol and carbohydrate ingestion on ultra-endurance exercise performance. *Int J Sport Nutr Exerc Metab* 2005;15:15.

61. Goforth HW Jr, et al. Persistence of supercompensated muscle glycogen in trained subjects after carbohydrate loading. *J Appl Physiol* 1997;82:342.

62. Gotshalk LA, et al. Creatine supplementation improves muscular performance in older men. *Med Sci Sports Exerc* 2002;34:537.

63. Goulet ED, et al. Effect of glycerol-induced hyperhydration on thermoregulatory and cardiovascular function and endurance performance during prolonged cycling in a 25 degrees C environment. *Appl Physiol Nutr Metab* 2006;31:101.

64. Grant KE, et al. Chromium and exercise training: effect on obese women. *Med Sci Sports Exerc* 1997;29:992.

65. Green AL, et al. The influence of oral creatine supplementation on metabolism during sub-maximal incremental treadmill exercise. *Proc Nutr Soc* 1993;53:84A.

66. Green AL, et al. Carbohydrate ingestion augments skeletal muscle creatine accumulation during creatine supplementation in humans. *Am J Physiol* 1996;271:E821.

67. Greenhauf PL. Creatine and its application as an ergogenic aid. *Int J Sports Nutr* 1995;5:S100.

68. Greenhaff PL, et al. Effect of oral creatine supplementation on skeletal muscle phosphocreatine resynthesis. *Am J Physiol* 1994;266:E725.

69. Halberstam M, et al. Oral vanadyl sulfate improves insulin sensitivity in NIDDM but not in obese nondiabetic subjects. *Diabetes* 1996;45:659.

70. Hallmark MA, et al. Effects of chromium and resistive training on muscle strength and body composition. *Med Sci Sports Exerc* 1996;28:139.

71. Hargreaves M, et al. Effect of muscle glycogen availability on maximal exercise performance. *Eur J Appl Physiol* 1997;75:188.

72. Harris RC, et al. The effect of oral creatine supplementation on running performance during maximal short term exercise in man. *J Physiol* 1993;467:74P.

73. Harris RK, et al. Elevation of creatine in resting and exercised muscle of normal subjects by creatine supplementation. *Clin Sci* 1992;83:367.

74. Hasten DL, et al. Effects of chromium picolinate on beginning weight training students. *Int J Sports Nutr* 1992;2:343.

75. Hatfield DL, et al. The effects of carbohydrate loading on repetitive jump squat power performance. *J Strength Cond Res* 2006;20:167.

76. Hathcock JN, Shao A. Risk assessment for coenzyme Q_{10} (ubiquinone). *Regul Toxicol Pharmacol* 2006;45:242.

77. Hawley JA. Effect of increased fat availability on metabolism and exercise capacity. *Med Sci Sports Exerc* 2002;34:1485.

78. Hellsten Y, et al. Effect of ribose supplementation on resynthesis of adenine nucleotides after intense intermittent training in humans. *Am J Physiol Regul Integr Comp Physiol* 2004;286:R182.

79. Heymsfield SB, et al. Garcinia cambogia (hydroxycitric acid) as a potential antiobesity agent: a randomized controlled trial. *JAMA* 1998; 280:1596.

80. Hitchins S, et al. Glycerol hyperhydration improves cycle time trial performance in hot humid conditions. *Eur J Appl Physiol* 1999;80:494.

81. Horton TJ, et al. Fuel metabolism in men and women during and after long-duration exercise. *J Appl Physiol* 1998;85:1823.

82. Indner WJ, et al. The effect of glycerol and desmopressin on exercise performance and hydration in triathletes. *Med Sci Sports Exerc* 1998;30:1263.

83. Ivy JL. Effect of pyruvate and dehydroxyacetone on metabolism and aerobic endurance capacity. *Med Sci Sports Exerc* 1998;6:837.

84. Izquierdo M, et al. Effects of creatine supplementation on muscle power, endurance, and sprint performance. *Med Sci Sports Exerc* 2002;34:332.

85. Jakobi JM, et al. Neuromuscular properties and fatigue in older men following acute creatine supplementation. *Eur J Appl Physiol* 2001; 84:321.

86. Janssen G, et al. Muscle carnitine level in endurance training and running a marathon. *Int J Sports Med* 1989;10:S153.

87. Jansson E. Sex differences in metabolic response to exercise. In: Saltin B, ed. *Biochemistry of Exercise* VI. Champaign, IL: Human Kinetics,1986.

88. Jenkins RR. Exercise, oxidative stress, and antioxidants: a review. *Int J Sports Nutr* 1993;3:356.

89. Jeukendrup AE, Aldred S. Fat supplementation, health, and endurance performance. *Nutrition* 2004;20:678.

90. Jeukendrup AE, et al. Metabolic availability of medium-chain triglycerides coingested with carbohydrate during prolonged exercise. *J Appl Physiol* 1995;79:756.

91. Jeukendrup AE, et al. Effect of endogenous carbohydrate availability on oral medium chain triglyceride oxidation during prolonged exercise. *J Appl Physiol* 1996;80:949.

92. Jeukendrup AE, et al. Effect of medium-chain triacylglycerol and carbohydrate ingestion during exercise on substrate utilization and subsequent cycling performance. *Am J Clin Nutr* 1998;67:397.

93. Jeukendrup AE, et al. Nutritional considerations in triathlon. *Sports Med* 2005;35:163.

94. Jowko E, et al. Creatine and beta-hydroxy-beta-methylbutyrate (HMB) additively increase lean body mass and muscle strength during a weight training program. *Nutrition* 2001;17:558.

95. Juhn MS, Tarnopolsky M. Potential side effects of oral creatine supplementation: a critical review. *Clin J Sports Med* 1998;8:298.

96. Kaats GR, et al. A randomized, double-masked, placebo-controlled study of the effects of chromium picolinate supplementation on body composition: a replication and extension of a previous study. *Curr Ther Res* 1998;57:747.

97. Karlic H, Lohninger A. Supplementation of L-carnitine in athletes: does it make sense? *Nutrition* 2004;20:709.

98. Kavouras SA, et al. Rehydration with glycerol: endocrine, cardiovascular, and thermoregulatory responses during exercise in the heat. *J Appl Physiol* 2006;100:442.

99. Kenney J, Carlberg KA. The effect of choline and myo-inositol on liver and carcass fat levels in aerobically trained rats. *Int J Sports Med* 1995;16:114.

100. Kersick R, et al. Effects of ribose supplementation prior and during intense exercise on anaerobic capacity and metabolic markers. *Int J Sports Nutr Exerc Metab* 2005;15:653.

101. Kilduff LP, et al. Effects of creatine on isometric bench-press performance in resistance-trained humans. *Med Sci Sports Exerc* 2002;34:1176.

102. Koh-Banerjee PH, et al. Effects of calcium pyruvate supplementation during training on bocy composition, exercise capacity, and metabolic responses to exercise. *Nutrition* 2005;21:312.

103. Koenigsberg PS, et al. Sustained hyperhydration with glycerol ingestion. *Life Sci* 1995;57:645.

104. Koopman R, et al. Combined ingestion of protein and carbohydrate improves protein balance during ultra-endurance exercise. *Am J Physiol Endocrinol Metab* 2004;287:E712.

105. Koopman R, et al. Combined ingestion of protein and free leucine with carbohydrate increases postexercise muscle protein synthesis in vivo in male subjects. *Am J Physiol Endocrinol Metab* 2005;288:E645.

106. Kovacs Em, Westerterp-Plantenga MS. Effects of (-)–hydroxycitrate on net fat synthesis as de novo lipogenesis. *Physiol Behav* 2006;23:88:371.

107. Kraemer WJ, et al. Hormonal responses to consecutive days of heavy-resistance exercise with or without nutritional supplementation. *J Appl Physiol* 1998;85:1544.

108. Kramer WJ, et al. The effects of amino acid supplementation on hormonal responses to resistance training overreaching. *Metabolism* 2006;55:282.

109. Kreider RB, et al. Effects of creatine supplementation on body composition, strength, and sprint performance. *Med Sci Sports Exerc* 1998;30:73.

110. Kreider RB, et al. Effects of oral d-ribose supplementation on anaerobic capacity and selected metabolic markers in healthy males. *Int J Sport Nutr Exerc Metab* 2003;13:87.

111. Kreider RB, et al. Long-term creatine supplementation does not significantly affect clinical markers of health in athletes. *Mol Cell Biochem* 2003;244:95.

112. Kriketos AD, et al. (-)-Hydroxycitric acid does not affect energy expenditure and substrate oxidation in adult males in a post-absorptive state. *Int J Obes Relat Metab Disord* 1999;23:867.

113. Laaksonen R, et al. Ubiquinone supplementation and exercise capacity in trained young and older men. *Eur J Appl Physiol* 1995;72:95.

114. Latzka WA, et al. Hyperhydration: tolerance and cardiovascular effects during uncompensable heat stress. *J Appl Physiol* 1998;84:1858.

115. Levenhagen DK, et al. Post-exercise nutrient intake is critical to recovery of leg glucose, and protein homeostasis in humans. *Am J Physiol Endocrinol Metab* 2001;280:E982.

116. Levenhagen DK, et al. Postexercise protein intake enhances whole-body and leg protein accretion in humans. *Med Sci Sports Exerc* 2002;34:828.

117. Lieberman HR, et al. Carbohydrate administration during a day of sustained aerobic activity improves vigilance, as assessed by normal ambulatory monitoring device, and mood. *Am J Clin Nutr* 2002;76:120.

118. Kim K, et al. (-)–Hydroxycitrate ingestion and endurance exercise performance. *J Nutr Sci Vitaminol* 2005;51:1.

119. Lukaski HC, et al. Chromium supplementation and resistance training effects on whole body and regional composition, strength, and trace element status of men. *Am J Clin Nutr* 1996;63:954.

120. Lynch NJ, et al. Effects of moderate dietary manipulation on intermittent exercise performance and metabolism in women. *Eur J Appl Physiol* 2000;81:197.

121. Lyons TP, et al. Effects of glycerol-induced hyperhydration prior to exercise in the heat on sweating and core temperature. *Med Sci Sports Exerc* 1990;22:477.

122. Magal M, et al. Comparison of glycerol and water hydration regimens on tennis-related performance. *Med Sci Sports Exerc* 2003;35:150.

123. Maher TJ. Safety concerns regarding supplemental amino acids: results of a study. In: Marrtiott BM, ed. *Food Components to Enhance Performance*. Washington, DC: Committee on Military Nutrition Research. National Academy Press, 1994.

124. Malm C, et al. Supplementation with ubiquinone-10 causes cellular damage during intense exercise. *Acta Physiol Scand* 1996;157:511.

125. Maughan RJ. Creatine supplementation and exercise performance. *Int J Sport Nutr* 1995;5:94.

126. Mihic S, et al. Acute creatine loading increases fat-free mass, but does not affect blood pressure, plasma creatine, or DK activity in men and women. *Med Sci Sports Exerc* 2000;32:291.

127. Miller SL, et al. Independent and combined effects of amino acids and glucose after resistance exercise. *Med Sci Sports Exerc* 2003;35:449.

128. Mujika I, et al. Creatine supplementation does not improve sprint performance in competitive swimmers. *Med Sci Sports Exerc* 1996; 28:1435.

129. Murray R, et al. Physiological responses to glycerol ingestion during exercise. *J Appl Physiol* 1991;71:144.

130. Nakai M, et al. Mechanism of insulin-like action of vanadyl sulfate: studies on interaction between rat adipocytes and vanadium compounds. *Biol Pharm Bull* 1995;18:719.

131. Odland LM, et al. Effect of oral creatine supplementation on muscle [PCr] and short-term maximum power output. *Med Sci Sports Exerc* 1997;29:216.

132. Op't Eijnde B, Hespel P. Short-term creatine supplementation does not alter the hormonal response to resistance training. *Med Sci Sports Exerc* 2001;33:449.

133. Op't Eijnde B, et al. No effects of oral ribose supplementation on repeated maximal exercise and de novo ATP resynthesis. *J Appl Physiol* 2001;91:2275.

134. Oyono-Enguelle S, et al. Prolonged submaximal exercise and L-carnitine in humans. *Eur J Appl Physiol* 1988;58:53.

135. Palmer GS, et al. Carbohydrate ingestion immediately before exercise does not improve 20 km time trial performance in well trained cyclists. *Int J Sports Med* 1998;19:415.

136. Parise G, et al. Effects of acute creatine monohydrate supplementation on leucine kinetics and mixed-muscle protein synthesis. *J Appl Physiol* 2001;91:1041.

137. Pearlman JP, Fielding RQ. Creatine monohydrate as a therapeutic aid in muscular dystrophy. *Nutr Rev* 2006;64(2Pt1):80.

138. Pitsiladis YP, Maughan RJ. The effects of alterations in dietary carbohydrate intake on the performance of high-intensity exercise in trained individuals. *Eur J Appl Physiol* 1999;79:433.

139. Pline KA, Smith CL. The effect of creatine intake on renal function. *Am Pharmacother* 2005;39:1093.

140. Poortmans JR, Francaux M. Long-term oral creatine supplementation does not impair renal function in healthy athletes. *Med Sci Sports Exerc* 1999;31:1108.

141. Porter DA, et al. The effect of oral coenzyme Q_{10} on the exercise tolerance of middle-aged, untrained men. *Int J Sports Med* 1995;16:421.

142. Prevost MC, et al. Creatine supplementation enhances intermittent work performance. *Res Q Exerc Sport* 1997;68:233.

143. Pritchard NR, Kaira PA. Renal dysfunction accompanying oral creatine supplements. *Lancet* 1998;351:1252.

144. Raben AB, et al. Serum sex hormones and endurance performance after a lacto-ovo-vegetarian and mixed diet. *Med Sci Sports Exerc* 1992;24:1290.

145. Rasmussen BB, Phillips SM. Contractile and nutritional regulation of human muscle growth. *Exerc Sport Sci Rev* 2003;31;127.

146. Rasmussen BB, et al. An oral essential amino acid-carbohydrate supplement enhances muscle protein anabolism after resistance exercise. *J Appl Physiol* 2000;88:386.

147. Rawson ES, Clarkson PM. Acute creatine supplementation in older men. *Int J Sports Med* 2000;21:75.

148. Rawson ES, et al. Effects of 30 days of creatine ingestion in older men. *Eur J Appl Physiol* 1999;80:139.

149. Redondo D, et al. The effect of oral creatine monohydrate supplementation on running velocity. *Med Sci Sports Exerc* 1994;26:S23.

150. Reed MJ, et al. Dietary lipids: an additional regulator of plasma levels of sex hormone binding globulin. *J Clin Endocrinol Metab* 1987;64:1083.

151. Rennie MJ, Tipton KD. Protein and amino acid metabolism during and after resistance exercise and the effects of nutrition. *Annu Rev Nutr* 2000;20:457.

152. Riedesel ML, et al. Hyperhydration with glycerol solutions. *J Appl Physiol* 1987;63:2262.

153. Roberts J. The effect of coenzyme Q_{10} on exercise performance. *Med Sci Sports Exerc* 1990;22:S87.

154. Robertson RJ, et al. Blood glucose extraction as a mediator of perceived exertion during prolonged exercise. *Eur J Appl Physiol* 1990;61:100.

155. Robinson TM, et al. Role of submaximal exercise in promoting creatine and glycogen accumulation in human skeletal muscle. *J Appl Physiol* 1999;87:598.

156. Romer LM, et al. Effects of oral creatine supplementation on high intensity, intermittent exercise performance in competitive squash players. *Int J Sports Med* 2001;24:546.

157. Roy BD, et al. Effect of glucose supplement timing on protein metabolism after resistance training. *J Appl Physiol* 1997;82:1882.

158. Roy BD, et al. Macronutrient intakes and whole body protein metabolism following resistance exercise. *Med Sci Sports Exerc* 2000;32:1412.

159. Saldanha Aoki M, et al. Carnitine supplementation fails to maximize fat mass loss induced by endurance training in rats. *Ann Nutr Metab* 2004;48:90.

160. Shao A, Hathcock JN. Risk assessment for creatine monohydrate. *Regul Toxicol Pharmacol* 2006;45:242.

161. Shomrat A, et al. Effects of creatine feeding on maximal exercise performance in vegetarians. *Eur J Appl Physiol* 2000;82:321.

162. Snow RJ, Murphy RM. Factors influencing creatine loading into human skeletal muscle. *Exerc Sport Sci Rev* 2003;31: 154.

163. Stanko RT, et al. Inhibition of lipid accumulation and enhancement of energy expenditure by the addition of pyruvate and dihydroxyacetone to a rat diet. *Metabolism* 1986;35:182.

164. Stanko RT, et al. Enhanced leg-exercise endurance with a high-carbohydrate diet and dihydroxyacetone and pyruvate. *J Appl Physiol* 1990;69:1651.

165. Stanko RT, et al. Enhancement of arm-exercise endurance capacity with dihydroxyacetone and pyruvate. *J Appl Physiol* 1990;68:119.

166. Stanko RT, et al. Body composition, energy utilization, and nitrogen metabolism with a 4.25-MJ/d low-energy diet supplemented with pyruvate. *Am J Clin Nutr* 1992;56:630.

167. Stanko RT, et al. Body composition, energy utilization and nitrogen metabolism with a severely restricted diet supplemented with dihydroxyacetone and pyruvate. *Am J Clin Nutr* 1992;55:771.

168. Starling RD, et al. Relationships between muscle carnitine, age and oxidative status. *Eur J Appl Physiol* 1995;71:143.

169. Starling RD, et al. Effect of inosine supplementation on aerobic and anaerobic cycling performance. *Med Sci Sports Exerc* 1996;28:1193.

170. Stensrud T, et al. L-Tryptophan supplementation does not improve running performance. *Int J Sports Med* 1992;13:481.

171. Steussi C, et al. L-carnitine and the recovery from exhaustive exercise: a randomized double-bline, placebo-controlled trial. *Eur J Appl Physiol* 2005;95:431.

172. Stevenson SW, Dudley GA. Dietary creatine supplementation and muscular adaptation to resistive overload. *Med Sci Sports Exerc* 2001;33:1304.

173. Suminski R, et al. The effect of amino acid ingestion and resistance exercise on growth hormone responses in young males. *Med Sci Sports Exerc* (abstr) 1993;25:S77.

174. Tarnopolsky MA, et al. Carbohydrate loading and metabolism during exercise in men and women. *J Appl Physiol* 1995;78:1360.

175. Tarnopolsky MA, et al. Gender differences in carbohydrate loading are related to energy intake. *J Appl Physiol* 2001;91:225.

176. Tegelman R, et al. Effects of a diet regimen on pituitary and steroid hormones in male ice hockey players. *Int J Sports Med* 1992;13:424.

177. Thompson KH, et al. Studies of vanadyl sulfate as a glucose-lowering agent in STZ-diabetic rats. *Biochem Biophys Res Commun* 1993;197:1549.

178. Tipton KD, et al. Acute response of net muscle protein balance reflects 24-h balance after exercise and amino acid ingestion. *Am J Physiol* 2003;284:E76.

179. Trappe SW, et al. The effects of L-carnitine supplementation on performance during swimming. *Int J Sports Med* 1994;15:181.

180. Trent LK, Thieding-Cancel D. Effects of chromium picolinate on body composition in a remedial conditioning program. *NHRC* publ 94-20, 1995.

181. Vandenberghe K, et al. Caffeine counteracts the ergogenic action of creatine loading. *J Appl Physiol* 1996;80:452.

182. Vandenberghe K, et al. Long-term creatine intake is beneficial to muscle performance during resistance training. *J Appl Physiol* 1997;83:2055.

183. Vandenberghe K, et al. Phosphocreatine resynthesis is not affected by creatine loading. *Med Sci Sports Exerc* 1999;31:236.

184. VanLeemputte M, et al. Shortening of muscle relaxation time after creatine loading. *J Appl Physiol* 1999;86:840.

185. van Loon LJC, et al. Effects of acute (—)-hydroxycitrate supplementation on substrate metabolism at rest and during exercise in humans. *Am J Clin Nutr* 2000;72:1445.

186. Van Schuylenbergh R, et al. Effects of oral creatine-pyruvate supplementation on cycling performance. *Int J Sports Med* 2003;24:144.

187. Vasankari TJ, et al. Increased serum and low-density-lipoprotein antioxidant potential after antioxidant supplementation in endurance athletes. *Am J Clin Nutr* 1997;65:1052.

188. Vierck JL, et al. The effects of ergogenic compounds on myogenic satellite cells. *Med Sci Sports Exerc* 2003;35:769.

189. Volek JS. Influence of nutrition on responses to resistance training. *Med Sci Sports Exerc* 2004;36:689.

190. Volek JS, et al. Response of testosterone and cortisol concentrations to high-intensity resistance exercise following creatine monohydrate supplementation. *J Strength Cond Res* 1996;10:292.

191. Volek JS, et al. Testosterone and cortisol in relationship to dietary nutrients and resistance exercise. *J Appl Physiol* 1997;82:49.

192. Volek JS, et al. Performance and muscle fiber adaptations to creatine supplementation and heavy resistance training. *Med Sci Sports Exerc* 1999;31:1147.

193. Volek JS, et al. Physiological responses to short-term exercise in the heat after creatine loading. *Med Sci Sports Exerc* 2001;33:1101.

194. Vukovich MD, et al. Carnitine supplementation: effect on muscle carnitine and glycogen content during exercise. *Med Sci Sports Exerc* 1994;26:1122.

195. Walker LJ, et al. Dietary carbohydrate, muscle glycogen content, and endurance performance in well-trained women. *J Appl Physiol* 2000;88:2151.

196. Walker LS, et al. Chromium picolinate effects on body composition and muscular performance in wrestlers. *Med Sci Sports Exerc* 1998;30:1730.

197. Wapnir PA, et al. Enhancement of intestinal water absorption and sodium transport by glycerol in rats. *J Appl Physiol* 1996;81:2523.

198. Warber JP, et al. The effect of choline supplementation on physical performance. *Int J Sport Nutr Exerc Metab* 2000;10:170.

199. Williams AG, et al. Effects of resistance exercise volume and nutritional supplementation on anabolic and catabolic hormones. *Eur J Appl Physiol* 2002;86:315.

200. Williams MM, et al. Effect of inosine supplementation on 3-mile treadmill run performance and V̇O₂ peak. *Med Sci Sports Exerc* 1990;22:517.

201. Willoughby DS, Rosene J. Effects of oral creatine and resistance training on myosin heavy chain expression. *Med Sci Sports Exerc* 2001;33:1674.

202. Willoughby DS, Rosene J. Effects of oral creatine and resistance training on myogenic regulatory factors expression. *Med Sci Sports Exerc* 2003;35:923.

203. Wiroth JB, et al. Effects of oral creatine supplementation on maximal pedaling performance in older adults. *Eur J Appl Physiol* 2001;84:533.

204. Wolfe RR. Regulation of muscle protein by amino acids. *J Nutr* 2002;132:3219S.

205. Wyss M, Kaddurah-Daouk R. Creatine and creatinine metabolism. *Physiol Rev* 2000;60:1107.

206. Yan Z, et al. Effect of low glycogen on glycogen synthase in human muscle during and after exercise. *Acta Physiol Scand* 1992;145:345.

207. Yuen VG, et al. Comparison of the glucose-lowering properties of vanadyl sulfate and bis (maltolato) oxovanadium (IV) following acute and chronic administration. *Can J Physiol Pharmacol* 1995;73:55.

208. Zuliani U, et al. The influence of ubiquinone (CoQ10) on the metabolic response to work. *J Sports Med Phys Fitness* 1989;29:57.

Part 6

Body Composition, Weight Control, and Disordered Eating Behaviors

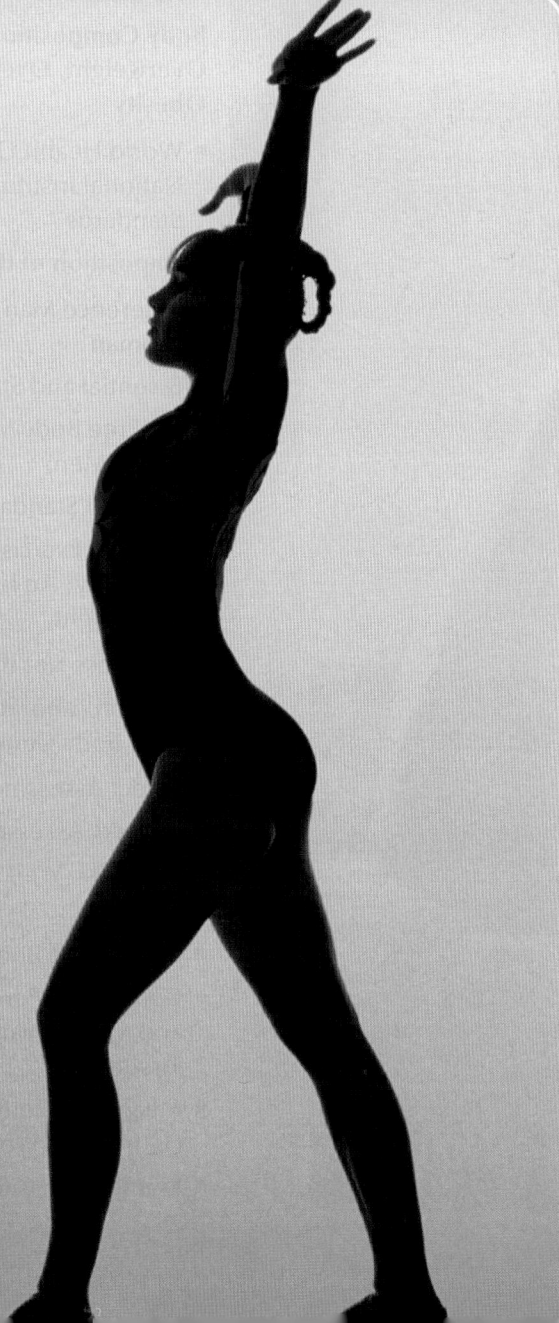

Chapter 13

Body Composition Assessment and Sport-Specific Observations

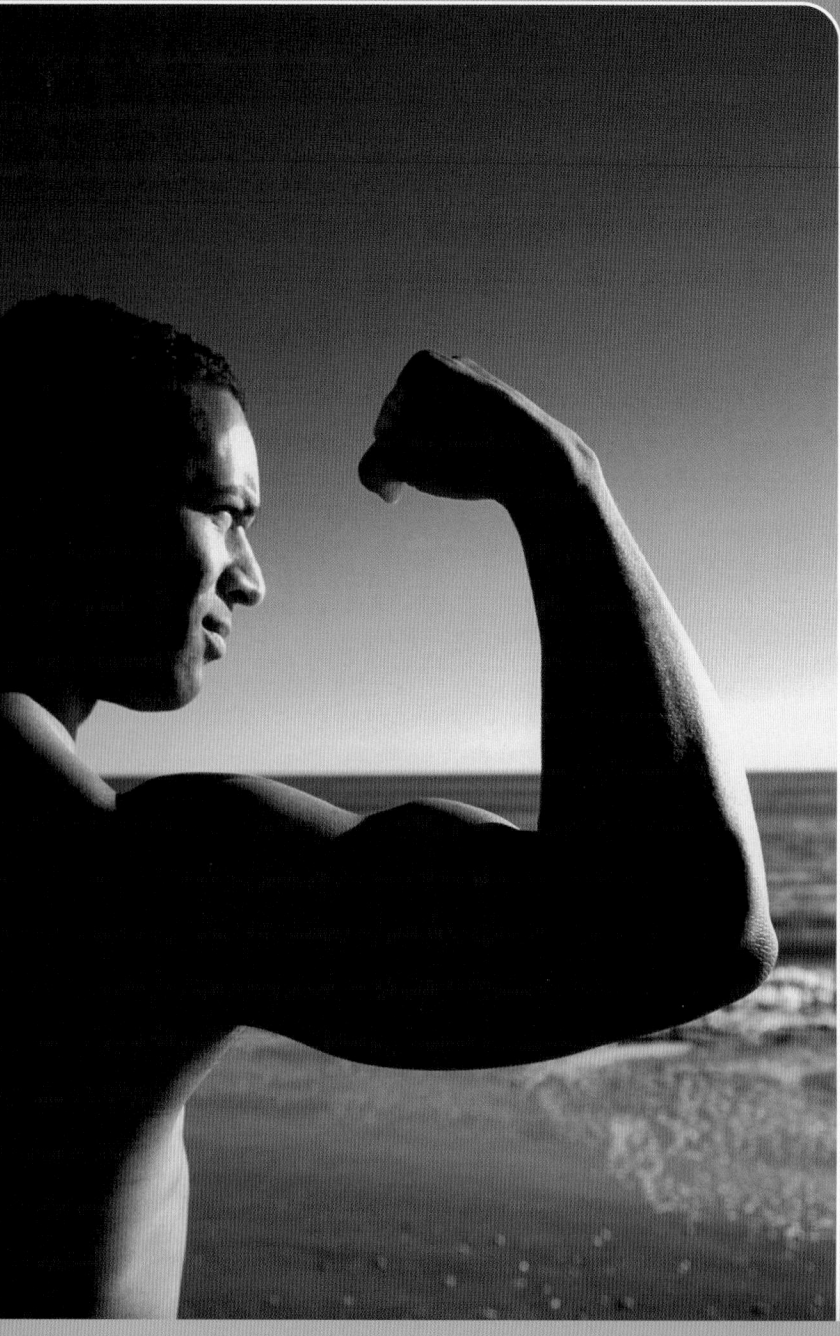

Skinfold Measurements

- The Caliper
- Usefulness of Skinfold Scores
- Skinfolds and Age
- User Beware

Girth Measurements

- Usefulness of Girth Measurements
- Predicting Body Fat from Girths

Regional Fat Distribution: Waist Girth and Waist/Hip Ratio

Bioelectrical Impedance Analysis

- Influence of Hydration and Ambient Temperature
- Applicability of Bioelectrical Impedance Analysis in Sports and Exercise Training

Near-Infrared Interactance

- Questionable Validity of Near Infrared Interactance

Computed Tomography, Magnetic Resonance Imaging, and Dual-Energy X-Ray Absorptiometry

Bod Pod

Estimating Body Fat Among Athletic Groups

Average Values for Body Composition in the General Population

Determining a Goal Body Weight

Physique of Champion Athletes

The Elite Athlete

- Olympic and Elite Athletes
- Field Event Athletes
- Female Endurance Athletes
- Male Endurance Athletes
- Triathletes
- Swimmers Versus Runners
- American Football Players
- A Worrisome Trend Among Less-Skilled and Younger Players
- Professional Golfers

Other Longitudinal Trends in Body Size

- Wrestlers
- Weightlifters and Bodybuilders

Test Your Knowledge

Answer these 10 statements about body composition assessment. Check your results using the scoring key at the end of the chapter. Repeat this test after you have read the chapter and compare your results.

1. **T F** The fundamental importance of the BMI is its ability to classify individuals by level of body fat and total muscle mass.
2. **T F** A male with a stature of 175.3 cm and body mass of 97.1 kg classifies as obese.
3. **T F** Men and women of superior athletic status generally possess similar values for body composition, particularly percentage body fat.
4. **T F** Total body fat exists in two storage sites called subcutaneous and intra-abdominal.
5. **T F** Archimedes' fundamental discovery explained the concept of specific gravity.
6. **T F** A male with a body density of 1.0719 has a body fat content of 10% of body mass and a fat mass of 5 kg.
7. **T F** A female with a waist girth of 38 inches falls just below the threshold value for increased risk for various diseases.
8. **T F** The average percentage body fat is 15% for college-age men and 25% for women.
9. **T F** A 120-kg (265-lb) shot-put athlete with 24% body fat wants to attain a body fat level of 15%. He must lose 40 lb of fat.
10. **T F** Among female athletes, bodybuilders possess the lowest percentage body fat.

Body Composition Assessment

The accurate appraisal of body composition serves an important role in a comprehensive program of total nutrition and physical fitness. There are six important reasons to assess an individual's body composition:

TABLE 13.1	Weight-for-Height Tables and Determination of Frame Size

A. Suggested Body Weights for Adults, with Recommended Adjustment for Age based on National Institutes of Health Recommendations[a]

Height[b]	Weight (lb)[c]	
	19–34 years	35 years
5'0"	97–128	108–138
5'1"	101–132	111–143
5'2"	104–137	115–148
5'3"	107–141	119–152
5'4"	111–146	122–157
5'5"	114–150	126–162
5'6"	118–155	130–167
5'7"	121–160	134–172
5'8"	125–164	138–178
5'9"	129–169	142–183
5'10"	132–174	146–188
5'11"	136–179	151–194
6'0"	140–184	155–199
6'1"	144–189	159–205
6'2"	148–195	164–210
6'3"	152–200	168–216
6'4"	156–205	173–222
6'5"	160–211	177–228
6'6"	164–216	182–234

[a]The lower weights more often apply to women who have less muscle and bone.

[b]Without shoes.

[c]Without clothes.

B. 1983 Sex-Specific Standards Proposed by the Metropolitan Life Insurance Company[d]

Men			
Height	Small Frame	Weight (lb)[d] Medium Frame	Large Frame
5'2"	128–134	131–141	138–150
5'3"	130–136	133–143	140–153
5'4"	132–138	135–145	142–156
5'5"	134–140	137–148	144–160
5'6"	136–142	139–151	146–164
5'7"	138–145	142–154	149–168
5'8"	140–148	145–157	152–172
5'9"	142–151	148–160	155–176
5'10"	144–154	151–163	158–180
5'11"	146–157	154–166	161–184
6'0"	149–160	157–170	164–188
6'1"	152–164	160–174	168–192
6'2"	155–168	164–178	172–197
6'3"	158–172	167–182	176–202
6'4"	162–176	171–187	181–207

Women			
Height	Small Frame	Weight (lb)[d] Medium Frame	Large Frame
4'10"	102–111	109–121	118–131
4'11"	103–113	111–123	120–134
5'0"	104–115	113–126	122–137
5'1"	106–118	115–129	125–140
5'2"	108–121	118–132	128–143
5'3"	111–124	121–135	131–147
5'4"	114–127	124–138	134–151
5'5"	117–130	127–141	137–155
5'6"	120–133	130–144	140–159
5'7"	123–136	133–147	143–163
5'8"	126–139	136–150	146–167
5'9"	129–142	139–153	149–170
5'10"	132–145	142–156	152–173
5'11"	135–148	145–159	155–176
6'0"	138–151	148–162	158–179

From Statistical Bulletin, Metropolitan Life Insurance Company, New York City.

[d]Weights at ages 25–59 years based on lowest comparative mortality. Weight in pounds according to frame size for men wearing indoor clothing weighing 5 lb, shoes with 1-in heels; for women, indoor clothing.

TABLE 13.1	Weight-for-Height Tables and Determination of Frame Size *(continued)*

C. How to Determine Frame Size from Elbow Breadth Based on Height.

The person's right arm extends forward perpendicular to the body, with arm bent so angle at the elbow forms 90°, with fingers pointing up and palm turned away from body. The greatest breadth across the elbow joint is measured with a sliding caliper along the axis of the upper arm. This records as elbow breadth. The table gives the **elbow breadth** *measurements for medium-framed men and women of various heights. Smaller measurements indicate a small frame size; higher measurements indicate a large frame size.*

Men	
Height in 1" Heels	**Medium-Framed Elbow Breadth**
5′2″–5′3″	2′1/2″–2′7/8″
5′4″–5′7″	2′5/8″–2′7/8″
5′8″–5′11″	2′3/4″–3′
6′0″–6′3″	2′3/4″–3′1/8″
>6′4″	2′7/8″–3′1/4″

Women	
Height in 1" Heels	**Medium-Framed Elbow Breadth**
4′10″–4′11″	2′1/4″–2′1/2″
5′0″–5′3″	2′1/4″–2′1/2″
5′4″–5′7″	2′3/8″–2′5/8″
5′8″–5′11″	2′3/8″–2′5/8″
>6′0″	2′1/2″–2′3/4″

1. Provides a starting point to base current and future decisions about weight loss and weight gain
2. Provides realistic goals about how to best achieve an "ideal" balance between the body's fat and nonfat compartments
3. Relates to general health status, thus playing an important role in establishing short *and* long-term health and fitness goals for *all* individuals
4. Monitors changes in the body's fat and fat-free components during exercise regimens of different durations and intensities and rehabilitation programs that use different modalities and treatment practices
5. Delivers an important message about the potential need to alter lifestyle, particularly the need to increase the quantity and quality of physical activity beginning in early adulthood and continuing throughout the life span, regardless of weight goals (to gain weight, reduce excess weight, or remain unchanged)
6. Allows the allied-health practitioner (sports nutritionist, dietician, personal trainer, coach, athletic trainer, physical therapist, chiropractor, physician, exercise leader) to interact with the individuals they deal with to provide quality information intimately related to nutrition, weight control, exercise, training, and rehabilitation

BODY COMPOSITION ASSESSMENT PROCEDURES

Weight-for-Height Tables

The weight-for-height tables serve as statistical landmarks based on the average ranges of body mass related to stature in which men and women aged 25 to 59 years have the lowest mortality rate. Weight-for-height tables *do not* consider specific causes of death or disease status before death (morbidity). In addition, many versions of the tables recommend different "desirable" weight ranges, with some considering frame size, age, and sex, whereas others do not. TABLE 13.1A AND B shows examples of two weight-for-height standards; Table 13.1A gives suggested body weights for adults with adjustment for age. Table 13.1B presents sex-specific standards proposed by the Metropolitan Life Insurance Company with consideration for bony frame size. Table 13.1C presents a convenient method to estimate sex-specific frame size using elbow breadth and stature.

LIMITATIONS OF WEIGHT-FOR-HEIGHT TABLES

The actuarial-based weight-for-height tables assess the extent of "overweightness" from sex and bony frame size. Such tables do not, however, provide reliable information about the relative *composition* of the human body. (The proper scientific terms expressed in SI units for *height* and *weight* are *stature* (cm) and *mass* (kg), and we have changed *weight* to *mass* and *height* to *stature* as long as it preserves readability.)

The popular weight-for-height tables have limited value as a standard to evaluate physique because "overweight" and "overfat" often describe different aspects of body composition for physically active men and women. Competitive athletes clearly illustrate this point; many possess high muscularity and exceed the average weight for their sex and height but otherwise possess a lean body composition. For these individuals, attempting to lose weight can impair exercise performance.

For example, many athletes weigh more than the average weight-for-height standards of life insurance company statistics—the "extra" weight due simply to additional muscle mass. According to Table 13.1A, for example, the desirable body mass for a 24-year-old professional football player 6 ft 2 in (188 cm) and 255 lb (116 kg) ranges between 148 lb (67.3 kg) and 195 lb (88.6 kg). Similarly, a young adult male of the same stature should weigh on average 187 lb (85 kg). Using either criterion, the player's "overweight" means he should reduce body mass at least 27 kg to the upper limit of the desirable weight range for a man of his stature. He must reduce an additional 3.6 kg to match his "average" American male counterpart. If the player followed these guidelines, he certainly would jeopardize his football career and possibly overall health. Some larger-sized persons are indeed "overweight," yet they may fall within a normal range for body fat without a need to reduce weight. The football player's total fat content equaled only 12.7% of body mass (compared with 15.0% body fat for untrained young men), even though he weighed 31 kg more than the average.

In the early 1940s, Navy physician and medical researcher Dr. Albert Behnke (1919–1990) assessed the body composition of 25 professional football players. From standards based on height and weight, 17 players failed to qualify for military service because their "overweight" status incorrectly indicated excessive fatness.[10] Carefully evaluating each player's body composition indicated the excess weight consisted primarily of muscle mass not fat mass. These observations clearly specified that the term "overweight" refers only to body mass greater than some standard, usually the average body mass for a given stature. Being above some "average," "ideal," or "desirable" body mass based on weight-for-height tables should not necessarily dictate whether someone should reduce weight. A more desirable strategy, particularly for physically active individuals, evaluates body composition by one of the techniques reviewed in this chapter.

The Body Mass Index: A Better Use for Mass and Stature

Clinicians and researchers use the body mass index (BMI), derived from body mass related to stature squared to evaluate the "normalcy" of body size. BMI has a somewhat higher yet still moderate association with body fat than estimates based only on stature and/or mass alone. Current classification standards for overweight and obese (next section) assume that the relationship between BMI and percentage body fat remains independent of age, gender, ethnicity, and race, but this may not be the case. For example, at a given BMI level Asians have greater body fat content than Caucasians and thus show greater risk for fat-related illness. Evidence also indicates a higher body fat percentage for a given BMI among Hispanic American women than for European American and African American women.[44] Failure to consider these sources of bias alters the proportion of individuals defined as obese by measured percentage body fat.[78,124]

$$BMI = Body\ mass,\ kg \div Stature,\ m^2$$

The importance of this easily obtained index illustrated in the bottom table of FIGURE 13.1 lies not in predicting overfatness but rather in its curvilinear relationship to all-cause mortality; as BMI increases so does risk for cardiovascular complications, including hypertension and stroke, type 2 diabetes, and renal disease.[22,125,133] The classification schema at the bottom of the figure indicates level of risk with each 5-unit increase in BMI. The lowest health risk category occurs for individuals with BMIs between 20 and 25, and the highest risk category includes individuals whose BMIs exceed 40. For women, 21.3 to 22.1 represents the desirable BMI range; the corresponding range for men is 21.9 to 22.4. An increased incidence of high blood pressure, diabetes, and coronary heart disease occurs when BMI values exceed 27.8 for men and 27.3 for women.

Limitations of BMI for Physically Active Individuals

As with weight-for-height tables, the BMI fails to consider the body's proportional composition or the all-important com-

ponent of body fat distribution referred to as fat patterning. Specifically, bone and muscle mass and even the increased quantity of plasma volume induced by exercise training affect the numerator (mass) of the BMI equation. A high BMI could lead to an incorrect interpretation of overfatness in relatively lean individuals with excessive muscle mass because of genetic makeup or exercise training. Healthy individuals who exercise regularly may lose body fat not reflected in body weight or BMI changes from an exercise-induced concurrent gain fat-free body mass.[54]

The possibility of misclassifying someone as overweight or "overfat" by BMI applies particularly to large-sized males, particularly field athletes, bodybuilders, weightlifters, upper-weight-class wrestlers, and professional football players (particularly offensive and defensive linemen). For example, the BMI for seven defensive linemen from a former National Football League (NFL) Super Bowl team averaged 31.9 (team BMI = 28.7), clearly signaling these professional athletes as overweight and placing them in the moderate category for mortality risk. Their body fat content, 18.0% for the linemen and 12.1% for the team, did not indicate excessive fatness, suggesting a misclassification when using BMI as a standard. Interestingly, the trend for excessively large BMIs still applies to the offensive and defensive linemen of the 2007 Super Bowl teams (TABLE 13.2). By any standard including the BMI for the reference man, they are classified as "obese" (overfat), with a relative "overweight" that exceeds 100 lb. While their levels of body fat most likely exceed the "normal" value of 15% of body fat for the reference man, their large body size includes a large lean mass component.

Misclassification of body weight relative to body fat also applied to the typical NFL player from 1920 to 1996. FIGURE 13.2 displays the average BMI for all 53,333 NFL roster players at 5-year intervals between 1920 and 1996. Average body fat content during the late 1970s through the 1990s fell below the range typically associated with normal males (see Table 13.8, p. 425). The body fat for football players evaluated by hydrostatic weighing (see page 410) included the NFL New York Jets, Washington Redskins, New Orleans Saints, and Dallas Cowboys. On average, all players from 1960 forward classify as overweight (based on weight-for-height using insurance company statistics). Up to 1989, the BMI for linebackers, skill players, and defensive backs represents the "low" category for disease risk, while the BMI for offensive and defensive linemen places these players at "moderate" risk. Thereafter, the BMI for linebackers changed from the low to moderate category, while the BMI for offensive and defensive linemen quickly approached "high" risk and since 1991 remained in that category. Unfortunately, the rate of increase in BMI for the largest NFL players (offensive and defensive linemen) shows no sign of declining, as was the case for the 2007 Super Bowl offensive and defensive linemen.

The extent of "largeness" is not limited to just pro players—it also includes Division I collegiate football athletes from the Big Ten Conference teams. Not surprisingly, of the 1124 roster players for the 2004–2005 season, 43% had BMIs that exceeded 30, and 14% had BMIs greater than 35 (which would characterize the latter group as severely obese). The three teams with the largest BMIs placed from first to last in the Big Ten

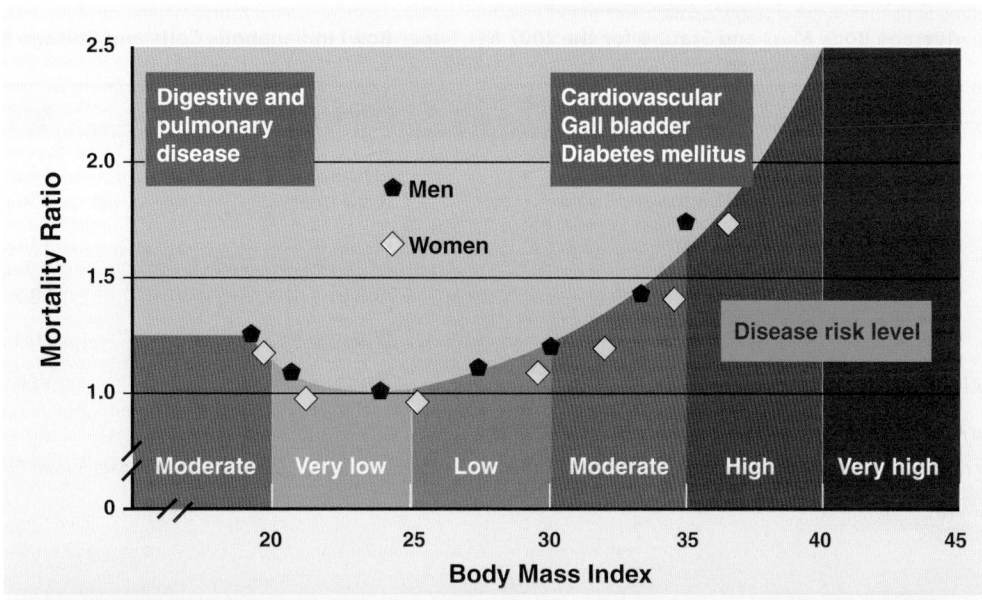

Body Mass Index, kg·m⁻²*													
19	20	21	22	23	24	25	26	27	28	29	30	35	40
Height, Inches					Body Weight , Pounds								
58	91	96	100	105	110	115	119	124	129	134	138	143	167	191
59	94	99	104	109	114	119	124	128	133	138	143	148	173	198
60	97	102	107	112	118	123	128	133	138	143	148	153	179	204
61	100	106	111	116	122	127	132	137	143	148	153	158	185	211
62	104	109	115	120	126	131	136	142	147	153	158	164	191	218
63	107	113	118	124	130	135	144	146	152	158	163	169	197	225
64	110	116	122	128	134	140	145	151	157	163	169	174	204	232
65	114	120	126	132	138	144	150	156	162	168	174	180	210	240
66	118	124	130	136	142	148	155	161	167	173	179	186	216	247
67	121	127	134	140	146	153	159	166	172	178	184	191	223	254
68	125	135	138	144	151	158	164	171	177	184	190	197	230	262
69	128	135	142	149	155	162	169	176	182	189	196	203	236	270
70	132	139	146	153	160	167	174	181	188	195	202	207	243	278
71	136	143	150	157	165	172	179	186	193	200	208	215	250	286
72	140	147	154	162	169	176	183	191	199	206	213	221	258	294
73	144	151	159	166	174	182	189	197	204	212	219	227	265	302
74	148	155	163	171	178	186	194	202	210	218	225	233	272	311
75	152	160	168	176	184	192	200	208	216	224	232	240	280	319
76	156	164	172	180	189	197	205	213	221	230	238	246	287	328

*The intersection of weight and height provides the BMI (kg·m⁻²). For an exact calculation of BMI, follow these steps:

Step 1. Multiply body weight (lb) by 0.45 to convert to kilograms.
Step 2. Multiply height (in) by 0.0254 to convert to meters.
Step 3. Multiply answer in step 2 by itself to obtain height in square meters (m²).
Step 4. To compute BMI, divide step 1 result (mass, kg) by step 3 result (m²).

FIGURE 13.1 ■ Curvilinear relationship based on American Cancer Society data between all-cause mortality and body mass index. (Modified from Bray GA. Pathophysiology of obesity. *Am J Clin Nutr* 1992;55:488S.)

TABLE 13.2   Average Body Mass and Stature for the 2007 NFL Super Bowl Indianapolis Colts and Chicago Bears Offensive and Defensive Linemen

Variable	Indianapolis Colts	Chicago Bears	Reference Man
Body mass	136.6 kg 301.3 lb	137.5 kg 302.2 lb	70.0 kg 154.0 lb
Stature	190.8 cm 1.908 m 75.1 in	192.8 cm 1.928 m 75.9 in	174.0 cm 1.740 m 68.5 in
BMI, kg/m^2	37.5	37.0	20.1
BMI classification[a]	Obese	Obese	Very low

From 2006 team rosters; [a]obese = BMI >30.0; normal weight = BMI 22.0–25.0.

Values for body mass given in pounds and kilograms, and stature in inches, centimeters, and meters. The reference man data is from Fig. 13.4

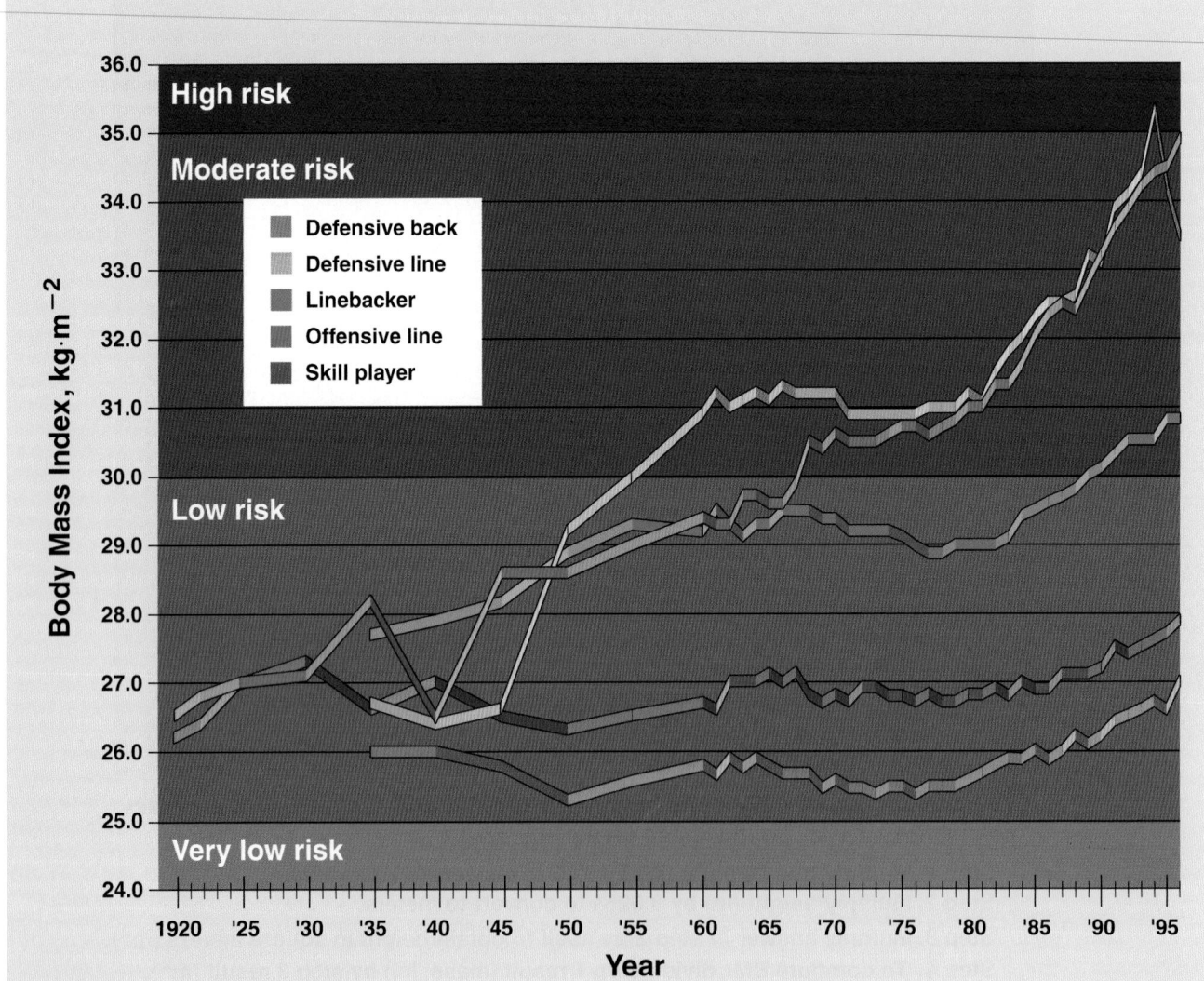

FIGURE 13.2 ■ Body mass index *(BMI)* for all roster players in the National Football League between 1920 and 1996 (N = 53,333). Categories include offensive and defensive linemen, linebackers, skill players (quarterbacks, receivers, backfield), and defensive backs. The four horizontal bands of color refer to Bray's classification in Figure 13.1 for relative disease risk levels. According to the 1998 federal guidelines for identification, evaluation, and treatment of overweight and obesity, offensive and defensive linemen from 1980 to present would classify as obese. (Data courtesy of F. Katch.)

standing, indicating the BMI team status does not relate necessarily to team performance or ranking. If such findings can be generalized, a common trend seems evident in collegiate football—the rising prevalence of players heavier than 300 lb. This does not bode well from a health perspective for either large-size professional or collegiate players.

BODY COMPOSITION DEFINITIONS: OVERWEIGHT, OVERFATNESS, AND OBESITY

Considerable confusion surrounds the precise meaning of the terms overweight, overfat, and obesity as applied to body composition. Each term often takes on a different meaning depending on the situation and context of use. The medical literature indicates that the term **overweight** refers to an overfat condition, despite the absence of accompanying body fat measures. Within this context, **obesity** refers to individuals at the extreme of the overfat continuum. This frame of reference delineates the body fat continuum by means of the body mass index.

Research and contemporary discussion among diverse disciplines emphasizes the need to distinguish between overweight, overfat, and obesity to ensure consistency in use and interpretation. In general, weight-for-height at a given age has provided the most convenient (and easily obtained) index to infer body fat and accompanying health risks. In proper context, however, the **overweight** condition simply refers to a body weight that exceeds some average for stature, and perhaps age, usually by some standard deviation unit or percentage. The overweight condition frequently accompanies an increase in body fat, but not always (e.g., male power athletes), and may or may not coincide with the comorbidities glucose intolerance, insulin resistance, dyslipidemia, and hypertension (e.g., physically fit overfat men and women).

When body fat measures are available (hydrostatic weighing, skinfolds, girths, bioelectrical impedance analysis [BIA], dual-energy x-ray absorptiometry [DXA]), one can more accurately place an individual's body fat level on a continuum from low to high, independent of body weight.

Overfatness then would refer to a condition in which body fat exceeds an age- and/or gender-appropriate average by a predetermined amount. In most situations, "overfatness" represents the correct term when assessing individual and group body fat levels.

The term **obesity** refers to the overfat condition that accompanies a constellation of comorbidities that include one or all of the following components of the "obese syndrome": glucose intolerance,[163] insulin resistance, dyslipidemia, type 2 diabetes, hypertension, elevated plasma leptin concentrations,[82] increased visceral adipose tissue,[103] and increased risk of coronary heart disease[95] and cancer.[23] Limited research suggests that excess body fat, not excess body weight per se, explains the relationship between above-average body weight and disease risk.[3,131,145,156] Such findings emphasize the importance of distinguishing the composition of excess body weight to determine an overweight person's disease risk.

Many men and women may be overweight or overfat, yet do not exhibit components of the **"obese syndrome."** For these individuals, we urge caution in using the term obesity (instead of overfatness) in all cases of excessive body weight. We acknowledge that these terms are often used interchangeably (as we at times do in this text) to refer to the same condition.

World Health Organization and National Institutes of Health Standards

In 1998, a 24-member expert panel convened by the National Institutes of Health (NIH: www.nih.gov) and National Heart, Lung and Blood Institute (NHLBI: www.nhlbi.nih.gov) adopted the single standards of the World Health Organization (WHO: www.who.int) and lowered the BMI demarcation for "overweight" (the preobese state) for all adults from 27 to 25. FIGURE 13.3 shows the current standards for identifying obesity (defined by BMI ≥ 30.0) for six heights (from 5 ft 6 in to 6 ft 3 in). Persons with a BMI of 30 average about 30 lb overweight. For example, a man 6 ft 0 in weighing 221 lb and a woman weighing 186 lb at 5 ft 6 in both have a BMI of 30, and both are approximately 30 lb overweight. The

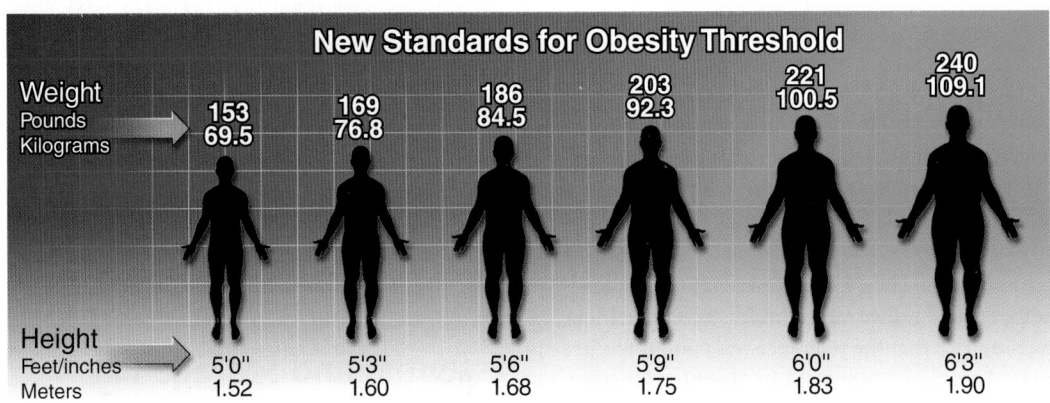

FIGURE 13.3 ■ New standards for the threshold of obesity.

revised standards place 65% of Americans in either the overweight or obese categories—up from 56% in 1994.[50,102,183,200]

The prevalence of obesity has nearly doubled in the United States over the past 30 years. For the first time, overweight persons (BMI > 25) outnumber those of desirable body weight. In terms of ethnicity and gender, significantly more black, Mexican, Cuban, and Puerto Rican men and women classify as overweight compared with white counterparts.[49] This study, by far the largest of its kind, concluded that overweight and obesity in the United States may account for 14% of all cancer deaths in men and 20% in women. We discuss the worldwide prevalence of overweight and obesity more fully in Chapter 14.

The following BMI-based classification can determine the adequacy of one's body weight:

Normal Weight: BMI ≤ 25.0
Overweight: 25.0–29.9
Obese: ≥ 30.0

Sample Computation of BMI

Male:

Stature = 175.3 cm, 1.753 m, (69 in)
Body mass = 97.1 kg (214.1 lb)
BMI = $97.1 \div (1.753)^2 = 31.6 \text{ kg} \cdot \text{in}^{-2}$

In this example, the BMI falls above the threshold of the upper range of BMI values and classifies the person as obese.

COMPOSITION OF THE HUMAN BODY

One approach to body composition assessment views the human body with three major structural components—muscle, fat, and bone. Marked sex differences in the relative amounts of these parameters make a convenient basis to compare men and women by applying the concept of reference standards developed by Dr. Behnke (FIG. 13.4). The standards incorporate the average physical dimensions from thousands of individuals measured in large-scale civilian and military anthropometric surveys to create a theoretical **reference man** and **reference woman**.[9]

Reference Man and Reference Woman

The reference man is taller and heavier, his skeleton weighs more, and he has a larger muscle mass and lower total fat content than the reference woman. Differences exist even when expressing the amount of fat, muscle, and bone as a percentage of body mass. This holds particularly true for body fat, which represents 15% of total body mass for the reference man and 27% for the female counterpart. The concept of reference standards does not mean that men and women should strive to achieve this body composition or that the reference man and reference woman are, in fact, "average," "normal," or "healthy." Instead, the model provides a useful frame of reference for statistical comparisons and interpretations of data from other studies of

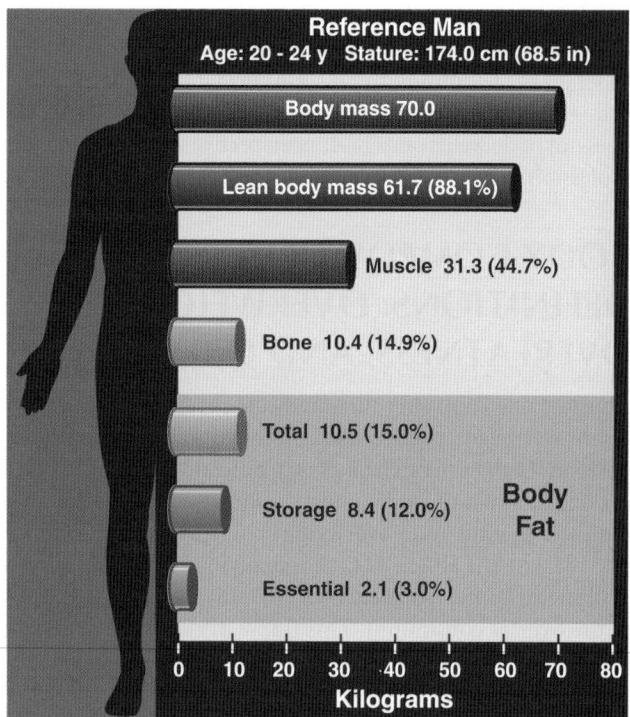

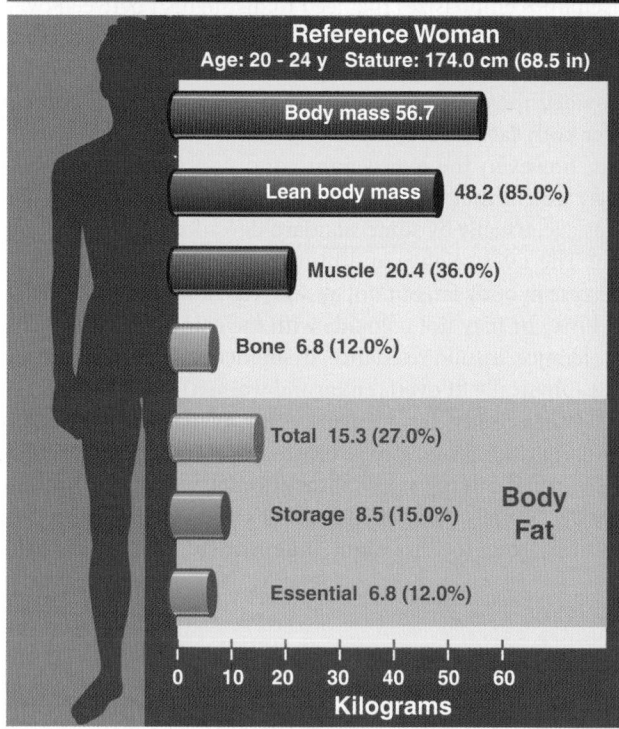

FIGURE 13.4 ■ Behnke's theoretical model for the reference man and reference woman. Values in parenthesis represent the specific value expressed as a percentage of total body mass.

diverse groups of athletes, individuals involved in physical training programs, and the underweight and obese.

Essential and Storage Fat

In the reference model, total body fat exists in two storage sites or depots called essential fat and storage fat.

Essential Fat

Essential fat consists of the fat stored in the marrow of bones, heart, lungs, liver, spleen, kidneys, intestines, muscles, and lipid-rich tissues of the central nervous system. *Normal physiologic functioning requires this fat.* In the female, essential fat includes additional **sex-specific essential fat**. Whether this fat provides reserve storage for metabolic fuel remains unclear. More than likely, sex-specific essential fat serves biologically important childbearing and other hormone-related functions. FIGURE 13.5 partitions the distribution of body fat for the reference woman. As part of the 5 to 9% sex-specific fat reserves, breast fat probably contributes no more than 4% of body mass for women whose body fat content varies from 14 to 35% of body mass.[93] This means that sites other than the breasts (lower body region that includes the pelvis, hips, and thighs) furnish a large proportion of sex-specific essential fat. Essential body fat apparently represents a biologically established range limit below which encroachment impairs health status.

Storage Fat

This major fat depot consists of fat accumulation in adipose tissue. This nutritional energy reserve contains about 83% pure fat in addition to 2% protein and 15% water within its

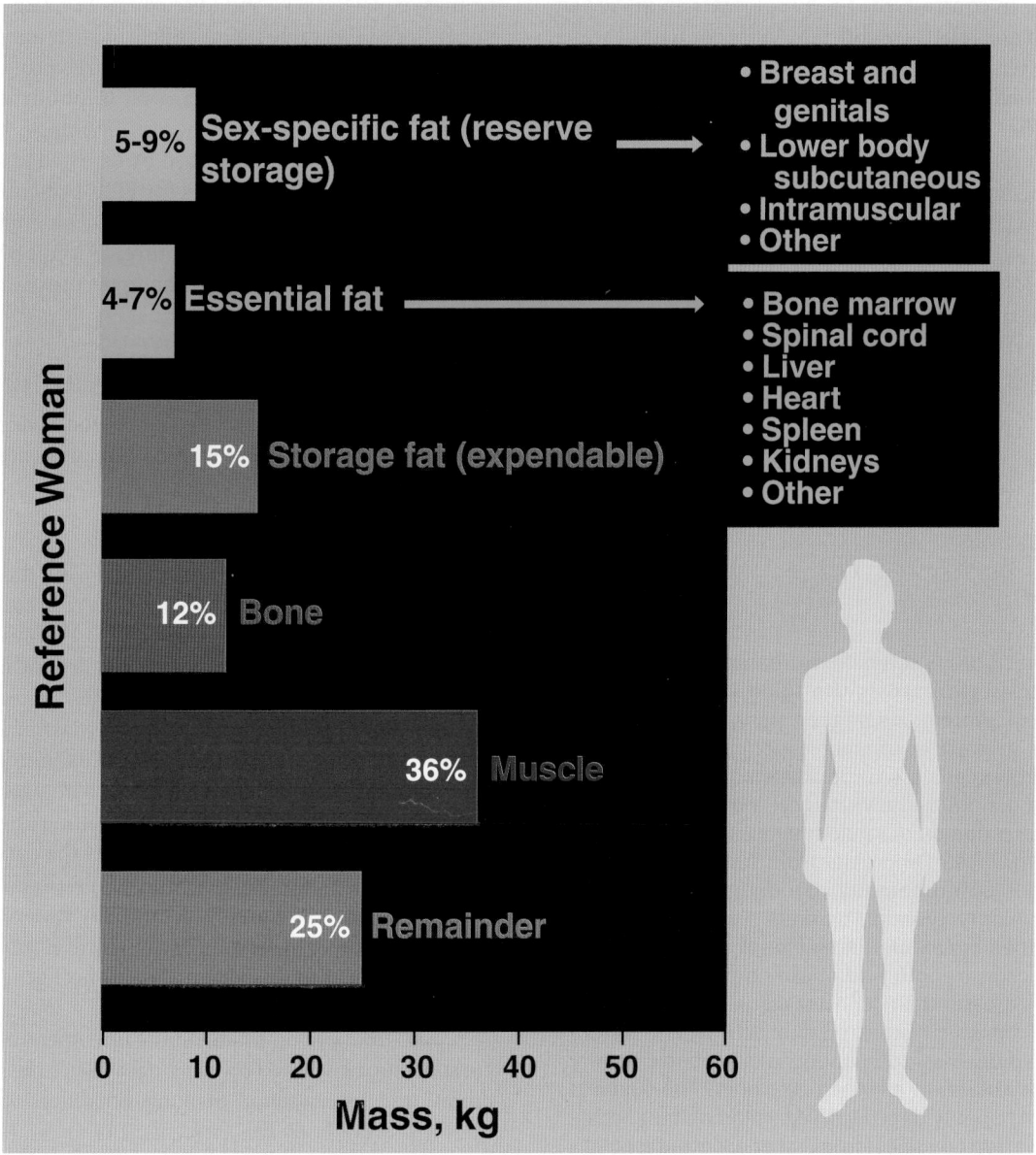

FIGURE 13.5 ■ Theoretical model for body fat distribution for a reference woman whose body mass equals 56.7 kg (stature = 163.8 cm) and body fat equals 23.6%. (From Katch VL, et al. Contribution of breast volume and weight to body fat distribution in females. *Am J Phys Anthropol* 1980;53:93.)

supporting structures. Storage fat includes the visceral fatty tissues that protect the various organs within the thoracic and abdominal cavities and the larger subcutaneous fat tissue volume deposited beneath the skin's surface. The reference man and reference woman have similar percentages of storage fat—approximately 12% of body mass in men and 15% in women.

Fat-Free Body Mass and Lean Body Mass (Men)

The terms *fat-free body mass* and *lean body mass* refer to specific entities: lean body mass (LBM) contains the small percentage of essential fat stores equivalent to approximately 3% of body mass. In contrast, fat-free body mass (FFM) represents the body devoid of *all* extractable fat. Behnke points out that FFM refers to an *in vitro* entity appropriate to carcass analysis. In contrast, the LBM represents an *in vivo* entity that remains relatively constant in its content of water, organic matter, and minerals throughout the adult's life span. *In normally hydrated, healthy adults, FFM and LBM differ only in the "essential" lipid-rich stores in bone marrow, brain, spinal cord, and internal organs.* Thus, LBM calculations include the small quantity of essential fat, whereas FFM computations exclude "total" body fat (FFM = Body mass − Fat mass).

Figure 13.4 reveals that LBM in men and the **minimal body mass** in women consist chiefly of essential fat (plus sex-specific fat for females), muscle, water, and bone. Whole-body density of the reference man with 12% storage fat and 3% essential fat equals 1.070 g · cm^{-3}, and the density of his FFM equals 1.094 g · cm^{-3}. If the reference man's total body fat percentage equals 15.0% (storage plus essential fat), the density of a hypothetical "fat-free" body attains the upper limit of 1.100 g · cm^{-3}.

Upper Limit for Fat-Free Body Mass

The FFM for Japanese elite sumo wrestlers (*seki-tori*) averages 109 kg.[100] These athletes share the distinction of being among the world's largest athletes with some American professional football players who weigh 159 kg (350 lb). It seems unlikely that athletes in this weight range would possess less than 15% body fat; the FFMs of the largest football players at 15% body fat theoretically would correspond to 135 kg. At 20% body fat, the FFM would be about 127 kg. But this value remains hypothetical in the absence of reliable data. Even for an exceptionally large professional basketball player (body mass, 138.3 kg [305 lb] and stature, 210.8 cm [83 in]), percentage body fat is unlikely to be less than 10% of body mass. Thus, fat mass equals 13.8 kg and FFM equals 114.2 kg—perhaps an upper limit FFM value for an athlete of such dimensions. The body composition of an exceptionally large professional football player (NFL Oakland Raiders; unpublished data, Dr. Robert Girandola, Department of Kinesiology, University of Southern California) determined by repeated trials of underwater weighing exceeds values for FFM presented in the research literature. The player whose body fat content equaled 11.3% (body mass, 141.4 kg; stature, 193 cm; BMI, 38.4 kg · in^{-2}) had a FFM of 125.4 kg, the uppermost value we have ever seen reported.

Minimal Standards for Leanness

A biologic lower limit seems to exist beyond which a person's body mass cannot decrease without impairing health status or altering normal physiologic functions.

Men

To calculate the lower fat limit in men (i.e., the LBM), subtract storage fat from body mass. For the reference man, LBM (61.7 kg) includes approximately 3% (2.1 kg) essential body fat. Encroachment into this reserve may impair normal physiologic function and capacity for vigorous exercise.

Low body fat values exist for world-class male endurance athletes and some conscientious objectors to military service who voluntarily reduce body fat stores with prolonged semi-starvation.[96] The low fat levels of marathon runners, ranging from 1 to 8% of body mass, likely reflect the combined effect of self-selection into the sport and adaptations to the severe training for distance running. A low body fat level reduces the energy cost of weight-bearing exercise; it also provides a more effective gradient to dissipate metabolic heat generated during intense physical activity.

TABLE 13.3 presents data on the physique status and body composition of selected professional athletes classified as "underfat" and "overweight." Striking differences occur between these groups in body size, percentage body fat, FFM, lean-to-fat ratio, and various girth measures. The defensive and offensive backs in football are "underfat" compared with the reference man (or any other nonathletic standard), whereas the linemen and shot putters are clearly "overweight" for

Sarcopenic Obesity: A Growing Concern

Sarcopenic obesity refers to decreases in muscle mass and increases in fat mass with aging. Inflammatory cytokines (e.g., protein and peptide signaling compounds that allow intercellular communication) produced mostly by visceral fat in adipose tissue accelerates muscle breakdown that maintains the vicious cycle that initiates and sustains the condition. A random sample of 378 men and 493 women 65 years and older from Tuscany, Italy were assessed for anthropometry, handgrip strength, and proinflammatory cytokine markers. Participants were cross classified by sex-specific tertiles of waist circumference and grip strength and obesity defined as a body mass index greater than 30. After adjusting for age, sex, education, smoking history, physical activity, and history of comorbid diseases, components of sarcopenic obesity were associated with elevated cytokines. The findings suggest that obesity directly affects inflammation, which negatively affects muscle strength that contributes to sarcopenic obesity. These results suggested that proinflammatory cytokines may be critical in the development and progression of sarcopenic obesity.[154]

| **TABLE 13.3** | Physique and Body Composition of "Underfat" Professional Football Players and "Overweight" Offensive and Defensive Professional Football Linemen and Shot Putters | | | | | | | |

Variable	Four Defensive Backs (All-Pro)				Offensive Back, All-Pro (N = 1)	Defensive Linemen, Dallas 1977 (N = 510)	Offensive Linemen, Dallas 1977 (N = 5)	Shot-Putters, Olympics (N = 13)
	1	2	3	4				
Age, y	27.1	30.2	29.4	24.0	32	31	29	24
Stature, cm	184.7	181.9	187.2	181.5	184.7	193.8	197.6	187.0
Mass, kg	87.9	87.1	88.4	88.9	90.6	116.0	116.5	112.3
Relative fat, %	3.9	3.8	3.8	2.5	1.4	18.6	13.2	14.8
Absolute fat, kg	3.4	3.3	3.4	2.2	1.3	21.6	15.4	16.6
Fat-free body mass, kg	84.5	83.8	85.0	86.7	89.3	94.4	101.1	95.7
Lean/fat ratio	24.85	25.39	25.00	39.41	68.69	4.37	6.57	5.77
Girths, cm								
Shoulders	122.1	119.0	120.5	117.2	121.8	129.5	122.5	133.3
Chest	101.6	101.0	99.5	107.5	102.0	116.5	109.9	118.5
Abdomen, avg	81.8	85.5	81.0	82.6	81.7	102.0	97.0	100.3
Buttocks	98.0	99.0	101.9	102.0	96.5	112.8	111.5	112.3
Thigh	61.0	61.0	58.5	64.0	63.2	66.2	69.3	69.4
Knee	39.5	41.3	41.1	38.0	41.0	44.8	45.8	42.9
Calf	37.6	38.8	38.8	37.8	41.3	43.5	42.4	43.6
Ankle	21.8	23.1	23.5	22.4	22.7	25.8	25.7	24.7
Forearm	31.8	29.1	31.1	31.8	33.5	33.5	34.8	33.7
Biceps	38.0	35.8	37.1	37.7	40.4	41.5	41.7	42.2
Wrist	18.5	17.2	17.4	17.5	18.0	19.3	19.3	18.9

From Katch FI, Katch VL. The body composition profile: techniques of measurement and applications. Clin Sports Med 1984;3:30,

their stature. Body mass in relation to stature (mass per unit size) for these athletic men represents the 90th percentile for nonathletic males.

Women

In contrast to the lower limit of body mass for the reference man, which includes about 3% essential fat, the lower limit for the reference woman includes about 12% essential fat. This theoretical lower limit termed minimal body mass equals 48.5 kg for the reference woman. Generally, body fat percentages for the leanest women in the population do not fall below 10 to 12% of body mass. This value probably represents the lower limit of fatness for most women in good health. *Behnke's theoretical concept of minimal body mass in women, which incorporates about 12% essential fat, corresponds to the lean body mass in men that includes 3% essential fat.*

UNDERWEIGHT AND THIN. The terms underweight and thin at times describe different physical conditions. Measurements in our laboratories have focused on the structural characteristics of apparently "thin" females.[92] Subjects were initially screened subjectively as appearing thin or "skinny." Each of the 26 women then underwent a thorough anthropometric evaluation that included measurement of skinfolds, circumferences, bone diameters, and percentage body fat and FFM from hydrostatic weighing.

Unexpectedly, the women's body fat averaged 18.2%, only about 7 percentage points below the average value of 25 to 27% typical for young adult women. Another striking finding included equivalence in four trunk and four extremity bone-diameter measurements in comparisons among the 26 thin-appearing women, 174 women who averaged 25.6% fat, and 31 women who averaged 31.4% body fat. *Thus appearing thin or skinny did not necessarily correspond to a diminutive frame size or an excessively low percentage body fat.*

LEANNESS, EXERCISE, AND MENSTRUAL IRREGULARITY: AN INORDINATE FOCUS ON BODY WEIGHT

In 1967, professional models weighed only 8% less than the average American woman; today, their weight averages 23% lower. In January 2007, the Council of Fashion Designers of

America CFDA: www.cfda.com) formulated guidelines as part of a new health initiative that targeted its models to emulate a healthy lifestyle, rather than one that promotes eating disorders. These nonbinding guidelines include the following:

1. Keep models younger than age 16 off the runway, and disallow models younger than 18 to work at fittings or photo shoots past midnight.
2. Educate those in the industry to identify the early warning signs of eating disorders.
3. Require models identified with eating disorders to receive professional help, and allow those models to continue only with approval from that professional.
4. Develop workshops on the causes and effects of eating disorders, and raise awareness of the effects of smoking and tobacco-related disease.
5. Provide healthy meals and snacks during fashion shows, while prohibiting alcohol and smoking.

The CFDA, in contrast to the fashion industry in Italy, does not mention the applicability of a BMI under 18.5 as a screening tool to determine the degree of underweight established by the World Health Organization (WHO). Some organizations (American Academy of Eating Disorders: www.aedweb.org) have called for even stricter guidelines than the WHO to target two distinct populations of young women (i.e., models and the millions of girls worldwide who try to emulate them).

As we discuss in Chapter 15, eating disorders and unrealistic weight goals have become common among females of all ages, particularly among athletes for whom the "norm" fosters striving for excessive leanness as a prerequisite for success. Physically active women, particularly participants in the "low-weight" or "appearance" sports such as distance running, body building, figure skating, diving, ballet, and gymnastics increase their chances of delayed onset of menstruation (after age 16 years), an irregular menstrual cycle (oligomenorrhea), or complete cessation of menses (amenorrhea).[30,193] Amenorrhea occurs in 2 to 5% of women of reproductive age in the general population, but reaches 10 to 15% among athletes and as high as 40% in some athletic groups. As a group, ballet dancers remain exceptionally lean, with greater incidence of menstrual dysfunction, eating disorders, and a higher mean age at menarche than age-matched, nondance females.[55,196] One third to one half of female athletes in endurance-type sports experience some menstrual irregularity. In premenopausal women, menstrual irregularity or absence of menstrual function increases risk of bone loss and musculoskeletal injury in vigorous exercise.[7,61]

A high level of chronic physical stress may disrupt the hypothalamic–pituitary–adrenal axis to modify the output of gonadotropin-releasing hormone to alter menstrual function (**exercise stress hypothesis**). A concurrent and more widely accepted hypothesis maintains that the body "senses" high physical stress and inadequate energy reserves to sustain a pregnancy; in such cases, ovulation ceases (**energy availability** or **energy drain hypothesis**). Some researchers argue that at least 17% body fat represents a "critical level" for onset of

menstruation, and 22% fat is the level required to maintain a normal cycle.[55] They reason that body fat below these levels triggers hormonal and metabolic disturbances that affect the menses. Research with animals has identified leptin, a hormone intimately linked to both body fat levels and appetite control (see Chapter 14), as a principal chemical signal that initiates puberty.[28,175] A linkage may thus exist between the onset of sexual maturity (and perhaps continued optimal sexual function) and the level of stored energy as reflected by accumulated body fat.

Leanness Not the Only Factor

Undoubtedly, the lean-to-fat ratio plays a key role in normal menstrual function, perhaps through peripheral fat's role that converts androgens to estrogens or through leptin production in adipose tissue. *Many physically active females fall below the supposed critical level of 17% body fat, but have normal menstrual cycles and maintain a high level of physiologic and performance capacity.* Conversely, some amenorrheic athletes have average body fat levels. We evaluated menstrual cycle regularity for 30 athletes and 30 nonathletes, all with less than 20% body fat.[90] Four of the athletes and three nonathletes ranging from 11 to 15% body fat maintained regular cycles, whereas seven athletes and two nonathletes had irregular cycles or were amenorrheic. For the total sample, 14 athletes and 21 nonathletes had regular menstrual cycles. These data indicate that normal menstrual function does not *require* a critical body fat level of 17 to 22%.

Potential causes of menstrual dysfunction include the complex interplay of physical, nutritional, genetic, hormonal, fat distribution, psychosocial, and environmental factors.[73,116,210] For physically active women, an intense exercise bout triggers the release of an array of hormones, some with antireproductive properties. The release of cortisol and other stress-related hormones with intense or prolonged exercise suggests that stimulation of the hypothalamic–pituitary–adrenal axis affects normal ovarian function.[33,118] It remains unclear whether regular intense exercise produces cumulative hormonal effects sufficient to disrupt the normal menses. In this regard, when injuries in young amenorrheic ballet dancers prevent them from exercising regularly, normal menstruation resumes, even though body weight remains low.[196] *Primary predisposing factors for reproductive endocrine dysfunction that affect physically active women include nutritional inadequacy and an exercise-induced energy deficit with heavy training.*[19,30,117] *Proper nutrition that emphasizes the maintenance of energy balance can prevent or reverse athletic amenorrhea without requiring the athlete to reduce exercise training volume or intensity.*

Proponents of this "energy deficit" explanation maintain that that exercise per se exerts no deleterious effect on the reproductive system other than the potential impact of its energy cost on creating a negative energy balance.[116,203] *In all likelihood, 13 to 17% body fat represents the minimal fat level for regular menstrual function.* The effects and risks of sustained amenorrhea on the reproductive system remain unknown. A gynecologist/endocrinologist should evaluate failure to menstruate or cessation of the normal cycle because it may reflect pituitary or thyroid gland malfunction or premature menopause.[6,115,162] As discussed in Chapter 2, prolonged menstrual dysfunction profoundly diminishes the density of the bone mass, which is not regained if and when menstruation resumes.

Delayed Onset of Menstruation and Cancer Risk

The delayed onset of menarche in chronically active young females may offer positive health benefits.[56] Female athletes who start training in high school or earlier show a lower lifetime occurrence of cancers of the breast and reproductive organs and non–reproductive-system cancers than less-active counterparts. Even among older women, regular exercise protects against reproductive cancers Women who exercise an average of 4 hours a week after menarche reduce breast cancer risk by 50% compared with age-matched inactive women. One proposed mechanism for reduced cancer risk links less total estrogen production (or a less potent estrogen form) over the athlete's lifetime with fewer ovulatory cycles because of the delayed onset of menstruation. Lower body fat levels in physically active individuals also may contribute to lowered cancer risk because peripheral fatty tissues convert androgens to estrogen.

COMMON LABORATORY METHODS TO ASSESS BODY COMPOSITION

Two general approaches determine the fat and fat-free components of the human body:

1. Direct measurement by chemical analysis of the animal carcass or human cadaver

2. Indirect estimation by hydrostatic weighing, simple anthropometric measurements, or other non-invasive procedures

Direct Assessment

One direct technique of body composition assessment literally dissolves the body in a chemical solution to determine the fat and fat-free components of the mixture. The other technique involves the physical dissection of fat, fat-free adipose tissue, muscle, and bone. Considerable research exists on the direct chemical assessment of body composition in various animal species, but few studies have directly determined human fat content.[52,127] These analyses are time consuming and tedious, require specialized laboratory equipment, and involve ethical questions and legal problems in obtaining cadavers for research purposes.

Direct assessment of body composition indicates that while considerable variation exists in total body fatness, the compositions of skeletal mass and lean and fat tissues remain relatively stable. The assumed constancy of these tissues enables researchers to develop mathematical equations to predict the body's fat percentage.

Indirect Assessment

Diverse indirect procedures commonly assess body composition. One involves Archimedes' principle applied to hydrostatic weighing (also referred to as *densitometry*, or *underwater weighing*). This method computes percentage body fat from whole-body density (the ratio of body mass to body volume). Other popular procedures to predict body fat use skinfold thickness and girth measurements, x-ray, total body electrical conductivity or impedance, near-infrared interactance, ultrasound, computed tomography, dual-energy x-ray absorptiometry, air plethysmography, and magnetic resonance imaging.

Case Study

Personal Health and Exercise Nutrition 13–1

How to Predict Percentage Body Fat from Body Mass Index

Body weight adjusted for height squared, referred to as body mass index (BMI; in kg · m^{-2}), in excess of 25 and 30 indicates overweight and obesity, respectively. The assumption underlying BMI guidelines lies in its supposed close association with body fatness and consequent morbidity and mortality. Several formulae predict percentage body fat (%BF) from BMI, which may provide a better indication of morbidity and mortality than BMI alone.

Measurement Variables

The following variables predict percentage body fat (%BF) from BMI:

- 1.00 ÷ BMI
- Age in years
- Sex: male, female
- Race: white, African American, Asian

Equation

Predict %BF with the following equation:

%BF = 63.7 − 864 × (1.00 ÷ BMI) − 12.1 × sex + 0.12 × age + 129 × Asian × (1 ÷ BMI) − 0.091 × Asian × age − 0.030 × African-American × age

where sex = 1 for male and 0 for female; Asian = 1 for Asians and 0 for other races; African American = 1 for African Americans and 0 for other races; age in years; BMI = body weight in kg ÷ stature in m^2

Examples

Example 1. African American male; age 30 years; BMI = 25

%BF = 63.7 − (864 × (1÷BMI)) − (12.1 × sex) + (0.12 × age) + (129 × Asian × (1 ÷ BMI)) − (0.091 × Asian × age) − (0.030 × African American × age)

= 63.7 − (864 × 0.04) − (12.1 × 1) + (0.12 × 30) + (129 × 0 × 0.04) − (0.091 × 0 × 30) − (0.030 × 1 × 30)

= 63.7 − (34.56) − (12.1) + (3.6) + (0) − (0) − (0.9)

= 19.7%

Example 2. Asian female; age 50 years; BMI = 30

%BF = 63.7 − (864 × (1 ÷ BMI)) − (12.1 × sex) + (0.12 × age) + (129 × Asian × (1÷ BMI)) − (0.091 × Asian × age) − (0.030 × African American × age)

= 63.7 − (864 × 0.0333) − (12.1 × 0) + (0.12 × 50) + (129 × 1 × 0.0333) − (0.091 × 1 × 50) − (0.030 × 0 × 50)

= 63.7 − (28.80) − (0) + (6.0) + (4.295) − (4.55) − (0)

= 40.7%

Example 3. Asian male; age 70 years; BMI = 28

%BF = 63.7 − (864 × (1 ÷ BMI)) − (12.1 × sex) + (0.12 × age) + (129 × Asian × (1÷ BMI)) − (0.091 × Asian × age) − (0.030 × African-American × age)

= 63.7 − (864 × 0.03571) − (12.1 × 1) + (0.12 × 70) + (129 × 1 × 0.03571) − (0.091 × 1 × 70) − (0.030 × 0 × 70)

= 63.7 − (30.853) − (12.1) + (8.4) + (4.61) − (6.37) − (0)

= 25.4%

Example 4. White Male; age = 55 years; BMI = 24.5

%BF = 63.7 − (864 × (1 ÷ BMI)) − (12.1 × sex) + (0.12 × age) + (129 × Asian × (1÷ BMI)) − (0.091 × Asian × age) − (0.030 × African American × age)

= 63.7 − (864 × 0.0408) − (12.1 × 1) + (0.12 × 55) + (129 × 0 × 0.0408) − (0.091 × 0 × 55) − (0.030 × 0 × 55)

= 63.7 − (35.25) − (12.1) + (6.6) + (0) − (0) − (0)

= 22.9%

Accuracy

The correlation coefficient between predicted %BF (using the above formulae) and measured %BF (using a four-compartment model to estimate body fat) is r = 0.89, with a standard error for estimating an individual's %BF equal to ±3.9% body fat units. This compares favorably with other body fat prediction methods that use skinfolds and girths.

Case Study *continued*

Predicted Percentage Fat at Given Critical BMI Values

Table 1 presents predicted %BF values for different threshold BMI values for men and women of different ethnicity. These data provide an approach for developing healthy percentage body fat ranges from guidelines based on the BMI.

Table 1   Predicted Percentage Body Fat by Sex and Ethnicity Related to BMI Healthy Weight guidelines

	Females			Males		
Age and BMI	**African Americans**	**Asians**	**White**	**African Americans**	**Asians**	**White**
20–39 y						
BMI <18.5	20%	25%	21%	8%	13%	8%
BMI ≥25	32%	35%	33%	20%	23%	21%
BMI ≥30	38%	40%	39%	26%	28%	26%
40–59 y						
BMI <18.5	21%	25%	23%	23%	13%	11%
BMI ≥25	34%	36%	35%	35%	24%	23%
BMI ≥30	39%	41%	42%	41%	29%	29%
60–79 y						
BMI <18.5	23%	26%	25%	11%	14%	13%
BMI ≥25	35%	36%	38%	23%	24%	25%
BMI ≥30	41%	41%	43%	29%	29%	31%

From Gallagher D, Heymsfield SB, et. al. Healthy percentage body fat ranges: an approach for developing guidelines based on body mass index. Am J Clin Nutr 2000;72:694.

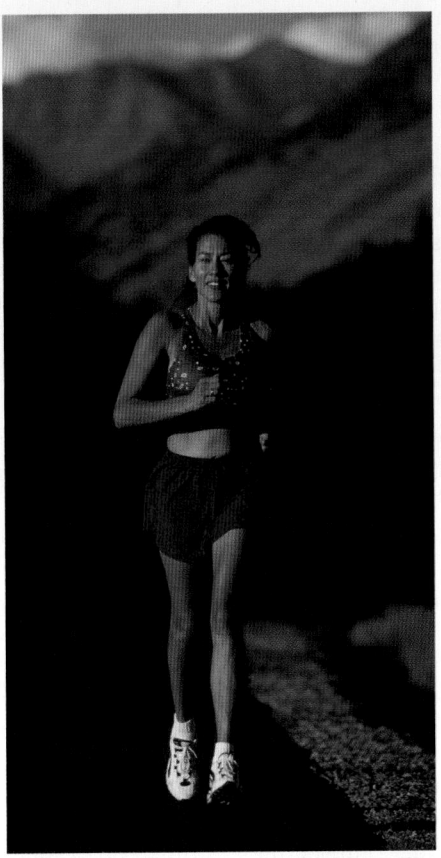

HYDROSTATIC WEIGHING (ARCHIMEDES' PRINCIPLE)

The Greek mathematician and inventor Archimedes (287–212 BC) discovered a fundamental principle currently applied to evaluate human body composition. An itinerant scholar of that time described the interesting circumstances surrounding the event:

> King Hieron of Syracuse suspected that his pure gold crown had been altered by substitution of silver for gold. The King directed Archimedes to devise a method for testing the crown for its gold content without dismantling it. Archimedes pondered over this problem for many weeks without succeeding, until one day he stepped into a bath filled to the top with water and observed the overflow. He thought about this for a moment, and then, wild with joy, jumped from the bath and ran naked through the streets of Syracuse shouting eureka, eureka, I have discovered a way to solve the mystery of the King's crown.

Archimedes reasoned that a substance such as gold must have a volume in proportion to its mass, and the way to measure the volume of an irregularly shaped object required submersion in water with collection of the overflow. Archimedes took lumps of gold and silver, each having the same mass as the crown, and submerged each in a container full of water. To his delight, he discovered the crown displaced more water than the lump of gold and less than the lump of silver. This could only mean the crown consisted of *both* silver and gold as the King suspected.

Essentially, Archimedes evaluated the specific gravity of the crown (ratio of the crown's mass to the mass of an equal volume of water) compared to the specific gravities of gold and silver. Archimedes probably also reasoned that an object submerged or floating in water becomes buoyed up by a counterforce equaling the weight of the volume of water it displaces. This buoyant force helps to support an immersed object against the downward pull of gravity. Thus, an object is said to lose weight in water. Because the object's loss of weight in water equals the weight of the volume of water it displaces, specific gravity refers to the ratio of the weight of an object in air divided by its loss of weight in water. The loss of weight in water equals the weight in air minus the weight in water.

Specific gravity = Weight in air ÷ Loss of weight in water

In practical terms, suppose a crown weighed 2.27 kg in air and 0.13 kg less (2.14 kg) when weighed underwater (FIG. 13.6). Dividing the weight of the crown (2.27 kg) by its loss of weight in water (0.13 kg) results in a specific gravity of 17.5. This ratio differs considerably from the specific gravity of gold, with a value of 19.3, so we too can conclude: "Eureka, the crown is a fraud!" The physical principle Archimedes discov-

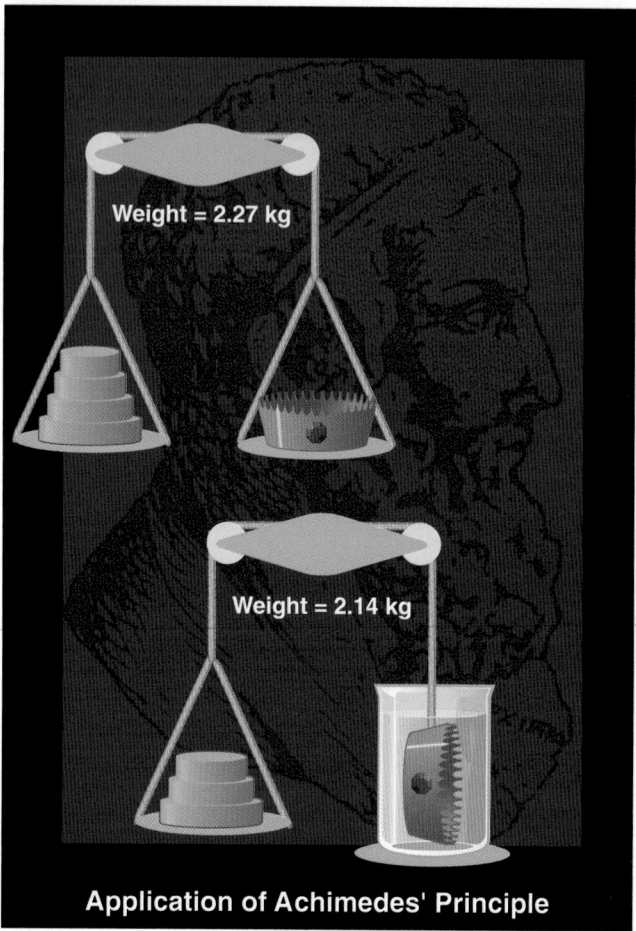

Application of Achimedes' Principle

FIGURE 13.6 ■ Archimedes' principle of buoyant force to determine the volume and subsequently the specific gravity of the king's crown.

ered allows us to apply water submersion or hydrodensitometry to determine the body's volume. Dividing a person's body mass by body volume yields body density (Density = Mass ÷ Volume) and from this an estimate of percentage body fat.

Computing Body Density

For illustrative purposes, suppose a 50-kg person weighs 2 kg when submerged in water. According to Archimedes' principle, loss of weight in water of 48 kg equals the weight of the displaced water. The volume of water displaced can easily be computed because we know the density of water at any temperature. In the example, 48 kg of water equals 48 L, or 48,000 cm^{-3} (1 g of water = 1 cm^{-3} by volume at 39.2°F). Measuring the person at the cold-water temperature of 39.2°F requires no density correction for water. In practice, researchers use warmer water and apply the appropriate density value for water at the particular temperature. The density of this person, computed as mass ÷ volume, equals 50,000 g (50 kg) ÷ 48,000 cm^{-3}, or 1.0417 g · cm^{-3}. The next step estimates percentage of body fat and the mass of fat and fat-free tissues.

Computing Percentage Body Fat and Mass of Fat and Fat-Free Tissues

An equation that incorporates whole-body density can estimate the body's fat percentage. This equation, derived from the premise that the densities of fat mass (all extractable lipid from adipose and other body tissues) and FFM (remaining lipid-free tissues and chemicals, including water) remain relatively constant (fat tissue, $0.90 \text{ g} \cdot \text{cm}^{-3}$; fat-free tissue, $1.10 \text{ g} \cdot \text{cm}^{-3}$). These consistencies remain even with large variations in total body fat and the fat-free tissue components of bone and muscle. The assumed densities for the components of the FFM at body temperature of 37°C (98.6°F) are water, $0.9937 \text{ g} \cdot \text{cm}^{-3}$ (73.8% of FFM); minerals, $3.038 \text{ g} \cdot \text{cm}^{-3}$ (6.8% of FFM); protein, $1.340 \text{ g} \cdot \text{cm}^{-3}$ (19.4% of FFM). The following equation, derived by Berkeley scientist Dr. William Siri (1919–2004), computes percentage body fat by incorporating the measured value of whole-body density:

Siri Equation
Percentage body fat = 495 ÷ Body density − 450

To estimate percentage body fat, substitute the body density value of $1.0417 \text{ g} \cdot \text{cm}^{-3}$ for the subject in the previous example in the Siri equation as follows:

$$\text{Percentage body fat} = 495 \div 1.0417 - 450$$
$$= 25.2$$

Compute mass of body fat by multiplying body mass by percentage fat:

$$\text{Fat mass (kg)} = \text{Body mass (kg)} \times [\text{Percentage fat} \div 100]$$
$$= 50 \text{ kg} \times 0.252$$
$$= 12.6$$

Compute FFM by subtracting the mass of fat from body mass:

$$\text{FFM (kg)} = \text{Body mass (kg)} - \text{Fat mass (kg)}$$
$$= 50 \text{ kg} - 12.6 \text{ kg}$$
$$= 37.4$$

In this example, 25.2%, or 12.6 kg, of the 50 kg body mass consists of fat, with the remaining 37.4 kg representing the FFM.

Possible Limitations of Hydrostatic Weighing

The generalized density values for fat-free ($1.10 \text{ g} \cdot \text{cm}^{-3}$) and fat ($0.90 \text{ g} \cdot \text{cm}^{-3}$) tissues represent averages for young and middle-aged adults. These assumed "constants" vary among individuals and groups, particularly the density and chemical composition of the FFM. Such variation limits accuracy of predicting percentage body fat from whole-body density. More specifically, a significantly larger average density of the FFM exists for blacks ($1.113 \text{ g} \cdot \text{cm}^{-3}$) and Hispanics ($1.105 \text{ g} \cdot \text{cm}^{-3}$) than whites ($1.100 \text{ g} \cdot \text{cm}^{-3}$).[62,139,155,168,177] Consequently, using the existing equations formulated on assumptions for whites to calculate body composition from whole-body density of blacks or Hispanics *overestimates* the FFM and *underestimates* percentage body fat.[35,41] The following modifications of

the Siri equation compute percentage body fat from body density measures for blacks.[192]

Modification of Siri equation for blacks:
Percentage body fat = [(4.858 ÷ Body density) − 4.394] × 100

Applying constant density values for the fat and fat-free tissues to growing children or aging adults also introduces errors in predicting body composition.[113] For example, the water and mineral contents of the FFM continually change during the growth period and the well-documented demineralization of osteoporosis with aging. Reduced bone density reduces the density of the fat-free tissue of young children and the elderly below the assumed constant of $1.10 \text{ g} \cdot \text{cm}^{-3}$, thus overestimating percentage body fat. For boys and girls, researchers have modified equations to predict body fat from whole-body density to adjust for density changes in FFM during childhood and adolescence (TABLE 13.4). Alterations in the density of the fat-free component may also occur in highly trained amateur and professional football players and champion distance runners and bodybuilders and affect estimation of percentage body fat from whole-body density (see below).

ADJUST FOR PERSONS WITH LARGE MUSCULOSKELETAL DEVELOPMENT. Chronic resistance training changes the density of the FFM, thus altering body fat estimation from whole-body density determinations.[130] White male weightlifters with considerable muscular development and nontrained controls were measured for body density, total body water, and bone mineral content. Comparisons included estimations of percentage body fat using the two-compartment model (assumed densities for the fat and fat-free compartments applied in the Siri equation) and a four-compartment model using the body's fat, water, mineral, and protein content and their associated densities. Percentage body fat estimated from body density (Siri equation) produced significantly higher values than percentage body fat estimated from the four-compartment model in weight trainers, but not in the untrained controls. A lower FFM density in weight trainers than controls ($1.089 \text{ vs } 1.099 \text{ g} \cdot \text{cm}^{-3}$) with the four-compartment model explained this discrepancy: it resulted from larger water and smaller mineral and protein fractions of the FFM in the resistance-trained men. For them, incorrect assumptions about density of the FFM underlying the Siri equation overestimated percentage body fat.

Regular weight-lifting increases muscularity disproportionately to changes in bone mass. A lower FFM density occurred because the density of their fat-free muscle ($1.066 \text{ g} \cdot \text{cm}^{-3}$ at 37°C) was less than the $1.1 \text{ g} \cdot \text{cm}^{-3}$ assumed in the Siri equation. Disproportionate increases in muscle mass relative to increases in bone mass reduce density of the FFM below $1.1 \text{ g} \cdot \text{cm}^{-3}$, thus overpredicting percentage body fat by the Siri equation.

Based on the revised densities of the FFM ($1.089 \text{ g} \cdot \text{cm}^{-3}$) and fat mass ($0.9007 \text{ g} \cdot \text{cm}^{-3}$), the researchers recommend modifying Siri's equation for more accurate appraisal with resistance-trained white males.

Modification for resistance-trained white males:
Percentage body fat = (521 ÷ Body density) − 478

TABLE 13.4	Percentage (%) Body Fat Estimated from Body Density (BD) Using Age- and Sex-Specific Conversion Constants to Account for Changes in the Density of the Fat-Free Body Mass as the Child Matures	
Age, years	**Boys**	**Girls**
7–9	% Fat = (5.38/BD − 4.97) × 100	% Fat = (5.43/BD − 5.03) × 100
9–11	% Fat = (5.30/BD − 4.89) × 100	% Fat = (5.35/BD − 4.95) × 100
11–13	% Fat = (5.23/BD − 4.81) × 100	% Fat = (5.25/BD − 4.84) × 100
13–15	% Fat = (5.08/BD − 4.64) × 100	% Fat = (5.12/BD − 4.69) × 100
15–17	% Fat = (5.03/BD − 4.59) × 100	% Fat = (5.07/BD − 4.64) × 100

From Lohman T. Applicability of body composition techniques and constants for children and youth. Exerc Sports Sci Rev 1986;14:325.

Measuring Body Volume by Hydrostatic Weighing

Hydrostatic weighing illustrates the most common application of Archimedes' principle to determine body volume. Body volume computes as the difference between body mass measured in air (M_a) and body weight measured during water submersion (W_w); *weight* is the correct term, because the body's mass remains unchanged under water. *Body volume equals loss of weight in water with the appropriate temperature correction for water density.*

FIGURE 13.7 illustrates the procedure for measuring body volume by hydrostatic weighing. The first step accurately assesses the subject's body mass in air, usually to the nearest ± 50 g. A diver's belt secured around the waist prevents the subject from floating toward the surface during submersion. Seated with the head out of the water, the subject makes a forced maximal exhalation while lowering the head beneath the water. The breath is held for several seconds as the underwater weight is recorded (minus the underwater weight of the diver's belt and chair). The subject repeats the procedure 8 to 12 times to obtain a dependable underwater weight score. Body volume calculation requires subtraction of the buoyant effect of the air remaining in the lungs after a forced exhalation (residual lung volume) measured immediately before, during, or after the underwater weighing. Without accounting for the residual lung volume, the computed whole-body density value would decrease because the lungs' air volume contributes to buoyancy. This would indeed make a person "fatter" when converting body density to percentage body fat.

Variations with Menstruation

Normal fluctuations in body mass (chiefly body water) related to the menstrual cycle generally do not affect body density and body fat assessed by hydrostatic weighing. However, some females experience noticeable increases in body water (>1.0 kg) during menstruation. Water retention of this magnitude affects body density and introduces a small error in computing percentage body fat.

Examples of Calculations

Data for two professional football players, an offensive guard and a quarterback, illustrate the sequence of steps to compute body density, percentage body fat, mass of fat, and FFM.

	Offensive guard	Quarterback
Body mass	110 kg	85 kg
Underwater weight	3.5 kg	5.0 kg
Residual lung volume	1.2 L	1.0 L
Water temperature correction factor	0.996	0.996

The loss of body weight in water equals body volume, so the body volume of the offensive guard becomes 110 kg − 3.5 kg = 106.5 kg, or 106.5 L; body volume for the quarterback (85 kg − 5.0 kg) equals 80.0 kg, or 80 L. Dividing body volume by the water temperature correction factor of 0.996 increases body volume slightly for both players (106.9 L for the guard and 80.3 L for the quarterback). By subtracting residual lung volume, the body volume of the offensive guard then becomes 105.7 L (106.9 L − 1.2 L) and for the quarterback, 79.3 L (80.3 L − 1.0 L).

Body density computes as mass ÷ volume. Body density for the offensive guard becomes 110 kg ÷ 105.7 L = 1.0407 kg · L^{-1}, or 1.0407 g · cm^{-3}. The corresponding density for the quarterback equals 85.0 kg ÷ 79.3 L or 1.0719 kg · L^{-1}, or 1.0719 g · cm^{-3}.

From the Siri equation, percentage body fat computes as follows:

Offensive guard:

$$495 \div 1.0407 - 450 = 25.6\%$$

Quarterback:

$$495 \div 1.0719 - 450 = 11.8\%$$

Total mass of body fat calculates as follows:
Offensive guard:

$$110 \text{ kg} \times 0.256 = 28.2 \text{ kg}$$

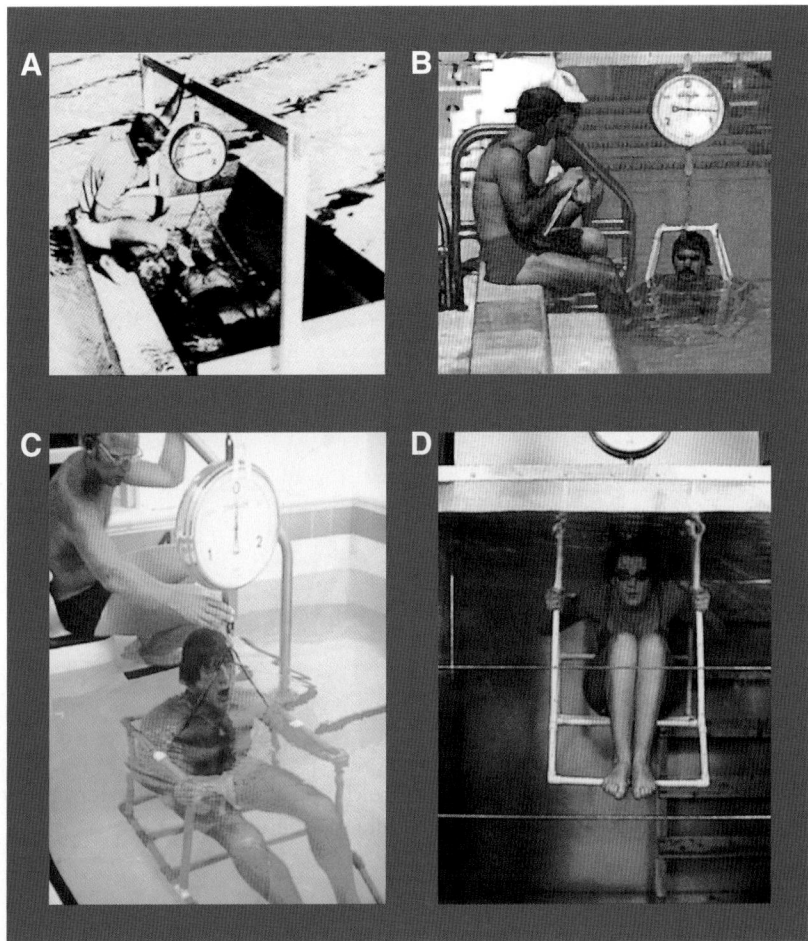

FIGURE 13.7 ■ Measuring body volume by underwater weighing. Prone and supine methods for underwater weighing with no difference in results, with residual lung volume measured before, during, or after the underwater weighing. Measurements taken **(A)** prone, **(B)** seated in a swimming pool, **(C)** seated in a therapy pool, and **(D)** upright in a stainless steel tank with Plexiglas front in the laboratory. For any method, subjects can use a snorkel with nose clip if apprehensive about submersion. Final calculation of underwater weight must account for these objects.

Quarterback:

$$85 \text{ kg} \times 0.118 = 10.0 \text{ kg}$$

FFM computes as follows:
Offensive guard:

$$110 \text{ kg} - 28.2 \text{ kg} = 81.8 \text{ kg}$$

Quarterback:

$$85 \text{ kg} - 10.0 \text{ kg} = 75.0 \text{ kg}$$

Body composition analysis illustrates that the offensive guard possesses more than twice the percentage body fat of the quarterback (25.6 vs 11.8%) and almost three times as much total fat (28.2 vs 10.0 kg). In contrast, the guard's FFM, which largely indicates muscle mass, exceeds the quarterback's FFM.

SKINFOLD MEASUREMENTS

Simple anthropometric procedures validly predict body fatness. The most common of these procedures measures skinfolds. The rationale for using skinfolds to estimate body fat comes from the relationships among three factors: (1) fat in the adipose tissue deposits directly beneath the skin (subcutaneous fat), (2) internal fat, and (3) whole-body density.

The Caliper

By 1930, a special pincer-type caliper accurately measured subcutaneous fat at selected body sites. The three calipers shown in FIGURE 13.8 operate on the same principle as a micrometer that measures distance between two points. Measuring skinfold thickness requires grasping a fold of skin

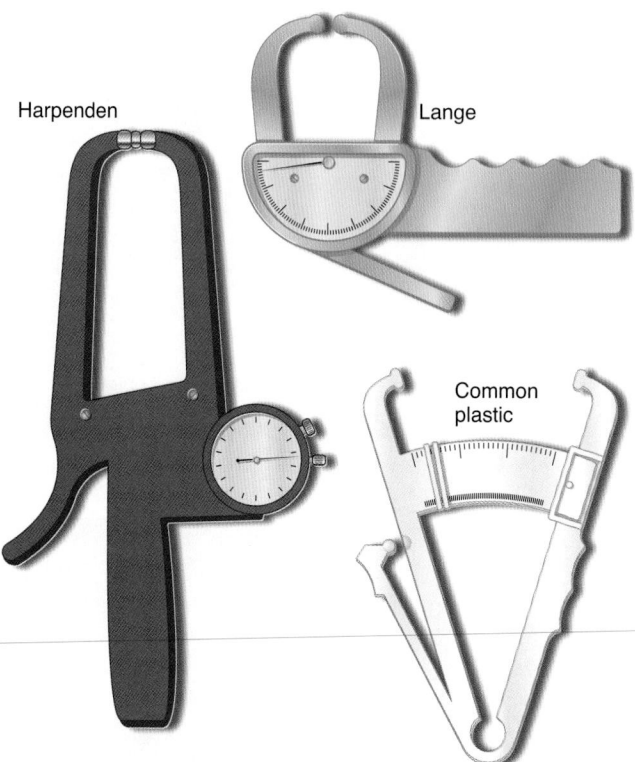

FIGURE 13.8 ■ Common calipers for skinfold measurements. The Harpenden and Lange calipers provide constant tension at all jaw openings.

and subcutaneous fat firmly with the thumb and forefingers, pulling it away from the underlying muscle tissue following the natural contour of the skinfold. The pincer jaws of calipers used for precise measurement exert a constant tension of $10 \text{ g} \cdot \text{mm}^{-2}$ at the point of contact with the caliper. The caliper dial indicates skinfold thickness in millimeters, which is recorded within 2 seconds after applying the full force of the caliper. This time limitation avoids excessive skinfold compression when taking the measurement. For research purposes, the investigator should have considerable experience in taking measurements and demonstrate consistency in duplicating values for the same subject made on the same day, consecutive days, or even weeks apart. A good rule of thumb to achieve consistency requires duplicate or triplicate practice measurements on at least 30 individuals who vary in body fat. This amount of careful attention to details usually ensures high reproducibility of measurement.

The Sites
The most common anatomic locations for skinfold measurement include the triceps, subscapular, suprailiac, abdominal, and upper thigh sites (FIG. 13.9). The tester takes a minimum

of two or three measurements at each site on the right side of the body with the subject standing. The average value represents the skinfold score.

1. **Triceps:** Vertical fold at the posterior midline of the upper arm, halfway between the tip of the shoulder and tip of the elbow; elbow remains in an extended, relaxed position
2. **Subscapular:** Oblique fold, just below the bottom tip of the scapula
3. **Suprailiac (iliac crest):** Slightly oblique fold, just above the hipbone (crest of ileum); the fold follows the natural diagonal line
4. **Abdominal:** Vertical fold 1 inch to the right of the umbilicus
5. **Thigh:** Vertical fold at the midline of the thigh, two thirds of the distance from the middle of the patella (kneecap) to the hip

Other sites include the **chest**: diagonal fold with its long axis directed toward the nipple, on the anterior axillary fold, as high as possible. The **biceps**: vertical fold at the posterior midline of the upper arm, and the **midaxillary**, a vertical fold on the midaxillary line at the level of the sternum's xiphoid process.

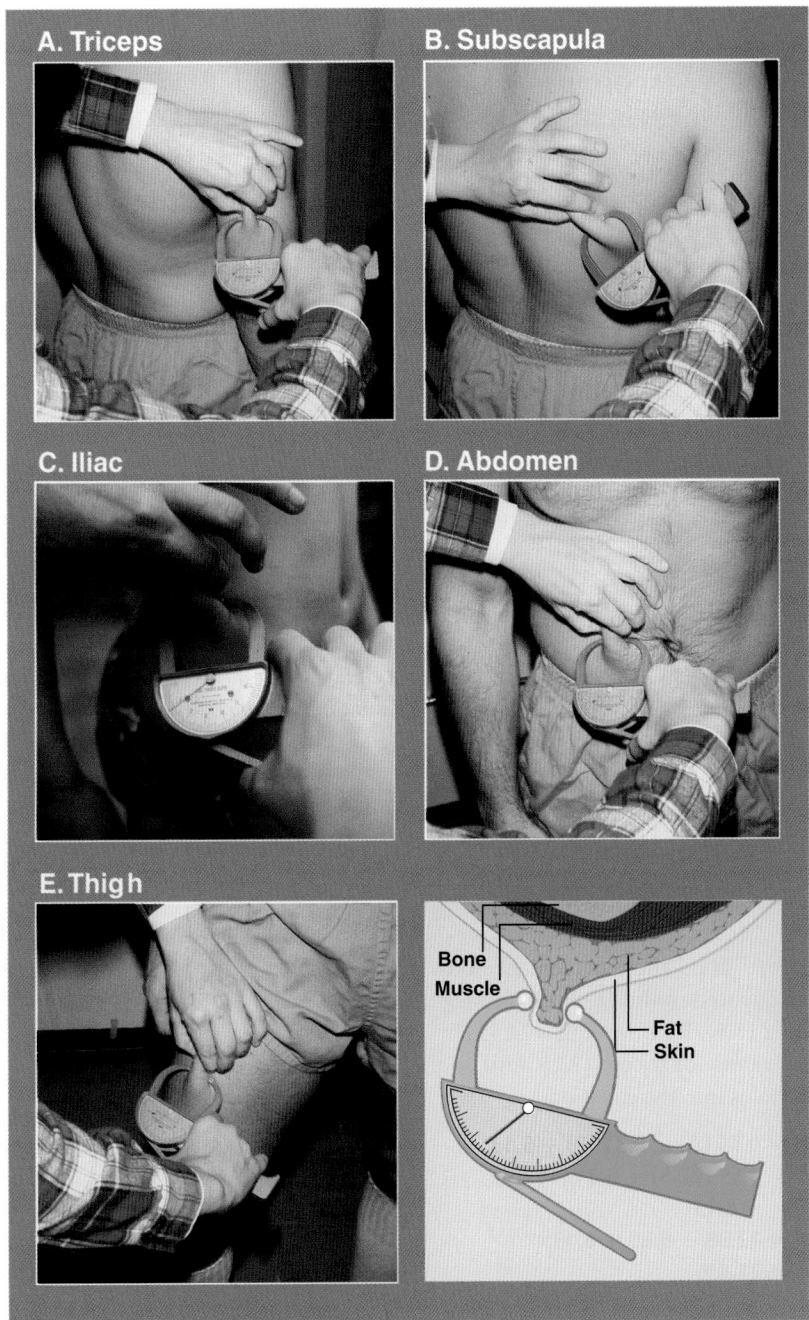

FIGURE 13.9 ■ Anatomic location of five common skinfold sites: **A.** Triceps. **B.** Subscapular. **C.** Iliac (suprailiac). **D.** Abdomen. **E.** Thigh. The *lower right* shows a schematic diagram for use of a skinfold caliper. Note the compression of a double layer of skin and underlying tissue during the measurement. Except for subscapular and suprailiac sites measured diagonally, take measurements in the vertical plane.

Usefulness of Skinfold Scores

Skinfold measurements provide consistent and meaningful information concerning body fat and its distribution. We recommend two ways to use skinfolds. The first sums the skinfold scores to indicate relative fatness among individuals. This "sum of skinfolds" and individual skinfold values reflect with some accuracy body fat changes "before" and "after" an intervention program. Evaluate these changes on either an absolute or a percentage basis.

One can draw the following three conclusions from the skinfold data in TABLE 13.5 obtained from a 22-year-old female college student before and after a 16-week exercise program:

1. Largest changes in skinfold thickness occurred at the suprailiac and abdominal sites.
2. Triceps skinfold showed the largest percentage decrease and the subscapular skinfold the smallest percentage decrease.
3. Total skinfold reduction at the five sites equaled 16.6 mm, or 12.6% below the "before" condition.

A second use of skinfolds incorporates population-specific statistical equations to predict body density or percentage body fat. The equations prove accurate for subjects similar in age, gender, training status, fatness, and race to the group for whom they were derived.[16,77,86,142,185] When meeting these criteria, predicted percentage body fat for an individual usually ranges between 3 to 5% body fat units of the value computed using hydrostatic weighing. The first and third skinfold equations in TABLE 13.6 accurately predict percentage body fat in men and women of diverse ages.

We have developed the following equations to predict body fat from triceps and subscapular skinfolds in young women and men[86–89]:

Young women, ages 17 to 26 years:

Percentage body fat = 0.55(A) + 0.31(B) + 6.13

Young men, ages 17 to 26 years:

Percentage body fat = 0.43(A) + 0.58(B) + 1.47

In both equations, A = triceps skinfold (mm) and B = subscapular skinfold (mm).

We computed the "before" and "after" percentage body fat of the woman who participated in the 16-week physical conditioning program (Table 13.5). Body fat equals 24.4% by substituting the pretraining values for triceps (22.5 mm) and subscapular (19.0 mm) skinfolds into the equation.

$$
\begin{aligned}
\text{Percentage body fat} &= 0.55\,(A) + 0.31\,(B) + 6.13 \\
&= 0.55\,(22.5) + 0.31\,(19.0) \\
&\quad + 6.13 \\
&= 12.38 + 5.89 + 6.13 \\
&= 24.4\%
\end{aligned}
$$

Substituting the posttraining values for triceps (19.4 mm) and subscapular (17.0 mm) skinfolds produced a body fat value of 21.1%.

$$
\begin{aligned}
\text{Percentage body fat} &= 0.55\,(19.4) + 0.31\,(17.0) \\
&\quad + 6.13 \\
&= 10.67 + 5.27 + 6.13 \\
&= 22.1\%
\end{aligned}
$$

Percentage body fat determined before and after a physical conditioning or weight-loss program provides a useful means to evaluate body composition alterations, often independent of body weight changes.

Skinfolds and Age

In young adults, subcutaneous fat constitutes approximately half of the body's total fat, with the remainder visceral and organ fat. With advancing age, a proportionately greater quantity of fat deposits internally than subcutaneously. Thus, the same skinfold score reflects *greater* total percentage body fat as one gets older. *For this reason, use age-adjusted generalized equations to predict body fat from skinfolds or girths in children and in older men and women.*[76,77,180]

For both fatter and leaner white and African American children the following two skinfold equations best predict percentage body fat:[17]

Percentage body fat = 9.02 + 1.09 (biceps, mm) + 0.42 (calf, mm)

Percentage body fat = 8.596 + 0.81 (biceps, mm) + 0.40 (triceps, mm) + 0.30 (subscapular, mm)

User Beware

The person taking skinfold measurements must develop expertise with the proper measurement techniques. Also, with extremely obese people skinfold thickness often exceeds the width of the caliper's jaws. The particular caliper used also contributes to measurement errors.[58] It often becomes difficult to determine which prediction equation to use because of

TABLE 13.5	Changes in Selected Skinfolds for a Young Woman during a 16-Week Exercise Program			
Skinfolds	**Before (mm)**	**After (mm)**	**Absolute Change (mm)**	**Percentage Change**
Triceps	22.5	19.4	−3.1	−13.8
Subscapular	19.0	17.0	−2.0	−10.5
Suprailiac	34.5	30.2	−4.3	−12.8
Abdomen	33.7	29.4	−4.3	−12.8
Thigh	21.6	18.7	−2.9	−13.4
Sum	**131.3**	**114.7**	**−16.6**	**−12.6**

TABLE 13.6 Body Composition Prediction Equations for Use With Athletes

Method	Sport	Gender	Equation
Skinfolds	All	Women (18–29 y)	$Db (g \cdot cc^{-1})^a = 1.096095 - 0.0006952$ (4 SKF) $+ 0.0000011$ (4 SKF)^2 $- 0.0000714$ (age)
	All	Boys (14–19 y)	$Db (g \cdot cc^{-1})^a = 1.10647 - 0.00162$ (subscapular SKF) $- 0.00144$ (abdomen SKF) 0.00077 (triceps SKF) $+ 0.00071$ (midaxillary SKF)
	All	Men (18–29 y)	$Db (g \cdot cc^{-1})^a = 1.112 - 0.00043499$ (7 SKF) $+ 0.00000055$ (7 SKF)^2 $- 0.00028826$ (age)
	Wrestling	Boys (high school)	$Db (g \cdot cc^{-1})^a = 1.0982 - 0.000815$ (3 SKF) $- 0.00000084$ (3 SKF)^2
BIA	All	Women (NR)	FFM (kg) $= 0.73$ (HT^2/R) $+ 0.23$ (X_c) $+ 0.16$ (BW) $+ 2.0$
	All	Women (college)	FFM (kg) $= 0.73$ (HT^2/R) $+ 0.116$ (BW) $+ 0.096$ (X_c) $- 4.03$
	All	Men (college)	FFM (kg) $= 0.734$ (HT^2/R) $+ 0.116$ (BW) $+ 0.096$ (X_c) $- 3.152$
	All	Men (19–40 y)	FFM (kg) $= 1.949 + 0.701$ (BW) $+ 0.186$ (HT^2/R)
	All	Women (18–23 y)	FFM (kg) $= 0.757$ (BW) $+ 0.981$ (neck C) $- 0.516$ (thigh C) $+ 0.79$
Anthropometry (girths)	Ballet	Girls/women (11–25 y)	FFM (kg) $= 0.73$ (BW) $+ 3.0$
	Wrestling	Boys (13–18 y)	$Db (g \cdot cc^{-1})^a = 1.12691 - 0.00357$ (arm C) $- 0.00127$ (AB C) $+ 0.00524$ (forearm C)
	Football	White men (18–23 y)	%BF $= 55.2 + 0.481$ (BW) $- 0.468$ (HT)

From Heyward VH, Stolarczyk LM. *Applied body composition assessment.* Champaign, IL: Human Kinetics, 1996.

Abbreviations: 4SKF (mm) = sum of four skinfolds: triceps + anterior suprailiac + abdomen + thigh; 7SKF (mm) = sum of seven skinfolds: chest + midaxillary + triceps + subscapular + abdomen + anterior suprailiac + thigh; HT, height (cm); R, resistance (Ω); Xc, reactance (Ω); BW, body weight (kg); C, circumference (cm); thigh C (cm) at the gluteal fold; AB C (cm), average abdominal circumference = [(AB$_1$ + AB$_2$)/2], where AB$_1$ (cm) = abdominal circumference anteriorly midway between the xiphoid process of the sternum and the umbilicus and laterally between the lower end of the rib cage and iliac crests, and AB$_2$ (cm) = abdominal circumference at the umbilicus level.

^{a}Use the following formulas to convert body density (Db) to %body fat (BF): men %BF = [(4.95/Db) − 4.50] × 100, women %BF = [(5.01/Db) − 4.57] × 100, boys (7–12 y) %BF = [(5.30/Db) − 4.89] × 100, boys (13–16 y) %BF = [(5.07/Db) − 4.64] × 100, boys (17–19 y) %BF = [(4.99/Db) − 4.55] × 100.

lack of standards to judge the results of different investigators. A prediction equation developed by one researcher (that shows high validity for the sample measured) may produce large prediction errors when applied to skinfolds from a dissimilar group.

GIRTH MEASUREMENTS

Apply a linen or plastic measuring tape lightly to the skin surface so the tape remains taut but not tight. This avoids skin compression that produces lower than normal scores. Make duplicate measurements at each site and average the scores. FIGURE 13.10 displays common anatomic landmarks for taking girths for anthropometric measurement and to predict body fatness.

Usefulness of Girth Measurements

The equations and constants presented in Appendix D for young and older men and women predict an individual's body fat within ±2.5 to 4.0% of the value from hydrostatic

weighing, provided the person resembles the original validation group. Such relatively small prediction errors make the equations particularly useful to those without access to laboratory facilities. Do not use the equations to predict fatness in individuals who appear excessively thin or fat or who participate regularly in strenuous sports or resistance training. Along with predicting percentage body fat, girths can analyze patterns of body fat distribution, including changes in fat distribution during weight loss.[83] Specific equations based on girths also accurately estimate the body composition of obese adults.[179,198] Not surprisingly, equations that use the more labile sites of fat deposition (e.g., waist and hips instead of upper arm or thigh in females and abdomen in males) provide the greatest accuracy for predicting *changes* in body composition.[54]

Predicting Body Fat from Girths

From the appropriate tables in Appendix D, substitute the corresponding constants A, B, and C in the formula shown at the bottom of each table. This requires one addition and two

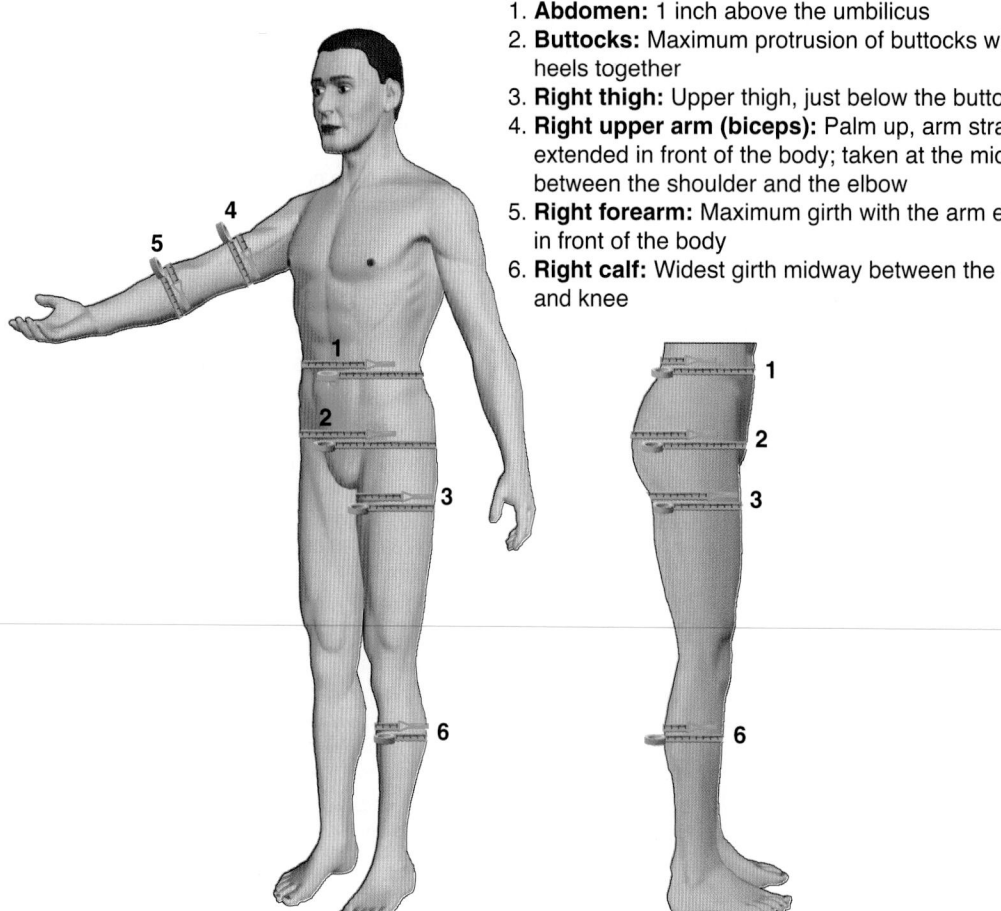

1. **Abdomen:** 1 inch above the umbilicus
2. **Buttocks:** Maximum protrusion of buttocks with the heels together
3. **Right thigh:** Upper thigh, just below the buttocks
4. **Right upper arm (biceps):** Palm up, arm straight and extended in front of the body; taken at the midpoint between the shoulder and the elbow
5. **Right forearm:** Maximum girth with the arm extended in front of the body
6. **Right calf:** Widest girth midway between the ankle and knee

FIGURE 13.10 ■ Landmarks for measuring various girths at six common anatomic sites (see text for descriptions).

subtraction steps. The following five-step example shows how to compute percentage body fat, fat mass, and FFM for a 21-year-old man who weighs 79.1 kg:

Step 1. Measure upper arm, abdomen, and right forearm girths with a cloth tape to the nearest tenth of an inch (0.24 cm): upper arm = 11.5 in (29.2 cm); abdomen = 31.0 in (78.7 cm); right forearm = 10.7 in (27.3 cm).

Step 2. Determine the three constants A, B, and C corresponding to the three girths from Appendix D: constant A corresponds to 11.5 in = 42.56; constant B corresponds to 31.0 in = 40.68; constant C corresponds to 10.7 in = 58.37.

Step 3. Compute percentage body fat by substituting the appropriate constants in the formula for young men shown at the bottom of Chart 1 in Appendix D.

$$\text{Percentage fat} = \text{Constant A} + \text{Constant B}$$
$$- \text{Constant C} - 10.2$$
$$= 42.56 + 40.68 - 58.37 - 10.2$$
$$= 83.24 - 58.37 - 10.2$$
$$= 24.87 - 10.2$$
$$= 14.7\%$$

Step 4. Calculate the mass of body fat as follows:

$$\text{Fat mass} = \text{Body mass} \times (\% \text{ fat} \div 100)$$
$$= 79.1 \text{ kg} \times (14.7 \div 100)$$
$$= 79.1 \text{ kg} \times 0.147$$
$$= 11.63 \text{ kg}$$

Step 5. Calculate FFM as follows:

$$\text{FFM} = \text{Body mass} - \text{Fat mass}$$
$$= 79.1 \text{ kg} - 11.63 \text{ kg}$$
$$= 67.5 \text{ kg}$$

Case Study

Personal Health and Exercise Nutrition 13–2

Predicting Percentage Body Fat of Hispanics

Despite the fact that Hispanics represent the second largest minority population in the United States, little validated research exists on body composition prediction equations for this group. The available research suggests the density of the fat-free body mass of Hispanic women differs from their white counterparts.

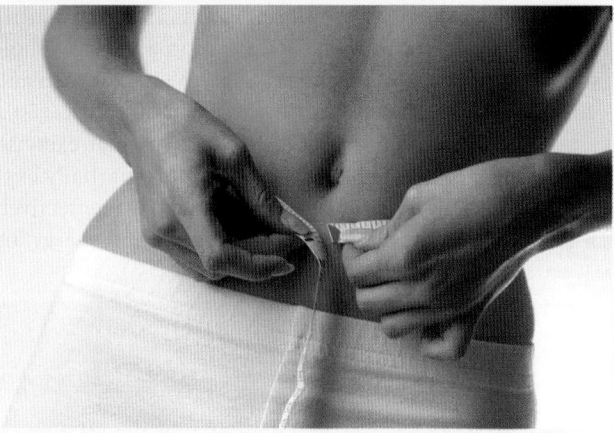

Variables

The generalized skinfold equations of Jackson and colleagues[76,77] have been used successfully with Hispanic men and women. The seven skinfold measurements for men and women include the five skinfold sites listed in FIGURE 13.9, page 413. For both males and females the chest skinfold is the diagonal fold, midway between the upper armpit and the nipple. The midaxillary skinfold is the horizontal fold directly below the armpit.

1. Abdomen
2. Thigh
3. Triceps
4. Subscapular
5. Suprailiac
6. Midaxillary
7. Chest

Equations

For both men and women: Db = body density in $g \cdot cm^{-3}$; $\Sigma 7SKF$ comprise chest + abdomen + thigh + triceps + subscapular + suprailiac + midaxillary skinfolds in mm.

Men (ages 18–61 years):

$$Db = 1.112 - [0.00043499 \times \Sigma 7SKF] + [0.00000055 \times (\Sigma 7SKF)^2] - [0.00028826 \times age]$$

To convert Db to %BF:

$$\%BF = 495 \div Db - 450$$

Women (ages 18–55 years):

$$Db = 1.0970 - [0.00046971 \times \Sigma 7SKF] + [0.00000056 \times (\Sigma 7SKF)^2] - [0.00012828 \times age]$$

To convert Db to %BF:

$$\%BF = 487 \div Db - 441$$

Examples

Example 1: Hispanic male, age 24 years

Skinfold data: chest = 15.0 mm; abdomen = 33.0 mm; thigh = 21.0 mm; triceps = 18 mm; subscapular = 19 mm; suprailiac = 30 mm; midaxillary = 12.0 mm

$$
\begin{aligned}
Db &= 1.112 - [0.00043499 \times \Sigma 7SKF] + \\
&\quad [0.00000055 \times (\Sigma 7SKF)^2] - [0.00028826 \times \\
&\quad age] \\
&= 1.112 - [0.00043499 \times 148] + [0.00000055 \\
&\quad \times 21904] - [0.00028826 \times 24] \\
&= 1.112 - 0.064378 + 0.012047 - 0.0069182 \\
&= 1.0528 \ g \cdot cm^{-3}
\end{aligned}
$$

$$
\begin{aligned}
\%BF &= 495 \div Db - 450 \\
&= 495 \div 1.0528 - 450 \\
&= 20.2
\end{aligned}
$$

Example 2: Hispanic female, age 30 years

Skinfold data: chest = 12.0 mm; abdomen = 30.0 mm; thigh = 18.0 mm; triceps = 20.0 mm; subscapular = 16.0 mm; suprailiac = 30 mm; midaxillary = 15.0 mm

$$
\begin{aligned}
Db &= 1.0970 - [0.00046971 \times \Sigma 7SKF] + \\
&\quad [0.00000056 \times (\Sigma 7SKF)^2] - [0.00012828 \times \\
&\quad age] \\
&= 1.0970 - [0.00046971 \times 141 + [0.00000056 \times \\
&\quad 19881] - [0.00012828 \times 30] \\
&= 1.0970 - 0.066229 + 0.011133 - 0.003848 \\
&= 1.0381 \ g \cdot cm^{-3}
\end{aligned}
$$

$$
\begin{aligned}
\%BF &= 487 \div Db - 441 \\
&= 487 \div 1.0381 - 441 \\
&= 28.2
\end{aligned}
$$

REGIONAL FAT DISTRIBUTION: WAIST GIRTH AND WAIST/HIP RATIO

Measures of waist girth and the ratio of waist girth to hip girth provide an important indication of disease risk.[65,132,161] FIGURE 13.11 shows two types of regional fat distribution. The increased health risk from fat deposition in the abdominal area (central or android-type obesity), particularly internal visceral deposits, may result from this tissue's active lipolysis with catecholamine stimulation. Fat stored in this region shows greater metabolic responsiveness than fat in the gluteal and femoral regions (peripheral or gynoid-type obesity). Increases in central fat more readily support processes that cause heart disease.

Over a broad range of BMI values, men and women with high waist circumference values possess greater relative risk for cardiovascular disease, type 2 diabetes, gallstones, cancer, and cataracts, the leading cause of blindness worldwide, than individuals with small waist circumference or with peripheral obesity.[81,152,182]

For men, the percentage of visceral fat increases progressively with age, whereas this fat deposition in women begins to increase at menopause onset. The waist/hip ratio poorly captures the specific effects of each girth measure. Waist and hip circumferences reflect different aspects of body composition and fat distribution. Each has an independent and often opposite effect on cardiovascular disease risk. Waist girth, the so-called malignant form of obesity that reflects central fat deposition, provides a reasonable indication of the accumulation of intra-abdominal (visceral) adipose tissue. This currently makes waist girth the trunk measure of clinical choice to evaluate health risks associated with obesity[65,132,161] when more precise assessments are impractical.[170]

TABLE 13.7 presents classification guidelines and associated disease risk for overweight and obesity based on BMI or waist girth. Men with a 102-cm (40 in) or larger waist and women with waist girth larger than 86 cm (35 in) maintain a high risk

for various diseases. Waist girths of 90 cm (35.4 in) for men and 83 cm (32.7 in) for women correspond to a BMI threshold of overweight (BMI, ≥25) while 100 cm (39 in) for men and 93 cm (37 in) for women reflect the obesity cutoff (BMI, ≥30).[212]

Documentation of a strong effect of regular exercise on reducing waist girth selectively in men may partially explain why physical activity reduces disease risk more effectively in men than in women. Both physical activity and energy intake

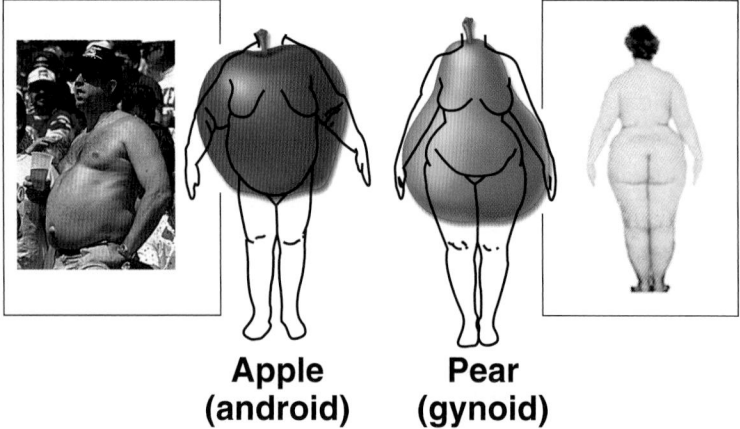

Waist-to-Hip Ratio

- Waist at navel while standing relaxed, not pulling in stomach
- Hips (largest girth around buttocks)
- Divide waist girth by hip girth

Ratio for significant health risk
Males: ≥0.95
Females: ≥0.80

Apple (android)   **Pear (gynoid)**

FIGURE 13.11 ■ Male (android pattern) and female (gynoid pattern) fat patterning, including waist-to-hip girth ratio threshold for significant health risk.

TABLE 13.7   Classifications of Overweight and Obesity by BMI, Waist Circumference, and Associated Disease Risk

| Classification | BMI, kg·m^{-2} | Disease Risk[a] Relative to Normal Weight and Normal Waist Circumference | |
		Men ≤102 cm Women ≤ 88 cm	Men >102 cm Women > 88 cm
Underweight	<18.5	NR	NR
Normal[b]	18.5–24.9	NR	NR
Overweight	25.0–29.9	Increased	High
Obesity, class			
I	30.0–34.9	High	Very high
II	35.0–39.9	Very high	Very high
III (morbid obesity)	≥40	Extremely high	Extremely high

[a]Disease risk for type 2 diabetes, hypertension, and cardiovascular disease. NR indicates no risk assigned at these BMI levels.

[b]Increased waist circumference can indicate increased risk even in persons of normal weight.

From Executive summary of the clinical guidelines on the identification, evaluation, and treatment of overweight and obesity in adults. Arch Intern Med 1998;158:1855.

A Risky Place to Store Fat

Central excess fat deposition, independent of excess fat storage in other anatomic areas, reflects an altered metabolic profile that increases risk of the following eight conditions:

1. Hyperinsulinemia (insulin resistance)
2. Glucose intolerance
3. Type 2 diabetes
4. Endometrial cancer
5. Hypertriglyceridemia
6. Hypercholesterolemia and negatively altered lipoprotein profile
7. Hypertension
8. Atherosclerosis

Risk Not Limited to Adults

For children and adolescents, central body fat distribution associates with higher blood cholesterol, triacylglycerol, and insulin levels and lower HDL cholesterol in addition to higher blood pressure and increased left ventricular wall thickness.

selectively predict waist-to-hip ratio in men but not in women. For men, higher energy intakes and higher energy expenditures associate (independent of BMI) with higher and lower waist/hip ratios, respectively.[181]

BIOLECTRICAL IMPEDANCE ANALYSIS

A small alternating current flowing between two electrodes passes more rapidly through hydrated fat-free body tissues and extracellular water than through fat or bone tissue. This occurs because of the greater electrolyte content (lower electrical resistance) of the fat-free component. Impedance to electric current flow relates to total body water content and in turn relates to FFM and percentage body fat.

With **bioelectrical impedance analysis (BIA),** a person lies on a flat nonconducting surface. Injector (source) elec-

trodes attach on the dorsal surfaces of the foot and wrist, and detector (sink) electrodes attach between the radius and ulna (styloid process) and at the ankle between the medial and lateral malleoli (FIG. 13.12). A painless, localized electric current (about 800 μA at a frequency of 50 kHz) is introduced, and the impedance (resistance) to current flow determined between the source and detector electrodes. Conversion of the impedance value to body density—adding body mass and stature, gender, age, and sometimes race, level of fatness, and several girths to the equation—computes percentage body fat from the Siri equation or another similar density conversion equation.

Influence of Hydration and Ambient Temperature

Hydration level, even small changes that occur with exercise, affects BIA accuracy, and may give inaccurate information about a person's body fat content.[101,135,151] Hypohydration and hyperhydration alter normal electrolyte concentrations, which in turn affect current flow independent of a real change in body composition. For example, a loss of body water through prior exercise sweat loss or voluntary fluid restriction decreases the impedance measure. This *lowers* the estimate of percentage body fat, whereas hyperhydration produces the opposite effect (*higher* fat estimate).

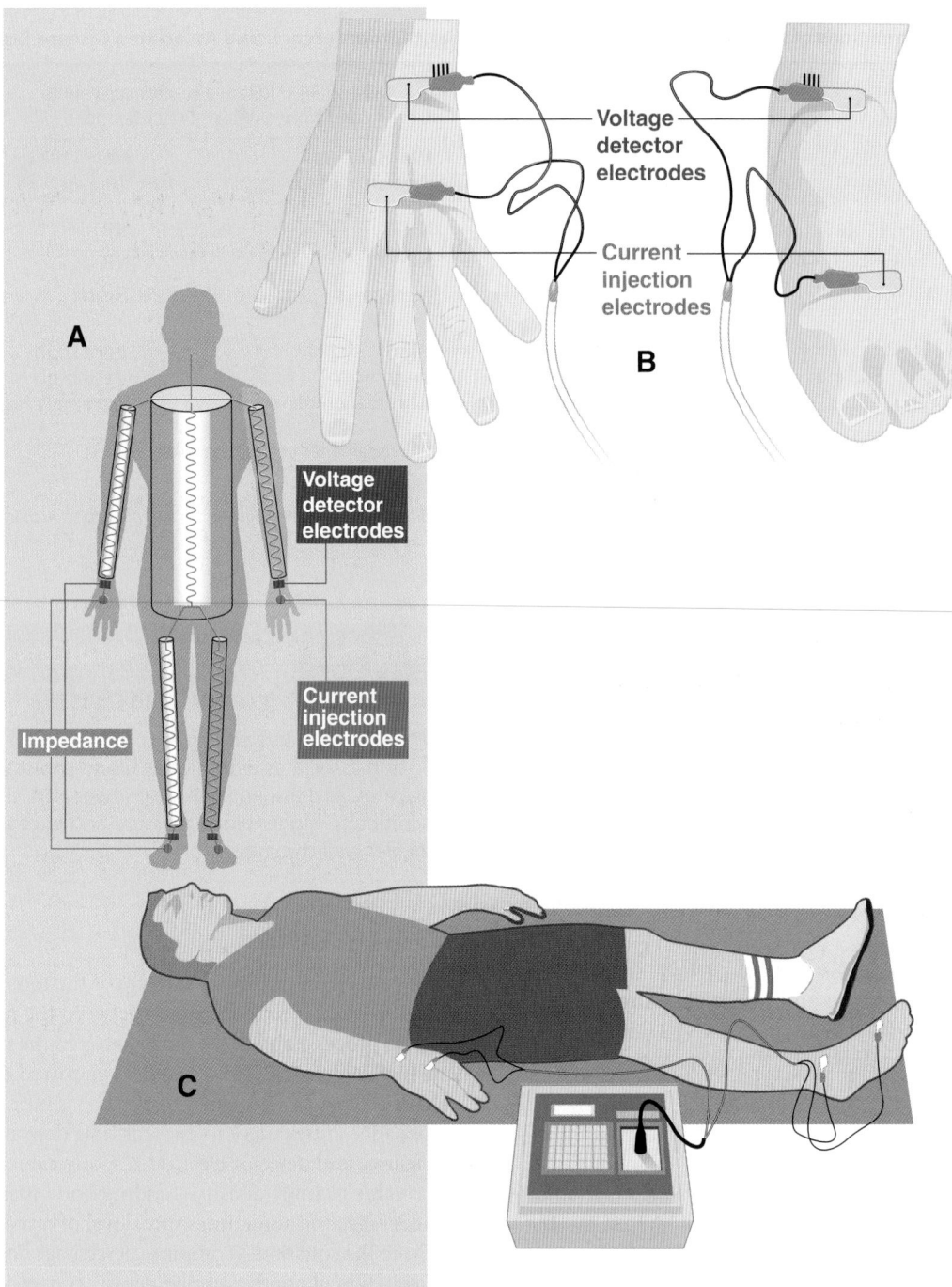

FIGURE 13.12 ■ Body composition assessment by bioelectrical impedance analysis. **A.** Four-surface electrode technique that applies current via one pair of distal (injection) electrodes while the proximal (detector) electrode pair measures electrical potential across the conducting segment. **B.** Standard placement of electrodes. **C.** Proper body position during whole-body impedance measurement.

Skin temperature (influenced by ambient conditions) also affects whole-body resistance and thus the BIA prediction of body fat. A *lower* predicted body fat value occurs in a warm environment (less impedance to electrical flow) than in a cold one.[5,27]

Even with normal hydration and environmental temperature, body fat predictions prove less satisfactory than hydrostatic weighing. BIA tends to *overpredict* body fat in lean and athletic subjects and *underpredict* body fat in obese subjects.[119,159] BIA often predicts body fat less accurately than girths and skinfolds.[18,40,169] Whether BIA can detect small changes in body composition during weight loss is also unclear.[105,134,143,150] In contrast to skinfold and girth measurements, conventional BIA technology cannot assess regional fat distribution.

At best, BIA provides a noninvasive, safe, and relatively easy and reliable means to assess total body water. Proper BIA use requires that experienced personnel make measurements under strictly standardized conditions, particularly those related to electrode placement and subject's body position, hydration status, previous food and beverage intake, skin temperature, and recent physical activity.[13,104,136,195] For example, ingestion of consecutive meals progressively decreases bioelectrical impedance (possibly the combined effect of increased electrolytes and a redistribution of extracellular fluid), which decreases the computed percentage body fat.[167] Level of body fatness and racial characteristics also influence predictive accuracy.[2,172,190,209] Fatness-specific BIA equations exist for obese and nonobese American Indian, Hispanic, and white men and women.[168,169] With proper measurement standardization the menstrual cycle does not affect body composition assessment by BIA.[122]

Applicability of BIA in Sports and Exercise Training

Coaches and athletes need a safe, easily administered, rapid, and valid tool to assess body composition and detect changes with caloric restriction or exercise training. A major limitation in achieving these goals concerns BIA's lack of sensitivity to detect small changes in body composition.[8,129,134,158] For example, sweat-loss dehydration or reduced glycogen reserves (and associated loss of glycogen-bound water) from prior exercise increase body resistance (impedance) to electrical current flow. Increased impedance underestimates FFM and overestimates percentage body fat measured by BIA. The tendency to overestimate body fat becomes more pronounced among black athletes.[68,158]

NEAR-INFRARED INTERACTANCE

Near-infrared interactance (NIR) applies technology developed by the U.S. Department of Agriculture to assess body composition of livestock and lipid content of various grains. The commercial versions to assess body composition in humans use principles of light absorption and reflection. A fiberoptic probe, or light "wand," emits a low-energy beam of near-infrared light into the single measuring site at the anterior midline surface of the biceps of the dominant arm. A detector within the same probe measures the intensity of the re-emitted light, expressed as optical density. Shifts in the wavelength of the reflected beam as it interacts with organic material in the arm added to the manufacturer's prediction equation (often including variables such as subject's body mass and stature, estimated frame size, sex, and physical activity level) rapidly computes percentage body fat and FFM. This safe, portable, and lightweight equipment requires minimal training to use and necessitates little physical contact

with the subject during measurement. These test administration aspects make NIR popular for body composition assessment in health clubs, hospitals, and weight-loss centers. The important question about the usefulness of NIR concerns its validity.

Questionable Validity of Near Infrared Interactance

Early research with animals indicated a significant relationship between spectrophotometric measures of light interactance at various sites on the body and body composition assessed by total body water.[34] Subsequent research with humans did not confirm the validity of NIR when compared to hydrostatic weighing and skinfold measurements. In fact, NIR may be *less accurate* than skinfolds in assessing percentage body fat.[29,63,74,186] It *overestimates* body fat in lean men and women and *underestimates* body fat in fatter subjects.[123]

Research has shown that skinfold measurement more accurately predicted percentage body fat based on hydrostatic weighing than did NIR. In more than 47% of the subjects, an error greater than 4% body fat units occurred with NIR, with the greatest errors at the extremes of body fatness. Furthermore, NIR produced large errors—standard error of estimate and total prediction error—when estimating percentage body fat for children[26] and youth wrestlers.[70] It significantly underestimated body fat in college football players.[69] *Available data do not support NIR as a robust, valid method to assess human body composition.*

COMPUTED TOMOGRAPHY, MAGNETIC RESONANCE IMAGING, AND DUAL-ENERGY X-RAY ABSORPTIOMETRY

Computed tomography (CT) and **magnetic resonance imaging (MRI)** produce images of body segments. With appropriate computer software, the CT scan gives pictorial and quantitative information for the total tissue area, total fat and muscle area, and thickness and volume of tissues within an organ.[57,128,189]

FIGURE 13.13A–C shows CT scans of the upper legs and a cross section at the midthigh in a professional walker who completed an 11,200-mile walk around the 50 United States in 50 weeks. Total cross section of muscle increased significantly, and subcutaneous fat decreased correspondingly in the midthigh region in the "after" scans.

Studies have demonstrated the efficiency of CT scans to evaluate the relationship between simple anthropometric measures (skinfolds and girths) at the abdominal region and total adipose tissue volume measured from single or multiple pictorial "slices" through the abdominal region.[4,160] Surprisingly, almost no relationship existed between "external" (subcutaneous) abdominal fat and "internal" (visceral) abdominal fat depots in men and women.

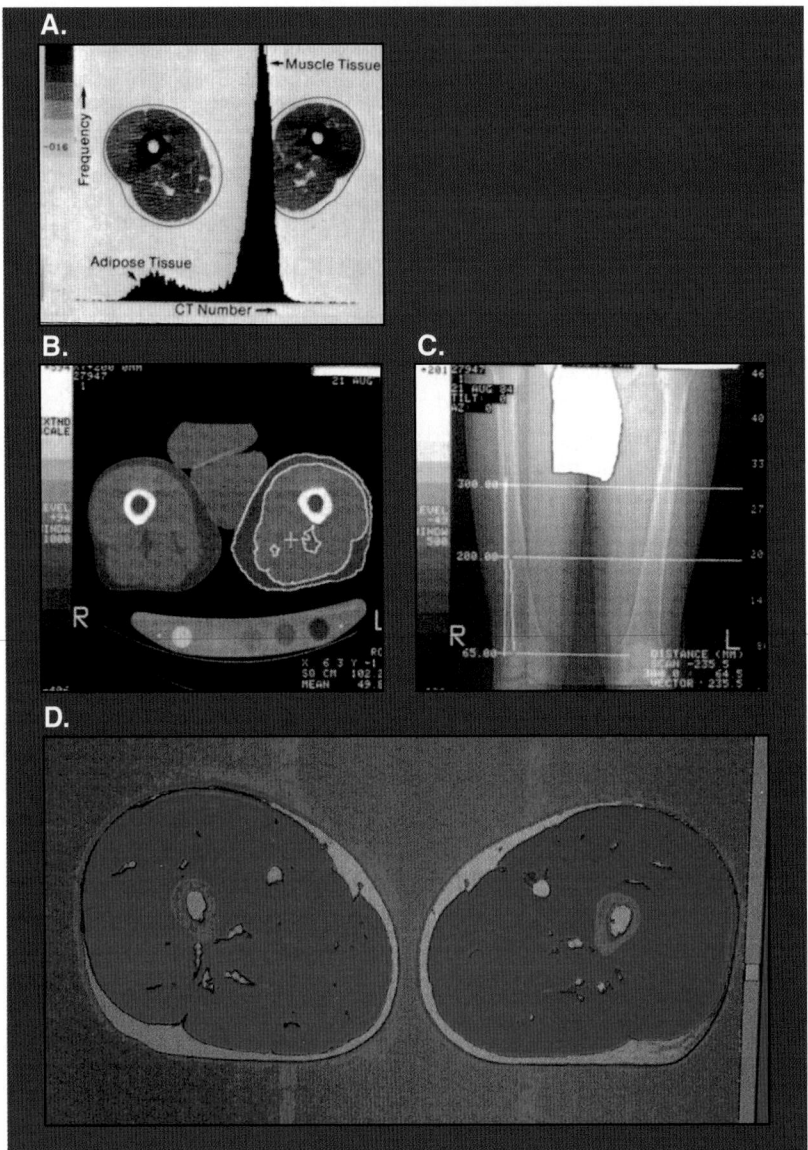

FIGURE 13.13 ■ Computed tomography (CT) and magnetic resonance imaging (MRI) scans. **A.** Plot of pixel elements (CT scan) illustrating the extent of adipose and muscle tissue in a thigh cross-section. The two other views show a cross section of the midthigh **(B)** and an anterior view of the upper leg **(C)** before a 1-year walk across the United States in a champion walker. **D.** MRI scan of the midthigh of a 30-year-old male middle-distance runner. (CT images courtesy of Dr. Steven Heymsfeld, St. Luke's Roosevelt Hospital Center, New York; MRI scan courtesy of J. Staab, Department of the Army, USARIEM, Natick, MA.)

The newer technology of MRI provides a rapid, safe technique to obtain accurate information about the body's tissue compartments.[85,110,174] FIGURE 13.13D displays a color-enhanced MRI transaxial image of the midthigh of a 30-year-old male middle-distance runner. Computer software subtracts fat and bony tissues *(lighter-colored areas)* to compute thigh muscle cross-sectional area *(blue area)*. With MRI, electromagnetic radiation (not ionizing radiation as in CT scans) in a strong magnetic field excites the hydrogen nuclei of the body's water and lipid molecules. The nuclei then project a detectable signal that rearranges under computer control to visually depict the body tissues. MRI effectively quantifies total and subcutaneous adipose tissue in individuals of varying degrees of body fatness. Combined with muscle mass analysis, MRI assesses changes in a muscle's lean and fat components following resistance training or during different stages of growth and aging,[80] including changes in muscle volume following spaceflight.[107]

Dual-energy x-ray absorptiometry (DXA), another high-technology procedure, reliably quantifies fat and nonbone regional lean body mass, including the mineral content of the body's deeper bony structures and muscle mass.[97,114,148,202] It has become the accepted clinical tool to assess spinal osteoporosis and related bone disorders.[21,42] For body composition analysis, DXA does not require the assumptions about the biologic constancy of the fat and fat-free components inherent with hydrostatic weighing.

With DXA, two distinct low-energy x-ray beams (short exposure with low radiation dosage) penetrate bone and soft tissue to a 30-cm depth. An entire DXA scan takes approximately 12 minutes. Computer software reconstructs the attenuated x-ray beams to produce an image of the underlying tissues and quantify bone mineral content, total fat mass, and FFM. Analyses also include selected trunk and limb regions for detailed study of tissue composition and possible relation to disease risk, including the effects of exercise training and detraining.[11,71,90,111,120,205] DXA provides a sensitive noninvasive tool to asses body composition and body composition changes in diverse populations.

BOD POD

A procedure to estimate body volume has been perfected to possibly replace the densitometry technique in groups ranging from infants to the elderly to collegiate wrestlers and exceptionally large athletes like professional football and basketball players.[31,48,121,149,184,211] The method has adapted air displacement plethysmography first reported in the late 1800s and in the 1950s using helium as the gas displaced. The subject sits inside a small chamber (marketed commercially as **BOD POD**, Life Measurement Instruments, Concord, CA). Measurement requires 2 to 5 minutes, and reproducibility of test scores within and across days is high ($r \geq 0.90$).

After being weighed to the nearest 5 g on an electronic scale, the subject sits comfortably in the 750-L volume, dual-chamber fiberglass shell (FIG. 13.14A). The molded front seat separates the unit into front and rear chambers. The electronics, housed in the rear of the chamber, include pressure transducers, breathing circuit, and an air circulation system. To ensure measurement accuracy, the person wears a tight-fitting swimsuit. This suit does not affect measurement reliability or accuracy compared to measurement in the nude.[188] Wearing a hospital gown reduces estimated percentage body fat by about 9% compared with the recommended swim suit.[46,47] Body volume becomes the chamber's initial volume

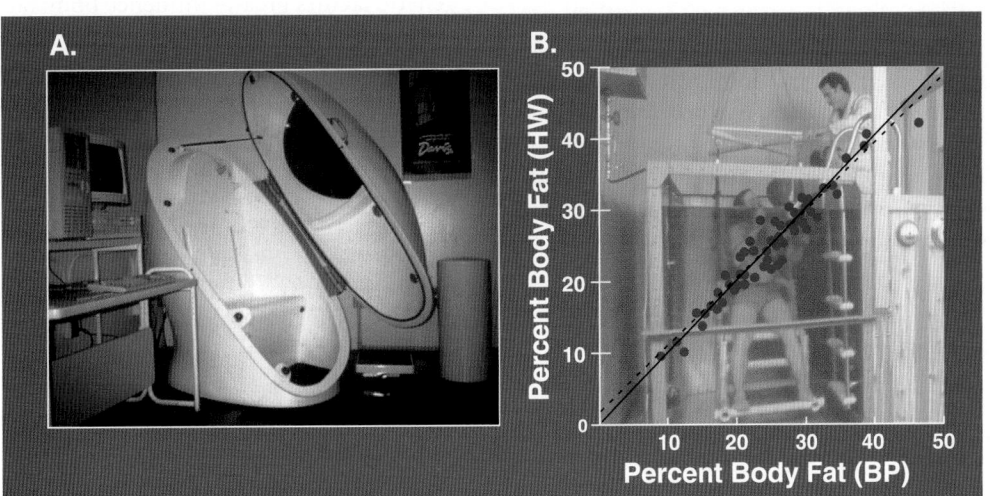

FIGURE 13.14 ■ **A.** BOD POD to measure human body volume. (Photo courtesy of Dr. Megan McCrory, Tufts University, Boston, MA.) **B.** Regression of percentage body fat assessed by hydrostatic weighing *(HW)* versus percentage body fat assessed by BOD POD *(BP)*. (Data from McCrory MA, et al. Evaluation of a new air displacement plethysmograph for measuring human body composition. *Med Sci Sports Exerc* 1995;27:1686)

minus the reduced chamber volume with the subject inside. The subject breathes into an air circuit for several breaths to assess thoracic gas volume, which when subtracted from measured body volume yields actual body volume. Body density computes as body mass (measured in air) ÷ body volume (measured in BOD POD). The Siri equation converts body density to percentage body fat. Figure 13.14B shows the relationship between percentage body fat assessed by hydrostatic weighing (HW) versus percentage body fat by BOD POD (BP). The subject pool comprised 42 men and 26 women ages 21 to 56 years who differed in ethnicity (47 non-Hispanic white, 10 Hispanic, 7 African American, 4 Asian American), body mass (52–129 kg), and stature (145–191 cm). A difference of only 0.3% (0.2% fat units) occurred between body fat determined by hydrostatic weighing and BOD POD; the validity correlation was r = 0.96 between the two methods. Other studies report similar results.[112,126]

ESTIMATING BODY FAT AMONG ATHLETIC GROUPS

Accurate body composition assessment enhances precision in determining a competitor's appropriate body weight for sports with specific weight classifications or that emphasize a "required" physical appearance. Valid body composition appraisal also provides an important first step for *identifying* potential eating disorders and *formulating* and *assessing* nutritional counseling.

Skinfolds and girth measurements and BIA have estimated body density and percentage body fat for diverse groups of athletes. Table 13.6 presented (1) generalized equations using these methods applied to athletes in all sports, and (2) sport-specific equations for ballet dancers, wrestlers, and football players. Additional equations for wrestlers and high school female gymnasts appear in Chapter 14. When sport-specific equations are unavailable, population-based generalized equations (accounting for age and sex) provide an acceptable alternative to estimate body fat.[29,68,76,137,166,176] The third skinfold equation in Table 13.6 estimates the body composition of adult male athletes; the second equation pertains to adolescent males, while the first equation has been recommended for adult and teenage female athletes.

AVERAGE VALUES FOR BODY COMPOSITION IN THE GENERAL POPULATION

TABLE 13.8 lists average values for percentage body fat in samples of men and women throughout the United States. Values representing ±1 standard deviation provide some indication of the variation or spread from the average; the column headed "68% Variation Limits" indicates the range for percentage body fat that includes one standard deviation, or

about 68 of every 100 persons measured. As an example, the average percentage body fat of 15.0% for young men from the New York sample includes the 68% variation limits ranging between 8.9 and 21.1% fat. Interpreting this statistically, for 68 of every 100 young men measured, percentage fat ranges between 8.9 and 21.1%. Of the remaining 32 young men, 16 possess more than 21.1% body fat, while 16 others have a body fat percentage below 8.9. *Percentage body fat for young adult men averages between 12 and 15%; the average fat value for women falls between 25 and 28%.* For comparative purposes, see the inset tables in Figure 13.16 on page 431 for percentage body fat values for various groups of male and female athletes.

Percentage body fat usually increases in adult men and women as they age. Individuals who maintain a vigorous physical activity profile throughout life slow the "average" or "normal" age-related fat accretion. Age-related body composition changes could occur because the aging skeleton becomes demineralized and porous, reducing body density because of decreased bone density. In contrast, regular physical activity maintains or increases bone mass while preserving muscle mass. Reduced physical activity provides another reason for the relative increase in body fat with age. A sedentary lifestyle increases storage fat and reduces muscle mass, even if the daily caloric intake remains essentially unchanged.

DETERMINING GOAL BODY WEIGHT

Excess body fat detracts from good health, physical fitness, and athletic performance. No one really knows the optimum body fat or body mass for a particular individual. Inherited genetic factors greatly influence body fat distribution and certainly affect the long-term programming of body size.[14,15] Women and men who exercise regularly have lower percentage body fat values than the population average. In contact sports and activities requiring muscular power, successful performance usually requires a large body mass with minimal body fat. In contrast, success in weight-bearing endurance activities requires a lighter body mass and less body fat. For these individuals, attaining a low body weight must not compromise lean tissue mass and energy reserves. *Proper assessment of body composition, not body weight, determines a physically active person's ideal body weight. For athletes, this **goal body weight** must coincide with optimizing sport-specific measures of physiologic function and exercise capacity.*

Suppose a 120-kg (265-lb) shot-put athlete, with 24% body fat, wishes to know how much fat weight to lose to attain a body fat composition of 15%. Compute a goal body weight based on the desired body fat level as follows:

Goal body weight = Fat-free body mass ÷ (1.00 − % fat desired)

TABLE 13.8 Average Values of Percentage Body Fat for Younger and Older Women and Men from Selected Studies

Study	Age Range, y	Stature, cm	Mass, kg	% Fat	68% Variation Limits
Younger women					
North Carolina, 1962	17–25	165.0	55.5	22.9	17.5–28.5
New York, 1962	16–30	167.5	59.0	28.7	24.6–32.9
California, 1968	19–23	165.9	58.4	21.9	17.0–26.9
California, 1970	17–29	164.9	58.6	25.5	21.0–30.1
Air Force, 1972	17–22	164.1	55.8	28.7	22.3–35.3
New York, 1973	17–26	160.4	59.0	26.2	23.4–33.3
North Carolina, 1975	—	166.1	57.5	24.6	—
Army Recruits, 1986	17–25	162.0	58.6	28.4	23.9–32.9
Massachusetts, 1998	17–31	165.2	57.8	21.8	16.7–27.9
Older women					
Minnesota, 1953	31–45	163.3	60.7	28.9	25.1–32.8
	43–68	160.0	60.9	34.2	28.0–40.5
New York, 1963	30–40	164.9	59.6	28.6	22.1–35.3
	40–50	163.1	56.4	34.4	29.5–39.5
North Carolina, 1975	33–50	—	—	29.7	23.1–36.5
Massachusetts, 1993	31–50	165.2	58.9	25.2	19.2–31.2
Younger men					
Minnesota, 1951	17–26	177.8	69.1	11.8	5.9–11.8
Colorado, 1956	17–25	172.4	68.3	13.5	8.3–18.8
Indiana, 1966	18–23	180.1	75.5	12.6	8.7–16.5
California, 1968	16–31	175.7	74.1	15.2	6.3–24.2
New York, 1973	17–26	176.4	71.4	15.0	8.9–21.1
Texas, 1977	18–24	179.9	74.6	13.4	7.4–19.4
Army recruits, 1986	17–25	174.7	70.5	15.6	10.0–21.2
Massachusetts, 1998	17–31	178.1	76.4	12.9	7.8–19.0
Older men					
Indiana, 1966	24–38	179.0	76.6	17.8	11.3–24.3
	40–48	177.0	80.5	22.3	16.3–28.3
North Carolina, 1976	27–50	—	—	23.7	17.9–30.1
Texas, 1977	27–59	180.0	85.3	27.1	23.7–30.5
Massachusetts, 1993	31–50	177.1	77.5	19.9	13.2–26.5

Fat mass

$$= 120 \text{ kg} \times 0.24$$
$$= 28.8 \text{ kg}$$

Fat-free body mass

$$= 120 \text{ kg} - 28.8 \text{ kg}$$
$$= 91.2 \text{ kg}$$

Goal body weight

$$= 91.2 \text{ kg} \div (1.00 - 0.15)$$
$$= 91.2 \text{ kg} \div 0.85$$
$$= 107.3 \text{ kg} (236.6 \text{ lb})$$

Desirable fat loss = Present body weight − Goal body weight

$$= 120 \text{ kg} - 107.3 \text{ kg}$$
$$= 12.7 \text{ kg} (28.0 \text{ lb})$$

If this athlete reduced 12.7 kg of body fat, his new body weight of 91.2 kg would contain fat equal to 15% of body mass. These calculations assume no change in FFM during weight loss. Moderate caloric restriction plus increased daily energy expenditure through regular exercise induce fat loss and conserve lean tissue. Chapter 14 discusses prudent yet effective approaches to lose body fat.

Summary

1. Standard weight-for-height tables reveal little about an individual's body composition. Studies of athletes clearly show that overweight does not coincide with excessive body fat.

2. Body mass index (BMI) relates more closely to body fat and health risk than simply body mass and stature. BMI fails to consider the body's proportional composition.

3. For the first time in the United States, overweight persons (BMI 25–29) outnumber individuals of desirable weight.

4. Total body fat consists of essential fat and storage fat. Essential fat contains fat present in bone marrow, nerve tissue, and organs; it is not a labile energy reserve, but instead an important component for normal biologic functions. Storage fat represents the energy reserve that accumulates mainly as adipose tissue beneath the skin and in visceral depots.

5. Storage fat averages 12% of body mass for men and 15% body mass for women. Essential fat averages 3% body mass for men and 12% for women. The greater essential fat for women probably relates to childbearing and hormonal functions.

6. A sumo wrestler has the largest fat-free body mass (FFM) reported in the literature (121.3 kg); this value most likely represents the upper limit for male athletes. Estimates place the upper limit for FFM for athletic women at 80 kg (176 lb).

7. Menstrual dysfunction often occurs in athletes who train hard and maintain low body fat levels. The precise interaction among the physiologic and psychologic stress of intense training and competition, hormonal balance, energy and nutrient intake, and body fat remains unknown.

8. The most popular indirect methods to assess body composition include hydrostatic weighing and prediction methods based on skinfolds and girths. Hydrostatic weighing determines body density with subsequent estimation of percentage body fat. Subtracting fat mass from body mass yields FFM.

9. Part of the error inherent in predicting body fat from whole-body density lies in the correctness of assumptions concerning the densities of the body's fat and fat-free components. These densities differ from assumed constants because of race, age, and athletic experience.

10. Common body composition assessments use prediction equations from relationships among selected skinfolds and girths and body density and percentage fat. These equations show population specificity because they most accurately predict body fat with subjects similar to those who participated in the equations' original derivation.

11. Hydrated fat-free body tissues and extracellular water facilitate electrical flow compared with fat tissue, because of the greater electrolyte content of the fat-free component. Bioelectrical impedance analysis (BIA) applies this fact to assess body composition.

12. Near infrared interactance should be used with caution to assess body composition because this methodology lacks verification of adequate validity.

13. Computed tomography (CT), magnetic resonance imaging (MRI), and dual-energy x-ray absorptiometry (DXA) indirectly assess body composition. Each has a unique application and special limitations for expanding knowledge of the compositional components of the live human body and its changes with regular exercise training.

14. The BOD POD air displacement method offers promise for body composition assessment because of the high reliability of body volume scores and relatively high validity.

15. Data from healthy young adults indicate that the average male possesses approximately 15% body fat and women about 25%. These values often provide a frame of reference for evaluating the body fat of individual athletes and specific athletic groups.

16. Goal body weight computes as FFM ÷ (1.00 − desired % body fat.)

Physique of Champion Athletes

Body composition differs considerably between athletes and nonathletes. Pronounced differences in physique also exist among sports participants of the same sex, including Olympic competitors, track and field specialists, wrestlers, football players, and highly proficient adolescent competitors. We now take a closer look at the physiques of elite athletes by sport category and competition level. Research may eventually discern the degree that body size and composition contribute to (and are prerequisite for) elite performance in specific sports.

THE ELITE ATHLETE

Different anthropometric methodologies have quantified physique status. Visual appraisal often describes individuals as small, medium, or large or thin (ectomorphic), muscular (mesomorphic), or fat (endomorphic). This approach termed *somatotyping* describes body shape by placing a person into a category such as thin or muscular. Visual appraisal does not quantify body dimensions such as size of the chest or shoulders, or how biceps development compares with that of the thighs or calves. Somatotyping has provided a valuable adjunct in the analysis of physique status of world-class athletes.[25,38] The remainder of this chapter focuses on body fat and FFM components of body composition.

Olympic and Elite Athletes

Early studies of Olympic competitors revealed that physique related to a high level of sports achievement.[36,98] TABLES 13.9 AND 13.10 list the anthropometric characteristics of male and female competitors in the 1964 Tokyo and 1968 Mexico City Olympics.[38,66] TABLE 13.11 lists anthropometric data (body mass, stature, and eight skinfolds) for male and female swimmers, divers, and water polo athletes at the 1992 Sixth World Championships in Australia.

Also of interest are the body size differences among different groups of athletes within a particular sport. FIGURE 13.15 *(top)* compares the body mass, stature, chest girth, and upper- and lower-limb lengths for 12 male swimmers rated "best" in the 200 + 400-m free-style with measures of less successful counterparts. The bottom of the figure also compares selected body size variables between the "best" 50, 100, 200-m breaststroke female swimmers and other swimmers. The best male swimmers are heavier and taller and have larger chest, upper-arm, and thigh girths and upper- and lower-limb lengths than counterparts not ranking among the top 12. The best female breaststroke swimmers are taller and heavier, but also possess larger arm spans, foot and arm lengths, and hand and wrist breadth than less successful competitors.

Gender Differences

Table 13.9 reveals that male basketball players, rowers, and weight-throwers were tallest and heaviest; they also possessed the largest FFM and percentage body fat. For example, weight-throwers in both Olympiads averaged 30% body fat, whereas 94 marathon and 133 long-distance runners averaged an exceptionally low 1.6% body fat. The largest body composition discrepancy within a particular sports category emerged in comparisons of the Tokyo wrestlers (12.7% body fat) and wrestlers in Mexico City (1.2% body fat). Age, stature, and FFM were similar in both groups, making this difference even more remarkable.

The most striking physical characteristic of female Olympians (Table 13.10) is their relatively low body fat. Except for the weight-throwers (about 31% body fat), competitors in the other sports groups approximated the 13.1% average body fat for all 676 female participants in both Olympiads.

TABLE 13.9	Age, Body Size, and Body Composition of Male Athletes in Selected Events Who Competed in the Tokyo and Mexico City Olympics							
Specialty	Event	Olympics	N	Age (y)	Stature (cm)	Mass (kg)	LBM[a] (kg)	Body fat[b] (%)
Sprint	100–200 m; 4 × 100 m; 110–m hurdles	Tokyo	172	24.9	178.4	72.2	64.9	10.1
		Mexico City	79	23.9	175.4	68.4	62.8	8.2
Long-distance running	3000, 5000, 10,000 m	Tokyo	99	27.3	173.6	62.4	61.5	1.4
		Mexico City	34	25.3	171.9	59.8	60.1	20.5
Marathon	42.2 km	Tokyo	74	28.3	170.3	60.8	59.2	2.7
Decathlon		Tokyo	26	26.3	183.2	83.5	68.5	18.0
		Mexico City	8	25.1	181.3	77.5	67.1	13.4
Jump	High, long, triple jump	Tokyo	89	25.3	181.5	73.2	67.2	8.2
		Mexico City	14	23.5	182.8	73.2	68.2	6.8
Weight	Shot, discus, hammer throwing	Tokyo	79	27.6	187.3	101.4	71.6	29.4
		Mexico City	9	27.3	186.1	102.3	70.7	30.9
Swimming	Free, breast, back, butterfly, medley	Tokyo	450	20.4	178.7	74.1	65.1	12.1
		Mexico City	66	19.2	179.3	72.1	65.6	9.0
Basketball		Tokyo	186	25.3	189.4	84.3	73.2	13.2
		Mexico City	63	24.0	189.1	79.7	73.0	8.4
Gymnastics	All events	Tokyo	122	26.0	167.2	63.3	57.0	9.9
		Mexico City	28	23.6	167.4	61.5	57.2	7.0
Wrestling	Bantam, featherweight	Tokyo	29	27.3	163.3	62.3	54.4	12.7
		Mexico City	32	22.5	166.1	57.0	56.3	1.2
Rowing	Single, double skulls; pairs, fours, eights	Tokyo	357	25.0	186.0	82.2	70.6	14.1
		Mexico City	85	24.3	185.1	82.6	69.9	15.4

Adapted from De Garay, et al. Genetic and anthropological studies of Olympic athletes. New York: Academic Press, 1974, and Hirata K. Physique and age of Tokyo Olympic champions. J Sports Med Phys Fitness 1966;6:207.

[a]*Calculated by Behnke's method: LBM = h × 0.204, where h = stature, dm (see ref. 9)*

[b]*Body fat (%) = (Body mass − LBM) ÷ Body mass × 100*

TABLE 13.10 **Age, Body Size, and Body Composition of Female Athletes Who Competed in the Tokyo and Mexico City Olympics in Selected Events**

Specialty	Event	Olympics	N	Age (y)	Stature (cm)	Mass (kg)	LBM[a] (kg)	Body fat[b] (%)
Sprint	100–200 m; 100-m hurdles	Tokyo	85	22.7	166.0	56.6	49.2	12.4
		Mexico City	28	20.7	165.0	56.8	49.0	13.7
Jump	High, long, triple jump	Tokyo	56	23.6	169.5	60.2	51.7	14.1
		Mexico City	12	21.5	169.4	56.4	51.7	8.4
Weight	Shot, discus, hammer throwing	Tokyo	37	26.2	170.4	79.0	52.3	33.8
		Mexico City	9	19.9	170.9	73.5	52.5	28.5
Swimming	Free, breast, back, butterfly, medley	Tokyo	272	18.6	166.3	59.7	49.8	16.6
		Mexico City	28	16.3	164.4	56.9	48.6	14.5
Diving	Spring, high	Tokyo	65	18.5	160.9	54.1	46.6	13.9
		Mexico City	7	21.1	160.4	52.3	46.3	11.5
Gymnastics	All events	Tokyo	102	22.7	157.0	52.0	44.4	14.7
		Mexico City	21	17.8	156.9	49.8	44.3	11.0

Adapted from De Garay, et al. Genetic and anthropological studies of Olympic athletes. New York: Academic Press, 1974, and Hirata K. Physique and age of Tokyo Olympic champions. J Sports Med Phys Fitness 1966;6:207.

[a] *Calculated by Behnke's method: LBM (lean body mass) = $h^2 \times 0.18$, where h = stature, dm (see ref. 9)*

[b] *Body fat (%) = (Body mass − LBM ÷ Body mass × 100)*

For aquatic athletes (Table 13.11), skinfolds at most sites were larger in females than in males. Prior studies established a relationship between certain aspects of body composition and swimming performance. A swimmer's morphology influences the horizontal components of lift and drag. Selected anthropometric variables play important roles in propulsive and resistive forces acting on the swimmer that affect forward movement. The combined influence of stroke length and stroke frequency on swimming velocity also relates to a swimmer's overall body size and shape. In well-trained freestyle swimmers, arm length, leg length, and hand and foot size—factors governed largely by genetics—influence stroke length and stroke frequency.

TABLE 13.12 presents additional anthropometric comparisons between male and female Olympians in five different sports (including swimming) at the 1976 Montreal Summer Olympics.

RATIO OF FAT-FREE BODY MASS TO FAT MASS. FIGURE 13.16 compares the ratios of FFM to fat mass (FFM/FM) derived from data in the world literature among male and female competitors. The inset tables present their average body mass, percentage body fat, fat weight, and FFM. Appendix E presents additional body composition data from various studies of male and female athletes. Such data help to evaluate typical variation in body fat within and between diverse athletic groups. Male marathon runners and gymnasts have the largest FFM/FM, while American football offensive and defensive lineman and shot-putters show the smallest ratios. Among women, bodybuilders have the largest FFM/FM values (equal to those of men), whereas the smallest ratios emerge for field event participants. Surprisingly, female gymnasts and ballet dancers rank about intermediate compared with other female sport participants.

TABLE 13.11 **Comparison of Body Mass, Stature, and Eight Skinfolds in Male and Female Swimmers, Divers, and Water Polo Athletes at the Sixth World Championships Held in Perth, Australia, in 1992**

	Mass (kg)	Stature (cm)	Tri[a]	Scap	Supra	Abd	Thi	Calf	Bic	Iliac
Males										
Swimming	78.4	183.8	7.0	7.9	6.3	9.4	9.6	6.5	3.7	9.2
Diving	66.7	170.9	6.8	7.9	6.0	9.6	9.6	6.0	3.8	8.5
Water polo	86.1	186.5	9.2	9.9	8.2	14.9	12.6	7.9	4.3	13.4
Females										
Swimming	63.1	71.5	12.1	8.8	7.3	12.1	19.1	11.4	5.9	9.8
Diving	53.7	61.2	11.4	8.5	6.8	11.1	18.2	9.7	4.9	7.9
Water polo	64.8	171.3	15.3	10.5	9.6	17.6	23.4	13.5	7.1	12.1

Modified from Mazza JC, et al. Absolute body size. In: Carter JE, Ackland TR, eds. Kinanthropometry in aquatic sports. A study of world class athletes. Human Kinetics Sport Science Monograph Series, vol. 5. Champaign, IL: Human Kinetics, 1994.

[a] *These abbreviations are for skinfolds (mm): Tri, triceps; Scap, subscapula; Supra, supraspinale; Abd, abdomen; Thi, thigh; Calf, midcalf; Bic, biceps; Iliac, iliac crest.*

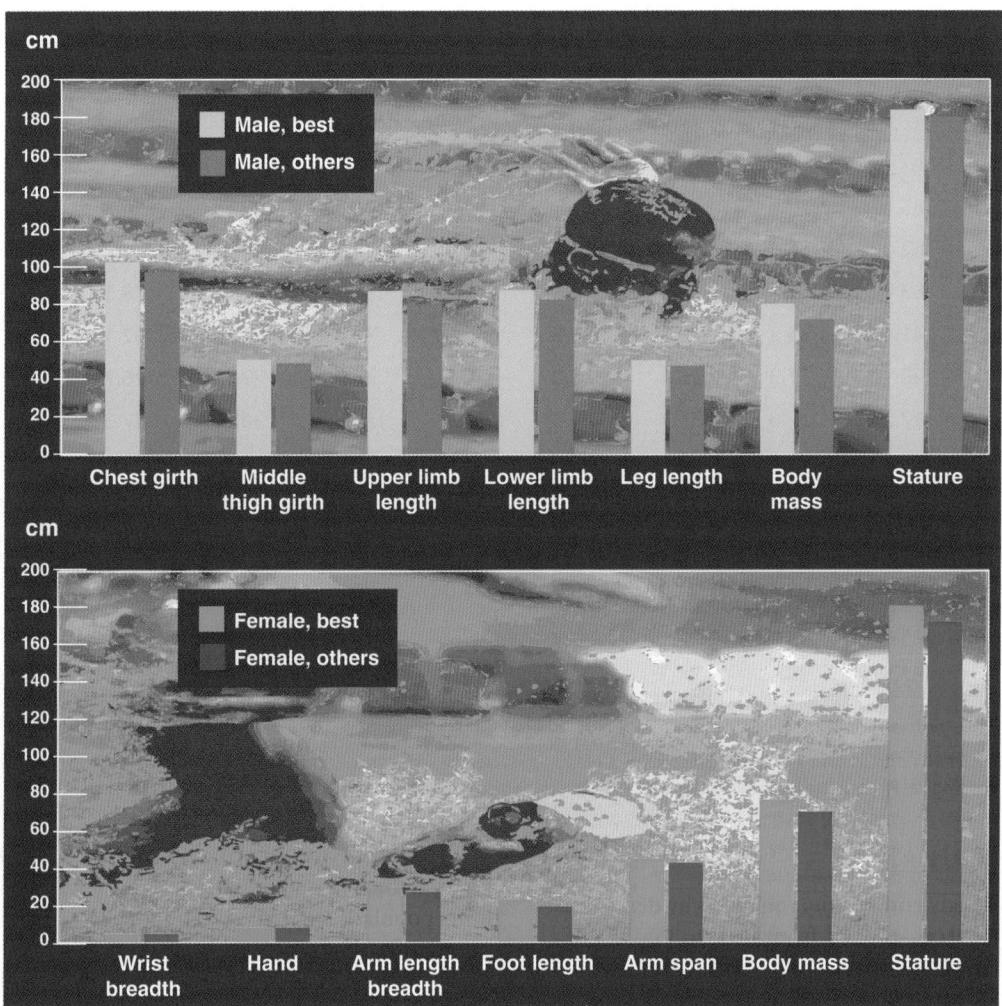

FIGURE 13.15 ■ *Top.* Comparison of 200- + 400-m free-style male swimmers for body mass, stature, chest girth, arm span (actual values divided by 4), and upper and lower limb lengths, categorized as best performers (top 12 ranks) with those of remaining competitors. *Bottom.* Comparison of differences in body size variables between the best 50-, 100-, and 200-m female breaststroke swimmers (top 12 ranks) and the rest of the competitors. *Y* axis in centimeters for all data except body mass (kilograms). (Modified from Mazza JC, et al. Absolute Body Size. In: Carter JE, Ackland TR, eds. *Kinanthropometry in Aquatic Sports: A Study of World Class Athletes.* Human kinetics sport science monograph series, vol 5. Champaign, IL: Human Kinetics, 1994.)

Percentage Body Fat Grouped by Sport Category

FIGURE 13.17 presents six classifications of sports activities based on common characteristics and performance requirements, with percentage body fat rankings within each category for male and female competitors (where applicable). This provides an overview of percentage body fat of athletes within a broad grouping of relatively similar sports.

Racial Differences in Physique Affect Athletic Performance

Black sprinters and high jumpers, for example, have longer limbs and narrower hips than their white counterparts.[173] From a mechanical perspective, a black sprinter with leg and arm size identical to a white sprinter would have a lighter, shorter, and slimmer body to propel. This might confer a more favorable power-to-body mass ratio at any given body size. Greater power output provides an advantage in jumping and sprint running events, where generating rapid energy for short durations is crucial to success. This advantage diminishes somewhat in the various throwing events. Compared with whites and blacks, Asian athletes have short legs relative to upper torso components, a dimensional characteristic beneficial in short and longer distance races and in weight-lifting. In fact, successful weightlifters of all races (compared with other athletic groups) have relatively short arms and legs for their stature.

TABLE 13.12   Selected Anthropometric Measurements in Males and Females Who Competed in Five Different Sports at the Montreal Olympic Games

Measurement[a]	Canoe		Gymnastics		Rowing		Swimming		Track	
	M	F	M	F	M	F	M	F	M	F
Stature, cm	185.4	170.7	169.3	161.5	191.3	174.3	178.6	166.9	179.1	168.5
Upper extremity L[a]	82.4	76.0	76.0	72.2	85.2	76.0	80.2	74.7	80.9	74.8
Lower extremity L[a]	88.0	81.8	78.9	76.5	91.7	82.3	84.1	78.1	86.9	80.3
Biacromial D	41.4	36.8	39.0	35.9	42.5	37.4	40.8	37.1	40.2	36.3
Billiac D	28.1	27.3	25.8	25.0	30.2	28.2	27.9	26.7	27.1	27.2
Arm relaxed G	32.2	27.6	30.7	24.3	31.7	27.6	30.6	27.3	29.1	24.5
Arm flexed G	35.3	29.6	33.9	25.9	34.9	29.3	33.3	28.2	32.2	26.4
Forearm G	29.3	25.4	27.5	23.2	30.3	25.5	27.4	23.9	27.9	23.3
Chest G	102.6	88.9	95.1	83.5	103.7	89.6	98.6	88.0	94.3	83.8
Waist G	80.6	69.8	72.8	63.2	84.0	70.8	79.3	69.4	77.7	67.4
Thigh G	54.6	54.0	51.0	49.9	60.2	57.5	55.4	52.8	55.0	53.9
Calf G	37.5	34.9	34.7	33.3	39.3	37.0	36.9	34.0	37.6	34.9

[a]L, length; D, diameter; G, girth; all values are in centimeters.

Adapted from Carter JE, et al. Anthropometry of Montreal Olympic athletes. In: Carter JEL, ed. Physical structure of Olympic athletes. Part 1: The Montreal Olympic Games Anthropological Project. Basal: Karger, 1982.

Field Event Athletes

FIGURE 13.18 shows body composition obtained by densitometry and anthropometry—ranked from high to low in percentage body fat, fat weight, FFM, and lean-to-fat ratio—for the 10 top American athletes in the discus, shot put, javelin, and hammer throw 2 years before the 1980 Moscow Olympics. For comparison, data include international elite middle- and long-distance runners (average treadmill $\dot{V}O_{2max}$= 76.9 mL · kg^{-1} · min^{-1}) and Behnke's reference man. TABLE 13.13 lists the corresponding data for girth and skinfold anthropometry. Shot-putters clearly possessed the largest overall size (body mass and girths), followed by athletes in discuss, hammer, and javelin.

Female Endurance Athletes

TABLE 13.14 presents data for body mass, stature, and body composition for 11 female long-distance runners of national and international caliber. The runners averaged 15.2% body fat (hydrostatic weighing), similar to reports of high school cross-country runners[20] and elite Kenyan female endurance runners who averaged 16.0% body fat,[12] but considerably lower than the 26% reported for sedentary females of the same age, stature, and body mass.[87] Compared with other female athletic groups, runners have relatively less fat than collegiate basketball players (20.9%),[164] competitive gymnasts (15.5%),[165] younger distance runners (18%),[98] swimmers (20.1%),[91] and tennis players (22.8%).[91]

Interestingly, the runners' average body fat equaled the 15% value generally reported for nonathletic males, and close to the quantity of essential fat proposed by Behnke's model for the reference woman. The 6 to 9% body fat levels of several ap-

parently healthy runners in Table 13.14 fall within the range reported for elite male endurance athletes. The leanest women in the population based on Behnke's reference standards have essential fat equal to 12 to 14% of body mass. This apparent discrepancy between estimated fat content of distance runners and the theoretical lower limit for body fat in women requires further study. Note the relatively high body fat (35.4%) of one of the best runners; other factors must override limitations to distance running imposed by excess fat.

Male Endurance Athletes

TABLE 13.15 presents the body composition of 11 male elite middle- and long-distance runners and 8 elite marathoners. A representative sample of 95 untrained college-aged men provides comparison data. The runners maintain extremely low body fat values that average 4.5% for the distance athletes and 4.3% for the marathoners, considering that essential fat constitutes about 3% of body mass. This agrees with values for elite Kenyan runners whose body fat averaged 6.6% (predicted from skinfold measures).[12] Clearly, these competitors represent the lower end of the lean-to-fat continuum for elite athletes.

Benefits of a Lean Physique

A lean physique most likely influences success in distance running. This makes sense for several reasons: First, effective heat dissipation during running maintains thermal balance—excess fat thwarts heat dissipation. Second, excess body fat represents "dead weight;" it adds directly to exercise energy cost without providing propulsive energy.

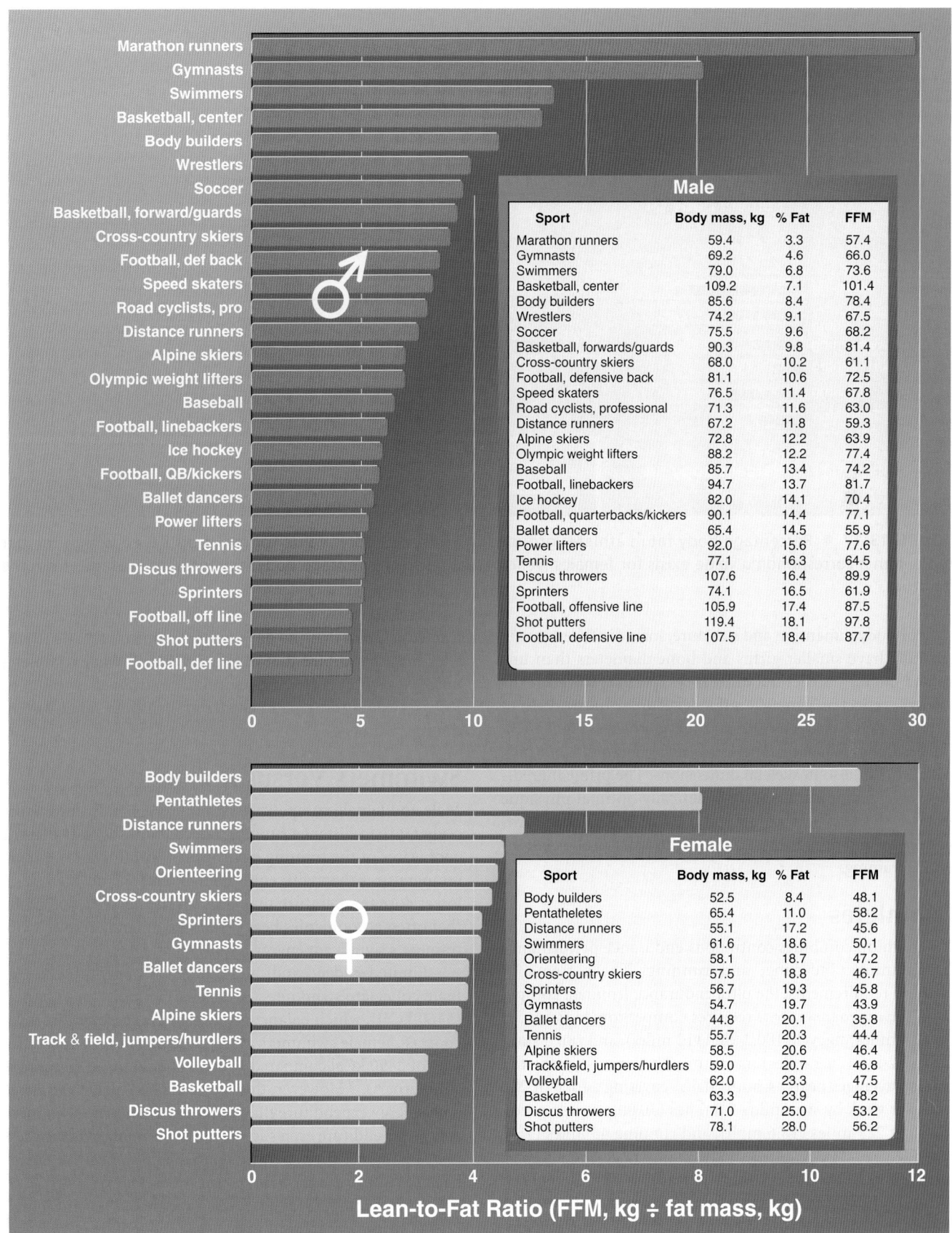

Male

Sport	Body mass, kg	% Fat	FFM
Marathon runners	59.4	3.3	57.4
Gymnasts	69.2	4.6	66.0
Swimmers	79.0	6.8	73.6
Basketball, center	109.2	7.1	101.4
Body builders	85.6	8.4	78.4
Wrestlers	74.2	9.1	67.5
Soccer	75.5	9.6	68.2
Basketball, forwards/guards	90.3	9.8	81.4
Cross-country skiers	68.0	10.2	61.1
Football, defensive back	81.1	10.6	72.5
Speed skaters	76.5	11.4	67.8
Road cyclists, professional	71.3	11.6	63.0
Distance runners	67.2	11.8	59.3
Alpine skiers	72.8	12.2	63.9
Olympic weight lifters	88.2	12.2	77.4
Baseball	85.7	13.4	74.2
Football, linebackers	94.7	13.7	81.7
Ice hockey	82.0	14.1	70.4
Football, quarterbacks/kickers	90.1	14.4	77.1
Ballet dancers	65.4	14.5	55.9
Power lifters	92.0	15.6	77.6
Tennis	77.1	16.3	64.5
Discus throwers	107.6	16.4	89.9
Sprinters	74.1	16.5	61.9
Football, offensive line	105.9	17.4	87.5
Shot putters	119.4	18.1	97.8
Football, defensive line	107.5	18.4	87.7

Female

Sport	Body mass, kg	% Fat	FFM
Body builders	52.5	8.4	48.1
Pentatheletes	65.4	11.0	58.2
Distance runners	55.1	17.2	45.6
Swimmers	61.6	18.6	50.1
Orienteering	58.1	18.7	47.2
Cross-country skiers	57.5	18.8	46.7
Sprinters	56.7	19.3	45.8
Gymnasts	54.7	19.7	43.9
Ballet dancers	44.8	20.1	35.8
Tennis	55.7	20.3	44.4
Alpine skiers	58.5	20.6	46.4
Track&field, jumpers/hurdlers	59.0	20.7	46.8
Volleyball	62.0	23.3	47.5
Basketball	63.3	23.9	48.2
Discus throwers	71.0	25.0	53.2
Shot putters	78.1	28.0	56.2

Lean-to-Fat Ratio (FFM, kg ÷ fat mass, kg)

FIGURE 13.16 ■ Comparison of the lean-to-fat ratios among male and female competitors in diverse sports. Values based on the average body mass and percentage body fat for each sport from various studies in the literature. The lean-to-fat ratio equals FFM (kg) ÷ fat mass (kg). The values in the inset tables represent averages for body composition if the literature contained two or more citations about a specific sport.

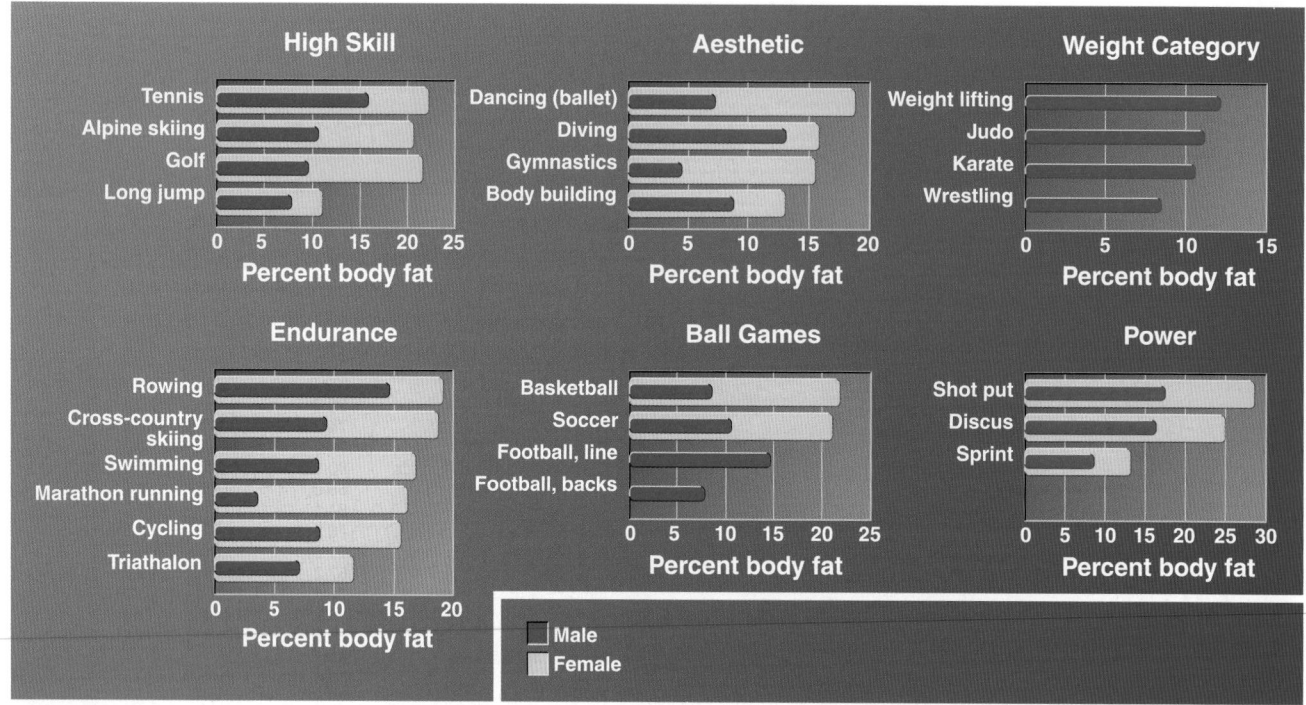

FIGURE 13.17 ■ Percentage body fat in athletes grouped by sport category. Value for males displayed within the bar *(red)* when a corresponding value exists for females *(yellow)*. Values for percentage body fat represent averages from the literature.

For body dimension and structure, male distance runners generally have smaller girths and bone diameters than untrained males.[38] Structural differences, particularly bone diameters, reflect a "genetic" influence similar to the distinct anthropometric characteristics of aquatic athletes (Fig. 13.15). The best long-distance runners possess a slight build, not only in stature but also in skeletal dimensions. The prime ingredients for a champion blends a genetically optimal physique profile with a lean body composition, a highly developed aerobic system, and proper psychologic attitude for prolonged, intensive training.

Triathletes

The triathlon combines continuous endurance performance in swimming, bicycling, and running. The extreme of triathlon requirements, the ultra endurance Ironman competition (www.ironman.com) requires competitors to swim 3.9 km (2.4 miles), bicycle 180.2 km (112 miles), and run a standard 42.2 km (26.2 miles) marathon. The serious triathlete's training averages nearly 4 hours daily, covering a total of 280 miles per week by swimming 7.2 miles (30:00 per mile pace), bicycling 227 miles (18.6 mph), and running 45 miles (7:42 per mile pace).[67] Percentage body fat of 6 male and 3 female participants in the 1982 Ironman Triathlon ranged between 5.0 and 11.3% for men and between 7.4 and 17.2% for women. Body fat averaged 7.1% for the top 15 male finishers, with a corresponding $\dot{V}O_{2max}$ value of 72.0 mL · kg^{-1} · min^{-1}. Triathletes have a body fat content and aerobic capacity comparable to other athletes in single endurance sports.[141] A study of 14 triathletes training for the 1984 Ironman competi-

tion concluded that the physique of male and female triathletes most resembled that of elite cyclists.[140] Male triathletes possess aerobic capacities similar to trained swimmers; $\dot{V}O_{2max}$ values for females cluster at the upper range for endurance runners.

Swimmers Versus Runners

Male and female competitive swimmers generally have more body fat than distance runners. Speculation suggests that the cool water of the training environment produces lower core temperatures than with equivalent-intensity land exercise. A lower core temperature may prevent the decreased appetite that often accompanies heavy training on land, despite swim training's significant energy requirement.

Limited evidence indicates similar daily energy intakes for male collegiate swimmers (3380 kCal) and distance runners (3460 kCal), which balances training energy expenditure. In contrast, female swimmers averaged a higher daily energy intake of 2490 kCal compared with 2040 kCal for their running counterparts.[79] However, the swimmers had higher estimated daily energy expenditure than did the runners. The swimmers' energy expenditure even surpassed energy intake placing them in a slightly *negative* energy balance. Thus, a positive energy balance (intake greater than output) does not explain typically higher percentage body fat levels in male (12%) and female (20%) swimmers than in male (7%) and female (15%) runners. Subsequent research from the same laboratory evaluated energy expenditure and fuel use of swimmers and runners during each form of training (45 minutes at 75–80% $\dot{V}O_{2max}$) and 2 hours' recovery.[51] The researchers hypothesized that dif-

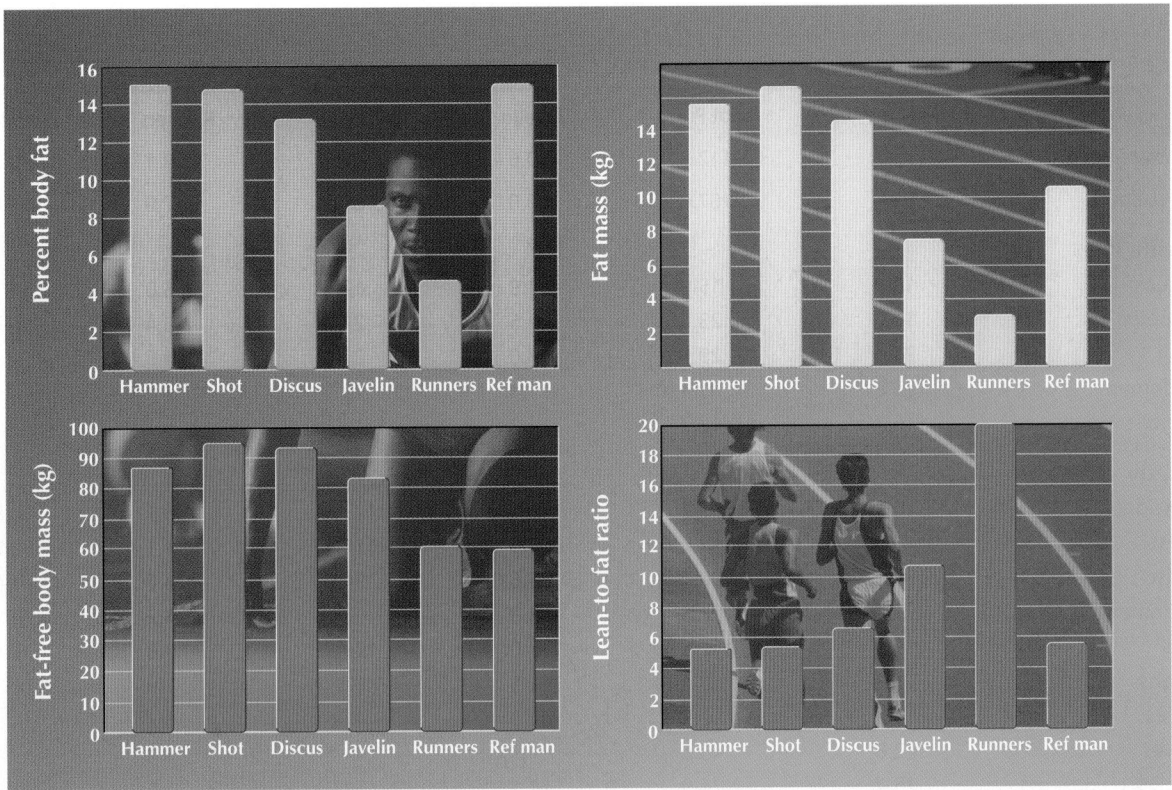

FIGURE 13.18 ■ Body composition (determined by hydrostatic weighing) of the 10 top American male athletes in the discus, shot put, javelin, and hammer throw. (Data collected by two of the authors [FK and VK] at a 1978 U.S. Olympic thrower's minicamp at the University of Houston, Houston, TX. Data include gold medalist Wilkins [discus] and world-record holder Powell [discus]. Data for the international elite middle- and long-distance runners from Pollock ML, et al. Body composition of elite class distance runners. *Ann NY Acad Sci* 1977;301:361. Reference man *[Ref man]* data from Behnke model.)

ferences in hormonal response and substrate catabolism between the two exercise modes accounted for body fat differences between groups. Thus, the small differences between activities in energy expenditure, substrate use, and hormone levels could *not* account for body fat differences.

American Football Players

The first detailed body composition analyses of American professional football players in the 1940s clearly demonstrated the inadequacy of determining a person's "optimal" body mass from height–weight standards.[197] The players as a group had body fat content that averaged only 10.4% of body mass, while FFM averaged 81.3 kg (179.3 lb). Certainly these men were heavy but not fat. The heaviest lineman weighed 118 kg (260 lb, 17.4% body fat, 215 lb FFM), whereas the lineman with the most body fat (23.2%) weighed 115.4 kg (252 lb). Body mass of a defensive back with the least fat (3.3%) was 82.3 kg (182 lb) with a FFM of 79.6 kg (175 lb).

TABLE 13.16 presents a clearer picture for body mass, stature, percentage body fat, and FFM of college and professional players grouped by position.[201,204] The *Pro, older* group consists of 25 players from the 1942 Washington Redskins, the first professional players measured for body composition by hydrostatic weighing. The *Pro, modern* group consists of 164 players from 14 teams in the NFL (69% veterans, 31% rookies). Some 107 members of the 1976 to 1978 Dallas Cowboys and New York Jets make up the third group. Four groups of collegiate players include candidates for spring practice at St. Cloud State College in Minnesota, the University of Massachusetts (UMass), and Division III Gettysburg College and teams from the University of Southern California (USC), 1973 to 1977, national champions and participants in two Rose Bowls. Body composition measurements for this data set included hydrostatic weighing with correction for measured residual lung volume.

One would generally expect modern-day professional players to have a larger body size at each position than a representative collegiate group. Although this occurred for comparison with the St. Cloud and UMass players, the USC players generally maintained a physique similar to modern professionals. With the exception of defensive linemen, the USC players at each position showed nearly the same fat content as current professionals. No USC player possessed more than 4.4 kg less FFM than that of the professionals at each position. The average defensive lineman in the NFL outweighed his USC counterpart in FFM by only 1.8 kg. Total body mass of the professional linemen significantly exceeded that of USC counterparts, primarily because professionals possessed 18.2% body fat versus the collegians 14.7%. These data suggest that

| | TABLE 13.13 | Skinfold and Girth Anthropometry of the Top 10 American Athletes in the Discus, Shot Put, Javelin, and Hammer Throw | | | | | |

Measurement[a]	Discus	Shot Put	Javelin	Hammer	Runners	Ref Man
Body mass, kg	108.2	112.3	90.6	104.2	63.1	70.0
Stature, cm	191.7	187.0	186.0	187.3	177.0	174.0
Skinfolds, mm						
Triceps	13.0	15.0	11.9	12.7	5.0	—
Scapular	18.0	23.8	12.5	21.5	6.4	—
Iliac	24.5	29.6	17.0	27.4	4.6	—
Abdomen	25.6	31.4	18.4	29.1	7.1	—
Thigh	16.4	15.7	13.3	17.3	6.1	—
Girths, cm						
Shoulders	129.8	133.3	121.5	127.4	106.1	110.8
Chest	113.5	118.5	104.6	111.3	91.1	91.8
Waist	94.1	99.1	86.6	94.8	74.6	77.0
Abdomen	97.5	101.5	87.8	98.0	74.2	79.8
Hips	110.4	112.3	102.0	108.7	87.8	93.4
Thighs	66.3	69.4	61.5	67.3	51.9	54.8
Knees	41.5	42.9	40.0	41.0	36.2[b]	36.6
Calves	42.6	43.6	39.5	41.5	35.4	35.8
Ankles	25.4	24.9	24.1	24.3	21.0	22.5
Biceps	41.8	42.2	37.7	39.9	28.2	31.7
Forearms	33.1	33.7	30.8	32.4	26.4	26.4
Wrists	18.7	18.9	18.2	18.4	16.0	17.3
Diameters, cm						
Biacromial	44.5	43.8	43.2	44.8	39.5	40.6
Chest	33.1	33.7	30.8	32.6	31.3	30.0
Bi-iliac	31.3	31.2	29.6	30.4	28.0	28.6
Bitrochanter	35.5	34.9	33.7	34.8	32.2	32.8
Knee	10.2	10.5	10.0	10.2	9.5	9.3
Wrist	6.3	6.2	6.0	6.2	5.6	5.6
Ankle	7.6	7.6	7.5	7.4	—	7.0
Elbow	7.6	7.6	7.6	7.2	—	7.0

[a]*Details about measurement procedures from Katch FI, Katch VL. The body composition profile: techniques of measurement and applications. Clin Sports Med, 1984;3:31. Data correspond to the athletic groups presented in Fig. 13.18.*

elite college and professional players maintain similar body size and body composition.

As a group, professional players of 70 years ago were lower in body fat (10.4%), shorter in stature, and lighter in total body mass and FFM than modern professionals. The exceptions, defensive and offensive backs and receivers, were almost identical to more-current players in body size and composition. The biggest differences in physique emerged for defensive linemen; modern players were 6.7 cm taller, 20 kg heavier, and 4.2 percentage points of body fat fatter and had 12.3 kg more FFM. Obviously, "bigness" was not an important factor in line play during the 1940s. To illustrate this point, the *top* of FIGURE 13.19 shows the average body weight for all ros-

ter players in the NFL (N = 51,333) over a 76-year period. From 1920 to 1985, offensive linemen were the heaviest; this changed beginning with the 1990 season, when defensive linemen achieved the same body mass as the offensive linemen and then surpassed them. While the body mass for offensive linemen appeared to level off at nearly 280 lb, defensive linemen continued to increase in weight, particularly from 1990 to 1996. At this time, they weighed an average of 16 lb more or double the weight gain for offensive linemen for the comparable period. On average, offensive linemen were 1.3 lb heavier per year from 1920 to 1996. At this rate of increase, they should attain 320 lb by the year 2008 (at an average height of 6 ft 8 in)! At this size, their BMI equals 35.6, classifying them as

TABLE 13.14	Body Composition of Female Endurance Runners					
Subjects (N)	Age (y)	Stature (cm)	Mass (kg)	FFM (kg)	Body Fat (kg)	Body Fat (%)
1[a]	24	172.7	52.6	49.5	3.1	5.9
2[b]	26	159.8	71.5	46.2	25.3	35.4
3[c]	28	162.6	50.7	47.6	3.1	6.1
4	31	171.5	52.0	47.3	4.7	9.0
5	33	176.5	61.2	50.8	10.4	17.0
6	34	166.4	52.9	44.8	8.1	15.2
7	35	168.4	55.0	48.7	6.3	11.6
8	36	164.5	53.1	44.3	8.8	16.6
9	36	182.9	61.5	50.4	11.1	18.1
10	36	182.9	65.4	55.7	9.7	14.8
11	37	154.9	53.6	44.0	9.6	18.0
Average	**32.4**	**169.4**	**57.2**	**48.1**	**9.1**	**15.2**

From Wilmore JH, Brown CH. Physiological profiles of women distance runners. Med Sci Sports 1974;6:178.

[a]World's best time in marathon (2:49:40) 1974.

[b]World's best time in 50-mile run (7:04:31); established 18 months after the body composition evaluation.

[c]Noted U.S. distance runner. Five consecutive national and international cross-country championships.

TABLE 13.15	Body Composition Characteristics of Elite Male Middle- and Long-Distance Runners and Elite Marathoners						
Group	Stature (cm)	Mass (kg)	Density (g · cm^{-3})	Body Fat (%)	FFM (kg)	Fat Mass (kg)	Sum 7 Skinfolds (mm)
Distance runners							
Brown	187.3	72.10	1.07428	10.8	64.31	7.79	53.0
Castaneda	178.6	63.34	1.09102	3.7	61.00	2.34	32.5
Crawford	171.8	58.01	1.09702	1.2	57.31	0.70	32.5
Geis	179.1	66.28	1.07551	10.2	59.52	6.76	49.0
Johnson	174.6	61.79	1.08963	4.35	9.13	2.66	35.5
Manley	177.8	69.10	1.09642	1.5	68.06	1.04	32.0
Ndoo	169.3	53.97	1.08379	6.7	50.35	3.62	33.5
Prefontaine	174.2	68.00	1.08842	4.8	64.74	3.26	38.0
Rose	175.6	59.15	1.08248	7.3	54.83	4.32	31.5
Tuttle	176.8	61.44	1.09960	0.2	61.32	0.12	31.5
Mean	**170.5**	**60.92**	**1.08916**	**4.5**	**58.18**	**2.74**	**34.5**
(standard deviation)	(5.0)	(5.30)	(0.00832)	(3.5)	(4.90)	(2.38)	(7.4)
Marathon runners							
Cusack	174.6	64.19	1.08096	7.9	59.12	5.07	45.5
Galloway	180.9	65.76	1.08419	6.6	61.42	4.34	43.0
Kennedy	167.0	56.52	1.09348	2.7	54.99	1.53	37.0
Moore	184.1	64.24	1.09193	3.3	62.12	2.12	37.0
Pate	179.6	57.28	1.09676	1.3	56.54	0.74	32.5
Shorter	178.4	61.17	1.09475	2.2	59.82	1.35	45.0
Wayne	172.1	61.61	1.07859	8.9	56.13	5.48	42.5
Williams	177.2	66.07	1.09569	1.8	64.88	1.19	41.5
Mean	**176.8**	**62.11**	**1.08954**	**4.3**	**59.38**	**2.73**	**40.5**
(standard deviation)	(5.6)	(3.66)	(0.00718)	(3.0)	(3.38)	(1.92)	(4.6)

Data from Pollock ML, et al. Body composition of elite class distance runners. Ann NY Acad Sci 1977;301:361.

TABLE 13.16   Body Compositions of Collegiate and Professional Football Players Grouped by Position

Position[a]	Level	N	Stature (cm)	Mass (kg)	Body Fat (%)	FFM (kg)
Defensive backs	St. Cloud[b]	15	178.3	77.3	11.5	68.4
	U Mass[c]	12	179.9	83.1	8.8	76.8
	USC[d]	15	183.0	83.7	9.6	75.7
	Gettysburg[e]	16	175.9	79.8	13.6	68.9
	Pro, modern[f]	26	182.5	84.8	9.6	76.7
	Pro, older[g]	25	183.0	91.2	10.7	81.4
Offensive backs	St. Cloud	15	179.7	79.8	12.4	69.6
and receivers	U Mass	29	181.8	84.1	9.5	76.4
	USC	18	185.6	86.1	9.9	77.6
	Gettysburg	18	176.0	78.3	12.9	68.2
	Pro, modern	40	183.8	90.7	9.4	81.9
	Pro, older	25	183.0	91.7	10.0	87.5
Linebackers	St. Cloud	7	180.1	87.2	13.4	75.4
	U Mass	17	186.1	97.1	13.1	84.2
	USC	17	185.6	98.8	13.2	85.8
	Gettysburg	—	—	—	—	—
	Pro, modern	28	188.6	102.2	14.0	87.6
Offensive linemen	St. Cloud	13	186.0	99.2	19.1	79.8
and tight ends	U Mass	23	187.5	107.6	19.5	86.6
	Gettysburg	15	182.6	110.4	26.2	81.0
	USC	25	191.1	106.5	15.3	90.3
	Pro, modern	38	193.0	112.6	15.6	94.7
Defensive linemen	St. Cloud	15	186.6	97.8	18.5	79.3
	U Mass	8	188.8	114.3	19.5	91.9
	USC	13	191.1	109.3	14.7	93.2
	Gettysburg	11	178.0	99.4	21.9	77.6
	Pro, modern	32	192.4	117.1	18.2	95.8
	Pro, older	25	185.7	97.1	14.0	83.5
All positions	St. Cloud	65	182.5	88.0	15.0	74.2
	U Mass	91	184.9	97.3	13.9	83.2
	USC	88	186.6	96.6	11.4	84.6
	Gettysburg	60	178.0	90.6	18.1	73.3
	Pro, modern	164	188.1	101.5	13.4	87.3
	Pro, older	25	183.1	91.2	10.4	81.3
	Dallas-Jets[h]	107	188.2	100.4	12.6	87.7

[a]Grouping according to Wilmore JH, Haskel WL. Body composition and endurance capacity of professional football players. J Appl Physiol 1972;33:564.

[b]Data from Wickkiser JD, Kelly JM. The body composition of a college football team. Med Sci Sports 1975;7:199.

[c]UMass data from Coach Robert Stull and F Katch, University of Massachusetts. Data collected during spring practice, 1985; %fat by densitometry.

[d]USC data from Dr. Robert Girandola, University of Southern California, Los Angeles, 1978, 1993.

[e]Data courtesy of Dr. Kristin Steumple, Department of Exercise and Sport Science, Gettysburg College, Gettysburg, PA, 2000.

[f]Data from Wilmore JH, et al. Football pros' strengths—and CV weakness—charted. Phys Sportsmed 1976;4:45.

[g]Data from Dr. A. R. Behnke.

[h]Data from Katch FI, Katch, VL. Body composition of the Dallas Cowboys and New York Jets football teams, unpublished, 1978.

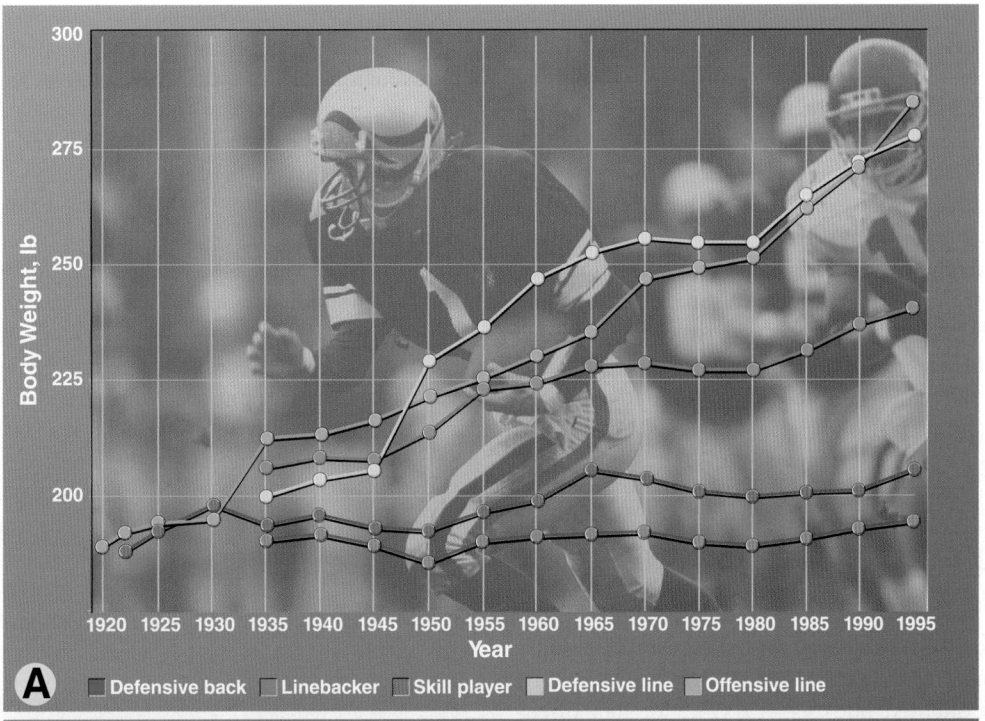

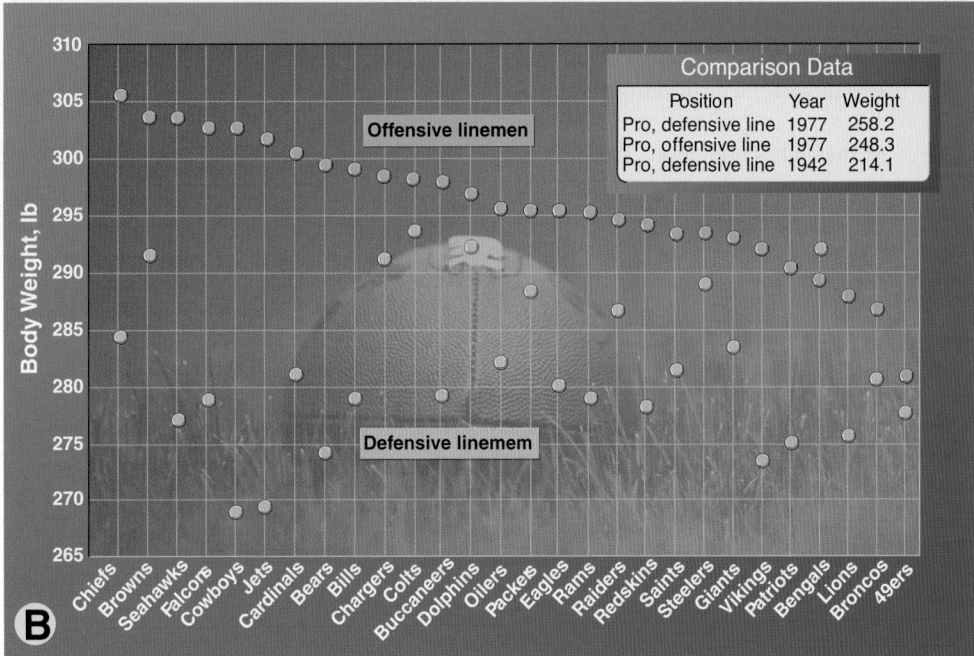

FIGURE 13.19 ■ **A.** Average body weights by position for all roster players in the NFL between 1920 and 1995. **B.** Average body weights of all roster offensive and defensive linemen in the NFL in 1994. Team rankings progress from the heaviest to lightest body weight for the team's offensive linemen. (From active team rosters for 28 NFL teams as of the first regular-season weekend, September 4–5, 1994.) Comparison of body weight data for the pro offensive and defensive line (1977) shown in the inset box combine data for the New York Jets and Dallas Cowboys football teams (collected by FK and VK). The 1942 data provided by Dr. Albert Behnke from his studies of the Washington Redskins. (Data courtesy of the National Football League public relations department.)

high for disease risk (Fig. 13.1). Even more eye opening was the body size of the 2007 Super Bowl team's 28 offensive and defensive linemen (Indianapolis Colts and Chicago Bears). BMI averaged 38.3 (body mass, 139.2 kg; stature, 194.7 cm), the largest yet reported for Super Bowl teams. Research must determine if such relatively homogenous groups of elite, physically active, overweight men experience greater morbidity and mortality than normal-weight peers.

The body weight of offensive and defensive linemen for each of the NFL teams during the 1994 season (*bottom of figure 13.19*) ranged from heaviest (Kansas City Chiefs; Super Bowl 1970) to lightest (San Francisco 49ers; Super Bowls 1990 and 1995). For the 1994 season (the date of the comparison in the bottom figure), the average body weight of the winning Super Bowl offensive line (Dallas Cowboys) ranked fifth highest of 28 teams.

A Worrisome Trend Among Less-Skilled and Younger Players

Exceptionally high BMIs also occur at less elite levels of collegiate competition. The average BMI of 33.1 for the Division III 1999 Gettysburg offensive line (N = 15) (29.9 for 2000 offensive line, N = 13)[171] and 31.7 for other National Collegiate Athletic Association (NCAA) Division III America football linemen (N = 26; 1994–1995) raises similar concerns about potential health risks for such large young men (stature, 1.84 m; body mass, 107.2 kg).[153] At the high school level, The BMI of *Parade Magazine's* (www.parade.com) All-America football teams increased dramatically beginning in the early 1970s through 1989 and then further increased in rate of gain to the year 2006. The plot in FIGURE 13.20 shows a clear shift at 1972 in

the slope of the regression line (*black line yellow data points*) relating BMI to year of competition compared with age-matched individuals from large-scale epidemiologic normative data (*red line*). Particularly disturbing are the most recently available 2006 data for the high school offensive and defensive linemen (not indicated in the figure) whose BMI averaged 33.7 (stature = 194.7 cm; mass = 131.2 kg). These values for stature and body mass for the high school players now are *almost identical* to the average values for the 2007 National Champion BCS (Bowl Championship Series) teams (University of Florida and Ohio State University) and 2007 Super Bowl teams (Indianapolis Colts and Chicago Bears)! For eight of the 18 high school All-America linemen who exceeded 300 lb, their BMI averaged 36.6 (body mass = 142.8 kg; stature =195.3 cm). Such data are consistent with the latest survey that indicates that 56% of 2168 NFL players in 2003–2004 were considered obese based on BMI classification.[60] The implications for the student athlete linemen's health risk (e.g., high blood pressure, insulin resistance, and type 2 diabetes) and long-term outlook remain to be determined, but certainly are not encouraging.[106]

The Interaction of Enhanced Training and Performance-Enhancing Drugs

The shift toward a higher BMI among high school football players probably relates to two factors: (1) improved nutrition and training and/or (2) the emerging prevalent use among high-school athletes of performance-enhancing drugs such as anabolic steroids.

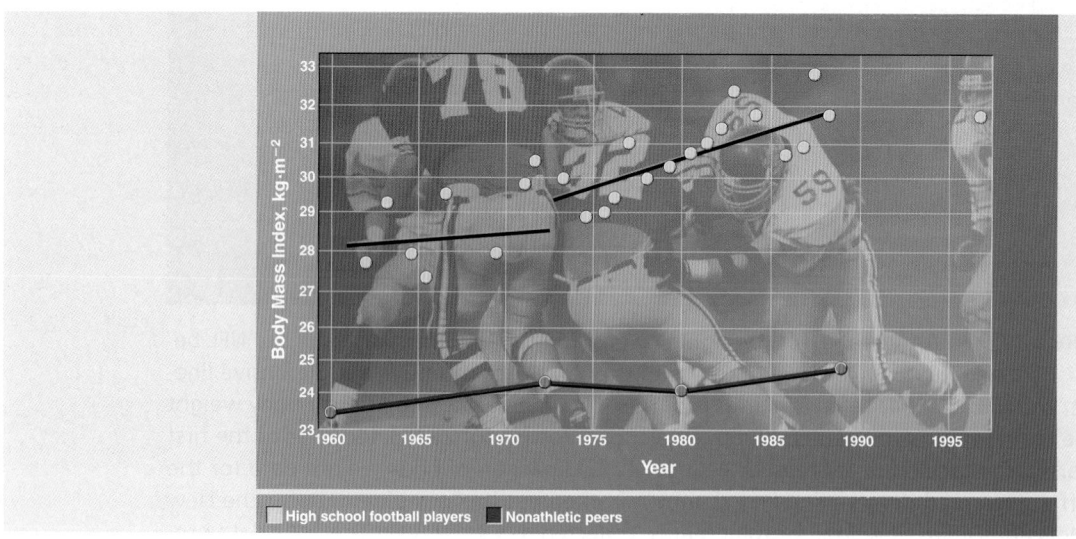

FIGURE 13.20 ■ Body mass index of *Parade Magazine's* All-America high school football players from 1960 to 2006. Comparison data are available for similar age high school students from 1960 to 1995. The 2006 data included 18 linemen who ranged in body mass from 104.3 to 153.3 kg and in stature from 188.0 to 203.2 cm. The lineman with the highest BMI of 38.7 weighed 153.3 kg (338 lb; stature = 198.1 cm; 6 ft 8 in).

Professional Golfers

Limited data exist on the body composition of professional golfers, although height and weight for tour PGA and Champions Tour are available from popular golf magazines. TABLE 13.17 lists the height, weight, and BMI for 2005 Champions Tour winners and PGA tour champions. Data for Behnke's reference man are included for comparison. Interestingly, little difference in the physical characteristics and BMI exists for the two groups of players. The projected mortality ratio for these high-skill athletes based on BMI rates as very low (Fig. 13.1). This contrasts to the high school and professional football players who classify as obese. For the obese NFL players, half fall in the severely obese range (BMI that reaches 35), and those with a BMI above 40 classify as morbidly obese.

OTHER LONGITUDINAL TRENDS IN BODY SIZE

To expand upon longitudinal trends in body size for elite athletes, we determined stature and body mass for two groups of professional athletes: (1) all National Basketball Association (NBA) players from 1970 to 1993 (number ranged from 156 to 400) and (2) professional Major League Baseball (MLB) players from 28 teams during the 1986, 1988, 1990, 1992, and 1995 seasons (5031 roster players).

For the NBA players (FIG. 13.21A), average body mass increased by 3.8 lb (1.7 kg) or 1.8% during the 23-year interval. Stature increased more slowly; it changed by only 1 inch, or less than 1%, over the same interval. The NBA players' BMI during this time remained within a narrow range of 0.8 BMI units from 23.6 to 24.4. The MLB players (shown in *red* in the same figure) reveal slightly higher mean values than did the basketball players. Compared with American professional and collegiate football players, baseball and basketball athletes have maintained BMIs within guidelines considered relatively healthful for minimizing mortality and disease risk.

One might question whether gross body size reflected by BMI relates to sports performance variables. For example, the graphs in Figure 13.21B show the BMI of National and American League Cy Young award winners and their earned run average over the 5-year comparison period. This comparison, while of interest, fails to delineate a clear relation between BMI and performance among the best pitchers in baseball.

Wrestlers

Wrestlers represent a unique athletic group who train intensely and attempt to keep a low body weight with as high a fat-free mass as possible.[24,37,146,147,157,178,207,208] The NCAA introduced rule changes for the 1998–1999 season in response to the deaths of three collegiate wrestlers in 1997 from excessive weight loss (largely from dehydration) to discourage dangerous weight-cutting practices and increase safe participation.[32,138] Another rule change included measures of urine specific gravity (ratio of the density of urine to the density of water) to assess hydration status to ensure euhydration of wrestlers at weight certification. Athletes with a urine specific gravity of 1.020 or less are considered euhydrated while those with specific gravity in excess of 1.020 cannot have their body fat assessed to determine minimum competitive wrestling weight for the season. Urine specific gravity reflects hydration status, but it does lag behind true hydration status in periods of rapid body fluid turnover during acute dehydration. Such a scenario would fail to detect a large number of dehydrated wrestlers.[144]

Weightlifters and Bodybuilders

Men

Resistance-trained athletes, particularly bodybuilders, Olympic weightlifters, and power weightlifters, exhibit remarkable muscular development and FFM and a relatively lean physique. Percentage body fat from underwater weighing averaged 9.3% in bodybuilders, 9.1% in power weightlifters, and 10.8% in Olympic weightlifters.[94] Considerable leanness exists for each group of athletes, even though height–weight tables classify up to 19% of these men as overweight. Groups did not differ in skeletal frame size, FFM, skinfolds, and bone diameters. The only differences occurred for shoulders, chest, biceps (relaxed and flexed), and forearm girths, with bodybuilders larger at each site. Bodybuilders exhibited nearly 16 kg more muscle than predicted for their size; power weightlifters, 15 kg; and Olympic weightlifters, 13 kg.

Women

Bodybuilding gained widespread popularity among women in the United States during the late 1970s. As women aggressively undertook the vigorous demands of resistance training, competition became more intense, and the level of achievement increased significantly. Bodybuilding success depends on a slim and lean appearance, with a well-defined yet en-

TABLE 13.17 Comparison of Height, Body Weight, and BMI for 2005 Champions Tour and PGA Golf Tour Champions

Group[a]	Height, cm	Weight, kg	BMI
PGA Tour (N = 33)	182.0	84.1	25.4
Champions Tour (N = 18)	181.0	85.8	26.2
Reference man[b]	174.0	70.0	23.1

[a]The Official Annual 2006 PGA TOUR and The Official Annual 2006 Champions Tour New York: Boston Hannah International Publishers, 2006.

[b]Source: Figure 13.4.

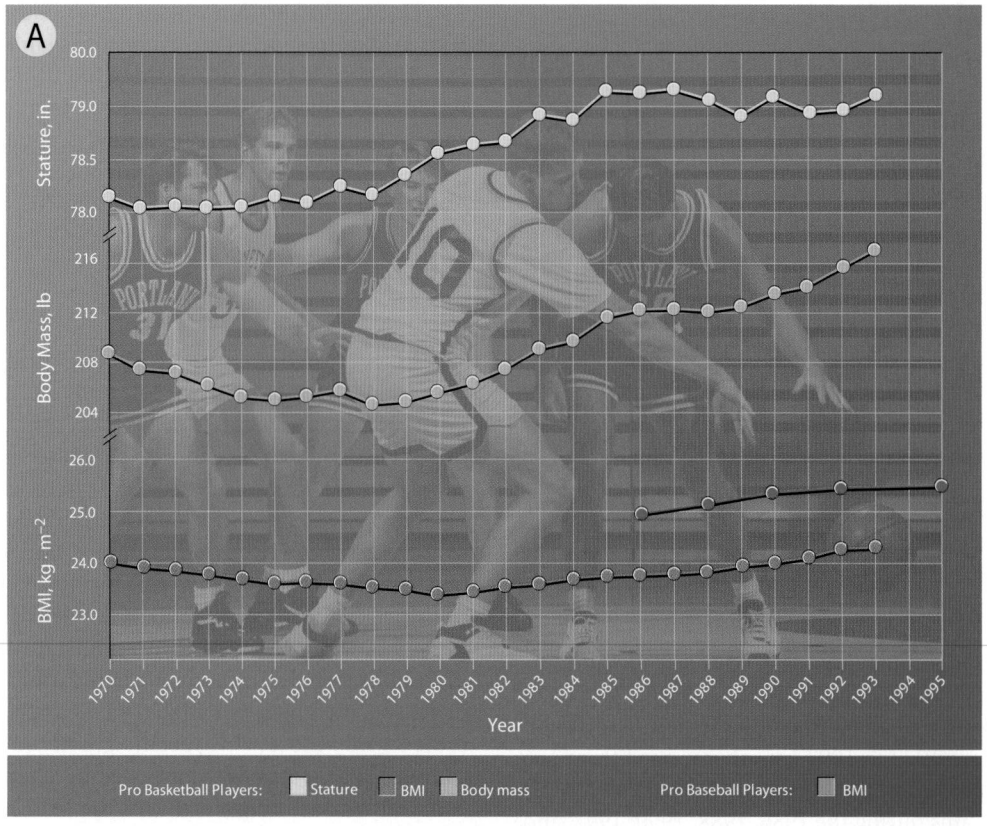

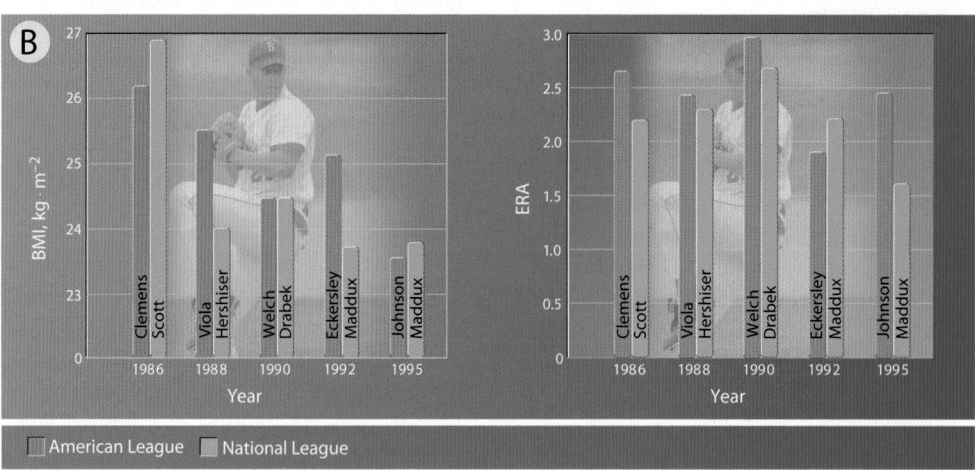

FIGURE 13.21 ■ **A.** BMI, body mass, and stature of professional NBA players (1970–1993) and BMI of Major League Baseball (MLB) players (1986–1995). **B.** BMI for American League and National League Cy Young award winners (best baseball pitcher) along with corresponding earned run average (ERA). (Data for NBA players from team rosters, compiled by F. Katch; MLB data from team rosters courtesy of Major League Baseball.)

larged musculature. These requirements raise interesting questions about the women's body composition. How lean do competitors become, and does a relatively large muscle mass accompany their low body-fat levels?

Body composition of 10 competitive female bodybuilders revealed an average of 13.2% body fat (range, 8.0–18.3%) and 46.6 kg of FFM.[53] Except for champion gymnasts, who also average about 13% body fat, bodybuilders were 3 to 4% shorter, 4 to 5% lighter, and had 7 to 10% less total fat mass than other top female athletes.

A Remarkable Physique Characteristic

A most striking compositional characteristic of the female bodybuilder is her dramatically large FFM/FM ratio of 7:1, which nearly doubles the 4.3:1 ratio for other female athletic groups. This difference presumably occurred without steroid use (assessed by questionnaire). Interestingly, 8 of the 10 bodybuilders reported normal menstrual function despite relatively low body fat.

Men Versus Women

TABLE 13.18 compares body composition, girths, and excess body mass of male and female bodybuilders. Excess body mass represents the difference between actual body mass and body weight-for-height from the Metropolitan Life Insurance tables. Overweight for the men corresponded to a 14.8-kg (18%) excess and for the women, a 1.2- kg (2.2%) excess. Obviously, excess body mass for these lean athletes primarily reflected FFM as increased skeletal muscle mass.

Contrasting the girth data allows comparisons of individuals (or groups) who differ in body size. The analysis shows that gender differences in girths, when scaled to body size (referred to as "adjusted" in the table), do not differ as much as the uncorrected girth values. Relative to body size, females exceed the male bodybuilders in seven of 12 body areas. *Women probably can alter muscle size to the same relative extent as males, at least when scaled to body size.* The larger hip size in women probably relates to greater fat stores in this location.

TABLE 13.18 Body Composition and Anthropometric Girths of Male and Female Bodybuilders

Sex	Age, y	Mass, kg	Stature, cm	Fat, %	FFM, kg	Excess Mass,[a] kg
Male (N = 18)	27.0	82.4	177.1	9.3	74.6	14.8
Female (N = 10)	27.0	53.8	160.8	13.2	46.6	1.2

Body Girth (cm)	Males Raw[b]	Males Adjusted[c]	Females Raw	Females Adjusted	% Difference Raw	% Difference Adjusted
Shoulders	123.1	37.1	101.7	36.7	17.4	1.1
Chest	106.4	32.1	90.6	32.7	14.9	21.9
Waist	82.0	24.7	64.5	23.3	21.3	5.7
Abdomen	82.3	24.8	67.7	25.1	15.3	21.2
Hips	95.6	28.8	87.0	31.4	9.0	29.0
Biceps relaxed	35.9	10.8	25.8	9.3	28.1	13.9
Biceps flexed	40.4	12.2	28.9	10.4	28.5	14.8
Forearm	30.7	9.2	24.0	8.7	21.8	5.4
Wrist	17.4	5.2	15.1	5.4	13.2	23.8
Thigh	59.6	17.9	53.0	19.1	11.1	26.7
Calf	37.3	11.2	32.4	11.7	13.1	24.5
Ankle	22.8	6.9	26.3	7.3	11.0	25.8

FFM, fat-free body mass.

[a]Body mass minus body mass estimated from height–weight tables. Abraham S, et al. Weight and height of adults 18 to 74 years of age. United States Vital and Health Statistics, series H, no. 211. Washington, DC: U.S. Government Printing Office, 1979.

[b]Actual girth measurement

[c]Girth size relative to body size using method of Behnke (see Ref. 9)

Summary

1. Body composition assessment reveals that athletes generally have physique characteristics unique to their specific sport. Field event athletes have relatively large fat-free body mass (FFM) and high percentage body fat; distance runners have the lowest FFM and fat mass.

2. Champion performance blends physique characteristics with highly developed physiologic support systems.

3. Male and female triathletes possess the body composition and aerobic capacity most similar to elite bicyclists.

4. American football players are among the heaviest of all athletes, yet maintain a relatively lean body composition. At the highest levels of competition, collegiate and professional football players attain similar body size and body composition.

5. Competitive male and female swimmers generally have higher body fat levels than distance runners, probably from self-selection related to economically exercising in the different environments rather than real metabolic effects caused by the environments.

6. Wrestlers undergo severe training and repeated bouts of short-term weight loss. Wrestlers should be discouraged from drastically reducing body fat if it brings them below 5%.

7. The FFM/FM ratio of female bodybuilders significantly exceeds the FFM/FM ratios of other elite female athletes.

8. Female bodybuilders can probably alter muscle size to almost the same *relative* extent as male bodybuilders.

Test Your Knowledge Answers

1. **False:** The importance of the BMI is not that it predicts body fat level (although it moderately relates to this variable) but rather its curvilinear relationship to all-cause mortality ratio. As BMI increases, so does the risk for cardiovascular complications including hypertension and stroke, diabetes, and renal disease. The lowest health risk category occurs for individuals with BMIs between 20 and 25, and the highest risk category includes individuals whose BMI exceeds 40.

2. **True:** His BMI = 31.6 kg per m^2 [97.1 ÷ (1.753)^2], which exceeds the upper range of BMI values (BMI: normal weight, <25.0; overweight, 25.0–29.9; obese, ≥30.0). This classifies him as obese.

3. **False:** In the general population, the average man is taller and heavier, his skeleton weighs more, and he has a larger muscle mass and lower total fat content than the typical woman. Differences exist even when expressing the amount of fat, muscle, and bone as a percentage of body mass. This holds particularly true for body fat, which represents 15% of total body mass for the man and 27% for his female counterpart. These differences in body composition emerge in comparisons among elite athletes in diverse sports. Among the leanest male competitors such as elite marathon runners body fat levels range between 3 and 5% while for female counterparts percentage body fat rarely falls below 12 to 15%.

This higher level of body fat among females across the entire fitness spectrum most likely relates to sex-specific essential fat that serves biologically important childbearing and other hormone-related functions.

4. **False:** The two sites for body fat deposition are essential fat and storage fat. Essential fat comprises fat stored in the marrow of bones, heart, lungs, liver, spleen, kidneys, intestines, muscles, and lipid-rich tissues of the central nervous system. In the female, essential fat also includes additional sex-specific essential fat. Storage fat consists of fat accumulation in adipose tissue. This includes the visceral fatty tissues that protect the various internal organs within the thoracic and abdominal cavities, and the larger subcutaneous fat tissue volume deposited beneath the skin's surface.

5. **True:** Archimedes showed that an object submerged or floating in water becomes buoyed up by a counterforce equaling the weight of the volume of water it displaces. This buoyant force helps to support an immersed object against the downward pull of gravity. Thus, an object is said to lose weight in water. Because the object's loss of weight in water equals the weight of the volume of water it displaces, specific gravity refers to the ratio of the weight of an object in air divided by its loss of weight in water.

6. **False:** From the Siri equation, percentage body fat computes as follows: $495 \div 1.0719 - 450 = 11.8\%$. Total mass of body fat equals 85 kg 0.118×10.0 kg.

7. **False:** Men with a 102-cm (40-in) or larger waist and women with waist girth larger than 86 cm (35 in) maintain a high risk for various diseases. Waist girths of 90 cm for men and 83 cm for women correspond to a BMI threshold of overweight (BMI, 25), while 100 cm for men and 93 cm for women reflect the obesity cutoff (BMI, 30).

8. **True:** Based on an average computed from data in diverse studies, percentage body fat for young adult men averages between 12 and 15%, whereas the average fat value for women ranges between 25 and 28%.

9. **False:** Given the data, desirable fat mass loss computes as follows:

Fat mass = 120 kg × 24% (0.24) body fat = 28.8 kg

Fat-free body mass = 120 kg − 28.8 kg = 91.2 kg

Goal body weight = 91.2 kg ÷ (1.00 − 0.15) = 91.2 kg
  ÷ 0.85 = 107.3 kg (236.6 lb)

Desirable fat loss = 120 kg − 107.3 kg = 12.7 kg (28.0 lb)

10. **True:** The body composition for 10 competitive female bodybuilders averaged 13.2% body fat (range, 8.0–18.3%) and 46.6 kg of FFM. Except for champion gymnasts, who also average about 13% body fat, bodybuilders were 3 to 4% shorter, were 4 to 5% lighter, and possessed 7 to 10% less total fat mass than other top female athletes. The bodybuilders' most striking compositional characteristic, a dramatically large FFM/FM ratio of 7:1, nearly double the 4.3:1 ratio for other female athletic groups.

References

1. Abe E, et al. Gender differences in FFM accumulation and architectural characteristics. *Med Sci Sports Exerc* 1998;30:1066.
2. Ainsworth BE, et al. Predictive accuracy of bioimpedance in estimating fat-free mass of African-American women. *Med Sci Sports Exerc* 1997;29:781.
3. Allison DB, et al. Annual deaths attributable to obesity in the United States. *JAMA* 1999;282:1530.
4. Ashwell M, et al. Obesity: new insight into the anthropometric classification of fat distribution shown by computed tomography. *Br Med J* 1985; 290:1692.
5. Baumgartner RN, et al. Bioelectric Impedance for Body Composition. In: Pandolf KB, Holloszy JO, eds. *Exercise and Sport Sciences Reviews.* Vol 18. Baltimore: Williams & Wilkins, 1990.
6. Beals KA, Manore MM. Behavioral, psychological, and physical characteristics of female athletes with subclinical eating disorders. *Int J Sport Nutr Exerc Metab* 2000;10:128.
7. Beckvid Henriksson G, et al. Women with menstrual dysfunction have prolonged interruption of training due to injury. *Gynecol Obstet Invest* 2000;49:41.
8. Bedogni G, et al. Comparison of bioelectrical impedance analysis and dual-energy x-ray absorptiometry for the assessment of appendicular body composition in anorexic women. *Eur J Clin Nutr* 2003;57:1068.
9. Behnke AR, Wilmore JH. *Evaluation and Regulation of Body Build and Composition.* Englewood Cliffs, NJ: Prentice Hall, 1974.
10. Behnke AR, et al. The specific gravity of healthy men. *JAMA* 1942;118:495.
11. Bemben DA, et al. Musculoskeletal responses to high- and low-intensity resistance training in early postmenopausal women. *Med Sci Sports Exerc* 2000;32:1949.
12. Billat V, et al. Training and bioenergetic characteristics in elite male and female Kenyan runners. *Med Sci Sports Exerc* 2003;35:297.
13. Bioelectrical impedance analysis in body composition measurement: National Institutes of Health technology assessment conference statement. *Am J Clin Nutr* 1996;64 (suppl):524S.
14. Bouchard C. Long-term programming of body size. *Nutr Rev* 1996;54:58.
15. Bouchard C, et al. Inheritance in the amount and distribution of human body fat. *Int J Obes* 1988;12:205.
16. Brandon LJ. Comparison of existing skinfold equations for estimating body fat in African American and white women. *Am J Clin Nutr* 1998;67:1115.
17. Bray GA, et al. Evaluation of body fat in fatter and leaner 10-y-old African American and white children: the Baton Rouge Children's Study. *Am J Clin Nutr* 2001;73:687.
18. Broeder CE, et al. Assessing body composition before and after resistance or endurance training. *Med Sci Sports Exerc* 1997;29:705.
19. Brooks-Gunn J, et al. The relation of eating problems and amenorrhea in ballet dancers. *Med Sci Sports Exerc* 1987;19:41.
20. Butts NK. Physiological profile of high school female cross-country runners. *Phys Sportsmed* 1983;10:103.
21. Cadarette SM, et al. Evaluation of decision rules for referring women for bone densitometry by dual-energy x-ray absorptiometry. *JAMA* 2001;286:57.
22. Calle EE, et al. Body-mass index and mortality in a prospective cohort of U.S. adults. *N Engl J Med* 1999;341:1097.
23. Calle EE, et al. Overweight, obesity, and mortality from cancer in a prospectively studied cohort of U.S. adults. *N Engl J Med* 2003;348:1625.
24. Carey D. The validity of anthropometric regression equations in predicting percent body fat in collegiate wrestlers. *J Sports Med Phys Fitness* 2000;40:254.
25. Carter JEL, Ackland TR. Kinanthropometry in Aquatic Sports: A Study of Worldclass Athletes. In: Carter JE, Ackland TR, eds. *Human Kinetics Sport Science Monograph Series.* Vol 5. Champaign, IL: Human Kinetics, 1994.
26. Cassady SL, et al. Validity of near infrared body composition analysis in children and adolescents. *Med Sci Sports Exerc* 1993;25:1185.
27. Caton JR, et al. Body composition by bioelectrical impedance: effect of skin temperature. *Med Sci Sports Exerc* 1988;20:489.
28. Chehab FF, et al. Early onset of reproductive function in normal female mice treated with leptin. *Science* 1997;275:88.
29. Clark RR, et al. A comparison of methods to predict minimal weight in high school wrestlers. *Med Sci Sports Exerc* 1993;25:1541.
30. Cobb KL, et al. Disordered eating, menstrual irregularity, and bone mineral density in female runners. *Med Sci Sports Exerc* 2003;35:711.
31. Collins MA, et al. Evaluation of the BOD POD for assessing body fat in collegiate football players. *Med Sci Sports Exerc* 1999;31:1350.
32. Committee refines wrestling safety rules. *NCAA News* 1998;35:1.

33. Constantine NW, Warren MP. Physical Activity, Fitness, and Reproductive Health in Women: Clinical Observations. In: Bouchard C, et al, eds. *Physical Activity, Fitness, and Health.* Champaign, IL: Human Kinetics, 1994.

34. Conway JM, et al. A new approach for the estimation of body composition: infrared interactance. *Am J Clin Nutr* 1984;40:1123.

35. Côté KD, Adams WC. Effect of bone density on body composition estimates in young adult black and white women. *Med Sci Sports Exerc* 1993;25:290.

36. Cureton TK. *Physical Fitness of Champion Athletes.* Urbana, IL: University of Illinois Press, 1951.

37. Dale KS, Landers DM. Weight control in wrestling: eating disorders or disordered eating? *Med Sci Sports Exerc* 1999;31:1382.

38. DeGaray AL, et al. *Genetic and Anthropological Studies of Olympic Athletes.* New York: Academic Press, 1974.

39. Diabetes Prevention Research Group. Reduction in the incidence of type 2 diabetes with lifestyle intervention or metformin. *N Engl J Med* 2002;346:393.

40. Eliakim A, et al. Assessment of body composition in ballet dancers: correlation among anthropometric measurements, bio-electrical impedance analysis, and dual-energy x-ray absorptiometry. *Int J Sports Med* 2000;21:598.

41. Ellis KJ, et al. Body composition of a young, multiethnic female population. *Am J Clin Nutr* 1997;65:724.

42. Engelen MP, et al. Dual-energy x-ray absorptiometry in the clinical evaluation of body composition and bone mineral density in patients with chronic obstructive pulmonary disease. *Am J Clin Nutr* 1998;68:1298.

43. Fahey T, et al. Body composition and V̇O₂max of exceptional weight-trained athletes. *J Appl Physiol* 1975;39:559.

44. Fernáandez JR, et al. Is percentage body fat differentially related to body mass index in Hispanic Americans, African Americans, and European Americans. *Am J Clin Nutr* 2003;77:71.

45. Fields DA, Goran MI. Body composition techniques and the four-compartment model in children. *J Appl Physiol* 2000;89:613.

46. Fields DA, et al. Validation of the BOD POD with hydrostatic weighing: influence of body clothing. *Int J Obes Relat Metab Disord* 2000;24:200.

47. Fields DA, et al. Comparison of BOD POD with the four-compartment model in adult females. *Med Sci Sports Exerc* 2001;33:1605.

48. Fields DA, et al. Body-composition assessment via air-displacement plethysmography in adults and children: a review. *Am J Clin Nutr* 2002;75:453.

49. Flegal KM, Troiano RP. Changes in the distribution of body mass index of adults and children in the US population. *Int J Obes Relat Metab Disord* 2000;24:807.

50. Flegal KM, et al. Prevalence and trends in obesity among US adults, 1999-2000. *JAMA* 2002;288:1723.

51. Flynn ML, et al. Fat storage in athletes: metabolic and hormonal responses to swimming and running. *Int J Sports Med* 1990;11:433.

52. Forbes RM, et al. The composition of the adult human body as determined by chemical analysis. *J Biol Chem* 1953;203:349.

53. Freedson PS, et al. Physique, body composition, and psychological characteristics of competitive female bodybuilders. *Phys Sportsmed* 1983;11:85.

54. Friedl KE, et al. Evaluation of anthropometric equations to assess body-composition changes in young women. *Am J Clin Nutr* 2001;73:268.

55. Frisch RE, et al. Delayed menarche and amenorrhea in ballet dancers. *N Engl J Med* 1980;303:17.

56. Frisch RE, et al. Lower lifetime occurrence of breast cancer and cancers of the reproductive system among former college athletes. *Am J Clin Nutr* 1987;45:328.

57. Goodpaster BH, et al. Composition of skeletal muscle evaluated with computed tomography. *Ann NY Acad Sci* 2000;904:18.

58. Gore CJ, et al. Skinfold thickness varies directly with spring coefficient and inversely with jaw pressure. *Med Sci Sports Exerc* 2000;32:540.

59. Gower BA, et al. Effects of weight loss on changes in insulin sensitivity and lipid concentrations in premenopausal African American and white women. *Am J Clin Nutr* 2002;76:923.

60. Harp JB, Hecht L. Obesity in the National Football League. *JAMA* 2005; 293:1061.

61. Hetland ML, et al. Running induces menstrual irregularities but bone mass is unaffected, except in amenorrheic women. *Am J Med* 1993;95:53.

62. Heyward VH, Stolarczyk LM. *Applied Body Composition Assessment.* Champaign, IL: Human Kinetics, 1996.

63. Hicks VL, et al. Validation of near-infrared interactance and skinfold methods for estimating body composition of American Indian women. *Med Sci Sports Exerc* 2000;32:531.

64. Hill JO, Peters JC. Environmental contributions to the obesity epidemic. *Science* 1998;280:1371.

65. Hiura Y, et al. Hypertriglyceridemic waist as a screening tool for CVD risk in indigenous Australian women. *Ethn Dis* 2003;13:80.

66. Hirata K. Physique and age of Tokyo Olympic champions. *J Sports Med Phys Fitness* 1966;6:207.

67. Holly RG, et al. Triathlete characterization and response to prolonged competition. *Med Sci Sports Exerc* 1986;18:123.

68. Hortobagyi T, et al. Comparison of four methods to assess body composition in black and white athletes. *Int J Sports* Nutr 1992;2:60.

69. Houmard JA, et al. Validity of a near-infrared device for estimating body composition in a college football team. *J Appl Sport Sci Res* 1991;5:53.

70. Housh TJ, et al. Validity of near-infrared interactance instruments for estimating percent body fat in youth wrestlers. *Pediatr Exerc Sci* 1996;8:69.

71. Houtkooper LB, et al. Comparison of methods for assessing body-composition changes over 1 y in postmenopausal women. *Am J Clin Nutr* 2000;72:401.

72. Hu FB, et al. Trends in the incidence of coronary heart disease and changes in diet and lifestyle in women. *N Engl J Med* 2000;343:530.

73. Hunter GR, et al. Fat distribution, physical activity, and cardiovascular risk factors. *Med Sci Sports Exerc* 1997;29:362.

74. Israel RG, et al. Validity of near-infrared spectrophotometry device for estimating human body composition. *Res Q Exerc Sport* 1989;60:379.

75. Istook E Jr. Research funding on major disease is not proportionate to taxpayers' needs. *J NIH Res* 1997;9:26.

76. Jackson AS, Pollock ML. Generalized equations for predicting body density of men. *Br J Nutr* 1978;40:497.

77. Jackson AS, et al. Generalized equations for predicting body density of women. *Med Sci Sports* 1980;12:175.

78. Jackson AS, et al. The effect of sex, age and race on estimating percentage body fat from body mass index: the Heritage Family Study. *Int J Obes* 2002;26:789.

79. Jang KT, et al. Energy balance in competitive swimmers and runners. *J Swim Res* 1987;3:19.

80. Janssen I, et al. Skeletal muscle mass and distribution in 468 men and women aged 18-88 yr. *J Appl Physiol* 2000;89:81.

81. Janssen I, et al. Body mass index and waist circumference independently contribute to prediction of nonabdominal, abdominal subcutaneous, and visceral fat. *Am J Clin Nutr* 2002;75:683.

82. Janssen I, et al. Fitness alters the associations of BMI and waist circumference with total and abdominal fat. *Obes Res* 2004;12:525.

83. Johnston FE. Body fat deposition in adult obese women. Part 1. Patterns of fat distribution. *Am J Clin Nutr* 1988;47:225.

84. Jurimae T, et al. Relationships between plasma leptin levels and body composition parameters measured by different methods in postmenopausal women. *Am J Hum Biol* 2003;15:628.

85. Kamba M, et al. Proton magnetic resonance spectroscopy for assessment of human body composition. *Am J Clin Nutr* 2001;73:172.

86. Katch FI, Katch VL. Measurement and prediction errors in body composition assessment and the search for the perfect prediction equation. *Res Q Exerc Sport* 1980;51:249.

87. Katch FI, McArdle WD. Prediction of body density from simple anthropometric measurements in college-age men and women. *Hum Biol* 1973;45:445.

88. Katch FI, McArdle WD. Validity of body composition prediction equations for college men and women. *Am J Clin Nutr* 1975;28:105.

89. Katch FI, Michael ED. Prediction of body density from skinfold and girth measurements of college females. *J Appl Physiol* 1968; 25:92.

90. Katch FI, Spiak DL. Validity of the Mellits and Cheek method for body-fat estimation in relation to menstrual cycle status in athletes and non-athletes below 22 percent fat. *Ann Hum Biol* 1984;11:389.

91. Katch FI, et al. Effects of physical training on the body composition and diet of females. *Res Q* 1969;40:99.

92. Katch FI, et al. The underweight female. *Phys Sportsmed* 1980;8:55.

93. Katch VL, et al. Contribution of breast volume and weight to body fat distribution in females. *Am J Phys Anthropol* 1980;53:93.

94. Katch VL, et al. Muscular development and lean body weight in body-builders and weightlifters. *Med Sci Sports* 1980;12:340.

95. Kenchaiah S, et al. Obesity and the risk of heart failure. *N Engl J Med* 2002;347:305.

96. Keys A, et al. *The Biology of Human Starvation.* Minneapolis, University of Minnesota Press, 1950.

97. Kim J, et al. Total-body skeletal muscle mass: estimation by a new dual-energy x-ray absorptiometry method. *Am J Clin Nutr* 2002;76:378.

98. Kohlraush W. Zusammenhang von Korperform und Leistung. Ergebnisse der anthropometrischen Messungen an der Athletern der Amsterdamer Olympiade. *Int Z Angrew Physiol* 1970;2:187.

99. Kohrt WM. Preliminary evidence that DEXA provides an accurate assessment of body composition. *J Appl Physiol* 1998;84:372.

100. Kondo M, et al. Upper limit of fat-free mass in humans: a study of Japanese sumo wrestlers. *Am J Hum Biol* 1994;6:613.

101. Koulmann N, et al. Use of bioelectrical impedance analysis to estimate body fluid compartments after acute variations of the body hydration level. *Med Sci Sports Exerc* 2000;32:857.

102. Kuczmarski RJ, Flegal KM. Criteria for definition of overweight in transition: background and recommendations for the United States. *Am J Clin Nutr* 2000;72:1074.

103. Kuk JL, et al. Waist circumference and abdominal adipose tissue distribution: influence of age and sex. *Am J Clin Nutr* 2005;81:1300

104. Kushner RF, et al. Clinical characteristics influencing bioelectrical impedance analysis measurements. *Am J Clin Nutr* 1996;64(suppl):423S.

105. Kyle UG, et al. Physical activity and fat-free and fat mass by bioelectrical impedance in 3853 adults. *Med Sci Sports Exerc* 2001;33:576.

106. Laurson KR, Eisenmann JC. Prevalence of overweight among high school football linemen. *JAMA* 2007;297:363.

107. LeBlanc A, et al. Muscle volume, MRI relaxation times (T2), and body composition after spaceflight. *J Appl Physiol* 2000;89:2158.

108. Lee CD, et al. Cardiorespiratory fitness, body composition, and all-cause and cardiovascular disease mortality in men. *Am J Clin Nutr* 1999;69:373.

109. Lee I-M, et al. U.S. weight guidelines: is it also important to consider cardiorespiratory fitness? *Int J Obes* 1998;22:S2.

110. Lee RC, et al. Total-body skeletal muscle mass: development and cross-validation of anthropometric prediction models. *Am J Clin Nutr* 2000;72:796.

111. Lehtonen-Veromaa M, et al. Influence of physical activity on ultrasound and dual-energy x-ray absorptiometry bone measurements in peripubertal girls: a cross-sectional study. *Calcif Tissue Int* 2000; 66:248.

112. Lockner DW, et al. Comparison of air-displacement plethysmography, hydrodensitometry, and dual-energy x-ray absorptiometry for assessing body composition of children 10 to 18 years of age. *Ann NY Acad Sci* 2000;904:72.

113. Lohman TG, Going SB. Multicomponent models in body composition research: opportunities and pitfalls. *Basic Life Sci* 1993;60:53.

114. Lohman TG, et al. Assessing body composition and changes in body composition: another look at dual-energy x-ray absorptiometry. *Ann NY Acad Sci* 2000;904:45.

115. Long TD, et al. Lack of menstrual cycle effects on hypothalamic-pituitary-adrenal axis response to insulin-induced hypoglycaemia. *Clin Endocrinol (Oxf)* 2000;52:781.

116. Loucks AB. Energy availability, not body fatness, regulates reproductive function in women. *Exerc Sport Sci Rev* 2003;31:144.

117. Loucks AB. Callister R. Induction and prevention of low-T3 syndrome in exercising women. *Am J Physiol* 1993;264:R924.

118. Loucks AB, et al. Hypothalamic-pituitary-thyroidal function in eumenorrheic and amenorrheic athletes. *J Clin Endocrinol Metabol* 1992;75:514.

119. Lukaski HC. Methods for the assessment of human body composition: traditional and new. *Am J Clin Nutr* 1987;46:537.

120. Maddalozzo GF, Snow CM. High intensity resistance training: effects on bone in older men and women. *Calcif Tissue Int* 2000;66:399.

121. McCrory MA, et al. Evaluation of a new air displacement plethysmograph for measuring human body composition. *Med Sci Sports Exerc* 1995;27:1686.

122. McKee JE, Cameron N. Bioelectrical impedance changes during the menstrual cycle. *Am J Hum Biol* 1997;9:155.

123. McLean K, Skinner JS. Validity of the Futrex-5000 for body composition determination. *Med Sci Sports Exerc* 1992;24:253.

124. Mei Z, et al. Validity of body mass index compared with other body-composition screening indexes for the assessment of body fatness in children and adolescents. *Am J Clin Nutr* 2002;75:978.

125. Meyer HE, et al. Body mass index and mortality: the influence of physical activity and smoking. *Med Sci Sports Exerc* 2002;34:1065.

126. Millard-Stafford ML, et al. Use of air displacement plethysmography for estimating body fat in a four-component model. *Med Sci Sports Exerc* 2001;33:1311.

127. Mitchell HH, et al. The chemical composition of the adult human body and its bearing on the biochemistry of growth. *J Biol Chem* 1945;158,625.

128. Mitsiopoulos N, et al. Cadaver validation of skeletal muscle measurement by magnetic resonance imaging and computerized tomography. *J Appl Physiol* 1998;85:115.

129. Miyatani M, et al. Validity of bioelectrical impedance and ultrasonographic methods for estimating the muscle volume of the upper arm. *Eur J Appl Physiol* 2000;82:391.

130. Modlesky CM, et al. Density of the fat-free mass and estimates of body composition in male weight trainers. *J Appl Physiol* 1996;80:2085.

131. Must A, et al. The disease burden associated with overweight and obesity. *JAMA* 1999;282:1523.

132. National Institutes of Health, National Heart, Lung, and Blood Institute. Clinical guidelines on the identification, evaluation and treatment of overweight and obesity in adults: the evidence report. *Obes Res* 1998;6(suppl):51S.

133. National Task Force on the Prevention and Treatment of Obesity. Obesity, overweight and health risk. *Arch Intern Med* 2000;160:898.

134. Nelson ME, et al. Analysis of body composition techniques and models for detecting change in soft tissue with strength training. *Am J Clin Nutr* 1996;63:678.

135. O'Brien C, et al. Bioelectrical impedance to estimate changes in hydration status. *Int J Sports Med* 2002;23:361.

136. Oppliger RA, et al. Bioelectrical impedance prediction of fat-free mass for high school wrestlers validated. *Med Sci Sports Exerc* 1991;23:S73.

137. Oppliger RA, et al. Body composition of collegiate football players: bioelectrical impedance and skinfolds compared to hydrostatic weighing. *J Orthop Sports Phys Ther* 1992;15:187.

138. Oppliger RA, et al. NCAA rule change improves weight loss among national championship wrestlers. *Med Sci Sports Exerc* 2006;38:963.

139. Ortiz O, et al. Differences in skeletal muscle and bone mineral mass between black and white females and their relevance to estimates of body composition. *Am J Clin Nutr* 1992;55:8.

140. O'Toole ML. Training for ultraendurance triathletes. *Med Sci Sports Exerc* 1989;21:209.

141. O'Toole M., et al. The ultraendurance triathlete: a physiological profile. *Med Sci Sports Exerc* 1987;19:45.

142. Peterson MJ, et al. Development and validation of skinfold-thickness prediction equations with a 4-compartment model. *Am J Clin Nutr* 2003;77:1186.

143. Phillips SM, et al. A longitudinal comparison of body composition by total body water and bioelectrical impedance in adolescent girls. *J Nutr* 2003;133:1419.

144. Popowski LA, et al. Blood and urinary measures of hydration status during progressive acute dehydration. *Med Sci Sports Exerc* 2001;33:747.

145. Quesenberry CP, et al. Obesity, health services use, and health care costs among members of a health maintenance organization. *Arch Intern Med* 1998;158:466.

146. Roemmich JN, Sinning WE. Weight loss and wrestling training: effects of nutrition, growth, maturation, body composition, and strength. *J Appl Physiol* 1997;82:1751.

147. Sady SP, et al. Physiological characteristics of high-ability prepubescent wrestlers. *Med Sci Sports Exerc* 1984;16:72.

148. Salamone LM, et al. Measurement of fat mass using DEXA: a validation study in elderly adults. *J Appl Physiol* 2000;89:345.

149. Sardinha LB, et al. Comparison of air displacement plethysmography with dual-energy absorptiometry and 3 field methods for estimating body composition in middle-aged men. *Am J Clin Nutr* 1998;68:786.

150. Sartorio A, et al. Changes of bioelectrical impedance after a body weight reduction program in highly obese subjects. *Diabetes Nutr Metab* 2000;13:186.

151. Saunders MJ, et al. Effects of hydration changes on bioelectrical impedance in endurance trained individuals. *Med Sci Sports Exerc* 1998;30:885.

152. Schaumberg DA, et al. Relations of body fat distribution and height with cataract in men. *Am J Clin Nutr* 2000;72:1495.

153. Schmidt WD. Strength and physiological characteristics of NCAA Division III American football players. *J Strength Cond Res* 1999;13:210.

154. Schrager MA, et al. Sarcopenic obesity and inflammation in the CHIANTI study. *J Appl Physiol* 2007;102:919.

155. Schutte JE, et al. Density of lean body mass is greater in blacks than whites. *J Appl Physiol* 1984;56:1647.

156. Schwimmer JB, et al. Health-related quality of life of severely obese children and adolescents. *JAMA* 2003;289:1851.

157. Scott JR, et al. Acute weight gain in collegiate wrestlers following a tournament weigh-in. *Med Sci Sports Exerc* 1994;26:1181.

158. Segal KR. Use of bioelectrical impedance analysis measurements as an evaluation for participating in sports. *Am J Clin Nutr* 1996;64 (suppl):469S.

159. Segal K, et al. Lean body mass estimation by bioelectrical impedance analysis: a four-site cross-validation study. *Am J Clin Nutr* 1988;47:7.

160. Seidell JC, et al. Abdominal fat depots measured with computed tomography: effects of degree of obesity, sex, and age. *Eur J Clin Nutr* 1988;42:805.

161. Seidell JC, et al. Waist and hip circumferences have independent and opposite effects on cardiovascular disease risk factors: the Quebec Family Study. *Am J Clin Nutr* 2001;74:315.

162. Shangold MM, et al. Evaluation and management of menstrual dysfunction in athletes. *JAMA* 1990;262:1665.

163. Sinha R, et al. Prevalence of impaired glucose tolerance among children and adolescents with marked obesity. *N Engl J Med* 2002;346: 802.

164. Sinning WE. Body composition, cardiorespiratory function, and rule changes in women's basketball. *Res Q* 1973;44:313.

165. Sinning WE, Lindberg GD. Physical characteristics of college age women gymnasts. *Res Q* 1972;43:226.

166. Sinning WE, et al. Validity of "generalized" equations for body composition analysis in male athletes. *Med Sci Sports Exerc* 1985;17:124.

167. Slinde F, Rossander-Hulthén L. Bioelectrical impedance effect of 3 identical meals on diurnal impedance variation and calculation of body composition. *Am J Clin Nutr* 2001;74:474.

168. Stolarczyk LM, et al. Predictive accuracy of bioelectrical impedance in estimating fat-free mass of Hispanic women. *Med Sci Sports Exerc* 1995;27:1450.

169. Stolarczyk LM, et al. The fatness-specific bioelectrical impedance analysis equations of Segal et al: are they generalizable and practical? *Am J Clin Nutr* 1997;66:8.

170. Stollk RP, et al. Ultrasound measurements of intraabdominal fat estimate the metabolic syndrome better than do measurements of waist circumference. *Am J Clin Nutr* 2003;77:857.

171. Stuempfle KJ, et al. Body composition relates poorly to performance tests in NCAA Division III football players. *J Strength Cond Res* 2003;17:238.

172. Sun SS, et al. Development of bioelectrical impedance analysis prediction equations for body composition with the use of a multicomponent model for use in epidemiologic surveys. *Am J Clin Nutr* 2003;77:331.

173. Tanner JM. *The physique of the Olympic Athlete.* London: Allen & Unwin, 1964.

174. Thomas EL, et al. Magnetic resonance imaging of total body fat. *J Appl Physiol* 1998;85:1778.

175. Thong FS, et al. Plasma leptin in female athletes: relationship with body fat, reproductive, nutritional, and endocrine factors. *J Appl Physiol* 2000;88:2037.

176. Thorland WG, et al. Midwest wrestling study: prediction of minimal weight for high school wrestlers. *Med Sci Sports Exerc* 1991;23:1102.

177. Thorland WG, et al. Estimation of body composition in black adolescent male athletes. *Pediatr Exerc Sci* 1993;5:116.

178. Tipton C.M, Oppliger RA. Nutritional and fitness considerations for competitive wrestlers. In: Simopoulos AP, Pavlou KN, eds. Nutrition and fitness for athletes. *World Rev Nutr Diet* 1993;71:84.

179. Tran ZV, Weltman A. Predicting body composition of men from girth measurements. *Hum Biol* 1988;60:167.

180. Tran ZV, Weltman A. Generalized equation for predicting body density of women from girth measurements. *Med Sci Sports Exerc* 1989;21:101.

181. Trichopoulou A, et al. Physical activity and energy intake selectively predict the waist-to-hip ratio in men but not in women. *Am J Clin Nutr* 2001;74:574.

182. Taai C-J, et al. Prospective study of abdominal obesity and gallstone disease in U S men. *Am J Clin Nutr* 2005;80:38.

183. US Department of Agriculture and US Department of Health and Human Services. Nutrition and your health: dietary guidelines for America. Washington, DC: US Government Printing Office, 2000 (Home and Garden bulletin no. 232.)

184. Utter AC, et al. Evaluation of air displacement for assessing body composition of collegiate wrestlers. *Med Sci Sports Exerc* 2003;35:500.

185. van der Ploeg GE, et al. Use of anthropometric variables to predict relative body fat determined by a four-compartment body composition model. *Eur J Clin Nutr* 2003;57:1009.

186. Vehrs P, et al. Reliability and concurrent validity of Futrex and bioelectrical impedance. *Int J Sports Med* 1998;19:560.

187. Vescovi JD, et al. Evaluation of the BOD POD for estimating percentage body fat in a heterogeneous group of human adults. *Eur J Appl Physiol* 2001;85:326.

188. Vescovi JD, et al. Effects of clothing on accuracy and reliability of air displacement plethysmography. *Med Sci Sports Med* 2002;34:282.

189. von Eyben FE, et al. Intra-abdominal obesity and metabolic risk factors: a study of young adults. *Int J Obes Relat Metab Disord* 2003;27:941.

190. Wagner DR, et al. Predictive accuracy of BIA equations for estimating fat-free mass of black men. *Med Sci Sports Exerc* 1997;29:969.

191. Wagner DR, et al. Validation of air displacement plethysmography for assessing body composition. *Med Sci Sports Exerc* 2000;32:1339.

192. Wagner DR, et al. Validity of two component models for estimating body fat of black men. *J Appl Physiol* 2001;90:649.

193. Walberg JL, Johnston CS. Menstrual function and eating behavior in female recreational weight lifters and competitive body builders. *Med Sci Sports Exerc* 1991;23:30.

194. Wang MQ, et al. Changes in body size of elite high school football players: 1963-1989. *Percept Mot Skills* 1993;76:379.

195. Ward IC, et al. Reliability of multiple frequency bioelectrical impedance analysis: an intermachine comparison. *Am J Hum Biol* 1997;9:63.

196. Warren MP. The effects of exercise on pubertal progression and reproductive function. *J Clin Endocrinol Metab* 1980;51:1150.

197. Welham WC, Behnke AR. The specific gravity of healthy men. *JAMA* 1942;118:498.

198. Weltman A, et al. Accurate assessment of body composition in obese females. *Am J Clin Nutr* 1988;48:1179.

199. Weyers AM, et al. Comparison of methods for assessing body composition changers during weight loss. *Med Sci Sports Exerc* 2002;34:497.

200. Wickelgren I. Obesity: how big a problem? *Science* 1998;280:1364.

201. Wickkiser JD, Kelly JM. The body composition of a college football team. *Med Sci Sports* 1975;7:199.

202. Williams MJ, et al. Regional fat distribution in women and risk of cardiovascular disease. *Am J Clin Nutr* 1997;65:855.

203. Williams NL. Lessons from experimental disruptions of the menstrual cycle in humans and monkeys. *Med Sci Sports Exerc* 2003;35:1564.

204. Wilmore JH, Haskell WL. Body composition and endurance capacity of professional football players. *J Appl Physiol* 1972;33:564.

205. Winters KM, Snow CM. Detraining reverses positive effects of exercise on the musculoskeletal system in premenopausal women. *J Bone Miner Res* 2000;15:2495.

206. Wolk A, et al. A prospective study of obesity and cancer risk. *Cancer Causes Control* 2001;12:2001.

207. Wroble RR, Moxley DP. Acute weight gain and its relationship to success in high school wrestlers. *Med Sci Sports Exerc* 1998;30: 949.

208. Wroble RR, Moxley DP. Weight loss patterns and success rates in high school wrestlers. *Med Sci Sports Exerc* 1998;30:625.

209. Yanovski JA, et al. Differences in body composition of black and white girls. *Am J Clin Nutr* 1996;64:833.

210. Yeager KK, et al. The female athlete triad: disordered eating, amenorrhea, and osteoporosis. *Med Sci Sports Exerc* 1993;25:775.

211. Yee AJ, et al. Calibration and validation of an air-displacement plethysmography method for estimating body fat in an elderly population: a comparison among compartmental methods. *Am J Clin Nutr* 2001;74:637.

212. Zhu S, et al. Waist circumference and obesity-associated risk factors among whites in the third National Health and Nutrition Examination Survey: clinical action thresholds. *Am J Clin Nutr* 2002;76: 743.

Additional Readings

Aghdassi E, et al. Estimation of body fat mass using dual-energy x-ray absorptiometry, bioelectric impedance analysis, and anthropometry in HIV-positive male subjects receiving highly active antiretroviral therapy. *J Parenter Enteral Nutr* 2007;31:135.

Aleman Mateo H, et al. Determination of body composition using air displacement plethysmography, anthropometry and bio-electrical impedance in rural elderly Mexican men and women. *J Nutr Health Aging* 2004;8:344.

Aleman-Mateo H, et al. Body composition by three-compartment model and relative validity of some methods to assess percentage body fat in Mexican healthy elderly subjects. *Gerontology* 2004;50:366.

Al-Nakeeb Y, et al. Body fatness and physical activity levels of young children. *Ann Hum Biol* 2007;34:1.

Anderson DE. Reliability of air displacement plethysmography. *J Strength Cond Res* 2007;21:169.

Andreacci JL, et al. Effect of a maximal treadmill test on percent body fat using leg-to-leg bioelectrical impedance analysis in children. *J Sports Med Phys Fitness* 2006;46:454.

Bosy-Westphal A, et al. Value of body fat mass vs anthropometric obesity indices in the assessment of metabolic risk factors. *Int J Obes (Lond)* 2006;30:475.

Davis JA, et al. Reliability and validity of the lung volume measurement made by the BOD POD body composition system. *Clin Physiol Funct Imaging* 2007;27:42.

Ellis KJ, et al. Body-composition assessment in infancy: air-displacement plethysmography compared with a reference 4-compartment model. *Am J Clin Nutr* 2007;85:90.

Garnett SP, et al. Relation between hormones and body composition, including bone, in prepubertal children. *Am J Clin Nutr* 2004;80:966.

Hill AM, et al. Estimating abdominal adipose tissue with DXA and anthropometry. *Obesity* (Silver Spring). 2007;15:504.

Himes JH. Long-term longitudinal studies and implications for the development of an international growth reference for children and adolescents. *Food Nutr Bull* 2006;27(4 suppl Growth Standard):S199 [Review].

Hoffman DJ, et al. Changes in body weight and fat mass of men and women in the first year of college: a study of the "freshman 15." *J Am Coll Health* 2006;55:41.

Kagawa M, et al. Body composition and anthropometry in Japanese and Australian Caucasian males and Japanese females. *Asia Pac J Clin Nutr* 2007;16(suppl 1):31.

Kagawa M, et al. New percentage body fat prediction equations for Japanese females. *J Physiol Anthropol* 2007;26:23.

Ketel IJ, et al. Superiority of skinfold measurements and waist over waist-to-hip ratio for determination of body fat distribution in a population-based cohort of Caucasian Dutch adults. *Eur J Endocrinol* 2007;156:655.

Kraemer M. A new model for the determination of fluid status and body composition from bioimpedance measurements. *Physiol Meas* 2006;27:901.

Larssoln I, et al. Body composition in the SOS (Swedish Obese Subjects) reference study. *Int J Obes Relat Metab Disord* 2004;28:1317.

Laurson KR, Eisenmann JC. Prevalence of overweight among high school football linemen. *JAMA* 2007;297:363.

Lim S, et al. Body composition changes with age have gender-specific impacts on bone mineral density. *Bone* 2004;35:792.

Luchsinger JA, et al. Measures of adiposity and dementia risk in elderly persons. *Arch Neurol* 2007;64:392.

Mahon AK, et al. Measurement of body composition changes with weight loss in postmenopausal women: comparison of methods. *J Nutr Health Aging* 2007;11:203.

McCarthy HD. Body fat measurements in children as predictors for the metabolic syndrome: focus on waist circumference. *Proc Nutr Soc* 2006;65:385 [Review].

Mei Z, et al. Do skinfold measurements provide additional information to body mass index in the assessment of body fatness among children and adolescents? *Pediatrics* 2007;119:e1306.

Midorikawa T, High REE in Sumo wrestlers attributed to large organ-tissue mass. *Med Sci Sports Exerc* 2007;39:688.

Miller JC, et al. DXA measurements confirm that parental perceptions of elevated adiposity in young children are poor. *Obesity* (Silver Spring) 2007;15:165.

Mok E, et al. Estimating body composition in children with Duchenne muscular dystrophy: comparison of bioelectrical impedance analysis and skinfold-thickness measurement. *Am J Clin Nutr* 2006;83:65.

Neovius MG, et al. Sensitivity and specificity of classification systems for fatness in adolescents. *Am J Clin Nutr* 2004;80:597.

Noreen EE, Lemon PW. Reliability of air displacement plethysmography in a large, heterogeneous sample. *Med Sci Sports Exerc* 2006;38:1505.

Norgan NG. Laboratory and field measurements of body composition. *Public Health Nutr* 2005;8A:1108 [Review].

Ode JJ, et al. Body mass index as a predictor of percent fat in college athletes and nonathletes. *Med Sci Sports Exerc* 2007;39:403.

Ostojic SM. Estimation of body fat in athletes: skinfolds vs bioelectrical impedance. *J Sports Med Phys Fitness* 2006;46:442.

Rance M, et al. Lower-limb and whole-body tissue composition assessment in healthy active older women. *Ann Hum Biol* 2006;33:89.

Ruhl CE, et al. Body mass index and serum leptin concentration independently estimate percentage body fat in older adults. *Am J Clin Nutr* 2007;85:1121.

Siegel MJ, et al. Total and intraabdominal fat distribution in preadolescents and adolescents: measurement with MR imaging. *Radiology* 2007;242:846.

Slattery ML, et al. Energy balance and rectal cancer: an evaluation of energy intake, energy expenditure, and body mass index. *Nutr Cancer* 2003;46:166

St-Onge MP, et al. Dual-energy x-ray absorptiometry-measured lean soft tissue mass: differing relation to body cell mass across the adult life span. *J Gerontol A Biol Sci Med Sci* 2004;59:796.

Tanaka S, et al. MR measurement of visceral fat: assessment of metabolic syndrome. *Magn Reson Med Sci* 2006;5:207.

Toscani M, et al. Estimation of truncal adiposity using waist circumference or the sum of trunk skinfolds: a pilot study for insulin resistance screening in hirsute patients with or without polycystic ovary syndrome. *Metabolism* 2007;56:992.

van Marken Lichtenbelt WD, et al. Body composition changes in body-builders: a method comparison. *Med Sci Sports Exerc* 2004;36:490.

Varady KA, et al. Validation of hand-held bioelectrical impedance analysis with magnetic resonance imaging for the assessment of body composition in overweight women. *Am J Hum Biol* 2007;19:429.

Warren M, et al. The relation between visceral fat measurement and torso level: is one level better than another? The Atherosclerosis Risk in Communities Study, 1990-1992. *Am J Epidemiol* 2006;163:352.

Zhang TM, et al. Assessment of total body fat percentage from regional spine and femur DXA measurements among Chinese women and men. *J Clin Densitom* 2007;10:55.

Zhu F, et al. Application of bioimpedance techniques to peritoneal dialysis. *Contrib Nephrol* 2006;150:119 [Review].

Zoico E, et al. High baseline values of fat mass, independently of appendicular skeletal mass, predict 2-year onset of disability in elderly subjects at the high end of the functional spectrum. *Aging Clin Exp Res* 2007;19:154.

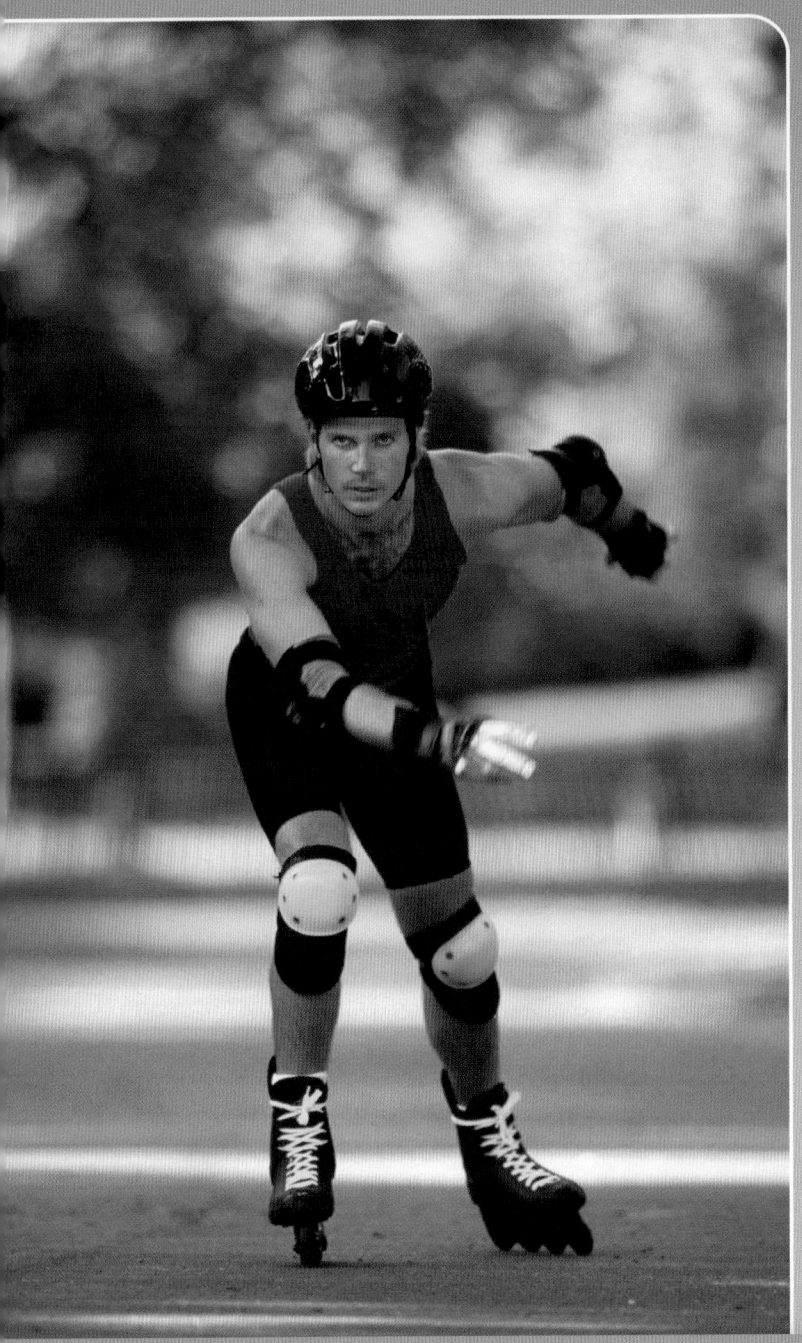

Chapter **14**

Energy Balance, Exercise, and Weight Control

The Appropriate Diet Plan: Well Balanced But Less of It

Maximizing Chances for Success with Dieting

- Personal Assessment: The Important First Step

- Behavioral Approaches Can Help: Modification of Eating Behaviors

Exercise for Weight Control

- Weight Gain: Not Simply a Problem of Gluttony

- Total Daily Energy Expenditure

- Effectiveness of Increasing Energy Expenditure

- The Ideal: Conserve Lean and Reduce Fat

- A Dose–Response Relationship

Maximizing Chances for Success with Increased Physical Activity: Modification of Exercise Behaviors

- Describe the Behavior for Modification

- Substitute Alternative Behaviors

- Maximize Success

Alternative Exercise Behaviors

Food Restriction Plus Increased Physical Activity

- Setting a Realistic Target Time

Spot Reduction Does Not Work

- Where on the Body Does Fat Loss Occur?

Possible Gender Difference in Exercise Effects on Weight Loss

Effects of Diet and Exercise on Body Composition During Weight Loss

Weight Loss Recommendations for Wrestlers and Other Power Athletes

- Adolescent Female Gymnasts

Gaining Weight: A Unique Dilemma for Physically Active Individuals

- Increase the Lean, Not the Fat

- How Much Lean Tissue Gain to Expect?

Test Your Knowledge

Answer these 10 statements about energy balance, exercise, and weight control. Use the scoring key at the end of the chapter to check your results. Repeat this test after you have read the chapter and compare your results.

1. **T F**   A global obesity epidemic currently exists.
2. **T F**   No "racial" differences exist in the prevalence of obesity; overfatness does not discriminate.
3. **T F**   Dietary approaches offer the best defense against regaining lost body weight.
4. **T F**   Weight gain is an inevitable consequence of aging.
5. **T F**   The most prudent approach to weight control combines moderate food restriction with increased daily physical activity.
6. **T F**   The body reduces basal energy expenditure during weight loss by food restriction.
7. **T F**   Very low calorie diets (VLCDs) offer the best and fastest method to successfully induce weight loss.
8. **T F**   Simply stated, excessive food intake produces weight gain.
9. **T F**   Increasing regular physical activity improves one's health status but does little for weight control because of the few number of calories expended during most physical activities.
10. **T F**   One must engage in aerobic exercises for weight loss; weight/resistance exercises offer little value.

The annual food intake for adults in the United States (National Agricultural Statistics Service: www.nass.usda.gov) averages above 900 kg (1985 lb) and includes approximately 116 kg of eggs, 87 kg of flour and cereal products, 51 kg of red meats (33 kg of poultry), 8 kg of fish and shellfish, 14 kg of cheese, 64 kg of caloric sweeteners, 41 kg of fats and oils, 314 kg of fruits and vegetables, 435 soft drinks, 9 L of wine and almost 100 L of beer and 10 L of liquor! Physically active men and women often consume 50% more of many of these same foods. Only when calories from food exceed daily energy requirements do excess calories store mainly as fat in adipose tissue. Slight but prolonged caloric excess produces substantial weight gain. Eating an extra 2 oz of roasted peanuts daily, for example, theoretically would produce a weight gain of about 7.3 kg (16 lb) in 1 year. Energy output must balance energy input to prevent such a caloric disparity. Unfortunately. energy balance is often not achieved, producing a national and global crisis in excess caloric consumption and an epidemic of overweightness and obesity.

A random-digit telephone survey of nearly 110,000 U.S. adults found that nearly 70% struggle to either lose weight (29% of men and 40% of women) or just maintain it.[148] Only one fifth of the 45 to 50 million Americans trying to lose weight follow the recommended combination of eating fewer calories and engaging in at least 150 minutes of moderate physical activity weekly. Those attempting weight loss spent nearly $40 billion in the year 2000 (projected to exceed $60 billion in 2008) on weight-reduction products and services, often engaging in potentially harmful dietary practices and drug use while ignoring sensible approaches to weight loss.[15,31,140] More than 2 million Americans collectively spend $150 million or more on over-the-counter appetite-suppressing diet pills that line the shelves of drugstores, health food and fitness centers, and supermarkets, not to mention sales via TV and radio marketing, mail order, and the Internet.

Despite the upswing in attempts at weight loss, Americans have become shamefully more overweight than a generation ago, with obesity increasing in all regions of the United States (FIG. 14.1).[109,110]

Some States Are Fatter Than Others

According to the latest 2005 data from the Centers for Disease Control Behavioral Risk Factor Surveillance Survey (www.cdc.gov/nccdphp/dnpa/obesity/trend/maps/), only four states in 2005 had obesity prevalence rates less than 20%, while 17 states had prevalence rates equal to or exceeding 25%—with Mississippi and West Virginia exceeding 30%!

Figure 14.1 compares national surveys of overweight and obesity prevalence among adults in the United States during the measurement periods 1990, 1998, and 2006. Current classification by the National Heart Lung and Blood Institute

(www.nhlbi.org) defines "overweight" as a BMI of 25 to 29.9 and "obesity" as a BMI equal to or greater than 30. These standards place the prevalence of overweight and obesity in adults at about 130 million Americans, or 65% of the population (including 35% of college students, up from 56% in 1982). Overweight occurrence particularly affects women and minority groups (Hispanic, African American, Pacific Islander). The major increase occurs from a near doubling of the obesity component to one in four Americans over the past two decades.[149,258] As of July 2006, about 31% of the adult population or 60+ million people classify as obese compared with only 14.5% in 1980; similar increases in obesity exist worldwide.[80,151,184,249]

A Significant and Expensive Risk to Health

The Centers for Disease Control and Prevention (www.cdc.gov) ranks obesity as a close second to cigarette smoking as the leading cause of preventable death in America. Fourteen percent of the money spent on health care for American men ages 50 to 69 went to obesity-related complications. If the body mass of the nation continues to increase at the current rate, obesity will account for about one in five health care dollars spent on middle-aged Americans by the year 2020.

On a worldwide basis, the thousands of consumer books published over the past 25 years that advocate fad and bizarre diets or exercise plans for weight loss share one common thread—most claim their easy-to-use plans guarantee results. If this were true, and a simple solution could maintain the "perfect" body size permanently, then the large number of overly fat Americans could be readily cured. Even when an advertising blitz popularizes a diet plan by "documenting" dramatic weight loss or enlisting testimonials and success stories from actors and athletes, such schemes often jeopardize the dieter's health. An additional negative effect of inappropriate strategies for weight loss entails the increased likelihood of impaired physiologic function and exercise performance.

WORLDWIDE EPIDEMIC

Increases in obesity worldwide have contributed to the rising tide of type 2 diabetes and cardiovascular disease, prompting the World Health Organization (WHO; www.who.int/en) and International Obesity Task Force (www.iotf.org) to declare a global **obesity epidemic**.[118,159] FIGURE 14.2 depicts the powerful effect of excess body weight in predicting death at older age. Overweight but not obese, nonsmoking men and women in their mid-30s to mid-40s die at least 3 years sooner than normal-weight counterparts—a risk as damaging to life expectancy as cigarette smoking.[122] Obese individuals can ex-

Obesity Trends Among U.S. Adults for 1990, 1998, and 2006

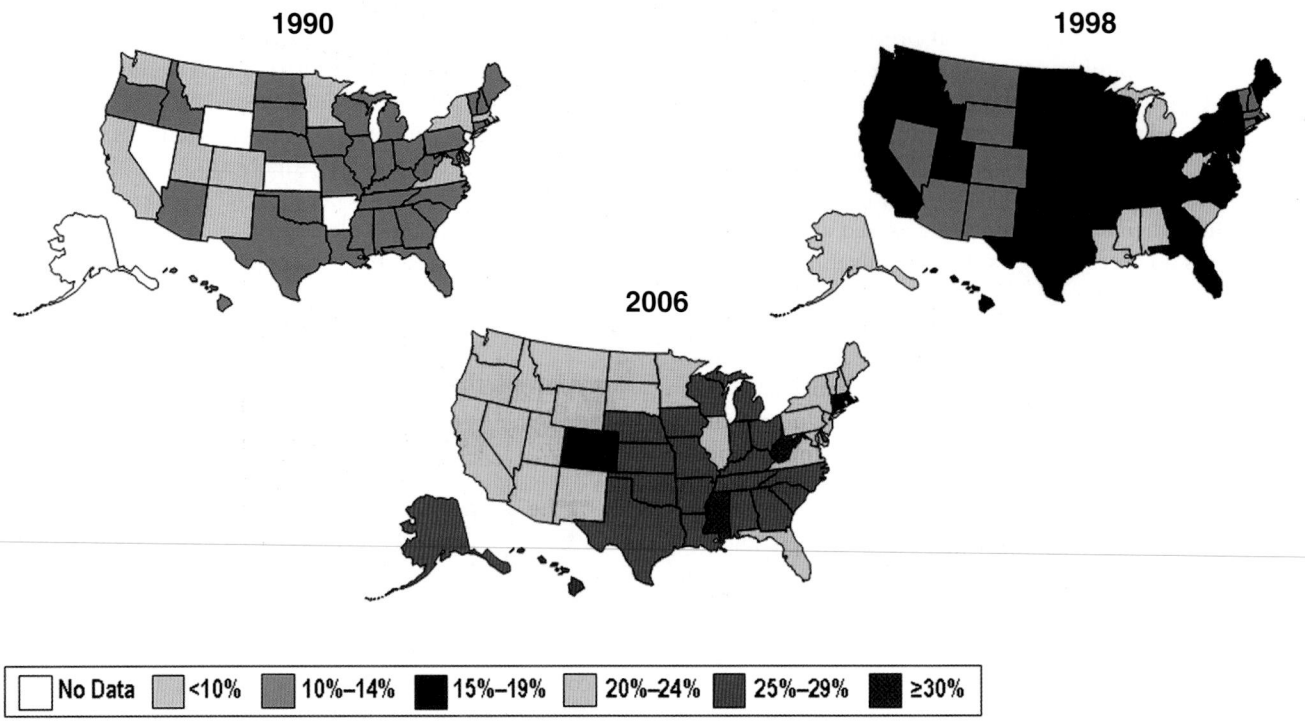

FIGURE 14.1 ■ During the past 20 years there has been a dramatic increase in obesity in the United States. In 2006, only four states had a prevalence of obesity less than 20%. Twenty-two states had a prevalence equal or greater than 25%; two of these states (Mississippi and West Virginia) had a prevalence of obesity equal to or greater than 30%. (Data source: CDC Behavioral Risk Factor Surveillance System; www.cdc.gov/nccdphp/dnpa/obesity/trends/map).

pect an approximately 7-year decrease in longevity. Correctly, physicians tell us to eat less and to increase the time we devote to exercising. In industrialized nations, economic factors operate to counter this advice: food continues to become cheaper and more fat laden, while most occupations have decreased their exertional demands.

Obesity Translates to Excess Body Fat

The term *obesity* refers to the overfat condition that accompanies a constellation of comorbidities that includes one or all of the following components of the "obese syndrome": glucose intolerance, insulin resistance, dyslipidemia, type 2 diabetes, hypertension, elevated plasma leptin concentrations, increased visceral adipose tissue, and increased risk of coronary heart disease and cancer.

FIGURE 14.3 illustrates the results of a national survey on the prevalence of overweight (defined at the time of this 1994

publication as a BMI ≥27) among adults in the United States compared with the government's objective for the year 2000. Between 1988 and 1991, one third of adults ages 20 to 74 years classified as overweight. This represents a dramatic increase from previous surveys, with obesity incidence particularly high among other minority groups (inset table). Based on the most recent estimate, more than 50% of non-Hispanic black women aged 40 years and older are obese and more than 80% are overweight.[48,52]

To help stem the obesity epidemic in the United States, the U.S. Preventive Services Task Force (www.ahrq.gov/clinic/uspstfix.htm), a government advisory group, urged physicians to weigh and measure all patients and recommend counseling and behavior therapy for individuals found to be obese. Specifically, the group recommended that doctors prescribe intensive behavior therapy at least twice a month (in indiviidual or group sessions) for up to 3 months under supervision of a health-professional team comprising psychologists, registered dietitians, and exercise specialists. These guidelines, which usually become the standard of care for medical practice, represented a major shift in how the health care system treats obesity and may prompt health

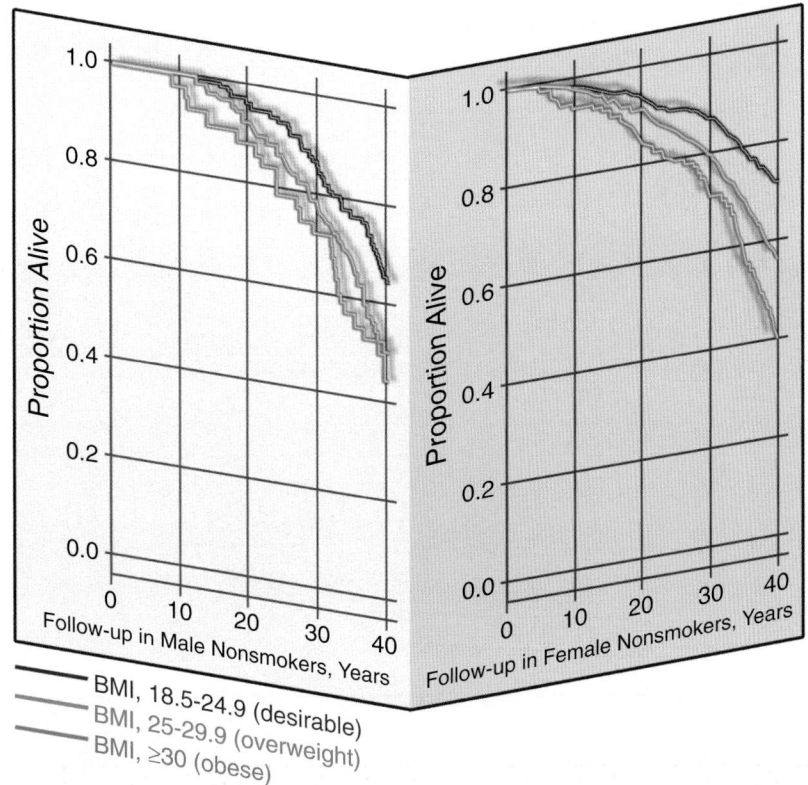

BMI, 18.5-24.9 (desirable)
BMI, 25-29.9 (overweight)
BMI, ≥30 (obese)

FIGURE 14.2 ■ Survival estimates for groups of women and men categorized by body mass index (BMI). (From Peeters A, et al. Obesity in adulthood and its consequences for life expectancy. *Ann Intern Med* 2003;138:24.)

plans and insurers to pay for obesity treatment, but that practice has not been popularly endorsed or widely implemented.

Caloric Intake Continues to Increase

Adult women now eat 335 more calories daily than in 1970, while the daily intake for men has increased by 168 calories. In 2000, this translated to an average yearly increase of 278 lb of food per capita intake. On the surface, some of this increase seems desirable because it includes increased vegetable intake. Nevertheless, nearly one third of the vegetables comprised iceberg lettuce, French fries, and potato chips. The grain component of this increase consisted of processed flour-based items such as pasta, tortillas, and hamburger buns, not the fiber-rich whole grain breads and cereals recommended. Highly processed, low-fiber carbohydrates have the equivalent nutritional value of table sugar.

Disturbingly Prevalent Among Children

FIGURE 14.4A shows the sharp rise in the percentage of U.S. children classified as overweight or obese from 1963 to 2000, while FIGURE 14.4B presents the revised United States growth charts for boys and girls age 2 to 20 years. Children experience as depressing a situation as adults because the prevalence of overweight in children (BMI ≥95th percentile for age and sex) or at risk for overweight (BMI ≥85th percentile and ≤95th percentile) has attained grim proportions.[38,119,156] The incidence of overweight among American youth has more than doubled in the last 15 years, with an ever-widening gap between the weights of individuals deemed overly fat and those considered thin. Data from the years 1999–2000 indicate that excess body fat among children continued on the upswing, including 15.3% of children ages 6 to 11 years of age, 15.5% ages 12 to 19 years, and 10.4% ages 2 to 5 years, up from an average of 5% in the early 1970s (Fig. 14.4A)—with the trend continuing.[38,177] The rapid rate of increase remains particularly prevalent among poor and minority children in whom excessive body fat represents the most common chronic disorder.[28,47,165] Similar results emerge from a study

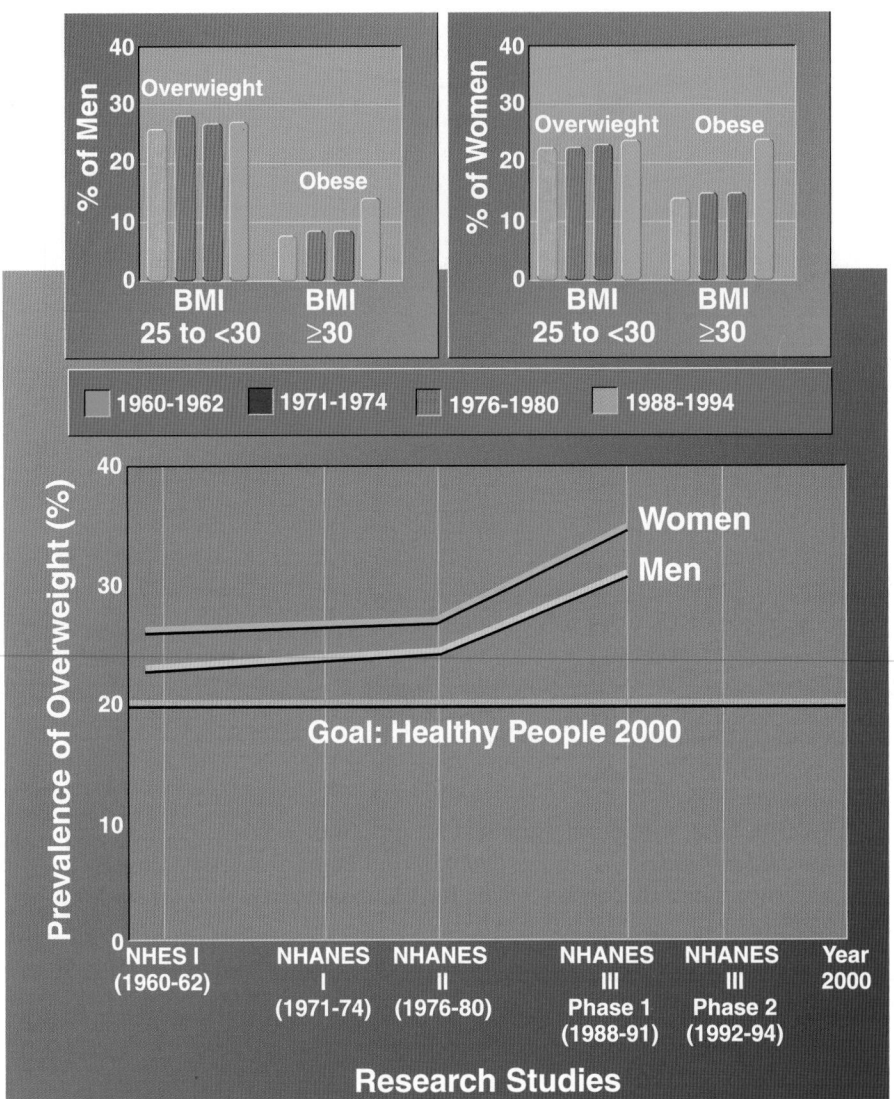

Group	Men (%)*		Women (%)*	
	Overweight	Severely overweight	Overweight	Severely overweight
White	24.4	7.8	24.6	9.6
Black	26.3	10.4	45.1	19.7
Mexican	31.2	10.8	41.5	16.7
Cuban	28.5	10.3	31.9	6.9
Puerto Rican	25.7	7.9	39.8	15.2

*Age-adjusted percentages of overweight and severely overweight persons aged 20-74 y living in the U.S.

FIGURE 14.3 ■ The fattening of America. Trends in age-adjusted prevalence of overweight in the U.S. population aged 20 through 74 years, compared with the *Healthy People 2000* objective for overweight. The *inset table* presents age-adjusted percentages of overweight and severely overweight persons aged 20 to 74 years from NHANES II (1976–1980) and NHANES I (1971–1974), categorized by ethnicity and gender. NHES, National Health Examination Survey; NHANES, National Health and Nutrition Examination Survey. (From Kuczmarski RJ, et al. Increasing prevalence of overweight among US adults. JAMA 1994;272:205; *inset table* from Kuczmarski Rj, et al. Prevalence of overweight and weight gain in the United States. Am J Clin Nutr 1992;55:495S.). The *top inset figure* shows change in the age-adjusted prevalence of overweight and obesity in men and women aged 20 to 74 years from 1960 to 1994. (From National Task Force on the Prevention and Treatment of Obesity. Overweight, obesity, and health risk. *Arch Intern Med* 2000;160:898.)

A

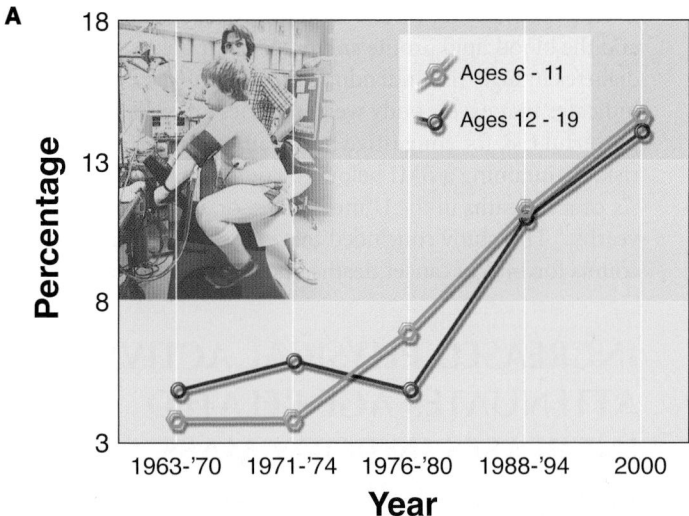

B

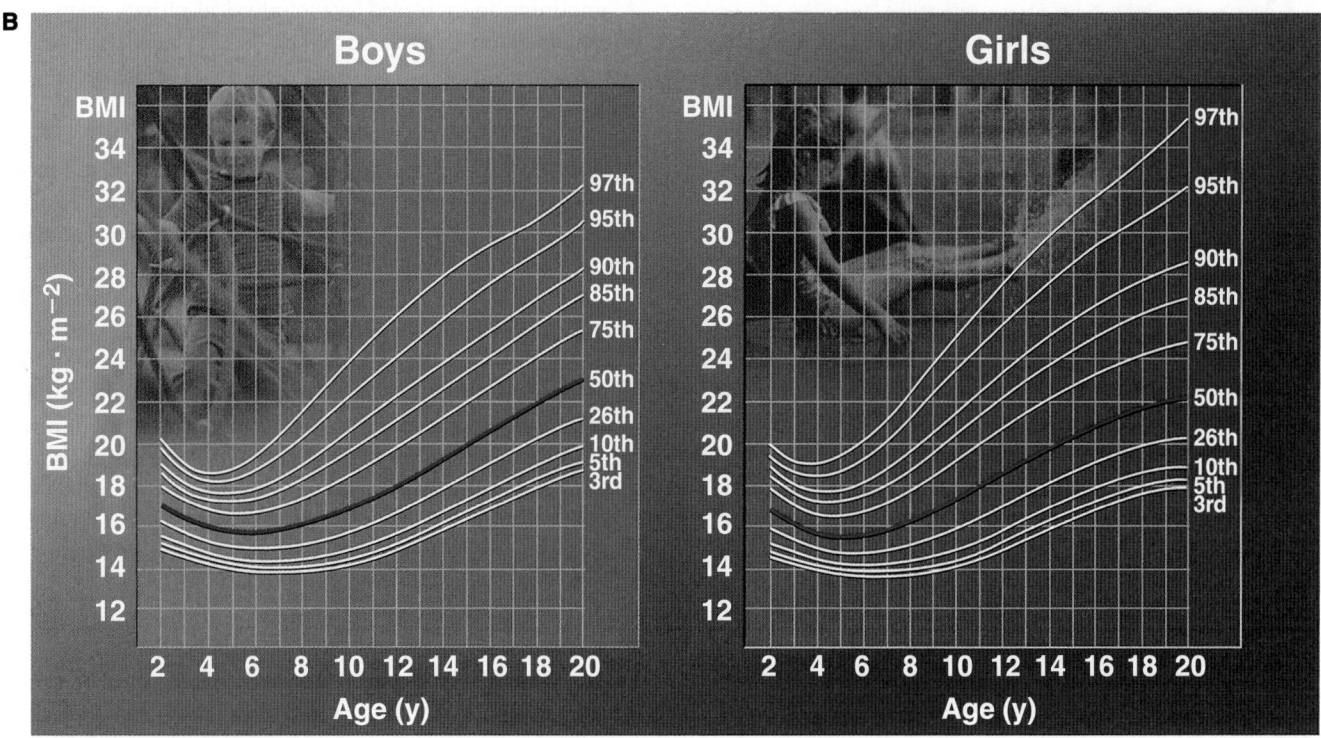

FIGURE 14.4 ■ **A.** A disturbing trend in the percentage of overweight young persons from 1963 to 2000. **B.** Body mass index-for-age percentiles for boys and girls ages 2 to 20 years. Developed by the National Center for Health Statistics in collaboration with the National Center for Chronic Disease Prevention and Health Promotion (2000). (From Kuczmarski RJ, et al. CDC growth charts: United States. *Advance Data* 2000; 314. From Vital and Health Statistics of the Center for Disease Control and Prevention/National Center for Health Statistics.)

Obesity Refers to Increased Disease Risk

According to the Centers for Disease Control and Prevention (www.cdc.gov/), which collects data on a sample of about 5000 people each year through in-person examinations, American children are continuing to become fat, with more than one third classifying as overweight. American men have also joined this group, but the percentage of overweight American women appears to have peaked. The percentage of overweight men rose to 71% in 2003–2004 from 67% in 1999–2000 while the obese percentage rose to 31% from 27.5%. For women, overweight and obese percentages held steady at 62% and 33%, respectively. This leveling off in women could signal a turning point in the nation's obesity problem.

of Australian children ages 7 to 15 years.[16] In the period from 1985 to 1997, the prevalence of overweight and obesity combined doubled and that of obesity tripled, far greater increases than in the previous 16 years.

A child or adolescent with a high BMI percentile ranking shows a significant risk of being overweight or obese at age 35, and that risk increases with the youth's age.[60] More than 60% of children between ages 5 and 10 years exhibit at least one risk factor for cardiovascular disease. Excessive fatness in youth represents even more of an adult health risk than obesity begun in adulthood. Overweight children and adolescents, regardless of final body weight as adults, exhibit greater risk for a broad range of illnesses as adults than children who maintain a normal body weight.[59,172]

Increased Calorie Intake and a Depressed Energy Output Spell Trouble

By 2025, 75% of the American population will classify as overweight, with about one third classified obese. More than likely, a sedentary lifestyle and ready availability of tasty, fatty, and calorie-rich foods served in increasingly "supersized" portions remain prime culprits for expressing unhealthy patterns of pre-existing susceptible genes in the fattening of Western civilization.

HEALTH RISKS OF OBESITY

Obesity (or excess body fat) represents the second leading cause of preventable death in America (cigarette smoking ranks first), with the cost of obesity-related diseases exceeding $110 billion annually in the year 2005. One trip to the doctor annually made by 25% of the total obese Americans population costs more than $810 million based on a doctor visit charge of $60. On the downside, the estimated number of annual deaths attributed to obesity per se ranges between 280,000 and 325,000.[25,112] Comorbidities include hypertension, elevated blood sugar, pulmonary dysfunction including asthma and sleep apnea, psychiatric problems (depression and eating disorders), postmenopausal breast cancer, pancreatic cancer (and diverse other cancers), gastrointestinal disorders including gallstones, and elevated total cholesterol and low high density lipoprotein (HDL) cholesterol levels, type 2 diabetes, and cardiovascular disease, with a somewhat stronger impact on diabetes risk.

On a positive note, increasing physical activity exerts a considerable influence in reducing risk for cardiovascular disease and a more moderate effect on diabetes risk. In essence, increased adiposity and reduced physical activity strongly and independently predict death.[76] These consequences heighten a sedentary, overweight individual's risks of poor health at any given level of excess weight. Unfortunately, the increasing prevalence of obesity has slowed the decline in coronary heart disease among middle-aged women.[75] Obese and overweight individuals with two or more heart disease risk factors should reduce excess weight. Overweight persons without other risk factors should at least maintain their current body weight.

Even a modest weight reduction improves insulin sensitivity and the blood lipid profile and prevents or delays the onset of diabetes in high-risk individuals. Epidemiologic evidence also indicates that excess body weight carries an independent and powerful risk for congestive heart failure. In terms of cancer risk, maintaining a BMI below 25 could prevent one of every six cancer deaths in the United States, or about 90,000 deaths yearly.[26] This study concluded that excess weight probably accounts for 14% of cancer deaths in men and 20% in women.

INCREASED PHYSICAL ACTIVITY ATTENUATES AGE-RELATED INCREASES IN BODY MASS AND FAT

Maintaining an increased level of physical activity attenuates the age-related increases in body weight and body fat.[190] Prospective 7-year survey data from male and female runners who maintained detailed records of body weight and abdominal and hip girths during 7 years of continuous run training confirmed that individuals who accumulated more running miles ($\leq$48 km · wk^{-1} or 29.8 mi · wk^{-1}) reduced the normal aging tendency to gain body weight (and increase BMI) and body fat more than less physically active runners ($\leq$24 km · wk^{-1} or 14.9 mi · wk^{-1}). For example, the yearly gain in body weight for males between the ages of 18 and 24 years who exceeded 48 km per week was 0.83 kg compared to a gain of 1.56 kg for the same age-group of men who ran less than 24 km per week. For female counterparts, the change in body weight over a 7-year interval was about three times less (0.39 kg · y^{-1}) in women who exceeded running 48 km · km^{-1} than women who ran less distance (0.91 kg · y^{-1}). These results and supportive data[171–174] indicte that increased physical activity maintained over protracted time periods is more important as an independent factor to minimize the increase in body size that occurs normally with aging than simply reducing body weight sometimes repeatedly over a relatively short time span of weeks or even a year to normalize any excess weight accumulation. The public health message seems clear—increased regular physical activity, not dieting and/or short-term exercise should become the important consideration in exercise prescription for weight control and good health. Stated somewhat differently, preventing the rise in BMI with aging may be more effectively achieved by preventing weight gain with longer-term, increased physical activity as a lifestyle choice than acutely deceasing BMI by weight loss in individuals already overweight or obese by BMI standards.

GENETICS PLAYS A ROLE IN BODY WEIGHT REGULATION

Body weight should be viewed as the end result of complex interactions between one's genes and environmental influ-

It Doesn't Take Much to Improve Health Status

A 5 to 10% weight loss often normalizes an obese person's serum cholesterol and triacylglycerol levels and reduces blood pressure and overall heart disease risk, including risk of congestive heart failure. Obesity now stands on a par with high cholesterol, hypertension, cigarette smoking, and sedentary lifestyle as a major heart attack risk factor in contrast to its former status as a contributing risk factor.

Disturbing Factors About Life Expectancy in the United States

Despite the fact that life expectancy in the United States has been extended by 30 years in the past century, it still lags behind 41 other countries, including Japan, most of Europe, Jordan, Guam, and the Cayman Islands. Other disturbing (and contributing) factors include:

- Adults in the United States have one of the highest obesity rates in the world. Nearly one third of adults above age 20 years are obese, while about two thirds are overweight.
- Significant racial disparities exist in that black Americans have an average life expectancy of 73.3 years, 5 years shorter than white counterparts.
- The slipping of the United States in international rankings of life expectancy may result from other countries' improvement in health care, nutrition, and lifestyles. Sadly, 45 million Americans lack health insurance, whereas Canada and many European countries have universal health care.
- A relatively high percentage of babies born in the United States die before their first birthday compared with other industrialized nations. Forty countries, including Cuba, Taiwan, and most of Europe, had lower infant mortality rates than the United States in 2004. The U.S. rate was 6.8 deaths for every 1000 live births. It was 13.7 for black Americans, the same as Saudi Arabia.
- The longest life expectancy occurs in the principality of Andorra, a tiny country in the Pyrenees mountains landlocked between France and Spain (83.5 years). The shortest life expectancies were clustered in Sub-Saharan Africa (Swaziland [34.1 years], followed by Zambia, Angola, Liberia, and Zimbabwe), a region that has been devastated by human immunodeficiency virus (HIV) and acquired immune deficiency syndrome (AIDS), and famine and civil strife.

Source: National Center for Health Statistics (www.cdc. gov/nchs)

ences, rather than simply the consequence of psychologic factors that affect eating behaviors. Research with twins, adopted children, and specific segments of the population attribute up to 80% of the risk of becoming obese to genetic factors. For example, newborns with large body weights become fat adolescents, particularly if the mother is overweight.[53] Reduced risk exists for an overweight toddler to grow into an obese adult if both parents are of normal weight. But for a child under age 10 (regardless of current weight) who has one or both obese parents, the child has more than double the normal risk of becoming an obese adult. Even among normal-weight prepubertal girls, body composition and regional fat distribution relate to the body composition characteristics of the mother and to a lesser extent the father.[164]

Genetic makeup does not necessarily cause excessive weight gain. In the presence of powerful environmental influences it lowers the threshold for gaining weight and contributes to variability in weight gain among individuals fed an identical daily caloric excess.[18,19] The impact of the environment on genetic predisposition largely explains the rapid increase in obesity in the United States over the last 30 years.

Racial Factors Contribute

The greater prevalence of obesity among black women (about 50%) compared with white women (33%) frequently has been attributed to racial differences in food and exercise habits and attitudes toward body weight. Studies of obese women whose weight averaged 224 pounds show that small differences in resting metabolism also contribute to the racial differences in obesity.[50,80] On average, black women burned nearly 100 fewer calories each day during rest than white counterparts; the slower rate of processing calories persists even after adjusting for differences in body mass and body composition. The greater energy economy of black women during exercise and throughout the day reflects an inherited trait because it persists both before and after weight loss.[178] This "racial" effect, which also exists among children and adolescents,[157,163] predisposes a black female to gain weight and more readily regain it after weight loss. A 100-kCal reduction in daily metabolism translates to nearly 1 lb of body fat gained each month. Such data suggest that black female athletes with weight problems may experience greater difficulty achieving and maintaining a goal body weight for competition than an overweight white counterpart.

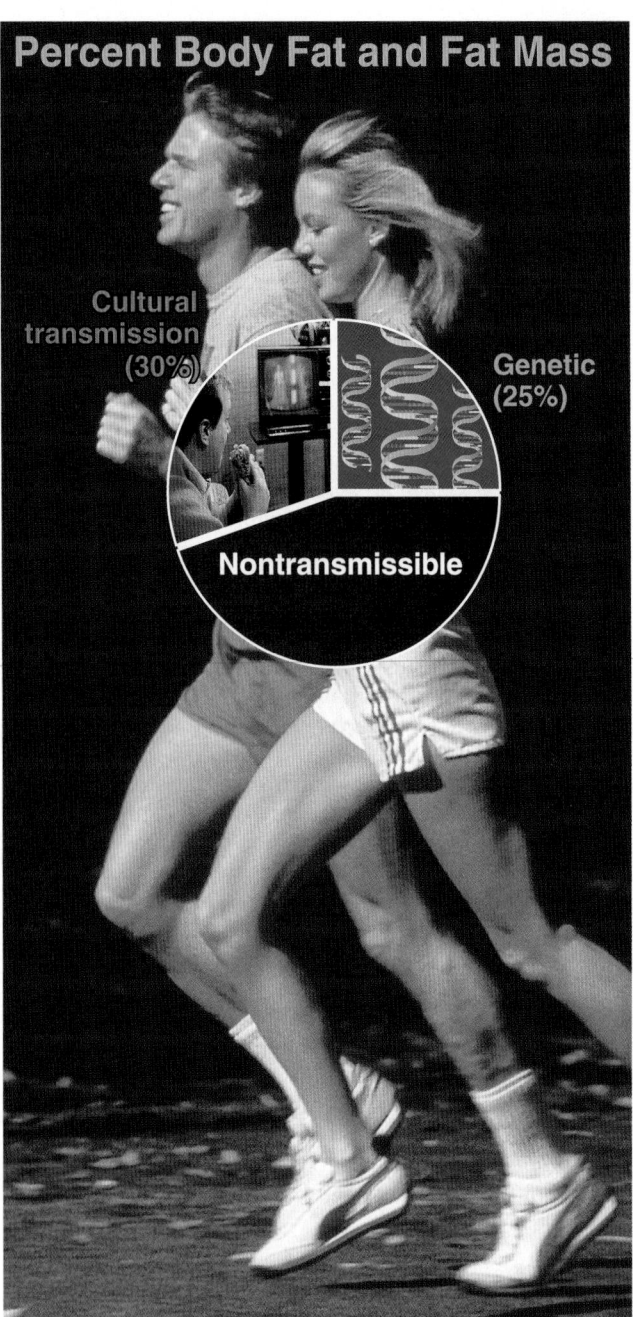

Percent Body Fat and Fat Mass

Cultural transmission (30%)

Genetic (25%)

Nontransmissible

FIGURE 14.5 ■ Total transmissible and genetically determined variance for body fat. (From Bouchard C, et al. Inheritance of the amount and distribution of human body fat. *Int J Obes* 1988;12:205.)

Not Simply a Lack of Willpower

The linkage of genetic and molecular abnormalities to obesity allows researchers to view overfatness as a disease rather than a psychologic flaw. Studies of a relatively large number of different types of relatives indicate that genetic factors that affect metabolism and appetite determine about 25% of the variation among people in percentage body fat and total fat mass. A larger percentage of variation relates to a transmissible (cultural) effect (unhealthy expression patterns of pre-existing genes; FIG. 14.5). In an obesity-producing environment—sedentary, stressful, easy access to high-fat foods—the genetically susceptible (obesity-prone) individual gains weight and possibly lots of it.[43,57] Athletes in weight-related sports who have a genetic propensity for obesity must constantly battle to achieve (and maintain) an optimal body weight and body composition for competitive performance.

POSSIBLE MECHANISMS FOR WEIGHT GAIN

Research with a strain of mice that balloon up to five times the size of normal mice provides evidence for a genetic "destiny" to gain body fat.[195] The mutation of a gene called obese (or simply *ob*) disrupts hormonal signals that regulate metabolism, fat storage, and appetite. This causes energy balance to tip toward fat accumulation.

The model in FIGURE 14.6 proposes that the *ob* gene normally activates in adipose tissue to stimulate production of a body fat-signaling, hormone-like protein (**ob protein** or **leptin**, first identified by Dr. Jeffrey Friedman and colleagues of the Howard Hughes Medical Institute at Rockefeller University in 1994; runews.rockefeller.edu/index.php?page=engine&id=214) that then enters the bloodstream.[63,123] This satiety signal molecule migrates to the ventromedial nucleus, the brain's hypothalamic area that controls appetite and metabolism. Normally, leptin depresses the urge to eat when food intake coincides with ideal fat stores. Depressed leptin receptor sensitivity signals the brain that the body lacks fat reserves, often triggering overeating. Leptin may affect target neurons in the hypothalamus to (1) stimulate production of chemicals that suppress appetite and/or (2) reduce the level of brain chemicals that stimulate appetite. These mechanisms would explain how body fat remains intimately "connected" to the brain (and appetite) via a physiologic pathway to regulate energy balance. In a way, the adipocyte serves an endocrine-like function. With a gene defective for either adipocyte leptin production and/or hypothalamic leptin sensitivity (as probably exists in humans), the brain cannot adequately assess adipose tissue status. This creates a persistent urge to eat.

The hormone–hypothalamic control mechanism fits nicely within the set-point theory (see page 464) to explain abnormal body fat accumulation. It also accounts for the extreme difficulty obese individuals have in sustaining significant body

Twelve Specific Health Risks of Excessive Body Fat

1. Impaired cardiac function from increased mechanical work and autonomic and left ventricular dysfunction
2. Hypertension, stroke, and deep-vein thrombosis
3. Increased insulin resistance in children and adults and type 2 diabetes (80% of these patients are overweight)
4. Renal disease
5. Sleep apnea, mechanical ventilatory constraints (particularly in exercise), and pulmonary disease from impaired function because of added effort to move the chest wall
6. Problems receiving anesthetics during surgery
7. Osteoarthritis, degenerative joint disease, and gout
8. Endometrial, breast, prostate, and colon cancers
9. Abnormal plasma lipid and lipoprotein levels
10. Menstrual irregularities
11. Gallbladder disease
12. Enormous psychological burden and social stigmatization and discrimination

fat loss. Short- or long-term exercise alone does not appear to affect leptin levels in humans. Changes in lifestyle that combine decreased dietary fat intake and increased physical activity reduce plasma leptin concentrations below the reduction expected from any change in body fat mass.[124,134]

Leptin alone does not determine obesity or explain why some people eat whatever they want and gain little weight, whereas others become obese with the same energy intake. Besides defective leptin production, defective receptor action (via a leptin receptor molecule on brain cells) increases resistance to satiety chemicals.[32] A specific gene, the uncoupling protein-2 *(UCP2)* gene, active in all human tissue adds another piece to the obesity puzzle. The *UCP2* gene activates a protein that stimulates the burning of excess calories as heat without coupling to other energy-consuming processes.[49] This futile metabolism blunts excess fat storage. Individual differences in gene activation and resultant alterations in metabolic activity lend credence to the common claim "Every little bit of excess food I eat turns to fat." Finding a drug that turns on the *UCP2* gene to synthesize more heat-generating protein could provide a pharmacologic "solution" to shed excess body fat. Specific drugs and drug combinations that inhibit brain chemicals that stimulate appetite may ultimately provide the long-term "cure" for the overly fat condition in a way similar to drug use to manage such chronic conditions as hypertension and diabetes.

PHYSICAL ACTIVITY: A CRUCIAL COMPONENT IN WEIGHT CONTROL

The standard dietary approach to weight loss that decreases caloric intake below the requirement for current weight maintenance generally helps obese patients lose about 0.5 kg per week.[175] Success at preventing weight regain remains relatively poor, averaging between 5 and 20%. Weight loss professionals now argue that regular physical activity, through either recreation or occupation, effectively contributes to preventing weight gain and thwarts the tendency to regain lost weight.[79,90,145,183] For example, individuals who maintain weight loss over time show greater muscle strength and engage in more physical activity than counterparts who regained lost weight.[181] Variations in physical activity alone accounted for more than 75% of the regained body weight. Such findings point to the need to identify and promote strategies that increase regular physical activity. Current national guidelines by the Surgeon General and Institute of Medicine, respectively, recommend a minimum of 30 to 60 minutes of moderate physical activity daily. We endorse an increase to at least 75 minutes of total daily exercise (over and above that required during "normal" living) to combat the prevalence of obesity in the U.S. population.

Older men and women who maintain active lifestyles thwart the "normal" pattern of fat gain in adulthood.[92,128] Middle-aged male distance runners remain leaner than sedentary counterparts.[185] Time spent in physical activity inversely relates to body fat level in young and middle-aged men who exercise regularly.[66,107] Surprisingly, no relationship emerged between the runners' body fat level and caloric intake. Thus, the greater level of body fat among active middle-aged men compared with younger, more active counterparts resulted from less vigorous training, not greater energy intake.

From age 3 months to 1 year, the total energy expenditure of infants who later became overweight averaged 21% less than infants with normal weight gain.[135] For children aged 6 to 9 years, percentage body fat inversely related to physical activity level in boys but not in girls.[10] Obese preadolescent children generally spend less time in physical activity or engage in lower-intensity physical activity than normal-weight peers.[33,173] By the time young girls reach adolescence many do no leisure-time physical activity. For girls, the decline in time spent in physical activity averaged nearly 100% among blacks and 64% among whites between ages 9 or 10 and 15 or 16.[88] By age 16 or 17, 56% of the black girls and 31% of the white girls reported no leisure-time physical activity. The 24-hour energy expenditure of young-adult Native Americans inversely related to body weight changes over a 2-year period.[132] A four times greater risk of gaining more than 7.5 kg occurred in individuals with low rather than high 24-hour energy expenditures.

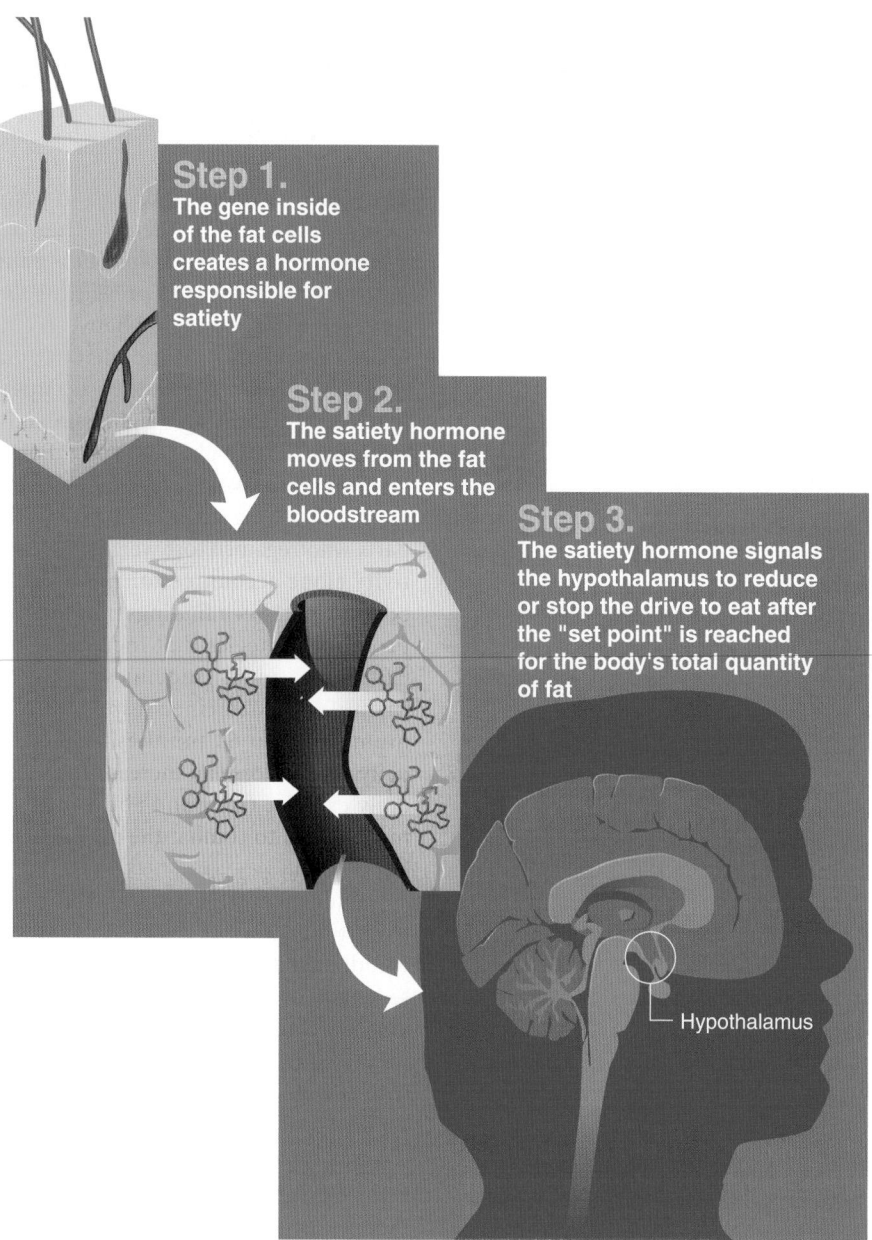

Step 1.
The gene inside of the fat cells creates a hormone responsible for satiety

Step 2.
The satiety hormone moves from the fat cells and enters the bloodstream

Step 3.
The satiety hormone signals the hypothalamus to reduce or stop the drive to eat after the "set point" is reached for the body's total quantity of fat

Hypothalamus

FIGURE 14.6 ■ A genetic model for obesity. A malfunction of the satiety gene markedly affects production of the satiety hormone leptin (after the Greek word *leptos,* thin). This disrupts the events that occur in *step 3* in the hypothalamus, the center that adjusts body fat level. (Model is based on research conducted at Rockefeller University, New York.) Two general categories of medication treat obesity in the United States: I. Those that decrease food intake by reducing appetite or increase satiety. These medications increase availability of anorexigenic neurotransmitters such as norepinephrine, serotonin, and dopamine in the central nervous system. II. Those that decrease macronutrient absorption in the digestive tract. The fat-fighting chemicals dexfenfluramine (trade name Redux) and fenfluramine (Pondimin) promote release of serotonin thus decreasing appetite. (On Sept. 15, 1997, the FDA asked manufacturers of these drugs to remove them from the market because of their potential for causing damage to heart valves.) Sibutramine (Meridia) alters brain chemicals to trick the body into feeling full, primarily by inhibiting the reuptake of the neurotransmitters norepinephrine and serotonin; orlistat (Xenical) facilitates weight loss by inhibiting intestinal absorption of about one third of ingested lipids.

Physical Activity and Decreased Mortality: A Little Is Good but More May Be Better

The largest prospective cohort of U.S. adults (527,265 men and women aged 50 to 71 years) enrolled in the NIH-AARP Diet and Health Study (www.dietandhealth.cancer.gov) examined the relationship between physical activity and mortality. Results showed that individuals who exercised a minimum of 20 minutes of vigorous activity either 1 to 3 times a month, 1 to 2 times weekly, 3 to 4 times a week, or 5 or more times per week showed a lower mortality relative risk (increased physical activity more effective) than to those who rarely exercised. These findings indicate that vigorous physical activity reduced the risk of premature mortality for women and men. (Data courtesy of Dr. Michael Leitzmann, U.S. National Cancer Institute.) Additional supportive data for lower mortality risk with higher levels of occupational physical activity come from a 24-year follow-up analysis of 47,405 Norwegian men and women.[78]

Biochemicals That Influence Eating Behaviors: Signals That Travel Among the Digestive Tract, Adipose Tissue, and Eating-Control Centers

- **Leptin:** Produced by adipocytes. Normal levels signal the hypothalamus to maintain food intake so body weight remains stable. Below-normal leptin levels signal the brain to increase appetite so that body fat levels increase. Leptin also elevates metabolic rate.
- **Peptide YY3-36 (PYY):** Produced by intestinal cells in response to food intake. It then travels to the hypothalamus to inhibit the urge to eat. Overweight persons normally make less of this satiety signal than persons of normal body weight.
- **Neuropeptide Y:** A transmitter protein of the nervous system that stimulates food intake and regulates metabolism and fat synthesis.
- **Ghrelin:** Exerts effects opposite to those of leptin. A powerful appetite-stimulating hormone (also slows energy output) produced in the stomach and small intestine. Only known natural appetite stimulant made outside the brain. Drugs that block this hormone would not only stimulate weight loss but also increase energy expenditure.
- **Melanocortin-4:** Possibly supplies the signal to stop eating. About 10% of obese patients show genetic mutations in the gene that regulates this compound.

Increasing Energy Output May Help as One Ages

For male runners 18 years of age and older, maintaining a lifestyle that included a regular but constant level of exercise did not fully forestall the tendency to add weight through middle age. FIGURE 14.7 shows the strong inverse association between distance run and BMI and waist circumference in all age categories. Active men were leaner than sedentary counterparts for each decade. Those who ran longer distances each week weighed less than those who ran shorter distances. The typical man who maintained a constant weekly running distance through middle age added 3.3 lb while waist size (presumably from intra-abdominal fat) increased about three fourths of an inch, regardless of distance run. Such findings suggest that by age 50, a physically active man can expect to weigh about 10 lb more (with a 2-inch larger waist) than he weighed at age 20, despite maintaining a constant level of physical activity. The reasons for this proclivity to gain weight and girth remain unknown. Perhaps, reduced testosterone and growth hormone levels induce age-related change in physique and increase abdominal and visceral fat. The researchers advise annually increasing weekly exercise by about 1.4 miles starting at age 30 to effectively counter weight gain with aging. One can achieve the same effect without additional exercise by modestly reducing energy intake while making more nutritious food selections.

WEIGHT LOSS: A UNIQUE DILEMMA FOR THE COMPETITIVE ATHLETE

For many "overweight" athletes whose competitive careers have ended, achieving a lighter body weight and favorable body composition (combined with proper nutritional practices) offers overall health benefits. For the athlete currently competing, successful performance depends on achieving an "ideal" body mass and body composition. In figure skating, ballet dancing, diving, gymnastics, and bodybuilding, success often requires a predefined "aesthetic look." To complicate matters, the relatively low intensity of training in some of these sports contributes little to fat loss.

Reduced Body Size Affects Exercise Performance

In weight-bearing competitive sports such as racewalking, running, cross-country skiing, and ice skating, energy cost re-

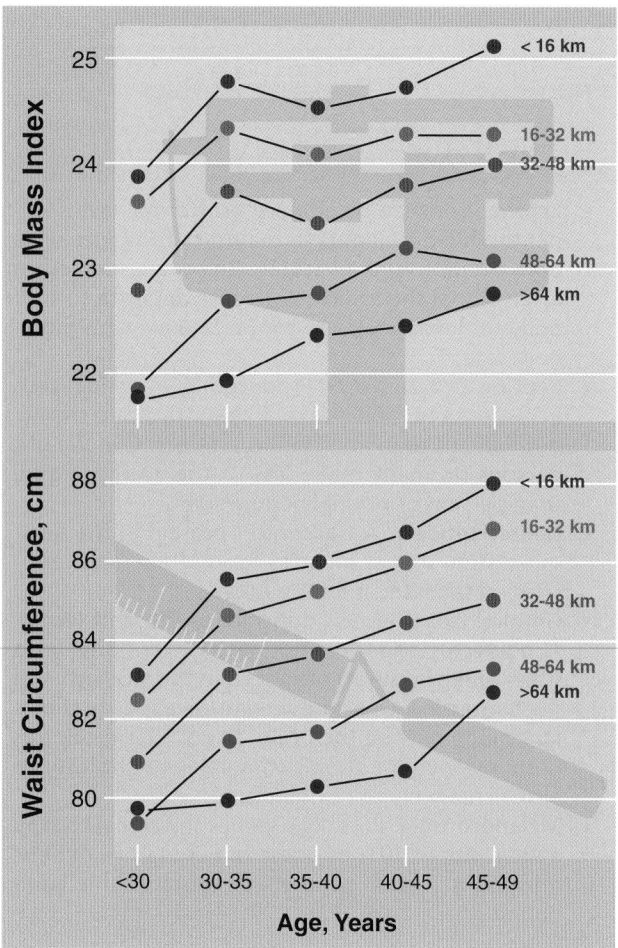

FIGURE 14.7 ■ Relationship of average body mass index (BMI, kg per m²) *(top)* and waist circumference *(bottom)* and age for men who maintained constant weekly running of varying distances. Analyses of these relationships indicate that men who annually increase their distance run by 1.39 miles (2.24 km) per week compensate for the anticipated weight gain during middle age. (From Williams PT. Evidence for the incompatibility of age-neutral overweight and age-neutral physical activity standards from runners. *Am J Clin Nutr* 1997;65:1391.)

lates directly to body mass. Consequently, achieving the lightest body weight without compromising physiologic function and metabolic capacity should improve performance. In weight-supported sports such as swimming, body weight reduction may not have as dramatic an affect on performance, although a smaller body size should reduce the drag forces that impede movement through the water.

A reasonable approach to enhance performance for some athletes involves reducing body weight, particularly fat mass. Pole-vaulters and jumpers who reduce body weight without compromising skill and power-output capacity achieve greater ease in overcoming the force of gravity. The same holds true

for runners, skaters, cyclists, and others who compete at high movement velocities. Not only does the resistance of gravity diminish with a lighter body weight, but also the impeding effects of the drag force created by air (or water) becomes less with a smaller body frontal surface area.

A Prudent Approach Most Effective

To reduce body size, a person can decrease weight in a relatively short time by restricting food and fluid intake and sweating excessively. Body weight loss in this situation occurs mainly from water loss and depletion of liver and muscle glycogen reserves. Longer-term attempts at weight loss through semistarvation increase the risk of depressing resting metabolism (making continued weight loss more difficult) and increasing loss of lean tissue, glycogen stores, and muscular strength and power.[137] Severe dehydration in trying to "make weight" also places these individuals at risk for heat injury. Combining moderate food restriction with additional daily physical activity offers the greatest flexibility for achieving fat loss, yet remaining well nourished for training and peak performance.

The potential to improve competitive performance with weight loss assumes that any lost weight does not adversely affect skill, strength, or power capacity. If these important determinants of performance deteriorate, the athlete does worse not better. The weight loss program must not adversely affect daily training. One should view weight loss from a longer-term perspective, because body fat's contribution to an energy deficit increases as the duration of weight loss progresses. No more than 1 or 2 lb (about 1% of body mass) should be lost each week to minimize adverse effects of weight loss on fat-free body mass (FFM), nutrient status, and exercise performance. Food composition tables or appropriate computer software should assess nutrient status to ensure maintenance of the predetermined daily caloric deficit and recommended carbohydrate, protein, and micronutrient intake. Concurrently, body composition evaluation can regularly assess the compositional characteristics of the weight lost.

THE ENERGY BALANCE EQUATION APPLIED TO WEIGHT LOSS

Guidelines for weight loss generally come from studies of sedentary, overly fat individuals. Although precise recommendations do not exist for physically active men and women or competitive athletes, the current understanding of prudent body fat loss should also apply to these individuals. As discussed in Chapter 7 and illustrated in Figure 7.1, the human body functions in accord with the laws of thermodynamics. If total daily food calories exceed daily energy expenditure, excess calories accumulate as fat in adipose tissue. Conversely, if energy expenditure exceeds the energy from food intake, body weight decreases.

Three methods unbalance the energy balance equation to produce weight loss:

1. Reduce caloric intake below daily energy requirements
2. Maintain daily caloric intake and increase energy expenditure through additional physical activity
3. Decrease daily caloric intake and increase daily energy expenditure

When considering the sensitivity of overall energy balance, note that if daily energy intake exceeds output by only 100 kCal, the surplus calories consumed in a year equal 36,500 kCal (365 × 100 kCal). Because each pound (454 g, or 0.45 kg) of body fat consists of about 87% lipid (454 g × 0.87 = 395 g × 9 kCal · g^{-1} = 3555 kCal [usually rounded to 3500 kCal] per 0.45 kg), this caloric excess causes a yearly gain of about 4.7 kg (10.3 lb) of body fat. In contrast, if daily food intake decreases by 100 kCal, and energy expenditure increases by 100 kCal (e.g., by jogging 1 extra mile each day), then the yearly caloric deficit equals about 9.5 kg (21 lb) of body fat. Whether shifting dietary composition toward higher carbohydrate content actually affects body fat gain or loss remains unresolved.[22,72,184]

A Prudent Recommendation

The objective of obesity therapy has changed dramatically over the past 15 years. The previous approach assigned a goal body weight that coincided with an "ideal" weight based on body stature and mass. Achievement of goal body weight heralded the weight-loss program's success. Currently, the WHO, the Institute of Medicine of the National Academy of Sciences (www.iom.edu), and the National Heart, Lung and Blood Institute (www.nhlbi.nih.gov) recommend that an obese person reduce initial body weight by 5 to 15%. This more realistic weight loss diminishes weight-related comorbidities and complications from hypertension, type 2 diabetes, and abnormal blood lipids and often exerts a positive effect on social–psychologic complications. Setting the initial weight loss goal beyond the 5 to 15% recommendation often gives patients an unrealistic and potentially unattainable target in light of current treatment methods.

DIETING TO TIP THE ENERGY BALANCE EQUATION

Many people believe that only calories from dietary lipids increase body fat. These individuals reduce lipid intake (generally a good idea) but often disproportionately increase carbohydrate and protein intakes so total caloric intake remains unchanged or even increases. Weight loss occurs whenever energy output exceeds energy intake regardless of the diet's macronutrient mixture, reaffirming the first law of thermodynamics. A prudent dietary approach to weight loss unbalances the energy balance equation by reducing daily energy intake 500 to 1000 kCal below daily energy expenditure. Moderately reduced food intake produces greater body fat loss in relation to the energy deficit than more severe energy restriction that exacerbates loss of FFM. In addition, individuals poorly tolerate a prolonged caloric restriction of more than 1000 kCal a day; this form of semistarvation increases the chances for poor nourishment and depletion of the all-important glycogen reserves. Total energy intake, not diet composition, determines the effectiveness of weight loss with reduced-energy diets.[54]

Suppose an overly fat man who consumes 3800 kCal daily and maintains body mass of 80 kg wishes to reduce 5 kg by dieting. He maintains his activity level but decreases food intake to create a daily caloric deficit of 1000 kCal. Thus, instead of consuming 3800 kCal, he takes in only 2800 kCal daily. In 7 days, the accumulated deficit equals 7000 kCal, or the energy equivalent of 0.9 kg (2 lb) of body fat. Actually, he would lose considerably more than 0.9 kg during the first week because initially the body's glycogen stores make up a substantial portion of the energy deficit. Stored glycogen contains fewer calories per gram and considerably more water than stored fat. For this reason, short periods of caloric restriction often encourage the dieter but produce a large percentage of water and carbohydrate loss per unit weight loss, with only a small decrease in body fat. As weight loss progresses, a larger proportion of body fat supports the energy deficit created by food restriction. To reduce body fat by an additional 1.4 kg, the dieter must maintain the reduced caloric intake of 2800 kCal for another 10.5 days; at this point, body fat theoretically decreases at a rate of 0.45 kg every 3.5 days.

Weight Loss Results Not Always Predictable

The mathematics of weight loss through caloric restriction seems straightforward, but the results do not always follow. One assumes that daily energy expenditure remains relatively unchanged throughout the dieting period. However, some dieters experience lethargy (often related to depletion of the body's glycogen stores); this decreases daily energy expenditure. The energy cost of physical activity also decreases proportionately with body weight reduction. This shrinks the energy output side of the energy balance equation. As we discuss in the next section, the body also "defends" itself against a depressed caloric intake by reducing resting metabolism, which further blunts the weight loss effort.

Set-Point Theory: A Case Against Dieting

One can reduce large amounts of weight in a relatively short time simply by not eating, but success remains short-lived, and eventually the urge to eat wins out and the lost weight returns. Some argue that the reason for this failure lies in a genetically determined "set point" that differs from what the dieter would like. The proponents of a **set-point theory** maintain that all persons (fat or thin) have a well-regulated internal control mechanism located deep within the lateral hypothalamus that tightly maintains a preset level of body weight and/or body fat. In a practical sense, this represents a person's body weight when not counting calories. Regular exercise and Food and Drug Administration (FDA)-approved antiobesity drugs (Xenical [orlistat], Meridia [sibutramine] and phentermine) may lower a person's set point, whereas

Higher Protein in Weight-Loss Diet Helps to Conserve Muscle Mass

Forty-six women (ages 28–80 years and BMI = 26–37) consumed a 750 kCal · d^{-1} energy deficit diet for 12 weeks that contained either 30% protein (high-protein [HP]) or 18% (normal protein [NP]).[100] The subjects were retrospectively placed into one of two obesity classifications—preobese (POB; BMI = 26–29.9) or obese (OB; BMI = 30–37). Both groups lost comparable amounts of body mass, but lean tissue loss expressed as (kg) was less in HP (–1.5 ± 0.3) than NP –2.8 ± 0.5), and POB versus OB (–1.2 ± 0.3 and –2.9 ± 0.4). The major effects of the protein content of the daily diet and obesity levels on LBM changes were independent and additive—POB-HP lost significantly less LBM than OB-NP. The implications of this research seem fairly clear—POB women of normal BMI who consumed a higher protein diet while reducing body mass over a 3-month interval conserved more LBM during weight loss than obese women who also reduced body mass on the higher protein diet.

sents the expected weight loss from the 450-kCal diet. The decline in resting metabolism (*middle figure*) conserved energy, causing the diet to become progressively less effective. More than half of the total weight loss occurred over the first 8 days of dieting; the remaining weight loss occurred during the final 16 days. A plateau in the theoretical weight-loss curve often frustrates and discourages dieters, causing them to abandon the program.

Further disconcerting news awaits those desiring permanent fat loss. When obese persons lose weight, adipocytes increase their level of the fat-storing enzyme lipoprotein lipase.[87] Unfortunately, this adaptation facilitates body fat synthesis, and the fatter the person before weight loss, the greater is the lipoprotein lipase production with weight loss. This observation supports the existence of a feedback mechanism between the brain and body fat levels and helps explain the great difficulties overweight persons encounter in maintaining weight loss.[63,72,193]

The set-point theory delivers unwelcome news to those with a set point tuned "too high." Fortunately, regular exercise may lower the set-point level. Concurrently, regular exercise conserves and even increases fat-free mass (FFM), raises resting metabolism (if FFM increases), and alters metabolism to facilitate fat breakdown.[71,99,111,169] These healthful adaptations

dieting exerts no effect. Each time body fat decreases below one's pre-established set point, internal adjustments and regulatory mechanisms resist the change and attempt to conserve and/or replenish body fat. For example, resting metabolism slows, and the individual becomes obsessed with food, unable to control the urge to eat. Even when a person overeats to gain weight above the normal level, the body resists this change by increasing resting metabolism and causing the person to lose interest in food.

RESTING METABOLISM DECREASES. Resting metabolism often decreases when dieting progressively produces weight loss.[45,99,111,182] This hypometabolism in response to caloric deficit often exceeds the decrease attributable to the loss of body mass or FFM. An overly reduced metabolism characterizes individuals attempting to lose weight, whether they dieted previously or whether they are fat or lean. Depressed metabolism conserves energy, causing the diet to become less effective despite a restricted caloric intake. This produces a weight-loss plateau at which further weight loss becomes considerably less than predicted from the mathematics of the restricted energy intake.

FIGURE 14.8 depicts the body's defense against deviations in body weight. This classic study carefully monitored body mass, resting oxygen uptake (minimal energy requirement), and caloric intake of six obese men for 31 days. During the prediet period, body mass and resting oxygen uptake stabilized with a daily food intake of 3500 kCal. When subjects then switched to 450-kCal low-calorie diet, body mass and resting metabolism decreased, and the percentage decline in metabolism exceeded the body mass decrease. The dashed line repre-

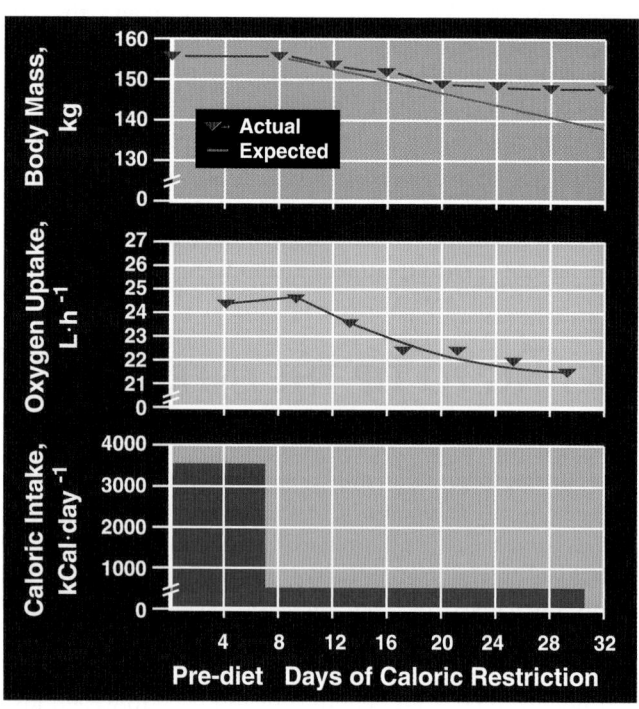

FIGURE 14.8 ■ Effects of two levels of caloric intake on changes in body mass and resting oxygen uptake. Failure to lose weight at a rate predicted from food restriction leaves the dieter frustrated and discouraged. (Adapted from Bray G. Effect of caloric restriction on energy expenditure in obese subjects. *Lancet* 1969;2:397.)

Case Study

Personal Health and Exercise Nutrition 14–1

How to Predict Percentage Body Fat for Overly Fat Men and Women from Girths

Estimating percentage body fat (%BF) in the overly fat by skinfold prediction becomes problematic because of difficulty securing accurate and repeatable measurements owing to an extensive mass of subcutaneous fat. In addition, with increasing levels of body fatness, the proportion of subcutaneous fat to total body fat changes, thereby affecting the relationship between skinfolds and body density (Db). The following factors limit skinfold use with the overly fat population:

1. Site selection and palpation of body landmarks are difficult.
2. Skinfold thickness may exceed caliper jaw aperture.
3. Variability in adipose tissue composition affects skinfold compressibility.
4. Poorer objectivity in skinfold measures as body fat increases.

Predicting Percentage Body Fat

Use the following equations to predict %BF in obese (>30%BF) women (ages 20 to 60 years and) and obese (>20%BF) men (ages 24–68 years).

Women

$$\%BF = 0.11077 \, (ABDO) - 0.17666 \, (HT) + 0.14354 \, (BW) + 51.03301$$

Men

$$\%BF = 0.31457 \, (ABDO) - 0.10969 \, (BW) + 10.8336$$

where ABDO = the average of (1) waist girth (taken horizontally at the level of the natural waist—narrowest part of the torso, as seen from the anterior) and (2) abdomen girth (taken horizontally at the level of the greatest anterior extension of the abdomen, usually, but not always, at the level of the umbilicus). Duplicate measurements are taken and averaged. BW = body weight in kg; and HT = stature in cm.

Examples
1: Overly Fat Woman

Data: waist girth = 115 cm; abdomen girth = 121 cm; HT = 165.1 cm; BW = 97.5 kg

$$\%BF = 0.11077 \, (ABDO) - 0.17666 \, (HT) + 0.14354 \, (BW) + 51.03301$$

$$= 0.11077 \, (115+121/2) - 0.17666 \, (165.1) + 0.14354 \, (97.5) + 51.03301$$

$$= 13.07 - 29.17 + 13.995 + 51.03301$$

$$= 48.9$$

2: Overly Fat Man

Data: waist girth = 131 cm; abdomen girth = 136 cm; BW = 135.6 kg

$$\%BF = 0.31457 \, (ABDO) - 0.10969 \, (BW) + 10.8336$$

$$= 0.31457 \, (131.0+136.0/2) - 0.10969 \, (135.6) + 10.8336$$

$$= 41.995 - 14.873 + 10.8336$$

$$= 37.9$$

Weltman A, et al. *Accurate assessment of body composition in obese females. Am J Clin Nutr* 1988;48:1179.

Tran ZV, Weltman A. *Predicting body composition of men from girth measurements. Hum Biol* 1988;60:167.

all augment the weight loss effort. Food intake declines initially with regular exercise for overly fat men and women. Eventually, as an active lifestyle continues and body fat reserves decrease, caloric intake balances daily energy requirements and body mass stabilizes at a new, lower level.

CHALLENGE TO THE SET-POINT PROPONENTS. Some research challenges the argument that individuals who lose weight necessarily maintain the initial depressed metabolism that predisposes them to weight regain.[179] Without doubt, energy restriction produces a transient state of hypometabolism if the dieter maintains the state of negative energy intake. This adaptive downregulation in resting metabolism does not persist when individuals lose weight but then re-establish (at their lower body weight) a balance in which energy intake equals energy expenditure. Consequently, research that fails to establish energy balance after a period of weight loss gives the inaccurate impression that individuals who lose weight necessarily battle a prolonged overcompensating reduction in resting energy expenditure until they return to their original body weight. Replication of these findings will support the contention that downregulation of resting metabolism is not a necessary characteristic of weight loss or a primary component to explain the tendency for weight regain.

Weight Cycling: Going No Place Fast

The futility of repeated cycles of weight loss and weight gain (referred to as the **yo-yo effect**) emerged from food efficiency studies that evaluated weight loss–weight gain as related to ingested calories in animals. Considerable debate exists on this subject,[13,67,82,115,130,192] but weight regain may occur more readily with repeated cycles of weight loss. For example, animals require twice the time to lose the same weight during a second period of caloric restriction and only one-third the time to regain it.[23]

Obesity raises the risk of heart disease, yet failure to keep off the lost weight may pose an additional risk. Initial reports indicated that repeated bouts of weight loss–weight regain increased the likelihood of death from a heart attack. The risk averaged almost 70% more for weight regainers than for those who maintained body weight.[83] In contrast, data from 6500 originally healthy Japanese American men revealed no ill effects from a repeated cycle of weight loss and regain.[77] The periods of rapid weight loss and regain common in dieters do not increase hypertension risk any more than the increased risk from being overweight or gaining weight in the first place.[24] Furthermore, repeated cycles of dieting do not induce adverse psychologic effects for stress level, anxiety, anger, and depression.[151]

If weight cycling should pose an additional health risk, one can only speculate on the potential long-term negative effects from repeated weight cycling so common among high school and collegiate athletes that compete in sports requiring a lean and/or low body mass. From a public health perspective, however, the risks from overweight and obesity far exceed those for weight cycling. The obese should not use the potential hazards of yo-yo dieting as an excuse to abandon efforts to reduce excess body fat. In particular, this includes efforts to increase "extra" physical activities of daily living and sports and recreational activities.

Extremes of Dieting: Potential Negative Consequences for the Physically Active Individual

Professional organizations have voiced strong opposition to certain dietary practices, particularly extremes of fasting and low-carbohydrate, high-fat, and high-protein diets. These practices remain troublesome to professionals in sports medicine and exercise physiology because of reports documenting that physically active individuals often exhibit bizarre and pathogenic weight-control behaviors and disordered eating patterns. Imprudent eating behaviors negatively affect body composition, energy reserves, and psychologic and physical well-being (see Chapter 15).

Low-Carbohydrate Ketogenic Diets

Low-carbohydrate ketogenic diets emphasize carbohydrate restriction while generally ignoring total calories and the diet's protein, cholesterol, and saturated fat content. Billed as a "diet revolution" and championed by the late Dr. Robert C. Atkins,[8] the diet was first promoted in the late 1800s and has appeared in various forms since. Long disparaged by the medical establishment, advocates maintain that restricting daily carbohydrate intake to 20 g or less for the initial 2 weeks, with some liberalization afterward, causes the body to mobilize significant fat for energy. This generates excess plasma ketone bodies—by-products of incomplete fat breakdown from inadequate carbohydrate catabolism—that supposedly suppress appetite. Theoretically, the ketones lost in the urine represent unused energy that should facilitate further weight-loss. Proponents claim that urinary energy loss becomes so great that dieters can eat all they want provided they restrict carbohydrates. Often not considered is the fact that restricting the carbohydrate-containing foods that most people eat creates a low-calorie diet that produces weight loss.

At best, energy lost by urinary ketone excretion equals only 100 to 150 kCal daily.[2] This accounts for a small weight loss of approximately 0.45 kg per month—not appealing when lipid intake as high as 70% of total calories represents the primary food source. Initial weight loss also results from dehydration from an extra solute load on the kidneys that increases water excretion. Water loss does not reduce body fat. A low-carbohydrate diet rapidly depletes glycogen reserves, which severely affects one's ability to train hard and compete. This diet also sets the stage for loss of lean tissue as the body recruits amino acids from muscle to maintain blood glucose (gluconeogenesis)—an undesirable side effect for a diet designed for body fat loss.

Although an estimated 30 to 40 million Americans attempted a low-carbohydrate diet in 2005, whether the ketogenic diet facilitates fat loss more than a well-balanced, low-calorie diet remains unclear. In general, weight loss relates principally to the diet's low caloric content and diet duration rather than reduced carbohydrate content.[21] Three recent controlled clinical trials compared the Atkins-type, low-carbohydrate diet with traditional low-fat diets for weight loss.[51,144,194] The low-carbohydrate diet was more effective in achieving a modest weight loss for severely overweight people. Some measures of heart health also improved as reflected by a more favorable blood lipid profile and glycemic control in those who followed the low-carbohydrate diets for up to 1 year.[154] Such findings add a measure of credibility to the use of low-carbohydrate diets and challenge conventional wisdom concerning the potential dangers from consuming a high-fat diet.

Importantly, Atkins-type, high-fat low-carbohydrate diets require systematic long-term evaluation (up to 5 years) for safety and effectiveness, particularly as related to the blood lipid profile. The diet, which places no limit on the amount of meat, fat, eggs, and cheese a person eats, may pose potential hazards. For example, low-carbohydrate, high-protein diets raise serum uric acid levels, potentiate the development of kidney stones, alter electrolyte concentrations to initiate cardiac arrhythmias, cause acidosis, aggravate existing kidney problems from the extra solute burden in the renal filtrate, deplete glycogen reserves to contribute to a fatigued state, decrease calcium balance and increase risk for bone loss, and cause dehydration. This diet is definitely contraindicated during pregnancy, because it retards fetal development from inadequate carbohydrate intake.

The South Beach Diet: A More Prudent Approach

In many ways, the currently popular South Beach diet, advocated by cardiologist Dr. Arthur Agatston, does not differ from the low-carbohydrate diet plan promoted by Atkins. Both individuals believe that refined carbohydrates and white flour greatly contribute to the nation's climbing obesity rate. Like the Atkins diet, the South Beach diet strictly limits intake of bread, potatoes, and other carbohydrates while permitting consumption of higher-fat red meat, cheese, and eggs. Advocates argue that most carbohydrate foods in the U.S. diet are of the high-glycemic variety that digest and absorb rapidly and raise blood glucose levels. This rise causes an insulin spike and rebound hypoglycemia that produces greater hunger and subsequently greater food intake that leads to weight gain. The increase in insulin stimulates greater storage of lipid within fat cells by downregulating hormone-sensitive lipase that helps to degrade lipid. In addition, the additional insulin increases the concentration of acetyl CoA carboxylase, which further promotes lipid storage. Keeping insulin levels depressed would theoretically allow more energy to be derived from lipid (and thus reduce body weight from the loss in lipid). In contrast to the Atkins diet that allows just about any fatty food with a low starch content, Dr. Agatston emphasizes moderate intake of unsaturated fats, like those in olive oil, fish, and nuts. The diet prohibits foods such as butter, margarine, bacon, or anything fried. Carbohydrates are permitted if they are of the slow-release unrefined, complex variety (relatively low glycemic index); these include multigrain bread, wild rice, lentils, and soy milk.

The first 2 weeks of the diet (phase 1) focus on stabilizing blood glucose by consuming only foods with the lowest glycemic indexes. Fiber-rich carbohydrates and unsaturated fatty acids are gradually reintroduced in phase 2 (until desired weight is reached) and phase 3 (maintenance). If weight gain occurs, the individual returns to phase 1. In essence, the effectiveness of the South Beach diet hinges on whether it reduces caloric intake, mainly by reducing cravings induced by dramatic swings in blood insulin. With the exception of the extreme nature of phase 1 of the diet plan, the South Beach diet appears more prudent than its Atkins counterpart because it offers more variety and promotes more healthful foods. Well-controlled research must now assess the long-term effectiveness of this dietary regimen for promoting successful weight loss and markers of overall health (e.g., high-protein diets stress kidney function and bone mass). For high-performance endurance athletes who train mainly above 65% of maximum effort, switching to a high-fat diet is ill advised because of the body's need to maintain glucose in the bloodstream and glycogen packed in the active muscles and liver storage depots. Fatigue during high-intensity exercise for more than 60 minutes duration occurs more rapidly when athletes have consumed high-fat meals than carbohydrate-rich meals. Refer to Chapter 12 for a thorough discussion of this topic.

High-Protein Diets

Low-carbohydrate, high-protein diets may shed pounds in the near term, but their long-term success remains questionable and they may even pose health risks.[44] Such diets have been commercially extolled as "last-chance diets." Earlier versions consisted of protein in liquid form advertised as "miracle liquid." Unknown to the consumer, the liquid protein mixture often contained a blend of ground-up animal hooves and horns, with pigskin mixed in a broth with enzymes and tenderizers to "predigest" it. Such collagen-based blends produced from gelatin hydrolysis (supplemented with small amounts of essential amino acids) often failed to contain the highest quality amino acid mixture and lacked required vitamins and minerals, particularly copper. A negative copper balance coincides with electrocardiographic abnormalities and rapid heart rate.[46] Protein-rich foods often contain high levels of saturated fat that increase heart disease and type 2 diabetes risk. Diets excessively high in animal protein increase urinary excretion of oxalate, a compound that combines primarily with calcium to form kidney stones.[133] High levels of urinary calcium with these diets also indicate decreased calcium balance and increased risk for bone loss. The diet's safety improves by adding high-quality protein with ample carbohydrate, essential fatty acids, and micronutrients.[114] Recently, a less extreme version of the high-protein, low-fat diet was shown to produce nutritional, weight loss, body composition, and metabolic benefits equal to and sometimes greater than a conventional high-carbohydrate, low-fat diet.[117] What remains to be answered is whether (1) relatively high-protein diets can be maintained permanently and (2) these diets can assist in maintaining the weight loss and metabolic improvements they achieve.

Some "experts" claim that extremely high protein intake suppresses appetite through reliance on fat mobilization and subsequent ketone formation. In addition, the elevated thermic effect of dietary protein, with a relatively low coefficient of digestibility (particularly for plant protein), ultimately reduces the net calories available from ingested protein compared with a well-balanced meal of equivalent caloric value. This point has some validity, but one must consider other factors when formulating a sound weight-loss program, particularly for the physically active individual. Important considerations include a high-protein diet's potential for (1) strain on liver and kidney function and accompanying dehydration, (2) electrolyte imbalance, (3) glycogen depletion, (4) lean-tissue loss, and (5) kidney stones and reduced calcium absorption.

Semistarvation Diets

Physically active individuals often "starve" themselves to lose weight. A therapeutic fast or very-low-calorie diet (VLCD) can benefit severe clinical obesity in which body fat exceeds 40 to 50% of body mass. The diet provides between 400 and 800 kCal daily as high-quality protein foods or liquid meal replacements. Dietary prescriptions usually last up to 3 months, but only as a "last resort" before undertaking more extreme medical approaches that include surgery. Dieting with a VLCD requires close supervision, usually in a hospital setting. Proponents maintain that severe food restriction breaks established dietary habits; this, in turn, improves prospects for long-term success. These diets also depress appetite to help compliance. Daily medications that accompany a VLCD usually include calcium carbonate or antihistamines for nausea, bicarbonate of soda and potassium chloride to maintain consistency of body fluids, mouthwash and sugar-free chewing gum for bad breath (from high ketone levels from fat catabolism), and bath oils for dry skin. Although surgical treatments such as gastric bypass (60,000 Americans in 2002 and 80,000 in 2003) induce a sustained weight loss, they are only prescribed for patients with a BMI of 40 or greater or a BMI of 35 to 40 accompanied by other obesity-related medical conditions.

For most individuals, semistarvation does not constitute an "ultimate diet" or the proper approach to weight control. Because a VLCD provides inadequate carbohydrate, the glycogen-storage depots in the liver and muscles deplete rapidly. This impairs physical tasks requiring either high-intensity aerobic effort or shorter-duration anaerobic power output. The continuous nitrogen loss with fasting and weight loss reflects and exacerbated lean tissue loss, which may occur disproportionately from critical organs like the heart. Finally, success rate remains relatively poor for prolonged fasting.

TABLE 14.1 summarizes the principles and main advantages and disadvantages of popular dietary approaches to weight loss. Most diets induce weight loss during the first several weeks, but body water makes up much of the lost weight. In addition, significant lean tissue loss occurs with dieting alone, particularly in the early phase of a VLCD.

THE APPROPRIATE DIET PLAN: WELL BALANCED BUT LESS OF IT

A calorie-counting approach to weight loss should provide an appropriate dietary plan that contains all the essential nutrients. If one maintains a caloric deficit, diet composition exerts little effect on the magnitude of weight lost. Reducing diets should contain the recommended micronutrients and protein, with reduced cholesterol and saturated and *trans* fatty acids. For the physically active person, the remainder should consist predominantly of unrefined, fiber-rich, complex carbohydrates. Calories do count; the trick lies in keeping within the daily limit specified by the rate of fat loss desired.

Two factors largely determine one's daily energy expenditure: (1) resting energy requirement and (2) energy expended in daily physical activities (see Fig. 14.9). Weight loss occurs if a true caloric deficit exists and energy output exceeds energy input. Short periods of caloric restriction often encourage the dieter, but do not produce the desired decrease in body fat. Instead, the lost weight consists largely of water and carbohydrate per unit of body weight lost. As weight loss progresses, a larger proportion of body fat provides energy to make up the caloric deficit created by food restriction.

MAXIMIZING CHANCES FOR SUCCESS WITH DIETING

We usually eat for two reasons. First, we consume food because of true hunger. This enables us to maintain the energy and building blocks to power the body's vital processes and sustain life. Second, we eat to satisfy appetite, which in America usually "turns on" at least three times daily. Human eating behavior intimately ties to both external (environmental) cues and internal (physiologic) cues that signal a real need for food intake. External "food cues" include the sight of food; its packaging, display, and advertising; the time and physical environment for eating; and the taste, smell, color, texture, and size of portions, which have increased steadily over the past 20 years (see Fig. 9.4).[139]

Personal Assessment: The Important First Step

Accurately assessing food intake and energy expenditure provides the framework for unbalancing the energy balance equation to favorably modify body mass and body composition.

Estimates of caloric intake from carefully obtained records of daily food intake (refer to Appendix F) usually fall within 10% of the actual number of calories consumed, an acceptable level of accuracy. For example, suppose the caloric value of daily food intake directly measured in the bomb calorimeter averages 2130 kCal. With a careful 3-day dietary

TABLE 14.1   Principles and Main Advantages and Disadvantages of Some Popular Weight Loss Methods

Method	Principle	Advantages	Disadvantages	Comments
Surgical procedure	Alteration of the gastro-intestinal tract changes capacity or amount of absorptive surface	Caloric restriction less necessary	Risks of surgery and postsurgical complications can include death	Radical procedures include stapling of the stomach and removal of a section of the small intestine (a jejunoileal bypass)
Fasting	No energy input, ensures negative energy balance	Rapid weight loss (which may be a disadvantage); reduced exposure to temptation	Ketogenic; a large portion of weight lost comes from lean body mass; nutrients lacking	Medical supervision mandatory and hospitalization recommended
Protein-sparing modified fast	Same as fasting except protein or protein with carbohydrate intake presumably helps preserve lean body mass	Same as in fasting	Ketogenic; nutrients lacking; some unconfirmed deaths have been reported, possibly from potassium depletion	Medical supervision mandatory; popular presentation in Lin's "The Last Chance Diet"
One-food-centered diets	Low-caloric intake favors negative energy balance	Being easy to follow has initial psychologic appeal	Being too restrictive means that nutrients are probably lacking; repetitious nature may cause boredom	No food or food combination known to "burn off" fat; examples include grapefruit diet and egg diet
Low-carbo-hydrate/high-fat diets	Increased ketone excretion removes energy-containing substances from the body; fat intake is often voluntarily decreased; a low calorie diet results	Inclusion of rich foods may have psychologic appeal; initial rapid loss of water may be an incentive	Ketogenic; high-fat intake contraindicated for heart and diabetes patients; nutrients lacking	Popular versions have been offered by Taller and Atkins; some called "Mayo," "Drinking Man's," and "Air Force" diets
Low-carbo-hydrate/high-protein diets	Low caloric intake favors negative energy balance	Initial rapid water loss an incentive Increased thermic effect of protein	Expense and repetitious nature may make diet difficult to sustain	Emphasizing meat makes the diet high in lipid; Pennington diet an example
High-carbo-hydrate/low-fat diets	Low caloric intake favors negative energy balance	Wise food selections can make the diet nutritionally sound	Initial water retention may be discouraging	Pritikin diet is an example

Modified and reprinted by permission from Reed PB. Nutrition: an applied science. Copyright 1980 by West-Publishing Co. All Rights Reserved.

Body Weight Stigma: No Benefit but the Opposite Effect

Stigmatizing overweight people by making them feel "bad" about themselves and their condition represents an unacceptable and ineffective form of motivation to lose weight that actually contributes to unhealthy behavior that adds to the problem of obesity. Surprisingly, family members (closely followed by health care professionals) represent the most common sources of weight stigmatization.

history to estimate caloric intake, the daily value falls between about 1920 and 2350 kCal.

Careful record keeping of food intake accomplishes two things: (1) it provides the dieter with an objective list of the foods actually consumed (rather than a "guesstimate" of food intake) and (2) it triggers the awareness of current eating habits and food preferences, an important aspect of the weight control process.

Psychological Factors Influence Eating Behavior

Depression, frustration, boredom, "uptight" or anxious feelings, guilt, sadness, and anger often trigger an urge to eat. A dieter must learn to make accurate appraisals of eating behavior, not only the quantity and frequency of eating but also specific circumstances linked to food intake. Self-analysis requires keen awareness of all aspects of food consumption. Once accomplished, a new set of desirable eating responses can substitute for previously learned "undesirable" behaviors.

Behavioral Approaches Can Help: Modification of Eating Behaviors

The first step in eating behavior modification involves describing the various eating behaviors of the person desiring to lose weight, not immediately changing the diet. The person keeps meticulous records and answers the following eight questions:

1. When were meals eaten?
2. In what place were meals eaten?
3. What was the mood, feeling, or psychological state during the meal?
4. How much time was spent eating?
5. What activities were engaged in during the meal (watching TV, driving a car, reading, during or after a workout)?
6. Who was present during the meal?
7. What food was eaten?
8. How much food was eaten?

This time-consuming and often annoying record keeping provides objective information concerning one's personal eating behaviors and reveals certain recurring patterns associated with eating. For example, the dieter may discover that (1) eating candy often accompanies feelings of depression, (2) snacking occurs while watching television, (3) hunger becomes prevalent at a particular time of day or after working out, (4) an ice-cream binge usually takes place after an argument, or (5) breakfast and lunch are never eaten at the kitchen table. Based on this analysis, the next step substitutes alternative behaviors to replace undesirable ones.

Substituting Alternative Behaviors

Many acceptable behaviors can replace an established set of undesirable ones. The box below lists some existing behaviors associated with overeating and possible substitute behaviors. Many of these recommended substitutions have been promulgated for the general population, but they also apply to recreational and competitive athletes. The major aim of this approach creates new, more positive associations to replace inappropriate eating behavior patterns.

Upgrading Control of Eating Behaviors

- **Make the act of eating a ritual.** Limit eating to one place in the house. No matter what foods you eat, follow a set routine. For example, use a place mat, set the table with silverware, and use the same dishes at each meal. Do this for main meals and snacks. One dieter who continually snacked between meals curbed this habit by dressing up in formal attire for each meal and snack—snacking between meals soon stopped. To discourage eating bread, take only one slice at a time and toast it before eating it. For each slice, get up from the table, unwrap the loaf and take out a slice, rewrap the loaf and replace it in the cupboard, toast the slice, and return to the table to eat it. Following an inconvenient routine to obtain some "special" food item often suppresses desire for the food.
- **Use smaller dishes.** The impetus to finish a meal may not be the food per se, but the desire to view an empty plate or glass. Also, try to always leave some food on the plate.
- **Eat slowly.** Fight the tendency to eat too rapidly by taking more time at meals. Cut food into smaller pieces and chew each piece 10 to 15 times before swallowing. Also, place the knife, spoon, or fork back on the table after each two or three bites, and allow a 1- or 2-minute rest pause between mouthfuls.
- **Reduce the lipid content of meals.** Simple modifications in food selection within the same food category dramati-

Substitutes for Undesirable Eating Behaviors

Established behavior patterns	Replacement behavior
Eating candy while driving	Singing along with the radio
Eating snacks while watching television	Sewing, painting, or writing letters
Feeling hungry at 4:00 PM	Going for a walk at 4:00 PM
Eating ice cream after an argument	Doing 20 repetitions of an exercise
Never eating breakfast or lunch at the kitchen table	Eating breakfast and lunch only at the kitchen table
Visiting the kitchen during TV commercials	Jogging in place; doing sit-ups
Food shopping on the way home before dinner	Do all food shopping and buying only what is on a list, after eating

---

TABLE 14.2   Checklist for Cutting Down on Dietary Lipid

- Substitute cold cuts with 1 g of fat per 1-oz serving for regular bologna, salami, or pickled beef.
- Substitute frozen yogurt or sherbet with 4 g or less of fat per 4-oz serving for high-fat ice cream.
- Substitute air-popped popcorn and pretzels for party chips.
- Substitute whole-grain breads and crackers for croissants and corn bread.
- Substitute a variety of cereals for high-fat granola preparations.
- Substitute cheese with less than 4 to 5 g of fat per ounce for high-fat cheeses.
- Substitute egg whites for egg yolks, or use a dehydrated egg substitute.
- Substitute light or fat-free mayonnaise for regular mayonnaise.
- Substitute 2% or 1% milk for whole milk.
- Substitute a variety of herbs or use low-calorie salad dressings or salsa instead of oil-rich or creamy salad dressings.
- Avoid frozen vegetables in rich sauces.
- Buy beef and pork with words "round" or "lean" in the name.
- Buy low-fat cake mixes.
- Do not add oil or butter to water when cooking pasta, macaroni, or oatmeal.
- Make hamburgers from ground round or ground sirloin.
- Substitute two egg whites for one whole egg in baking.
- Substitute evaporated skim milk for cream in recipes.
- Replace 1/4 of the fat in your favorite recipe with applesauce.

---

cally affect the meal's caloric density. TABLE 14.2 presents a convenient checklist for cutting down on the intake of dietary lipid; TABLE 14.3 provides appropriate low-calorie substitutions within various food categories.

- **Follow a Food Plan.** Following a highly structured daily food plan (what, when, and where food will be eaten) reduces the risk of eating high-calorie "impulse" foods.

Developing New Techniques to Control Eating

Many useful techniques can control eating behaviors once undesirable environmental cues and associated behaviors have been identified and replaced or modified. Delaying, substituting, and avoiding represent three behavioral strategies for interrupting poor eating behaviors:

- **Delaying.** Add time or steps between the links in the behavior chain:
  - Slow down the eating pace
  - Take a roundabout way to the kitchen
  - Purchase single-portion packages of snacks
  - Put off unplanned eating as long as possible—mail a letter, read a book, mow the lawn, or do sit-ups or pushups
- **Substituting.** Break the behavior chain with activities incompatible with eating:
  - Pleasant activities—read, go for a walk, listen to music, do hobbies, surf the Internet
  - Required activities—plan the budget, pay bills, do errands, clean the house

- **Avoiding.** Keep yourself out of situations in which food is visible or easily accessible:
  - Stay out of the kitchen or other areas associated with eating
  - Do not combine eating with other activities such as reading, TV watching, driving, or working out
  - When finished eating, remove dishes and food from the table
  - Scrape excess food directly into the garbage

EXERCISE FOR WEIGHT CONTROL

A sedentary lifestyle consistently emerges as an important factor in weight gain for children, adolescents, and adults.

Weight Gain: Not Simply a Problem of Gluttony

Conventional wisdom views excessive food intake as the prime cause of the overly fat condition. Most persons believe that the only way to reduce unwanted body fat entails caloric restriction by dieting. This overly simplistic strategy partly accounts for the dismal success in maintaining weight loss over the long term, refocusing debate on the contribution of food intake to obesity.[65,149]

In the United States, per capita caloric intake has not increased enough to account for the steady rise in the national

TABLE 14.3   Substituting Foods with Lower Calorie Content

The chart below can help you plan your meals while following the simple guidelines for healthful eating. When you select a variety of foods from those listed in the far left column, you'll be eating foods that are low in fats and/or high in dietary fiber.

Type of Food	Select Most Often	Select Moderately	Select Least Often
Animal protein	Lean cuts of beef/pork Salmon, halibut (broiled) Canned tuna in water Poultry (w/o skin) Egg Crab	Untrimmed beef and pork Canned tuna in oil Poultry (with skin) Lobster, shrimp Canadian bacon	Fatty beef, lamb, pork Luncheon meats/hot dogs Fried chicken Fried fish Liver, kidneys
Dairy	Nonfat yogurt Nonfat milk (or 1/2%) Nonfat dry milk Nonfat frozen yogurt	Reduced fat and part-skim cheeses Low-fat cottage cheese Low-fat milk Low-fat yogurt 95% Fat-free frozen yogurt	Whole-milk cheese (cheddar, muenster) Whole milk Sour cream, ice cream Cream, half-and-half
Vegetable protein	Dried beans and peas (kidney, lima, and soy beans; lentils; split peas) Tofu (bean curd)	Raw or dry-roasted nuts and seeds Peanut and other butters (moderate amounts)	Oil-processed nuts and seeds
Vegetables	Raw, fresh vegetables Fresh or frozen, slightly cooked vegetables	Canned vegetables Canned tomatoes or vegetable juice	Vegetables in cream or butter sauces Fried vegetables
Fruits	Fresh, raw fruit Dried fruit Frozen and fresh fruit juices	Canned fruit packed in juice Canned fruit juices Frozen fruit	Fruit-flavored beverages Canned fruit packed in syrup Avocados Olives
Grain products	Shredded wheat, oats Whole-grain cereals Whole-grain breads Brown rice Wheat bran, oat bran Bagels Fig bars	Refined cereals Enriched white breads Refined pastas White rice Granolas Toast with margarine Plain cookies	Cookies, cakes, pies Sweetened cereals Tortilla chips Oil-processed crackers Cream-filled doughnuts Croissants, doughnuts
Other	Popcorn (air-popped)	Low-fat salad dressing Low-fat mayonnaise Pretzels	Fat-rich salad dressing Mayonnaise Gravies, cream sauce Potato chips

From Wardlaw GM, et al. Contemporary nutrition issues and insights. 2nd ed. St. Louis, MO: Mosby, 1992.

body mass over the last century, a weight gain equivalent to 30 lb for a 6-foot man. Only in the past decade has daily energy intake increased above the level in the early part of the 20th century. The observation that overly fat persons often eat the same or even less than thinner people holds true for a large number of overly fat adults over a broad age range as they become less active and slowly add weight. Excess weight gain often parallels reduced physical activity rather than increased caloric intake. Current estimates indicate that 27% of U.S. adults engage in no daily physical activity and another

28% do not regularly take part in physical activity.[110] Among active endurance-trained men, body fat inversely relates to energy expenditure (low body fat, high energy expenditure and vice versa); no relationship emerges between body fat and food intake.[107] Surprisingly, physically active people who eat the most generally weigh the least and exhibit the highest levels of fitness.

Excessive food intake does not fully explain the rise in obesity among children. Obese infants do not characteristically consume more calories than recommended dietary standards. For children ages 4 to 6 years, a reduced level of physical activity primarily accounted for their daily energy expenditure 25% lower than the energy intake recommendation for this age.[27] More specifically, 50% of boys and 75% of girls in the United States fail to engage in even moderate physical activity three or more times weekly. Children ages 6 to 17 years have consumed 4% fewer calories over the past 25 years, yet the prevalence of childhood obesity continues to increase dramatically. In contrast, physically active children tend to be leaner than less active counterparts. For preschool children, no relationship emerged between total energy intake, or the fat, carbohydrate, and protein composition of the diet and percentage body fat.[7] Time-in-motion photography to document activity patterns of elementary school students showed that overweight children remained less physically active than their normal-weight peers; excess body weight did not relate to food intake. Overly fat high school girls and boys actually consumed fewer calories than their nonobese peers.[85,138] Excessive fatness and incidence of type 2 diabetes relate directly to the number of hours spent watching television (a consistent marker of inactivity) among individuals of all ages.[4,76] For example, 3 hours of television viewing a day led to a twofold increase in obesity and a 50% increase in diabetes.[76] Each 2-hour per day increment of TV watching coincided with a 23% increase in obesity and a 14% rise in diabetes risk. Family structure (e.g., with or without sibldings and number of siblings; one-parent vs two-parent familiies) also interact to influence children's physical activity and television viewing time.[9] Excessive television watching, playing video games, and otherwise remaining physically inactive particularly characterizes minority teens.[55,136] Minimizing time devoted to these behaviors helps to combat childhood fat gain.

Total Daily Energy Expenditure

Total daily energy expenditure (TDEE) consists of the sum of all the anabolic and catabolic chemical reactions within the body. Three general factors influence TDEE (see Fig. 6.8).

- **Factor 1.** Resting metabolic rate refers to the sum of metabolic processes for maintenance of normal body function and regulatory balance during rest. It includes basal and sleeping conditions plus the added metabolic cost of arousal. Resting metabolism generally accounts for 60 to 75% of TDEE, depending on daily level of physical activity.
- **Factor 2.** Energy expended during physical activity and recovery profoundly affects variability among individuals in

TDEE. World-class athletes nearly double their daily caloric output with 3 to 4 hours of arduous training. Most persons can sustain metabolic rates 10 times the resting level during "big muscle" activities such as fast walking, running, cycling, and swimming. Under typical circumstances, physical activity accounts for between 15 and 30% of the TDEE.
- **Factor 3.** Thermogenic effect of food consumed (TEF) refers to the effect of food consumption on energy metabolism. TEF (also called dietary-induced thermogenesis) consists of two components. One component, obligatory thermogenesis, results from the energy required to digest, absorb, and assimilate food nutrients. The second component, facultative thermogenesis, results from sympathetic nervous system activation from food ingestion and its stimulating effect on metabolism.[146]

Effectiveness of Increasing Energy Expenditure

Regular physical activity plays a central role in protecting against weight gain. Men and women of all ages who maintain a physically active lifestyle (or become involved in regular exercise programs) maintain a more desirable level of body composition than less active counterparts. For overweight adult women, a dose–response relationship exists between the amount of exercise and long-term weight loss.[81] Obese adolescents and adults improve body composition and visceral fat distribution from regular moderate physical activity or more vigorous exercise that improves cardiovascular fitness.[61,103,106] For obese boys and girls, the most favorable body composition changes occur with (1) low-intensity, long-duration exercise; (2) aerobic exercise combined with high-repetition resistance training; and (3) exercise programs combined with a behavior-modification component.[61,103] For those who lose weight, regular exercise facilitates weight-loss maintenance better than programs relying solely on dieting.[1,3,91,121,152,187] This positive effect occurs partly because regular exercise counteracts the typical postdiet decline in fat oxidation in those who lose weight by only energy restriction.[168]

Even for currently active individuals, additional exercise unbalances the energy balance equation for weight loss, favorably alters body composition and body fat distribution,[95,141,142,161] and further improves physical fitness.[14,142,166] Additional spin-off from regular physical activity includes (1) slowing of the age-related loss in muscle mass, (2) improvement in obesity-related comorbidities, (3) decreased mortality, and (4) beneficial effects on existing chronic diseases.[20,64,98,104,155,167,178]

Regular Exercise Increases Daily Energy Expenditure

Some truth exists to the notion that one must perform an extraordinary amount of exercise to lose body fat. The statistics reveal that just to lose 0.45 kg (1 lb) of body fat a person has to chop wood for 10 hours, golf for 20 hours, perform mild calisthenics for 22 hours, play ping-pong for 28 hours or volleyball for 32 hours, or run 35 miles. Understandably, such a commitment seems overwhelming to the person who plans to reduce by 10 or 15 kg or more. From a longer-term perspective, if the person walked an extra 3.5 miles (about 350 kCal) 2 days a week (700 kCal), it would take about 5 weeks, or 10 walking days, to lose 0.45 kg of body fat (3500 kCal). Assuming one continued to walk year-round, walking 2 days a week reduces body fat by 4.5 kg during the year provided food intake remains fairly constant. Exercise produces cumulative calorie-expending effects; 0.45-kg body fat loss occurs when the caloric deficit equals 3500 kCal, regardless of whether the deficit occurs rapidly or systematically over time.

During low-to-moderate exercise (as performed by most persons who exercise for weight control), recovery metabolism—the so-called recovery afterglow—contributes minimally to total energy expenditure because recovery occurs rapidly. In addition, regular exercise causes faster adjustments in postexercise energetics, reducing the total recovery oxygen consumption.[150] Calories burned *during* physical activity represent the most important factor in total exercise energy expenditure, not calories expended for recovery.

The Ideal: Conserve Lean and Reduce Fat

Regular physical activity, with or without dietary restriction, protects against weight gain and favorably changes body mass and body composition.[34,35,141] This occurs because exercise training enhances fat mobilization from adipose depots and increases fat breakdown by the active muscles.[105] In addition, exercise retains skeletal muscle protein (maintains positive nitrogen balance), while simultaneously retarding protein breakdown. The protein-sparing effect of regular exercise partly explains why more of the weight lost comes from fat in a program that uses exercise than in one using only food restriction. Those with the largest amount of excess fat lose body weight and fat more readily with exercise than their leaner counterparts.[11] Even without dietary restrictions, exercise provides positive "spin-off" to favorably alter body composition by reducing body fat and maintaining or even increasing FFM.

Best Types of Physical Activities

When using exercise to lose weight, consider the **FITT** acronym: **F**requency, **I**ntensity, **T**ime, and **T**ype of exercise. Ideal aerobic activities having moderate-to-high caloric cost include brisk walking and hiking, running, rope skipping, stair stepping, circuit-resistance training, cycling, and swimming. TABLE 14.4 lists the "top 12" physical activities for energy expenditure. Many recreational sports and games also create an effective caloric deficit for weight loss, but precise quantification and regulation of energy expenditure remain difficult with these activities. No selective effect exists for running, walking, or bicycling; each effectively burns sufficient calories to favorably alter body composition. For low-impact walking as the sole means of exercising, energy expenditure increases by adding hand, wrist, or ankle weights or using

TABLE 14.4	"Top 12" Exercises Ranked by Relative Strenuousness (kCal expended per min)
kCal·min^{-1}	Activity
25.9	Roller skiing, V-Skate technique, 11.2 mph, trained athletes
23.3	In-line skiing, double-pole technique, 11.2 mph, trained athletes
22.0	Skiing, cross-country, hard snow, uphill (5° grade), maximum effort, trained
19.3	Swimming, Mini-Gym Swim Bench, 45 strokes per min (freely chosen)
18.2	Rowing, mechanically braked rowing ergometer; stroke rate = 28–32 per min, 1750 kg-m·min^{-1}, athletes
18.1	Rowing, "all out" for 6 min on a rowing ergometer
18.0	Running, 10.9 mph (5.5 min per mile pace)
18.0	Race walking, competition, 8.5 mph, men
17.2	Marathon running, 5:03 min per mile pace, trained
17.1	Running, shallow water (1.3 m depth), no vest, maximal effort
17.0	Forestry, ax-chopping, fast
16.0	Skin-diving, vigorous

Data source: Katch FI, et al. Calorie expenditure charts. Fitness Technologies Press. 1132 Lincoln Avenue. Ann Arbor MI, 1996. Used by permission.

race-walking techniques. An extra 300-kCal daily caloric expenditure induced by moderate jogging daily for 30 minutes theoretically produces a 0.45-kg fat loss in about 12 days, or a yearly caloric deficit equivalent to the energy in 13.6 kg of body fat.

RESISTANCE TRAINING. Resistance training provides an important adjunct to aerobic training to promote weight loss and weight maintenance. The energy expended in circuit resistance training—continuous exercise using low resistance and high repetitions—averages about 9 kCal per minute. Consequently, this exercise mode burns substantial calories during a typical 30- to 60-minute workout. Even conventional resistance training that involves less total energy expenditure affects muscular strength and FFM more positively during weight loss than programs that rely solely on food restriction.[12,171] Individuals who maintain high muscular strength levels tend to gain less weight than weaker counterparts.[97] In addition, standard resistance training performed regularly reduces coronary heart disease risk, improves glycemic control, favorably modifies the lipoprotein profile, and increases resting metabolic rate (if FFM increases).[126,127,129,158] TABLE 14.5 illustrates the effects of 12 weeks of either endurance training or resistance training on nondieting young men. Endurance training

TABLE 14.5 Changes in Body Composition after 12 Weeks of Either Resistance Training or Endurance Training						
	Controls		Resistance Trained		Endurance Trained	
Variable	Pretreatment	Posttreatment	Pretreatment	Posttreatment	Pretreatment	Posttreatment
Relative body fat (%)	20.1±8.5	20.2±8.5	21.8±6.2	18.7±6.6[a]	18.4±7.9	16.5±6.4[a]
Fat mass (kg)	16.2±10.8	16.3±10.5	17.2±7.6	14.8±6.2[a]	14.4±7.9	12.8±7.1[a]
Fat-free body mass (kg)	64.3±5.4	64.4±6.6	61.9±8.3	64.4±9.0[a]	64.1±8.2	64.7±8.6
Total body mass (kg)	80.5±8.1	80.7±8.5	79.1±8.3	79.2±7.6	78.5±8.2	77.5±7.9

From Broeder CE, et al. Assessing body composition before and after resistance or endurance training. Med Sci Sports Exerc 1997;29:705.

[a]Significant difference between pre- and posttest measurements (P ≤.05).

All values means ±SD.

significantly reduced percentage body fat by reducing fat mass (−1.6 kg; no change in FFM), while resistance training significantly decreased body fat mass (−2.4 kg) and increased the FFM (+2.4 kg). Conserving and/or increasing FFM maintains a relatively high level of resting metabolism, independent of age.[17,39,40,101,143,191] This reduces the body's tendency to store calories, which augments the effectiveness of the weight loss program. For athletes, maintaining FFM during weight reduction counters the potential negative effects of weight loss on exercise performance.

A Dose–Response Relationship

Some individuals believe that light aerobic exercise induces more effective weight loss because fat contributes a greater percentage of total calories burned in exercise compared with more intense physical activity in which carbohydrate represents the primary fuel. Fat combustion does provide a greater percentage of the total energy metabolism during light versus intense aerobic exercise (see Chapter 5). However, a larger total quantity of fat combustion occurs in higher-intensity aerobic exercise performed for an equivalent duration. The total number of calories expended to create the exercise energy deficit, not the percentage mixture of macronutrients oxidized, determines the effectiveness of exercise in weight loss

A direct dose-response relationship exists between time spent exercising and weight lost. The person who exercises by walking burns considerable calories simply by extending exercise duration. Also, a proportional relationship exists between the energy cost of weight-bearing exercise like walking and body mass; thus, the overweight person expends considerably more calories walking than does someone of average body weight.

MAXIMIZING CHANCES FOR SUCCESS WITH INCREASED PHYSICAL ACTIVITY: MODIFICATION OF EXERCISE BEHAVIORS

A person burns additional calories through physical activity simply by extending exercise duration, perhaps at a lower in-

tensity. Another effective calorie-burning strategy replaces daily periods of inactivity with additional physical activity requiring greater energy expenditure.

Describe the Behavior for Modification

Any hope of changing the profile of daily physical activity depends on an accurate appraisal of daily activities. The first step in exercise behavior modification determines the daily pattern of physical activity, including the minimal requirements of sleeping, eating, going to the bathroom, and bathing. The next step substitutes more strenuous activities for those that rate low in energy expenditure. Appendix F illustrates an activity profile from daily records of time spent in various activities for 3 consecutive days. The records should describe the activity, its duration, and estimated energy requirements.

Substitute Alternative Behaviors

Various options exist to increase energy expenditure within the time allotted to daily routines. The important consideration involves determining when and how to make changes with alternative exercise behaviors.

Maximize Success

Four techniques can help to maximize success when using exercise for weight loss.

1. **Progress slowly.** Add additional exercise gradually. Over time, more opportunities to add physical activity become apparent.
2. **Include variety.** Rather than performing the same exercise repeatedly in a given time, vary the exercise and number of repetitions. For a competitive athlete, the added physical activity for weight loss need not be in the specific sport.
3. **Become goal oriented.** Set a specific and realistic goal for increasing physical activity. Three ways generally add additional exercise using goal-oriented behavior: (1) exercise for a certain length of time, (2) continue to exercise until you reach a predetermined number of repetitions or distance, or (3) manipulate exercise duration and repetitions or distance.

4. **Be systematic.** Set aside certain times during the day to exercise. Do not allow outside factors (e.g., watching television, shopping, housework) to interfere with daily physical activity.

ALTERNATIVE EXERCISE BEHAVIORS

1. When driving to school, work, or the gym, park one-half mile away and walk the remaining distance; brisk walking to and from the car each day, 5 days a week, burns the caloric equivalent of about 3.2 kg of body fat in 1 year.
2. When taking public transportation, depart several stops early and walk the remaining distance.
3. When traveling relatively short distances, walk, jog, or bicycle instead of driving.
4. Skip the restaurant for lunch; instead, "brown bag" it and then participate in some form of physical activity for 15 to 30 minutes.
5. Wake up an hour early and take a brisk walk, cycle, row, rollerblade, or swim before breakfast.
6. Replace the cocktail hour or the evening beer with 20 minutes of exercise.
7. Replace coffee breaks with exercise breaks.
8. Walk up and down several flights of stairs after each hour at work or school.
9. Sweep the sidewalks in front of your house, apartment, or dorm.
10. Allow time for exercise when going on a family outing. Get out of the car before reaching your destination; let a friend or family member drive the rest of the way while you walk or jog.
11. Instead of eating at an intermission at sporting events, walk around the stadium or arena; climb up and down stairs instead of using an elevator or escalator.
12. Replace the hired help and undertake some of these tasks yourself:
    - Garden
    - Mow the lawn
    - Paint
    - Wash and wax the car
    - Rake leaves
    - Shovel snow
    - Run in place, jump rope, jog up and down stairs, or perform vigorous calisthenics during television commercials.

FOOD RESTRICTION PLUS INCREASED PHYSICAL ACTIVITY

Success stories exist for those with considerable excess body fat, despite the difficulties encountered losing weight.[69,91] Among lifetime members of a commercial weight loss organization that promotes prudent caloric restriction, behavior modification, group support, and moderate physical activity, over half maintained their original weight loss goal after 2 years, and more than one third had done so after 5 years.[108] Combinations of exercise and dietary restraint with more unrefined, low-glycemic carbohydrates and less lipids offer considerably more flexibility for achieving a negative caloric balance than either exercise alone or diet alone.[39,42,70,96,113,131,174] Body fat losses of up to 2 lb (0.9 kg) each week fall within acceptable limits, but a steady 0.5 to 1.0 lb a week loss may be even more desirable.

Setting a Realistic Target Time

Suppose 20 weeks represents the target time to achieve a 9-kg (20-lb) fat loss. With this goal, the weekly energy deficit must average 3500 kCal, or a daily average of 500 kCal (3500 kCal ÷ 7d). By dieting, the person reduces daily caloric intake by 500 kCal for 5 months (3500 kCal weekly deficit) to achieve the desired 9-kg fat loss. Instead, if the dieter performed an additional one-half hour of moderate exercise equivalent to 350 "extra" kCal 3 days per week, then the weekly caloric deficit increases by 1050 kCal (3 days × 350 kCal per exercise session). Consequently, weekly food intake could decrease to only 2400 kCal (about 350 kCal per day) instead of 3500 kCal to achieve the desired 0.45-kg weekly fat loss. Increasing the number of weekly exercise days from 3 to 5 requires reducing daily food intake by only 250 kCal. If duration of the 5-day per week extra exercise lengthens from 30 minutes to 1 hour, then the desired weight loss occurs without reducing food intake because the extra physical activity produces the entire 3500-kCal deficit.

If intensity of the 1-hour exercise performed 5 days per week increased by only 10% (cycling at 22 instead of 20 mph; running a mile in 9 instead of 10 minutes; swimming each 50 yards in 54 seconds instead of 60 seconds), the number of weekly exercise calories burned increases by 350 kCal (3500 kCal per week × 10%). This new weekly deficit of 3850 kCal, or 550 kCal per day, would then permit the "dieter" to increase daily food intake by 50 kCal and still lose a pound of fat each week, a clear example of "eat more, weigh less"!

The effective use of physical activity by itself or in combination with mild dietary restriction unbalances the energy balance equation to produce meaningful weight loss. This combined approach reduces feelings of intense hunger and psychologic stress more than does weight loss exclusively by caloric restriction. In addition, prolonged dieting increases the chances of developing a variety of nutritional deficiencies that hinder exercise training and competitive performance. Combining exercise with weight loss produces desirable reductions in blood pressure at rest and in situations that typically elevate blood pressure such as intense physical activity and emotional distress.[153]

SPOT REDUCTION DOES NOT WORK

The notion of spot reduction comes from the belief that increasing a muscle's activity facilitates fat mobilization from the adipose tissue in close proximity to the muscle. Exercising

Regardless of the approach to weight loss, a statement from the National Task Force on the Prevention and Treatment of Obesity best sums up the difficulty in solving the overly fat condition on a long-term basis: "Obese individuals who undertake weight loss efforts should be ready to commit to lifelong changes in their behavioral patterns, diet, and physical activity."[114]

a specific body area should selectively reduce more fat from that area than if different muscle groups exercised at the same caloric intensity. Advocates of selective spot reduction recommend large numbers of sit-ups or side-bends for a person with excessive abdominal fat. Whereas the promise of spot reduction with exercise offers aesthetic and health-risk benefits, critical evaluation of the research evidence does not support its effectiveness.

To examine the claims for spot reduction, researchers compared the girths and subcutaneous fat stores of the right and left forearms of high-caliber tennis players.[62] As expected, the girth of the dominant or playing arm exceeded that of the nondominant arm because of modest muscular hypertrophy from the exercise overload of tennis. Measurements of skinfold thickness indicated that years of playing tennis did not reduce subcutaneous fat in the playing arm. Another study evaluated fat biopsy specimens from the abdominal, subscapular, and buttock sites before and after 27 days of sit-up exercise training.[86] The daily number of sit-ups increased from 140 at the end of the first week to 336 on day 27. Despite this impressive amount of localized "spot" exercise, adipocytes in the abdominal region were no smaller than in unexercised buttocks or subscapular control regions.

Undoubtedly, a negative energy balance created through regular exercise reduces total body fat because exercise stimulates mobilization of fatty acids through hormones that act on fat depots throughout the body. Body areas of greatest body fat concentration and/or lipid-mobilizing enzyme activity supply the greatest amount of this energy. Selective exercise does not cause significantly more fatty acid release from the fat pads directly over the active muscles.

Where on the Body Does Fat Loss Occur?

Changes in body fat and fat distribution in obese women at successive 2.3-kg (5-lb) increments of weight loss over a 14-week period addressed the frequently asked question. "Where on the body does fat loss occur when weight is lost?" Caloric restriction and a 45-minute, 3-day per week exercise program affected weight loss.[89] FIGURE 14.9 displays the changes in body composition, skinfolds, and girths in the three sub-

groups that reduced body mass by 2.3, 4.5, and 9.1 kg. A 4.5-kg weight loss produced approximately twice as much change in overall body composition as a loss of 2.3 kg *(top graph)*. The corresponding change in body composition almost tripled when weight loss doubled from 4.5 to 9.1 kg. Skinfolds *(middle graph)* and girths *(bottom graph)* in the trunk region decreased about twice as much as those in the extremities. Decreases in body fat with exercise training and/or caloric restriction preferentially occur in upper-body subcutaneous fat and deep abdominal fat rather than the more "resistant" fat depots in gluteal and femoral regions.[34,36,93,116]

POSSIBLE GENDER DIFFERENCE IN EXERCISE EFFECTS ON WEIGHT LOSS

An interesting question concerns the possibility of a gender difference in the responsiveness of weight loss to regular exercise.[41,95,180] A meta-analysis of 53 research studies on this topic concluded that men generally respond more favorably than women to the effects of exercise on weight loss.[11] One possible explanation involves gender differences in body fat distribution and gender-related differences from an increased energy intake in response to exercise and a lower energy expenditure in exercise for women compared to men.[41] The mobilization capacity of triacylglycerols for energy depends on anatomic location. Fat distributed in the upper body and abdominal regions (central fat) shows an active lipolysis to sympathetic nervous system stimulation and preferentially mobilizes for energy during exercise.[5,6,147,176] The greater distribution of upper-body adipose tissue in men than in women may contribute to their greater sensitivity to lose fat with regular exercise. The final answer to this intriguing question awaits further research.

EFFECTS OF DIET AND EXERCISE ON BODY COMPOSITION DURING WEIGHT LOSS

TABLE 14.6 summarizes the benefits of exercise for weight loss. Addition of exercise to a weight loss program favorably modifies the composition of the weight lost in the direction of greater fat loss.[12,34,35] In a pioneering study in this area, three groups of adult women maintained a 500-kCal daily caloric deficit during 16 weeks of weight loss.[196] The diet group reduced daily food intake by 500 kCal, whereas women in the exercise group maintained daily energy intake but increased energy output by 500 kCal with a supervised walking and conditioning program. The women using diet plus exercise created the daily 500 kCal deficit by reducing food intake by 250 kCal and increasing exercise energy output by 250 kCal. No difference emerged among the three groups for weight loss; each group lost approximately 5 kg. This finding highlights that a caloric deficit reduces body weight regardless of

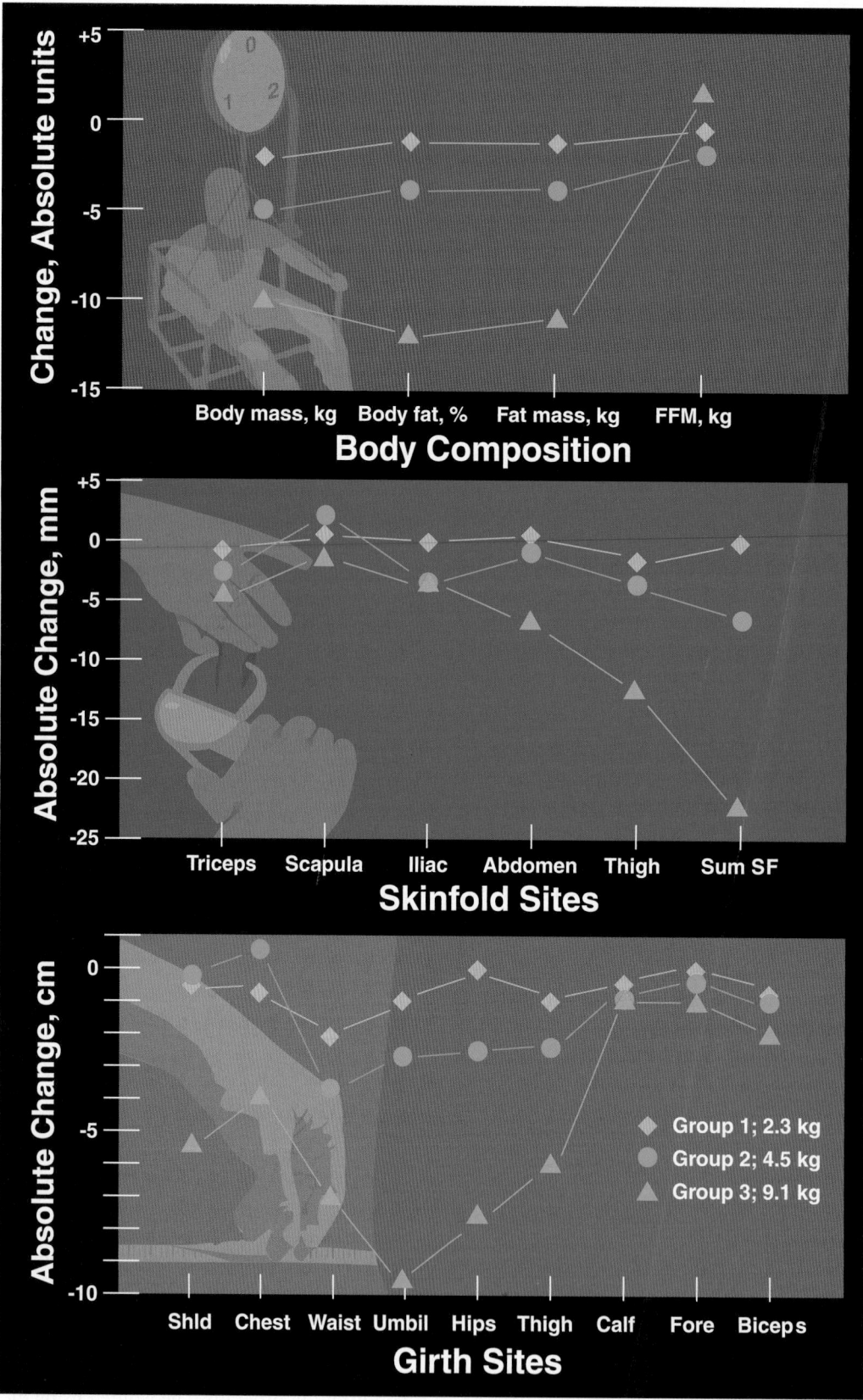

FIGURE 14.9 ■ Changes in body composition *(top)*, skinfolds *(middle)*, and girths *(bottom)* with specified amounts of weight loss. Abbreviations for girths: *Shld,* shoulders; *Umbil,* umbilicus abdomen; *Fore,* forearm; *SF,* skinfolds. Figures 13.10 and 13.11 illustrate the anatomic sites for skinfold and girth measurement. (Data from King AC, Katch FL. Changes in body density, fatfold and girths at 2.3 kg increments of weight loss. *Hum Biol* 1986;58:708.

TABLE 14.6	Benefits of Adding Exercise to Dietary Restriction for Weight Loss

- Increases the overall size of the energy deficit
- Facilitates fat mobilization and oxidation, especially from visceral adipose tissue depots
- Increases the relative loss of body fat by preserving the fat-free body mass
- By conserving and even increasing the fat-free body mass, blunts the drop in resting metabolism that frequently accompanies weight loss
- Requires less reliance on caloric restriction to create energy deficit
- Contributes to the long-term success of the weight loss effort
- Provides unique and significant health-related benefits
- May provide moderate suppression of appetite

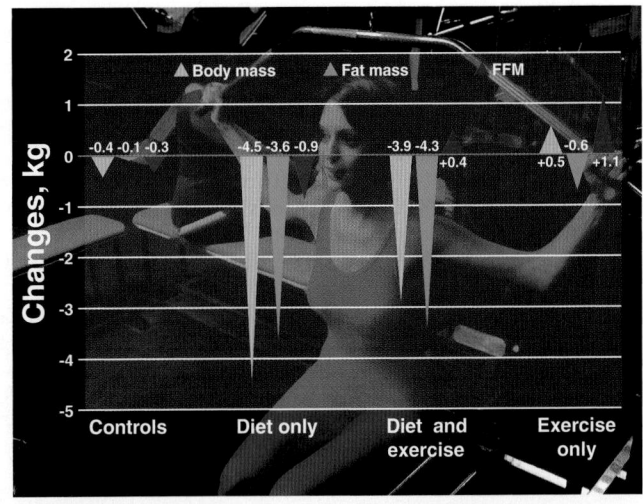

FIGURE 14.10 ■ Changes in body composition with resistance exercise and diet in obese females. (From Ballor DI, et al. Resistance weight training during caloric restriction enhances lean body weight maintenance. *Am J Clin Nutr* 1988;47:190.)

the method used to create the energy imbalance. An interesting observation for weight loss concerned FFM. The exercise group increased FFM by 0.9 kg, and the combination group increased FFM by 0.5 kg, but the dieters lost 1.1 kg of lean tissue! For body fat reduction, combining diet and exercise proved most effective.

FIGURE 14.10 displays body composition changes for 40 obese women placed into one of four groups: (1) control, with no exercise and no diet; (2) diet only, no exercise (DO); (3) diet plus resistance exercise (D + E); and (4) resistance exercise only, no diet (EO). The exercise groups trained 3 days a week for 8 weeks. They performed 10 repetitions for each of 3 sets of eight strength exercises. Body mass decreased for DO (−4.5 kg) and D + E (−3.9 kg) groups, compared with EO (+0.5 kg) and controls (−0.4 kg). Importantly, FFM increased significantly for EO (+1.1 kg), whereas the DO group lost 0.9 kg of FFM. Clearly, augmenting a calorie-restriction program with resistance exercise training preserves FFM compared with dietary restriction alone.

WEIGHT LOSS RECOMMENDATIONS FOR WRESTLERS AND OTHER POWER ATHLETES

Weightlifters, gymnasts, and other athletes in sports requiring large muscular strength and power in relation to body mass often must lose body fat without negatively affecting exercise performance. For these athletes, an increase in relative muscular strength and short-term power output capacity should improve competitive performance. The following discussion focuses on wrestlers but applies to all physically active individuals who desire to reduce body fat without negatively affecting health, safety, and exercise capacity.

To reduce injury and medical complications from short- and longer-term periods of weight loss and dehydration, the American College of Sports Medicine (ACSM; www.acsm. org), National Collegiate Athletic Association (NCAA; www.ncaa.org), and the American Medical Association (AMA; www.ama-assn.org) recommend assessing each wrestler's body composition. The National Federation of State High School Associations (www.nfhs.org) required the adoption of weight certification beginning with the 2005 season. This assessment takes place several weeks before the competitive season to determine a **minimal wrestling weight** based on percentage body fat. Five percent body fat (determined using hydrostatic weighing or population-specific skinfold equations) represents the lowest acceptable level for safe wrestling competition.[29,120,160] For wrestlers under 16 years of age, 7% body fat level represents the recommended lower limit. The hydrostatic weighing or skinfold assessment of body fat recommended by the NCAA has recently been cross-validated by the more-rigorous four-component body composition assessment and found acceptable in terms of accuracy and precision.[29] Importantly, percentage body fat must be determined in the euhydrated state, because dehydration of between 2 and 5% body weight through fluid restriction and exercise in a hot environment (techniques commonly used by wrestlers) violates the assumptions necessary for accurate and precise prediction of minimal wrestling weight. TABLE 14.7 outlines a practical application to determine minimal wrestling weight and an appropriate competitive weight class. The ACSM also recommends that weight-loss, if war-

---

TABLE 14.7 **Using Anthropometric Equations to Predict a Minimal Wrestling Weight and to Select a Competitive Weight Class**

A. To predict body density (BD), use one of the following equations: (For each skinfold, record the average of at least three trials in mm.)

1. Lohman equation[a]
   BD = 1.0982 − (0.00815 × [triceps + subscapular + abdominal skinfolds])
     + (0.00000084 × [triceps + subscapular + abdominal skinfolds]^2)
2. Katch and McArdle equation[b]
   BD = 1.09448 − (0.00103 × triceps skinfold) − (0.00056 × subscapular skinfold) − (0.00054 × abdominal skinfold)
3. Behnke and Wilmore equation[c]
   BD = 1.05721 − (0.00052 × abdominal skinfold) + (0.00168 × iliac diameter) + (0.00114 × neck circumference)
     + (0.00048 × chest circumference) + (0.00145 × abdominal circumference)
4. Thorland equation[d]
   BD = 1.0982 − (0.000815 × [triceps + abdominal skinfolds]) + (0.00000084 × [triceps + abdominal skinfolds])

B. To determine fat percentage, use the Brožek equation:

% Fat = [4.570 ÷ BD − 4.142] × 100

C. To determine fat-free weight and to identify a minimum weight class, follow the examples below:

1. Jonathan, a 15 year-old wrestler who weighs 132 lb, has a body density of 1.075 g·cc^{-1} and hopes to compete in the 119-lb weight class.
2. Jonathan's percentage fat is (4.570 ÷ 1.075 − 4.142) × 100 = 10.9%
3. Jonathan's fat weight and fat-free weight are:
   a. 132.0 lb × 0.109 = 14.4 lb fat weight
   b. 132.0 lb − 14.4 lb fat = 117.6 lb fat-free weight

D. To calculate a minimal wrestling weight:

1. Realize that the recommended minimum body weight for those 15 years and younger contains 93% (0.93) fat-free weight and 7% fat (0.07).
2. Divide the wrestler's calculated fat-free weight by the greatest allowable fraction of fat-free weight to estimate minimal wrestling weight: 117.6 ÷ (93/100) = 117.6 ÷ 0.93 = 126.5 lb.

E. To allow for a 2% error, perform the following calculations:

1. 126.5 minimal weight × 0.02 = 2.5 lb error allowance
2. 126.5 lb − 2.5 lb = 124.0 lb minimum wrestling weight

F. Conclusion: Jonathan cannot wrestle in the 119-pound weight class; rather he must compete in the 125-pound class.

From Tipton CM. Making and maintaining weight for interscholastic wrestling. Gatorade Sports Science Exchange. 1990;2(22).

[a]*Lohman TG. Skinfolds and body density and their relationship to body frames: a review. Hum Biol 1981;53:181.*

[b]*Katch FI, McArdle WD. Prediction of body density from simple anthropometric measurements in college-age men and women. Hum Biol 1973;l45:445.*

[c]*Behnke AR, Wilmore JH. Evaluation and regulation of body build and composition. Englewood Cliffs, NJ: Prentice Hall, 1974.*

[d]*Thorland W, et al. New equations for prediction of a minimal weight in high school wrestlers. Med Sci Sports Exerc 1989;21:S72.*

---

ranted, should progress gradually and not exceed a 1- to 2-lb loss per week. At the same time, the athlete should continue to consume a nutritious diet.

Adolescent Female Gymnasts

As with wrestlers, coaches must establish a safe minimal competitive body weight for female gymnasts, many of whom use disordered eating behaviors to achieve weight loss (see Chapter 15). Based on an cross-validation analyses of 11 skinfold equations for predicting percentage body fat, the following equation most accurately estimates body composition in female high school gymnasts.[74,162] This prediction equation can assess body composition in the preseason (1 standard error of estimate equals ±2.4% body fat); for fe-

male gymnasts, body weight should contain no less than 14 to 16% body fat.

Female High School Gymnasts

% Body Fat = [457 ÷ 1.0987−0.00122 (Σ triceps, subscapular, suprailiac skinfolds in mm)
  + 0.00000263 (Σ triceps, subscapular, suprailiac skinfolds in mm)^2] − 414.2

TABLE 14.8 presents general guidelines and recommendations for athletes who wish to lose weight (specifically body fat) without jeopardizing health, safety, and exercise capacity and training responsiveness. These recommendations were originally formulated for athletes in the high-power sports, but they apply to other athletes as well.

TABLE 14.8   Recommendations to High-Power Athletes Who Want to Lose Weight

Many athletes will lose weight one way or another in an attempt to increase relative strength and power for their sport. These recommendations help the athlete lose weight in a way that minimizes health risks and maximizes sport performance and training.

1. **Arrange for qualified personnel (exercise physiologist, nutritionist, physician, or athletic trainer) to do the following:**
   a. Determine % body fat and fat-free body mass.
   b. Calculate minimal weight at 5% fat (males) or 12% (females).
   The difference between present weight and minimal weight is the amount of weight that can be lost.

2. **Begin weight loss early, before the competitive season begins and progress slowly to maximize fat loss and minimize muscle and water loss; maximum rate of weight loss. should be 0.5–1.0 kg (1–2 lb) per week.**

3. **Increase energy expenditure by doing aerobic training at least twice per week before and early in the competitive season.**

4. **Decrease the intake of calories by reducing dietary lipid, protein, and carbohydrate, but DO NOT totally eliminate any one of these three. Consume at least 1500 calories per day to prevent vitamin and mineral deficiencies. Specific recommendations include:**
   a. Cut out desserts, butter and margarine, sauces, gravy, and dressings.
   b. Eat foods high in complex carbohydrates (fruits, vegetables, whole-grain cereals).
   c. Grill, bake, broil, or boil food; do not fry.

5. **Weigh in before and after each practice session to keep track of body water loss. Specifically:**
   a. Do not restrict water during intense training, especially in hot training environments.
   b. Consume water, sports drinks, or other fluids after practice to restore at least 80% of the weight lost in a practice session.
   c. Drink fluids low in calories (e.g., skim milk rather than whole milk).

From Horswill CA. Does rapid weight loss by dehydration adversely affect high-power performance? Gatorade Sports Science Exchange 1991;3(30).

GAINING WEIGHT: A UNIQUE DILEMMA FOR PHYSICALLY ACTIVE INDIVIDUALS

Gaining weight to enhance body composition and exercise performance in activities requiring muscular strength and power or aesthetic appearance poses a unique problem not easily resolved. Most persons focus on weight loss to reduce excess body fat and improve overall health and appearance. Weight (fat) gain per se occurs all too readily by tilting the body's energy balance to favor greater caloric intake. Weight gain for active individuals should represent muscle mass and accompanying connective tissue. Generally, this form of weight gain occurs if increased caloric intake—carbohydrates for adequate energy and protein sparing plus the amino acid building blocks for tissue synthesis—accompanies a resistance exercise program.

Individuals attempting to increase muscle mass often fall easy prey to health food and diet supplement manufacturers who market "high-potency, tissue-building" substances—chromium, boron, vanadyl sulfate, β-hydroxy-β-methyl butyrate, and numerous protein and amino acids mixtures—none of which reliably increases muscle mass. Of the hundreds of products marketed in the health and bodybuilding literature to enhance exercise performance, most focus on augmenting muscular development.[58,125] Chapters 11 and 12 discussed the efficacy of many of these compounds and chemicals. Commercially prepared mixtures of powdered protein, predigested amino acids, or special high-protein "cocktails" do not promote muscle growth any more effectively than protein consumed in a well-balanced diet.[30] If an athlete experiences difficulty achieving the recommended protein intake through normal food intake—because of lifestyle, eating habits, and time requirements of training and competition—then high-quality protein supplements should prove beneficial.

Increase the Lean, Not the Fat

Endurance training usually increases FFM only slightly, but the overall effect reduces body weight from the calorie-burning and possible appetite depressing effects of this exercise type. In contrast, heavy muscular overload through resistance training, supported by adequate energy and protein intake (with sufficient recovery), greatly increases muscle mass and strength. Adequate energy intake during such training ensures that no catabolism of the protein available for muscle growth occurs from an energy deficit. Intense aerobic training should not coincide with resistance training designed to increase muscle mass.[68,94] More than likely, the added energy (and perhaps protein) demands of concurrent aerobic and resistance training impose a limit on muscle growth with resistance training. A prudent recommendation increases daily protein intake to about 1.6 g per kg of body mass during the resistance-training period.[102] Diverse sources of plant and animal proteins should be consumed; relying solely on animal protein (high in saturated fatty acids and cholesterol) potentially increases heart disease risk.

If all calories consumed in excess of the energy requirement of resistance training sustained muscle growth, then 2000 to 2500 extra kCal could supply each 0.5-kg increase in lean tissue. In practical terms, 700 to 1000 kCal added to the well-balanced daily meal plan supports a weekly 0.5- to 1.0-kg gain in lean tissue plus the additional energy needs for training. The ideal situation presupposes that all extra calories synthesize lean tissue.

How Much Lean Tissue Gain to Expect?

Many factors increase lean tissue accretion with resistance training, including energy balance, type of training program, and the individual's genetic makeup. A 1-year program of intense resistance training for young athletic men generally increases body mass by about 20%, the major portion consisting of lean tissue. The rate of lean tissue gain rapidly plateaus as training progresses beyond the first year. For athletic women, first-year gains in lean tissue mass average 50 to 75% of the absolute values for the men, probably owing to women's smaller initial lean body mass. Individual differences in the daily amount of nitrogen incorporated into body protein (and protein incorporated into muscle) may also limit gains in muscle tissue and explain differences among people in muscle mass increases with resistance training. FIGURE 14.11 presents eight specific factors that affect the responsiveness of lean tissue synthesis to resistance training.

Individuals with relatively high androgen/estrogen ratios and greater percentages of fast-twitch muscle fibers probably

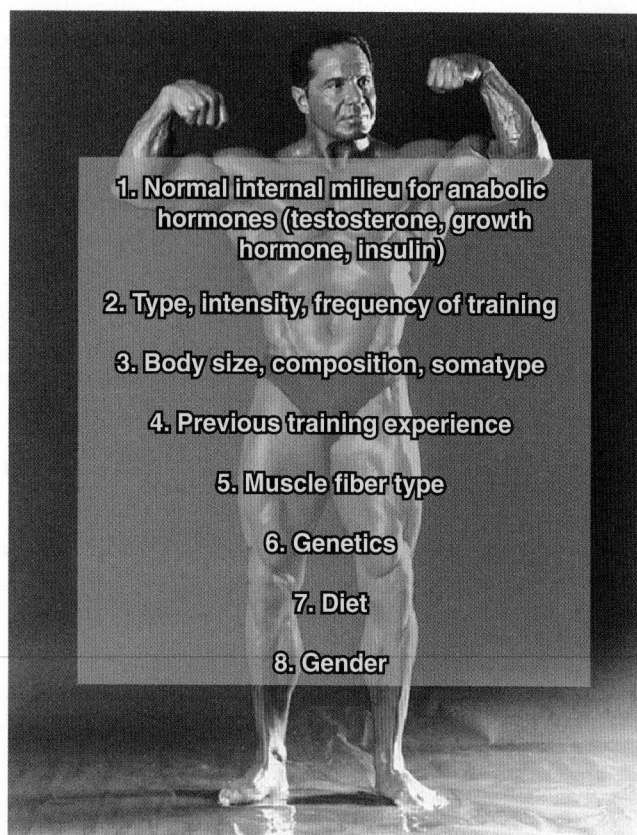

FIGURE 14.11 ■ Specific factors affecting the magnitude of lean tissue synthesis with resistance training. (Photo courtesy of Bill Pearl.)

increase lean tissue to the greatest extent in response to resistance training. Muscle mass increases occur most readily at the start of training in individuals with the largest relative FFM (FFM corrected for stature and body fat).[170] Regularly monitoring body mass and body fat verifies whether the combination of training and additional food intake increases lean tissue and not body fat.

Case Study

Personal Health and Exercise and Nutrition 14–2

Weight Loss and Exercise Prescription

About 300,000 adult Americans die each year from obesity-related diseases. Heart disease, high blood pressure, and type 2 diabetes directly link to excess body weight and insufficient aerobic exercise. Regular aerobic exercise reduces risks of some diseases by 50% or more.

Exercise prescription for weight loss in overweight individuals emphasizes frequency and duration that progresses to 45 to 60 minutes each day. Exercise intensity becomes a consideration only when the individual achieves sufficient weight loss and a fitness level suitable for cardiovascular conditioning.

Exercise Prescription

Initial focus of a prudent exercise prescription for weight loss centers on progressively increasing exercise volume (and caloric expenditure) with relatively low-intensity physical activity. Walking or running energy expenditure proportionally increases with speed. For example, a 70-kg person walking at 3.5 mph (17 minutes per mile pace) burns about 3.3 net kCal per minute, that is, calories above the resting level. If the same person runs at 7 mph (8.5 minutes per mile pace), net calories burn four times faster. For each mile covered, the runner burns twice as many calories as the walker and covers each mile twice as fast. This accounts for the fourfold greater rate of energy expenditure. These calculations are based on net energy expenditure values—the energy expenditure due to the exercise itself—in contrast to gross energy expenditure, which includes the resting value. The resting energy expenditure should not be counted toward weight (fat) loss, because these calories are burned whether or not the person exercises.

Interestingly, nearly the same energy expenditure occurs for running and walking a given distance (about 100 kCal per mile for a 70-kg person); this refers to the gross energy expenditure and not net values. Because walkers take longer to cover a mile than runners, they burn more calories associated with the resting component, which results in similar total kCal per mile. For weight loss purposes, however, consider only the net caloric expenditure in exercise. Thus, one must evaluate the payoff between increasing speed of walking/running and increasing exercise duration (and/or frequency) to increase total net energy expenditure. In practice, prudent exercise for the untrained, overweight individual emphasizes duration and frequency, particularly in the early stages of the program.

Subject Data and History

Female, single with no children; cigarette smoker (10 years); secretary in big office; family history of diabetes (father, type 2 diabetes) and heart disease (mother, grandmother).

Age: 35 years

Body weight: 199 lb (90.3 kg)

Height: 5 ft 6 in (1.676 m)

BMI: 32.1

Percentage body fat: 37%

Fat weight (FW): 73.6 lb (33.4 kg)

Fat-free body mass (FFM): 125.44 lb (56.9 kg)

Physical examination: Knee problems make walking/running difficult; no other obvious medical problems.

Exercise experience: Has not exercised for past 10 years except for occasional weekend biking, which she enjoys; she dislikes walking/running/swimming; very sedentary throughout life; family of nonexercisers.

Laboratory data:

- Normal lipid profile
- Normal blood glucose
- Daily caloric intake of about 3200 kCal
- High lipid intake (>38% of total kCal)
- Normal blood pressure

General impressions: Obese female with four risk factors (sedentary; obesity; smoking; family history of heart disease). Person needs lifestyle modification.

Case Questions

1. Give a preliminary assessment
2. Recommend a body weight goal
3. Formulate a prudent exercise prescription

Answers to Questions

1. Sedentary, overly fat woman (without specific symptoms) who needs to lose body fat. Individual has four heart disease risk factors that place her in a moderate-to-high risk category. She needs lifestyle modifications that include beginning an exercise program, reducing caloric intake and modifying the types of foods consumed, and starting a smoking cessation program.

2. Initially, this woman should be encouraged to lose a modest amount of weight of about 10 lb over a 5-

Case Study *continued*

to 10-week period. Such weight loss will favorably modify her risk profile and empower her to realize that she really can lose weight. Over the long term, a reduction in body weight to a corresponding 28% body fat level becomes a desirable goal.

Goal body weight = FFM ÷ (1.00 − desired %BF)
$$= 125.4 ÷ (1.00 − 0.28)$$
$$= 125.4 ÷ 0.72$$
$$= 174 \text{ lb (rounded)}$$

Goal fat loss = Current body weight − goal body weight
$$= 199 − 174 = 25 \text{ lb}$$

3. a. She should check with her physician or health care provider for clearance before beginning an exercise program. She chooses stationary bicycle riding as her primary exercise activity. After a 2-week adaptation period of shorter-duration exercise 3 to 5 days a week, exercise frequency is set at 6 days per week; the exercise duration goal is 60 minutes per session.

   b. Set intensity of exercise between 50% (lower level) and 70% (upper level) using the heart rate reserve method.

   Resting heart rate determined in the morning before rising: 85 bpm
   Maximum heart rate (HR_{max} [bpm]) by use of the following formula:

HR_{max} = 200 − 0.5 × (age in years)
$$= 200 − 0.5 × (35)$$
$$= 183 \text{ bpm}$$

   c. Target heart rates using heart rate reserve method calculate as follows:

Target HR = (intensity percentage) (HR_{max} − HR_{rest}) + HR_{rest}

Lower target HR = (0.5) (183 − 85) + 85
$$= 134 \text{ bpm}$$

Upper target HR = (0.7) (183 − 85) + 85
$$= 154 \text{ bpm}$$

During the first few sessions of exercise on the stationary cycle ergometer the person determines that she can exercise comfortably at a heart rate between 140 and 147 bpm at 75

watts (450 kg-m · min^{-1}). This then becomes the initial exercise intensity.

   d. Estimate the net exercise energy expenditure as follows:

Gross exercise oxygen consumption ($\dot{V}O_2$)

Gross exercise $\dot{V}O_2$, mL·kg^{-1}·min^{-1}
$$= 7 + (1.8 \text{ [work rate, kg·m·min}^{-1}] ÷ \text{body weight, kg)}$$
$$= 7 + (1.8 \text{ [450]} ÷ 90.3)$$
$$= 16.1 \text{ mL·kg}^{-1}·\text{min}^{-1}$$

Net exercise oxygen consumption ($\dot{V}O_2$)

Net exercise $\dot{V}O_2$, mL·kg^{-1}·min^{-1}
= Gross exercise $\dot{V}O_2$, mL·kg^{-1}·min^{-1} − Resting $\dot{V}O_2$
i.e., of 3.5 mL·kg^{-1}·min^{-1}
$$= 16.1 − 3.5$$
$$= 12.6 \text{ mL·kg}^{-1}·\text{min}^{-1}$$

CALORIE CONVERSION

Convert net exercise $\dot{V}O_2$ in mL · kg^{-1} · min^{-1} to mL · min^{-1} by multiplying by body weight in kg

$$= 12.6 × 90.3$$
$$= 1138 \text{ mL · min}^{-1}$$

Divide by 1000 to convert to L · min^{-1}.

$$= 1138 ÷ 1000$$
$$= 1.14 \text{ L · min}^{-1}$$

Multiply the L · min^{-1} value by 5 to convert oxygen consumption to kCal (1 L O_2 = 5 kCal)

$$= 1.14 × 5.0$$
$$= 5.7 \text{ kCal · min}^{-1}$$

Multiply kCal · min^{-1} by time of exercise

5.7 kCal • min^{-1} × 60 min = 342 kCal per exercise session

This woman expends approximately 342 kCal per exercise session, representing about a 0.59-lb fat loss per week from exercise alone (342 kCal × 6 d = 2052 kCal; 2052 kCal ÷ 3500 kCal = 0.59). This ideally complements a dietary modification that restricts energy intake by 500 to 750 kCal daily. Combining these modifications in diet and exercise behaviors produces nearly 2 lb of weight loss per week.

Franklin BA, et al. ACSMs guidelines for exercise testing and prescription. 6th ed. Baltimore: Lippincott Williams & Wilkins, 2000:214.

Miller WC, et al. Predicting max HR and the HR–$\dot{V}O_2$ relationship for exercise prescription in obesity. Med Sci Sports Exerc 1993;25:1077.

Summary

1. Slight but prolonged caloric excesses produce substantial weight gain. To prevent such a caloric disparity, energy output must balance energy input.

2. Nearly 70% of Americans struggle to lose weight (29% of men and 40% of women), yet only one fifth use the recommended combination of eating fewer calories and exercising regularly.

3. Almost 65% of the U.S. population classify as either overweight (BMI 25.0–29.9) or obese (BMI ≥30). Of this total, 30.5% classify as obese. The obesity epidemic contributes significantly to the rising tide of type 2 diabetes, cancer, and cardiovascular disease.

4. Among U.S. youth, obesity has more than doubled in the last 15 years, with an ever-widening gap between the weights of individuals deemed overly fat and those considered thin. Excessive body fatness becomes particularly prevalent among poor and minority children.

5. Genetic factors probably account for 25 to 30% of excessive body fat accumulation.

6. Genetic predisposition does not necessarily cause obesity, but given the right environment, the genetically susceptible individual gains body fat. Substantial alterations in the population's gene pool (which requires millions of years) cannot explain the dramatic worldwide obesity epidemic.

7. A defective gene for adipocyte leptin production and/or hypothalamic leptin insensitivity (plus defects in production and/or sensitivity to other chemicals) causes the brain to assess adipose tissue status improperly. This creates a chronic state of positive energy balance.

8. The standard dietary approach to weight loss that decreases caloric intake below the requirement for current weight maintenance generally helps obese patients to lose about 0.5 kg per week. Success in preventing weight regain is relatively poor, averaging between 5 and 20% of those who lose weight. Typically, one third to two thirds of the lost weight returns within a year and almost all of it within 5 years.

9. Reducing body fat generally improves exercise performance because it directly increases relative (per unit body size) muscular strength and power and aerobic capacity. Reduced drag force, which impedes forward movement in air and water, also represents a positive effect of weight loss on exercise performance.

10. Three methods unbalance the energy-balance equation to produce weight loss: (1) reduce energy intake below daily energy expenditure, (2) maintain normal energy intake and increase energy output, and (3) decrease energy intake and increase energy expenditure.

11. A caloric deficit of 3500 kCal, created through either diet or exercise, represents the calories in 0.45 kg (1.0 lb) of adipose tissue.

12. Appropriate modification of eating and exercise behaviors increases one's chance for successful weight loss.

13. Prudent dieting effectively promotes weight loss. Disadvantages of extremes of semistarvation include loss of fat-free mass (FFM), lethargy, possible malnutrition, and depressed resting metabolism (as long as one maintains an energy deficit).

14. Repeated cycles of weight loss–weight regain (yo-yo effect) may increase the body's ability to conserve energy, thus making weight loss with subsequent dieting less effective. From a public health perspective, the risks from obesity far exceed those from weight cycling.

15. Daily energy expenditure consists of the sum of resting metabolism, thermogenic influences (particularly the thermic effect of food), and energy generated during physical activity. Physical activity most profoundly affects the variability among humans in daily energy expenditure.

16. The calories burned in exercise accumulate. Regular extra physical activity creates a considerable energy deficit over time.

17. The precise role of exercise in appetite suppression or stimulation remains unclear, but moderate increases in physical activity may blunt appetite and depress energy intake of a previously sedentary, overweight person. Most athletes eventually consume enough calories to counterbalance training's added caloric expenditure.

18. Combining exercise with caloric restriction offers a flexible and effective means for weight loss. Exercise enhances fat mobilization and catabolism. Regular aerobic exercise retards lean tissue loss; resistance training increases the FFM.

19. Rapid weight loss during the first few days of a caloric deficit mainly reflects loss of body water and stored glycogen; greater fat loss occurs per unit of weight lost as caloric restriction continues.

20. Selective exercise of specific body areas proves no more effective for localized fat loss than more-general physical activity. Areas of greatest fat concentration and/or lipid-mobilizing enzyme activity supply the most energy for exercise, regardless of the area exercised.

21. Differences in body fat distribution partially explain the gender difference in exercise-induced weight loss. Fat deposited in the upper body and abdominal regions (male-pattern obesity) responds readily to neurohumoral stimulation and preferentially mobilizes in exercise com-

Summary *continued*

pared with fat deposited in gluteal and femoral regions (female-pattern obesity).

22. Physically active individuals should add weight as lean body tissue (muscle mass). This occurs most readily with a modest increase in caloric intake plus resistance training.

23. Seven hundred to 1000 extra kCal per day supports a weekly 0.5- to 1.0-kg gain in lean tissue and the energy requirements of resistance training. Individual physiologic variations and training factors affect gains in muscle mass.

Test Your Knowledge Answers

1. **True:** The World Health Organization and the International Obesity Task Force have declared a global obesity epidemic. Obesity now represents the second leading cause of preventable deaths (smoking first) in the United States (300,000 deaths yearly) at a total yearly cost of $140 billion, or approximately 10% of the U.S. health care expenditures. Overweight, but not obese, nonsmoking men and women in their mid-30s to mid-40s die at least 3 years sooner than normal-weight counterparts, a risk just as damaging to life expectancy as cigarette smoking. Obese individuals can expect a about a 7-year decrease in life expectancy.

2. **False:** There is greater prevalence of obesity among black women (about 50%) than among white women (33%). Studies of obese black and white women show small differences in resting metabolism; on average, black women burn nearly 100 fewer calories each day during rest than whites. This slower rate of processing calories persists even after adjusting for differences in body mass and body composition. The greater energy economy of black women during exercise and throughout the day most likely reflects an inherited trait, as it persists both before and after weight loss. This effect, which also exists among children and adolescents, predisposes a black female to gain weight and regain it following weight loss.

3. **False:** The standard dietary approach to weight loss that decreases caloric intake below the requirement for current weight maintenance generally helps obese patients lose about 0.5 kg per week. Success at preventing weight regain is relatively poor, averaging between 5 and 20%. Regular physical activity, through either recreation or occupation, effectively contributes to preventing weight gain and thwarts the tendency to regain lost weight.

4. **False:** Older men and women who maintain active lifestyles impede the "normal" pattern of fat gain observed in most adults. Research shows that time spent in physical activity inversely relates to body fat level in young and middle-aged men who exercise

regularly. The greater level of body fat among active middle-aged men compared with younger, more active counterparts resulted from less vigorous training, not greater energy intake.

5. **True:** Combining moderate food restriction with additional daily physical activity offers the greatest flexibility for achieving fat loss. This combination also enables the individual to remain well nourished for exercise training and peak performance.

6. **True:** Resting metabolism decreases when food restriction progressively produces weight loss. This hypometabolism often exceeds the decrease attributable to the loss of body mass or fat-free body mass. Depressed metabolism conserves energy, causing the diet to become less effective despite a restricted caloric intake. This produces a weight-loss plateau at which further weight loss becomes considerably less than predicted from the mathematics of the restricted energy intake.

7. **False:** For most individuals, semistarvation with a very low calorie diet (VLCD) does not compose an "ultimate diet" or the proper approach to weight control. Because a VLCD provides inadequate carbohydrate, the glycogen-storage depots in the liver and muscles deplete rapidly. This impairs physical tasks requiring either high-intensity aerobic effort or shorter-duration anaerobic power output. The continuous nitrogen loss with fasting and weight loss reflects and exacerbated lean tissue loss, which may occur disproportionately from critical organs like the heart. The success rate remains poor for prolonged VLCD use.

8. **False:** Excess weight gain often parallels reduced physical activity rather than increased caloric intake. Approximately 27% of U.S. adults engage in no daily physical activity, and another 28% do not regularly take part in physical activity. Among active endurance-trained men, body fat inversely relates to energy expenditure (low body fat, high energy expenditure and vice versa); no relationship emerges between body fat and food intake. Surprisingly, physically active people who eat the

most generally weigh the least and exhibit the highest levels of fitness. Also, excessive food intake does not fully explain the rise in obesity among children. Obese infants do not characteristically consume more calories than recommended dietary standards. For children ages 4 to 6 years, a reduced level of physical activity primarily accounts for their 25% lower daily energy expenditure than the energy intake recommendation for this age.

9. **False:** Regular physical activity plays an important role in protecting against weight gain. Men and women of all ages who maintain a physically active lifestyle (or become involved in regular exercise programs) maintain a more desirable level of body composition. For overweight adult women, a

dose–response relationship exists between the amount of exercise and long-term weight loss.

10. **False:** Resistance training provides an important adjunct to aerobic training in programs of weight loss and weight maintenance. The energy expended in circuit resistance training (continuous exercise using low resistance and high repetitions) averages about 9 kCal per minute. This exercise mode, therefore, can "burn" substantial calories during a typical 30- to 60-minute workout. Even conventional resistance training that involves less total energy expenditure affects muscular strength and fat-free body mass during weight loss more positively than programs that rely solely on food restriction.

References

1. American College of Sports Medicine. Position statement on proper and improper weight loss programs. *Med Sci Sports Exerc* 1993;15:9.
2. American Medical Association. A critique of low-carbohydrate ketogenic weight and reduction regimens (a review of Dr. Atkins' diet revolution). *JAMA* 1973;224:1418.
3. Anderson JW, et al. Long-term weight-loss maintenance: a meta-analysis of US studies. *Am J Clin Nutr* 2001;74:579.
4. Anderson RE, et al. Relationship of physical activity and television watching with body weight and level of fatness among children. *JAMA* 1998;279:938.
5. Arner P, et al. Adrenergic regulation of lipolysis in situ at rest and during exercise. *J Clin Invest* 1991;32:423.
6. Arner P, et al. Expression of lipoprotein lipase in different human subcutaneous adipose tissue regions. *J Lipid Res* 1991;32:423.
7. Atkin L-M, Davies PSW. Diet composition and body composition in preschool children. *Am J Clin Nutr* 2000;72:15.
8. Atkins RC. *Dr Atkins' New Diet Revolution.* New York: Avon, 1997.
9. Bagley S, et al. Family structure and children's television viewing and physiocal activity. *Med Sci Sports Exerc* 2006;38:910.
10. Ball EJ, et al. Total energy expenditure, body fatness, and physical activity in children aged 6-9 y. *Am J Clin Nutr* 2001;74:524.
11. Ballor DL, Keesey RE. A meta-analysis of the factors affecting changes in body mass, fat mass and fat-free mass in males and females. *Int J Obes* 1991;15:717.
12. Ballor DL, Poehlman ET. Exercise training enhances fat-free mass preservation during diet-induced weight loss: a meta-analytical finding. *Int J Obes* 1994;18:35.
13. Blackburn GL, et al. Weight cycling: the experience of human dieters. *Am J Clin Nutr* 1989;49:1105.
14. Blair SN, et al. Influences of cardiorespiratory fitness and other precursors on cardiovascular disease and all-cause mortality in men and women. *JAMA* 1996;276:205.
15. Blank HM, et al. Use of nonprescription weight loss products: results from a multistate survey. *JAMA* 2001;286:930.
16. Booth ML, et al. Changes in the prevalence of overweight and obesity among young Australians, 1969-1997. *Am J Clin Nutr* 2003;77:29.
17. Bouchard C, et al. Long-term exercise training with constant energy intake. Part I. Effect on body composition and selected metabolic variables. *Int J Obes* 1990;14:57.
18. Bouchard C, et al. The response to long term feeding in identical twins. *N Engl J Med* 1990;322:1477.
19. Bouchard C, et al. The response to exercise with constant energy intake in identical twins. *Obes Res* 1994;2:400.
20. Boule NG, et al. Effect of exercise on glycemic control and body mass in type 2 diabetes mellitus: a meta-analysis of controlled clinical trials. *JAMA* 2001;286:1218.
21. Bravata DM, et al. Efficacy and safety of low-carbohydrate diets: a systematic review. *JAMA* 2003;289:1767.
22. Bray GA, Popkin BM. Dietary fat intake does affect obesity! *Am J Clin Nutr* 1998;68:1157.
23. Brownell KD, et al. The effects of repeated cycles of weight loss and regain in rats. *Physiol Behav* 1986;38:459.
24. Byers T, et al. Weight cycling, weight gain, and risk of hypertension in women. *Am J Epidemiol* 1999;150:573.
25. Calle EE, et al. Body-mass index and mortality in a prospective cohort of U.S. adults. *N Engl J Med* 1999;341:1097.
26. Calle EE, et al. Overweight, obesity, and mortality from cancer in a prospectively studied cohort of U.S. adults. *N Engl J Med* 2003;348:1625.
27. Carpenter WH, et al. Total energy expenditure in 4 to 6 year old children. *Am J Physiol* 1993;27:E706.
28. Centers for Disease Control and Prevention. Update: prevalence of overweight among children, adolescents, and adults: United States, 1988-1994. *MMWR* 1997;46:199.
29. Clark RR, et al. Minimum weight prediction methods cross-validated by the four-component model. *Med Sci Sports Exerc* 2004;36:639.
30. Clarkson M. Dietary Supplements and Pharmacological Agents for Weight Loss and Gain. In: Lamb DR, Murray R, eds. *Perspectives in Exercise Science and Sports Medicine.* Vol 10. Exercise, Nutrition, and Weight Control. Carmel, IN: Cooper Publishing, 1998.
31. Cleland R, et al. *Commercial Weight Loss Products and Programs: What Consumers Stand to Gain and Lose.* Washington, DC: Federal Trade Commission, Bureau of Consumer Protection, 1998.
32. Considine RV, et al. Serum immunoreactive-leptin concentrations in normal-weight and obese humans. *N Engl J Med* 1996;334:292.
33. DeLany JP, et al. Energy expenditure in preadolescent African American and white boys and girls: the Baton Rouge Children's Study. *Am J Clin Nutr* 2002;75:705.
34. Dengel DR, et al. Effects of weight loss by diet alone or combined with aerobic exercise on body composition in older obese men. *Metabolism* 1994;43:867.
35. Després J-P. Physical Activity and Adipose Tissue. In: Bouchard C, et al. eds. *Physical Activity, Fitness, and Health.* Champaign, IL: Human Kinetics, 1994.

36. Després J-P, et al. Loss of abdominal fat and metabolic response to exercise training in obese women. *Am J Physiol* 1991;261:E159.

37. Diabetes Prevention Research Group. Reduction in the incidence of type 2 diabetes with lifestyle intervention or metformin. *N Engl J Med* 2002;346:393.

38. Dietz WH, Robinson TN. Overweight children and adolescents. *N Engl J Med* 2005;352:2100.

39. DiPietro L. Physical activity, body weight, and adiposity: an epidemiologic perspective. *Exerc Sport Sci Rev* 1995;23:275.

40. Dolezal BA, Potteiger JA. Concurrent resistance and endurance training influence basal metabolic rate in nondieting individuals. *J Appl Physiol* 1998;85:695.

41. Donnelly JE, Smith BK. Is exercise effective for weight loss with *ad libitum* diet? Energy balance, compensation, and gender differences. *Exerc Sport Sci Rev* 2005;33:169.

42. Ebbeling CB, Rodriguez NR. Effect of exercise combined with diet therapy on protein utilization in obese children. *Med Sci Sports Exerc* 1999;31:378.

43. Eck Clemens LH, et al. The effect of eating out on quality of diet in premenopausal women. *J Am Diet Assoc* 1999;99:4421.

44. Eisenstein J, et al. High-protein weight loss diets: are they safe and do they work? A review of the experimental and epidemiological data. *Nutr Rev* 2002;60:189.

45. Elliot DL, et al. Sustained depression of the resting metabolic rate after massive weight loss. *Am J Clin Nutr* 1989;49:93.

46. Fisler JS. Cardiac effects of starvation and semi-starvation diets: safety and mechanisms of action. *Am J Clin Nutr* 1992;56:230S.

47. Flegal KM, Troiano RP. Changes in the distribution of body mass index of adults and children in the US population. *Int J Obes Relat Metab Disord* 2000;24:807.

48. Freedman CS, et al. Trends and correlates of class 3 obesity in the United States from 1990 through 2000. *JAMA* 2002;288:1758.

49. Fleury C, et al. Uncoupling protein-2: a novel gene linked to obesity and hyperinsulinemia. *Nat Genet* 1997;15:269.

50. Foster GD, et al. Resting energy expenditure in obese African American and Caucasian women. *Obes Res* 1997;5:1.

51. Foster GD, et al. A randomized trial of a low-carbohydrate diet for obesity. *N Engl J Med* 2003;348:2082.

52. French SA, et al. Predictors of weight change over two years among a population of working adults: the Healthy Worker Project. *Int J Obes* 1994;18:145.

53. Frisancho AR. Prenatal compared with parental origins of adolescent fatness. *Am J Clin Nutr* 2000;72:1186.

54. Golay A, et al. Similar weight loss with low- or high-carbohydrate diets. *Am J Clin Nutr* 1996;63:174.

55. Gordon-Larsen, P, et al. Adolescent physical activity and inactivity vary by ethnicity: the National Longitudinal Study of Adolescent Health. *J Pediatr* 1999;135:301.

56. Gower BA, et al. Effects of weight loss on changes in insulin sensitivity and lipid concentrations in premenopausal African American and white women. *Am J Clin Nutr* 2002;76:923.

57. Grundy SM. Multifactorial causation of obesity: implications for prevention. *Am J Clin Nutr* 1998;67(suppl):563S.

58. Grunewald K, Bailey R. Commercially marketed supplements for bodybuilding athletes. *Sports Med* 1993;15:90.

59. Gunnell DJ, et al. Childhood obesity and adult cardiovascular mortality: a 57-y follow-up study based on the Boyd Orr cohort. *Am J Clin Nutr* 1998;67:1111.

60. Guo SS, et al. Predicting overweight and obesity in adulthood from body mass index values in childhood and adolescence. *Am J Clin Nutr* 2002;76:653.

61. Gutin B, et al. Effect of exercise intensity on cardiovascular fitness, total body composition, and visceral adiposity of obese adolescents. *Am J Clin Nutr* 2002;75:818.

62. Gwinup G, et al. Thickness of subcutaneous fat and activity of underlying muscles. *Ann Intern Med* 1971;74:408.

63. Halaas JL, et al. Weight-reducing effects of the plasma protein encoded by the obese gene. *Science* 1995;269:543.

64. Hansen RD, Allen BJ. Habitual physical activity, anabolic hormones, and potassium content of fat-free mass in post menopausal women. *Am J Clin Nutr* 2002;75:314.

65. Harnack LJ, et al. Temporal trends in energy intake in the United States: an ecologic perspective. *Am J Clin Nutr* 2000;71:1478.

66. Heath GW, et al. A physiological comparison of younger and older endurance-trained athletes. *J Appl Physiol* 1981;51:634.

67. Heitmann BL, Garby L. Composition (lean and fat tissue) of weight changes in adult Danes. *Am J Clin Nutr* 2002;75:834.

68. Hennessy LC, Watson AWS. The interference effects of training for strength and endurance simultaneously. *J Strength Cond Res* 1994;8:12.

69. Heshka S, et al. Weight loss with self-help compared with a structured commercial program: a randomized trial. *JAMA* 2003;289:1792.

70. Hill JO, et al. Evaluation of an alternating-calorie diet with and without exercise in the treatment of obesity. *Am J Clin Nutr* 1989;50:248.

71. Hill JO, et al. Exercise and Moderate Obesity. In: Bouchard C, et al., eds. *Physical Activity, Fitness, and Health.* Champaign, IL: Human Kinetics, 1994.

72. Hirsch J, et al. Diet composition and energy balance in humans. *Am J Clin Nutr* 1998;67(suppl):551S.

73. Hortobagyi T, et al. Comparison of four methods to assess body composition in black and white athletes. *Int J Sports Nutr* 1992;2:60.

74. Housh TJ, et al. Validity of skinfold estimates of percent fat in high school female gymnasts. *Med Sci Sports Exerc* 1996;28:1331.

75. Hu FB, et al. Trends in the incidence of coronary heart disease and changes in diet and lifestyle in women. *N Engl J Med* 2000;343:530.

76. Hu F, et al. Television watching and other sedentary behaviors in relation to risk of obesity and type 2 diabetes mellitus in women. *JAMA* 2003;289:1785.

77. Iribarren C, et al. Association of weight loss and weight fluctuation with mortality among Japanese American men. *N Engl J Med* 1995;333:686.

78. Iversen SG, et al. Occupational physical activity, overweight, and mortality: a follow-up study of 47,405 Norwegian women and men. *Res Q Exerc Sport* 2007;78:151.

79. Jakicic JM, Gallagher KI. Exercise considerations for the sedentary, overweight adult. *Exerc Sport Sci Rev* 2003;31:91.

80. Jakicic JM, Wing RR. Differences in resting energy expenditure in African American versus Caucasian overweight females. *Int J Obes* 1998;22:236.

81. Jakicic JM, et al. Effects of intermittent exercise and use of home exercise equipment on adherence, weight loss, and fitness in overweight women. *JAMA* 1999;282:1554.

82. Jeffery RW. Does weight cycling present a risk? *Am J Clin Nutr* 1996;63(suppl):452S.

83. Jeffrey R, et al. Weight cycling and cardiovascular risk factors in obese men and women. *Am J Clin Nutr* 1992;55:641.

84. Johnson MJ, et al. Loss of muscle mass is poorly reflected in grip strength performance in healthy young men. *Med Sci Sports Exerc* 1994;26:235.

85. Johnson ML, et al. Relative importance of inactivity and overeating in energy balance in obese high school girls. *Am J Clin Nutr* 1986;44:779.

86. Katch FI, et al. Effects of situp exercise training on adipose cell size and adiposity. *Res Q Exerc Sport* 1984;55:242.

87. Kern PA, et al. The effects of weight loss on the activity and expression of adipose-tissue lipoprotein lipase in very obese humans. *N Engl J Med* 1990;322:1053.

88. Kimm S, et al. Decline in physical activity in black and white girls during adolescence. *N Engl J Med* 2002;347:709.

89. King AC, Katch FI. Changes in body density, fatfolds and girths at 2.3 kg increments of weight loss. *Hum Biol* 1986;58:708.

90. King G, et al. Relationship of leisure-time physical activity and occupational activity to the prevalence of obesity. *Int J Obes* 2001;25:606.

91. Klem ML, et al. A descriptive study of individuals successful at long-term maintenance of substantial weight loss. *Am J Clin Nutr* 1997;66:239.

92. Kohrt WM, et al. Body composition of healthy sedentary and trained, young and older men and women. *Med Sci Sports Exerc* 1992;24:832.

93. Kohrt WM, et al. Exercise training improves fat distribution patterns in 60- to 70-year-old men and women. *J Gerontol* 1992;47:M99.

94. Kraemer WJ, et al. Compatibility of high-intensity strength and endurance training on hormonal and skeletal muscle adaptations. *J Appl Physiol* 1995;78:976.

95. Kraemer WJ, et al. Influence of exercise training on physiological and performance changes with weight loss in men. *Med Sci Sports Exerc* 1999;31:1320.

96. Lahti-Koski M, et al. Associations of body mass index and obesity with physical activity, food choices, alcohol intake, and smoking in the 1982-1997 Finrisk Studies. *Am J Clin Nutr* 2002;75:809.

97. Larew K, et al. Muscle metabolic function, exercise performance, and weight gain. *Med Sci Sports Exerc* 2003;35:230.

98. Lee I-M, et al. Physical activity and coronary heart disease in women: is "no pain no gain" passé? *JAMA* 2001;285:1447.

99. Leibel R, et al. Changes in energy expenditure resulting from altered body weight. *N Engl J Med* 1995;332:621.

100. Leidy HJ et al. Higher protein intake preserves lean mass and satiety with weight loss in pre-obese and obese women. *Obesity* 2007;15:421.

101. Lemmer JT, et al. Effects of strength training on resting metabolic rate and physical activity: age and gender comparisons. *Med Sci Sports Exerc* 2001;33:532.

102. Lemon PWR. Do athletes need more dietary protein and amino acids? *Int J Sports Nutr* 1995;5:S39.

103. LeMura LM, Maziekas MT. Factors that alter body fat, body mass, and fat-free mass in pediatric obesity. *Med Sci Sports Exerc* 2002; 34:487.

104. Manson JE, et al. Walking compared with vigorous exercise for the prevention of cardiovascular events in women. *N Engl J Med* 2002; 347:716.

105. Martin WA. Effect of acute and chronic exercise on fat metabolism. *Exerc Sport Sci Rev* 1996;24:203.

106. Mayo MJ, et al. Exercise-induced weight loss preferentially reduces abdominal fat. *Med Sci Sports Exerc* 2003;35:207.

107. Meredith CN, et al. Body composition and aerobic capacity in young and middle-aged endurance-trained men. *Med Sci Sports Exerc* 1987;19:557.

108. Miller-Kovach K, et al. Weight maintenance among Weight Watchers lifetime members. *FASEB J* 1998;282:1519.

109. Mokdad AH, et al. The spread of the obesity epidemic in the United States, 1991-1998. *JAMA* 1999;282:1519.

110. Mokdad AH, et al. The continuing epidemics of obesity and diabetes in the United States. *JAMA* 2001;286:1195.

111. Molé PA, et al. Exercise reverses depressed metabolic rate produced by severe caloric restriction. *Med Sci Sports Exerc* 1989;21:29.

112. Must A, et al. The disease burden associated with overweight and obesity. *JAMA* 1999;282:1523.

113. National Institutes of Health, National Heart, Lung, and Blood Institute. Obesity evaluation initiative, clinical guidelines and the identification, evaluation, and treatment of overweight and obesity in adults. Bethesda, MD: National Institutes of Health, June, 1998.

114. National Task Force on the Prevention and Treatment of Obesity. Very-low-calorie diets. *JAMA* 1993;270:976.

115. National Task Force on the Prevention and Treatment of Obesity. Weight cycling. *JAMA* 1994;272:1196.

116. Nicklas BJ. Effects of endurance exercise on adipose tissue metabolism. *Exerc Sport Sci Rev* 1997;25:77.

117. Keogh JB, et al. Long-term weight maintenance and cardiovascular risk factors are not different following weight loss on carbohydrate-restricted diets high in either monounsaturated fat or protein in obese hyperinsulinaemic men and women. *Br J Nutr* 2007;97:405.

118. Obesity: preventing and managing the global epidemic: report of a WHO consultation. Geneva, Switzerland: World Health Organization; 2000. WHO Technical Report series, 894.

119. Ogden CL, et al. Prevalence and trends in overweight among US children and adolescents, 1999-2000. *JAMA* 2002;288:1728.

120. Oppliger RA, et al. NCAA rule change improves weight loss among national championship wrestlers. *Med Sci Sports Exerc* 2006;38:963.

121. Pavlou KN, et al. Exercise as an adjunct to weight loss and maintenance in moderately obese subjects. *Am J Clin Nutr* 1989;49:1115.

122. Peeters A, et al. Obesity in adulthood and its consequences for life expectancy. *Ann Intern Med* 2003;138:24.

123. Pellymounter MA, et al. Effects of the *obese* gene product on body weight reduction in *ob/ob* mice. *Science* 1995;269:540.

124. Pérusse L, et al. Acute and chronic effects of exercise on leptin levels in humans. *J Appl Physiol* 1997;83:5.

125. Philen RD, et al. Survey of advertising for nutritional supplements in health and bodybuilding magazines. *JAMA* 1992;268:1008.

126. Poehlman ET, Melby C. Resistance training and energy balance. *Int J Sports Nutr* 1998;8:143.

127. Poehlman ET, et al. Effect of resistance training and endurance training on insulin sensitivity in nonobese, young women. *J Clin Endocrinol Metab* 2000;85:2463.

128. Pollock ML, et al. Twenty-year follow-up of aerobic power and body composition of older track athletes. *J Appl Physiol* 1997;82:1508.

129. Prabhakaran B, et al. Effect of 14 weeks of resistance training on lipid profile and body fat percentage in premenopausal women. *Br J Sports Med* 1999;33:190.

130. Prentice AM, et al. Effects of weight cycling on body composition. *Am J Clin Nutr* 1992;56:209S.

131. Racette SB, et al. Effects of aerobic exercise and dietary carbohydrate on energy expenditure and body composition during weight reduction in obese women. *Am J Clin Nutr* 1995;61:486.

132. Ravussin E, et al. Reduced rate of energy expenditure as a risk factor for body-weight gain. *N Engl J Med* 1988;318:467.

133. Reddy ST, et al. Effect of low-carbohydrate, high-protein diets on acid-base balance, stone-forming propensity, and calcium metabolism. *Am J Kidney Dis* 2002;40:265.

134. Reseland JE, et al. Effect of long-term changes in diet and exercise on plasma leptin concentrations. *Am J Clin Nutr* 2001;73:240.

135. Roberts SB, et al. Energy expenditure and intake in infants born to lean and overweight mothers. *N Engl J Med* 1988;318:461.

136. Robinson TN. Reducing children's television viewing to prevent obesity: a randomized clinical trial. *JAMA* 1999;282:1562.

137. Roemmich JN, Sinning WE. Weight loss and wrestling training: effects of nutrition, growth, maturation, body composition, and strength. *J Appl Physiol* 1997;82:1751.

138. Rolland-Cachera MF, Bellisle F. No correlation between adiposity and food intake: why are working class children fatter? *Am J Clin Nutr* 1986;44:779.

139. Rolls BJ, et al. Portion size of food affects energy intake in normal-weight and overweight men and women. *Am J Clin Nutr* 2002;76:1207.

140. Rosenbaum M, et al. Obesity. *N Engl J Med* 1997;337:396.

141. Ross R, et al. Exercise alone is an effective strategy for reducing obesity and related comorbidities. *Exerc Sport Sci Rev* 2000;28:165.

142. Ross R, et al. Reduction in obesity and related comorbid conditions after diet-induced weight loss or exercise-induced weight loss in men. *Ann Intern Med* 2000;133:92.

143. Ryan SS, et al. Resistive training increases fat-free mass and maintains RMR despite weight loss in postmenopausal women. *J Appl Physiol* 1995;79:818.

144. Samaha FF, et al. A low-carbohydrate as compared with a low-fat diet in severe obesity. *N Engl J Med* 2003;348:2074.

145. Schoeller D, et al. How much physical activity is needed to minimize weight gain in previously obese women? *Am J Clin Nutr* 1997;66:551.

146. Schoeller DA, et al. The importance of clinical research: the role of thermogenesis in human obesity. *Am J Clin Nutr* 2001;73:511.

147. Schwartz RS, et al. The effect of intensive endurance exercise training on body fat distribution in young and older men. *Metabolism* 1991;40:545.

148. Serdula MK, et al. Prevalence of attempting weight loss and strategies for controlling weight. *JAMA* 1999;282:1359.

149. Shepard TY, et al. Occasional physical inactivity combined with a high-fat diet may be important in the development and maintenance of obesity in human subjects. *Am J Clin Nutr* 2001;73:703.

150. Short KR, Sedlock DA. Excess postexercise oxygen consumption and recovery rate in trained and untrained subjects. *J Appl Physiol* 1997;83:153.

151. Simkin-Silverman L, et al. Lifetime weight cycling and psychological health in normal-weight and overweight women. *Int J Eating Disord* 1998;24:175.

152. Skender MI, et al. Comparison of 2-year weight loss trends in behavioral treatments of obesity: diet, exercise, and combination interventions. *J Am Diet Assoc* 1996;96:342.

153. Steffen PR, et al. Effects of exercise and weight loss or blood loss on blood pressure during daily life. *Med Sci Sport Exerc* 2001;33:1635.

154. Stern L, et al. The effects of low-carbohydrate versus conventional weight loss diets in severely obese adults: one-year follow-up of randomized trial. *Arch Intern Med* 2004;140:778.

155. Stewart KJ. Exercise training and the cardiovascular consequences of type 2 diabetes and hypertension: plausible mechanisms for improving cardiovascular health. *JAMA* 2002;288:1622.

156. Strauss RS, Pollack HA. Epidemic increase in childhood overweight, 1986–1998. *JAMA* 2001;286:2845.

157. Sun M, et al. A longitudinal study of resting energy expenditure relative to body composition during puberty in African American and white children. *Am J Clin Nutr* 2001;73:308.

158. Tanasescu M, et al. Exercise type and intensity in relation to coronary heart disease in men. *JAMA* 2002;288:1994.

159. Taubes G. As obesity rates rise, experts struggle to explain why. *Science* 1998;280:1367.

160. Tcheng T, Tipton CM. Iowa wrestling study: anthropometric measurements and the prediction of a "minimal" body weight for high school wrestlers. *Med Sci Sports* 1973;5:1.

161. Technology Assessment Conference Panel. Methods for voluntary weight loss and control. Technology Assessment Conference statement. *Ann Intern Med* 1992;116:942.

162. Thorland WG, et al. Estimation of body density in adolescent athletes. *Hum Biol* 1984;56:439.

163. Torshakovec AM, et al. Age, sex, ethnicity, body composition, and resting energy expenditure of obese African American children and adolescents. *Am J Clin Nutr* 2002;75:867.

164. Treuth MS, et al. Familial resemblance of body composition in prepubertal girls and their biological parents. *Am J Clin Nutr* 2001;74:529.

165. Troiano RP, Flegal KM. Overweight children and adolescents: description, epidemiology, and demographics. *Pediatrics* 1998;101:497.

166. Tuomilehto J, et al. Prevention of type 2 diabetes mellitus by changes in lifestyle among subjects with impaired glucose tolerance. *N Engl J Med* 2001;344:1343.

167. US Department of Health and Human Services. Physical activity and health: a report of the Surgeon General. Atlanta, GA: Centers for Disease Control and Prevention, 1996.

168. VanAnggel-Leijssen DPC, et al. Short term effects of weight loss with or without low-intensity exercise training on fat metabolism in obese men. *Am J Clin Nutr* 2001;73:523.

169. VanDale D, Saris WHM. Repetitive weight loss and weight regain: effects on weight reduction, resting metabolic rate, and lipolytic activity before and after exercise and/or diet treatment. *Am J Clin Nutr* 1989;49:409.

170. VanEtten LMLA, et al. Effect of body build on weight-training-induced adaptations in body composition and muscular strength. *Med Sci Sports Exerc* 1994;26:515.

171. VanEtten LMLA, et al. Effect of an 18-wk weight-training program on energy expenditure and physical activity. *J Appl Physiol* 1997;82:298.

172. VanHorn L, Greenland P. Prevention of coronary artery disease is a pediatric problem. *JAMA* 1997;278:1779.

173. Vincent SD, et al. Activity levels and body mass index of children in the United States, Sweden, and Australia. *Med Sci Sports Exerc* 2003;35:1367.

174. Wadden TA. Characteristics of Successful Weight Loss Maintenance. In: PiSunyer FX, Allison DB, eds. *Obesity Treatment: Establishing Goals, Improving Outcomes, and Establishing the Research Agenda.* New York: Plenum Press, 1995.

175. Wadden TA, Foster GD. Behavioral treatment of obesity. *Med Clin North Am* 2000;84:441.

176. Wahrenberg H, et al. Adrenergic regulation of lipolysis in human fat cells during exercise. *Eur J Clin Invest* 1991;21:534.

177. Wang Y, Beydoun MA. The obesity epidemic in the United States: gender, age, socioeconomic, racial/ethnic, and geographic characteristics: a systematic review and meta-regression analysis. *Epidemiol Rev* 2007;29:6.

178. Wei M, et al. Relationship between low cardiorespiratory fitness and mortality in normal-weight, overweight, and obese men. *JAMA* 1999;282:1547.

179. Weinsier RL, et al. Do adaptive changes in metabolic rate favor weight regain in weight-reduced individuals? An examination of the set-point theory. *Am J Clin Nutr* 2000;72:1088.

180. Weinsier RL, et al. Energy expenditure and free-living physical activity in black and white women: comparison before and after weight loss. *Am J Clin Nutr* 2000;71:138.

181. Weinsier RL, et al. Free-living activity energy expenditure in women successful and unsuccessful at maintaining a normal body weight. *Am J Clin Nutr* 2002;75:499.

182. Weyer C, et al. Energy metabolism after 2 y of energy restriction: the Biosphere 2 experiment. *Am J Clin Nutr* 2000;72:946.

183. Wier L, et al. Determining the amount of physical activity needed for long-term weight control. *Int J Obes* 2001;25:613.

184. Willett WC. Is dietary fat a major determinant of body fat? *Am J Clin Nutr* 1998;67(suppl):555S.

185. Williams PT. Relationship of distance run per week to coronary heart disease risk factors in 8,283 male runners: the National Runners Health Study. *Arch Intern Med* 1997;157:191.

186. Williams PT. Nonlinear relationships between weekly walking distance and adiposity in 27,567 women. *Med Sci Sports Exer* 2005;37:1893.

187. Williams PT, Pate RR. Cross-sectional relationships of exercise and age to adiposity in 60,617 male runners. *Med Sci Sports Exer* 2005;37:1329.

188. Williams PT, Satariano WA. Relationships of age and weekly running distance to BMI and circumferences in 41,582 physically active women. *Obes Res* 2005;13:1370.

189. Williams PT, Thompson PD. Dose-dependent effects of training and detraining on weight in 6406 runners during 7.4 years. *Obesity* (Silver Spring) 2006;14:1975.

190. Williams PT. Maintaining vigorous activity attenuates 7-yr weight gain in 8340 runners. *Med Sci Sports Exer* 2007;39:801.

191. Wilmore JH. Increasing physical activity: alterations in body mass and composition. *Am J Clin Nutr* 1996;63(suppl):456S.

192. Wing RR. Weight cycling in humans: a review of the literature. *Ann Behav Med* 1992;14:113.

193. Wroble RR, Moxley DP. Weight loss patterns and success rates in high school wrestlers. *Med Sci Sports Exerc* 1998;30:625.

194. Yancy WS Jr, et al. A low-carbohydrate, ketogenic diet versus a low-fat diet to treat obesity and hyperlipidemia: a randomized, controlled trial. *Ann Intern Med* 2004;140:769.

195. Zhang Y, et al. Positional cloning of the mouse obese gene and its human homologue. *Nature* 1994;372:425.

196. Zuti WB, Golding LA. Comparing diet and exercise as weight reduction tools. *Phys Sportsmed* 1976;4:49.

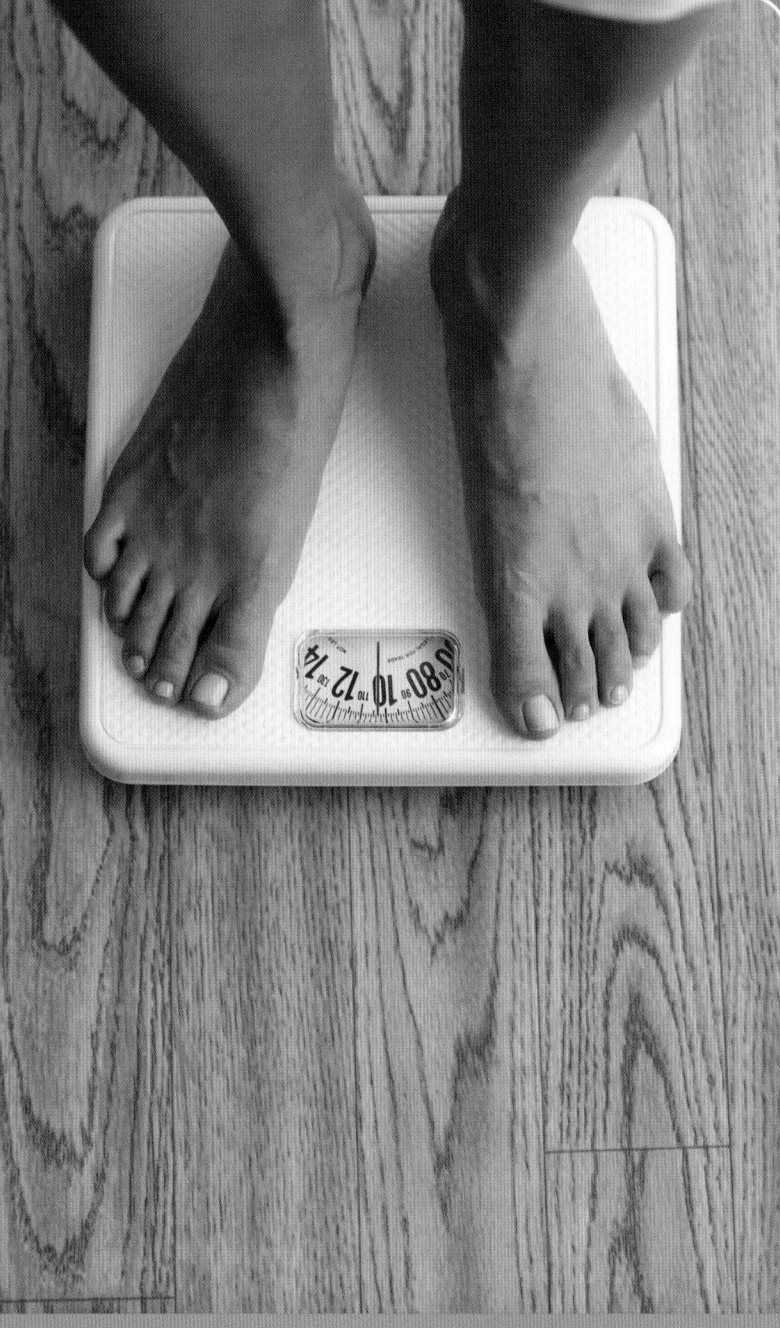

Chapter 15

Disordered Eating

Test Your Knowledge

Answer these 10 statements about disordered eating. Use the scoring key at the end of the chapter to check your results. Repeat this test after you have read the chapter and compare your results.

1. **T F** The Miss America contestants are a prime example of the perfect reference woman for body fat and body mass.
2. **T F** In general, athletes are at no greater risk for disordered eating behaviors than nonathletes.
3. **T F** A unique subclass of disordered eating behaviors most likely exists among female athletes.
4. **T F** Disordered eating behaviors do not appear to afflict men.
5. **T F** Two major characteristics of anorexia nervosa include an obsession with food and excessive exercise.
6. **T F** The primary goal in treating anorexia nervosa is normalizing eating behaviors.
7. **T F** Two major characteristics of bulimia nervosa include an obsession with weight loss and excessive exercise.
8. **T F** Forced hospitalization is the primary treatment for eating disorders.
9. **T F** Exercise treatment is not useful for anorexia nervosa, but it has proven useful in treating bulimia nervosa.
10. **T F** Muscle dysmorphia refers to severe muscle weakness induced by repetitive purging behaviors.

EATING DISORDERS VERSUS DISORDERED EATING

Eating disorders and *disordered eating* do not describe the same phenomenon. Anorexia nervosa or bulimia nervosa represent *eating disorder* illnesses that seriously interfere with one's daily activities. In contrast, *disordered eating* represents a temporary or mild change in eating behavior. Often, disordered eating patterns occur either after an illness or stressful event, or relate to a dietary change intended to improve health or appearance. Disordered eating activities rarely persist and do not require professional intervention. In contrast, persistent disordered eating behaviors can lead to a diagnosed eating disorder.

For individuals with an eating disorder, the focus on food becomes a source of consistent stress and anxiety and requires professional intervention. Eating disorders include a spectrum of emotional illnesses that range from self-imposed starvation to chronic binge eating. These illnesses produce severe distortions of the eating process and often lead to life-threatening physical and psychological consequences.

Many people have eaten to the point of discomfort during a Thanksgiving or Christmas dinner. Stuffing oneself at a holiday meal or going on an occasional food restriction plan does not constitute an eating disorder. According to the *Manual of Clinical Dietetics*, "*a defining characteristic of an eating disorder is a persistent inability to eat in moderation.*"

A Continuum

The American Psychiatric Association's *Diagnostic and Statistical Manual of Mental Disorders (DSM-IV)* places eating disorders into three categories, with small but significant areas of overlap,[23] These categories form a continuum with self-starvation at one end and compulsive overeating at the other end (FIGURE 15.1 and TABLE 15.1).

Anorexia nervosa occurs at the self-starvation end of the continuum. Anorexia, a self-imposed starvation syndrome triggered by many factors, includes a severely distorted body image. Anorectics are at war with their bodies even when they are dangerously underweight while severely restricting food intake (the major symptom of anorexia nervosa).

Binge eating or compulsive overeating lies at the opposite end of the continuum of eating disorders. People with this disorder chronically consume massive quantities of food and are typically overfat; however, not all overfat people binge eat. The diagnosis of binge-eating disorder is based on a person having an average of two binge-eating episodes per week for 6 continuous months. Bulimia nervosa occurs in the middle of the eating disorder continuum. These individuals compulsively gorge themselves and then purge to eliminate the ingested food.

History

Anorexia nervosa, while considered a relatively recent disorder, has a history that dates back many centuries.[14,70,94] Examples of self-starvation appeared in the Hellenistic era (circa 323–146 BC). Holy or saintly anorexics abused their bodies, rejected marriage, and sought religious asylum, where unfortunately many perished. During the Victorian era, large numbers of mothers and daughters avoided food for fear of giving the impression their physical appetite linked to their appetite for sex. It was commonly believed that

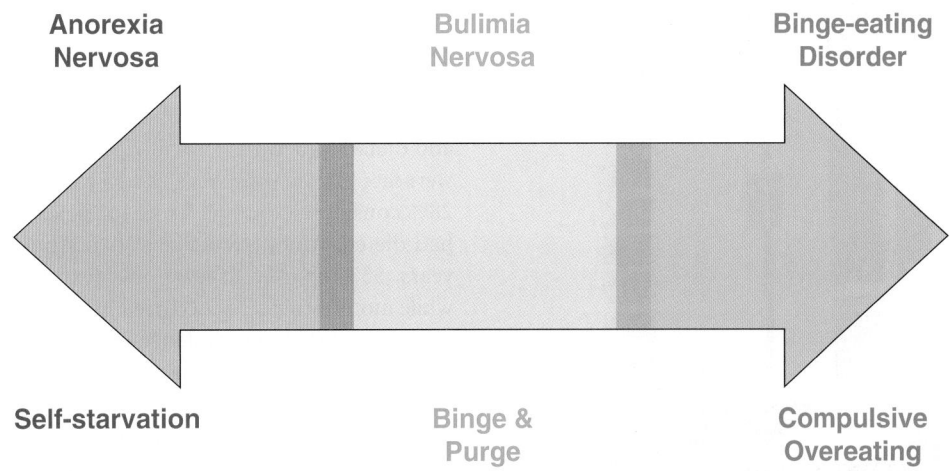

FIGURE 15.1 ■ The continuum of eating disorders.

women who consumed too much food had a greater sexual appetite!

Richard Morton (1637–1698) generally receives credit for the first medical description in 1689 of a wasting (anorectic) disease often associated with tuberculosis.[113] In the early 1800s, scattered reports emerged in the English medical literature about eating disorders, and two neurologists in 1873 separately described the condition now called anorexia nervosa. Ernest Charles Lasègue, a student friend of renowned French physiologist Claude Bernard, wrote of women's refusal of food "that may be indefinitely prolonged," and Sir William Gull, (physician to Queen Victoria of England), studied women who refused food (Gull is credited as the first person to "officially" use the term anorexia nervosa instead of anorexia-hysteria coined by Lasègue). Lasègue's book chronicled the stages of this disease in young French girls.

It was not until the early 1970s that the American media began to write about eating disorders. Beginning in 1974, articles described how young women refused to eat but without really explaining the seriousness of the illness. In 1983, the popular folksinger Karen Carpenter died of anorexia nervosa, bringing intense media scrutiny about the history and seriousness of eating disorders in general and anorexia nervosa in particular. This watershed event prompted other actresses and public figures to speak out about their battles to achieve thinness.

The first published photo of a person suffering from anorexia nervosa appeared in a 1932 issue of the *New England Journal of Medicine* (FIG. 15.2). Before the common usage of the term "anorexia nervosa," the disease was known as "long-term fasting" or "self-starvation."

In 1978, noted psychologist Hilde Bruch published *The Golden Cage*, a book based on 70 cases mostly from young women's testimonials during her three decades of clinical ex-

TABLE 15.1	**Distinguishing Characteristics of Eating Disorders**		
Factor	**Anorexia Nervosa**	**Bulimia Nervosa**	**Binge-Eating Disorder**
Body Weight	Below normal (<85% of recommended weight)	Usually normal	Above normal
Binge eating	Possible	Yes, at least twice for 3 months	Yes, at least twice for 6 months
Purging	Possible	Yes, at least twice for 3 months	No
Restrict food intake	Yes	Yes	Yes
Body image	Dissatisfaction with body and distorted image of body size	Dissatisfaction with body and distorted image of body size	Dissatisfaction with body
Fear of being fat	Yes	Yes	Not excessive
Self-esteem	Low	Low	Low
Menstrual abnormalities	Absence of at least 3 consecutive periods	No	No

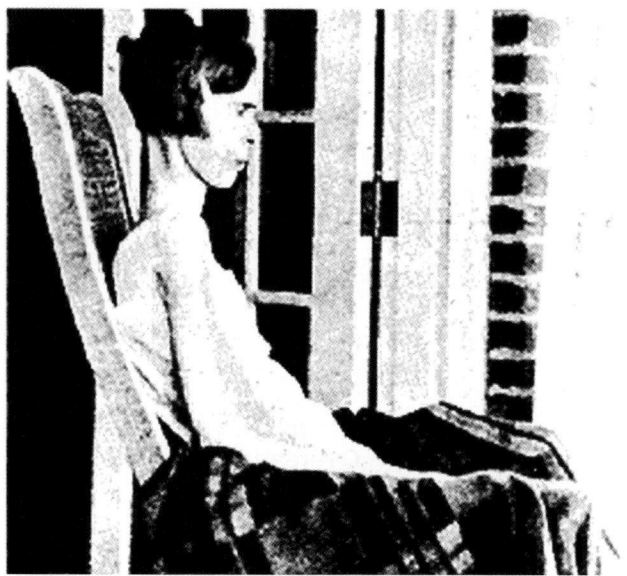

FIGURE 15.2 ■ The first published photo of an anorectic in an American medical journal. (From Fasting girls. *N Engl J Med* 1932;207.

AN INORDINATE FOCUS ON BODY WEIGHT

Among 3000 middle-school children studied for body image and dietary practices, 55% of eighth-grade girls believed they were fat (13% actually were), and 50% had dieted. For the boys, 28% considered themselves fat (13% actually were), and 15% had dieted. Among 869 Australian schoolgirls ages 14 to 17 years, 335 reported at least one disordered eating behavior, while monthly bingeing occurred in 8% and vomiting in 27%.[38] TABLE 15.2 lists the prevalence of monthly unhealthy and extreme weight reduction practices of these teenage girls. Of the group, 57% practiced "unhealthy dieting" and 36% practiced dieting behaviors considered extreme—crash dieting, fasting, and use of diet pills, diuretics, laxatives, and cigarettes.

Disordered eating behaviors generally affect females between the ages of 15 and 35, although women in their 30s, 40s, and 50s may account for up to one third of eating disorders in the United States. The prevalence in the general population ranges from 1 to 5% of female high school and college students to as high as 12 to 15% for females in medical and graduate schools.[24,43,44,73,89,116] Thin body preoccupation and social pressure represent important risk factors for the development of eating disorders in adolescent girls.[65,114] Childhood traits reflecting obsessive–compulsive personality also appear to be important risk factors.[1] Adolescent girls who experience physical and sexual dating violence show a relatively high rate of abnor-

perience in treating eating disorders.[13] Bruch also claimed the disease had become an increasing problem in American colleges and universities. Research now confirms this supposition, particularly in women's individual sports (gymnastics, swimming and diving, dance) where thinness and "looking good" remain a premium (discussed more fully in Chapter 14). Fortunately, many private and public institutions now focus their research efforts on the causes and etiology of eating disorders.

Prevalence and Incidence of Eating Disorders

The term *prevalence* of eating disorders refers to the estimated population of people afflicted with an eating disorder at any given time. The term *incidence* refers to the annual diagnosis rate or number of new cases diagnosed yearly. These two statistics differ; a short-lived disease such as flu can have high annual incidence but low prevalence, and a life-long disease such as diabetes can have a low annual incidence but high prevalence.

Over a lifetime, an estimated 0.5% to 3.7% of females suffer from anorexia nervosa and 1.1% to 4.2% from bulimia nervosa.[24,38] Community surveys estimate that between 2% and 5% of Americans experience binge-eating disorder in any 6-month period.[40] The mortality rate among people with anorexia nervosa averages 0.6% a year or approximately 5.6% per decade—about 12 times higher than the annual death rate due to all causes of death among females ages 15 to 24 years in the general population.[45]

TABLE 15.2	Prevalence of Unhealthy and Extreme Weight-Reduction Practices among Teenage Girls
Behavior (monthly)	**Prevalence (%)**
No dairy[a]	16
No meats[a]	18
No starchy foods[a]	13
Slimming biscuit use	15
Slimming drink use	11
Skipping meals	46
Fad dieting	14
"Crash" dieting[b]	22
Fasting[b]	21
Diet pills	5
Diuretic use[b]	2
Laxative use[b]	5
Cigarette use[b]	12

From Grigg M, et al. Disordered eating and unhealthy weight-reduction practices among adolescent females. Prevent Med 1996;25:745.

[a]These foods eliminated and not compensated for with a balanced diet (e.g., a balanced vegetarian diet).

[b]Extreme dieting defined as "crash" dieting, fasting, or use of diet pills, diuretics, laxatives, and cigarettes.

mal weight control behaviors such as laxative use and/or vomiting.[81,95] Contrary to the conventional belief of many health professionals, African American women are not immune from eating disorders. A survey of African American college women found a prevalence of eating disorders similar to that among white peers; 2% had a full-blown eating disorder, and 23% showed some eating disorder symptoms. Cultural differences in the view of attractiveness—thin African American women are often considered unattractive—often causes some African American women to gain weight by binge eating.[71]

FIGURE 15.3 displays the relationship between the girls' actual body weight classification (determined by body mass index [BMI]) and perceived body weight. Regardless of objective weight categorization, 47% of all girls actively tried to lose weight, including 19% of underweight girls and 56% of normal-weight girls. When asked to categorize their current weight, 63% considered themselves overweight, yet only 16% actually were; 28% seemed "just right" (55% were of normal weight), and 9% concluded they were underweight (30% actually were). Such findings take on additional significance because previous attempts at dieting often develop into a full-blown eating disorder.

Miss America and BMI—Undernourished Role Models?

In 1967, only an 8% difference in body weight existed between professional models and the average American woman. Today, a model's body weight averages 23 lb below the national average for women (5 ft 11in, 117 lb vs 5 ft 4 in, 140 lb). This makes the BMI of most fashion models lower than that of all but 2% of American women. A focus on thinness has become particularly apparent among Miss America contestants.

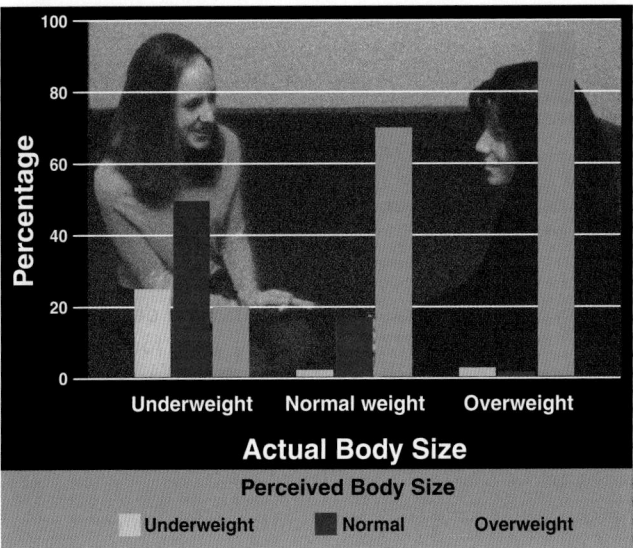

FIGURE 15.3 ■ Perception of current body weight and actual body weight classification determined by BMI in 851 teenage girls. (From Grigg M, et al. Disordered eating and unhealthy weight reduction practices among adolescent females. *Prevent Med* 1996;25:745.)

Many consider Miss America beauty pageant contestants to possess the ideal combination of beauty, grace, and talent. Each competitor survives the rigors of state and local contests, thus satisfying judges that finalists have "ideal qualities" worthy of role-model status. To some extent, the consummate image of the Miss America physique shapes society's generalized "ideal" for female size and shape. The contest, televised worldwide to millions of viewers, reinforces this notion. However, does such an image project or reinforce an unhealthful message to those who attempt to emulate these women?

FIGURE 15.4 shows the BMIs of Miss America contestants from available data between 1922 and 1999 (excluding 1927–1933, when the pageant was not held). The *lower horizontal dashed line* designates the World Health Organization (WHO) cutoff for undernutrition established at a BMI of 18.5.[124] The *upper horizontal line* represents the BMI for Behnke's standard for the reference woman (Fig. 13.6; stature, 1.638 m; body mass, 56.7 kg; BMI, 21.1). The downward slope of the regression line from 1922 to 1999 shows a clear tendency for relative undernutrition from the mid-1960s to approximately 1990. Using the WHO cutoff, the BMIs of 30% (N = 14) of the 47 Miss America winners fell below 18.5. Raising the BMI cutoff to 19.0 adds another 18 women, or a total of 48% of

Bigger Models? Slim Chance!

Recent deaths of several high-profile models (22-year-old popular Uruguayan model suffered a heart attack believed the result of a 10-year struggle with anorexia nervosa; a 21-year-old Brazilian, 5-ft 7-in model who weighed only 88 lb died during a runway shoot), have caused some clothes designers to require that models submit proof they do not suffer from eating disorders.

The Council of Fashion Designers of America (CFDA) recently recommended that model agencies (1) do not hire women under age 16, (2) supply their models with healthy snacks backstage at shoots, and (3) provide them with nutrition and fitness education. But CFDA failed to endorse recommendations by nutritionist and scientists that any model with a BMI below 18.5 not be allowed to walk the runway. In the fashion industry, thin remains in; fashion ideals are set by the highest social classes and fashion magazine editors, who believe that clothes on skinny girls (size 2–4) look better. The industry preys on women who fantasize they might look like a model if they wear the clothes. Even though more than half of American women wear a size 14 or larger, they want to be smaller or at least try to look that way, and the fashion industry promotes this dream. Twenty years ago a current size 2 dress was a size 6 and a current size 8 was a size 12. This size distortion (that occurs only with women's clothing) is designed to sell more cloths to women who desire to be smaller when in reality they are actually considerably larger.

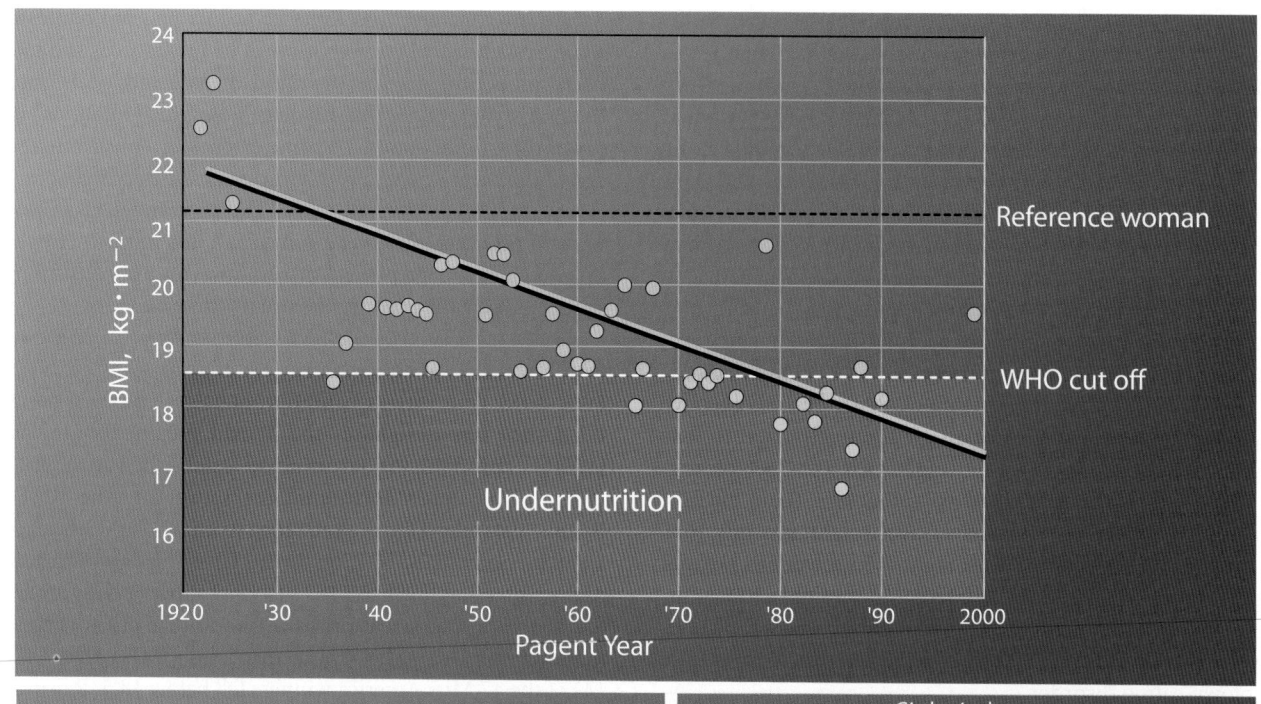

FIGURE 15.4 ■ BMI of 47 Miss America pageant contestants from 1922 to 1999. The *top horizontal dashed black line* represents the BMI for Behnke's reference woman (21.1 kg · m⁻²). The *bottom horizontal dashed white line* designates the WHO's BMI demarcation for undernutrition (18.5 kg · m⁻²). The *left inset table* shows the available data for age, height (in), and weight (lb) for the contest winners. The *right inset table* shows selected girths for 24 Miss America winners from 1926 to 1965.

the winners with undesirable values. Approximately 24% of the BMIs of contest winners ranged between 20.0 and 21.0, and no winner after 1924 had a BMI greater than 21!

Interestingly, 1965 was the last year that we could locate girth measurements from official press releases or newspaper coverage of the contest. We compared the percentage difference between Miss America girth averages with corresponding values for the reference woman (*bottom row* of *right inset*

table). For the average bust, waist, and hip values (35.1 in, 24.0 in, 35.4 in, respectively), Miss America's bust measurement exceeded the reference woman's measurement by 2.6 inches (8%) but fell 7% below the waist value (−1.8 in) and 5% (−1.7 in) below the value for the hips. Unfortunately, no contemporary BMI data exist from 1966 to 2004 to compare the "modern" Miss America's physique status with historical data. If the Miss America contest indeed serves as a subtle promoter of the

Case Study

Personal Health and Exercise Nutrition 15–1

How to Calculate Recommended (Optimal) Body Weight

A major objective in determining an individual's body composition relates to recommending an "optimal" body weight (OBW). Usually this refers to a recommended weight for health considerations, occupational and sport performance requirements, or simply aesthetics (self-assessment based on appearance). OBW computation is based on comparison with an optimal percentage body fat (OPT%BF). Determining OPT%BF becomes subjective because no absolute standards by age, fitness, ethnicity, or any other variable are available. Several body composition reference classifications can serve as guidelines for setting OPT%BF levels for different ages (Table 1). Selecting the OPT%BF should reflect the person's current OPT%BF and his or her personal objectives.

Table 1 Body Composition Classification by Age According to Percentage Body Fat from Typical Data in the Research

Age, y	Below Average	Average	Above Average
Males			
≤19	12–17	17–22	22–27
20–29	13–18	18–23	23–28
30–39	14–19	19–24	24–29
40–49	15–20	20–25	25–30
≥50	16–20	21–26	26–31
Females			
≤19	17–22	22–27	27–32
20–29	18–23	23–28	28–33
30–39	19–24	24–29	29–34
40–49	20–25	25–30	30–35
≥50	21–26	26–31	31–36

Procedures

1. Determine body weight (BW) in kilograms and %BF using available valid techniques (see Chapters 13 and 14).
2. Calculate body fat weight (FW) in kilograms.

$$FW = BW \times \%BF$$

where %BF is expressed in decimal form (e.g., 23.0% = 0.23)

3. Determine fat-free body mass (FFM) in kilograms.

$$FFM = BW - FW$$

4. Select an optimal body weight (OBW) expressed in decimal form (e.g., 15.0% = 0.15).
5. Compute OBW in kilograms.

$$OBW = FFM \div (1.00 - OPT\%BF)$$

Example Calculations

1. Data: Female; age 19 years; body weight = 66.0 kg; %BF from hydrostatic weighing = 30.0% (decimal form = 0.30); OPT%BF chosen = 25.0% (0.25).

Calculate FW in kilograms:

2. FW = BW × %BF
   = 66.0 kg × 0.30
   = 19.8 kg (43.7 lb)

Determine FFM in kilograms:

3. FFM = BW—FW
   = 66.0 kg—19.8 kg
   = 46.2 kg (101.9 lb)

Select OPT%BF expressed in decimal form:

4. %BF = 0.25

Compute OBW in kg:

5. OBW = FFM ÷ (1.00 − %BF)
   = 46.2 kg ÷ (1.00 − 0.25)
   = 61.6 kg (135 lb)

Computing Recommended Fat Loss

From the above calculations, the amount of fat loss in kilograms required to reach OBW (at the chosen OPT%BF of 25.0%) computes as:

Fat loss = BW − OBW
= 66.0 kg − 61.6 kg
= 4.4 kg (9.7 lb)

"ideal" female size and shape, then the more recent message delivered to impressionable teenagers overemphasizes that "thin is in," regardless of the potential negative nutritional and long-term health implications.[29]

Female Athletes at Greater Risk

Most studies documenting disordered eating behaviors among athletes rely on anonymous self-report surveys or inventories, with relatively little data from in-depth interviews. Generalizations come mainly from "snapshots" of small numbers of high school and college athletes in specific sports without considering the athletes' skill level, experience, and achievement status. Notwithstanding these limitations in research strategy, female athletes clearly face a unique set of circumstances that make them particularly vulnerable to disordered eating behaviors. These behaviors flourish when strong negative aesthetic connotations about excess body fat blend with the athlete's belief that *any* body fat dooms success. Thirty years ago, female gymnasts weighed about 21 lb more than today's counterparts.

Clinical observations indicate a prevalence between 15 and 70% for eating disorders among athletes, with some groups at higher risk than others. More specifically, eating disorders and unrealistic weight goals (and general dissatisfaction with one's body) occur most frequently among female athletes in the aesthetic sports such as ballet, bodybuilding, diving, figure skating, cheerleading, and gymnastics, in which success often coincides with extreme leanness.[11,35,41,48,51,79,87,105–107,118,127] An inordinate preoccupation with eating also occurs among adolescent female swimmers.[8,25,120,122] Controversy exists as to the prevalence of eating disorders among endurance runners,[18,78] but recent data show a nearly 26% prevalence of eating disorders as indicated by elevated scores on the Eating Disorders Inventory.[19]

Coaches often compound the problem.[97] Sixty-seven percent of female collegiate gymnasts reported that their coaches said they weighed too much, and 75% of these athletes used weight-loss strategies involving vomiting or laxative or diuretic use.[90,91] Weight reduction attempts averaged 85% in female and 93% in male weight-class athletes.[30] Between 27 and 37% of women in aesthetic, endurance, and weight-class sports experienced menstrual disorders, compared with only 5% in other sports. Unfortunately, reducing body weight significantly below normal levels also coincides with inadequate nutrient intake.[58]

Among athletes classified "at risk" for developing an eating disorder, 92% met the criteria for anorexia nervosa, bulimia nervosa, or anorexia athletica (see pp. 502, 507 and 509).[88] Eighty-five percent of the athletes dieted, compared with 27% of controls. Adolescent dancers and figure skaters exhibited more frequent patterns of disordered eating than other athletic groups and nonathletes.[12] In a survey of female college athletes, 14% of the women reported self-induced vomiting, while 16% indicated laxative use for weight control.[91] Among female college gymnasts, all were trying to diet and 25% reported self-induced vomiting.[90] Other studies also indicate high incidence of disordered eating behaviors

among female gymnasts.[74,80,83,120] However, prevalence rates did not differ from age-matched, nonathletic controls.

Risk factors for disordered eating among athletes include[112]:

1. Pressure to optimize performance and/or modify appearance
2. Psychologic factors, such as low self-esteem, poor coping skills, perceived loss of control, perfectionism, obsessive–compulsive traits, depression, anxiety, and history of sexual/physical abuse
3. Underlying chronic diseases related to caloric use (e.g., diabetes)

Preoccupation with body weight and associated eating disorders among female gymnasts during college abates considerably after retirement from the sport.[75] TABLE 15.3 presents data on eating disorder symptoms from former college gymnasts approximately 15 years postcompetition. These women scored below published average values *(norms)* for each variable measured. Nonathletic controls and gymnasts scored similarly on all variables except asceticism and body dissatisfaction, on which gymnasts scored significantly lower. The former gymnasts also maintained nutrient intakes within the recommended range and possessed greater bone mineral density at multiple body sites than controls.[58] One must determine if findings from former gymnasts of 15 to 25 years ago apply to contemporary gymnasts, for whom exaggerated leanness and small body structure now seem to play a more important part in competitive success.

TABLE 15.4 summarizes findings of 23 studies of eating patterns of athletes. In general, the incidence of eating disor-

---

TABLE 15.3 Eating Disorders Inventory Scores from Normative Data (Norms), Former Gymnasts, and Control Subjects

	Norms (N = 205)	Gymnasts (N = 22)	Controls (N = 22)
Drive for thinness	5.5	3.3	4.0
Bulimia	1.2	0.6	1.0
Body dissatisfaction	12.2	7.9	14.1*
Ineffectiveness	2.3	1.2	2.3
Perfectionism	6.2	5.0	4.3
Interpersonal distrust	2.0	1.6	2.5
Interoceptive awareness	3.0	0.9	1.4
Maturity fears	2.7	1.8	2.0
Asceticism	3.4	2.4	4.5*
Impulse regulation	2.3	0.7	0.9
Social insecurity	3.3	1.4	3.1

* Significantly different from gymnasts, P ≤ 0.05.

From O'Connor PJ, et al. Eating disorder symptoms in former female college gymnasts: relations with body composition. Am J Clin Nutr 1996;64:840.

TABLE 15.4   Summary of Selected Studies of Eating Disorders in Athletes

Study (ref. #)	Sport	Subjects	Measures[a]	Outcome
9	Female and male athletes from 8 sports	695 athletes (55% female) from 8 sports. Mean age, 19 y (range, 16–25)	41-item questionnaire mailed to coaches in 21 colleges in the midwest; coaches administered it to athletes	59% lost weight by "excessive" exercise, 24% by consuming less than 600 kCal/d, 12% by fasting, 11% by using fad diets, 6% by vomiting, 4% by using laxatives, and 1% by using enemas; relatively few gender differences, but trend for males to use exercise and females to use dieting to lose weight
10	Female athletes from 7 sports	79 female athletes in sports emphasizing leanness (ballet, bodybuilding, cheerleading, gymnastics) or sports with no emphasis (swimming, track and field, volleyball); 101 nonathlete controls	EDI	No overall differences between athletes and controls; athletes in sports emphasizing leanness had a higher percentage of elevated scores than athletes in other sports
12	Ballet dancers	55 female dancers in national and regional companies	EAT-26	33% had anorexia or bulimia in the past; 50% of amenorrheic subjects reported anorexia compared with 13% of women with normal cycles
21	Various sports	64 female athletes in "thin-build" sports (e.g., gymnastics); 62 females in "normal-build" sports (e.g., volleyball); 64 female univ. student controls	EDI	Overall EDI scores not different among groups; athletes in thin-build sports had greater weight concerns, more body dissatisfaction, and more dieting than normal-build athletes and controls, even though body weights were lower
25	Swimmers	487 girls and 468 boys, ages 9–18, at a competitive swimming camp	Questionnaire on dieting and weight-control practices	15.4% of the girls (24.8% of the postmenarchal girls) and 3.6% of boys used pathogenic weight loss techniques; girls were more likely than boys to perceive themselves heavier than they were
27	Wrestlers, swimmers, Nordic skiers	26 male wrestlers, 21 male swimmers, and cross-country skiers	EAT-40, restraint questionnaire, body image assessment	Higher EAT scores in wrestlers due to higher scores on weight fluctuation and dieting; no overall differences in estimates of body size; a small subsample of wrestlers who scored high on restraint and EAT scores had distortions of body size
28	Dancers	21 female university dancers and 29 female university controls	EAT-40	33% of dancers and 14% of controls scored in the range symptomatic of anorexia on the EAT; difference in overall EAT scores not significant
32	Ballet dancers	10 female ballet dancers with stress fractures, 10 dancers without fractures, and 10 nondancer controls	EAT-26, structured interview on DSM-III criteria for eating disorders	Nonsignificant trend for stress-fracture dancers to have higher EAT scores than other 2 groups; greater incidence of eating disorders in stress-fracture group

(continues)

TABLE 15.4　Summary of Selected Studies of Eating Disorders in Athletes *(continued)*

Study (ref. #)	Sport	Subjects	Measures[a]	Outcome
35	Ballet dancers	35 female ballet students ages 11–14, followed 2–4 y	EDI	At follow-up, 26% of subjects had anorexia nervosa and 14% had bulimia nervosa or a "partial syndrome"; the "drive for thinness" and "body dissatisfaction" scales of the EDI predicted eating disorders at follow-up
41	Ballet dancers	55 white and 11 black female dancers in national and regional companies (mean age, 24.9 y)	EAT-26	15% of white dancers reported anorexia and 19% report bulimia; none of the black dancers reported anorexia or bulimia
42	Ballet dancers	32 female ballet dancers from 4 national US companies, 17 dancers from national company in China (mean age, 24.6 y)	Variation in EAT-26, subjects given description of eating disorders and asked if they had the problem	American dancers from less-selected companies had more eating problems, more anorectic behaviors and more female obesity than the highly-selected American or Chinese dancers
48	Majorettes	11 varsity majors	24-hour dietary recall on eating and weight practices; no standardized measures	Based on clinical observations, all subjects had distorted body image due to low weight standards. Subjects reported eating and drinking little for several days prior to weighings, high levels of exercise and using sauna, diet pills, and diuretics
Unpublished data	Runners	4551 (1911 females, 2640 males) respondents to survey in *Runners World* magazine	EAT-26 questions on eating and diet concerns	Mean EAT score = 9.0 for males, 14.1 for females; 8% of males and 24% of females scored ≥20 on EAT; 15% of males who ran ≥45 mi/wk scored ≥20, compared with 7% of males who ran less; 24% of females who ran ≥40 mi/wk scored ≥20, compared with 23% of those who ran less
55	Jockeys	10 male jockeys from England (mean age, 22.9 y; mean weight, 108.5 lb)	EDI, EAT-26	Poor response rate to full battery of tests (from 58 stables, only 10 subjects responded); mean EAT score was 14.9, higher than expected in young males; most reported food avoidance, saunas, and laxative abuse; diuretics and appetite suppressants were used; binges were common, but vomiting was unusual
59	Athletes from unspecified sports	126 female athletes from unspecified sports, 590 students from other groups (e.g., sororities, classes)	EDI questionnaire with eating disorder diagnosis questions	Athletes had generally lower scores on all eating disorders measures than other groups, but statistical tests not performed
65	Female athletes from different sports	87 female athletes from track, swimming, gymnastics, and ballet; 41 females with eating disorders, 120 female high school and junior high controls	Self-reports of dieting, vomiting, and eating disorders	Frequent dieting, vomiting, and self-reported anorexia more common in athletes than normal controls but less common than eating disorders subjects, but no statistical comparisons performed

(continues)

TABLE 15.4   Summary of Selected Studies of Eating Disorders in Athletes *(continued)*

Study (ref. #)	Sport	Subjects	Measures[a]	Outcome
79	Obligatory runners and weightlifters	15 males and 15 females in each of 3 groups; obligatory runners, obligatory weightlifters, and sedentary controls	Body size estimation 3 subscales on EDI	Runners and weightlifters had more eating disturbances than controls; females had more eating pathologies than males
90	Gymnasts	42 female college gymnasts	Questionnaire on dieting and weight control practices	All subjects were dieting (50% for appearance, 50% for performance); 62% used at least 1 pathogenic weight method (e.g., vomiting, diet pills, fasting); 66% were told they were too heavy by coaches
91	Varsity level female athletes from 10 sports	182 female varsity athletes	Questionnaire on dieting and weight control practices	32% engaged in at least 1 pathogenic weight-control practice; the percentages were 14% for vomiting, 16% for laxatives, 25% for diet pills, 5% for diuretics, 20% for regular binges, and 8% for excessive weight loss
92	Ice skaters	17 male (mean age, 21.1 y) and 23 female (mean age, 17.6 y) figure skaters from mid-Atlantic training facility	EAT-40	Mean EAT scores were 29.3 for women and 10 for men; 48% of the women and no man had EAT scores in anorectic range (>30)
99	Wrestlers	63 male college wrestlers and 378 high school wrestlers	Questionnaire on dieting and weight control practices	63% of college and 43% of high school wrestlers were preoccupied with food during the season (19% and 14% in the off-season); 41% of college and 29% of high school wrestlers reported eating out of control between matches; 52% of college and 26% of high school wrestlers reported fasting at least once a week
120	Female athletes from 7 sports	82 female athletes from gymnastics, cross-country, basketball, golf, volleyball, swimming, and tennis; 52 nonathlete controls	EAT-40, EDI	None of athletes scored in disturbed range; no overall differences between athletes and controls; cross-country runners showed less and gymnasts showed more eating disturbance than controls, but only on selected scales
121	Runners	125 female distance runners, 25 nonrunning controls	EAT-26, EDI	No greater incidence of eating problems in runners than in controls; elite runners more likely than other runners to have problems

From Brownell KD, Rodin J. Prevalence of eating disorders in athletes. In: Brownell KD, et al., eds. Eating, body weight and performance in athletes. Philadelphia: Lea & Febiger, 1992.

[a]*EAT-40, Eating Attitudes Test containing 40 questions in which subjects rate how well a statement applies to them on a 6-point scale; EAT-26, 26-question modification of EAT-40; EDI, Eating Disorder Inventory containing 64 questions with 8 subscales to assess behaviors and attitudes related to body image, eating behaviors, and dieting.*

ders is greater among athletes than in nonathletic comparison groups or general population. Future research should investigate the extent to which eating disorders permeate the competitive athletic scene among junior and senior high school female participants.

A study in conjunction with the National Collegiate Athletic Association clearly shows a greater prevalence of eating disorders among female athletes than male counterparts.[50] Among women, 1.1% met the clinical diagnostic criteria for bulimia nervosa; none met the criteria for anorexia nervosa, but 9.2% showed subclinical bulimia and subclinical anorexia. For the male athletes, none met the diagnostic criteria for anorexia, bulimia, or subclinical anorexia, and only 0.01% presented with subclinical bulimia.

Anorexia Athletica

The cluster of personality traits among athletes often shares a commonalty with patients with clinical eating disorders. The same traits that make an athlete excel in sports—compulsive, driven, dichotomous thinker, perfectionist, competitive, compliant and eager to please ("coachable"), and self-motivated—increase risk for developing an eating disorder.[46,82,101] More than likely, the greatest risk exists for individuals whose normal, genetically determined body size and shape deviate from the "ideal" imposed by the sport. The term **anorexia athletica** describes the continuum of subclinical eating behaviors of physically active individuals who fail to meet the criteria for a true eating disorder, but who exhibit at least one unhealthy weight-control method or disordered eating pattern.[3,74,75] This includes fasting, vomiting (termed "instrumental vomiting" when used to make weight), and use of diet pills, laxatives, or diuretics (water pills).

A study of Norwegian elite female athletes aged 12 to 35 years examined risk factors and triggers for eating disorders.[108] TABLE 15.5 lists the criteria to identify anorexia athletica. Based on the Eating Disorder Inventory (EDI), 117 of 522 athletes classified as "at risk." Follow-up with this subgroup revealed a significant incidence of anorexia nervosa (N = 7), bulimia nervosa (N = 42), and anorexia athletica (N = 43). TABLE 15.6 provides selected characteristics for sport-specific groupings from the 92 athletes with eating disorders; characteristics included weekly training volume and percentage of each athletic subgroup with high inventory scores. Interestingly, the athletes traced their eating disorder to one of three causes: (1) prolonged periods of dieting and fluctuations in body weight (37%), (2) new coach (30%), and (3) injury or illness (23%). All of the athletes and controls (athletes without eating disorders) dieted to enhance performance. Sixty-seven percent of athletes with an eating disorder dieted on their coach's recommendation, while 75% of control athletes dieted because of a coach's influence. This latter finding reveals that most female athletes, whether or not they engaged in disordered eating behaviors, remained impressionable to an authority figure, attempting to please coaches by following through on their recommendations.

For many athletes, disordered eating patterns coincide with the competitive season and abate when the season ends.

TABLE 15.5	Criteria for Identifying Anorexia Athletica	
Common Features	**Anorexia Athletica**
Weight loss[a]	+
Delayed puberty[b]	(+)
Menstrual dysfunction[c]	(+)
GI complaints	+
Absence of medical illness or affective disorder explaining the weight reduction	+
Disturbance in body image	(+)
Excessive fear of becoming obese	+
Purging[d]	(+)
Binging[d]	(+)
Compulsive exercising[d]	(+)
Restricted caloric intake[e]	+

+, criteria that all athletes had to meet; (+), anorexia athletica athletes met one or more of the listed criteria.
[a] >5% expected body weight.
[b] No menstrual flow at age 16 (primary amenorrhea).
[c] Primary, secondary, or oligomenorrhea.
[d] Defined in DSM-III-R(1).
[e] Use of diets at or below 1200 kCal for unspecified durations.

For them, the preoccupation with body weight may not reflect true underlying pathology, but rather a desire to achieve optimum physiologic function and competitive status.[20] For a small number of athletes, the season never "ends," and they develop a clinical eating disorder.

Eating Disorders Also Afflict Men

Although most people consider eating disorders a "female problem," an increasing number of men share this affliction. The question remains unanswered whether this increased number results from an actual increase in disease incidence or because more men with the condition now seek treatment. In one New York hospital treatment center, the percentage of male patients admitted with eating disorders rose steadily from 4% in 1988 to 13% in 1995. Men currently represent 6 to 10% of individuals with eating disorders, with the greatest prevalence among models, dancers, men abused during childhood, and gays.

Body weight-dependent sports such as wrestling, horse racing, lightweight rowing, distance running, and bodybuilding potentially create conditions to develop patterns of disordered eating, particularly purging.[4,27,55,99] Of 25 lower-weight-category collegiate wrestlers (BMI, 21.1) and 59 lightweight rowers (BMI, 21.0), 52% reported bingeing; 8% of the rowers and 16% of the wrestlers showed pathologic EDI profiles.[115] The 52% rate for bingeing behavior represents approximately twice the incidence in the normal male population. A survey of Michigan high school wrestlers showed that 72% engaged in at least one potentially harmful weight loss practice over the season, regardless of grade or success level.[56] Fasting and various

Sport Groups[a]	N	Age, y[b]	BMI	Training Volume, km · wk⁻¹	% with High EDI[c]
Technical sports	13	19 (14–30)	21 (17–26)	14 (12–19)	21
Endurance sports	24	22 (15–28)	20 (15–22)	21 (19–26)	20
Aesthetic sports	22	17 (12–24)	18 (15–21)	18 (17–23)	40
Weight-dependent sports	11	21 (15–23)	21 (17–23)	14 (11–16)	37
Ball game sports	21	20 (17–27)	21 (19–27)	15 (12–17)	14
Total sample	92	20 (13–28)	21 (15–27)	17 (12–26)	22
Athletic controls	30	20 (13–28)	22 (18–24)	15 (10–22)	0

TABLE 15.6 Characteristics of the Eating Disordered Athlete Representing the Different Sport Groups

Thirty control subjects represented a random sample of athletes without elevated scores on the Eating Disorder Inventory (EDI) who were matched on age, community of residence, and sport. At-risk subjects were classified by EDI scores above the mean for anorectic patients on the drive for thinness and body dissatisfaction subscales of the EDI.

From Sundgot-Borgen J. Eating disorders in female athletes. Sports Med 1994;17:176.

[a]**Technical:** alpine skiing, bowling, golf, high jump, horseback riding, long jump, rifle shooting, sailing sky diving; **Endurance:** biathlon, cross country-skiing, cycling, middle-distance and long-distance running, orienteering, race walking, rowing, speed skating, swimming: **Aesthetic:** diving, figure skating, gymnastics rhythmical gymnastics, sports dance; **Weight-dependent:** judo, karate, wrestling; **Ball games:** badminton, bandy (land hockey on ice), basketball, soccer, table tennis, team handball, tennis, volleyball, underwater rugby.

[b]Values for age, BMI, and training volume are given as means with ranges in parentheses.

[c]Based on N = 522.

dehydration methods provided the primary methods for rapid weight loss. Wrestlers who lost weight each week were the most likely to binge eat. Fifty percent of the wrestlers lost more than 5 lb and 27% lost 10 lb. Two percent of the wrestlers reported weekly use of laxatives, diet pills, or diuretics, and another 2% used vomiting to loose weight. With the changes in rules governing weight loss of wrestlers during the season, these practices are likely to no longer be prevalent.

MUSCLE DYSMORPHIA: "THE ADONIS COMPLEX"

A change has taken place in the way many men view the ideal male physique. Austrian, French, and American men project the "ideal" man's body as possessing about 28 lb more muscle than their own.[86] This mismatched perception coincides with the increased number of men who use anabolic steroids, experience eating disorders, and suffer from body obsession. An important component of body obsession relates to **muscle dysmorphia,** or the "Adonis complex," the pathologic preoccupation with muscle size and overall muscularity. These individuals view themselves as small and frail, when in reality, many are large and muscular.

In many ways, muscle dysmorphia and anorexia nervosa share common traits; a history of depression and anxiety, a hyperculturization of body image and unrealistic shame about one's body, and self-destructive behaviors. Both anorectic and dysmorphic groups act on their bodies for acceptance and use their bodies as a way to control their lives. They often endanger their health by excessive exercising, bingeing-and-purging rituals, steroid abuse, and inordinate reliance of nutritional

and dietary supplements to alter their appearance.[6,7,66] A large number of these men binge eat or inordinately focus on consuming low-fat, high-protein diets.

Characteristics of Muscle Dysmorphia Among Body Builders[76,93]

1. Respond that they are totally or mostly dissatisfied with their body
2. Have higher rates of current or past major mood, anxiety, or eating disorders
3. Spend more than 3 hours daily thinking about their muscularity
4. Avoid activities and people because of their perceived body defect
5. Report little or no control over compulsive weightlifting and dietary patterns
6. Relinquish activities that were formerly enjoyable

No formal diagnostic criteria exist to identify an individual at risk for muscle dysmorphia. TABLE 15.7 proposes some characteristic features exhibited by those with the disorder.

THE EXERCISE ADDICT

To some extent, cultural influences create similarities between anorexia nervosa and addictive exercise behaviors. Approximately 50% of women with eating disorders compulsively overexercise. Someone who exercises excessively—

TABLE 15.7 **Signs and Symptoms of Muscle Dysmorphia**

- Preoccupation with the idea that he is not sufficiently lean and muscular. Behaviors associated with this preoccupation include frequent weighing; constant checking of appearance in mirrors/windows, persistent criticism of body weight, size, and/or shape; wearing baggy clothing to camouflage the body; or, conversely, modifying clothing to accentuate muscularity (such as adding extra buttons to make a shirt sleeve look tighter).

- Preoccupation with muscularity causes clinically significant distress or impairment of social, occupational, or other important areas of life functioning (e.g., personal relationships), as demonstrated by at least two of the following:
  1. Frequently gives up important social, occupational, or recreational activities because of a compulsive need to maintain exercise and dietary regimens.
  2. Avoids situations where the body would be exposed to others (e.g., at the beach or swimming pool) or endures such situations, only with marked distress or intense anxiety.
  3. Preoccupation about the inadequacy of body size of muscularity causes significant distress or impairment in social, occupational, or other important areas of life.
  4. Continues to exercise, diet, or use performance-enhancing drugs/supplements despite knowledge of adverse physical and/or psychological consequences.

- Engages in excessive exercise, demonstrates preoccupation with food, follows strict dietary regimens (e.g., avoiding specific foods or groups of foods, maintaining excessively low-fat or high-protein diets), or abuses steroids and/or dietary supplements, particularly those aimed at increasing body size (e.g., creatine, HMB, DHEA, androstendione) and/or decreasing body fat (ephedrine, Ma Huang, Guarana).

From Pope HG Jr, et al. Muscle dysmorphia: an unrecognized form of body dysmorphic disorder. Psychosomatics 1997;38:548.

---

referred to as an **exercise addict** or exercise dependent—often does whatever it takes to make additional time to exercise. A rigid daily schedule of working-out often takes place at the expense of family, career, and interpersonal relationships. Sense of worth becomes inextricably tied to the volume of exercise accomplished. Disruption of the daily exercise routine often triggers conventional withdrawal symptoms that include anxiety, restlessness, and mood swings, traits that diminish only when exercise resumes. Typical regimens for the exercise-dependent individual include early morning and afternoon runs, an aerobics class in the evenings, and participation in two or more aerobics classes on weekends. Missing a planned exercise session often produces extreme frustration, culminating in food restraint. Eventually, life becomes unmanageable from a fanatical drive to exercise or a relentless pursuit to achieve a high fitness level. Compulsive exercisers often display the same psychological characteristics as bulimics and anorectics. Some clinicians, therefore, see the need to include *exercise addiction* as a separate diagnostic category. Inclusion might help to identify potentially harmful psychological behaviors associated with an eating disorder.

FIGURE 15.5 compares scores for exercise dependence among female dancers, marathon and ultramarathon runners, and field hockey players. The key comparison variable, the negative addiction scale, reflects an inordinate level of exercise dependence. It consists of 14 equally weighted motivational, emotional, and behavioral components of running behavior. Dancers and runners scored significantly higher on exercise dependence than field hockey participants, with dancers achieving the highest scores. The researchers concluded that

exercise-dependent athletes, particularly dancers, manifest a number of self-destructive behaviors. These findings highlight the need to carefully monitor females who participate in sports with above-normal levels of addictive exercise behavior (see Fig. 15.9). Compulsive exercise behavior, coupled with preoccupation to achieve an "ideal physique" for competition, should serve as a "wake-up call" to seek professional counseling or clinical intervention.

Not Simply an Athletic Problem

One of our laboratories administered the 26 six-point, forced-choice items of the Eating Attitudes Test (EAT-26) to evaluate eating behaviors in women (nonathletes) enrolled a university-sponsored fitness center. An EAT score of 20 or higher identifies individuals with one of the following conditions: (1) an eating disorder that meets strict diagnostic criteria; (2) a "partial syndrome" indicating marked dietary restriction, weight preoccupation, bingeing, vomiting, and other symptoms of clinical significance, but fails to meet all diagnostic criteria for an eating disorder; and (3) "obsessive dieters" or "weight-preoccupied" individuals who express concerns about weight and shape but do not present the abnormal concerns of those with the "partial syndrome." Of the 100 women, 24 scored higher on EAT (average score, 30.5; BMI = 22.2) than the remaining 76 women, whose score averaged 6.8 (BMI = 22.4).

Women with high EAT scores focused more on extreme exercise behaviors. A disturbing aspect concerns the relatively large percentage of "nonathlete" women with either high or

Case Study

Personal Health and Exercise Nutrition 15–2

Eating Attitudes Test (EAT-26) for Eating Disorders

The Eating Attitudes Test (EAT-26) was the screening instrument used in the 1998 National Eating Disorders Screening Program, and is probably the most widely used standardized measure of symptoms and concerns characteristic of eating disorders.

The EAT-26 alone does not yield a specific diagnosis of an eating disorder. Neither the EAT-26, nor any other screening instrument has been established as highly efficient as the sole means for identifying eating disorders. However, studies have shown that the EAT-26 can be an efficient screening instrument as part of a two-stage screening process in which those who score at or above a cut-off score of 20 are referred for a diagnostic interview. If you score above 20 on the EAT-26, please contact your doctor or an eating disorders treatment specialist for a follow-up evaluation.

Age: _____ Sex: _____ Height: _____ feet _____ inches

Current Weight: _____ Highest Weight:_____ Lowest Adult Weight: _____

Education: if currently enrolled in college/university, are you a:

☐ Freshman ☐ Sophomore ☐ Junior ☐ Senior ☐ Grad Student

If not enrolled in school, level of education completed:

☐ Jr. High/Middle School ☐ High School ☐ College ☐ Post College

Ethnic/Racial Group:

☐ African American ☐ Asian American ☐ European American ☐ Hispanic ☐ American Indian ☐ Other

Do you participate in athletics at any of the following levels:

☐ Intramural ☐ Intercollegiate ☐ Recreational ☐ High School

PLEASES CHECK A RESPONSE FOR EACH OF THE FOLLOWING STATEMENTS:

	Always	Usually	Often	Sometimes	Rarely	Never
1. Am terrified about being overweight.	3	2	1	0	0	0
2. Avoid eating when I am hungry.	3	2	1	0	0	0
3. Find myself preoccupied with food.	3	2	1	0	0	0
4. Have gone on eating binges that I feel I may not be able to stop.	3	2	1	0	0	0
5. Cut my food into small pieces.	3	2	1	0	0	0
6. Aware of the calorie content of foods I eat.	3	2	1	0	0	0
7. Particularly avoid food with a high carbohydrate content (bread, rice, potatoes, etc.).	3	2	1	0	0	0
8. Feel that others would prefer I ate more.	3	2	1	0	0	0
9. I vomit after eating.	3	2	1	0	0	0
10. Feel extremely guilty after eating.	3	2	1	0	0	0
11. Am preoccupied with a desire to be thinner.	3	2	1	0	0	0
12. Think about burning up calories when I exercise.	3	2	1	0	0	0
13. Other people think I'm too thin.	3	2	1	0	0	0
14. Am preoccupied with the thought of having fat on my body.	3	2	1	0	0	0

Case Study *continued*

	Always	Usually	Often	Sometimes	Rarely	Never
15. Take longer than others to eat my meals.	3	2	1	0	0	0
16. Avoid foods with sugar in them.	3	2	1	0	0	0
17. Eat diet foods.	3	2	1	0	0	0
18. Feel that food controls my life.	3	2	1	0	0	0
19. Display self-control around food.	3	2	1	0	0	0
20. Feel that others pressure me to eat.	3	2	1	0	0	0
21. Give too much time and thought to food.	3	2	1	0	0	0
22. Feel uncomfortable after eating sweets.	3	2	1	0	0	0
23. Engage in dieting behavior.	3	2	1	0	0	0
24. Like my stomach to be empty.	3	2	1	0	0	0
25. Have the impulse to vomit after meals.	3	2	1	0	0	0
26. Enjoy trying new rich foods.	3	2	1	0	0	0

PLEASE RESPOND TO EACH OF THE FOLLOWING QUESTIONS:

1. Have you gone on eating binges and you feel that you may not be able to stop? (Eating much more than most people would eat under the circumstances.)

   ☐ No   ☐ Yes, If YES, on average, how many times per month in the last 6 months? _____

2. Have you ever made yourself sick (vomited) to control your weight or shape?

   ☐ No   ☐ Yes, If YES, on average, how many times per month in the last 6 months? _____

3. Have you ever used laxatives, diet pills, or diuretics (water pills) to control your weight or shape?

   ☐ No   ☐ Yes, If YES, on average, how many times per month in the last 6 months? _____

4. Have you ever been treated for an eating disorder?

   ☐ No   ☐ Yes, If YES, when? _____

5. Have you recently thought of or attempted suicide?

   ☐ No   ☐ Yes, If YES, when? _____

Scoring System for the EAT-26

Responses for each item (No. 1–26) are weighted from 0 to 3, with a score of 3 assigned to the responses farthest in the "symptomatic" direction, a score of 2 for the immediately adjacent response, a score of 1 for the next adjacent response, and a 0 score assigned to the three responses farthest in the "asymptomatic" direction.

Total Score: Add the values circled for questions 1–26 above:
TOTAL _____

Items are assigned to three subscales as follows:

Dieting subscale items: 1, 6, 7, 10, 11, 12, 14, 16, 17, 22, 23, 24, 25

   Subscale Score: _____

Bulimia and Food Preoccupation subscale items: 3, 4, 9, 18, 21, 26

   Subscale Score: _____

Oral control subscale items: 2, 5, 8, 13, 15, 19, 20

   Subscale Score: _____

To determine subscale scores, add together all item scores for that particular subscale.

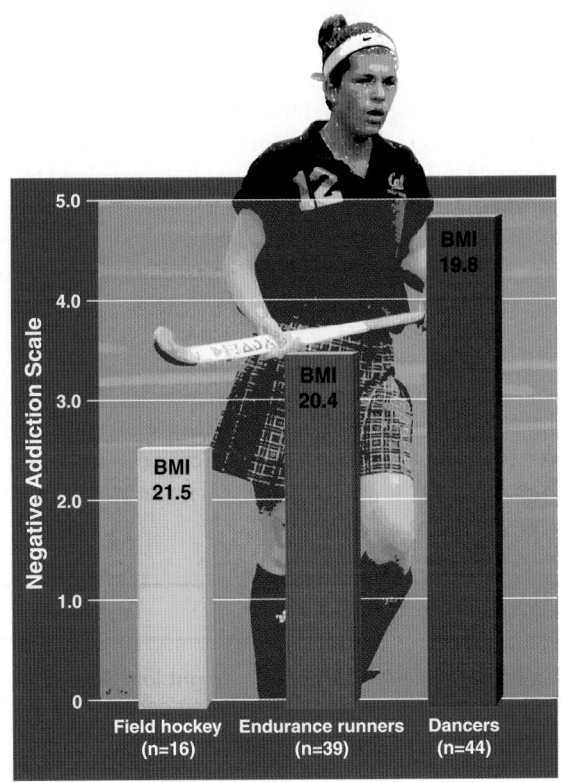

FIGURE 15.5 ■ Comparison of exercise dependence scores among collegiate female ballet and modern dancers, marathon and ultramarathon (greater than 50-mile distances) runners, and field hockey athletes. The dancers scored significantly higher than the runners; the field hockey athletes scored significantly lower in exercise dependence than both of these groups. Interestingly, the dancers had the lowest mean BMI (19.8), followed by the runners (20.4) and field hockey athletes (21.5). Self-destructive behaviors included perseverance in training despite serious injury, prioritization of physical activity over other responsibilities, and significant mood disturbances. (From Sachs ML, Pearman D. Running addiction: a depth interview examination. *J Sport Behav* 1979;2:143.)

low EAT scores who display compulsive exercise behaviors similar to those of gymnasts, dancers, and others preoccupied with eating and weight management. The exercise addict syndrome probably affects many college-age women and is not just a characteristic unique to competitive athletes.

CLINICAL EATING DISORDERS

Psychiatrists traditionally limit the definition of eating disorders to behaviors that produce negative health effects or drive a person to seek treatment. Anorexia nervosa, bulimia nervosa, and binge eating represent the three eating disorders included in the *Diagnostic and Statistical Manual of Mental Disorders* (DSM-IV), the American Psychiatric Association's official roster of psychiatric illnesses.[23]

Anorexia Nervosa

Anorexia nervosa, originally described in ancient writings, represents an unhealthy physical and mental state. This "nervous loss of appetite," particularly common and increasing in prevalence among adolescent girls and young women, is characterized by four factors: (1) distortions of body image, (2) a crippling obsession with body size, (3) preoccupation with dieting and thinness, and (4) refusal to eat enough food to maintain a minimally normal body weight. A relentless pursuit of thinness (present in about 1 to 2% of the general population) culminates in severe undernutrition, altered body composition characterized by depletion of fat and fat-free body mass (FFM), and cessation of menstruation (amenorrhea) in females. Body weight decreases below normal for age and stature. Anorexia nervosa represents the third most common medical illness in girls aged 15 to 19 years. Persons with anorexia actually perceive themselves as fat despite their emaciation. Such distorted perceptions and persistent disturbance in eating behavior frequently persist into recovery, despite improvement in eating behavior and psychological symptoms to produce extreme feelings of vulnerability and personal inadequacy.[53] *Denial and secrecy become a large part* *of the problem.* Many anorectics do not believe they suffer from starvation—they do eat, but consume far less food than adequate to maintain energy balance.[52,57,117]

Compulsive exercise behaviors go hand-in-hand with anorexia nervosa.[16,122] Rather than starve or vomit, the anorectic fanatically expends as many calories as possible through physical activity. A common misconception about anorectics concerns their state of hunger. In reality, they often remain continually hungry; their ability to overcome the urge to eat provides a sense of self-power and control. If untreated, between 6 and 21% of anorectics die prematurely from suicide, heart disease, or infections. In about one third of patients the disease becomes chronic, marked by frequent relapses that often require hospitalization.[84] TABLE 15.8 lists the clinical criteria for diagnosing anorexia nervosa.

Weight gain becomes a primary goal in the treatment of anorexia nervosa. Interestingly, when patients regain weight through hospitalization or out-patient supervision, most of the weight is gained in the trunk region rather than the extremities, with up to 70% of the regained weight as fat.[49,77,128] For example, at the end of treatment that produced an 11.9-kg weight gain (pretreatment fat, 9.8%; posttreatment fat, 22.6%), the ratio of FFM/fat mass averaged 3.4:1, with fat representing 55% of the gained weight.[88]

A 9-month longitudinal study serially assessed body composition in ambulatory anorectic women.[39] Patients exhibited an abnormal body composition during times of low body weight and after weight gain compared with a control group of normal-weight women. At low body weight, anorectic women possessed trunk fat as a percentage of total body fat similar to controls, but extremity fat percentage remained lower than in controls. After a modest 4.1-kg weight gain, the percentage of extremity fat changed little, but trunk fat percentage increased significantly. In contrast to results with other groups of women, estrogen therapy provided no protection against the gain in trunk fat with spontaneous weight gain in anorectic women. Researchers do not know whether anorexia nervosa patients with the most distress about weight gain in recovery (particularly abdominal fat) have the highest ratio of truncal fat to peripheral fat or gain the greatest quantity of truncal fat when they regain weight.[68]

Adolescent girls hospitalized with anorexia nervosa had significant body wasting as indicated by extremely low body fat and a low FFM as reflected by total body nitrogen (TABLE 15.9).[54] Triceps skinfold thickness provided the most significant anthropometric predictor of percentage body fat. This skinfold measure explained 68% of the variation in body fat, while body weight accurately indicated total body nitrogen and thus protein depletion in these patients.

Physical Consequences of Anorexia Nervosa

Death often results from prolonged starvation in about 7% of anorectic patients over a 10-year period; 18 to 20% die within 30 years. A range of other profound physical ailments also occur, including cardiac abnormalities (e.g., arrhythmias, heart block), electrolyte disturbances, impaired kidney function, decreased bone mineral density, gastrointestinal dysfunction (e.g., bleeding, ulceration, bloating, constipation), and anemia. Many effects such as depressed basal metabolic rate (BMR) and leptin concentrations, not fully explained by body composition changes,[85] reflect predictable outcomes from energy conservation as the body defends against prolonged caloric deprivation. FIGURE 15.6 depicts anorexia nervosa's potential physical and medical consequences.

COMMON SIGNS AND SYMPTOMS. Anorexia nervosa usually begins with a normal attempt to lose weight through dieting. As dieting progresses, the individual continues to eat less until the person consumes practically no food. Food restriction eventually becomes an obsession, and the anorectic achieves no satisfaction with any

---

TABLE 15.8 DSM-IV Clinical Criteria for Anorexia Nervosa (Code No. 307.1)

1. Refusal to maintain body weight at or above a minimally normal weight for age and height (e.g., weight loss leading to maintenance of body weight less than 85% of expected or failure to make expected weight gain during period of growth, leading to body weight less than 85% of expected).

2. Intense fear of gaining weight or becoming fat, even though underweight.

3. Disturbance in the way one's body weight or shape is experienced, undue influence of body weight or shape on self-evaluation, or denial of the seriousness of the current low body weight.

4. In post-menarchal females, amenorrhea i.e., the absence of at least three consecutive menstrual cycles. A woman is considered to have amenorrhea if her periods occur only following hormone (e.g., estrogen) administration.

Specify type:

1. *Restricting type:* During the current episode of anorexia nervosa, the person has not regularly engaged in binge-eating or purging behavior (i.e., self-induced vomiting or the misuse of laxatives, diuretics, or enemas).

2. *Binge-eating/purging type:* During the current episode of anorexia nervosa, the person has regularly engaged in binge-eating or purging behavior (i.e., self-induced vomiting or the misuse of laxatives, diuretics, or enemas).

Eating disorders criteria–DSM-IV: Selected Portions of the Diagnostic and Statistical Manual of Mental Disorders, Fourth Edition, relating to Eating Disorders. Copyright © 2000 American Psychiatric Association.

TABLE 15.9 Comparison of Body Compositions of Female Adolescents with Anorexia Nervosa and Healthy Controls

	Age, y	Body Weight, kg	BMI	%Fat	%TBN	FFM, kg	Trunk fat, kg	Leg fat, kg
Anorexia nervosa	15.5	40.2	15.3	13.8	73	34.5	2.1	2.6
Healthy controls	15.1	57.3	21.2	26.3	75	41.2	6.6	7.1

From Kerrvish KP, et al. Body composition in adolescents with anorexia nervosa. Am J Clin Nutr 2002;75:31.

%TBN, percentage total body nitrogen predicted for age; FFM, fat-free body mass

amount of weight loss. The person denies the accompanying extreme emaciation as weight loss progresses. Some anorectic persons cannot ignore the intense hunger accompanying near-total food deprivation; this causes episodes of bingeing and subsequent purging. The warning signs listed in TABLE 15.10 can help coaches and trainers identify athletes with anorexia nervosa.

Bulimia Nervosa

The term *bulimia*, literally meaning "ox hunger," refers to "gorging" or "insatiable appetite." At one time, some believed that **bulimia nervosa** reflected a manifestation of anorexia nervosa owing to similarities and overlap in the two condi-

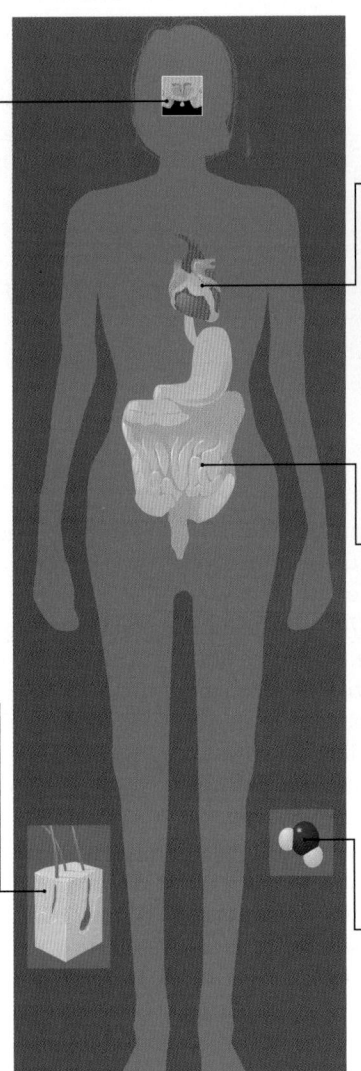

Neuroendocrine
- Loss of monthly menstrual cycle (amenorrhea)
- Cold intolerance (hands and feet)
- Lowered core temperature (related to abnormal temperature regulation and low body fat)
- Lowered BMR
- Reduced sexual desire
- Low estrogen levels leading to brittle bones (from mineral depletion) and stress fractures
- Decline in neurotransmitters (serotonin and epinephrine)
- Euthyroid sick syndrome: low to normal T-4, low to normal T-3, elevated reverse T-3

Skin and hair
- Lanugo (soft, downy hair growth over the body that traps air and increases insulation)
- Dry, scaly, and itchy skin
- Thinning, dull, and brittle hair
- Dry and brittle nails
- Yellowing skin

Cardovascular
- Hypotension
- Decreased resting heart rate (bradycardia)
- Cardiac arrythmias (from electrolyle imbalance)
- Diminished cardiac mass (particularly left ventricle)
- Anemia

Digestive
- Constipation
- Dental problems
- Decreased gastric emptying
- Abdominal pain and distension (related to GI tract disuse atrophy)

Fluid
- Dehydration

FIGURE 15.6 ■ Physical and medical consequences of anorexia nervosa.

TABLE 15.10 **Common Signs and Symptoms of Anorexia Nervosa**

General
- Appetite loss
- Fatigue
- Inability to exercise (due to fatigue and weakness)
- Impaired memory
- Anxiety
- Depression

Skin
- Dry
- Cool
- Mottled/blue
- Bruises
- Self-inflicted cuts
- Scalp hair loss
- Lanugo (baby) hair

Abdominal
- Heartburn
- Nausea
- Pain
- Cramping
- Constipation
- Early satiety
- Vomiting, bloating

Musculoskeletal
- Aching joints/muscles
- Fractures of spine, hip, wrist

Mouth
- Sores
- Cracking around lips
- Tooth decay
- Gum disease
- Parotid gland enlargement
- Adenopathy
- Bad breath

Circulatory
- Cool
- Blue feet and hands
- Low blood pressure
- Dizziness
- Fainting
- Dehydration
- Shortness of breath
- Swelling

Reproduction
- Infertility
- Oligomenorrhea
- Amenorrhea
- Decreased libido

Urinary
- Frequency, especially at night
- Diminished urine output

---

tions. For example, some anorectics experience bulimic episodes, while some bulimics experience episodes of anorexia. Based on more careful examination of the disorders, bulimia nervosa emerged in the late 1970s as a separate classification of eating disorder. The disease, far more common than anorexia nervosa, is characterized by frequent episodes of binge eating, followed by purging, laxative abuse, fasting, or extreme exercise and intense feelings of guilt or shame. Approximately 2 to 4% of adolescents and adults in the general population (mainly female, including about 5% of college women) are bulimic. A large percentage of the total is obese and enrolled in self-help or commercial weight loss programs. A sex difference probably exists in the emotional triggers for overindulgence in food. Compared with men, women with a weight problem exhibit greater binge eating during periods of negative emotions—anxiety, frustration, depression, or anger.[110]

Unlike the continual semistarvation with anorexia nervosa, bulimia nervosa includes binge eating of calorically dense food—often at night and usually between 1000 to 10,000 calories within several hours. Fasting, self-induced vomiting, taking laxatives or diuretics, or compulsively exercising solely to avoid weight gain takes place after the binge episode.[33,62]

Anorectics revel in their sense of control over eating, while striving toward a perceived level of physical perfection. In contrast, bulimics lose control; they recognize their impulsive behavior as abnormal. Eating extreme quantities of food often becomes a means to reduce stress, and purging provides the only way to regain control for their inability to stop eating voluntarily. Considerable variation exists in the type of food consumed during binge episodes. Some bulimics, who often attempt dieting with healthful eating, binge on large quantities of unhealthful, "forbidden" foods (cookies, chips, and chocolates). Others binge on food consumed regularly but only in extreme quantities. Some bulimics even overeat lower-calorie, diet-type foods, while others purge after every meal, regardless of what or how much they eat. *Bulimics span the gamut between normal body weight and overweight (or a history of overweight); this represents a striking difference between anorectics and bulimics.* While obvious physical characteristics exist for anorexia nervosa, many bulimic characteristics remain behavioral.

TABLE 15.11	DSM-IV Criteria for Bulimia Nervosa (Code No. 307.51)

1. Recurrent episodes of binge eating. An episode of binge eating is characterized by both of the following: (1) Eating, in a discrete period of time (e.g., within any 2-hour period), an amount of food that is definitely larger than most people would eat during a similar period of time and under similar circumstances. (2) A sense of lack of control over eating during the episode (e.g., a feeling that one cannot stop eating or control what or how much one is eating).
2. Recurrent inappropriate compensatory behavior in order to prevent weight gain, such as self-induced vomiting; misuse of laxatives, diuretics, enemas or other medications; fasting or excessive exercise.
3. The binge eating and inappropriate compensatory behaviors both occur, on average, at least twice a week for 3 months.
4. Self-evaluation is unduly influenced by body shape and weight.
5. The disturbance does not occur exclusively during episodes of anorexia nervosa.

Specify type:

1. *Purging type:* During the current episode of bulimia nervosa, the person has regularly engaged in self-induced vomiting or the misuse of laxatives, diuretics or enemas.
2. *Nonpurging type:* During the current episode of bulimia nervosa, the person has used inappropriate compensatory behaviors, such as fasting or excessive exercise, but has not regularly engaged in self-induced vomiting or the misuse of laxatives, diuretics or enemas.

Eating disorders criteria–DSM-IV: Selected Portions of the Diagnostic and Statistical Manual of Mental Disorders, Fourth Edition, relating to Eating Disorders. Copyright © 2000 American Psychiatric Association.

Most persons with bulimia nervosa meet standards for major depressive disorders—loss of interest, low mood, shortened attention span, disrupted sleep patterns, and suicidal thoughts. Bulimics also abuse alcohol and drugs at a higher rate than the general population. TABLE 15.11 lists the DSM–IV clinical criteria for diagnosing bulimia nervosa.

Purging and Calories: You Can't Expel the Total

A study that measured the amount and caloric value of food from a binge that remained in the stomach after vomiting found that on average, 1209 kCal were retained after a binge meal that contained 3530 kCal.

Physical Consequences of Bulimia Nervosa

FIGURE 15.7 depicts the diverse physical symptoms and disorders suffered by persons with bulimia nervosa.

DANGER SIGNALS AND INDICATIONS. Difficulty exists in diagnosing bulimia nervosa because many bulimics function well without noticeable signs. Bulimics remain conscious of what and how much they eat and generally never eat to excess in public. For the most part, they express feelings of perfectionist behavior, depression, low self-esteem, being out of control, and dissatisfaction with body size and shape. Often, those closest to the bulimic remain unaware of the problem. Another disturbing aspect of bulimia nervosa concerns substance abuse. In a comparison of women with anorexia nervosa and women with bulimia nervosa, the bulimics abused alcohol, amphetamines, barbiturates, marijuana, tranquilizers, and cocaine to a greater extent.[123] Independent of the diagnosis of either anorexia or bulimia, (1) the magnitude of caloric restriction predicted amphetamine use, (2) severity of binge eating predicted tranquilizer use, and (3) severity of purging predicted alcohol, cocaine, and cigarette use.

Warning Signs of Bulimia Nervosa

- Excessive concern about body weight, body size, and body composition
- Frequent gains and losses in body weight
- Visits to the bathroom following meals
- Fear of not being able to control eating
- Eating when depressed
- Compulsive dieting after binge-eating episodes
- Severe shifts in mood (depression, loneliness)
- Secretive binge eating, but never overeating in front of others
- Frequent criticism of one's body size and shape
- Experiencing personal or family problems with alcohol or drugs
- Irregular menstrual cycle (oligomenorrhea)

Binge-Eating Disorder

Binge-eating disorder (BED), first described in 1959, identified specific eating behavior patterns in a subgroup of obese patients undergoing treatment to lose weight. The affliction is characterized by recurrent episodes of binge eating. These occur often without subsequent purging or abusing laxatives to compensate for overeating common to bulimia nervosa and anorexia nervosa. Psychiatrists define the disorder as episodes of binge eating at least twice a week for at least 6 months and that cause significant emotional distress. Individuals with BED eat more rapidly than normal until they can no longer consume additional food. Such high levels of food intake exceed the physiologic drive of hunger. Binge eating, undertaken in private because of embarrassment, occurs with feelings of guilt, depression, or self-disgust. Binge eaters suffer greater self-

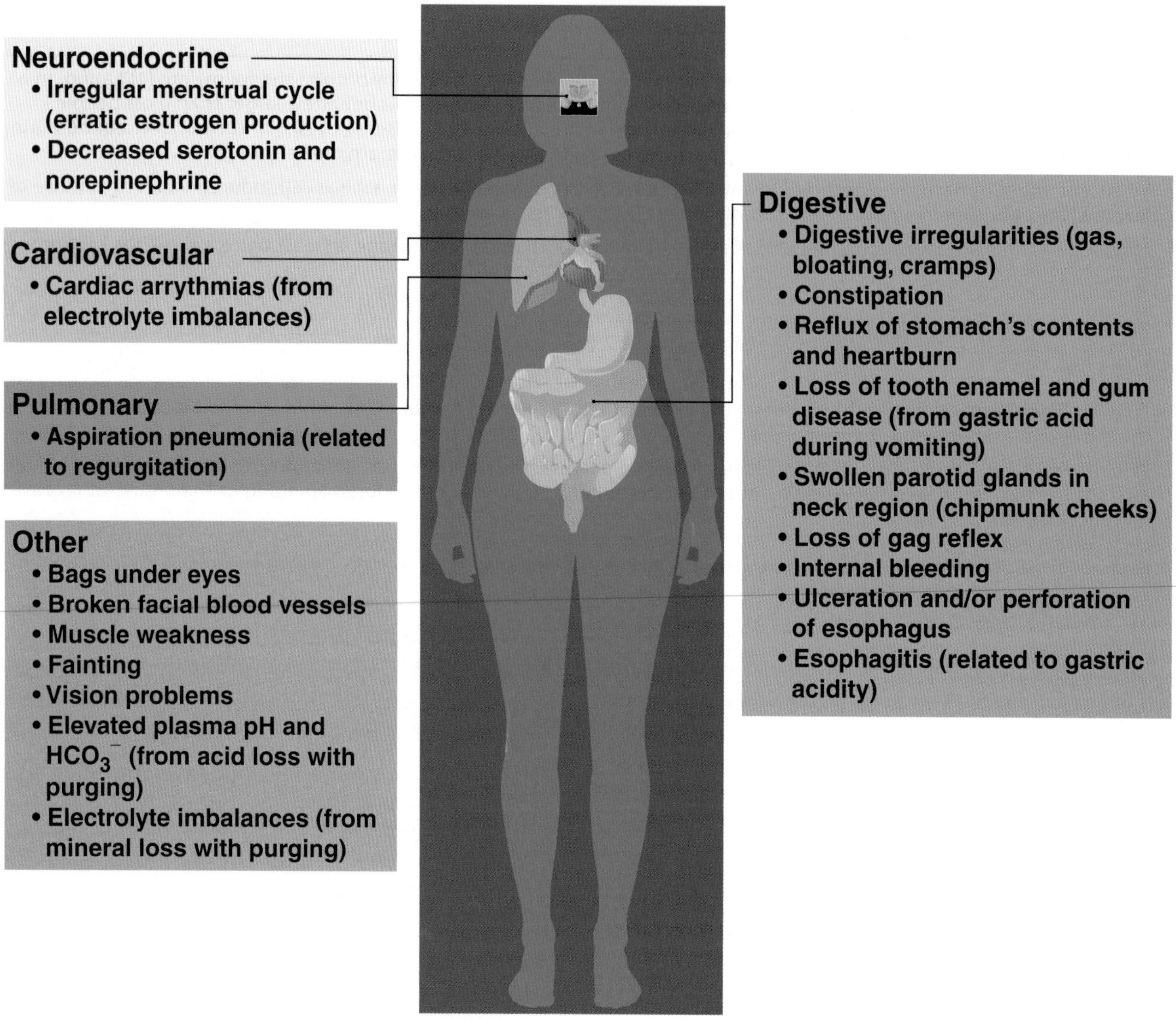

Neuroendocrine
- **Irregular menstrual cycle (erratic estrogen production)**
- **Decreased serotonin and norepinephrine**

Cardiovascular
- **Cardiac arrythmias (from electrolyte imbalances)**

Pulmonary
- **Aspiration pneumonia (related to regurgitation)**

Other
- **Bags under eyes**
- **Broken facial blood vessels**
- **Muscle weakness**
- **Fainting**
- **Vision problems**
- **Elevated plasma pH and HCO$_3^-$ (from acid loss with purging)**
- **Electrolyte imbalances (from mineral loss with purging)**

Digestive
- **Digestive irregularities (gas, bloating, cramps)**
- **Constipation**
- **Reflux of stomach's contents and heartburn**
- **Loss of tooth enamel and gum disease (from gastric acid during vomiting)**
- **Swollen parotid glands in neck region (chipmunk cheeks)**
- **Loss of gag reflex**
- **Internal bleeding**
- **Ulceration and/or perforation of esophagus**
- **Esophagitis (related to gastric acidity)**

FIGURE 15.7 ■ Physical and medical consequences of bulimia nervosa.

anger, shame, lack of control, and frustration than nonbingeing obese individuals.[17,31,47,63] They also experience relatively higher rates of sexual abuse and physical abuse and bullying by peers than the general population.[102] Studies in the early 1980s identified BED in 20 to 50% of obese patients.[37,62] Not only did these individuals exhibit difficulties with binge eating, but they also regained lost weight faster than obese non–binge eaters, and they more likely failed in treatment.[64] As an outgrowth of these early clinical observations, diagnostic criteria developed in the early 1990s helped to identify BED (TABLE 15.12).

A feature distinguishing BED from anorexia nervosa and bulimia nervosa is that persons seeking treatment for BED are often overweight or obese. Approximately 2% of the U.S. population (1 to 2 million people) and about 30% of Americans treated for obesity experience BED,[72] although incidence rate decreases on the basis of personal interview rather than questionnaire to assess its prevalence.[103] Current research does not support earlier beliefs that minorities were somehow "protected" from BED.[96] For example, comparisons between Caucasian and minority females showed similar scores on measures of eating disorder symptomology and general psychopathology.[60]

Ten to 15% of mildly obese people who enroll in self-help or commercial weight loss programs meet the criteria for BED. Those with body weight in excess of 20% of ideal weight exhibit the highest prevalence of BED and develop their obesity at a younger age than their non–binge-eating obese counterparts. Women experience BED at a 50% higher rate than do men. Women also report greater binge-eating episodes in response to negative emotions such as anxiety, anger and frustration, and depression. Men and women presenting for BED treatment score similarly on measures of eating disturbance, body shape and weight concerns, interpersonal problems, and self-esteem; men experience more psychiatric disturbance and less emotional eating.[98]

The causes of BED remain unknown. Up to 50% of bingers suffer depression, which may contribute to the disorder. Individuals with BED experience higher lifetime rates of

TABLE 15.12 **DSM-IV Eating Disorders Not Otherwise Specified (Code No. 307.50)**

Includes disorders of eating that do not meet the criteria for any specific eating disorder. Examples include:

1. For females, all of the criteria for anorexia nervosa are met except that the individual has regular menses.
2. All of the criteria for anorexia nervosa are met except that, despite significant weight loss the individual's current weight is in the normal range.
3. All of the criteria for bulimia nervosa are met except that the binge eating and inappropriate compensatory mechanisms occur at a frequency of less than twice a week or for duration of less than 3 months.
4. The regular use of inappropriate compensatory behavior by an individual of normal body weight after eating small amounts of food (e.g., self-induced vomiting after the consumption of two cookies).
5. Repeatedly chewing and spitting out, but not swallowing, large amounts of food.
6. Binge-eating disorder: recurrent episodes of binge eating in the absence of the regular use of inappropriate compensatory behaviors characteristic of bulimia nervosa.

Eating disorders criteria–DSM-IV: Selected Portions of the Diagnostic and Statistical Manual of Mental Disorders, Fourth Edition, relating to Eating Disorders. Copyright © 2000 American Psychiatric Association.

major depression, panic disorder, bulimia nervosa, borderline personality disorder, and avoidant personality disorder.[126] Moderately obese men and women with BED experience greater relative risk for psychiatric disorders than their obese counterparts without the disorder.[125]

Exercise Plus Behavior Therapy Intervention Helps

To investigate the role of exercise and behavior therapy in treating BED, two groups of women participated in identical exercise programs for 6 months.[61] One group also received behavior therapy with the exercise program. Pre- and post-treatment evaluations included exercise level, binge-eating frequency, and depressive symptoms. The results favored the group receiving exercise plus behavioral treatment for BED. At posttreatment, 81% of these subjects remained free from binge-eating episodes. They also exercised more frequently each week and thus expended greater energy.

CAUSE OR EFFECT? THE ROLE OF SPORT IN EATING DISORDERS

Does dedication to training for a specific sport induce development of an eating disorder, or do individuals with potentially pathologic concerns about body size and shape gravitate (self-select) to the sport? The **attraction to sport hypothesis** maintains that individuals with an existing eating disorder (or at high risk for developing one) find reward by participating in aesthetic-type sports that emphasize an excessively lean appearance. When training commences early in life (as in gymnastics and ballet dancing), it becomes difficult to make the case for the attraction to the sport hypothesis; that is, because the young girls participated because of the sport's focus on leanness and appearance. For these girls, disordered eating behaviors probably develop progressively as the young athlete realizes an inherent incompatibility between the sport's body-type requirements and genetic predisposition for body size and structure. Research must determine whether the inordinate focus of many athletes on food intake and leanness reflects a continuum of graded psy-

chologic disturbance that ultimately leads to a full-blown eating disorder.

TABLE 15.13 presents a brief questionnaire to evaluate the degree of restraint a person feels over issues concerning food choices, diet planning, and body-weight maintenance. Often, individuals tending toward disordered eating patterns exhibit extreme concern over what they eat and how it affects body weight. If they "give in" (because of a perceived lack of self-control) and eat "bad" foods believed to contribute to weight gain, they often reduce the resulting stress by purging or excessive exercise. The questions in Table 15.13 do not determine whether or not an eating disorder exists, but raise awareness about dietary restraint patterns and behaviors that ultimately may lead to an eating disorder.

EATING DISORDERS AFFECT EXERCISE PERFORMANCE

An athlete with an eating disorder faces a paradox: Behavior necessary to achieve a body weight for success in certain sports—semistarvation, purging, excessive exercising—adversely affects health, energy reserves, and physiologic function and the ability to train and compete at an optimal level. In Chapter 14, we noted that athletes often reduce body fat to improve exercise power output relative to body mass and to reduce drag forces that impede forward movement through air and water. For persons with eating disorders, chronic restriction of energy intake (as in anorexia nervosa) or reduced energy availability through purging (as in bulimia nervosa) rapidly depletes glycogen reserves. As emphasized throughout this text, the normally limited quantity of muscle and liver glycogen provides rapid energy for high-intensity anaerobic and aerobic exercise. Consequently, even short periods of disordered eating may deplete glycogen reserves, which profoundly affects capacity to train and recover. The reduced protein (and carbohydrate) intake usually accompanying an eating disorder also contributes to lean tissue loss. A subpar intake of vitamins and minerals required for energy metabo-

---

TABLE 15.13   How Do You Rate in Terms of Eating Restraint?

Circle the number that best describes your feelings or behaviors related to the question.

1. **How often are you dieting?**
   0 = never
   1 = rarely
   2 = sometimes
   3 = often
   4 = always

2. **What is the maximum amount of weight (in pounds) that you have ever lost within one month?**
   0 = 0–4
   1 = 5–9
   2 = 10–14
   3 = 15–19
   4 = 20+

3. **What is the most weight (in pounds) you have ever gained within a week?**
   1 = 1.1–2.0
   2 = 2.1–3.0
   3 = 3.1–5.0
   4 = 5.1+

4. **In a typical week, how much does your weight (pounds) fluctuate?**
   0 = 0–1.0
   1 = 1.1–2.0
   2 = 2.1–3.0
   3 = 2.1–5.0
   4 = 5.1+

5. **Would a weight fluctuation of 5 pounds affect the way you live your life?**
   0 = not at all
   1 = slightly
   2 = moderately
   3 = very much

6. **Do you eat sensibly in front of others and splurge alone?**
   0 = never
   1 = rarely
   2 = often
   3 = always

7. **Do you give too much time and thought to food?**
   0 = never
   1 = rarely
   2 = often
   3 = always

8. **Do you have feelings of guilt after overeating?**
   0 = never
   1 = rarely
   2 = often
   3 = always

9. **How conscious are you of what you are eating?**
   0 = not at all
   1 = slightly
   2 = moderately
   3 = extremely

10. **How many pounds over your desired weight were you at your maximum weight?**
    0 = 0–1
    1 = 1–5
    2 = 6–10
    3 = 11–20
    4 = 21+

Add up the numbers you have circled and select the category that best describes you.
   0–15 Relatively unrestrained
   16–23 Moderately restrained
   24–35 Highly restrained

From Herman CP, Policy J. Restrained eating. In: Stunkard AJ, ed. Obesity. Philadelphia: WB Saunders, 1980.

---

lism and tissue growth and repair facilitates poor exercise performance and increases injury potential.

EATING DISORDERS AFFECT BONE MINERAL DENSITY

Dual-energy x-ray absorptiometry (DXA; see Chapter 13) has evaluated skeletal and regional body composition characteristics in anorexia nervosa. In one study, body mass averaged 44.4 kg (97.9 lb) for 10 anorectic women. FIGURE 15.8 shows an anorectic female (*left two images*) and a typical female whose body fat percentage averaged 25% of her 56.7-kg (125-lb) body mass. Although FFM of the anorectic women approached the normal average of 43.0 kg, body fat equaled only 7.5%, a value more than three times less than that for comparison groups of typical young women. These women were anorectic for at least 1 year, and amenorrhea duration averaged 3.1 years (range, 1–8 years). The *inset table* compares regional bone mineral densities (BMD, g · cm^{-2}) of

anorectic women and 287 normal-weight women aged 20 to 40 years. The values in the *right column* represent the percentage for BMD for the anorectic group relative to the comparison group. Total-body BMD averaged 10% lower, the L2-L4 region of the lumbar spine averaged 27% less, and the femoral neck 13% lower than in comparable BMDs in the normal women. Spine BMD in the young anorectic group equaled the average BMD in 70-year-old women! Diminished BMD in anorexia nervosa, in addition to reducing skeletal size, may render these young women particularly vulnerable to osteoporotic fractures at a relatively young age.

MANAGEMENT OF EATING DISORDERS IN ATHLETES

Eating disorders do not just go away; there is no simple cause and no simple solution. Eating disorders represent not only a problem but also an attempted solution to a problem. In its mildest aspect, the disorder often stems from poor nu-

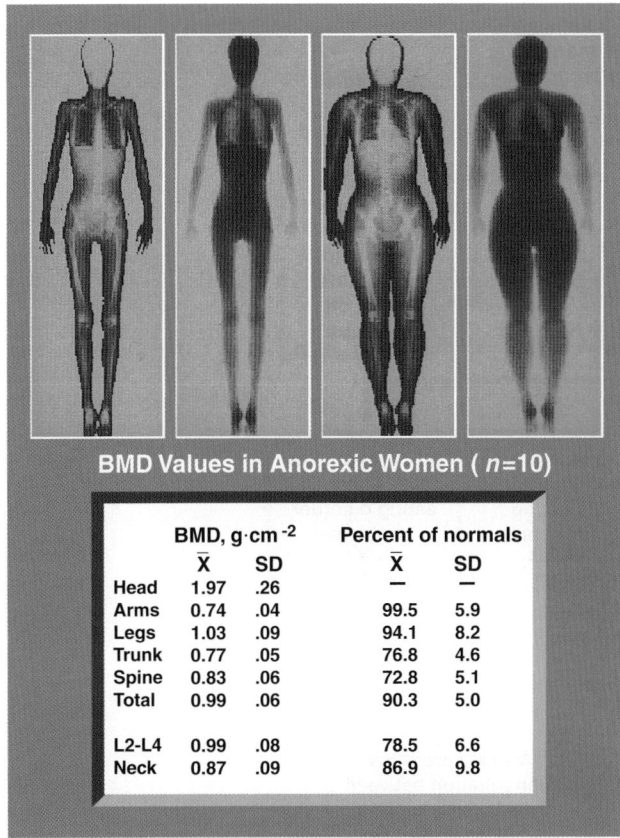

BMD Values in Anorexic Women (_n_=10)

	BMD, g·cm^{-2}		Percent of normals	
	X̄	SD	X̄	SD
Head	1.97	.26	—	—
Arms	0.74	.04	99.5	5.9
Legs	1.03	.09	94.1	8.2
Trunk	0.77	.05	76.8	4.6
Spine	0.83	.06	72.8	5.1
Total	0.99	.06	90.3	5.0
L2-L4	0.99	.08	78.5	6.6
Neck	0.87	.09	86.9	9.8

FIGURE 15.8 ■ Example of an anorectic female *(two left images)* and a typical female *(two right images)* whose body fat percentage averages 25% of body mass of 56.7 kg (125 lb). The average anorectic subject weighed 44.4 kg (97.9 lb) and had 7.5% body fat estimated by dual-energy x-ray absorptiometry (DXA) from the fat percentages at the arms, legs, and trunk regions. The values in the *right column of the inset table* present percentage values for bone mineral density (BMD) for different regional body areas in the anorectic group compared to 287 normal females ages 20 to 40 years. (Photo courtesy of RB Mazes, Department of Medical Physics, University of Wisconsin, Madison, WI, and the Lunar Radiation Corporation, Madison, WI. Data from Mazes RB, et al. Skeletal and body composition effects of anorexia nervosa. Paper presented at the international symposium on in vivo body composition studies. Toronto, Ontario, Canada, June 20–23, 1989.)

tritional information. Left untreated, abnormal eating behaviors often blossom into chronic eating disorders. Familial vulnerability also exists because the relatives of people with eating disorders exhibit higher risk of developing a disorder.[62] The relatives also show higher rates of depression and obsessive–compulsive disorders than the general population.

Disordered eating behaviors frequently produce nutritional problems in addition to the loss of tooth enamel from stomach acid during vomiting in bulimic patients. Effective treatment fo-

cuses primarily on the psychologic realm and attempts to reverse the negative effects of disordered eating behaviors. Depending on the patient's age, disorder severity, and its affect on health and well-being, therapy takes place either on an outpatient basis or in a hospital setting. With teenage athletes, the parents must become involved. Individuals with eating disorders frequently resist outside attempts at intervention and treatment. No single approach or theory has proved helpful in treating those with eating disorders. Often treatments that appear to have a high likelihood of success give opposite results.

Successful treatment usually involves a team approach using psychotherapeutic, medical, nutritional, and family support. FIGURE 15.9 outlines an intervention model for disordered eating behaviors in an athletic setting. The process consists of four steps:

Step 1. Identify and isolate the contributing factors.
Step 2. Formulate appropriate goals for intervention and prevention.
Step 3. Formulate long-term strategies to deal with the problem.
Step 4. Initiate long-term programs to address the situation.

FIGURE 15.10 illustrates the multidisciplinary approach to manage disordered eating behaviors in athletes at the University of Texas at Austin, an early leader in confronting eating disorders among athletes. This Division I collegiate-level athletic program prohibits coaches from weighing female athletes or talking to them about body weight or body composition; these responsibilities reside with the sports medicine staff. The important components include

- *Education* to provide information concerning the eating disorder and its consequences
- *Self-monitoring* to provide a clear understanding of current eating behaviors and patterns
- *Meal planning* to help gain control of eating patterns and establish a healthful pattern of eating

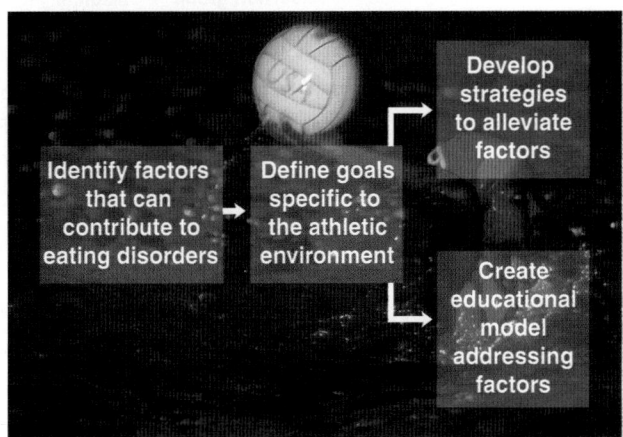

FIGURE 15.9 ■ Model intervention for dealing with disordered eating behaviors in an athletic setting. (From Ryan R. Management of eating problems in athletic settings. In: Brownell KD, et al, eds. *Eating, Body Weight and Performance in Athletes.* Philadelphia: Lea & Febiger, 1992.)

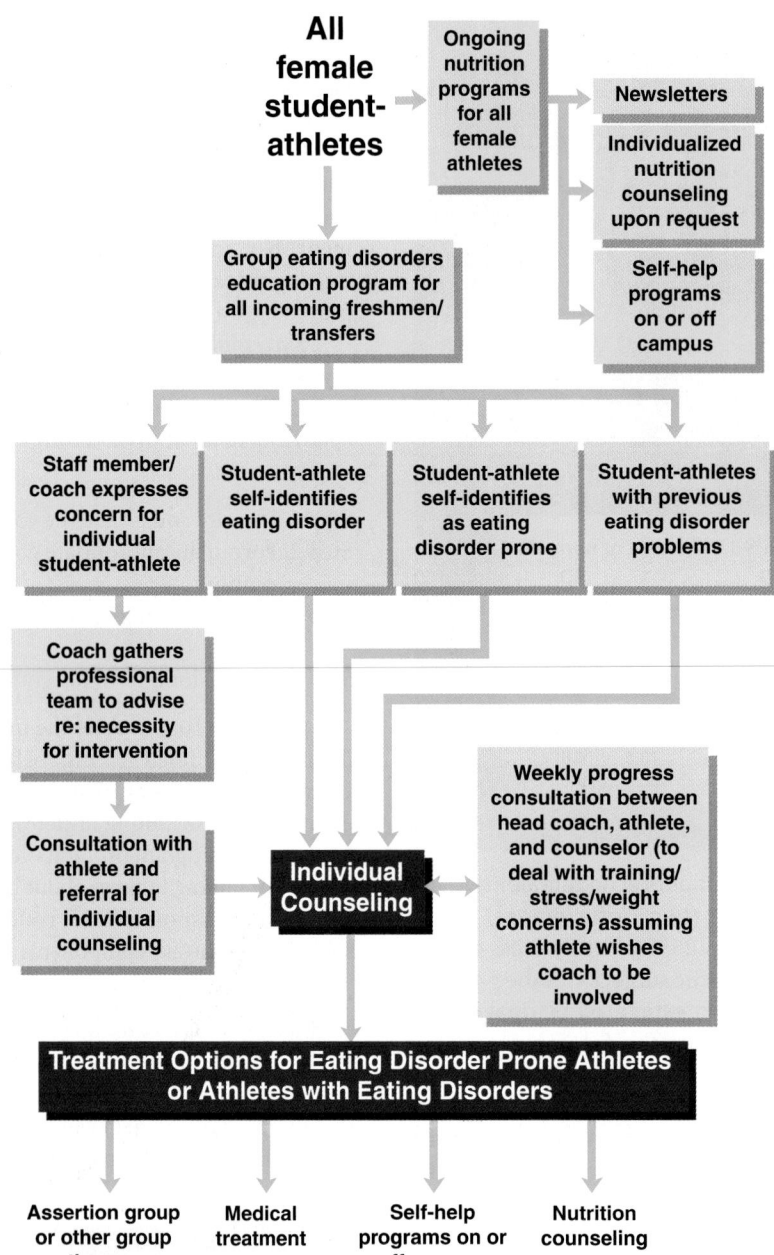

FIGURE 15.10 ■ Flow chart to prevent eating disorders and provide service for athletes who suffer from eating disorders. (From Ryan R. Management of eating problems in athletic settings. In: Brownell KD, et al, eds. *Eating, Body Weight and Performance in Athletes.* Philadelphia: Lea & Febiger, 1992.)

College Women at Risk for An Eating Disorder May Benefit from Online Intervention

An Internet-based intervention program may prevent some high risk, college-age women from developing an eating disorder.[111] Researchers conducted a randomized, controlled trial of 480 women identified in preliminary interviews at risk for developing an eating disorder. The trial included an 8-week, Internet-based, cognitive-behavioral program called "Student Bodies." The intervention aimed to reduce the participants' concerns about body weight and shape, enhance body image, promote healthy eating and weight maintenance, and increase knowledge about the risks associated with eating disorders.

The program contained reading and other assignments that included keeping an online body-image journal and participation in an online discussion group moderated by clinical psychologists. Participants were interviewed immediately at the end of the online program and annually for up to 3 years to determine attitudes toward their weight and shape and to detect and measure the onset of eating disorders.

The intervention achieved greatest success among overweight women with BMIs of 25 or greater at the start of the program. For these women in the intervention group, none developed an eating disorder after 2 years, while 11.9% of the women with comparable baseline BMIs in the control group developed an eating disorder.

The program helped women who exhibited symptoms of an eating disorder at the start of the program such as self-induced vomiting; laxative, diet pill, or diuretic use; or excessive exercise. Of those with these characteristics in the intervention group, 14% developed an eating disorder within 3 years in contrast to 30% with these characteristics in the control group. The intervention enabled high-risk women to become less concerned about their weight and shape, while helping them to better understand healthier eating and nutrition practices. This study was the first to show that eating disorders can be prevented among high-risk groups, and additional evidence that an inordinate focus on body weight and shape are causal risk factors leading to an eating disorder. Interestingly, the rate at which the women stayed with the program remained high—nearly 80% of the online program's Web pages were read—suggesting the participants were motivated to succeed.

COMMON SENSE GUIDELINES FOR COACHES AND TRAINERS CONCERNING EATING DISORDERS

Coaches and athletic trainers can play an important role in the lives of athletes with symptoms of disordered eating. Follow these 10 common sense guidelines whenever possible—they can make a difference.

1. Do not urge athletes to eat, do not watch them eat, refrain from discussing food, and forego discussions about body weight. Becoming involved with coaches concerning food and body weight provides a way for the athlete to "manipulate" the coaching and training staff; it refocuses attention on concerns the athlete feels about food or body weight.
2. Stay free from guilt about the athlete's attitudes and behaviors toward food or body weight. Solving an eating disorder ultimately remains the athlete's responsibility; your role provides support to the athlete (and parent) and, if appropriate, encourages counseling. Coaches and trainers should not permit concerns about food and body size to go unnoticed—they must exercise professional judgment in offering advice about external counseling.
3. Coaches and trainers should not counsel athletes about eating disorders. Reserve that role for a psychologist, psychiatrist, or other trained specialist in eating disorders.

4. Do not focus extra attention on the athlete with an eating disorder. This exacerbates the condition and does little to resolve issues concerning food or body weight.
5. Be prepared to "ignore" the athlete in matters of food or body weight; do not become so involved that teammates notice that the athletes receives "extra" attention about an eating disorder.
6. Refrain from telling the athlete about "successful" athletes or friends who overcame an eating disorder. Do not ask questions such as: "How are you feeling?" "How is your weight today?" "Did you eat a good breakfast?" "Are you getting enough to eat?"
7. Trust the athlete to develop her or his own standards and values rather than insisting the athlete emulate yours.
8. Encourage the athlete to develop initiative, become self-sufficient, and make decisions. Give choices, but not solutions to problems. This encourages independence and autonomy.
9. Show extreme patience when dealing with athletes who exhibit symptoms of disordered eating. No quick cures or fixes exist, so do not expect them.
10. Never give up on an athlete who displays symptoms of disordered eating. Be firm but fair; be tolerant but decisive, and show respect, not contempt or disapproval.

THERAPEUTIC METHODS TO TREAT EATING DISORDERS

Various therapeutic methods treat eating disorders and give patients a sense of balance, purpose, and future. One approach, **cognitive–behavioral therapy,** particularly effective in treating bulimia nervosa, focuses on teaching the patient to identify, monitor, and modify dysfunctional attitudes, core beliefs, and eating habits to lessen binges and "retrain" normal hunger and satiety responses.[26,104,109] An important component of this therapeutic approach teaches individuals to change misconceptions and reasoning errors and develop coping strategies for modifying dysfunctional responses to stressful situations.

Interpersonal psychotherapy helps the patient and family examine interpersonal relationships to positively affect problem areas. The therapist emphasizes the importance of body fat for return of menses and normalization of reproductive functions. For younger patients, the therapist stresses the effects of low body weight on maturation, growth, and bone mass. Paradoxically, the therapist needs to recognize that a normalization of body fat may increase the patient's fat phobia, which initially led her to her pursue extreme thinness.[89]

Pharmacologic treatment (e.g., Prozac [fluoxetine] and other antidepressants) helps some individuals. Trials of diverse classes of psychotropic medications to improve mood and augment weight gain in patients with anorexia nervosa have generally showed little effect.[2,68] Psychiatrists have recently prescribed two drugs Zonegran (Zonisamide) and Topamax (topiramate), approved to treat epilepsy and migraine headaches, for persons whose overeating meets the criteria for binge-eating disorder. These drugs require careful use but do help to reduce the frequency of binges for a subset of patients.[69] Widespread use of such pharmacologic treatment requires further research.

No one best treatment presently exists; combined multi-faceted, multidisciplinary approaches using individuals with expertise in areas of psychiatry, eating disorders, body image issues, medicine, and nutrition often work best. Improvement occurs slowly, with relapses and setbacks common. Achieving success often remains difficult for (1) individuals with eating disorders of long duration, (2) patients who have previously failed treatment, or (3) persons with a history of disturbed family relationships and poor individual adjustment.

Physical Activity May Prove Beneficial in Treatment of Bulimia Nervosa

Researchers evaluated 16 weeks of regular physical activity versus an equivalent time of nutritional counseling or cognitive behavioral therapy in treating bulimia nervosa.[109] Normal-weight female patients with bulemia randomly received either treatment or control conditions; a second control group contained healthy females. Nutritional counseling educated patients about sound principles of nutrition, nutritional needs, and the relationship between dieting and overeating. Meal-planning techniques established and maintained regular eating patterns. Cognitive behavioral therapy focused on enabling patients to (1) identify feelings and events related to bingeing episodes and how such episodes affected emotional status, (2) identify and modify core beliefs that influence bulimic behavior, (3) apply behavior modification techniques to combat bulimic behavior and develop more healthful strategies to deal with disturbing thoughts and emotions, and (4) develop general problem-solving skills. Exercise consisted of a 1-hour weekly group session of moderate physical activities to promote physical fitness, reduce feelings of fatness and bloating associated with eating, foster a more positive body image, and prevent binging and purging. These subjects were also urged to exercise at least 35 minutes twice a week on their own. FIGURE 15.11 compares the different treatments with respect to the EDI subscales of "Body dissatisfaction," "Bulimia," and "Drive for thinness" pre- and posttreatment and at 6- and 18-month follow-ups. Nutritional counseling proved no more effective than cognitive–behavioral therapy. More striking was the superior effect of regular physical activity compared with cognitive behavior therapy in reducing the pursuit of thinness, feelings of body dissatisfaction, and frequency of bingeing, purging, and laxative abuse. The augmented self-regulation with physical activity may result from the effects of exercise on reducing bulimic patients' bodily tensions and improving stress tolerance.

ATHLETICS MUST CHANGE FROM WITHIN

The following quote highlights the proactive role professionals in exercise nutrition, sports medicine, and athletics play in

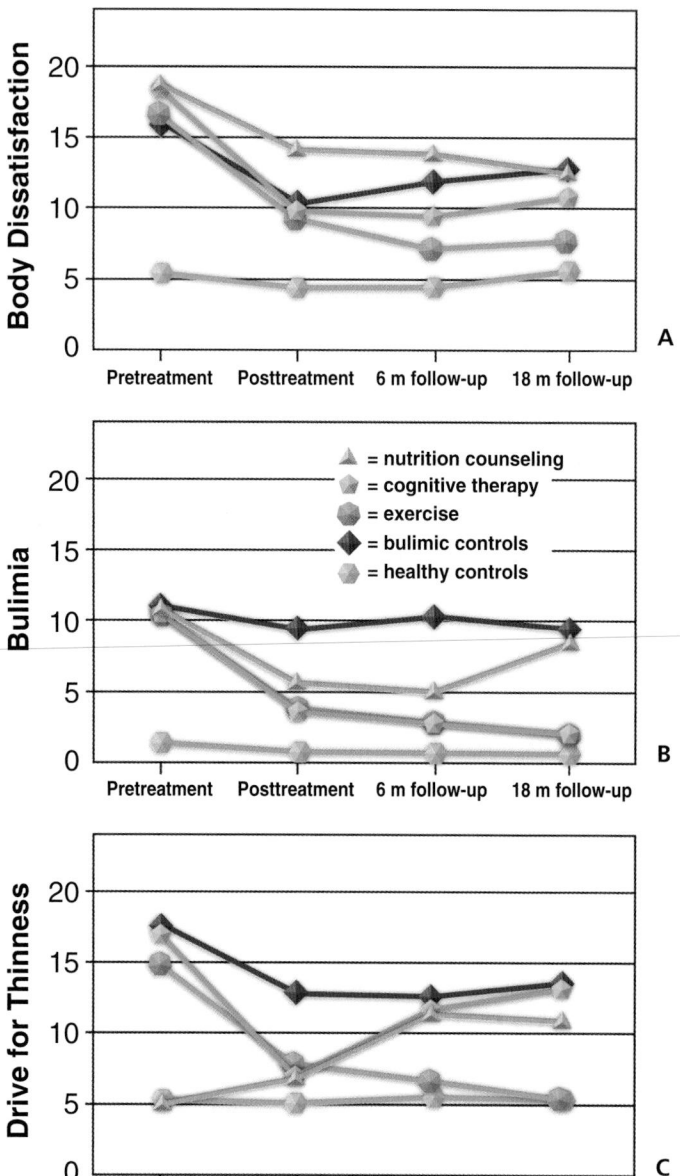

FIGURE 15.11 ■ Exercise, cognitive therapy, and nutritional counseling in treating bulimia nervosa. **A.** Mean scores on the Eating Disorders Index "Body dissatisfaction" subscale at pretreatment, posttreatment, and 6- and 18-month follow-up. **B.** Mean scores on the Eating Disorders Index "Bulimia" subscale. **C.** Mean scores on the Eating Disorders Index "Drive for thinness" subscale. (From Sundgot-Borgen J, et al. The effect of exercise, cognitive therapy, and nutritional counseling in treating bulimia nervosa. *Med Sci Sports Exerc* 2002;34:190.)

affecting the negative potential for certain sports to contribute to disordered eating among participants:[34]

"Finally, it is important to comment briefly on the need for reflection regarding the evolving aesthetic ideals for weight and shape in some sports. Particularly in those where the premium is placed on appearance and where adjudicators prevail (diving, figure skating, gymnastics and dance), questions should be raised

from within the sports community regarding the potentially destructive standards for shape and weight. When these standards seriously compromise the health and well being of all but the small minority who are constitutionally gaunt, it is a matter for sincere concern for all of those involved with the sport."

FUTURE RESEARCH

TABLE 15.14 lists 10 areas for future research about eating and weight control behaviors in athletes.[15] More focused and careful investigations with large representative samples, better measurement tools, and a longitudinal approach should provide a clearer understanding of the actual scope of disordered eating among athletes in general and specific athletic groups in particular. Appropriate research design becomes crucial in determining whether a cause-and-effect relationship exists between athletic participation and disordered eating. Better profiling of men and women with the greatest likelihood of encountering problems requires knowledge of the following seven factors:

1. Role and interaction of sport-specific risk
2. Age risk

TABLE 15.14 **Ten Research Needs Concerning the Prevalence of Eating Disorders in Athletes**

1. Carry out large-scale, epidemiologic studies using consistent measures to define the prevalence of eating disorders in various athletic populations.

2. Studies on prevalence should have the proper control groups. These should include athletes from sports with equivalent training but less emphasis on weight.

3. Examine both anorexia nervosa and bulimia nervosa, in addition to the range of behaviors and attitudes associated with eating disturbances.

4. Identify sports that bring the greatest risk for eating and weight problems.

5. Identify the psychological predisposing factors that place individual athletes at risk.

6. Identify the physiological factors that place an individual athlete at risk. Examples might be genetic predisposition to be heavy, low metabolic rate, and extreme energy efficiency.

7. Examine sex differences in the prevalence and development of eating disorders. This would involve studies of males and females in sports in which weight is emphasized (e.g., gymnastics, figure skating, and distance running).

8. Within sports, study athletes at varying levels of training and proficiency.

9. Study young athletes early in their training to identify early risk factors.

10. Validate self-report measures with athletes and identify the conditions under which self-reports of eating disturbances are most likely to be accurate.

From Brownell KD, Rodin J. Prevalence of eating disorders in athletes. In: Brownell KD, et al., eds. Eating, body weight and performance in athletes. Philadelphia: Lea & Febiger, 1992.

3. Gender risk
4. Training risk
5. Skill level and proficiency risk
6. Genetic risk
7. Psychosocial risk

Intensive education must focus on upgrading the knowledge of the coaching staff. These professionals need to maintain continual vigilance for signs and symptoms of eating disorders among their athletes.

FIGURE 15.12 provides an overview of general and sport-specific factors that can lead to eating disorders in athletes. Parents, coaches, athletic trainers, and teammates should look for the seven "high-risk" factors. *We recommend that coaches tilt the balance between good health and athletic success in the direction of good health.*

They should formulate prudent and realistic perceptions about what constitutes desirable body size and body shape. Advising an athlete without objective information about body composition (e.g., realistic target body fat levels, desirable FFM and lean/fat ratio, healthy body mass index, and appropriate appraisals of body image and current eating behaviors) often provides the blueprint for disaster. In gymnastics and classical ballet, achieving extremes of thinness should not become a goal, even when considering the participant's health and safety. Of course, this approach requires rearrangement of priorities concerning aesthetic and performance parameters. The perpetual struggle to emulate an ideal that rewards thinness often forms the root cause of acute and chronic eating disorder medical problems.

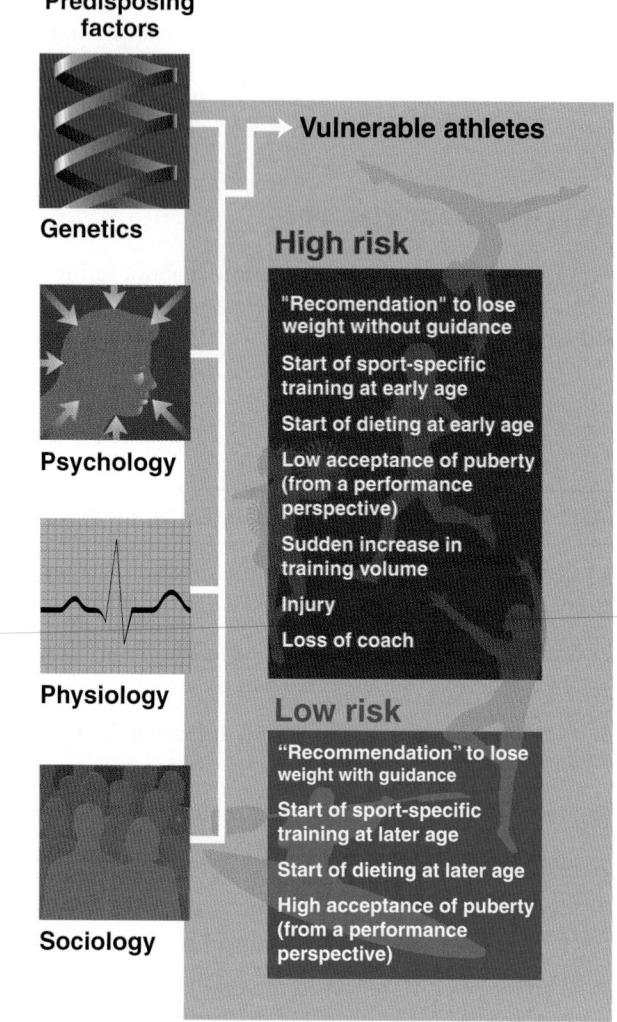

FIGURE 15.12 ■ General and sport-specific factors that lead to eating disorders in athletes. (Modified from Sundgot-Borgen J. Eating disorders in female athletes. *Sports Med* 1994;17:176.)

Summary

1. Eating disorders describe a broad spectrum of complex behaviors, core attitudes, coping strategies, and conditions that share the commonalty of an emotionally based, inordinate, and pathologic focus on body shape and body weight. An estimated 8 million people in the United States exhibit eating disorders, and approximately 90% are females.

2. Miss America contestants exhibit an image of extreme thinness. Thirty percent of contestant winners fall below the World Health Organization's cutoff for undernutrition (BMI <18.5). Raising the BMI cutoff to 19.0 adds another 18 women or a total of 48% of the winners with undesirable values. Approximately 24% of contest winners' BMIs ranged between 20.0 and 21.0, and no winner after 1924 had a BMI that equaled the BMI of the reference woman.

3. Athletes face a unique set of circumstances that makes them vulnerable to eating disorders. These behaviors flourish when the strong negative aesthetic connotations associated with excess body fat blend with the athlete's belief that any body fat spells doom for success.

4. Estimates of the prevalence of eating disorders range between 15 and 62% among female athletes, with the greatest prevalence among athletes in the aesthetic sports (ballet, bodybuilding, diving, figure skating, cheerleading, and gymnastics) in which success often coincides with extreme leanness.

5. Anorexia athletica describes the continuum of subclinical eating behaviors of physically active individuals who fail to meet the criteria for a true eating disorder but exhibit at least one unhealthy method of weight control.

6. Unhealthy weight control habits include fasting, vomiting, and use of diet pills, laxatives, or diuretics.

7. Approximately 50% of women with eating disorders compulsively overexercise. The term *exercise addict* describes someone who exercises excessively often doing "whatever it takes" to make additional time in the day to exercise more.

8. Many men project the ideal body as possessing about 28 lb more muscle than their own. This mismatch in perception has coincided with an increase in the number of men using anabolic steroids, experiencing eating disorders, and suffering from body obsession.

9. Body obsession encompasses a broad range of body-image concerns, but an important component relates to muscle dysmorphia or a pathologic preoccupation with muscularity.

10. Anorexia nervosa, present in about 1 to 2% of the general population, represents a crippling obsession with body size, a preoccupation with dieting and thinness, and a refusal to eat enough food to maintain a minimally normal body weight.

11. For anorectics, body weight decreases significantly below normal for age and stature, oftentimes leading to death.

12. Frequent episodes of binge eating followed by purging and intense feelings of guilt or shame characterize bulimia nervosa. Approximately 2 to 4% of all adolescents and adults in the general population suffer from bulimia nervosa.

13. Binge-eating disorder frequently occurs among obese patients undergoing treatment for weight loss.

14. Disordered eating behaviors—semistarvation, purging, excessive exercising—are used to achieve a body weight for success in certain "aesthetic" sports.

15. Eating disorders may be prevented among high-risk individuals with an Internet-based intervention program that includes continuous monitoring and feedback.

16. Four steps constitute an intervention strategy for disordered eating behaviors in athletes: (1) identify and isolate the contributing factors, (2) formulate appropriate goals for intervention and prevention, (3) formulate long-term strategies to deal with the problem, and (4) initiate a long-term program to address the situation.

17. Cognitive–behavioral therapy, interpersonal psychotherapy, and pharmacologic treatment currently treat eating disorders to give patients a sense of balance, purpose, and future. No one best treatment exists; combined approaches using individuals with expertise in psychiatry, eating disorders, body image issues, medicine, and nutrition often work best.

Test Your Knowledge Answers

1. **False:** In point of fact, Miss America contestants may represent an undernourished role model. The BMI of Miss America contestants generally falls below 18.5, a cutoff below the WHO standard that characterizes relative undernutrition.

2. **False:** Clinical observations indicate a prevalence of between 15 and 60% for disordered eating among athletes, with some groups at higher risk than others. More specifically, disordered eating patterns and unrealistic weight goals (and general dissatisfaction with one's body) occur most frequently among female athletes in the aesthetic sports such as ballet, body building, diving, figure skating, cheerleading, and gymnastics, in which success often coincides with extreme leanness. An inordinate preoccupation with eating also occurs among adolescent female swimmers. Controversy exists as to the prevalence of eating disorders among endurance runners.

3. **True:** The term *anorexia athletica* describes the continuum of subclinical eating behaviors of physically active individuals who fail to meet the criteria for a true eating disorder, but who exhibit at least one unhealthy weight control method. This includes fasting, vomiting (termed "instrumental vomiting" when used to make weight), and use of diet pills, laxatives, or diuretics (water pills).

4. **False:** Most persons consider eating disorders a "female problem," yet an increasing number of men share this affliction. An unanswered question concerns whether this increased number results from an increase in disease incidence or because more men seek treatment. In one New York hospital treatment center, the percentage of male patients admitted with eating disorders rose steadily from 4% in 1988 to 13% in 1995. Men currently represent about 6 to 10% of individuals with eating disorders, with the greatest prevalence among models, dancers, men abused during childhood, and gays.

5. **False:** Anorexia nervosa, particularly common and increasing in prevalence among adolescent girls and young women, is characterized by distortions of body image, a crippling obsession with body size, a preoccupation with dieting and thinness, and a refusal to eat enough food to maintain a minimally normal body weight. A relentless pursuit of thinness culminates in severe undernutrition, altered body composition characterized by depletion of fat and fat-free body mass, and cessation of menstruation (amenorrhea) in females. Body weight decreases below normal for age and stature.

6. **False:** Weight gain becomes a primary goal in the treatment of anorexia nervosa.

7. **False:** Bulimia nervosa, far more common than anorexia nervosa, is characterized by frequent episodes of bingeing calorically dense food (often at night and usually between 1000 to 10,000 calories), followed within several hours by purging, laxative abuse, fasting, or extreme exercise. Intense feelings of guilt or shame accompany these behaviors.

8. **False:** The main components in treating eating disorders include education (providing information concerning the eating disorder and its consequences); self-monitoring (providing a clear understanding of current eating behaviors and patterns); and meal planning (helping to gain control of eating patterns and establish a healthful pattern of eating).

9. **True:** Exercise has proven useful to treat bulimia nervosa. Regular physical activity reduces the pursuit of thinness, feelings of body dissatisfaction, and the frequency of bingeing, purging, and laxative abuse. The augmented self-regulation may result from the effects of exercise to reduce bulimic patients' bodily tensions and improve stress tolerance.

10. **False:** Muscle dysmorphia or the "Adonis complex" encompasses the pathologic preoccupation with muscle size and overall muscularity. These individuals view themselves as small and frail when in reality many are large and muscular. In many ways, muscle dysmorphia and anorexia nervosa share common traits; these include a history of depression and anxiety, a hyperculturization of body image and unrealistic shame about one's body, and self-destructive behaviors.

References

1. Anderluh MB, et al. Childhood obsessive-compulsive personality traits in adult women with eating disorders: defining a broader eating disorder phenotype. *Am J Psychiatry* 2003;160:242.
2. Attia E, et al. Does fluoxetine augment the inpatient treatment of anorexia nervosa? *Am J Psychiatry* 1998;155:548.
3. Bachner-Melman R, et al. How anorexic-like are the symptom and personality profiles of aesthetic athletes? *Med Sci Sports Exerc* 2006;38:628.
4. Baum A. Eating disorders in the male athlete. *Sports Med* 2006;36:1.
5. Benninghoven D, et al. Body image in patients with eating disorders and their mothers, and the role of family functioning. *Compr Psychiatry* 2007;48:118.
6. Beals KA, Hill AK. The prevalence of disordered eating, menstrual dysfunction, and low bone mineral density among US collegiate athletes. *Int J Sport Nutr Exerc Metab* 2006;16:1.
7. Beals KA. Disordered eating among athletes: a comprehensive guide for health professionals. Champaign, IL: Human Kinetics, 2004.
8. Benson J.E, et al. Eating problems and calorie intake levels in Swiss adolescent athletes. *Int J Sports Med* 1990;11:249.

9. Black DR, Burckes-Miller ME. Male and female college athletes: use of anorexia nervosa and bulimia nervosa weight loss methods. *Res Q* 1988;59:252.

10. Borgen JS, Corbin CB. Eating disorders among female athletes. *Phys Sportsmed* 1987;15:89.

11. Brooks-Gunn H, et al. Attitudes toward eating and body weight in different groups of female adolescent athletes. *Int J Eating Disord* 1988;7:748.

12. Brooks-Gunn JM, et al. The relation of eating problems and amenorrhea in ballet dancers. *Med Sci Sports Exerc* 1987;19:41.

13. Bruch H. *Golden Cage: The Enigma of Anorexia Nervosa.* Pocket Star, New York. 1979.

14. Brumberg JJ. *Fasting Girls: The History of Anorexia Nervosa.* New York: Penguin Books, 1988.

15. Brownell KD, Rodin J. Prevalence of Eating Disorders in Athletes. In: Brownell KD, et al, eds. Eating, Body Weight and Performance in Athletes. Philadelphia: Lea & Febiger, 1992.

16. Casper RC, et al. Total daily energy expenditure and activity level in anorexia nervosa. *Am J Clin Nutr* 1991;53:1143.

17. Chua JL, et al. Negative mood-induced overeating in obese binge eaters: an experimental study. Int J Obes Relat Metab Disord 2004;28:606.

18. Clark N, et al. Nutrition education for elite female runners. *Phys Sportsmed* 1988;16:124.

19. Cobb KL, et al. Disordered eating, menstrual irregularity, and bone mineral density in female runners. *Med Sci Sports Exerc* 2003;35:711.

20. Dale KS, Landers DM. Weight control in wrestling: eating disorders or disordered eating? *Med Sci Sports Exerc* 1999;31:1382.

21. Davis C, Cowles M. A comparison of weight and diet concerns and personality factors among female athletes and non-athletes. *J Psychosom Res* 1989;33:527.

22. De La Torre DM, Snell BJ. Use of the preparticipation physical exam in screening for the female athlete triad among high school athletes. *J Sch Nurs* 2005;21:340.

23. *Diagnostic and Statistical Manual of Mental Disorders.* DSM-IV-TR. 4th ed. (Text Revision). Arlington, VA: American Psychiatric Association, 2000.

24. Drewnowski A, et al. Bulimia in college women: incidence and recovery rates. *Am J Psychol* 1988;145:753.

25. Dummer GD, et al. Pathogenic weight control behavior of young, competitive swimmers. *Phys Sportsmed* 1987;15:75.

26. Eldredge KL. The effects of extending cognitive-behavioral therapy for binge eating disorder among initial treatment nonresponders. *Int J Eating Disord* 1997;21:347.

27. Enns MP, et al. Body composition, body size estimation and attitudes toward eating in male college athletes. *Psychosom Med* 1987;49:56.

28. Evers CL. Dietary intake and symptoms of anorexia nervosa in female university dancers. *J Am Diet Assoc* 1987;87:66.

29. Field AE, et al. Exposure to mass media and weight concerns among girls. *Pediatrics* 1999;103:E36.

30. Fogelholm M, Hilloskorpi H. Weight and diet concerns in Finnish female and male athletes. *Med Sci Sports Exerc* 1999;31:229.

31. Friederich HC, et al. Treatment outcome in people with subthreshold compared with full-syndrome binge eating disorder. *Obesity* 2007;15:283.

32. Frusztajer NT, et al. Nutrition and the incidence of stress fractures in ballet dancers. *Am J Clin Nutr* 1990;51:79.

33. Garfinkel PE. Kaplan AS. Anorexia Nervosa: Diagnostic Conceptualizations. In: Brownell KD, Foreyt JP, eds. Handbook of Eating Disorders. New York: Basic Books, 1986.

34. Garner DM, Rosen LW. Eating disorders among athletes: research and recommendations. *J Appl Sports Sci Res* 1991;5:100.

35. Garner DM, et al. A prospective study of eating disturbances in the ballet. *Psychother Psychosom* 1987;48:170.

36. Genazzani AD, et al. Diagnostic and therapeutic approach to hypothalamic amenorrhea. *Ann NY Acad Sci* 2006;1092:103.

37. Gormally J, et al. The assessment of binge eating severity among obese persons. *Addict Behav* 1982;7:47.

38. Grigg M, et al. Disordered eating and unhealthy weight reduction practices among adolescent females. *Prevent Med* 1996;25:745.

39. Grinspoon S, et al. Changes in regional fat redistribution and the effects of estrogen during spontaneous weight gain in women with anorexia nervosa. *Am J Clin Nutr* 2001;73:865.

40. Grucza RA, et al. Prevalence and correlates of binge eating disorder in a community sample. *Compr Psychiatry* 2007;48:124.

41. Hamilton LH, et al. Sociocultural influences on eating disorders in professional female ballet dancers. *Int J Eating Disord* 1985;4:465.

42. Hamilton LH, et al. The role of selectivity in the pathogenesis of eating problems in ballet dancers. *Med Sci Sports Exerc* 1988;20:560.

43. Herzog DB, et al. Eating disorders and social maladjustment in female medical students. *J Nerv Ment Disord* 1985;173:734.

44. Herzog DB, et al. Frequency of bulimic behaviors and associated social maladjustments in female graduate students. *J Psychol Res* 1986;20:355

45. Hill AJ. *Obesity* and eating disorders. *Obes Rev* 2007;8(suppl 1):151.

46. Hopkinson RA, Lock J. Athletics, perfectionism, and disordered eating. *Eat Weight Disord* 2004;9:99.

47. Hrabosky JI, et al. Overvaluation of shape and weight in binge eating disorder. *J Consult Clin Psychol* 2007;75:175.

48. Humphries LL, Gruber JJ. Nutrition behaviors of university majorettes. *Phys Sportsmed* 1986;14:91.

49. Iketani T, et al. Altered body fat distribution after recovery of weight in patients with anorexia nervosa. *Int J Eating Disord* 1999;26:275.

50. Johnson C, et al. Athletes and eating disorders: the national collegiate athletic association study. *Int J Eating Disord* 1999;26:179.

51. Joy E. Team management of the female athlete triad. *Phys Sportsmed* 1997;25:95.

52. Kaye WH, et al. Caloric intake necessary for weight maintenance in anorexia nervosa: nonbulimics require greater caloric intake than bulimics. *Am J Clin Nutr* 1986;44:443.

53. Kerr J. Characteristics common to females who exhibit anorexic or bulimic behavior: a review of current literature. *J Clin Psychol* 1991;47:846.

54. Kerrvish KP, et al. Body composition in adolescents with anorexia nervosa. *Am J Clin Nutr* 2002;75:31.

55. King MB, Mezey G. Eating behavior of male racing jockeys. *Psychol Med* 1987;17:249.

56. Kiningham RB, Gorenflo DW. Weight loss methods of high school wrestlers. *Med Sci Sports Exerc* 2001;33:810.

57. Kinoy BP. Eating disorders: New Directions in Treatment and Recovery. New York: Columbia University Press, 1994.

58. Kirchner EM, et al. Bone mineral density and dietary intake of female college gymnasts. *Med Sci Sports Exerc* 1995;27:543.

59. Kurtzman FD, et al. Eating disorders among selected female student populations at UCLA. *J Am Diet Assoc* 1989;89:45.

60. Le Grange D, et al. Eating and general psychopathology in a sample of Caucasian and ethnic minority subjects. *Int J Eating Disord* 1997;21:285.

61. Levine MD, et al. Exercise in the treatment of binge eating disorder. *Int J Eating Disord* 1996;19:171.

62. Lilenfeld D, et al. A controlled family study of anorexia nervosa and bulimia nervosa: psychiatric disorders in first-degree relatives and effects of proband comorbidity. *Arch Gen Psychiatry* 1998;55:603.

63. Marcus MD. Binge Eating in Obesity. In: Fairburn CG, Wilson GT, eds. *Binge Eating: Nature, Assessment, and Treatment.* New York: Guilford Press, 1993.

64. Marcus MD, et al. Binge eating and dietary restraint in obese patients. *Addict Behav* 1985;10:163.

65. Mallick MJ, et al. Behavioral and psychological traits of weight-conscious teenagers: a comparison of eating-disordered patients and high- and low-risk groups. *Adolescence* 1987;22:157.

66. Marzano-Parisoli MM. The contemporary construction of a perfect body image: bodybuilding, exercise addiction, and eating disorders. *Quest* 2001;53:216.

67. Mathieu J. Disordered eating across the life span. *J Am Diet Assoc* 2004;104:1208.

68. Mayer L. Body composition and anorexia nervosa: does physiology explain psychology? *Am J Clin Nutr* 2001;73:851.

69. McElroy SL, et al. Topiramate in the treatment of binge eating disorder. *Am J Psychiatry* 2003;160:255.

70. Morton R: Origins of Anorexia nervosa. *Eur Neurol* 2004;52:191.

71. Mulholland AM, Mintz LB Prevalence of eating disorders among African American women. *J Consult Psychol* 2001;48:111.

72. National Institutes of Health. Binge eating disorders. NIH Publication. no. 94-3589. Washington, DC: U.S. Department of Health and Human Services, 1993.

73. Nichols JF, et al. Prevalence of the female athlete triad syndrome among high school athletes. *Arch Pediatr Adolesc Med* 2006;160:137.

74. O'Conner P, et al. Eating disorder symptoms in female college gymnasts. *Med Sci Sports Exerc* 1995;26:550.

75. O'Connor PJ, et al. Eating disorder symptoms in former female college gymnasts: relations with body composition. *Am J Clin Nutr* 1996;64:840.

76. Olivardia R, et al. Muscle dysmorphia in male weightlifters: a case-control study. *Am J Psychiatry* 2000;157:1291.

77. Orphanidou CI, et al. Changes in body composition and fat distribution after short-term weight gain in patients with anorexia nervosa. *Am J Clin Nutr* 1997;65:1034.

78. Owens RG, Slade PD. Running and anorexia nervosa: an empirical study. *Int J Eating Disord* 1987;6:771.

79. Pasman L, Thompson JK. Body image and eating disturbance in obligatory runner, obligatory weightlifter, and sedentary individuals. *Int J Eating Disord* 1988;7:759.

80. Patton GC. The spectrum of eating disorder in adolescence. *J Psychosom Res* 1988;32:579.

81. Perkins DF, Luster T. The relationship between sexual abuse and purging: findings from community-wide surveys of female adolescents. *Child Abuse Negl* 1999;23:371.

82. Pernick Y, Nichols JF, Rauh , et al. Disordered eating among a multiracial/ethnic sample of female high-school athletes. *J Adolesc Health* 2006;38:689.

83. Petrie TA, Stoever S. The incidence of bulimia nervosa and pathogenic weight control behaviors in female collegiate gymnasts. *Res Quart Exerc Sport* 1993;64:238.

84. Pike KM. Long-term course of anorexia nervosa: response, relapse, remission, and recovery. *Clin Psychol Rev* 1998;18:447.

85. Polito A, et al. Basal metabolic rate in anorexia nervosa: relation to body composition and leptin concentrations. *Am J Clin Nutr* 2000;71:1495.

86. Pope HG Jr, et al. Body image perception among men in three countries. *Am J Psychiatry* 2000;157:1297.

87. Powers P, Johnson C. Targeting eating disorders in elite athletes. Part I. *Eating Disord Rev* 1996;7:4.

88. Probst M, et al. Body composition of anorexia nervosa patients assessed by underwater weighing and skinfold-thickness measurements before and after weight gain. *Am J Clin Nutr* 2001;73:190.

89. Pyle RL, et al. Maintenance treatment and 6-month outcome for bulimic patients who respond to initial treatment. *Am J Psychiatry* 1990;147:871.

90. Rosen LW, Hough DO. Pathogenic weight control behaviors among female gymnasts. *Phys Sportsmed* 1988;16:140.

91. Rosen LW, et al. Pathogenic weight control behavior in female athletes. *Phys Sportsmed* 1986;14:79.

92. Rucinski A: Relationship of body image and dietary intake of competitive ice skaters. *J Am Diet Assoc* 1989;89:98.

93. Schnirring L. When to suspect muscle dysmorphia: bringing the "Adonis complex" to light. *Phys Sportsmed* 2000;28:19.

94. Silverman JA. Marce Louis-Victor, 1828-1864: anorexia nervosa's forgotten man. *Psychol Med* 1989;19:833.

95. Silverman JG, et al. Dating violence against adolescent girls and associated substance use, unhealthy weight control, sexual risk behavior, pregnancy, and suicidality. *JAMA* 2001;286:572.

96. Smith DE. Binge eating in ethnic minority groups. *Addict Behav* 1995;20:695.

97. Sossin K. Nutrition beliefs, attitudes, and resource use of high school wrestling coaches. *Int J Sport Nutr* 1997;7:219.

98. Spurrell EB, et al. Age of onset for binge eating: are there different pathways to binge eating? *Int J Eat Disord* 1997;21:55.

99. Steen SN, Brownell KD. Current patterns of weight loss and regain in wrestlers: has the tradition changed? *Med Sci Sports Exerc* 1990;22:762.

100. Steen SN, McKinney S. Nutrition assessment of college wrestlers. *Phys Sportsmed* 1986;14:100.

101. Striegel-Moore RH. Risk factors for eating disorders. *Ann NY Acad Sci* 1997;817:98.

102. Striegel-Moore RH, et al. Abuse, bullying, and discrimination as risk factors for binge eating disorder. *Am J Psychiatry* 2002;159:1902.

103. Stunkard AJ, et al. Binge eating disorder and the night-eating syndrome. *Int J Obes Relat Metab Disord* 1996;20:1.

104. Sunday SR, Halmi KA. Micro- and macroanalyses of patterns within a meal in anorexia and bulimia nervosa. *Appetite* 1996;26:21.

105. Sundgot-Borgen J, Torstveit MK. Prevalence of eating disorders in elite athletes is higher than in the general population. *Clin J Sport Med* 2004;14:25.

106. Sundgot-Borgen J. Eating disorders among female athletes. *Phys Sportsmed* 1987;15:89.

107. Sundgot-Borgen J. Eating disorders in female athletes. *Sports Med* 1994;17:176.

108. Sundgot-Borgen J. Risk and trigger factors for the development of eating disorders in female elite athletes. *Med Sci Sports Exerc* 1994;26:414.

109. Sundgot-Borgen J, et al. The effect of exercise, cognitive therapy, and nutritional counseling in treating bulimia nervosa. *Med Sci Sport Exerc* 2002;34:190.

110. Tanofsky MB, et al. Comparison of men and women with binge eating disorder. *Int J Eating Disord* 1997;21:49.

111. Taylor CB, et al. Prevention of eating disorders in at-risk college-age women. *Arch Gen Psychiatry* 2006;63:881.

112. Team Physician Consensus Statement. Female athlete issues for the team physician: a consensus statement. *Med Sci Sports Exerc* 2003;35:1785.

113. Trail RR. Richard Morton (1637-1698). *Med Hist* 1970;14:166.

114. The McKnight Investigators. Risk factors for the onset of eating disorders in adolescent girls: results of the McKnight Longitudinal Risk Factor Study. *Am J Psychiatry* 2003;160:248.

115. Thiel A, et al. Subclinical eating disorders in male athletes: a study of the low weight category in rowers and wrestlers. *Acta Psychiatry Scand* 1993;88:259.

116. Thome JL, Espelage D. Relations among exercise, coping, disordered eating, and psychological health among college students. *Eat Behav* 2004;5:337.

117. Thompson RA, Sherman RT. *Helping Athletes with Eating Disorders.* Champaign, IL: Human Kinetics Publishers, 1993.

118. Tofler IR, et al. Physical and emotional problems of elite female gymnasts. *N Engl J Med* 1996;335:281.

119. Unoka Z, et al. Early maladaptive schemas and body mass index in subgroups of eating disorders: a differential association. *Compr Psychiatry* 2007;48:199.

120. Warren BJ, et al. Disordered eating patterns in competitive female athletes. *Int J Eating Disord* 1990;9:565.

121. Weight L, Noakes T. Is running an analog of anorexia? A survey of the incidence of eating disorders in female distance runners. *Med Sci Sports Exerc* 1987;19:213.

122. Wichmann S, Martin DR. Eating disorders in athletes: weighing the risks. *Phys Sportsmed* 1993;21:126.

123. Wiederman MW, Pryor T. Substance use among women with eating disorders. *Int J Eating Disord* 1996;20:163.

124. World Health Organization. Obesity: preventing and managing the global epidemic. Report of a WHO consultation presented at the World Health Organization; June 3–5, 1997, Geneva, Switzerland. Publication WHO/NUT/NCD/98.1.

125. Yanovski SZ. Binge eating disorder: current knowledge and future directions. *Obes Res* 1993;1:306.

126. Yanovski SZ, et al. Association of binge eating disorder and psychiatric comorbidity in obese subjects. *Am J Psychiatry* 1993;50:1472.

127. Yeager KK, et al. The female athlete triad: disordered eating, amenorrhea and osteoporosis. *Med Sci Sports Exerc* 1993;25:775.

128. Zamboni M, et al. Body fat distribution before and after weight gain in anorexia nervosa. *Int J Obes* 1997;21:33.

Additional Readings

American Dietetic Association. Position of the American Dietetic Association: Nutrition intervention in the treatment of anorexia nervosa, bulimia nervosa, and other eating disorders. *J Am Diet Assoc* 2006;106:2073.

Anderson DA, et al. Effect of response format on endorsement of eating disordered attitudes and behaviors. *Int J Eat Disord* 2007;40:90.

Bandini S, et al. Factors affecting dropout in outpatient eating disorder treatment. *Eat Weight Disord* 2006;11:179.

Beals KA, Meyer NL. Female athlete triad update. *Clin Sports Med* 2007;26:69 [Review].

Bomba M, et al. Endocrine profiles and neuropsychologic correlates of functional hypothalamic amenorrhea in adolescents. *Fertil Steril* 2007; 87:876.

Doyle AC, et al. Psychosocial and physical impairment in overweight adolescents at high risk for eating disorders. *Obesity* 2007;15:145.

Fisak B Jr, et al. Challenging previous conceptions of vegetarianism and eating disorders. *Eat Weight Disord* 2006;11:195.

Hinrichsen H, et al. Core beliefs and social anxiety in the eating disorders. *Eat Weight Disord* 2007;12:e14.

Hrabosky JI, Grilo CM. Body image and eating disordered behavior in a community sample of Black and Hispanic women. *Eat Behav* 2007;8:106.

Kim JY, et al. The impacts of *Obesity* on psychological well-being: a cross-sectional study about depressive mood and quality of life. *J Prev Med Pub Health* 2007;40:191.

Leung N, Price E. Core beliefs in dieters and eating disordered women. *Eat Behav* 2007;8:65.

Luce KH, et al. Eating disorders and alcohol use: group differences in consumption rates and drinking motives. *Eat Behav* 2007;8:177.

Piran N, Robinson S. The association between disordered eating and substance use and abuse in women: a community-based investigation. *Women Health* 2006;44:1.

Sossin K. Body image, disordered eating and the school environment. *School Nurse News* 2006;23:11.

Warner C, et al. Disordered eating in entry-level military personnel. *Mil Med* 2007;172:147.

Nutritive Values for Common Foods, Alcoholic and Nonalcoholic Beverages, and Specialty and Fast-Food Items[a]

This appendix has three parts. Part 1 lists nutritive values for common foods, Part 2 lists nutritive values for alcoholic and nonalcoholic beverages, and Part 3 presents nutritive values for specialty and fast-food items. The nutritive values of foods and alcoholic and nonalcoholic beverages, expressed in 1-ounce (28.4 g) portions, allow comparisons among different food categories. Thus, for example, the protein content of 1.55 g for 1 ounce of banana nut bread can be compared directly to the protein content of 6.28 g for 1 ounce of processed American cheese.

PART 1

Nutritive Values for Common Foods

The foods are grouped into categories and are listed in alphabetical order within each category. The categories include breads, cakes and pies, cookies, candy bars, chocolate, desserts, cereals, cheese, fish, fruits, meats, eggs, dairy products, vegetables, and typical salad bar entries. An additional section labeled Variety consists of food items such as soups, sandwiches, salad dressings, oils, some condiments, and other "goodies." The nutritive value for each food is expressed per ounce or 28.4 g of that food item. The specific values for each food include the caloric content (kCal) for 1 ounce, protein, total lipid, carbohydrate, calcium, iron, vitamin B_1, vitamin B_2, fiber content, and cholesterol.

[a]The information about the nutritive value of the foods comes from a variety of sources. This includes primarily data from Watt, BK, Merrill, AL. *Composition of Foods—Raw, Processed and Prepared*, Washington, DC: U.S. Department of Agriculture, 1963; Adams C, and Richardson, M. *Nutritive Value of Foods*. Washington, DC: Government Printing Office, 1981; Pennington JAT, and Douglass JP. Bowes & Church's Food Values of Portions Commonly Used. 18th ed. Baltimore: Lippincott Williams & Wilkins, 2005. Other sources include a comprehensive database maintained by the University of Massachusetts, the consumer relations departments of manufacturers, and journal articles that evaluated specific foods items. NA indicates data not available.

BREADS

	kCal	Protein (g)	Lipid (g)	CHO (g)	Ca (mg)	Fe (mg)	B₁ (mg)	B₂ (mg)	Fiber (g)	Cholesterol (mg)
Banana nut	91	1.55	4.00	12.7	10.0	0.470	0.054	0.046	0.66	18.3
Boston brown—canned	60	1.26	0.39	13.2	25.8	0.567	0.038	0.025	1.34	1.9
Cornmeal muffin—recipe	91	1.89	3.15	13.2	41.6	0.567	0.069	0.069	1.00	14.5
Croutons—dry	105	3.69	1.04	20.5	35.0	1.020	0.099	0.099	0.09	0
Cracked wheat	74	2.63	0.99	14.2	18.1	0.755	0.108	0.108	1.50	0
Cracked wheat—toast	88	3.00	1.17	16.9	21.6	0.899	0.100	0.128	1.82	0
French—chunk	81	2.67	1.10	14.3	31.6	0.875	0.130	0.097	0.57	0
Italian	78	2.55	0.25	16.0	4.7	0.756	0.116	0.066	0.47	0
Mixed grain	74	2.27	1.05	13.6	30.6	0.907	0.113	0.113	1.78	0
Mixed grain—toast	80	2.47	1.15	14.8	33.3	0.986	0.099	0.123	1.97	0
Oatmeal	74	2.37	1.25	13.6	17.0	0.794	0.130	0.075	1.10	0
Oatmeal—toast	80	2.47	1.36	14.8	18.5	0.863	0.110	0.081	1.20	0
Pita pocket	78	2.94	0.42	15.6	23.2	0.685	0.129	0.061	0.45	0
Pumpernickel	71	2.60	0.98	13.6	20.4	0.777	0.097	0.147	1.67	0
Pumpernickel—toast	78	2.86	1.08	15.0	22.5	0.857	0.088	0.162	1.87	0
Raisin—	77	2.15	1.12	15.0	28.4	0.879	0.093	0.176	0.68	0
Raisin—toasted	92	2.57	1.34	17.6	33.8	1.080	0.081	0.209	0.81	0
Rye—light	74	2.40	1.04	13.6	22.7	0.771	0.116	0.090	1.87	0
Rye—light—toast	84	2.73	1.18	15.5	25.8	0.876	0.107	0.103	2.15	0
Vienna	79	2.72	1.10	14.4	31.2	0.873	0.130	0.100	0.91	0
White	76	2.35	1.10	13.8	35.7	0.806	0.133	0.088	0.54	0
White—toast	84	2.67	1.26	15.7	40.6	0.915	0.121	0.103	0.64	0
Whole wheat	69	2.84	1.22	12.9	20.2	0.964	0.100	0.059	2.10	0
Whole wheat—toasted	79	3.42	1.47	14.4	22.5	1.090	0.090	0.066	2.74	0
Bread crumbs—dry grated	111	3.69	1.42	20.7	34.6	1.160	0.099	0.099	1.15	1.4
Bread crumbs—soft	76	2.35	1.10	13.9	35.9	0.806	0.134	0.088	0.54	0
Bread sticks wo/salt	109	3.40	0.82	21.3	7.9	0.255	0.017	0.020	0.43	0
Bread sticks w/salt	86	2.67	0.89	16.4	13.0	0.243	0.016	0.024	0.41	0

CAKES AND PIES

	kCal	Protein (g)	Lipid (g)	CHO (g)	Ca (mg)	Fe (mg)	B₁ (mg)	B₂ (mg)	Fiber (g)	Cholesterol (mg)
Cakes										
Angel food cake	67	1.71	0.09	15.2	23.5	0.123	0.014	0.057	0	0
Boston cream pie	61	0.59	1.89	10.4	6.1	0.142	0.002	0.043	0	4.7
Carrot cake	103	1.05	5.32	13.2	6.9	0.304	0.030	0.035	0	14.6
Cheesecake	86	1.54	5.45	8.1	15.9	0.136	0.009	0.037	0	52.4
Choc cupcake/choc frosting	97	1.24	3.29	16.5	16.9	0.575	0.029	0.041	0	15.2
Coffee cake	91	1.78	2.70	14.8	17.3	0.480	0.054	0.059	0	18.5
Dark fruitcake	109	1.32	4.62	16.5	27.0	0.791	0.053	0.053	0	13.2
Gingerbread cake	91	1.15	2.86	15.2	12.2	0.706	0.042	0.038	0	7.8
Pound cake	113	1.89	4.72	14.2	18.9	0.472	0.047	0.057	0	30.2
Sheet cake—plain	104	1.32	3.96	15.8	18.1	0.429	0.046	0.049	0	20.1
Sheet cake—white frosting	104	0.94	3.28	18.0	14.3	0.281	0.030	0.037	0	16.4
Sponge cake	83	2.01	1.27	16.0	10.8	0.524	0.043	0.046	0	58.8
White cake/coconut	109	1.30	4.05	17.0	13.7	0.454	0.041	0.053	0	1.2

CAKES AND PIES—*continued*

	kCal	Protein (g)	Lipid (g)	CHO (g)	Ca (mg)	Fe (mg)	B₁ (mg)	B₂ (mg)	Fiber (g)	Cholesterol (mg)
Cakes—cont'd										
White cake/white frosting	104	1.20	3.59	16.8	13.2	0.399	0.080	0.052	0	1.2
Yellow cake/chocolate frosting	101	1.03	4.48	15.9	9.5	0.509	0.020	0.058	0	15.6
Pies										
Apple pie	73	0.66	3.14	10.7	5.0	0.300	0.031	0.023	0	0
Apple pie—fried	85	0.73	4.67	10.7	4.0	0.312	0.030	0.020	0	4.7
Banana cream pie	46	0.90	1.85	6.7	21.0	0.156	0.022	0.042	0	2.2
Blueberry pie	68	0.72	3.05	9.9	4.7	0.377	0.031	0.025	0	0
Boston cream pie	61	0.59	1.89	10.4	6.1	0.142	0.002	0.043	0	4.7
Cherry pie	74	0.77	3.19	10.9	6.6	0.569	0.034	0.025	0	0
Cherry pie—fried	83	0.68	4.74	10.7	3.7	0.233	0.020	0.020	0	4.3
Chocolate cream pie	50	1.20	2.04	6.9	25.9	0.175	0.024	0.049	0	2.4
Coconut cream pie	57	1.03	2.79	7.2	24.0	0.198	0.021	0.042	0	2.5
Coconut custard pie	66	1.69	3.85	6.3	25.0	0.304	0.029	0.055	0	31.4
Cream pie	85	0.56	4.29	11.0	8.6	0.205	0.011	0.028	0	1.5
Custard pie	55	1.43	2.65	6.3	23.1	0.269	0.026	0.050	0	27.6
Lemon meringue pie	72	0.95	2.90	10.7	5.1	0.283	0.020	0.028	0	27.7
Mincemeat pie	70	0.65	2.13	12.8	6.9	0.360	0.028	0.024	0	0
Peach pie	73	0.63	3.14	10.9	4.8	0.340	0.031	0.028	0	0
Pecan pie	120	1.30	4.87	18.9	7.2	0.380	0.045	0.034	0	28.1
Pumpkin pie	52	1.28	2.23	7.3	30.0	0.373	0.019	0.042	0	15.5
Strawberry chiffon pie	65	0.85	3.46	8.0	7.7	0.254	0.022	0.023	0	7.1

COOKIES

	kCal	Protein (g)	Lipid (g)	CHO (g)	Ca (mg)	Fe (mg)	B₁ (mg)	B₂ (mg)	Fiber (g)	Cholesterol (mg)
Animal cookies	120	1.90	2.89	22.0	3.0	0.918	0.080	0.130	0	0.1
Brownies w/nuts	135	1.84	8.93	15.6	12.8	0.567	0.070	0.070	0	25.5
Butter cookies	130	1.76	4.82	20.2	36.3	0.170	0.011	0.017	0	4.1
Fig bars	106	1.02	1.93	21.4	20.2	0.689	0.039	0.037	0	13.7
Lady fingers	102	2.19	2.19	18.3	11.6	0.515	0.019	0.039	0	101.0
Oatmeal raisin cookies	134	1.64	5.45	19.6	9.8	0.600	0.049	0.044	0	1.1
Peanut butter cookies	145	2.36	8.27	16.5	12.4	0.650	0.041	0.041	0	13.0
Sandwich type cookies	138	1.42	5.67	20.6	8.5	0.992	0.064	0.050	0	0
Shortbread cookies	137	1.77	7.09	17.7	11.5	0.709	0.089	0.080	0	23.9
Sugar cookies	139	1.18	7.09	18.3	29.5	0.532	0.053	0.035	0	17.1
Vanilla wafers	131	1.42	4.96	20.6	11.3	0.567	0.050	0.070	0	17.7

CANDY BARS

	kCal	Protein (g)	Lipid (g)	CHO (g)	Ca (mg)	Fe (mg)	B₁ (mg)	B₂ (mg)	Fiber (g)	Cholesterol (mg)
Almond Joy	151	1.69	7.82	18.5	2.0	0.778	0	0	0	0
Sugar-coated almonds	146	3.10	9.12	14.6	39.6	0.775	0.042	0.156	0	0

CANDY BARS—*continued*

	kCal	Protein (g)	Lipid (g)	CHO (g)	Ca (mg)	Fe (mg)	B₁ (mg)	B₂ (mg)	Fiber (g)	Cholesterol (mg)
Bittersweet chocolate	141	1.90	9.73	15.7	13.0	1.040	0.015	0.050	0	0
Caramel—plain or chocolate	115	1.00	2.99	22.0	41.9	0.399	0.010	0.050	0	1.0
Chocolate candy kisses	154	2.10	8.98	15.9	52.9	0.499	0.020	0.080	0	0
Chocolate-coated almonds	161	3.92	12.70	8.0	47.8	1.090	0.052	0.186	0	0
Chocolate-covered coconut	133	0.91	7.10	17.5	8.4	0.614	0.008	0.016	0	0
Chocolate-covered mints	116	0.50	2.99	23.0	16.0	0.299	0.010	0.020	0	0
Chocolate-covered peanuts	159	5.00	11.70	9.8	32.9	0.689	0.086	0.043	0	0
Chocolate-covered raisins	111	1.06	2.71	20.6	12.2	0.663	0.034	0.025	0	0
Chocolate fudge	115	0.56	2.78	21.0	22.0	0.299	0.010	0.030	0	1.0
Chocolate fudge with nuts	114	1.06	4.99	18.8	22.0	0.299	0.016	0.030	0	7.4
English toffee	195	0.89	16.90	9.8	0	0.177	0.470	0.044	0	0
Gum drops	98	0	0.20	24.8	2.0	0.100	0	0	0	0
Hard candy	109	0	0	27.6	6.0	0.100	0	0	0	0
Jelly beans	104	0	0.10	26.4	1.0	0.299	0	0	0	0
Kit Kat	138	1.98	7.25	16.5	42.9	0.369	0.020	0.073	0	0
Krackle	149	2.00	8.09	16.9	50.0	0.400	0.017	0.075	0	0
Malted milk balls	135	2.30	6.99	17.8	62.9	0	0	0	0	0
M&M's plain chocolate	140	1.95	6.08	19.5	46.7	0.449	0.015	0.073	0	0
M&M's peanut chocolate	144	3.23	7.25	16.5	35.4	0.402	0.016	0.056	0	0
Mars bar	136	2.27	6.24	17.0	48.2	0.312	0.014	0.093	0	0
Milk chocolate—plain	145	2.00	8.98	16.0	49.9	0.399	0.020	0.100	0	6.0
Milk chocolate w/almonds	150	2.90	10.40	15.0	60.9	0.559	0.030	0.130	0	4.5
Milk chocolate w/peanuts	155	4.89	11.70	10.0	31.9	0.679	0.112	0.065	0	3.0
Milk chocolate + rice cereal	140	2.00	6.99	18.0	47.9	0.200	0.010	0.080	0	6.0
Milky Way	123	1.53	4.25	20.3	40.6	0.232	0.013	0.070	0	6.6
Mr. Goodbar	151	3.62	9.05	13.9	39.2	0.567	0.030	0.072	0	4.2
Reese's peanut butter cup	151	3.65	9.07	13.9	21.7	0.430	0.020	0.032	0	1.6
Snickers	134	3.08	6.62	17.0	32.4	0.227	0.013	0.050	0	0
Vanilla fudge	118	0.70	3.15	22.0	29.9	0.030	0.006	0.025	0	10.0
Vanilla fudge with nuts	122	1.00	5.01	18.3	25.0	0.159	0.017	0.026	0	8.5

CHOCOLATE

	kCal	Protein (g)	Lipid (g)	CHO (g)	Ca (mg)	Fe (mg)	B₁ (mg)	B₂ (mg)	Fiber (g)	Cholesterol (mg)
Baking chocolate	145	3.49	15.00	7.5	22.0	1.900	0.015	0.099	0	0
Bittersweet chocolate	141	1.90	9.73	15.7	13.0	1.040	0.015	0.050	0	0
Milk chocolate—plain	145	2.00	8.98	16.0	49.9	0.399	0.020	0.100	0	6.0
Semi-sweet chocolate chips	143	1.17	10.20	16.2	8.5	0.967	0.017	0.023	0	0
Dark chocolate—sweet	150	1.00	9.98	16.0	7.0	0.599	0.010	0.040	0	0
Chocolate cupcake/ chocolate frosting	97	1.24	3.29	16.5	16.9	0.575	0.029	0.041	0	15.2
Chocolate candy kisses	154	2.10	8.98	15.9	52.9	0.499	0.020	0.080	0	0
Chocolate chip cookies	122	1.54	5.94	18.9	11.0	0.540	0.068	0.155	0	3.4

CHOCOLATE—continued

	kCal	Protein (g)	Lipid (g)	CHO (g)	Ca (mg)	Fe (mg)	B₁ (mg)	B₂ (mg)	Fiber (g)	Cholesterol (mg)
Chocolate coated almonds	161	3.92	12.70	8.0	47.8	1.090	0.052	0.186	0	0
Chocolate coated peanuts	159	5.00	11.70	9.8	32.9	0.689	0.086	0.043	0	0
Chocolate covered mints	116	0.50	2.99	23.0	16.0	0.299	0.010	0.020	0	0
Chocolate covered raisins	111	1.06	2.71	20.6	12.2	0.663	0.034	0.025	0	0
Chocolate cream pie	50	1.20	2.04	6.9	25.9	0.175	0.024	0.049	0	2.4
Chocolate fudge	115	0.56	2.78	21.0	22.0	0.299	0.010	0.030	0	1.0
Chocolate fudge with nuts	114	1.06	4.99	18.8	22.0	0.299	0.016	0.030	0	7.4
Cake flour-baked value	103	2.08	0.28	22.4	4.5	1.250	0.154	0.096	0	0
Reese's peanut butter cup	151	3.65	9.07	13.9	21.7	0.430	0.020	0.032	0	1.6
Chocolate pudding/recipe	42	0.88	1.25	7.3	27.3	0.142	0.005	0.039	0	4.3
Chocolate pudding instant	34	0.85	0.818	5.9	28.4	0.065	0.009	0.039	0	3.1

DESSERTS AND BREAKFAST PASTRIES

	kCal	Protein (g)	Lipid (g)	CHO (g)	Ca (mg)	Fe (mg)	B₁ (mg)	B₂ (mg)	Fiber (g)	Cholesterol (mg)
Apple brown betty	43	0.30	1.60	7.40	5.4	0.130	0.016	0.012	0	3.8
Apple cobbler	55	0.53	1.74	9.57	8.8	0.206	0.023	0.019	0	0.3
Apple crisp	53	0.33	1.93	9.09	7.4	0.278	0.018	0.013	0	0
Apple dumpling	55	0.32	2.37	8.64	7.1	0.253	0.012	0.013	0	0
Banana nut bread	91	1.60	4.00	12.70	10.0	0.470	0.054	0.046	0	18.3
Bread + raisin pudding	60	1.20	2.47	8.54	27.7	0.304	0.030	0.048	0	24.4
Cheesecake	86	1.50	5.45	8.10	15.9	0.136	0.009	0.037	0	52.4
Cherry cobbler	44	0.53	1.37	7.52	8.5	0.391	0.019	0.021	0	0.3
Cherry & cream cheese torte	79	1.28	3.96	10.00	28.5	0.266	0.015	0.052	0	11.2
Vanilla milkshake	32	0.98	0.841	5.09	34.5	0.026	0.013	0.052	0	3.2
Cream puff w/custard fill	72	1.24	4.54	6.83	16.4	0.276	0.015	0.040	0	58.8
Chocolate eclair w/custard fill	79	1.20	4.43	8.96	18.6	0.258	0.019	0.041	0	50.4
Gelatin salad	17	0.43	0	3.99	0.5	0.024	0.002	0.002	0	0
Peach cobbler	28	0.50	1.35	7.96	7.6	0.197	0.018	0.017	0	0.3
Peach crisp	34	0.31	1.06	6.18	4.8	0.203	0.010	0.010	0	0
Crepe, unfilled	49	2.06	1.32	7.07	25.0	0.475	0.045	0.070	0.21	43.0
Pancakes—plain	63	2.10	2.10	9.45	28.4	0.525	0.063	0.074	0.42	16.8
Croissant	117	2.32	6.02	13.40	10.0	1.040	0.085	0.065	0.54	6.5
Danish pastry—plain	109	1.99	5.97	12.90	29.8	0.547	0.080	0.085	0	24.4
Danish pastry w/fruit	102	1.74	5.67	12.20	7.41	0.567	0.070	0.061	0	24.4
Doughnut—cake type	119	1.33	6.75	13.90	13.0	0.454	0.068	0.068	0	11.3
Doughnut—jelly filled	99	1.48	3.84	13.00	12.2	0.349	0.052	0.044	0	0
Doughnut—yeast-raised	111	1.89	6.28	12.30	8.0	0.661	0.132	0.057	0	9.9
Chocolate pudding	42	0.88	1.25	7.28	27.3	0.142	0.005	0.039	0	4.3
Tapioca pudding	38	1.43	1.44	4.85	29.7	0.120	0.012	0.052	0	27.3
Vanilla pudding	32	0.99	1.10	4.50	33.1	0.089	0.009	0.046	0	4.1
Chocolate pudding—instant	34	0.85	0.82	5.89	28.4	0.065	0.009	0.039	0	3.1
Rice pudding	33	0.86	0.86	5.80	28.6	0.107	0.021	0.039	0	3.2
Butterscotch pudding pop	47	1.19	1.29	7.80	37.8	0.020	0.015	0.055	0	0.5
Chocolate pudding pop	49	1.34	1.34	8.20	42.8	0.179	0.015	0.055	0	0.5
Vanilla pudding pop	46	1.19	1.29	7.80	37.8	0.020	0.015	0.055	0	0.5

CEREALS (WITHOUT MILK)

	kCal	Protein (g)	Lipid (g)	CHO (g)	Ca (mg)	Fe (mg)	B₁ (mg)	B₂ (mg)	Fiber (g)	Cholesterol (mg)
All-Bran	70	3.99	0.50	21.0	23.00	4.49	0.369	0.429	8.490	0
Alpha Bits	111	2.20	0.60	24.6	7.99	1.80	0.399	0.399	0.650	0
Apple Jacks	110	1.50	0.10	25.7	2.99	4.49	0.399	0.399	0.200	0
Bran Buds	73	3.95	0.68	21.6	18.90	4.52	0.371	0.439	7.860	0
Bran Chex	90	2.95	0.81	22.6	16.80	4.51	0.347	0.150	5.200	0
Buc Wheats	110	2.00	1.00	24.0	59.90	8.09	0.674	0.764	2.000	0
C.W. Post—plain	126	2.54	4.44	20.3	13.70	4.50	0.380	0.438	0.643	0
C.W. Post w/raisins	123	2.45	4.05	20.3	14.00	4.51	0.358	0.413	0.660	0
Cap'n Crunch	120	1.46	2.60	22.9	4.60	7.53	0.506	0.544	0.709	0
Cap'n Crunchberries	118	1.46	2.35	23.0	8.91	7.32	0.478	0.543	0.324	0
Cap'n Crunch—peanut butter	125	2.03	3.64	21.5	5.67	7.37	0.486	0.567	0.324	0
Cheerios	110	4.24	1.77	19.4	47.30	4.44	0.394	0.394	3.000	0
Cocoa Krispies	109	1.50	0.39	25.2	4.73	1.81	0.394	0.394	0.354	0
Cocoa Pebbles	117	1.35	1.49	24.7	5.40	1.75	0.405	0.405	0.312	0
Corn Bran	98	1.97	1.02	23.9	32.30	9.60	0.299	0.551	5.390	0
Corn Chex	111	2.00	0.10	24.9	2.99	1.80	0.399	0.070	0.499	0
Corn flakes—Kellogg's	110	2.30	0.09	24.4	1.00	1.80	0.367	0.424	0.594	0
Corn flakes—Post Toasties	110	2.30	0.09	24.4	1.00	0.70	0.367	0.424	0.594	0
Corn grits—enriched yellow dry	105	2.49	0.33	22.5	0.55	1.10	0.182	0.107	3.270	0
Corn grits—enriched ckd	17	0.41	0.06	3.7	0.12	0.18	0.028	0.018	0.527	0
Cracklin' Oat Bran	108	2.60	4.16	19.4	18.90	1.80	0.378	0.425	4.280	0
Cream of Rice	15	0.24	0.01	3.3	0.93	0.05	0.012	0	0.163	0
Cream of Wheat	16	0.42	0.07	3.4	6.27	1.27	0.028	0.008	0.395	0
Crispy Wheat 'n Raisins	99	2.00	0.46	23.1	46.80	4.48	0.396	0.396	1.320	0
Farina—cooked	14	0.41	0.02	3.0	0.49	0.14	0.023	0.015	0.389	0
Fortified Oat Flakes	105	5.32	0.41	20.5	40.20	8.09	0.354	0.413	0.827	0
40% Bran Flakes—Kellogg's	91	3.60	0.54	22.2	13.80	8.14	0.369	0.430	0.850	0
40% Bran Flakes—Post	92	3.20	0.45	22.3	12.70	4.50	0.374	0.435	3.800	0
Froot Loops	111	1.70	1.00	25.0	2.99	4.49	0.399	0.399	0.299	0
Frosted Mini-Wheats	102	2.93	0.27	23.4	9.15	1.83	0.366	0.457	2.160	0
Frosted Rice Krispies	109	1.30	0.10	25.7	1.00	1.80	0.399	0.399	0.998	0
Fruit & Fiber w/apples	90	2.99	1.00	22.0	9.98	4.49	0.374	0.424	4.190	0
Fruit & Fiber w/dates	90	2.99	1.00	21.0	9.98	4.49	0.374	0.424	4.190	0
Fruitful Bran	92	2.50	0	22.5	8.34	6.75	0.313	0.354	4.170	0
Fruity Pebbles	115	1.10	1.50	24.4	2.99	1.80	0.399	0.399	0.226	0
Golden Grahams	109	1.60	1.09	24.1	17.40	4.50	0.363	0.436	1.670	0
Granola—homemade	138	3.49	7.69	15.6	17.70	1.12	0.170	0.072	2.970	0
Granola—Nature Valley	126	2.89	4.92	18.9	17.80	0.95	0.098	0.048	2.960	0
Grape Nuts	100	3.28	0.11	23.2	10.90	1.22	0.398	0.398	1.840	0
Grape Nuts Flakes	102	2.99	0.30	23.2	11.00	4.49	0.399	0.399	1.900	0
Honey & Nut Corn Flakes	113	1.80	1.50	23.3	2.99	1.80	0.399	0.399	0.299	0
Honey Bran	96	2.51	0.57	23.2	13.00	4.54	0.405	0.405	3.160	0
Honey Comb	111	1.68	0.52	25.3	5.15	1.80	0.387	0.387	0.387	0
Honey Nut Cheerios	107	3.09	0.69	22.8	19.80	4.47	0.344	0.430	0.790	0
King Vitamin	115	1.49	1.62	24.0	NA	17.10	0.124	1.430	0.135	0
Kix	109	2.49	0.70	23.3	34.80	8.06	0.398	0.398	0.398	0
Life	104	5.22	0.52	20.3	99.20	7.47	0.612	0.644	0.902	0
Lucky Charms	111	2.57	1.06	23.1	31.90	4.52	0.354	0.443	0.624	0
Malt-O-Meal	14	0.43	0.03	3.1	0.59	1.13	0.057	0.028	0.354	0
Maypo—cooked	1	0.02	0.01	0.1	0.52	0.04	0.003	0.003	0.012	0

CEREALS (WITHOUT MILK) — *continued*

	kCal	Protein (g)	Lipid (g)	CHO (g)	Ca (mg)	Fe (mg)	B_1 (mg)	B_2 (mg)	Fiber (g)	Cholesterol (mg)
Nutri-Grain—barley	106	3.11	0.21	23.4	7.60	1.00	0.346	0.415	1.660	0
Nutri-Grain—corn	108	2.30	0.68	24.0	0.68	0.60	0.338	0.405	1.750	0
Nutri-Grain—rye	102	2.48	0.21	24.0	5.67	0.80	0.354	0.425	2.160	0
Nutri-Grain—wheat	102	2.45	0.32	24.0	7.73	0.80	0.387	0.451	1.800	0
Oatmeal—prepared	18	0.73	0.29	3.1	2.42	0.19	0.032	0.006	0.497	0
Rolled Oats	109	4.55	1.78	19.0	14.70	1.19	0.206	0.038	3.090	0
Instant Oatmeal w/apples	26	0.74	0.30	5.0	30.00	1.15	0.091	0.053	0.552	0
Instant Oatmeal w/bran & raisins	23	0.71	0.28	4.4	25.20	1.10	0.081	0.092	0.480	0
Instant Oatmeal w/maple	30	0.84	0.35	5.8	29.60	1.16	0.097	0.059	0.530	0
Instant Oatmeal w/cinnamon & spice	31	0.85	0.34	6.2	30.30	1.17	0.099	0.60	0.510	0
Instant Oatmeal w/raisins & spice	29	0.77	0.32	5.7	29.60	1.18	0.092	0.065	0.556	0
100% Bran	77	3.57	1.42	20.7	19.80	3.49	0.687	0.773	8.380	0
100% Natural	135	3.02	6.02	18.0	48.90	0.83	0.085	0.150	3.390	0
100% Natural—w/apples	130	2.92	5.32	19.0	42.80	0.79	0.090	0.158	1.300	0
100% Natural—w/raisins & dates	128	2.89	5.23	18.7	41.20	0.80	0.077	0.165	1.080	0
Product 19	108	2.75	0.17	23.5	3.44	18.00	1.460	1.720	0.369	0
Puffed Rice	111	1.79	0.20	25.5	2.03	0.30	0.030	0.028	0.227	0
Puffed Wheat	104	4.25	0.24	22.4	7.09	1.35	0.047	0.070	5.430	0
Quisp	117	1.42	2.08	23.6	8.50	5.96	0.510	0.718	0.378	0
Raisin Bran—Kellogg's	91	3.07	0.46	21.4	14.50	13.90	0.293	0.332	3.410	0
Raisin Bran—Post	86	2.68	0.55	21.4	13.70	4.56	0.373	0.430	3.190	0
Raisins, Rice & Rye	96	1.60	0.06	24.2	6.16	3.45	0.308	0.370	0.308	0
Ralston—cooked	15	0.62	0.09	3.2	1.57	0.18	0.022	0.020	0.370	0
Rice Chex	112	1.49	1.00	25.2	3.88	1.79	0.400	0.298	1.840	0
Rice Krispies	109	1.86	0.20	24.2	3.91	1.76	0.391	0.391	0.312	0
Roman Meal—dry	91	4.07	0.60	20.4	18.40	1.31	0.142	0.069	0.905	0
Roman Meal—cooked	17	0.77	0.11	3.9	3.45	0.25	0.028	0.014	0.877	0
Shredded Wheat	102	3.09	0.71	22.5	11.00	1.20	0.070	0.080	3.100	0
Shredded wheat	97	3.06	0.45	16.4	11.20	0.89	0.082	0.075	2.900	0
Special K	111	5.58	0.10	21.3	7.97	4.48	0.399	0.399	0.266	0
Sugar Corn Pops	108	1.40	0.10	25.6	0.10	1.80	0.399	0.399	0.100	0
Sugar Frosted Flakes	108	1.46	0.08	25.7	0.81	1.78	0.405	0.405	0.446	0
Sugar Smacks	106	2.00	0.50	24.7	2.99	1.80	0.369	0.429	0.319	0
Super Golden Crisp	106	1.80	0.26	25.6	6.01	1.80	0.344	0.430	0.430	0
Team	111	1.82	0.48	24.3	4.05	1.73	0.371	0.425	0.270	0
Total	105	2.84	0.60	22.3	172.00	18.00	1.460	1.720	2.060	0
Trix	108	1.50	0.40	24.9	5.99	4.49	0.399	0.399	0.184	0
Wheat & Raisin Chex	97	2.68	0.21	22.6	NA	4.04	0.263	0.315	1.890	0
Wheat Chex	104	2.77	0.68	23.3	11.00	4.50	0.370	0.105	2.100	0
Wheat germ—toasted	108	8.25	3.09	14.0	12.50	2.19	0.474	0.233	3.910	0
Wheat germ w/brown sugar, honey	107	6.19	2.30	17.2	8.98	1.93	0.349	0.180	3.390	0
Wheatena—cooked	16	0.58	0.13	3.4	1.28	0.16	0.002	0.006	0.385	0
Wheaties	99	2.74	0.51	22.6	43.00	4.50	0.391	0.391	2.540	0
Whole wheat berries	16	0.54	0.11	3.2	1.70	0.17	0.023	0.006	0.680	0
Whole wheat cereal—cooked	18	0.58	0.11	3.9	1.99	0.18	0.020	0.014	0.457	0

CHEESE

	kCal	Protein (g)	Lipid (g)	CHO (g)	Ca (mg)	Fe (mg)	B_1 (mg)	B_2 (mg)	Fiber (g)	Cholesterol (mg)
American—processed	106	6.28	8.84	0.45	174	0.110	0.008	0.111	0	27.0
American cheese food—cold pack	94	5.23	6.78	2.36	145	0.240	0.009	0.274	0	18.0
American cheese spread	82	5.16	6.00	2.48	159	0.090	0.014	0.380	0	16.0
Blue	100	6.09	8.14	0.66	150	0.090	0.008	0.395	0	21.0
Brick	105	6.40	8.40	0.79	191	0.130	0.004	0.159	0	27.0
Brie	95	5.87	7.84	0.13	52	0.140	0.020	0.147	0	28.0
Camembert	85	5.60	6.86	0.13	110	0.094	0.008	0.138	0	20.0
Caraway	107	7.13	8.27	0.87	191	0.100	0.009	0.196	0	25.0
Cheddar	114	7.05	9.38	0.36	204	0.197	0.008	0.106	0	29.9
Cheshire	110	6.60	8.66	1.36	182	0.060	0.013	0.198	0	28.9
Colby	112	6.73	9.08	0.73	194	0.216	0.004	0.171	0	27.0
Cottage	29	3.54	1.20	0.76	17	0.040	0.006	0.115	0	4.2
Cottage—lowfat 2%	26	3.90	0.55	1.03	20	0.045	0.007	0.052	0	2.4
Cottage—lowfat 1%	21	3.51	0.29	0.77	18	0.040	0.006	0.115	0	1.3
Cottage—dry curd	24	4.89	0.12	0.52	9	0.065	0.007	0.004	0	2.0
Cottage—w/fruit	35	2.80	0.96	3.78	14	0.031	0.005	0.115	0	3.1
Cream	99	2.10	9.87	0.75	23	0.337	0.005	0.056	0	30.9
Edam	101	7.07	7.79	0.40	207	0.125	0.010	0.274	0	25.0
Feta	75	4.49	6.19	1.16	140	0.180	0.040	0.315	0	25.0
Fontina	110	7.25	8.62	0.44	156	0.060	0.006	NA	0	32.9
Gjetost	132	2.74	8.32	12.00	113	0.130	0.009	0.170	0	25.0
Gorgonzola	111	6.99	8.98	0	149	0.120	0.010	0.512	0	25.0
Gouda	101	7.06	7.72	0.63	198	0.070	0.009	0.232	0	31.9
Gruyere	117	8.44	9.05	0.10	286	0.060	0.017	0.095	0	30.9
Liederkranz	87	4.99	7.99	0	110	0.120	0.010	0.389	0	21.0
Limburger	93	5.67	7.59	0.14	141	0.040	0.023	0.227	0	26.0
Monterey jack	106	6.93	8.56	0.19	212	0.200	0.004	0.119	0	26.0
Mozzarella—skim, low moist	80	7.60	4.67	0.89	207	0.076	0.006	0.150	0	15.0
Mozzarella—whole milk, regular	80	5.50	5.75	0.63	147	0.050	0.004	0.106	0	22.0
Mozzarella—whole milk, moist	90	6.10	7.19	0.43	163	0.060	0.005	0.119	0	25.0
Muenster	104	6.40	8.42	0.32	203	0.125	0.004	0.178	0	27.0
Neufchatel	74	2.82	6.70	0.83	21	0.080	0.004	0.113	0	22.0
Parmesan—hard	111	10.00	7.30	0.91	335	0.230	0.010	0.453	0	19.0
Parmesan—grated	129	11.80	8.50	1.06	389	0.270	0.013	0.527	0	22.0
Pimento processed	106	6.26	8.82	0.49	174	0.120	0.008	0.404	0	27.0
Port du salut	100	6.73	7.99	0.16	84	0.140	0.004	0.151	0	34.9
Provolone	100	7.13	7.54	0.61	214	0.146	0.005	0.248	0	20.0
Ricotta—part skim	39	3.23	2.25	1.45	77	0.126	0.006	0.052	0	8.8
Ricotta—whole milk	49	3.19	3.68	0.86	59	0.108	0.004	0.024	0	14.3
Romano	110	9.00	7.63	1.03	301	0.230	0.010	0.339	0	28.9
Romano—grated	128	10.50	8.86	1.20	350	0.270	0.013	0.394	0	32.9
Roquefort	105	6.10	8.93	0.57	188	0.172	0.010	0.512	0	26.0
Swiss	107	8.03	7.79	0.96	272	0.050	0.006	0.074	0	26.0
Swiss processed	95	7.00	6.97	0.60	219	0.170	0.004	0.078	0	24.0

FISH

	kCal	Protein (g)	Lipid (g)	CHO (g)	Ca (mg)	Fe (mg)	B₁ (mg)	B₂ (mg)	Fiber (g)	Cholesterol (mg)
Bass—freshwater raw	32	5.36	1.05	0	22.7	0.422	0.028	0.009	0	19.3
Bluefish—baked/broiled	45	7.43	1.42	0	2.6	0.174	0.022	0.030	0	17.9
Bluefish—fried in crumbs	58	6.44	2.78	1.33	2.3	0.151	0.017	0.023	0	17
Bluefish—raw	35	5.67	1.20	0	2.0	0.136	0.016	0.023	0	16.7
Carp—raw	36	5.05	1.59	0	11.6	0.352	0.013	0.011	0	18.7
Catfish—channel—raw	33	5.16	1.20	0	11.3	0.275	0.013	0.030	0	16.4
Cod—baked w/butter	37	6.46	0.94	0	5.7	0.139	0.025	0.022	0	17.0
Cod—batter-fried	56	5.56	2.92	2.13	22.7	0.142	0.011	0.011	0	15.6
Cod—baked/broiled	30	6.46	0.24	0	4.0	0.139	0.025	0.022	0	15.6
Cod—poached	29	6.24	0.24	0	4.0	0.139	0.025	0.022	0	15.6
Cod—steamed	29	6.24	0.24	0	4.0	0.139	0.025	0.022	0	15.9
Cod—smoked	22	5.19	0.17	0	4.0	0.113	0.023	0.020	0	14.2
Cod—Atlantic—raw	23	5.05	0.19	0	4.5	0.108	0.022	0.018	0	12.2
Cod liver oil	255	0	28.40	0	0	0	0	0	0	162.0
Eel—smoked	94	5.27	7.88	0.23	26.9	0.198	0.040	0.099	0	19.8
Haddock—breaded/fried	58	5.67	3.00	2.33	11.3	0.384	0.020	0.033	0.01	18.3
Haddock—smoked	33	7.14	0.27	0	13.9	0.397	0.013	0.014	0	21.8
Haddock—raw	22	5.36	0.20	0	9.4	0.298	0.010	0.010	0	16.2
Herring—pickled	74	4.03	5.10	2.73	21.8	0.346	0.010	0.039	0	3.7
Herring—smoked/ kippered	62	6.97	3.52	0	23.8	0.428	0.036	0.090	0	22.7
Herring—canned w/liquid	59	5.64	3.86	0	41.7	0.879	0.007	0.051	0	27.5
Mackerel—fried	49	7.00	2.35	0	4.3	0.445	0.045	0.116	0	19.8
Mackerel—Atlantic— baked/broiled	74	6.78	5.05	0	4.3	0.445	0.045	0.117	0	21.3
Mackerel—Atlantic—raw	58	5.27	3.94	0	3.4	0.462	0.050	0.088	0	19.8
Mackerel—Pacific—raw	45	6.12	2.84	0	2.3	0.567	0.043	0.096	0	22.7
Northern pike—raw	25	5.47	0.20	0	16.2	0.156	0.017	0.018	0	11.0
Ocean perch—breaded/ fried	62	5.34	3.67	2.33	30.7	0.400	0.033	0.037	0.03	15.3
Pollock—baked/broiled	28	6.60	0.31	0	19.3	0.149	0.014	0.057	0	19.8
Pollock—poached	36	6.60	0.31	0	17.0	0.149	0.010	0.050	0	19.8
Salmon—broiled/baked	61	7.74	3.10	0	2.0	0.157	0.061	0.048	0	24.7
Coho salmon—steamed/ poached	52	7.77	2.14	0	8.22	0.252	0.057	0.031	0	13.9
Smoked salmon— Chinook	33	5.17	1.22	0	03.0	0.240	0.007	0.029	0	6.7
Atlantic salmon— small can	36	5.05	1.62	0	3.1	0.204	0.057	0.097	0	17.0
Pink salmon—raw	33	5.64	0.98	0	11.3	0.218	0.040	0.057	0	14.7
Sardines	59	7.00	3.24	0	108.0	0.826	0.023	0.064	0	40.4
Sea trout steelhead—raw	30	4.73	1.02	0	4.8	0.077	0.023	0.057	0	23.5
Sea trout steelhead— cooked	37	6.07	1.42	0	5.7	0.088	0.024	0.064	0	32.3
Shad—baked with bacon	57	6.58	3.20	0	6.8	0.170	0.037	0.074	0	17.0
Smelt—rainbow—raw	28	4.99	0.69	0	17.0	0.255	0.016	0.034	0	19.8
Snapper—baked or broiled	36	7.46	0.49	0	11.3	0.068	0.015	0.021	0	13.3
Snapper—raw	28	5.81	0.38	0	9.1	0.051	0.013	0.017	0	10.5
Sole/flounder—baked w/butter	40	5.34	2.00	0	5.3	0.093	0.023	0.032	0	22.7
Sole/flounder—baked/ broiled	33	6.84	0.43	0	5.3	0.093	0.023	0.032	0	19.3

FISH—*continued*

	kCal	Protein (g)	Lipid (g)	CHO (g)	Ca (mg)	Fe (mg)	B₁ (mg)	B₂ (mg)	Fiber (g)	Cholesterol (mg)
Sole/flounder—batter-fried	83	4.47	5.10	4.07	16.7	0.239	0.057	0.042	0.01	15.0
Sole/flounder—breaded/fried	53	4.96	2.55	2.54	11.3	0.128	0.037	0.034	0	15.0
Sole/flounder—steamed	26	5.67	0.33	0	4.5	0.079	0.017	0.027	0	14.7
Sole/flounder—raw	26	5.33	0.34	0	5.1	0.102	0.025	0.022	0	13.6
Lemon sole—raw	23	4.85	0.21	0	4.8	0.088	0.026	0.023	0	17.0
Lemon sole—fried w/crumbs	56	4.56	3.12	2.64	26.9	0.176	0.020	0.023	0	18.4
Lemon sole—steamed	26	5.84	0.26	0	6.0	0.147	0.026	0.026	0	17.0
Swordfish—raw	34	5.61	1.14	0	1.1	0.230	0.010	0.027	0	11.0
Swordfish—broiled/baked	44	7.20	1.46	0	1.7	0.295	0.012	0.033	0	14.2
Trout—baked/broiled	43	7.47	1.22	0	24.3	0.690	0.024	0.064	0	20.7
Tuna—oil pack	56	8.26	2.34	0	3.8	0.395	0.010	0.030	0	5.0
Tuna—water pack	37	8.38	0.14	0	3.4	0.409	0.010	0.033	0	16.0
Tuna—raw	31	6.63	0.27	0	4.5	0.207	0.123	0.013	0	12.8
Whiting—flour/bread-fried	54	5.13	1.56	1.98	11.3	0.198	0.023	0.020	0	18.4

FRUITS

	kCal	Protein (g)	Lipid (g)	CHO (g)	Ca (mg)	Fe (mg)	B₁ (mg)	B₂ (mg)	Fiber (g)	Cholesterol (mg)
Apple w/peel	16	0.055	0.100	4.31	2.05	0.051	0.005	0.004	0.709	0
Apple slices w/peel—fresh	17	0.054	0.100	4.33	2.06	0.052	0.005	0.004	0.709	0
Apple juice—canned/bottled	13	0.017	0.032	3.32	1.94	0.105	0.006	0.005	0.034	0
Apple juice—frozen concentrate	47	0.144	0.105	11.60	5.78	0.258	0.003	0.015	0.089	0
Applesauce—sweetened	22	0.052	0.052	5.67	1.11	0.111	0.003	0.008	0.397	0
Apricot—fresh halves	14	0.397	0.110	3.15	4.02	0.154	0.009	0.011	0.538	0
Apricot halves—light syrup	18	0.150	0.013	4.67	3.34	0.110	0.005	0.006	0.319	0
Apricot nectar—canned	16	0.104	0.025	4.08	2.03	0.108	0.003	0.004	0.170	0
Avocado—average	46	0.563	0.340	2.10	3.07	0.284	0.030	0.035	2.720	0
Banana—fresh slices	26	0.293	0.136	6.63	1.74	0.088	0.013	0.028	0.578	0
Blackberries—canned	26	0.370	0.040	6.54	5.98	0.184	0.008	0.011	1.011	0
Blackberries—fresh	15	0.205	0.110	3.62	9.06	0.158	0.008	0.011	1.910	0
Blackberries—frozen	18	0.334	0.122	4.45	8.26	0.173	0.008	0.013	1.460	0
Blueberries—fresh	16	0.190	0.108	4.00	1.76	0.047	0.014	0.014	0.763	0
Blueberries-frozen unsweetened	14	0.119	0.181	3.46	2.19	0.051	0.009	0.010	0.658	0
Boysenberries—frozen	14	0.314	0.075	3.46	7.73	0.240	0.015	0.010	1.100	0
Sour cherries—frozen	13	0.260	0.124	3.13	3.66	0.150	0.012	0.010	0.384	0
Sweet cherries—fresh	20	0.340	0.272	4.69	4.10	0.110	0.014	0.017	0.430	0
Sweet cherries—frozen	25	0.325	0.037	6.34	3.39	0.099	0.008	0.013	0.224	0
Cranberries—whole—raw	14	0.110	0.057	3.58	2.09	0.057	0.009	0.006	1.190	0
Cranberry/apple juice	19	0.015	0.090	4.82	2.02	0.017	0.001	0.006	0.070	0
Cranberry juice cocktail	16	0.009	0.015	4.03	0.90	0.043	0.002	0.002	0.085	0
Date—whole—each	78	0.557	0.127	20.80	9.22	0.342	0.026	0.028	2.300	0

FRUITS— *continued*

	kCal	Protein (g)	Lipid (g)	CHO (g)	Ca (mg)	Fe (mg)	B_1 (mg)	B_2 (mg)	Fiber (g)	Cholesterol (mg)
Figs—medium—fresh	21	0.215	0.085	5.44	10.20	0.102	0.017	0.014	1.050	0
Fig—dried—each	72	0.864	0.330	18.50	40.80	0.634	0.020	0.025	3.140	0
Fruit cocktail—heavy syrup	21	0.111	0.020	5.36	1.78	0.081	0.005	0.005	0.280	0
Fruit cocktail—light syrup	16	0.114	0.020	4.23	1.80	0.082	0.005	0.005	0.284	0
Grapefruit half—pink/red	9	0.157	0.028	2.18	3.00	0.034	0.010	0.006	0.369	0
Grapefruit half—white	10	0.195	0.029	2.38	3.36	0.017	0.010	0.006	0.368	0
Grapefuit sections/fresh	9	0.179	0.028	2.29	3.33	0.025	0.010	0.006	0.370	0
Grapefruit sections—canned	17	0.160	0.028	4.38	4.02	0.114	0.010	0.006	0.313	0
Grapefruit juice—fresh	11	0.142	0.029	2.60	2.53	0.056	0.011	0.006	0.113	0
Grapefruit juice—sweetened	13	0.164	0.026	3.15	2.27	0.102	0.011	0.007	0.076	0
Grapefruit juice—unsweetened	11	0.148	0.028	2.54	1.95	0.057	0.012	0.006	0.077	0
Grapefruit juice—frozen concentrate	41	0.548	0.137	9.86	7.67	0.140	0.041	0.022	0.383	0
Grapes—Thompson	20	0.188	0.163	5.03	3.01	0.073	0.026	0.016	0.333	0
Grape juice—bottled/canned	17	0.158	0.021	4.25	2.47	0.068	0.007	0.010	0.141	0
Grape juice—frozen concentrate	51	0.184	0.088	12.60	3.68	0.102	0.015	0.026	0.492	0
Grape juice—prep frozen	15	0.053	0.026	3.62	1.13	0.029	0.004	0.007	0.142	0
Kiwi fruit	17	0.280	0.127	4.22	7.46	0.112	0.007	0.015	0.962	0
Lemon—fresh wo/peel	8	0.313	0.083	2.64	7.33	0.171	0.011	0.006	0.582	0
Lemon juice—fresh	7	0.107	0.081	2.45	2.09	0.009	0.008	0.003	0.099	0
Lemon juice—bottled	6	0.114	0.081	1.84	3.02	0.036	0.012	0.003	0.085	0
Lime—fresh	9	0.199	0.055	2.99	9.30	0.169	0.008	0.006	0.228	0
Lime juice—fresh	8	0.124	0.029	2.56	2.54	0.009	0.006	0.003	0.113	0
Lime juice—bottled	6	0.115	0.115	1.84	3.46	0.069	0.009	0.001	0.099	0
Loganberries—fresh	20	0.430	0.088	3.69	8.50	0.181	0.014	0.010	1.760	0
Loganberries—frozen	16	0.430	0.089	3.68	7.33	0.181	0.014	0.010	1.760	0
Mango—fresh—slices	19	0.146	0.077	4.83	2.92	0.360	0.016	0.016	0.997	0
Mango—fresh—whole	19	0.145	0.078	4.82	2.88	0.356	0.016	0.016	1.010	0
Cantaloupe—cubes	10	0.250	0.079	2.37	3.19	0.060	0.006	0.006	0.284	0
Casaba melon—cubes	8	0.255	0.028	1.75	1.50	0.113	0.017	0.006	0.284	0
Honeydew melon—cubes	10	0.128	0.028	2.60	1.67	0.020	0.022	0.005	0.307	0
Melon balls—mixed—frozen	9	0.239	0.023	2.25	2.79	0.008	0.005	0.006	0.295	0
Mixed fruit—dried	69	0.697	0.139	18.20	10.60	0.767	0.012	0.045	1.220	0
Mixed fruit—frozen—thawed	28	0.397	0.052	6.87	2.04	0.079	0.005	0.010	0.386	0
Nectarine	14	0.267	0.129	3.34	1.25	0.044	0.005	0.012	0.554	0
Orange	13	0.266	0.035	3.33	11.30	0.029	0.025	0.011	0.680	0
Orange sections—fresh	13	0.266	0.035	3.34	11.30	0.029	0.025	0.011	0.680	0
Mandarin oranges—canned	17	0.113	0.011	4.61	2.03	0.101	0.015	0.012	0.478	0
Orange juice—fresh	13	0.199	0.057	2.95	3.09	0.057	0.025	0.008	0.113	0
Oranged juice—frozen concentrate	45	0.679	0.059	10.80	9.05	0.099	0.079	0.018	0.313	0

FRUITS—*continued*

	kCal	Protein (g)	Lipid (g)	CHO (g)	Ca (mg)	Fe (mg)	B₁ (mg)	B₂ (mg)	Fiber (g)	Cholesterol (mg)
Orange juice—frozen	13	0.191	0.016	3.05	2.50	0.031	0.023	0.005	0.057	0
Papaya—whole fresh	11	0.173	0.040	2.78	6.71	0.028	0.008	0.009	0.482	0
Papaya—slices fresh	12	0.174	0.040	2.77	6.68	0.060	0.008	0.009	0.482	0
Papaya nectar—canned	16	0.049	0.043	4.12	2.72	0.098	0.002	0.001	0.170	0
Peaches—fresh	12	0.199	0.026	3.14	1.30	0.031	0.005	0.012	0.489	0
Peach slices—frozen/ thawed	27	0.177	0.037	6.80	0.91	0.105	0.004	0.010	0.467	0
Peach halves—heavy syrup	21	0.130	0.028	5.67	1.05	0.077	0.003	0.007	0.315	0
Peach halves—light syrup	15	0.126	0.010	4.13	1.05	0.101	0.002	0.007	0.402	0
Peach halves—dried	68	0.020	0.216	17.40	8.07	1.150	0	0.060	2.330	0
Peach nectar—canned	15	0.076	0.006	3.95	1.48	0.054	0	0.004	0.170	0
Pears—Bartlett	17	0.111	0.113	4.29	3.24	0.070	0.006	0.011	0.779	0
Pear halves—heavy syrup	21	0.057	0.036	5.42	1.44	0.061	0.004	0.006	0.395	0
Pear halves—light syrup	16	0.054	0.007	4.30	1.44	0.082	0.003	0.005	0.395	0
Pear nectar—canned	17	0.030	0.003	4.47	1.25	0.073	0	0.004	0.204	0
Pineapple slices—heavy syrup	22	0.098	0.034	5.72	3.91	0.108	0.025	0.007	0.270	0
Pineapple slices—light syrup	15	0.103	0.034	3.81	3.91	0.110	0.026	0.007	0.268	0
Pineapple—frozen sweetened	24	0.113	0.029	6.29	2.55	0.113	0.028	0.009	0.496	0
Pineapple juice—frozen concentrate	51	0.369	0.029	12.60	11.00	0.255	0.065	0.017	0.255	0
Plums	16	0.223	0.176	3.69	1.29	0.030	0.012	0.027	0.550	0
Plums—canned—heavy syrup	25	0.102	0.028	6.59	2.53	0.238	0.005	0.010	0.434	0
Plums—canned—light syrup	18	0.105	0.029	4.61	2.70	0.243	0.005	0.011	0.444	0
Prunes—dried	68	0.739	0.145	17.80	14.50	0.702	0.023	0.046	2.700	0
Prune juice—bottled	20	0.172	0.009	4.95	3.43	0.334	0.005	0.020	0.310	0
Raisins—seedless	85	0.914	0.130	22.50	13.90	0.594	0.044	0.025	1.670	0
Raspberries—fresh	14	0.256	0.157	3.27	6.22	0.162	0.009	0.026	1.770	0
Raspberries—canned w/liquid	26	0.235	0.034	6.62	2.99	0.120	0.006	0.009	1.200	0
Raspberries—frozen	29	0.197	0.044	7.42	4.30	0.184	0.005	0.013	1.300	0
Rhubarb—raw—diced	6	0.253	0.056	1.29	39.50	0.062	0.006	0.009	0.737	0
Rhubarb—cooked w/sugar	33	0.111	0.013	8.85	41.10	0.060	0.005	0.006	0.624	0
Strawberries—fresh	9	0.173	0.105	2.00	4.00	0.108	0.006	0.019	0.736	0
Strawberries—frozen	10	0.120	0.030	2.59	4.38	0.213	0.006	0.010	0.736	0
Tangerine—fresh	13	0.179	0.054	3.17	4.05	0.028	0.030	0.006	0.574	0
Tangerines—canned— light syrup	17	0.127	0.028	4.61	2.03	0.105	0.015	0.012	0.453	0
Watermelon	9	0.175	0.121	2.04	2.24	0.048	0.023	0.006	0.114	0

MEATS

	kCal	Protein (g)	Lipid (g)	CHO (g)	Ca (mg)	Fe (mg)	B_1 (mg)	B_2 (mg)	Fiber (g)	Cholesterol (mg)
Beef chuck—pot roasted	108	7.20	8.64	0	3.67	0.840	0.020	0.065	0	29.0
Beef chuck—pot roasted lean	77	8.80	4.34	0	3.67	1.040	0.024	0.080	0	30.0
Beef round—pot roasted lean & fat	74	8.44	4.20	0	1.67	0.920	0.020	0.069	0	27.0
Beef round—pot roasted lean	63	8.97	2.74	0	1.33	0.980	0.021	0.074	0	27.0
Ground beef—lean	77	7.00	5.34	0	3.00	0.600	0.013	0.060	0	24.7
Ground beef—regular	82	6.67	5.94	0	3.00	0.700	0.010	0.053	0	25.3
Sirloin steak—lean	57	8.10	2.53	0	2.33	0.700	0.026	0.056	0	21.7
T-bone steak—lean & fat	92	6.80	6.97	0	2.67	0.720	0.026	0.059	0	23.7
Beef lunchmeat—thin-sliced	50	7.96	1.09	1.62	2.99	0.759	0.023	0.054	0	12.0
Beef lunchmeat—loaf/roll	87	4.06	7.42	0.82	2.99	0.659	0.030	0.062	0	18.0
Beef rib—oven roasted—lean	68	7.70	3.90	0	3.34	0.740	0.023	0.060	0	22.7
Beef round—oven roasted—lean	54	8.14	2.12	0	1.67	0.834	0.028	0.076	0	23.0
Beef rump roast—lean only	51	8.40	1.89	0	1.13	0.567	0.026	0.049	0	19.6
Beef brains—pan-fried	56	3.57	4.50	0	2.67	0.630	0.037	0.074	0	566.0
Beef heart	47	8.17	1.59	0.12	1.67	2.130	0.040	0.436	0	54.7
Beef kidney	41	7.23	0.97	0.27	5.00	2.070	0.054	1.150	0	110.0
Beef liver—fried	61	7.57	2.27	2.23	3.00	1.780	0.060	1.170	0	137.0
Beef tongue—cooked	80	6.27	5.87	0.09	2.00	0.960	0.009	0.009	0	30.4
Beef tripe—raw	28	4.14	1.12	0	36.00	0.553	0.002	0.047	0	26.9
Beef tripe—pickled	17	3.29	0.40	0	25.00	0.389	0	0.028	0	15.0
Corned beef—canned	71	7.67	4.24	0	5.67	0.590	0.006	0.042	0	24.3
Corned beef hash—canned	49	2.35	1.29	2.82	3.74	0.567	0.016	0.052	0.153	17.0
Beef—dried/cured	47	8.24	1.10	0.44	2.00	1.280	0.050	0.230	0	45.9
Beef & vegetable stew	26	1.85	1.27	1.74	3.36	0.336	0.017	0.020	0.393	8.2
Beef stew—canned	22	1.64	0.88	2.06	2.66	0.368	0.008	0.014	0.150	1.7
Burrito—beef & bean	63	3.40	2.84	6.48	26.70	0.437	0.042	0.047	0.810	8.4
Tostada w/beans & beef	49	2.72	3.06	2.98	27.50	0.319	0.012	0.036	0.583	9.1
Beef + macaroni + tomato	24	1.25	0.73	3.16	3.81	0.300	0.024	0.021	0.291	2.8
Beef enchilada	69	3.09	3.26	3.69	60.20	0.418	0.017	0.039	0.465	8.9
Frankfurter—beef	92	3.20	8.36	0.68	3.48	0.378	0.014	0.029	0	13.4
Frankfurter—beef & pork	91	3.20	8.26	0.73	2.98	0.328	0.056	0.034	0	14.4
Beef pot pie—frozen	52	1.99	2.73	4.77	2.42	0.436	0.022	0.018	0.109	5.0
Beef pie—recipe	70	2.84	4.05	5.27	3.92	0.513	0.039	0.039	0.155	5.7
Beef taco	75	4.94	4.80	3.67	30.90	0.469	0.010	0.049	0.407	16.2
Chicken meat—all-fried	62	8.67	2.59	0.48	4.86	0.383	0.024	0.056	0.002	26.5
Chicken meat—all-roasted	54	8.20	2.10	0	4.25	0.342	0.020	0.050	0	25.3
Chicken meat—all-stewed	50	7.74	1.90	0	4.05	0.330	0.014	0.046	0	23.5
Boned chicken w/broth	47	6.17	2.26	0	3.99	0.439	0.004	0.037	0	17.6
Chicken—dark meat—fried	68	8.22	3.30	0.74	5.06	0.423	0.026	0.070	0.002	27.3
Chicken—dark meat—roasted	58	7.76	2.75	0	4.25	0.377	0.020	0.064	0	26.3
Chicken—dark meat—stewed	55	7.37	2.55	0	4.05	0.385	0.016	0.057	0	24.9

MEATS — continued

	kCal	Protein (g)	Lipid (g)	CHO (g)	Ca (mg)	Fe (mg)	B₁ (mg)	B₂ (mg)	Fiber (g)	Cholesterol (mg)
Chicken—light meat—fried	54	9.31	1.57	0.12	4.45	0.322	0.020	0.036	0	25.3
Chicken—light meat—roasted	49	8.77	1.28	0	4.25	0.302	0.018	0.033	0	23.9
Chicken—light meat—stewed	45	8.18	1.17	0	3.64	0.265	0.012	0.033	0	21.7
Chicken breast—no skin	47	8.80	0.99	0	4.29	0.295	0.020	0.032	0	24.0
Chicken breast meat—stewed	43	8.20	0.86	0	3.58	0.250	0.012	0.034	0	21.8
Chicken drumstick—batter fried	76	6.22	4.45	2.36	4.73	0.382	0.032	0.061	0.008	24.4
Chicken drumstick—roasted	61	7.69	3.16	0	3.27	0.376	0.020	0.061	0	26.2
Chicken wing—batter-fried	92	5.64	6.19	3.10	5.79	0.365	0.030	0.043	0.012	22.6
Chicken wing—flour-fried	91	7.40	6.28	0.67	4.43	0.354	0.017	0.039	0.009	23.0
Chicken wing—roasted	83	7.48	5.53	0	4.17	0.359	0.012	0.037	0	24.2
Chicken gizzards—simmered	44	7.73	1.04	0.32	2.58	1.180	0.008	0.070	0	54.9
Chicken hearts—simmered	52	7.49	2.23	0.03	5.27	2.560	0.017	0.206	0	68.7
Chicken livers—simmered	44	6.90	1.55	0.25	4.05	2.400	0.043	0.496	0	179.0
Chicken roll—light meat	45	5.52	2.08	0..69	11.90	0.274	0.018	0.037	0	13.9
Chicken frankfurter	73	3.67	5.52	1.93	27.00	0.567	0.019	0.033	0	28.4
Chicken a la king	54	3.12	3.93	1.93	14.70	0.289	0.012	0.049	0.154	25.6
Chicken + noodles	43	2.60	2.13	3.07	3.07	0.278	0.006	0.020	0.142	12.2
Chicken chow mein	29	2.60	1.25	1.13	6.58	0.284	0.009	0.026	0.466	8.5
Chicken curry	26	2.21	1.53	0.64	2.52	0.170	0.009	0.019	0.033	5.3
Chicken frankfurter	72	3.67	5.52	1.93	27.00	0.567	0.019	0.033	0	28.4
Chicken pot pie—frozen	53	1.84	2.84	5.08	3.70	0.382	0.020	0.020	0.210	4.9
Chicken roll—light meat	45	5.52	2.08	0.69	11.90	0.274	0.018	0.037	0	13.9
Chicken salad w/celery	97	3.82	8.90	0.47	5.92	0.239	0.012	0.028	0.109	17.3
Chicken patty sandwich	79	4.48	4.06	6.10	7.95	0.338	0.052	0.047	0.244	12.3
Chicken broth—from dry	2	0.16	0.13	0.17	1.74	0.009	0	0.004	0.001	0.1
Chicken broth—from cube	2	0.11	0.04	0.18	0.04	0.014	0.001	0.003	0	0.1
Chicken noodle soup	9	0.48	0.29	1.10	2.00	0.092	0.006	0.007	0.085	0.8
Tostada w/beans/chicken	45	3.50	2.06	3.38	29.30	0.305	0.013	0.034	0.668	9.6
Chicken taco	63	5.60	3.03	3.67	31.60	0.237	0.014	0.043	0.407	16.5
Chicken enchilada	64	3.38	2.48	3.69	60.50	0.359	0.018	0.036	0.465	9.1
Turkey dark meat—roasted	53	8.10	2.05	0	9.11	0.662	0.018	0.070	0	24.0
Turkey white meat—roasted	44	8.48	0.91	0	5.47	0.380	0.017	0.037	0	19.6
Turkey breast—barbecued	40	6.39	1.40	0	2.00	0.120	0.010	0.030	0	16.0
Turkey gizzards	46	8.34	1.10	0.17	4.32	1.540	0.009	0.093	0	65.6
Turkey hearts	50	7.58	1.73	0.58	3.72	1.950	0.019	0.250	0	64.0
Turkey livers	48	6.80	1.69	0.97	3.02	2.210	0.015	0.404	0	177.0
Turkey loaf	31	6.38	0.45	0	2.00	0.113	0.011	0.030	0	11.6
Turkey roll	41	5.27	2.03	0.15	11.40	0.358	0.025	0.064	0	11.9
Turkey bologna	56	3.86	4.27	0.27	23.40	0.432	0.015	0.047	0	28.0
Turkey frankfurter	64	4.05	5.22	0.42	36.50	0.485	0.023	0.050	0	24.6
Turkey ham	36	5.37	1.49	0.42	2.49	0.776	0.020	0.075	0	15.9
Turkey pastrami	37	5.22	1.75	0.43	2.49	0.403	0.022	0.075	0	14.9
Turkey salami	55	4.62	3.89	0.15	5.47	0.463	0.029	0.075	0	22.9
Turkey pot pie—frozen	51	1.80	2.75	4.65	7.79	0.256	0.020	0.020	0.110	2.4

EGGS

	kCal	Protein (g)	Lipid (g)	CHO (g)	Ca (mg)	Fe (mg)	B₁ (mg)	B₂ (mg)	Fiber (g)	Cholesterol (mg)
Egg white, cooked	13	2.68	0	0.33	3.20	0.008	0.002	0.072	0	0
Egg yolk, cooked	108	4.76	8.73	0.07	44.40	1.620	0.044	0.121	0	355.0
Egg, fried in butter	56	3.54	3.45	0.38	15.70	0.536	0.018	0.148	0	129.0
Egg, hard cooked	40	3.52	2.79	0.34	13.80	0.474	0.014	0.132	0	113.0
Egg, poached	40	3.50	2.79	0.34	13.80	0.474	0.014	0.132	0	113.0
Egg, scrambled milk + butter	40	2.88	2.57	0.61	23.90	0.412	0.013	0.106	0	93.9
Egg raw—large	40	3.52	2.79	0.34	13.80	0.474	0.017	0.139	0	113.0
Egg white—raw	13	2.68	0	0.33	3.20	0.008	0.002	0.075	0	0
Egg yolk, raw	108	4.76	8.73	0.07	44.40	1.620	0.051	0.126	0	355.0
Egg substitute, frozen	45	3.20	3.15	0.91	20.80	0.562	0.034	0.110	0	0.5
Egg substitute, powder	125	15.60	3.66	6.12	90.70	0.879	0.062	0.493	0	162.0

DAIRY PRODUCTS

	kCal	Protein (g)	Lipid (g)	CHO (g)	Ca (mg)	Fe (mg)	B₁ (mg)	B₂ (mg)	Fiber (g)	Cholesterol (mg)
Milk—1% lowfat	12	0.93	0.30	1.36	34.9	0.014	0.011	0.047	0	1.16
Milk—2% lowfat	14	0.94	0.56	1.36	34.5	0.012	0.011	0.047	0	2.56
Milk—skim	10	0.97	0.05	1.38	34.9	0.012	0.010	0.040	0	0.46
Milk—whole	17	0.93	0.95	1.32	33.8	0.014	0.010	0.046	0	3.83
Buttermilk	12	0.94	0.25	1.35	33.0	0.014	0.010	0.044	0	1.04
Milk—instant nonfat dry	102	9.96	0.21	14.80	349.0	0.088	0.117	0.496	0	5.00
Canned skim milk—evaporated	22	2.11	0.06	3.22	82.0	0.078	0.013	0.088	0	1.11
Canned whole milk—evaporated	38	1.91	2.20	2.81	73.9	0.054	0.014	0.090	0	8.33
Carob flavor mix—powder	106	0.47	0.05	26.50	0	1.300	0.002	0	4.020	0
Chocolate milk—1%	18	0.92	0.28	2.96	32.5	0.068	0.010	0.047	0.425	0.79
Chocolate milk—2%	20	0.91	0.57	2.95	32.2	0.068	0.010	0.046	0.425	1.93
Chocolate milk—whole	24	0.90	0.96	2.94	31.8	0.068	0.010	0.046	0.425	3.52
Hot cocoa—with whole milk	25	1.03	1.03	2.93	33.8	0.088	0.012	0.049	0.340	3.74
Instant breakfast w/2% milk	25	1.52	0.47	3.50	31.0	0.807	0.040	0.048	0	1.82
Instant breakfast w/1% milk	23	1.51	0.25	3.50	31.3	0.807	0.040	0.048	0	1.00
Instant breakfast w/skim milk	22	1.55	0.04	3.50	31.4	0.804	0.039	0.041	0	0.40
Instant breakfast w/whole milk	28	1.51	0.82	3.47	30.4	0.807	0.040	0.047	0	3.33
Egg nog	38	1.08	2.12	3.84	36.8	0.057	0.010	0.054	0	16.60
Kefir	20	1.13	0.55	1.07	42.6	0.060	0.055	0.054	0	1.22
Malt powder—chocolate flavored	107	1.49	1.08	24.80	17.6	0.648	0.049	0.057	0.540	1.35
Malted milk powder	117	3.12	2.30	21.50	85.0	0.209	0.143	0.260	0.405	5.40
Malted milk drink—chocolate	25	1.00	0.95	3.19	32.5	0.064	0.014	0.047	0.043	3.64

DAIRY PRODUCTS—*continued*

	kCal	Protein (g)	Lipid (g)	CHO (g)	Ca (mg)	Fe (mg)	B₁ (mg)	B₂ (mg)	Fiber (g)	Cholesterol (mg)
Chocolate milkshake	36	0.96	1.05	5.80	32.0	0.088	0.016	0.069	0.035	3.70
Strawberry milkshake	32	0.95	0.80	5.35	32.0	0.030	0.013	0.055	0.024	3.10
Vanilla milkshake	32	0.98	0.84	5.09	34.5	0.026	0.013	0.052	0.019	3.20
Ovaltine powder—chocolate flavored	102	2.00	0.85	23.70	134.0	6.190	0.719	0.772	0.013	0
Ovaltine powder—malt flavored	104	2.53	0.24	23.60	106.0	5.820	0.772	1.010	0.040	0
Ovaltine drink—chocolate flavored	24	1.02	0.94	3.12	41.9	0.510	0.067	0.104	0.001	3.53
Ovaltine drink—malt flavored	24	1.06	0.89	3.10	39.7	0.480	0.072	0.124	0.003	3.53
Milk—goat	20	1.00	1.17	1.27	37.9	0.014	0.014	0.039	0	3.25
Milk—sheep	31	1.70	1.99	1.52	54.8	0.028	0.018	0.100	0	0
Milk—soybean	9	0.78	0.54	0.51	1.2	0.163	0.046	0.020	0	0
Ice cream—regular-vanilla	57	1.02	3.05	6.76	37.5	0.026	0.011	0.070	0	12.60
Ice cream—rich-vanilla	67	0.79	4.54	6.13	28.9	0.019	0.008	0.054	0	16.90
Ice cream—soft-serve	62	1.15	3.69	6.28	38.7	0.070	0.013	0.073	0	25.00
Creamsicle ice cream bar	44	0.52	1.33	7.56	19.8	0	0.009	0.034	0	0
Drumstick ice cream bar	88	1.23	4.68	10.20	31.7	0.047	0.009	0.043	0	0
Fudgesicle ice cream bar	35	1.48	0.08	7.22	50.0	0.039	0.012	0.070	0	0
Ice milk	40	1.12	1.22	6.28	38.0	0.039	0.016	0.075	0	3.90
Ice milk—soft serve—3% fat	36	1.30	0.75	6.22	44.4	0.045	0.019	0.088	0	2.10
Yogurt—coffee-vanilla	24	1.40	0.35	3.90	48.5	0.020	0.012	0.057	0	1.42
Yogurt—lowfat with fruit	29	1.24	0.31	5.37	43.0	0.020	0.010	0.050	0	1.25
Yogurt—lowfat-plain	18	1.49	0.43	2.00	51.8	0.022	0.012	0.060	0	1.75
Yogurt—nonfat milk	16	1.62	0.05	2.17	56.5	0.025	0.014	0.066	0	0.50
Yogurt—whole milk	17	0.98	0.92	1.32	34.3	0.014	0.008	0.040	0	3.68

VEGETABLES

	kCal	Protein (g)	Lipid (g)	CHO (g)	Ca (mg)	Fe (mg)	B₁ (mg)	B₂ (mg)	Fiber (g)	Cholesterol (mg)
Alfalfa sprouts	9	1.13	0.200	1.07	9.5	0.272	0.021	0.036	1.030	0
Artichoke hearts—marinated	28	0.680	0.250	2.18	6.5	0.270	0.010	0.029	1.780	0
Asparagus—raw spears	6	0.865	0.063	1.05	6.4	0.193	0.032	0.035	0.395	0
Asparagus—canned spears	5	0.606	0.184	0.70	3.9	0.177	0.017	0.025	0.454	0
Bamboo shoots—sliced—raw	8	0.738	0.088	1.47	3.8	0.143	0.043	0.020	0.738	0
Bamboo shoots—sliced, canned	5	0.489	0.113	0.91	2.2	0.090	0.007	0.007	0.706	0
Bean sprouts—fresh raw	9	0.861	0.050	1.68	3.8	0.258	0.024	0.035	0.736	0
Bean sprouts—boiled	6	0.576	0.025	1.19	3.4	0.185	0.014	0.029	0.572	0
Bean sprouts—stir fried	14	1.220	0.059	3.00	3.7	0.549	0.040	0.050	0.777	0
Black beans—cooked	37	2.500	0.152	6.72	7.8	0.593	0.069	0.017	2.540	0

VEGETABLES—continued

	kCal	Protein (g)	Lipid (g)	CHO (g)	Ca (mg)	Fe (mg)	B_1 (mg)	B_2 (mg)	Fiber (g)	Cholesterol (mg)
Green beans—raw uncooked	9	0.515	0.034	2.02	10.6	0.363	0.024	0.030	0.644	0
Green beans—fresh—cooked	10	0.535	0.082	2.24	13.2	0.363	0.021	0.027	0.737	0
Green beans—frozen—cooked	8	0.386	0.038	1.73	12.8	0.233	0.014	0.021	0.880	0
Green beans—canned/drained	6	0.326	0.028	1.28	7.6	0.256	0.004	0.016	0.378	0
Red kidney beans—dry	94	6.690	0.234	16.90	40.5	2.330	0.150	0.062	6.160	0
Lima beans—dry large	96	6.080	0.194	18.00	22.9	2.130	0.144	0.057	8.600	0
Lima beans—fresh—cooked	35	1.930	0.090	6.70	9.0	0.695	0.040	0.027	2.670	0
Lima beans—dry small	98	5.790	0.397	18.20	18.4	2.270	0.136	0.048	8.500	0
Lima beans—canned/drained	27	1.530	0.100	5.20	8.0	0.487	0.010	0.013	2.420	0
Beans/w/franks—canned	40	1.900	1.860	4.37	13.6	0.490	0.016	0.016	1.950	1.7
Pork & beans—canned	32	1.500	0.413	5.95	17.4	0.470	0.013	0.017	1.560	1.9
Navy beans—dry, cooked	40	2.460	0.162	7.77	19.9	0.703	0.057	0.017	2.490	0
Pinto beans—dry, cooked	39	2.320	0.148	7.28	13.6	0.741	0.053	0.026	3.230	0
Refried beans—canned	30	1.770	0.303	5.24	13.2	0.500	0.014	0.016	2.470	0
Soybeans—dry	118	10.400	5.650	8.55	78.5	4.450	0.248	0.247	1.570	0
White beans—dry	95	5.990	0.334	17.70	36.0	2.190	0.210	0.059	0.766	0
White beans—dry, cooked	40	2.550	0.182	7.32	20.7	0.808	0.067	0.017	2.230	0
Yellow wax beans—raw	9	0.515	0.034	2.02	10.6	0.294	0.024	0.030	0.644	0
Yellow wax beans—raw	10	0.535	0.082	2.24	13.2	0.363	0.021	0.027	0.726	0
Yellow wax beans—frozen	8	0.386	0.038	1.73	12.8	0.233	0.014	0.021	0.880	0
Beets—cooked	9	0.300	0.014	1.90	3.1	0.176	0.009	0.004	0.539	0
Beets—pickled slices	18	0.227	0.028	4.63	3.1	0.116	0.006	0.014	0.587	0
Broccoli—raw chopped	8	0.844	0.097	1.49	13.5	0.251	0.019	0.034	0.934	0
Broccoli—raw spears	8	0.845	0.098	1.49	13.5	0.250	0.018	0.034	0.935	0
Broccoli—frozen cooked spears	8	0.879	0.034	1.51	14.5	0.173	0.015	0.023	0.826	0
Brussels sprouts—raw	12	0.960	0.084	2.54	11.6	0.396	0.039	0.026	1.260	0
Brussels sprouts—cooked	11	1.090	0.145	2.45	10.2	0.342	0.030	0.023	1.220	0
Brussels sprouts—frozen cooked	12	1.030	0.112	2.36	7.0	0.210	0.029	0.032	1.230	0
Cabbage—raw, shredded	7	0.340	0.049	1.52	13.0	0.162	0.015	0.009	0.680	0
Cabbage—cooked	6	0.272	0.070	1.35	9.5	0.110	0.016	0.016	0.661	0
Bok choy—raw, shredded	4	0.425	0.057	0.62	30.0	0.227	0.011	0.020	0.486	0
Bok choy—cooked	3	0.442	0.045	0.51	26.3	0.295	0.009	0.018	0.454	0
Red cabbage—raw	8	0.393	0.073	1.74	14.6	0.142	0.018	0.009	0.648	0
Red cabbage—cooked	6	0.299	0.057	1.32	10.6	0.102	0.010	0.006	1.567	0
Carrot—whole, raw	12	0.291	0.055	2.87	7.5	0.142	0.028	0.017	1.906	0
Carrot—grated, raw	12	0.289	0.052	2.88	7.7	0.142	0.027	0.016	0.907	0
Carrots—sliced, cooked	13	0.309	0.050	2.97	8.7	0.176	0.010	0.016	0.992	0
Carrots—frozen, cooked	10	0.338	0.031	2.34	8.2	0.136	0.008	0.010	1.050	0
Carrots—canned, drained	7	0.183	0.054	1.57	7.4	0.181	0.005	0.009	0.435	0
Carrot juice	11	0.267	0.041	2.63	6.7	0.130	0.026	0.015	0.385	0
Cauliflower—raw	7	0.561	0.051	1.39	7.9	0.164	0.022	0.016	0.720	0
Cauliflower—cooked	7	0.530	0.050	1.31	7.8	0.119	0.018	0.018	0.622	0

VEGETABLES—*continued*

	kCal	Protein (g)	Lipid (g)	CHO (g)	Ca (mg)	Fe (mg)	B₁ (mg)	B₂ (mg)	Fiber (g)	Cholesterol (mg)
Cauliflower—frozen, cooked	5	0.457	0.061	1.06	4.9	0.116	0.010	0.015	0.535	0
Celery—raw—chopped	5	0.189	0.033	1.03	10.4	0.137	0.009	0.009	0.472	0
Swiss chard—raw	5	0.510	0.057	1.06	14.5	0.510	0.011	0.025	0.512	0
Swiss chard—cooked	6	0.533	0.023	1.17	16.5	0.642	0.010	0.024	0.616	0
Collards—fresh	5	0.445	0.062	1.07	33.0	0.299	0.009	0.018	0.590	0
Collards—fresh, cooked	4	0.313	0.043	0.75	22.0	0.116	0.005	0.012	0.798	0
Collards—frozen, cooked	10	0.840	0.115	2.02	59.5	0.317	0.013	0.033	0.794	0
Corn—kernels raw	24	0.913	0.335	5.38	0.6	0.147	0.057	0.017	1.220	0
Corn on the cob—cooked	31	0.943	0.363	7.14	0.6	0.173	0.061	0.020	1.190	0
Corn—cooked from frozen	23	0.857	0.020	5.80	0.6	0.085	0.020	0.020	1.190	0
Corn—canned, drained	23	0.743	0.283	5.26	1.4	0.142	0.009	0.014	0.398	0
Corn—canned cream style	21	0.494	0.119	5.14	0.9	0.108	0.007	0.015	0.354	0
Cucumber slices w/peel	4	0.153	0.037	0.82	4.0	0.079	0.009	0.006	0.329	0
Eggplant—cooked	8	0.236	0.066	1.88	1.7	0.099	0.022	0.006	1.060	0
Escarole/curly endive—chopped	5	0.354	0.057	0.95	14.7	0.235	0.023	0.022	0.369	0
Garbanzo/chickpeas—dry	103	5.470	1.720	17.20	29.9	1.770	0.135	0.060	5.390	0
Garbanzo/chickpeas—cooked	47	2.500	0.735	7.78	13.8	0.819	0.033	0.018	1.920	0
Jerusalem artichoke—raw	22	0.567	0.004	4.95	4.0	0.964	0.057	0.017	0.369	0
Kale—fresh, chopped	14	0.935	0.198	2.84	38.0	0.482	0.031	0.037	1.650	0
Kohlrabi—raw slices	8	0.482	0.028	1.76	6.9	0.113	0.014	0.006	0.405	0
Kohlrabi—cooked	8	0.510	0.030	1.96	7.0	0.113	0.011	0.006	0.395	0
Leeks—chopped raw	17	0.425	0.085	4.00	16.7	0.594	0.017	0.008	0.668	0
Leeks—cooked, chopped	9	0.230	0.057	2.16	8.5	0.310	0.007	0.006	0.927	0
Lentils—dry	96	7.960	0.273	16.20	14.6	2.550	0.135	0.069	3.400	0
Lentils—cooked from dry	33	2.560	0.106	5.73	5.3	0.944	0.048	0.020	1.430	0
Lentils—sprouted, raw	30	2.540	0.156	6.30	7.0	0.909	0.065	0.036	1.150	0
Lettuce—butterhead	4	0.367	0.062	0.66	9.5	0.085	0.017	0.017	0.397	0
Lettuce—iceberg	4	0.286	0.054	0.59	5.4	0.142	0.013	0.009	0.347	0
Lettuce—romaine	5	0.459	0.057	0.67	10.2	0.312	0.028	0.028	0.482	0
Mushrooms—raw sliced	7	0.593	0.119	1.32	1.4	0.352	0.029	0.127	0.508	0
Mushrooms—cooked	8	0.614	0.134	1.46	1.7	0.494	0.020	0.085	0.625	0
Mushrooms—canned, drained	7	0.530	0.082	1.40	3.1	0.224	0.017	0.063	0.596	0
Mustard greens—fresh	7	0.764	0.057	1.39	29.4	0.414	0.023	0.031	0.764	0
Mustard greens—cooked	4	0.640	0.068	0.60	21.0	0.316	0.012	0.018	0.587	0
Okra pods—cooked	9	0.530	0.048	2.04	17.9	0.128	0.037	0.016	0.624	0
Okra slices—cooked	11	0.589	0.085	2.32	27.1	0.190	0.028	0.035	0.709	0
Onions—chopped, raw	10	0.335	0.074	2.07	7.1	0.105	0.017	0.003	0.454	0
Onion slices—raw	10	0.335	0.074	2.08	7.2	0.105	0.017	0.003	0.454	0
Onion—dehydrated flakes	91	2.530	0.122	23.70	72.9	0.446	0.022	0.018	2.510	0
Onion rings—frozen, heated	115	1.520	7.570	10.80	8.8	0.482	0.079	0.040	0.240	0
Parsley—freeze dried	81	8.910	1.420	11.90	40.5	15.200	0.304	0.648	22.000	0
Parsley—fresh chopped	9	0.624	0.085	1.96	36.9	1.760	0.023	0.031	1.550	0
Parsnips—sliced raw	21	0.341	0.085	5.09	10.0	0.167	0.026	0.014	1.280	0
Fresh peas—uncooked	23	1.530	0.113	4.10	7.0	0.416	0.075	0.037	1.380	0
Peas—cooked	24	1.520	0.060	4.43	7.8	0.438	0.073	0.042	1.360	0
Peas—frozen, cooked	22	1.460	0.078	4.04	6.7	0.443	0.080	0.050	1.280	0
Peas—edible pods—fresh	12	0.794	0.057	2.15	12.1	0.589	0.043	0.023	0.794	0
Split peas—dry	97	6.970	0.328	17.10	15.5	1.250	0.206	0.061	4.030	0

VEGETABLES—*continued*

	kCal	Protein (g)	Lipid (g)	CHO (g)	Ca (mg)	Fe (mg)	B₁ (mg)	B₂ (mg)	Fiber (g)	Cholesterol (mg)
Peas + carrots—frozen, cooked	14	0.875	0.120	2.87	6.4	0.266	0.064	0.020	1.170	0
Green chili pepper—raw	11	0.557	0.057	2.68	5.0	0.340	0.026	0.026	0.504	0
Red chili peppers—raw/chopped	11	0.567	0.057	2.68	4.9	0.340	0.026	0.026	0.454	0
Jalapeno peppers—canned chopped	7	0.225	0.170	1.39	7.5	0.792	0.008	0.014	0.850	0
Baked potato with skin	31	0.653	0.028	7.16	2.8	0.386	0.030	0.009	0.660	0
Baked potato—flesh only	26	0.556	0.029	6.10	1.5	0.100	0.030	0.006	0.436	0
Potato skin—oven baked	56	1.220	0.029	13.20	9.8	1.080	0.035	0.034	1.130	0
Potato + peel—microwaved	30	0.692	0.028	6.83	3.1	0.350	0.034	0.009	0.660	0
Peeled potato—boiled	24	0.485	0.029	5.67	2.1	0.088	0.028	0.005	0.426	0
French fries—oven heated	63	0.980	2.480	9.64	2.3	0.380	0.035	0.009	0.567	0
French fries—frozen—vegetable oil	90	1.140	4.690	11.20	5.7	0.215	0.050	0.008	0.567	0
Cottage-fried potatoes	62	0.975	2.320	9.64	2.8	0.425	0.034	0.009	0.567	0
Hash-brown potatoes	30	0.343	1.980	3.02	1.1	0.115	0.010	0.003	0.567	0
Mashed potatoes prep/milk	22	0.548	0.166	4.98	7.4	0.077	0.025	0.011	0.405	0.5
Mashed potatoes—milk & margarine	30	0.533	1.200	4.74	7.3	0.074	0.024	0.014	0.405	0.5
Potato pancakes	88	1.730	4.700	9.85	7.8	0.451	0.039	0.035	0.563	34.7
Potatoes au gratin mix	26	0.653	1.170	3.65	23.5	0.090	0.006	0.023	0.487	1.4
Scalloped potatoes—recipe	24	0.813	1.040	3.05	16.2	0.163	0.020	0.026	0.289	3.4
Potato chips	148	1.590	10.000	14.70	7.0	0.339	0.040	0.006	1.360	0
Potato flour	100	2.260	0.226	22.60	9.3	4.880	0.119	0.040	0.317	0
Pumpkin—canned	10	0.311	0.080	2.28	7.4	0.394	0.007	0.015	0.519	0
Red radishes	4	0.170	0.151	1.01	5.7	0.082	0.001	0.013	0.624	0
Rutabaga—cooked cubes	10	0.314	0.053	2.19	12.0	0.133	0.020	0.010	0.434	0
Sauerkraut—canned liquid	5	0.258	0.040	1.21	8.7	0.417	0.006	0.006	0.529	0
Soybeans—mature, raw	37	3.700	1.900	3.17	19.4	0.599	0.096	0.033	0.656	0
Spinach—cooked from fresh	7	0.843	0.074	1.06	38.4	1.010	0.027	0.067	0.702	0
Summer squash—raw slices	6	0.334	0.061	1.23	5.7	0.130	0.018	0.010	0.425	0
Zucchini squash—cooked	5	0.181	0.014	1.11	3.6	0.099	0.012	0.012	0.567	0
Acorn squash—boiled/mashed	10	0.190	0.023	2.49	7.5	0.159	0.028	0.002	0.680	0
Butternut squash/baked—cube	12	0.256	0.026	2.97	11.6	0.170	0.020	0.005	0.794	0
Spaghetti squash—baked/boiled	8	0.187	0.073	1.83	6.0	0.095	0.010	0.006	0.794	0
Winter squash—boiled	10	0.319	0.050	2.40	5.2	0.136	0.018	0.006	0.794	0
Sweet potato—baked in skin	29	0.487	0.032	6.89	8.0	0.129	0.020	0.036	0.850	0
Candied sweet potatoes	39	0.246	0.920	7.91	7.3	0.324	0.005	0.012	0.545	0
Tofu (soybean curd)	22	2.290	1.360	0.53	29.7	1.520	0.023	0.015	0.343	0
Tomato—fresh whole	6	0.251	0.060	1.23	2.1	0.136	0.017	0.014	0.415	0
Tomatoes—whole canned	6	0.265	0.070	1.22	7.4	0.171	0.013	0.009	0.298	0

VEGETABLES—*continued*

	kCal	Protein (g)	Lipid (g)	CHO (g)	Ca (mg)	Fe (mg)	B₁ (mg)	B₂ (mg)	Fiber (g)	Cholesterol (mg)
Tomato sauce—canned	9	0.376	0.047	2.04	3.9	0.218	0.019	0.016	0.425	0
Tomato paste—canned	24	1.070	0.249	5.33	9.9	0.848	0.044	0.054	1.210	0
Tomato juice—canned	5	0.215	0.017	1.20	2.6	0.164	0.013	0.009	0.220	0
Turnip cubes—raw	8	0.255	0.028	1.76	8.5	0.085	0.011	0.009	0.587	0
Mixed vegetables—frozen, cooked	17	0.812	0.043	3.70	7.2	0.232	0.020	0.034	1.120	0
Vegetable juice cocktail	6	0.178	0.026	1.29	3.1	0.119	0.012	0.008	0.178	0
Water chestnuts—raw	30	0.398	0.027	6.77	3.2	0.170	0.040	0.057	0.869	0
Watercress—fresh	3	0.650	0.033	0.37	33.4	0.050	0.025	0.033	0.719	0
White yams—raw	34	0.438	0.049	7.90	8.7	0.153	0.032	0.009	0.822	0

SALAD BAR

	kCal	Protein (g)	Lipid (g)	CHO (g)	Ca (mg)	Fe (mg)	B₁ (mg)	B₂ (mg)	Fiber (g)	Cholesterol (mg)
Alfalfa sprouts	8.59	1.130	0.196	1.070	9.45	0.272	0.021	0.036	1.030	0
Artichoke hearts, marinated	28.00	0.680	2.250	2.180	6.50	0.270	0.010	0.029	1.780	0
Asparagus	6.35	0.867	0.062	1.050	6.35	0.193	0.032	0.035	0.432	0
Avocado	45.70	0.563	4.340	2.100	3.07	0.284	0.030	0.035	2.720	0
Bacon, regular	163.00	8.640	14.000	0.164	2.98	0.482	0.195	0.080	0	23.9
Bean sprouts	8.50	0.861	0.050	1.680	3.82	0.258	0.024	0.035	0.7365	0
Beets	8.67	0.300	0.013	1.900	3.00	0.176	0.009	0.004	0.567	0
Beets, canned, diced	9.00	0.260	0.040	2.040	4.34	0.517	0.003	0.012	0.590	0
Broccoli, raw	7.73	0.844	0.097	1.490	13.50	0.251	0.019	0.034	0.934	0
Cabbage	6.48	0.340	0.049	1.520	13.00	0.162	0.015	0.009	0.680	0
Cabbage, red	7.70	0.393	0.073	1.740	14.60	0.142	0.018	0.009	0.648	0
Carrots, grated	12.40	0.289	0.052	2.880	7.73	0.142	0.027	0.016	0.907	0
Cauliflower	6.80	0.561	0.051	1.390	7.94	0.164	0.022	0.016	0.720	0
Celery	4.54	0.189	0.030	1.030	10.40	0.137	0.009	0.009	0.472	0
Chicken salad	96.70	3.820	8.900	0.469	5.92	0.239	0.012	0.028	0.109	17.3
Crab, cooked	23.90	5.050	0.561	0.140	12.90	0.104	0.012	0.044	0	18.0
Croutons, dry bread cubes	105.00	3.690	1.040	20.500	35.00	1.020	0.099	0.099	0.085	0
Cucumber slices	3.69	0.153	0.037	0.824	3.99	0.079	0.009	0.006	0.329	0
Egg, chopped	40.40	3.520	2.790	0.338	13.80	0.475	0.014	0.133	0	113
Escarole/curly endive	4.82	0.354	0.057	0.953	14.70	0.235	0.023	0.022	0.369	0
Garbanzo/chickpeas, cooked	46.50	2.500	0.735	7.780	13.80	0.819	0.033	0.018	1.920	0
Green pepper, sweet	6.80	0.244	0.130	1.500	1.70	0.357	0.024	0.014	0.454	0
Ham salad	51.50	5.000	3.000	0.880	2.00	0.280	0.244	0.072	0	16
Ham, minced	74.20	4.620	5.860	0.526	2.70	0.216	0.203	0.054	0	20.2
Leeks	17.30	0.425	0.085	4.000	16.70	0.594	0.017	0.008	0.688	0
Lettuce, butterhead	3.69	0.366	0.062	0.658	9.47	0.085	0.017	0.017	0.370	0
Lettuce, iceberg	3.69	0.287	0.054	0.592	5.37	0.142	0.013	0.009	0.370	0
Lettuce, loose leaf	5.11	0.369	0.085	0.992	19.20	0.397	0.014	0.023	0.391	0
Lettuce, Romaine	4.54	0.459	0.057	0.673	10.20	0.312	0.028	0.028	0.482	0
Lobster meat	27.80	5.800	0.168	0.364	17.20	0.111	0.020	0.019	0	20.3

SALAD BAR—*continued*

	kCal	Protein (g)	Lipid (g)	CHO (g)	Ca (mg)	Fe (mg)	B₁ (mg)	B₂ (mg)	Fiber (g)	Cholesterol (mg)
Mushrooms, raw	7.09	0.593	0.119	1.320	1.42	0.352	0.029	0.127	0.508	0
Onions	9.57	0.335	0.074	2.070	7.09	0.105	0.017	0.003	0.454	0
Parmesan cheese, grated	129.00	11.800	8.500	1.060	389.00	0.270	0.013	0.109	0	22.0
Peas, cooked	22.30	1.460	0.078	4.040	6.73	0.443	0.080	0.050	1.280	0
Sesame seed kernels, dried	167.00	7.480	15.500	2.660	37.20	2.210	0.204	0.024	1.950	0
Shrimp, boiled	28.00	5.930	0.306	0	11.00	0.876	0.009	0.009	0	55.3
Spinach, fresh	6.23	0.810	0.099	0.992	28.00	0.770	0.022	0.054	0.947	0
Sunflower seeds, dry	162.00	6.460	14.000	5.320	32.90	1.920	0.650	0.070	1.970	0
Tomatoes	5.51	0.252	0.061	1.230	1.89	0.135	0.017	0.014	0.416	0
Tuna salad	53.00	4.550	2.630	2.670	4.84	0.282	0.009	0.019	0.340	3.73
Turkey meat	41.30	5.270	2.030	0.149	11.40	0.358	0.025	0.064	0	11.9

VARIETY

	kCal	Protein (g)	Lipid (g)	CHO (g)	Ca (mg)	Fe (mg)	B₁ (mg)	B₂ (mg)	Fiber (g)	Cholesterol (mg)
Chips & crackers										
Doritos—nacho flavor	139	2.20	6.79	18.00	17.0	0.399	0.040	0.030	1.10	0
Doritos—taco flavor	140	2.60	6.59	17.60	44.9	0.699	0.080	0.090	1.10	0
Potato chips—sour cream & onion	153	2.40	9.48	14.60	21.0	0.474	0.040	0.055	1.35	1.0
Wheat cracker—thin	124	3.19	4.96	17.70	10.6	1.060	0.142	0.106	1.84	0
Whole wheat crackers	124	3.19	5.32	17.70	10.6	1.850	0.070	0.106	2.94	0
Condiments										
Catsup	30	0.52	0.11	7.17	6.2	0.228	0.026	0.020	0.45	0
Mustard	21	1.34	1.25	1.81	23.8	0.567	0.024	0.057	0.11	0
Soy sauce	14	1.46	0.02	2.40	4.7	0.567	0.014	0.036	0	0
Deli meats										
Bologna—beef	89	3.32	8.04	0.56	3.7	0.394	0.016	0.036	0	16.0
Bratwurst	92	4.05	7.90	0.84	13.8	0.292	0.070	0.064	0	17.8
Keilbasa sausage	88	3.76	7.70	0.61	12.0	0.414	0.064	0.061	0	18.5
Knockwurst sausage	87	3.37	7.88	0.05	2.9	0.258	0.097	0.040	0	16.3
Liverwurst	93	4.00	8.10	0.63	7.9	1.810	0.077	0.291	0	44.1
Pepperoni sausage	140	5.94	12.50	0.80	2.8	0.397	0.09	0.07		9.79
Polish sausage	92	3.99	8.13	0.46	3.0	0.409	0.142	0.042	0	20.0
Salami—beef	72	4.17	5.69	0.70	2.47	0.567	0.036	0.073	0	17.3
Salami—pork & beef	72	3.94	5.70	0.64	3.68	0.755	0.068	0.106	0	18.5
Salami—turkey	55	4.62	3.89	0.15	5.47	0.463	0.029	0.075	0	22.9
Salami—dry—beef & pork	120	6.49	9.75	0.74	2.84	0.425	0.170	0.082	0	22.7
Turkey pastrami	37	5.22	1.75	0.43	2.49	0.403	0.022	0.075	0	14.9
Mexican foods										
Beef taco	75.2	4.94	4.80	3.67	30.9	0.469	0.01	0.049	0.407	16.2
Beef enchilada	69.0	3.09	3.26	3.69	60.2	0.418	0.017	0.039	0.465	8.93
Cheese enchilada	78.0	3.12	4.2	3.78	108.0	0.324	0.015	0.050	0.465	10.2
Chicken enchilada	63.6	3.38	2.48	3.69	60.5	0.359	0.018	0.036	0.465	9.10
Corn tortilla, enriched, regular	61.4	1.89	0.964	12.30	39.7	0.567	0.047	0.028	2.27	0

VARIETY—*continued*

	kCal	Protein (g)	Lipid (g)	CHO (g)	Ca (mg)	Fe (mg)	B₁ (mg)	B₂ (mg)	Fiber (g)	Cholesterol (mg)
Mexican Foods—*continued*										
Corn torilla, enriched, thin	61.0	1.64	0.95	12.30	39.8	0.567	0.046	0.028	2.26	0
Corn tortilla, fried	82.2	2.08	2.84	12.30	39.7	0.567	0.047	0.028	2.27	0
Enchirito	60.4	3.15	2.75	3.31	51.5	0.410	0.015	0.037	0.748	9.18
Flour tortilla	84	2.07	2.15	15.50	17.0	0.440	0.102	0.062	0.800	0
Refried beans, canned	30.3	1.77	0.303	5.24	13.2	0.500	0.014	0.016	2.47	0
Nuts & seeds										
Almonds—dried, chopped	167	5.65	14.80	5.78	75.5	1.040	0.060	0.220	3.36	0
Almonds—whole toasted	167	5.77	14.40	6.48	80.0	1.400	0.037	0.170	3.99	0
Sunflower seeds—dry	162	6.46	14.00	5.32	32.9	1.920	0.650	0.070	1.97	0
Oils & shortening										
Cocoa butter oil	251	0	28.40	0	0	0	0	0	0	0
Corn oil	251	0	28.40	0	0	0.001	0	0	0	0
Cottonseed oil	251	0	28.40	0	0	0	0	0	0	0
Olive oil	251	0	28.40	0	0.1	0.109	0	0	0	0
Palm oil	251	0	28.40	0	0.1	0.003	0	0	0	0
Palm kernel oil	251	0	28.40	0	0	0	0	0	0	0
Peanut oil	251	0	28.40	0	0	0.008	0	0	0	0
Safflower oil	251	0	28.40	0	0	0	0	0	0	0
Sesame oil	250	0	28.40	0	0	0	0	0	0	0
Soybean oil	251	0	28.40	0	0	0.007	0	0	0	0
Sunflower oil	251	0	28.40	0	0	0	0	0	0	0
Walnut oil	251	0	28.40	0	0	0	0	0	0	0
Wheat germ oil	250	0	28.40	0	0	0	0	0	0	0
Vegetable shortening	251	0	28.40	0	0	0	0	0	0	0
Pasta & noodles										
Spaghetti, cooked firm, hot	41	1.42	0.142	8.53	3.1	0.454	0.051	0.028	0.482	0
Spaghetti, cooked tender, hot	31	1.01	0.111	6.48	3.0	0.405	0.04	0.022	0.425	0
Whole wheat spaghetti, cooked	35	1.53	0.113	7.49	4.3	0.244	0.048	0.020	1.040	0
Spaghetti + sauce + cheese, canned	22	0.68	0.227	4.42	4.5	0.318	0.040	0.032	0.284	0.3
Spaghetti + sauce + cheese, homemade	30	1.02	1.02	4.20	9.07	0.260	0.028	0.020	0.284	0.9
Spaghetti + sauce + meat, canned	30	1.36	1.13	4.42	6.01	0.374	0.017	0.020	0.312	2.6
Spaghetti + sauce + meat, homemade	38	2.17	1.37	4.46	14.20	0.423	0.029	0.034	0.314	10.2
Spaghetti sauce, homemade	23	0.77	1.25	2.95	6.70	0.380	0.026	0.017	0.343	0
Spaghetti sauce, canned	31	0.52	1.35	4.52	7.97	0.184	0.016	0.017	0.343	0
Spaghetti meat sauce,	30	1.03	1.30	3.72	4.95	0.385	0.028	0.022	0.193	2.3
Spaghetti sauce, dry, packet	79	1.70	0.28	18.20	48.20	0.765	NA	0.162	0.057	0
Spaghetti sauce + mushrooms, packet	85	2.84	2.55	13.90	113.00	0.510	NA	0.136	0.085	0
Egg noodles, cooked	35	1.17	0.35	6.60	3.19	0.400	0.039	0.023	0.624	8.9

VARIETY—continued

	kCal	Protein (g)	Lipid (g)	CHO (g)	Ca (mg)	Fe (mg)	B₁ (mg)	B₂ (mg)	Fiber (g)	Cholesterol (mg)
Pasta & noodles—continued										
Chow mein noodles, dry	139	3.72	6.93	16.40	8.82	0.252	0.032	0.019	1.100	3.2
Spinach noodles, dry	108	3.97	1.08	20.20	11.60	1.290	0.278	0.133	1.930	0
Spinach noodles, cooked	32	1.13	0.36	5.97	3.37	0.429	0.043	0.027	0.569	0
Chicken + noodles, recipe	43	2.60	2.13	3.07	3.07	0.278	0.006	0.020	0.142	12.2
Chicken + noodles, frozen	32	2.17	1.30	2.49	15.70	0.393	0.009	0.018	0.022	8.0
Noodles-ramen-beef, cooked	28	0.76	0.94	4.17	NA	NA	NA	NA	0.500	NA
Noodles, ramen, chicken, cooked	25	0.76	0.85	3.63	NA	NA	NA	NA	0.512	NA
Noodles, ramen, oriental	26	0.74	1.07	3.83	NA	NA	NA	NA	0.512	NA
Lasagna, frozen entree	38	2.32	1.71	2.61	34.00	0.343	0.026	0.045	0.194	12.4
Pizza										
Pizza—cheese	69	3.54	2.13	9.21	52.00	0.378	0.080	0.069	0.510	13.2
Pizza—mozzarella	80	7.60	4.67	0.89	207.00	0.076	0.006	0.097	0	15.0
Pizza—Canadian bacon	52	6.82	2.36	0.38	3.00	0.229	0.231	0.055	0	16.3
Pizza—pepperoni	140	5.94	12.50	0.81	2.80	0.397	0.090	0.070	0	9.8
Pizza—onion	10	0.34	0.07	2.07	7.10	1.105	0.017	0.003	0.450	0
Popcorn										
Popcorn—plain, air popped	106	3.50	1.42	21.30	3.50	0.709	0.106	0.035	4.600	0
Popcorn—cooked in oil/salted	142	2.32	7.99	15.50	7.70	0.696	0.026	0.052	3.090	0
Popcorn—syrup-coated	109	1.60	0.81	24.30	1.60	0.405	0.106	0.016	0.810	0
Rice										
Brown—dry	102	2.13	0.54	21.90	9.04	0.510	0.096	0.014	0.965	0
Brown—cooked	34	0.709	0.17	7.23	3.40	0.170	0.026	0.006	0.483	0
White—regular, dry	103	1.90	0.11	22.80	6.74	0.828	0.125	0.009	0.340	0
White—regular, cooked	31	0.567	0.03	6.86	2.84	0.397	0.03	0.003	0.102	0
White—converted, dry	105	2.10	0.15	23.00	17.00	0.828	0.124	0.010	0.624	0
White—converted, cooked	30	0.599	0.02	6.60	5.35	0.227	0.03	0.003	0.180	0
White—instant, dry	106	2.13	0.06	23.40	1.42	1.300	0.125	0.008	0.737	0
White—instant, prepared	31	0.624	0.03	6.86	0.85	0.227	0.037	0.003	0.216	0
Wild—cooked	26	1.02	0.06	5.39	1.42	0.312	0.031	0.045	0.709	0
Rice bran	78	3.77	5.44	14.40	21.50	5.500	0.64	0.070	6.150	0
Rice polish	75	3.43	3.62	16.40	19.40	4.560	0.521	0.051	0.680	0
Salad dressings										
Blue cheese salad dressing	143	1.37	14.80	2.09	22.90	0.057	0.003	0.028	0.020	7.6
Caesar's salad dressing	126	2.66	12.70	0.67	44.40	0.239	0.007	0.025	0.050	33.9
French dressing	150	0.16	16.00	1.81	3.55	0.113	0	0	0.220	0
Italian dressing—low calorie	15	0.02	1.18	1.37	0.59	0.059	0	0	0.080	1.7

VARIETY—continued

	kCal	Protein (g)	Lipid (g)	CHO (g)	Ca (mg)	Fe (mg)	B₁ (mg)	B₂ (mg)	Fiber (g)	Cholesterol (mg)
Salad dressings—continued										
Mayonnaise	203	0.31	22.60	0.77	5.67	0.168	0.005	0.012	0	16.8
Imitation mayonnaise	66	0	5.67	3.78	0	0	0	0	0	7.6
Ranch salad dressing	104	0.86	10.70	1.31	28.40	0.075	0.010	0.040	0	11.1
Russian salad dressing	140	0.45	14.50	3.00	5.44	0.174	0.014	0.014	0.080	18.4
1000 island dressing	107	0.26	10.10	4.30	3.52	0.170	0.006	0.009	0.060	7.3
1000 island dressing— low calorie	45	0.22	3.00	4.58	3.12	1.174	0.006	0.008	0.340	3.4
Vinegar & oil dressing	124	0	14.20	0	0	0	0	0	0	0
Salads, prepared										
Chicken salad w/celery	97	3.82	8.90	0.47	5.92	0.239	0.012	0.028	0.110	17.3
Cole slaw	20	0.36	0.74	3.52	12.80	0.166	0.019	0.017	0.570	2.3
Egg salad	68	2.91	6.01	0.45	14.50	0.525	0.019	0.070	0	97.4
Ham salad spread	62	2.46	4.39	3.01	2.24	0.168	0.123	0.034	0.030	10.4
Macaroni salad—no cheese	75	0.54	6.66	3.52	5.50	0.229	0.020	0.014	0.270	4.9
Potato salad w/mayo + eggs	41	0.76	2.32	3.16	5.44	0.185	0.022	0.017	0.420	19.3
Tuna salad	53	4.55	2.53	2.67	4.84	0.282	0.009	0.019	0.340	3.7
Waldorf salad	85	0.72	8.33	2.62	8.82	0.196	0.020	0.013	0.720	4.3
Sandwiches										
Avocado & cheese— white	64	2.02	4.00	5.39	43.1	0.418	0.057	0.059	0.98	4.4
Avocado & cheese— whole wheat	62	2.14	3.97	5.24	37.8	0.477	0.047	0.05	1.76	4.3
BLT —whole wheat	68	2.49	3.77	6.45	11.4	0.570	0.077	0.043	1.55	4.1
BLT—white	70	2.30	3.77	6.70	18.2	0.489	0.092	0.055	0.43	4.2
Grilled cheese—wheat	91	4.22	5.37	7.10	87.4	0.565	0.057	0.076	1.59	11.8
Grilled cheese— part WW	95	4.39	5.82	6.59	103.0	0.526	0.067	0.093	0.61	13.3
Grilled cheese—white	97	4.22	5.79	6.88	103.0	0.441	0.068	0.092	0.30	13.3
Chicken salad—wheat	80	3.00	4.25	8.13	14.7	0.679	0.066	0.046	1.88	6.2
Chicken salad—white	85	2.83	4.63	8.05	22.7	0.552	0.080	0.060	0.39	7.1
Corn dog	84	2.55	5.10	6.97	8.7	0.495	0.072	0.043	0.03	9.5
Corned beef & swiss on rye	83	5.26	4.59	4.90	63.8	0.768	0.044	0.078	0.97	16.4
English muffin (egg/ cheese/bacon)	74	3.70	3.70	6.37	40.5	0.637	0.095	0.103	0.32	43.8
Egg salad—wheat	79	2.60	4.56	7.44	17.0	0.744	0.063	0.059	1.67	48.8
Egg salad—soft white	83	2.41	4.90	7.25	24.5	0.636	0.075	0.074	0.30	41.6
Ham—rye bread	59	3.84	2.09	6.10	12.0	0.474	0.182	0.073	1.24	7.1
Ham—whole wheat	59	3.79	2.04	6.84	12.4	0.617	0.164	0.060	1.54	6.1
Ham—soft white	61	3.74	2.08	6.60	18.6	0.504	0.186	0.073	0.29	6.7
Ham & swiss—rye	68	4.65	3.23	5.08	63.5	0.389	0.147	0.079	0.99	10.8
Ham & cheese— wheat	67	4.20	3.23	5.72	40.5	0.527	0.136	0.066	1.27	9.7
Ham & cheese—soft white	69	4.20	3.36	5.43	48.0	0.428	0.152	0.078	0.23	10.6
Ham salad—wheat	75	2.45	4.02	7.83	11.5	0.569	0.104	0.045	1.52	5.6
Ham salad—white	78	2.25	4.26	7.71	17.5	0.454	0.119	0.057	0.28	6.2
Hotdog/frankfurter & bun	87	2.80	5.10	7.04	19.6	0.570	0.095	0.062	0.40	7.6

VARIETY—*continued*

	kCal	Protein (g)	Lipid (g)	CHO (g)	Ca (mg)	Fe (mg)	B₁ (mg)	B₂ (mg)	Fiber (g)	Cholesterol (mg)
Sandwiches—*continued*										
Patty melt—gound beef/rye	91	5.09	6.07	3.96	36.5	0.533	0.040	0.072	0.81	17.1
Peanut butter & jam—whole wheat	92	3.40	3.85	12.30	15.4	0.751	0.070	0.045	2.29	0
Peanut butter & jam—white	98	3.29	4.14	12.80	23.4	0.632	0.085	0.059	0.85	0
Reuben grilled	58	3.43	3.38	3.53	43.6	0.633	0.030	0.052	0.80	10.4
Roast beef—whole wheat	64	4.00	2.52	6.71	12.3	0.760	0.061	0.054	1.53	6.2
Roast beef—white	67	3.97	2.63	6.46	18.5	0.665	0.072	0.066	0.27	6.9
Tuna salad—wheat	72	3.29	3.29	8.03	13.0	0.667	0.057	0.040	1.74	5.5
Tuna salad—white	76	3.18	3.47	7.92	19.6	0.555	0.068	0.052	0.44	6.2
Turkey—whole wheat	62	4.09	2.33	6.67	11.6	0.554	0.056	0.044	1.53	6.0
Turkey—white	64	4.07	2.42	6.41	17.8	0.435	0.066	0.055	0.27	6.7
Turkey & ham—rye	58	3.74	2.12	6.18	12.3	0.743	0.060	0.079	1.23	8.4
Turkey & ham—whole wheat	59	3.71	2.07	6.90	12.6	0.846	0.060	0.064	1.54	7.2
Turkey & ham—white	60	3.65	2.10	6.67	18.8	0.762	0.071	0.078	0.28	8.0
Turkey & ham & cheese on rye	68	4.22	3.46	5.04	44.2	0.616	0.050	0.083	0.99	12.1
Turkey & ham & cheese—wheat	67	4.14	3.25	5.77	40.5	0.716	0.051	0.070	1.27	10.6
Turkey & ham & cheese—white	69	4.13	3.38	5.48	48.3	0.636	0.059	0.082	0.23	11.6
Sauces										
Bordelaise sauce	24	0.33	1.46	1.10	3.80	0.179	0.008	0.010	0.01	3.8
Hot chili sauce, red pepper	5	0.25	0.17	1.10	2.51	0.137	0.003	0.026	2.29	0
Teriyaki sauce	24	1.69	0.09	4.52	6.30	0.488	0.008	0.020	0	0
Seafood										
Anchovy—raw	37	5.78	1.37	0	41.7	0.921	0.016	0.073	0	19.6
Frog legs—raw meat	21	4.65	0.085	0	5.1	0.539	0.040	0.070	0	14.2
Lobster meat—cooked	28	5.80	0.17	0.36	17.2	0.111	0.020	0.019	0	20.3
Scampi—fried in crumbs	69	6.07	3.49	3.26	19.0	0.357	0.037	0.039	0.04	50.2
Shrimp—boiled	28	5.93	0.31	0	11.0	0.876	0.009	0.009	0	55.3
Squid (calamari)—fried in flour	50	5.10	2.12	2.20	11.0	0.287	0.016	0.130	0	73.7
Soups										
Cream of celery	20	0.38	1.27	2.00	9.04	0.141	0.007	0.011	0.09	3.2
Chicken, chunky	20	1.43	0.75	1.95	2.71	0.195	0.010	0.020	0.03	3.4
Chicken + dumpling	23	1.30	1.28	1.39	3.34	0.144	0.004	0.017	0.10	7.6
Chicken gumbo	13	0.60	0.32	1.89	5.53	0.201	0.006	0.009	0.05	0.9
Chicken-noodle—chunky	14	1.50	0.70	0.24	2.84	0.170	0.009	0.020	0.09	2.1
Chili with beans	32	1.62	1.56	3.38	13.20	0.973	0.014	0.030	0.91	4.8
Clam chowder—New England	19	1.08	0.75	1.90	21.40	0.169	0.008	0.027	0.11	2.5
Minestrone—chunky	15	0.60	0.33	2.45	7.20	0.209	0.006	0.014	0.12	0.6
Cream of mushroom	29	0.46	2.15	2.10	7.23	0.119	0.007	0.019	0.06	0.4
Mushroom—barley	14	0.43	0.51	1.69	2.82	0.113	0.006	0.020	0.17	0

VARIETY—continued

	kCal	Protein (g)	Lipid (g)	CHO (g)	Ca (mg)	Fe (mg)	B₁ (mg)	B₂ (mg)	Fiber (g)	Cholesterol (mg)
Soups—continued										
Onion—canned	13	0.87	0.40	1.89	6.10	0.156	0.008	0.006	0.11	0
Oyster stew	14	0.49	0.89	0.94	4.96	0.227	0.005	0.008	0	3.1
Pea—prepared w/milk	27	1.40	0.79	3.59	19.30	0.224	0.017	0.030	0.07	2.0
Cream of potato	17	0.39	0.53	2.59	4.52	0.107	0.008	0.008	0.10	1.5
Split pea + ham	22	1.31	0.47	3.17	3.90	0.253	0.014	0.011	0.19	0.8
Tomato—canned	19	0.47	0.43	3.75	3.05	0.396	0.020	0.011	0.11	0
Tomato-beef-noodle	32	1.00	0.97	4.78	3.95	0.252	0.019	0.020	0.03	0.9
Tomato bisque prepared w/milk	22	0.71	0.75	3.32	21.00	0.099	0.013	0.030	0.01`	2.5
Turkey—chunky	16	1.23	0.53	1.69	6.00	0.229	0.010	0.029	0.12	1.1
Turkey noodle	16	0.88	0.45	1.95	2.60	0.212	0.017	0.014	0.03	1.1
Cream vegetable— dry mix	126	2.27	6.84	14.80	1.42	0.539	1.470	0.127	0.22	1.2
Vegetable	16	0.49	0.45	2.77	4.96	0.249	0.012	0.010	0.37	0
Miscellanous										
Garlic cloves	42	1.80	0.14	9.38	51.30	0.482	0.057	0.030	0.47	0
Gelatin salad/desert	17	0.43	0	3.99	0.50	0.024	0.002	0.002	0.02	0
Quiche lorraine	97	2.09	7.73	4.67	34.00	0.226	0.018	0.052	0.09	45.9
Spinach souffle	45	2.29	3.84	0.59	47.90	0.279	0.019	0.064	0.79	38.4

PART 2

Nutritive Values for Alcoholic and Nonalcoholic Beverages

The nutritive values for alcoholic and nonalcoholic beverages are expressed in 1-ounce (28.4-g) portions. We have also included the nutritive values for the minerals calcium, iron, magnesium, phosphorus, and potassium and the vitamins thiamine (B₁), riboflavin (B₂), niacin, and cobalamin (B₁₂). The alcoholic beverages contain no cholesterol or fat.

ALCOHOLIC BEVERAGES (1 OUNCE)

				Minerals					Vitamins			
	kCal	Protein (g)	CHO (g)	Ca (mg)	Fe (mg)	Mg (mg)	P (mg)	K (mg)	B₁ (mg)	B₂ (mg)	Niacin (mg)	B₁₂ (mg)
Beer, regular	12	0.072	1.1	1.4	0.009	1.83	3.50	7.09	0.002	0.007	0.128	0.005
Beer, light	8	0.057	0.4	1.4	0.011	1.42	3.44	5.13	0.003	0.008	0.111	0.002
Brandy	69	0	10.6	2.5	0.012		1.01	1.01	0.002	0.002	0.004	0
Champagne	22	0.043	0.6	1.6	0.093	2.40	1.90	22.60	0	0.003	0.019	0
Dessert wine, dry	36	0.057	1.2	2.3	0.068	2.55	2.55	26.20	0.005	0.005	0.060	0
Dessert wine, sweet	44	0.057	3.3	2.3	0.057	2.55	2.64	26.20	0.005	0.005	0.060	0
Gin, rum, vodka, scotch, whiskey, 80 proof	64	0	0	0	0.010	0	0	1.01	0	0	0	0
Gin, rum, vodka, scotch, whiskey, 86 proof	71	0	0	0	0.012	0	1.16	0.55	0.002	0.002	0.004	0

ALCOHOLIC BEVERAGES (1 OUNCE) — *continued*

	kCal	Protein (g)	CHO (g)	Minerals					Vitamins			
				Ca (mg)	Fe (mg)	Mg (mg)	P (mg)	K (mg)	B₁ (mg)	B₂ (mg)	Niacin (mg)	B₁₂ (mg)
Gin, rum, vodka, scotch, whiskey, 90 proof	74	0	0	0	0.010	0	0	0.86	0	0	0	0
Sherry, dry	28	0.024	0.3	2.1	0.052	1.96	2.60	17.80	0.002	0.002	0.024	0
Sherry, medium	40	0.066	2.3	2.3	0.071	2.27	1.89	23.60	0.002	0.008	0.035	0
Vermouth, dry	34	0.028	1.6	2.0	0.096	1.42	1.89	11.30	NA	NA	0.011	0
Vermouth, sweet	44	0.014	4.5	1.7	0.099	1.13	1.65	8.50	NA	NA	0.011	0
Wine, dry white	19	0.029	0.2	2.6	0.093	2.62	1.67	17.40	0	0.001	0.019	0
Wine, medium white	19	0.028	0.2	2.5	0.085	3.03	3.84	22.60	0.001	0.001	0.019	0
Wine, red	20	0.055	0.5	2.2	0.122	3.60	3.84	31.50	0.001	0.008	0.023	0.004
Wine, rosé	20	0.055	0.4	2.4	0.108	2.74	4.08	28.10	0.001	0.004	0.020	0.002
Creme de menthe	105	0	11.8	0	0.023	0	0	0	0	0	0.001	0
Bloody mary	22	0.153	0.9	1.9	0.105	2.10	4.02	41.40	0.010	0.006	0.123	0
Bourbon and soda	26	0	0	1.0	0.244	0.24	0.48	0.48	0	0	0.005	0
Daiquiri	52	0	1.9	0.9	0.043	0.47	1.89	6.14	0.004	0.	0.012	0
Manhattan	64	0	0.9	0.5	0.025	0.01	1.99	7.46	0.003	0.001	0.026	0
Martini	63	0	0.1	0.4	0.024	0.40	0.81	5.26	0	0	0.004	0
Pina colada	53	0.120	8.0	2.2	0.062		2.01	20.10	0.008	0.004	0.033	0
Screwdriver	23	0.160	2.5	2.1	0.023	2.26	3.86	43.30	0.018	0.004	0.046	0
Tequila	31	0.099	2.4	1.7	0.077	1.98	2.80	29.30	0.010	0.005	0.054	0
Tom collins	16	0.013	0.4	1.3	NA	0.38	0.12	2.30	0	0	0.004	0
Whiskey sour	42	0	3.7	0.3	0.021	0.26	1.60	5.08	0.003	0.002	0.006	0
Coffee + cream liqueur	93	0.784	5.9	4.2	0.036	0.60	13.90	9.05	0	0.016	0.022	0
Coffee liqueur	95	0	13.3	0.5	0.016	0.54	1.64	8.18	0.001	0.003	0.040	0

NON ALCOHOLIC BEVERAGES (1 OUNCE)

	kCal	Protein (g)	CHO (g)	Minerals					Vitamins			
				Ca (mg)	Fe (mg)	Mg (mg)	P (mg)	K (mg)	B₁ (mg)	B₂ (mg)	Niacin (mg)	B₁₂ (mg)
Hot cocoa with whole milk	25	1.030	2.9	33.8	0.088	6.350	30.60	54.400	0.012	0.049	0.041	0.099
Cocoa mix + water—diet	7	0.561	1.3	13.3	0.110	4.870	19.80	59.800	0.006	0.030	0.024	0
Coffee—brewed	0.2	0.016	0.1	0.5	0.113	1.590	0.32	15.400	0	0.002	0.063	0
Coffee—instant dry powder	1.4	0.016	0.3	0.8	0.019	1.100	2.05	67.70	0	0	0.061	0
Coffee—capuchino	9.2	0.059	1.6	1.0	0.022	1.330	3.84	17.600	0	0	0.048	0
Coffee—Swiss mocha	7.7	0.078	1.3	1.1	0.036	1.360	4.37	17.900	0	0	0.039	0
Coffee whitener— nondairy,	38.5	0.284	3.2	2.6	0.009	0.060	18.20	54.1	0	0	0	0
liquid powder	155	1.360	15.6	6.3	0.326	1.200	120.00	230.0	0	0.047	0	0
Cola beverage, regular	12	0	3.0	0.7	0.009	0.230	3.52	0.306	0	0	0	0
Diet cola— w/aspartame	0	0	0	1.0	0.009	0.319	2.40	0	0.001	0.007	0	0
Club soda	0	0	0	1.4	0.012	0.319	0	0.479	0	0	0	0

NONALCOHOLIC BEVERAGES (1 OUNCE)—continued

	kCal	Protein (g)	CHO (g)	Minerals						Vitamins			
				Ca (mg)	Fe (mg)	Mg (mg)	P (mg)	K (mg)	B₁ (mg)	B₂ (mg)	Niacin (mg)	B₁₂ (mg)
Cream soda	15	0	3.8	1.5	0.015	0.229	0	0.306	0	0	0	0
Diet soda-avg assorted	0	0	0.0	1.1	0.011	0.200	3.03	0.559	0	0	0	0
Egg nog—commercial	38	1.080	3.8	36.8	0.057	5.250	31.00	46.900	0.010	0.054	0.030	0.127
Five Alive citrus	13	0.135	3.1	1.7	0.021	1.950	2.70	34.000	0.015	0.003	0.060	0
Fruit flavored soda pop	13	0	3.2	1.1	0.020	0.305	0.15	1.520	0	0	0.002	0
Fruit punch drink—canned	13	0.015	3.4	2.1	0.058	0.610	0.31	7.160	0.006	0.006	0.006	0
Gatorade	5	0	1.3	2.8	NA	NA	0	2.840	NA	NA	NA	0
Ginger ale	10	0.008	2.5	0.9	0.051	0.232	0.08	0.387	0	0	0	0
Grape soda carbonated	12	0	3.2	0.9	0.024	0.305	0	0.229	0	0	0	0
Kool-Aid w/ NutraSweet	0	0	0	0	0	0.028	0	0	0	0	0	0
Kool-Aid w/sugar added	12	0	3.0	0	0	0	0	0	0	0	0	0
Lemon-lime soda	12	0	3.0	0.7	0.019	0.154	0.08	0.308	0	0	0.004	0
Lemonade drink from dry	11	0	2.9	7.6	0.016	0.322	3.65	3.540	0	0	0.004	0
Lemonade frozen conc	51	0.078	13.3	1.9	0.205	1.420	2.46	19.200	0.007	0.027	0.020	0
Limeade frozen conc	53	0.052	14.0	1.4	0.029	7.800	1.69	16.800	0.003	0.003	0.028	0
Chocolate milkshake	36	0.962	5.8	32.0	0.088	4.700	28.90	56.800	0.016	0.069	0.046	0.097
Strawberry milkshake	32	0.952	5.4	32.0	0.030	3.600	28.40	51.700	0.013	0.055	0.050	0.088
Vanilla milkshake	32	0.982	5.1	34.5	0.026	3.500	29.00	49.300	0.013	0.052	0.052	0.101
Orange drink/ carbonated	14	0	3.5	1.5	0.018	0.305	0.31	0.686	0	0	0	0
Pepper-type soda	12	0	2.9	0.9	0.010	0.077	3.16	0.154	0	0	0	0
Root beer	12	0.008	3.0	1.5	0.014	0.306	0.15	0.230	0	0	0	0
Pineapple grapefruit drink	13	0.068	3.3	2.0	0.087	1.700	1.59	17.500	0.009	0.005	0.076	0
Pineapple orange drink	14	0.352	3.3	1.5	0.076	1.590	1.13	13.200	0.009	0.005	0.059	0
Tang orange juice crystals	13	0.170	0.06	3.1	4.57	0.002	0.02	0.008	0	0	0	0
Tonic water/Quinine water	10	0	2.5	0.4	0.019	0.077	0	0.077	0	0	0	0
Tea-brewed	0	0.001	0.1	0	0.006	0.796	0.16	10.500	0	0.004	0.012	0
Herbal tea, brewed	0	0	0	0.6	0.022	0.319	0	2.390	0.003	0.001	0	0
Perrier water	0	0	0	3.8	0	0.148	0	0	0	0	0	0
Poland Springs bottled water	0	0	0	0.4	0.001	0.239	0	0	0	0	0	0

Note: Alcoholic beverages contain no fat or cholesterol; light beer contains 0.5 g fiber and regular beer contains 1.2 g fiber per 8 oz. serving. All of the other nonmixed alcoholic beverages have no fiber.

Note: Other nonalcoholic beverages are listed in the sections on fruits and vegetables.

PART 3

Nutritive Values For Specialty and Fast-Food Items

Nutrient information was kindly provided by the manufacturer or its representative, and is reproduced from their literature. Unlike Parts 1 and 2, nutritive values are not given for 1-ounce portions but for actual amounts of the foods sold commercially. To make a direct comparison of the kCal values and the various nutrients, we recommend that the weight of the food and its nutrients be expressed relative to 1-ounce (28.4-g) portions.

Arby's

MARKET FRESH™ SALADS	Serving Weight (g)	kCal	kCals from fat	Fat – Total (g)	Saturated Fat (g)	Trans Fat (g)	Cholesterol (mg)	Sodium (mg)	Total CHO (g)	Dietary Fiber (g)	Sugars (g)	Proteins (g)
Light Buttermilk Ranch Dressing	64	112	57	6	1	0.14	1	472	13	1	5	1
Almonds, Toasted Sliced	14	81	76	8	1	0.01	0	0	2	1	0	4
Buttermilk Ranch Dressing	64	325	304	34	5	0.67	28	657	4	0	2	1
Chicken Club Salad	366	487	229	25	8	0.5	178	1220	31	4	3	32
Garlic & Cheese Croutons	14	77	42	5	1	0.05	1	116	7	0	0	2
Martha's Vineyard Salad™	330	277	71	8	4	0	72	451	24	4	17	26
Raspberry Vinaigrette	64	194	123	14	2	0	0	387	18	0	16	0
Southwest Ranch Dressing	64	296	279	31	5	0	21	692	4	0	1	1
Santa Fe Salad™	365	477	189	21	6	0.5	53	1131	42	6	6	29
Santa Fe Salad™ w/ Grilled Chicken	350	283	77	9	4	0	72	521	21	6	8	29
Tortilla Strips	14	71	27	3	0	0	0	25	9	1	0	1

MARKET FRESH™ SANDWICHES & WRAPS	Serving Weight (g)	kCal	kCals from fat	Fat – Total (g)	Saturated Fat (g)	Trans Fat (g)	Cholesterol (mg)	Sodium (mg)	Total CHO (g)	Dietary Fiber (g)	Sugars (g)	Proteins (g)
Corned Beef Reuben Wrap	280	577	264	29	8	0.5	83	1721	42	1	6	38
Roast Turkey Reuben Wrap	280	581	241	27	6	0	94	1301	43	1	6	48
Roast Ham & Swiss Sandwich	359	705	279	31	8	0.5	63	2103	75	5	19	36
Chicken Salad w/ Pecans Sandwich	322	769	351	39	10	0	74	1240	79	9	17	30
Chicken Salad w/ Pecans Wrap	277	638	342	38	10	1	74	1199	48	8	3	30
Corned Beef Reuben Sandwich	309	606	293	33	9	0.5	83	1849	55	3	6	34
Roast Beef & Swiss Sandwich	339	777	372	41	13	1.5	89	1743	73	5	16	37
Roast Turkey & Swiss Sandwich	359	725	270	30	8	0.5	91	1788	75	5	17	45
Roast Turkey Ranch & Bacon Sandwich	382	834	341	38	11	0.5	109	2258	75	5	17	49
Roast Turkey Ranch & Bacon Wrap	317	700	332	37	11	1	109	2215	44	4	3	49
Roast Turkey Reuben Sandwich	309	611	270	30	8	0.5	94	1429	56	3	6	44
Southwest Chicken Wrap	254	567	265	29	9	1	88	1451	42	4	3	36
Ultimate BLT Sandwich	294	779	407	45	11	0.5	51	1571	75	6	18	23
Ultimate BLT Wrap	249	648	398	44	11	1	51	1530	45	5	4	23

SHAKES & DESSERTS	Serving Weight (g)	kCal	kCals from fat	Fat – Total (g)	Saturated Fat (g)	Trans Fat (g)	Cholesterol (mg)	Sodium (mg)	Total CHO (g)	Dietary Fiber (g)	Sugars (g)	Proteins (g)
Strawberry Banana Swirl Shake	482	567	140	16	9	0.5	39	425	87	0	79	15
Apple Turnover	128	377	146	16	5	6.5	0	201	65	2	41	4
Cherry Turnover	128	377	137	15	5	6	0	201	65	2	41	4
Chocolate Chip Cookie	45	202	89	10	4	2	15	213	26	1	16	2
Chocolate Shake - Large	510	660	154	17	10	0.5	43	455	110	1	106	17
Chocolate Shake - Regular	397	507	121	13	8	0	34	357	83	0	81	13
Jamocha Shake - Large	510	647	154	17	10	0.5	43	509	107	1	102	17
Jamocha Shake - Regular	397	498	121	13	8	0	34	393	81	0	78	13
Strawberry Shake - Large	510	646	154	17	10	0.5	43	464	107	1	101	16
Strawberry Shake - Regular	397	498	121	13	8	0	34	363	81	0	77	13
Vanilla Shake - Large	468	555	154	17	10	0.5	43	445	83	0	82	16
Vanilla Shake - Regular	369	437	121	13	8	0	34	350	66	0	65	13

ARBY'S CHICKEN NATURALS®	Serving Weight (g)	kCal	kCals from fat	Fat – Total (g)	Saturated Fat (g)	Trans Fat (g)	Cholesterol (mg)	Sodium (mg)	Total CHO (g)	Dietary Fiber (g)	Sugars (g)	Proteins (g)
Popcorn Chicken - Large	184	531	233	26	6	1	59	1666	39	3	0	35
Popcorn Chicken Shakers™	240	585	239	27	6	1	59	2795	51	3	9	36
Popcorn Chicken - Regular	126	365	160	18	4	0.5	40	1145	27	2	0	24
BBQ Dipping Sauce	28	44	1	0	0	0	0	343	11	0	8	0
Buffalo Dipping Sauce	28	10	5	1	0	0	0	790	2	0	1	0
Chicken Bacon & Swiss - Crispy	214	624	264	29	7	0	68	1320	52	2	13	36
Chicken Bacon & Swiss - Grilled	209	462	151	17	4	0	25	1333	38	2	9	38
Chicken Cordon Bleu Sandwich - Crispy	243	650	283	31	6	0.5	74	1548	49	2	11	40
Chicken Cordon Bleu Sandwich - Grilled	238	488	169	19	4	0	32	1561	35	2	7	42
Chicken Fillet Sandwich - Crispy	238	576	266	30	5	0	52	901	50	3	11	30
Chicken Fillet Sandwich - Grilled	233	414	153	17	3	0	9	913	36	3	7	32
Chicken Tenders - 3 piece	131	379	166	18	3	0	42	1188	28	2	0	25
Chicken Tenders - 5 piece	218	630	277	31	5	0	70	1977	47	3	0	42
Honey Mustard Dipping	28	129	106	12	2	0	9	151	6	0	5	0

ARBY'S® TOASTED SUBS

	Serving Weight (g)	kCal	kCals from fat	Fat – Total (g)	Saturated Fat (g)	Trans Fat (g)	Cholesterol (mg)	Sodium (mg)	Total CHO (g)	Dietary Fiber (g)	Sugars (g)	Proteins (g)
Classic Italian Toasted Sub	379	828	410	46	13	0.5	89	2496	69	3	5	37
French Dip & Swiss Toasted Sub	337	622	180	20	7	1.5	79	3397	68	3	2	37
Philly Beef Toasted Sub	281	739	331	37	9	1	85	1881	64	3	4	32
Turkey Bacon Club Toasted Sub	341	619	159	18	4	0	82	2052	65	3	4	42

SIDES & SIDEKICKERS®

	Serving Weight (g)	kCal	kCals from fat	Fat – Total (g)	Saturated Fat (g)	Trans Fat (g)	Cholesterol (mg)	Sodium (mg)	Total CHO (g)	Dietary Fiber (g)	Sugars (g)	Proteins (g)
Mozzarella Sticks - Regular (4)	137	426	254	28	13	1	45	1370	38	2	5	18
Bronco Berry Dipping Sauce®	57	122	0	0	0	0	0	36	30	0	28	0
Cheddar Fries - Medium	170	465	253	28	6	2	2	1311	51	5	0	6
Cheddar Cheese Sauce - side	21	30	18	2	1	0.5	1	181	2	0	0	0
Cool Ranch Sour Cream Dipping Sauce	43	158	142	16	4	0	0	277	2	0	1	1
Curly Fries - Large	198	631	337	37	7	1	0	1476	73	7	0	8
Curly Fries - Medium	125	397	212	24	4	0	0	928	46	4	0	5
Curly Fries - Small	106	338	181	20	4	0	0	791	39	4	0	4
Homestyle Fries - Large	213	566	331	37	7	1	0	1029	82	6	1	6
Homestyle Fries - Medium	142	377	221	25	4	0.5	0	686	55	4	1	4
Homestyle Fries	142	377	221	25	4	0.67	0	686	55	4	1	4
Homestyle Fries - Small	113	302	177	20	4	0.5	0	549	44	3	1	3
Jalapeno Bites® - Large (10)	220	611	383	43	18	1.5	56	1052	58	4	5	11
Jalapeno Bites® - Regular (5)	110	305	191	21	9	1	28	526	29	2	3	5
Ketchup Packet	14	13	0	0	0	0	0	158	3	0	3	0
Loaded Potato Bites® - Large (10)	224	707	398	44	14	1.5	27	1601	54	5	0	23
Loaded Potato Bites® - Reg (5)	112	353	199	22	7	0.5	13	800	27	2	0	11
Mozzarella Sticks - Large (8)	273	849	507	56	26	2	90	2730	75	4	9	36
Onion Petals - Large	283	828	511	57	9	1	2	831	88	5	18	10
Onion Petals - Regular	113	331	205	23	4	0	1	332	35	2	7	4
Potato Cakes (2)	100	246	166	18	4	1	0	391	26	2	0	2
Potato Cakes (3)	150	369	249	28	5	1.5	0	587	39	3	0	3
Tangy Southwest Sauce®	57	333	312	35	5	0.5	29	371	5	0	4	1

Other

	Serving Weight (g)	kCal	kCals from fat	Fat – Total (g)	Saturated Fat (g)	Trans Fat (g)	Cholesterol (mg)	Sodium (mg)	Total CHO (g)	Dietary Fiber (g)	Sugars (g)	Proteins (g)
Spicy Cajun Fish Sandwich	246	603	287	32	7	0	68	883	61	3	9	21
Fish Sandwich	239	543	225	25	6	0	55	956	61	3	9	21

ARBY'S® ROAST BEEF SANDWICHES & MELTS

	Serving Weight (g)	kCal	kCals from fat	Fat – Total (g)	Saturated Fat (g)	Trans Fat (g)	Cholesterol (mg)	Sodium (mg)	Total CHO (g)	Dietary Fiber (g)	Sugars (g)	Proteins (g)
Kids Meal - Junior Roast Beef Sandwich	125	272	92	10	4	0	29	740	34	2	5	16
Arby's Melt	146	302	110	12	4	1	30	921	36	2	5	16
Arby's Sauce	14	15	1	0	0	0	0	177	4	0	1	0
Bacon Beef 'n Cheddar Sandwich	212	521	239	27	9	1.5	64	1573	45	2	9	27
BBQ Bacon \'n Jack 2for	169	360	141	16	5	0.5	38	1175	42	2	10	19
Beef 'n Cheddar Sandwich	195	445	185	21	6	1.5	51	1274	44	2	8	22
French Dip & Swiss Sandwich	224	473	160	18	7	1	79	1679	38	3	2	32
Ham & Swiss Melt Sandwich	138	275	51	6	2	0	27	1118	35	1	6	18
Horsey Sauce	14	62	45	5	1	0	5	173	3	0	1	0
Large Roast Beef Sandwich	281	547	256	28	12	1.5	102	1869	41	3	6	42
Medium Roast Beef Sandwich	210	415	186	21	9	1	73	1379	34	2	5	31
Regular Roast Beef	154	320	123	14	5	0.5	44	953	34	2	5	21
Mayonnaise Packet	14	105	103	11	2	0	9	74	0	0	0	0
Sourdough Ham Melt	165	380	118	13	3	0	31	1280	39	2	5	19
Sourdough Roast Beef Melt	166	355	126	14	5	1	30	1047	40	2	4	18
Super Roast Beef	198	398	174	19	6	0.5	44	1060	40	2	10	21
Swiss Melt	146	303	111	12	4	1	29	919	37	2	6	16
SpicyThree Pepper Sauce®	14	22	8	1	0	0	0	140	3	0	3	0

KIDS MEAL

	Serving Weight (g)	kCal	kCals from fat	Fat – Total (g)	Saturated Fat (g)	Trans Fat (g)	Cholesterol (mg)	Sodium (mg)	Total CHO (g)	Dietary Fiber (g)	Sugars (g)	Proteins (g)
Kids Meal - Junior Roast Beef Sandwich	125	272	92	10	4	0	29	740	34	2	5	16
Fruit Cup	57	35	2	0	0	0	0	0	9	1	8	0
Market Fresh™Mini Ham & Cheese Sandwich	112	228	43	5	1	0	23	916	28	2	6	14
Market Fresh™ Mini Turkey & Cheese Sandwich	112	235	40	4	1	0	33	798	28	2	6	17
Kids Meal - Chicken Tenders - 2 piece	100	289	127	14	2	0	32	907	21	1	0	19

BREAKFAST

	Serving Weight (g)	kCal	kCals from fat	Fat – Total (g)	Saturated Fat (g)	Trans Fat (g)	Cholesterol (mg)	Sodium (mg)	Total CHO (g)	Dietary Fiber (g)	Sugars (g)	Proteins (g)
Bacon & Egg Croissant	120	337	195	22	10	0	187	651	23	1	3	11
Bacon Biscuit	95	340	191	21	6	0	13	1028	29	1	3	9
Bacon, Egg & Cheese Biscuit	158	461	251	28	8	0	169	1446	30	1	4	17
Bacon, Egg & Cheese Croissant	133	378	202	22	10	0	198	850	23	1	3	14
Bacon, Egg & Cheese Sourdough	173	437	146	16	5	0	174	1220	40	2	5	20
Bacon, Egg, & Cheese Wrap	193	515	257	29	8	0.5	165	1367	50	2	2	16
Biscuit - Plain	82	273	139	15	4	0	1	786	28	1	3	5
Blueberry Muffin	85	320	108	12	2	0	20	490	49	1	26	4
Breakfast Syrup	28	78	0	0	0	0	0	25	20	0	11	0
Chicken Biscuit	132	417	203	23	5	0	17	1240	39	1	3	15
Croissant	57	190	90	10	6	0	30	190	21	1	2	3
Egg & Cheese Sourdough	164	392	112	12	3	0	166	1058	40	2	5	17
French Toastix	124	312	119	13	2	0	0	492	44	1	11	6
Sausage, Egg & Cheese Biscuit	185	557	340	38	11	0	187	1579	30	1	3	18
Sausage, Egg & Cheese Sourdough	191	514	246	27	8	0	186	1232	40	2	5	19
Ham & Cheese Croissant	113	274	108	12	7	0	53	842	22	1	3	13
Ham Biscuit	125	316	151	17	4	0	13	1240	29	1	4	13
Ham, Egg & Cheese Biscuit	188	437	211	23	6	0	169	1658	31	1	4	20
Ham, Egg & Cheese Croissant	213	434	216	24	10	0	343	1282	25	1	4	22
Ham, Egg & Cheese Sourdough	296	679	318	35	11	0	354	2104	42	2	6	34
Ham, Egg, & Cheese Wrap	242	568	275	31	10	1	183	1929	51	2	3	24
Sausage & Egg Croissant	147	433	284	32	13	0	206	784	23	1	3	12
Sausage Biscuit	122	436	279	31	9	0	32	1160	28	1	3	10
Sausage Gravy Biscuit	238	961	614	68	14	0	12	3755	107	1	19	7
Sausage Patty	51	210	180	20	7	0	40	480	0	0	0	6
Sausage, Egg & Cheese Croissant	160	475	290	32	13	0	216	982	23	1	3	15
Sausage, Egg & Cheese Wrap	239	689	404	45	15	1	202	1849	50	2	2	21

Burger King
Core Menu Items August 7, 2007

Nutrition: Menu Items	Serving Size (g)	kCal	Total Fat (g)	Saturated Fat (g)	Trans Fat (g)	Cholesterol (mg)	Sodium (mg)	Total CHO (g)	Dietary Fiber (g)	Total Sugars (g)	Protein (g)
Whopper Sandwiches											
WHOPPER® Sandwich	290	670	39	11	1.5	51	1020	51	3	11	28
w/o mayo	269	510	22	9	1	80	880	51	3	11	28
WHOPPER® Sandwich with Cheese	315	760	47	16	1.5	115	1450	52	3	11	33
w/o mayo	294	600	30	14	1.5	100	1310	52	3	11	32
DOUBLE WHOPPER® Sandwich	373	900	57	19	2	175	1090	51	3	11	47
w/o mayo	352	740	39	17	2	160	950	51	3	11	47
DOUBLE WHOPPER® Sandwich w/Cheese	398	990	64	24	2.5	195	1520	52	3	11	52
w/o mayo	376	830	47	22	2	180	1380	52	3	11	52
TRIPLE WHOPPER® Sandwich	456	1130	74	27	3	255	1160	51	3	11	67
w/o mayo	434	980	57	24	2.5	240	1020	51	3	11	66
TRIPLE WHOPPER® Sandwich w/Cheese	480	1230	82	32	3.5	275	1590	52	3	11	71
w/o mayo	459	1070	65	29	3	260	1450	52	3	11	71
WHOPPER JR.® Sandwich	158	370	21	6	0.5	50	570	31	2	6	15
w/o mayo	147	290	12	4.5	0	40	490	31	2	6	15
WHOPPER JR.® Sandwich with Cheese	170	410	24	8	1	60	780	32	2	6	18
w/o mayo	149	330	16	7	0.5	55	710	31	2	6	17
Bacon (1 Strip)	2.5	15	1	0	0	5	50	0	0	0	1

Fire-Grilled Burgers	Serving Size (g)	kCal	Total Fat (g)	Saturated Fat (g)	Trans Fat (g)	Cholesterol (mg)	Sodium (mg)	Total CHO (g)	Dietary Fiber (g)	Total Sugars (g)	Protein (g)
Hamburger	121	290	12	4.5	0	40	560	30	1	6	15
Cheeseburger	133	330	16	7	0.5	55	780	31	1	6	17
Double Hamburger	164	410	21	9	1	85	600	30	1	6	25
Double Cheeseburger	189	500	29	14	1.5	105	1030	31	1	6	30
Bacon Cheeseburger	138	360	18	8	0.5	60	870	31	1	6	19
Bacon Double Cheeseburger	194	530	31	14	1.5	110	1130	32	1	6	32
BK™ Double Stacker	190	610	39	16	1.5	125	1100	32	1	5	34
BK™ Triple Stacker	250	800	54	23	2	185	1450	33	1	5	48
BK™ Quad Stacker	311	1000	68	30	3	240	1800	34	1	6	62
The Angus Steak Burger	273	640	33	10	1.5	185	1260	55	3	10	33

Chicken, Fish, & Veggie	Serving Size (g)	kCal	Total Fat (g)	Saturated Fat (g)	Trans Fat (g)	Cholesterol (mg)	Sodium (mg)	Total CHO (g)	Dietary Fiber (g)	Total Sugars (g)	Protein (g)
TENDERGRILL® Chicken Sandwich	258	450	10	2	0	75	1210	53	4	9	37
with Mayo	258	510	19	3.5	0.5	75	1180	49	4	7	37
w/o Sauce	244	400	7	1.5	0	70	1090	49	4	7	36
TENDERCRISP® Chicken Sandwich	313	790	44	8	4	70	1640	68	5	9	33
Original Chicken Sandwich	219	660	40	8	2.5	70	1440	52	4	5	24
w/o Mayo	190	450	17	4	2	50	1250	52	4	5	23
CHICK'N CRISP™ Sandwich	144	480	31	5	2	45	870	36	1	4	15
w/o Mayo	122	320	13	2.5	1.5	30	730	36	1	4	15
CHICKEN TENDERS® Kid's Meal 4 pc	62	170	10	2.5	1.5	25	480	11	0	0	9
CHICKEN TENDERS® 5 pc	77	210	12	3	2	35	600	13	0	0	12
CHICKEN TENDERS® Big Kid's Meal 6 pc	92	250	15	3.5	2.5	40	720	16	0	0	14
CHICKEN TENDERS® 8 pc	123	340	20	5	3	55	960	21	<1	1	19

Chicken, Fish, & Veggie—continued

	Serving Size (g)	kCal	Total Fat (g)	Saturated Fat (g)	Trans Fat (g)	Cholesterol (mg)	Sodium (mg)	Total CHO (g)	Dietary Fiber (g)	Total Sugars (g)	Protein (g)
Barbecue Dipping Sauce (1 oz)	28	40	0	0	0	0	310	11	0	10	0
Honey Mustard Dipping Sauce (1 oz)	28	90	6	1	0	10	180	8	0	7	0
Sweet and Sour Dipping Sauce (1 oz)	28	45	0	0	0	0	55	11	0	10	0
Ranch Dipping Sauce (1 oz)	28	140	15	2.5	0	5	95	1	0	1	1
BK™ CHICKEN FRIES 6 pc	85	260	15	3.5	3	35	650	18	2	1	12
9 pc	128	390	23	5	4.5	50	980	26	3	1	18
12 pc	170	520	31	7	6	65	1300	35	4	2	25
Buffalo Dipping Sauce (1 oz)	28	80	8	1.5	0	5	350	2	0	1	0
BK BIG FISH® Sandwich	249	640	32	6	2.5	65	1450	67	3	9	24
w/o Tartar Sauce	220	470	13	3	2	50	1240	65	3	7	23
BK VEGGIE® Burger**	215	420	16	2.5	0	10	1100	46	7	8	23
w/ Cheese	228	470	20	5	0	20	1320	47	7	9	25
w/o Mayo	205	340	8	1	0	0	1030	46	7	8	23

Side Orders

	Serving Size (g)	kCal	Total Fat (g)	Saturated Fat (g)	Trans Fat (g)	Cholesterol (mg)	Sodium (mg)	Total CHO (g)	Dietary Fiber (g)	Total Sugars (g)	Protein (g)
MOTT'S® Strawberry Flavored Apple Sauce	113	90	0	0	0	0	0	23	<1	21	0
Onion Rings - Small	43	140	7	1.5	1	0	210	18	2	2	2
Onion Rings - Medium	91	310	15	3.5	2.5	0	440	37	3	4	4
Onion Rings - Large	130	440	22	4.5	4	0	620	53	5	6	6
Onion Rings - King	150	500	25	5	4.5	0	720	62	5	7	7
Zesty Onion Ring Dipping Sauce (1 oz)	28	150	15	2.5	0	15	210	3	<1	2	0
CHEESY TOTS™ - Small (6 pc)	77	210	12	4.5	2	20	650	20	2	1	7
CHEESY TOTS™ - Medium (9 pc)	115	320	18	7	3	30	970	30	2	2	10
CHEESY TOTS™ - Large (12 pc)	153	430	24	9	4	40	1300	40	3	2	14

	Serving Size (g)	kCal	Total Fat (g)	Saturated Fat (g)	Trans Fat (g)	Cholesterol (mg)	Sodium (mg)	Total CHO (g)	Dietary Fiber (g)	Total Sugars (g)	Protein (g)
French Fries - Small (Salted)	74	230	13	3	3	0	380	26	2	1	2
French Fries - Medium (Salted)	116	360	20	4.5	4.5	0	590	41	4	1	4
French Fries - Large (Salted)	160	500	28	6	6	0	820	57	5	1	5
French Fries - King (Salted)	194	600	33	8	7	0	990	69	6	2	6
French Fries - Small (Salt not added)	74	230	13	3	3	0	240	26	2	1	2
French Fries - Medium (Salt not added)	116	360	20	4.5	4.5	0	380	41	4	1	4
French Fries - Large (Salt not added)	160	500	28	6	6	0	530	57	5	1	5
French Fries - King (Salt not added)	194	600	33	8	7	0	640	69	6	2	6

Salads (w/out dressing or garlic parmesan croutons)

	Serving Size (g)	kCal	Total Fat (g)	Saturated Fat (g)	Trans Fat (g)	Cholesterol (mg)	Sodium (mg)	Total CHO (g)	Dietary Fiber (g)	Total Sugars (g)	Protein (g)
Side Garden Salad	98	15	0	0	0	0	0	3	1	1	1
TENDERGRILL™ Chicken Garden Salad	292	240	9	3.5	0	80	720	8	4	3	33
TENDERCRISP™ Chicken Garden Salad	306	410	22	6	3.5	70	1080	26	5	5	29
Garden Salad (no chicken)	184	90	5	2.5	0	15	125	7	3	3	5

Salad Dressings & Toppings & Condiments

	Serving Size (g)	kCal	Total Fat (g)	Saturated Fat (g)	Trans Fat (g)	Cholesterol (mg)	Sodium (mg)	Total CHO (g)	Dietary Fiber (g)	Total Sugars (g)	Protein (g)
KEN'S® Light Italian Dressing (2 oz)	57	120	11	1.5	0	0	440	5	0	4	0
KEN'S® Ranch Dressing (2 oz)	57	190	20	3	0	20	560	2	0	1	1
KEN'S® Creamy Caesar Dressing (2 oz)	57	210	21	4	0	25	610	4	0	3	3
KEN'S® Honey Mustard Dressing (2 oz)	57	270	23	3	0	20	520	15	0	14	1
KEN'S® Fat Free Ranch Dressing (2 oz)	57	60	0	0	0	0	740	15	2	5	0

Salads (w/out dressing or garlic parmesan croutons)

	Serving Size (g)	kCal	Total Fat (g)	Saturated Fat (g)	Trans Fat (g)	Cholesterol (mg)	Sodium (mg)	Total CHO (g)	Dietary Fiber (g)	Total Sugars (g)	Protein (g)
Garlic Parmesan Croutons	14	60	2	0	0	0	120	9	0	1	1
Ketchup (Packet)	10	10	0	0	0	0	125	3	0	2	0
Mayonnaise (Packet)	12	80	9	0.5	0	10	75	1	0	0	0

Desserts

	Serving Size (g)	kCal	Total Fat (g)	Saturated Fat (g)	Trans Fat (g)	Cholesterol (mg)	Sodium (mg)	Total CHO (g)	Dietary Fiber (g)	Total Sugars (g)	Protein (g)
Dutch Apple Pie	108	300	13	3	3	0	270	45	1	23	2
HERSHEY®'S Sundae Pie	79	310	19	12	0	10	220	32	1	22	3

Breakfast

	Serving Size (g)	kCal	Total Fat (g)	Saturated Fat (g)	Trans Fat (g)	Cholesterol (mg)	Sodium (mg)	Total CHO (g)	Dietary Fiber (g)	Total Sugars (g)	Protein (g)
CROISSAN'WICH® Egg & Cheese	115	300	17	6	2	145	740	26	<1	5	12
CROISSAN'WICH® Sausage & Cheese	106	370	25	9	2	50	810	23	<1	4	14
CROISSAN'WICH® Sausage, Egg & Cheese	159	470	32	11	2.5	180	1060	26	<1	5	19
CROISSAN'WICH® Ham, Egg & Cheese	149	340	18	6	2	160	1230	26	1	6	18
CROISSAN'WICH® Bacon, Egg & Cheese	122	340	20	7	2	155	890	26	<1	5	15
DOUBLE CROISSAN'WICH™ w/Sausage, Egg, & Cheese	215	680	51	18	3	220	1590	26	1	6	29
DOUBLE CROISSAN'WICH™ w/Bacon, Egg, & Cheese	142	430	27	10	2	175	1250	27	<1	6	21
DOUBLE CROISSAN'WICH™ w/Ham, Egg, & Cheese	196	420	23	9	2	185	2210	27	1	7	27
DOUBLE CROISSAN'WICH™ w/Sausage, Bacon, Egg & Cheese	179	550	39	14	2.5	200	1420	27	1	6	25
DOUBLE CROISSAN'WICH™ w/Ham, Bacon, Egg & Cheese	169	420	24	9	2	180	1600	27	1	7	24

Item											
DOUBLE CROISSAN'WICH™ w/Ham, Sausage, Egg & Cheese	206	550	37	14	2.5	205	2040	27	1	6	28
Enormous Omelet Sandwich	266	730	45	16	1	330	1940	44	2	8	37
Ham Omelet Sandwich	139	330	14	5	0	90	1130	35	1	9	16
Sausage Biscuit	118	390	26	8	5	35	1020	28	1	2	12
Ham, Egg, & Cheese Biscuit	156	390	22	7	5	145	1410	31	1	4	16
Sausage, Egg, & Cheese Biscuit	183	530	37	12	6	175	1490	31	1	4	20
Bacon, Egg & Cheese Biscuit	146	410	25	8	5	150	1320	31	1	4	16
Hash Browns – Small	84	260	17	4.5	5	0	500	25	2	0	2
Hash Browns – Medium	140	430	28	8	9	0	830	42	4	0	4
Hash Browns – Large	202	620	40	11	13	0	1200	60	6	1	5
CHEESY TOTS™ - See Side Orders											
Cini-minis	108	390	18	5	4	20	560	51	2	19	7
Vanilla Icing (for Cini-minis)	28	110	3	0.5	0.5	0	40	21	0	20	0
French Toast Sticks (3 piece)	65	240	13	2.5	2	0	260	26	1	6	4
French Toast Sticks (5 piece)	109	390	22	4.5	3	0	440	43	2	9	7
French Toast Kid's Meal (with syrup)	494	680	24	6	3	10	590	100	3	55	15
Grape Jam	12	30	0	0	0	0	0	7	0	6	0
Strawberry Jam	12	30	0	0	0	0	0	7	0	6	0
Breakfast Syrup	28	80	0	0	0	0	20	21	0	14	0

Footnote for "Saturated Fat* (g)": Does Not Include Trans Fat
Footnote for BK VEGGIE® Burger**: **Burger King Corporation makes no claim that the BK VEGGIE® Burger or any other of its products meets the requirements of a vegan or vegetarian diet. The patty is cooked in the microwave.
Footnote for "Salt not added–French Fries": To reduce sodium, you can order French fries without added salt
CHEESY TOTS™ is a trademark of H.J. Heinz Company and used under license by Burger King Corporation.

Carl's Jr.

CHARBROILED BURGERS	Serving Size (g)	kCal	kCals from fat	Total Fat (g)	Saturated Fat (g)	Cholesterol (mg)	Sodium (mg)	Total CHO (g)	Dietary Fiber (g)	Sugars (g)	Protein (g)
The Original Six Dollar Burger™	430	1010	600	68	27	150	1980	60	3	18	40
The Western Bacon Six Dollar Burger™	382	1130	600	66	28	150	2540	83	4	19	47
The Bacon Cheese Six Dollar Burger™	409	1070	670	76	30	170	1910	50	3	10	46
The Guacamole Bacon Six Dollar Burger™	447	1140	760	85	29	160	2010	54	6	11	43
The Double Six Dollar Burger™	602	1520	990	111	47	265	2760	60	3	18	69
The Low Carb Six Dollar Burger™	267	490	330	37	15	130	1290	6	2	4	33
Famous Star™ with Cheese	278	660	340	39	12	85	1260	53	3	10	27
Super Star® with Cheese	385	930	520	59	21	160	1600	54	3	10	47
Philly Cheesesteak Burger	297	830	480	55	17	125	1510	52	3	9	40
Western Bacon Cheeseburger®	241	710	290	33	12	85	1480	70	3	15	32
Double Western Bacon Cheeseburger™	323	970	470	52	21	155	1820	71	3	15	52
Jalapeño Burger™	286	720	410	45	8	90	1320	50	3	10	27
Big Hamburger	209	470	160	17	6	60	1060	54	3	13	24
Kid's hamburger	195	460	160	17	6	60	1060	53	2	13	24

CHICKEN & OTHER CHOICES	Serving Size (g)	kCal	kCals from fat	Total Fat (g)	Saturated Fat (g)	Cholesterol (mg)	Sodium (mg)	Total CHO (g)	Dietary Fiber (g)	Sugars (g)	Protein (g)
Charbroiled BBQ Chicken™ Sandwich	239	360	40	4.5	1	60	1150	48	4	12	34
Charbroiled Chicken Club™ Sandwich	264	550	210	25	7	95	1410	43	4	9	40
Charbroiled Santa Fe Chicken™ Sandwich	264	610	290	32	8	100	1540	43	4	10	37
Bacon Swiss Crispy Chicken™ Sandwich	318	720	310	35	8	85	1750	64	3	9	35
Chicken Breast Strips (3 pieces)	129	420	220	25	3.5	50	1210	28	1	1	23
Chicken Breast Strips (5 pieces)	215	710	370	41	6	80	2020	46	2	1	38
Spicy Chicken Sandwich	213	560	260	30	6	40	1480	59	2	7	15
Carl's Catch™ Fish Sandwich	291	660	280	31	5	30	1290	75	3	14	22

SIDES	Serving Size (g)	kCal	kCals from fat	Total Fat (g)	Saturated Fat (g)	Cholesterol (mg)	Sodium (mg)	Total CHO (g)	Dietary Fiber (g)	Sugars (g)	Protein (g)
French Fries (Kids)	79	250	110	12	2.5	0	150	32	3	0	4
French Fries (Small)	92	290	120	14	3	0	180	37	3	0	5

SIDES—*continued*

	Serving Size (g)	kCal	kCals from fat	Total Fat (g)	Saturated Fat (g)	Cholesterol (mg)	Sodium (mg)	Total CHO (g)	Dietary Fiber (g)	Sugars (g)	Protein (g)
French Fries (Medium)	147	460	200	22	4.5	0	280	59	5	1	7
French Fries (Large)	198	620	260	29	6	0	380	80	7	1	10
Onion Rings	128	430	190	21	4	0	550	53	2	5	6
Fried Zucchini	139	320	170	19	5	0	850	31	0	0	6
Fish & Chips	258	630	250	28	5	10	990	68	3	4	26
CrissCut® Fries	139	410	220	24	5	0	950	43	4	0	5
Chicken Stars™ (4 pieces)	57	170	100	11	3	25	320	10	1	0	9
Chicken Stars™ (6 pieces)	85	260	150	16	4	35	470	14	1	1	13
Chicken Stars™ (9 pieces)	127	380	220	24	6	55	710	21	1	1	20

SALADS – WITHOUT DRESSINGS

	Serving Size (g)	kCal	kCals from fat	Total Fat (g)	Saturated Fat (g)	Cholesterol (mg)	Sodium (mg)	Total CHO (g)	Dietary Fiber (g)	Sugars (g)	Protein (g)
Charbroiled Chicken Salad	417	260	60	7	3.5	75	710	16	5	8	34
Side Salad	139	50	20	2.5	1.5	5	60	5	2	3	3

SALAD DRESSINGS – 2 OZ PACKETS

	Serving Size (g)	kCal	kCals from fat	Total Fat (g)	Saturated Fat (g)	Cholesterol (mg)	Sodium (mg)	Total CHO (g)	Dietary Fiber (g)	Sugars (g)	Protein (g)
House Dressing	57	220	200	22	3.5	20	440	2	0	2	1
Blue Cheese Dressing	57	320	310	34	7	20	410	1	0	1	2
Thousand Island Dressing	57	250	20	2	3.5	20	480	7	0	3	0
Low Fat Balsamic Dressing	57	35	15	1.5	0	0	480	5	0	3	0

BREAKFAST

	Serving Size (g)	kCal	kCals from fat	Total Fat (g)	Saturated Fat (g)	Cholesterol (mg)	Sodium (mg)	Total CHO (g)	Dietary Fiber (g)	Sugars (g)	Protein (g)
Breakfast Burger™	309	830	420	47	15	275	1580	65	3	13	37
Sourdough Breakfast Sandwich	193	460	190	21	9	280	1050	39	2	4	28
Sunrise Croissant™ Sandwich	172	560	370	41	15	290	970	27	1	5	20
Bacon & Egg Burrito	208	570	300	33	11	515	990	37	1	1	30
Loaded Breakfast Burrito	328	820	460	51	16	595	1530	52	2	3	38
Steak & Egg Burrito	322	660	320	35	13	545	1690	44	0	4	40

BREAKFAST—*continued*	Serving Size (g)	kCal	kCals from fat	Total Fat (g)	Saturated Fat (g)	Cholesterol (mg)	Sodium (mg)	Total CHO (g)	Dietary Fiber (g)	Sugars (g)	Protein (g)
French Toast Dips® – No Syrup (5 pcs)	129	430	160	18	2.5	0	530	58	1	15	9
Hash Brown Nuggets	108	330	190	21	4.5	0	460	32	3	1	3

DESSERTS	Serving Size (g)	kCal	kCals from fat	Total Fat (g)	Saturated Fat (g)	Cholesterol (mg)	Sodium (mg)	Total CHO (g)	Dietary Fiber (g)	Sugars (g)	Protein (g)
Chocolate Chip Cookie	71	350	160	18	7	20	330	46	1	27	3
Chocolate Cake	85	300	100	12	3	30	350	48	1	37	3
Strawberry Swirl Cheesecake	99	290	150	17	9	55	230	30	0	20	6

HAND-SCOOPED ICE CREAM SHAKES & MALTS™	Serving Size (g)	kCal	kCals from fat	Total Fat (g)	Saturated Fat (g)	Cholesterol (mg)	Sodium (mg)	Total CHO (g)	Dietary Fiber (g)	Sugars (g)	Protein (g)
Vanilla Shake	397	710	300	33	23	100	230	86	0	76	14
Chocolate Shake	397	710	300	33	23	100	290	85	1	71	14
Strawberry Shake	397	700	300	33	23	100	240	84	0	75	14
OREO® Cookie Shake	397	720	340	37	24	100	350	79	1	64	16
Vanilla Malt	414	780	310	35	24	105	300	99	0	84	17
Chocolate Malt	414	780	310	35	24	105	360	98	1	79	17
Strawberry Malt	414	770	310	35	24	105	310	97	0	83	17
OREO® Cookie Malt	414	790	350	39	25	105	420	91	1	72	18

Dairy Queen

Burgers	Serving Size (g)	kCal	kCals from fat	Total Fat (g)	Saturated Fat (g)	Trans Fat (g)	Cholesterol (mg)	Sodium (mg)	Total CHO (g)	Dietary Fiber (g)	Sugars (g)	Proteins (g)	Percent Daily Value Vitamin A	Percent Daily Value Vitamin C	Percent Daily Value Calcium	Percent Daily Value Iron
DQ® Homestyle® Burger	142	350	130	14	7	0.5	50	400	33	1	8	17	6	0	4	15
DQ® Homestyle® Cheeseburger	156	400	160	18	9	0.5	65	640	34	1	9	19	12	0	10	15
DQ® Homestyle® Double Cheeseburger	226	640	310	34	18	1	130	950	34	1	9	34	15	0	20	25
DQ® Homestyle® Bacon Double Cheeseburger	245	730	370	41	21	1	150	1270	35	1	9	41	15	0	20	25
DQ® Ultimate® Burger	259	780	430	48	22	1.5	155	1110	33	1	8	41	20	20	20	45
1/4 lb. FlameThrower® GrillBurger™	245	780	480	54	14	3	90	1490	41	2	9	33	20	15	25	20
1/2 lb. FlameThrower® GrillBurger™	344	1030	650	73	23	4	145	2020	41	2	9	53	25	15	30	30
Classic GrillBurger™	212	470	200	23	7	2.5	40	1020	42	2	12	24	20	6	15	20
Classic GrillBurger™ with Cheese	231	560	270	30	11	2.5	60	1160	42	2	12	29	25	6	30	20
1/2 lb. GrillBurger™	297	670	330	37	12	3.5	80	1310	42	2	12	42	20	6	15	30
1/2 lb. GrillBurger™ with Cheese	330	820	430	49	19	3.5	115	1510	47	2	12	51	25	6	45	30
Bacon Cheddar GrillBurger™	229	650	330	37	13	2.5	80	1480	41	2	11	36	10	0	30	20
Mushroom Swiss GrillBurger™	210	630	350	40	11	3	65	950	39	2	8	29	4	0	30	20

Hot Dogs	Serving Size (g)	kCal	kCals from fat	Total Fat (g)	Saturated Fat (g)	Trans Fat (g)	Cholesterol (mg)	Sodium (mg)	Total CHO (g)	Dietary Fiber (g)	Sugars (g)	Proteins (g)	Percent Daily Value Vitamin A	Percent Daily Value Vitamin C	Percent Daily Value Calcium	Percent Daily Value Iron
All-Beef Hot Dog	115	300	130	15	6	0	30	870	30	1	5	11	4	0	8	15
All-Beef Chili Cheese Dog	150	380	220	24	11	0.5	55	1100	24	1	4	16	10	2	15	10

Sandwiches/Baskets

	Serving Size (g)	kcal	kCals from fat	Total Fat (g)	Saturated Fat (g)	Trans Fat (g)	Cholesterol (mg)	Sodium (mg)	Total CHO (g)	Dietary Fiber (g)	Sugars (g)	Proteins (g)	Percent Daily Value Vitamin A	Percent Daily Value Vitamin C	Percent Daily Value Calcium	Percent Daily Value Iron
Crispy Chicken Sandwich	198	540	260	29	5	2.5	45	700	47	1	6	23	10	6	4	25
Grilled Chicken Sandwich	177	350	140	16	2.5	0	55	780	49	1	6	23	10	6	4	10
Chicken Strip Basket™, 4-piece*	446	1030	480	54	9	10	75	2400	105	8	7	37	2	2	15	40
Chicken Strip Basket™, 6-piece*	531	1270	600	67	11	12	110	2910	121	10	8	51	2	2	15	50

Salads

	Serving Size (g)	kcal	kCals from fat	Total Fat (g)	Saturated Fat (g)	Trans Fat (g)	Cholesterol (mg)	Sodium (mg)	Total CHO (g)	Dietary Fiber (g)	Sugars (g)	Proteins (g)	Percent Daily Value Vitamin A	Percent Daily Value Vitamin C	Percent Daily Value Calcium	Percent Daily Value Iron
Crispy Chicken Salad – no dressing	424	420	200	22	7	2	70	960	90	6	9	28	130	80	80	25
Grilled Chicken Salad – no dressing	424	270	100	11	5	0	80	1160	92	4	9	32	130	80	70	15
Side Salad – no dressing																

Salad Dressings

	Serving Size (g)	kcal	kCals from fat	Total Fat (g)	Saturated Fat (g)	Trans Fat (g)	Cholesterol (mg)	Sodium (mg)	Total CHO (g)	Dietary Fiber (g)	Sugars (g)	Proteins (g)	Percent Daily Value Vitamin A	Percent Daily Value Vitamin C	Percent Daily Value Calcium	Percent Daily Value Iron
DQ® Honey Mustard Dressing	57	260	190	21	3.5	0	20	370	18	0	11	1	0	0	2	6
DQ® Blue Cheese Dressing	57	210	180	20	4	0	5	700	4	0	2	2	0	0	6	0
DQ® Ranch Dressing	57	310	300	33	5	0	25	390	3	0	2	1	0	0	2	0
Fat Free Italian Dressing	43	10	0	0	0	0	0	390	3	0	1	0	0	0	0	0

Fries/Onion Rings

	Serving Size (g)	kCal	kCals from fat	Total Fat (g)	Saturated Fat (g)	Trans Fat (g)	Cholesterol (mg)	Sodium (mg)	Total CHO (g)	Dietary Fiber (g)	Sugars (g)	Proteins (g)	Percent Daily Value Vitamin A	Percent Daily Value Vitamin C	Percent Daily Value Calcium	Percent Daily Value Iron
DQ® Small French Fries	140	360	150	16	3	2.5	0	760	50	5	0	4	0	2	2	6
DQ® Medium French Fries	196	510	210	23	4	3.5	0	1070	70	7	1	6	0	4	2	8
DQ® Large French Fries	280	730	290	33	6	5	0	1530	100	10	1	8	0	6	4	10
DQ® Regular Onion Rings	113	470	270	30	6	7	0	740	45	3	7	6	0	30	4	6
DQ® Large Onion Rings	142	590	330	37	7	9	0	930	56	4	9	7	0	15	4	8

Cones

	Serving Size (g)	kCal	kCals from fat	Total Fat (g)	Saturated Fat (g)	Trans Fat (g)	Cholesterol (mg)	Sodium (mg)	Total CHO (g)	Dietary Fiber (g)	Sugars (g)	Proteins (g)	Percent Daily Value Vitamin A	Percent Daily Value Vitamin C	Percent Daily Value Calcium	Percent Daily Value Iron
DQ® Vanilla Soft Serve, ½ cup	94	150	45	5	3	0	15	70	22	0	19	3	6	0	15	4
DQ® Chocolate Soft Serve, ½ cup	94	150	45	5	3.5	0	15	75	22	0	17	4	10	0	10	4
Small Vanilla Cone	142	240	70	7	4.5	0	20	115	32	0	27	6	10	2	20	6
Medium Vanilla Cone	199	340	90	10	6	0	30	160	54	0	38	8	15	2	25	8
Large Vanilla Cone	284	480	130	15	9	0.5	45	230	76	0	55	11	20	2	35	10
Small Chocolate Cone	142	240	70	7	5	0	20	115	32	0	25	6	15	0	15	8
Medium Chocolate Cone	199	340	90	10	7	0	30	160	54	0	34	9	15	2	25	10
Small Dipped Cone	156	340	140	16	10	1	20	120	36	1	31	6	10	2	20	8
Medium Dipped Cone	220	490	210	23	15	1.5	30	170	61	1	43	8	15	2	25	10
Large Dipped Cone	312	670	280	31	21	2.5	40	210	83	0	62	13	8	0	30	15

Royal Treats®

	Serving Size (g)	kCal	kCals from fat	Total Fat (g)	Saturated Fat (g)	Trans Fat (g)	Cholesterol (mg)	Sodium (mg)	Total CHO (g)	Dietary Fiber (g)	Sugars (g)	Proteins (g)	Percent Daily Value Vitamin A	Percent Daily Value Vitamin C	Percent Daily Value Calcium	Percent Daily Value Iron
Banana Split	374	530	120	14	10	0	30	180	98	3	77	8	15	35	25	10
Peanut Buster® Parfait	304	710	270	30	16	0	30	380	96	2	74	16	15	2	35	20
Brownie Earthquake™	304	740	250	28	15	0	60	370	149	1	87	10	15	2	25	15

Malts, Shakes, and Arctic Rush™

	Serving Size (g)	kCal	kCals from fat	Total Fat (g)	Saturated Fat (g)	Trans Fat (g)	Cholesterol (mg)	Sodium (mg)	Total CHO (g)	Dietary Fiber (g)	Sugars (g)	Proteins (g)	Percent Daily Value Vitamin A	Percent Daily Value Vitamin C	Percent Daily Value Calcium	Percent Daily Value Iron
Small Chocolate Malt	427	650	140	15	10	0	50	310	112	0	96	14	20	2	45	15
Medium Chocolate Malt	567	900	190	21	13	0.5	65	460	157	0	134	19	30	4	60	20
Large Chocolate Malt	854	1300	280	31	20	1	95	670	224	0	191	28	45	4	100	30
Small Chocolate Shake	406	560	130	14	9	0	45	280	95	0	82	12	20	2	45	15
Medium Chocolate Shake	550	780	180	20	13	0.5	60	380	133	0	115	17	30	4	60	20
Large Chocolate Shake	811	1130	260	29	19	1	90	500	188	0	163	25	45	4	90	25
Small Arctic Rush™ Slush	453	240	0	0	0	0	0	0	48	0	48	0	0	0	0	0
Medium Arctic Rush™ Slush	595	310	0	0	0	0	0	0	63	0	63	0	0	0	0	0

MooLatté® Frozen Blended Coffee

	Serving Size (g)	kCal	kCals from fat	Total Fat (g)	Saturated Fat (g)	Trans Fat (g)	Cholesterol (mg)	Sodium (mg)	Total CHO (g)	Dietary Fiber (g)	Sugars (g)	Proteins (g)	Percent Daily Value Vitamin A	Percent Daily Value Vitamin C	Percent Daily Value Calcium	Percent Daily Value Iron
Cappuccino MooLatté® – 16 oz.	411	500	170	18	15	0	30	170	73	0	65	7	15	2	25	6
Cappuccino MooLatté® – 24 oz.	602	710	220	24	18	0.5	50	260	107	0	95	11	20	2	40	10
Mocha MooLatté® – 16 oz.	427	590	210	23	15	0	30	200	84	0	74	8	15	2	25	10

	Serving Size (g)	kCal	kCals from fat	Total Fat (g)	Saturated Fat (g)	Trans Fat (g)	Cholesterol (mg)	Sodium (mg)	Total CHO (g)	Dietary Fiber (g)	Sugars (g)	Proteins (g)	Percent Daily Value Vitamin A	Percent Daily Value Vitamin C	Percent Daily Value Calcium	Percent Daily Value Iron
Mocha MooLatté® – 24 oz.	623	840	280	31	20	0.5	45	300	121	1	106	12	20	2	40	15
French Vanilla MooLatté® – 16 oz.	433	570	160	18	14	0	30	170	90	0	76	7	15	2	25	6
French Vanilla MooLatté® – 24 oz.	623	770	210	24	18	0.5	45	260	123	0	106	11	20	2	40	10
Caramel MooLatté® – 16 oz.	448	630	170	19	16	0	35	260	103	0	50	8	15	2	30	6
Caramel MooLatté® – 24 oz.	651	840	280	31	20	0.5	45	300	121	1	106	12	20	2	40	15

Sundaes

	Serving Size (g)	kCal	kCals from fat	Total Fat (g)	Saturated Fat (g)	Trans Fat (g)	Cholesterol (mg)	Sodium (mg)	Total CHO (g)	Dietary Fiber (g)	Sugars (g)	Proteins (g)	Percent Daily Value Vitamin A	Percent Daily Value Vitamin C	Percent Daily Value Calcium	Percent Daily Value Iron
Small Strawberry Sundae	192	280	60	7	4.5	0	20	130	50	1	45	5	10	45	20	6
Medium Strawberry Sundae	248	370	90	10	7	0	30	170	63	1	56	7	15	45	25	8
Large Strawberry Sundae	333	510	130	15	9	0	45	240	83	1	73	10	20	45	40	10
Small Chocolate Sundae	163	280	60	7	4.5	0	20	130	49	0	42	5	10	2	20	8
Medium Chocolate Sundae	234	410	90	10	7	0	30	190	72	0	61	7	15	2	25	10
Large Chocolate Sundae	333	580	130	15	9	0	45	262	100	0	86	10	20	2	35	15

Novelties

	Serving Size (g)	kCal	kCals from fat	Total Fat (g)	Saturated Fat (g)	Trans Fat (g)	Cholesterol (mg)	Sodium (mg)	Total CHO (g)	Dietary Fiber (g)	Sugars (g)	Proteins (g)	Percent Daily Value Vitamin A	Percent Daily Value Vitamin C	Percent Daily Value Calcium	Percent Daily Value Iron
DQ® Sandwich	85	190	45	5	3	0	10	95	32	1	18	4	2	0	8	2
Chocolate Dilly® Bar	87	240	140	15	9	0	15	70	24	1	20	4	6	0	10	0
Buster Bar®	148	480	280	31	15	0	20	220	45	2	35	11	8	0	20	6
StarKiss®	85	80	0	0	0	0	0	10	21	0	21	0	0	0	0	0
DQ® Fudge Bar – no sugar added	66	50	0	0	0	0	0	70	13	0	3	4	6	0	10	0
DQ® Vanilla Orange Bar – no sugar added	66	60	0	0	0	0	0	40	17	0	2	2	2	0	6	0

Blizzard® Treats

Blizzard® Treats	Serving Size (g)	kcal	Kcals from fat	Total Fat (g)	Saturated Fat (g)	Trans Fat (g)	Cholesterol (mg)	Sodium (mg)	Total CHO (g)	Dietary Fiber (g)	Sugars (g)	Proteins (g)	Vitamin A Percent Daily Value	Vitamin C Percent Daily Value	Calcium Percent Daily Value	Iron Percent Daily Value
Small Oreo®† Cookies Blizzard®	283	560	190	21	10	0	40	430	83	1	64	11	20	2	35	15
Medium Oreo®† Cookies Blizzard®	334	690	230	26	12	0.5	45	560	103	1	77	13	20	2	40	15
Large Oreo®† Cookies Blizzard®	500	1000	330	37	18	1.0	70	770	148	2	113	19	30	4	60	25
Small Choc. Chip Cookie Dough Blizzard®	319	720	250	28	14	3.0	50	370	105	1	78	12	30	2	35	15
Medium Choc. Chip Cookie Dough Blizzard®	446	1030	360	40	20	4.5	70	530	151	1	112	17	40	4	50	20
Large Choc. Chip Cookie Dough Blizzard®	560	1320	470	52	27	6.0	90	680	193	2	144	21	45	4	60	25
Small Banana Split Blizzard®	297	460	130	14	9	0	40	210	73	1	62	10	20	10	35	10
Medium Banana Split Blizzard®	382	580	150	17	11	0.5	50	260	97	1	91	12	25	15	40	15
Large Banana Split Blizzard®	527	810	210	23	15	1.0	70	360	134	1	113	16	30	25	60	
Small Reese's®†† Peanut Butter Cup Blizzard®	305	600	190	21	16	0	40	220	87	0	76	14	25	0	40	10
Medium Reese's®†† Peanut Butter Cup Blizzard®	383	790	250	28	22	0.5	50	280	114	0	99	18	30	0	50	15
Large Reese's®†† Peanut Butter Cup Blizzard®	514	1050	340	38	29	1	70	370	152	0	133	25	45	0	70	20
Small Strawberry CheeseQuake™ Blizzard®	283	530	190	21	13	1	85	320	76	<1	62	10	30	0	40	10
Medium Strawberry CheeseQuake™ Blizzard®	376	730	260	29	18	1	120	440	105	<1	84	13	40	0	50	15
Large Strawberry CheeseQuake™ Blizzard®	510	990	350	39	24	1.5	160	600	143	<1	114	18	55	0	70	20

DQ® Blizzard® Cakes

	Serving Size (g)	kCal	kCals from fat	Total Fat (g)	Saturated Fat (g)	Trans Fat (g)	Cholesterol (mg)	Sodium (mg)	Total CHO (g)	Dietary Fiber (g)	Sugars (g)	Proteins (g)	Percent Daily Value Vitamin A	Percent Daily Value Vitamin C	Percent Daily Value Calcium	Percent Daily Value Iron
Oreo® Cookies Blizzard® Cake, **8", ⅛ of Cake	220	490	180	20	12	1	30	250	67	1	51	8	15	0	25	10
Reese's® PB Cup Blizzard® Cake, **8", ⅛ of Cake	220	490	180	20	13	0	30	190	67	1	54	9	15	0	25	10
Chocolate Xtreme Blizzard® Cake, **8", ⅛ of Cake	249	660	280	31	20	1.5	40	340	85	2	68	10	20	0	25	15

DQ® Cakes

	Serving Size (g)	kCal	kCals from fat	Total Fat (g)	Saturated Fat (g)	Trans Fat (g)	Cholesterol (mg)	Sodium (mg)	Total CHO (g)	Dietary Fiber (g)	Sugars (g)	Proteins (g)	Percent Daily Value Vitamin A	Percent Daily Value Vitamin C	Percent Daily Value Calcium	Percent Daily Value Iron
8" Round Cake, **⅛ of Cake	209	410	140	16	11	1	30	220	60	<1	47	8	15	2	25	8

*Includes four or six breaded chicken strips, small French fries, Texas toast and gravy. **Undecorated
www.dairyqueen.com

Hardee's

Breakfast	Serving Size (g)	kCal	kCals from Fat	Total Fat (g)	Saturated Fat (g)	Cholesterol (mg)	Sodium (mg)	Total CHO (g)	Dietary Fiber (g)	Sugars (g)	Protein (g)
Loaded Breakfast Burrito	258	780	460	51	20	495	1620	38	2	2	40
Made from Scratch Biscuit	109	370	210	23	5	0	890	35	0	3	5
Egg Biscuit	152	450	260	29	6	205	940	35	0	4	11
Bacon Biscuit	120	430	250	28	7	10	1110	35	0	4	8
Sausage Biscuit	142	530	340	38	10	30	1240	36	0	4	11
Country Ham Biscuit	144	440	240	26	6	35	1710	36	0	3	14
Breaded Chicken Fillet Biscuit	226	600	310	34	7	55	1680	50	1	3	24
Breaded Country Steak Biscuit	180	620	370	41	11	35	1360	44	0	3	16
Breaded Pork Chop Biscuit	222	690	380	42	8	40	1330	48	1	4	29
Sausage & Egg Biscuit	185	610	390	44	11	235	1290	36	0	4	17
Country Steak & Egg Biscuit	223	690	420	47	11	235	1800	44	0	4	22
Bacon, Egg & Cheese Biscuit	174	560	340	38	11	225	1360	37	0	4	16
Ham, Egg & Cheese Biscuit	220	560	320	35	10	245	1800	37	0	5	23
Loaded Omelet Biscuit	198	640	400	44	14	245	1510	37	0	5	21
Monster Biscuit	212	710	460	51	17	70	2250	37	0	4	24
Biscuits "N" Gravy	251	530	310	34	8	10	1550	47	0	6	8
Sunrise Croissant with Ham	164	430	230	26	10	250	1050	28	0	5	23
Sunrise Croissant with Bacon	138	450	260	29	12	240	900	28	0	5	19
Sunrise Croissant with Sausage	161	550	340	38	15	265	1030	29	0	5	22
Sunrise Croissant	57	210	90	10	4	5	200	26	0	4	4
Frisco Breakfast Sandwich	185	420	180	20	7	240	1340	37	2	2.7	24
Loaded Omelet	89	270	190	21	9	245	620	2	0	2	16
Loaded Biscuit "N" Gravy Breakfast Bowl	326	770	490	54	14	245	1950	49	1	7	20
Low Carb Breakfast Bowl	208	620	450	50	21	325	1380	6	2	2	36
Pancake Platter	135	300	45	5	1	25	830	55	2	12	8
Big Country Breakfast Platter – Country Ham	377	970	470	53	12	460	2600	90	3	12	33
Big Country Breakfast Platter – Bacon	355	980	500	56	13	435	2080	90	3	13	28
Big Country Breakfast Platter – Sausage	374	1060	570	64	15	455	2140	91	4	13	30
Big Country Breakfast Platter – Chicken	458	1140	540	61	13	480	2580	105	4	12	44

Breakfast—continued

	Serving Size (g)	kCal	kCals from Fat	Total Fat (g)	Saturated Fat (g)	Cholesterol (mg)	Sodium (mg)	Total CHO (g)	Dietary Fiber (g)	Sugars (g)	Protein (g)
Big Country Breakfast Platter – Breaded Pork Chop	455	1220	620	68	13	465	2230	102	4	13	48
Big Country Breakfast Platter – Country Steak	412	1150	610	68	16	455	2260	98	4	12	36
Hash Rounds – small	83	260	150	16	4	0	360	25	2	1	3
Hash Rounds – medium	114	350	200	22	5	0	490	34	3	1	4

Lunch & Dinner

	Serving Size (g)	kCal	kCals from Fat	Total Fat (g)	Saturated Fat (g)	Cholesterol (mg)	Sodium (mg)	Total CHO (g)	Dietary Fiber (g)	Sugars (g)	Protein (g)
1/3 LB** Thickburger	349	910	570	64	21	110	1560	53	3	13	30
1/3 LB** Cheeseburger	254	680	350	39	19	90	1450	52	2	11	29
1/3 LB** Mushroom 'N' Swiss Thickburger	276	720	380	42	21	100	1570	48	2	7	35
1/3 LB** Bacon Cheese Thickburger	334	910	570	64	24	115	1550	50	3	10	33
1/3 LB** Low Carb Thickburger	245	420	280	32	12	115	1010	5	2	3	30
1/2 LB** Six Dollar Burger	412	1060	660	73	28	150	1950	58	3	18	40
1/2 LB** Grilled Sourdough Thickburger	381	1030	690	77	28	155	1910	42	2.8	5.4	42
2/3 LB** Double Thickburger	471	1250	810	90	35	195	2160	54	3	13	51
2/3 LB** Double Bacon Cheese Thickburger	463	1300	870	97	38	205	2200	50	3	10	54
2/3 LB** Monster Thickburger	413	1420	970	108	43	230	2770	46	2	9	60
Charbroiled Chicken Club Sandwich	277	560	270	30	8	95	1430	32	3	7	39
Charbroiled BBQ Chicken Sandwich	242	340	40	4	1	60	1070	40	3	13	33
Low Carb Charbroiled Chicken Club Sandwich	250	370	190	21	7	90	1170	10	2	5	35
Big Chicken Fillet Sandwich	351	800	330	37	6	90	1890	76	3	9	41
Spicy Chicken Sandwich	159	470	230	25	5	40	1220	46	2	6	13
Regular Roast Beef	137	330	150	16	7	40	860	29	2	2	19
Big Roast Beef	199	470	210	23	10	60	1290	38	2	3	29
Hot Ham 'N' Cheese	191	420	170	18	10	55	1600	39	2	4	30
Big Hot Ham 'N' Cheese	244	520	210	24	13	85	2190	40	2	4	40
Hot Dog	152	420	270	30	12	55	1200	22	1	4	16
1/4 LB** Double Cheeseburger	186	510	240	26	5	90	1120	38	1	9	28

Lunch & Dinner—*continued*	Serving Size (g)	kCal	kCals from Fat	Total Fat (g)	Saturated Fat (g)	Cholesterol (mg)	Sodium (mg)	Total CHO (g)	Dietary Fiber (g)	Sugars (g)	Protein (g)
1/4 LB** Double Hamburger	161	420	170	19	5	70	670	37	1	9	23
Cheeseburger	131	350	140	16	4	45	780	36	1	8	17
Hamburger	118	310	110	12	4	35	560	36	1	8	14
3 Piece Chicken Strips	145	380	190	21	4	55	1360	27	1	1	22
5 Piece Chicken Strips	241	630	310	34	6	90	2260	45	2	1	37
Kids Meal - Hamburger	197	560	210	24	6	35	710	67	4	8	18
Kids Meal - Cheeseburger	210	600	250	27	6	45	930	68	4	8	21
Kids Meal - 2 Chicken Strips	175	500	230	25	5	35	1050	50	3	1	19

Sides	Serving Size (g)	kCal	kCals from Fat	Total Fat (g)	Saturated Fat (g)	Cholesterol (mg)	Sodium (mg)	Total CHO (g)	Dietary Fiber (g)	Sugars (g)	Protein (g)
American Cheese slice (large)	16	60	45	5	4	15	260	1	0	1	3
American Cheese slice (small)	12	50	35	4	3	10	200	1	0	0	2
Swiss Cheese slice	16	50	35	4	3	15	230	0	0	0	4
Bacon - 2 strips	9	45	30	4	1	10	150	0	0	0	3
Au Jus Sauce	85	10	0	0	0	0	320	2	0	1	0
Fried Chicken Breast	148	370	130	15	4	75	1190	29	0	0	29
Fried Chicken Wing	66	200	70	8	2	30	740	23	0	0	10
Fried Chicken Thigh	121	330	130	15	4	60	1000	30	0	0	19
Fried Chicken Leg	69	170	60	7	2	45	570	15	0	0	13
French Fries-Kids	79	250	100	12	3	0	150	32	3	0	4
French Fries-Small	126	390	170	19	4	0	240	51	4	1	6
French Fries-Medium	166	520	220	24	5	0	320	67	5	1	8
French Fries-Large	193	610	260	28	6	0	370	78	6	1	10
Crispy Curls - Small	109	340	150	17	4	0	840	43	4	0	4
Crispy Curls - Medium	132	410	180	20	5	0	1020	52	4	0	5
Crispy Curls - Large	153	480	210	23	6	0	1190	60	5	0	6
Cole Slaw (small = 1 serving)	113	170	90	10	2	10	140	20	2	16	1

Sides—*continued*	Serving Size (g)	kCal	kCals from Fat	Total Fat (g)	Saturated Fat (g)	Cholesterol (mg)	Sodium (mg)	Total CHO (g)	Dietary Fiber (g)	Sugars (g)	Protein (g)
Mashed Potatoes (small = 1 serving)	142	90	15	2	0	0	410	17	0	1	1
Peach Cobbler	180	280	60	7	2	0	230	56	1	45	1
Chicken Gravy	43	20	5	1	0	0	220	3	0	1	0
Honey Mustard - Dipping Sauce	28	110	80	9	1.5	10	220	6	0	4	0
Ranch Dressing - Dipping Sauce	28	160	150	16	3	15	240	2	0	1	0
BBQ Sauce - Dipping Sauce	28	45	0	0	0	0	290	10	1	7	1
Sweet N Sour - Dipping Sauce	28	45	0	0	0	0	85	10	0	9	0
Mayonnaise (Packet)	12	90	80	9	1.5	5	70	1	0	0	0
Hot Sauce (Packet)	7	0	0	0	0	0	210	0	0	0	0
Horseradish Sauce (Packet)	7	25	20	2	0	5	35	1	0	1	0
Ketchup (Packet)	9	10	0	0	0	0	105	2	0	2	0

Desserts	Serving Size (g)	kCal	kCals from Fat	Total Fat (g)	Saturated Fat (g)	Cholesterol (mg)	Sodium (mg)	Total CHO (g)	Dietary Fiber (g)	Sugars (g)	Protein (g)
Chocolate Chip Cookie	68	290	100	11	5	20	270	44	0	26	4
Apple Turnover	85	290	140	15	5	5	350	36	1	11	2
Single Scoop Ice Cream Cone†	126	285	120	13	8	47	140	37	0	26	6
Single Scoop Ice Cream Bowl†	113	235	115	13	8	47	85	27	0	22	5
Vanilla Shake (Hand-Dipped) (regular)	16 fl oz	710	300	33	23	100	240	87	0	73	14
Chocolate Shake (Hand-Dipped) (regular)	16 fl oz	700	300	34	24	100	290	85	1	55	15
Strawberry Shake (Hand-Dipped) (regular)	16 fl oz	700	300	33	23	100	240	86	0	76	14
Hardee's Vanilla Malt (Hand-Dipped) 16 fl oz	16 fl oz	770	310	35	24	105	320	97	0.4	79	17
Hardee's Strawberry Malt (Hand-Dipped) 16 fl oz	16 fl oz	775	310	35	24	105	310	98	0.4	84	17
Hardee's Chocolate Malt (Hand-Dipped) 16 fl oz	16 fl oz	780	320	35	24	105	355	97	1.6	79	17

Jack In the Box

Breakfast	Serving Weight (g)	kCal	kCals from fat	Fat – Total (g)	Saturated Fat (g)	Trans Fat (g)	Cholesterol (mg)	Sodium (mg)	Potassium (mg)	Total CHO (g)	Dietary Fiber (g)	Sugars (g)	Protein (g)
Bacon, Egg & Cheese Biscuit	149	430	220	25	8	5	220	1100	140	34	1	3	17
Bacon Breakfast Jack®	113	300	120	14	5	0.5	215	730	180	29	1	4	16
Blueberry French Toast Sticks (4)	121	450	180	20	4.5	4.5	0	550	115	59	3	15	8
Breakfast Jack®	125	290	110	12	4.5	0	220	760	210	29	1	4	17
Chicken Biscuit	154	450	220	24	6	6	30	980	170	42	2	2	15
Ciabatta Breakfast Sandwich	278	710	320	36	10	1	440	1730	440	63	3	4	36
Extreme Sausage® Sandwich	213	670	430	48	17	1.5	290	1300	370	31	2	5	29
Hash Brown (1)	57	150	90	10	2.5	3	0	230	190	13	2	0	1
Meaty Breakfast Burrito	183	480	260	29	10	1	350	1210	300	29	2	1	25
Original French Toast Sticks (4)	121	470	210	23	5	5	25	450	120	58	4	14	7
Sausage Biscuit	131	440	260	29	8	5	35	870	340	32	2	3	12
Sausage Breakfast Jack®	154	450	250	28	10	1	245	840	250	29	1	4	20
Sausage Croissant	174	580	350	39	13	4	255	770	260	37	2	5	21
Sausage, Egg & Cheese Biscuit	234	740	490	55	17	6	280	1430	310	35	2	3	27
Spicy Chicken Biscuit	169	460	200	22	5	7	40	1020	260	44	2	2	21
Supreme Croissant	151	450	230	25	9	3.5	235	860	240	36	1	5	20
Ultimate Breakfast Sandwich	249	570	240	27	10	1	445	1700	370	49	2	8	34

Burgers

	Serving Weight (g)	kcal	Kcals from fat	Fat – Total (g)	Saturated Fat (g)	Trans Fat (g)	Cholesterol (mg)	Sodium (mg)	Potassium (mg)	Total CHO (g)	Dietary Fiber (g)	Sugars (g)	Protein (g)
Bacon Ultimate Cheeseburger	338	1090	700	77	30	3	140	2040	540	53	2	12	46
Bacon 'n' Cheese Ciabatta Burger	395	1120	690	76	28	3	135	1670	660	66	4	9	45
Hamburger	118	310	130	14	6	1	40	600	250	30	1	6	16
Hamburger with Cheese	131	350	160	17	8	1	50	790	270	30	1	7	18
Hamburger Deluxe	169	370	190	21	7	1	45	560	330	31	2	6	17
Hamburger Deluxe with Cheese	194	460	250	28	11	1	70	930	360	33	2	7	21
Jumbo Jack®	261	600	310	35	12	1.5	45	940	380	51	3	11	21
Jumbo Jack® with Cheese	286	690	370	42	16	1.5	70	1310	410	54	3	12	25
Junior Bacon Cheeseburger	131	430	230	25	9	1	60	820	270	30	1	6	20
Single Bacon 'n' Cheese Ciabatta Burger	308	870	490	54	18	1.5	90	1550	490	66	4	8	31
Sirloin Cheese Burger (Real Swiss & Grilled Onions)	421	1070	630	71	25	1.5	180	1850	680	61	4	10	53
Sirloin Bacon 'n' Cheese Burger (American Cheese & Red Onions)	422	1120	660	73	24	2.5	190	2620	790	63	4	11	54
Sourdough Jack®	245	710	460	51	18	3	75	1230	430	36	3	7	27
Sourdough Ultimate Cheeseburger	291	950	660	73	29	4.5	125	1360	490	36	2	7	38
Ultimate Cheeseburger	323	1010	640	71	28	3	125	1580	480	53	2	12	40

SHAKES & DESSERTS

	Serving Weight (g)	kcal	Kcals from fat	Fat – Total (g)	Saturated Fat (g)	Trans Fat (g)	Cholesterol (mg)	Sodium (mg)	Potassium (mg)	Total CHO (g)	Dietary Fiber (g)	Sugars (g)	Protein (g)
Cheesecake	103	310	140	16	9	1	55	220	180	34	0	23	7
Chocolate Ice Cream Shake – 16oz cup	414	880	400	45	31	2	135	330	840	107	1	94	14
Chocolate Ice Cream Shake – 24oz cup	576	1230	520	58	39	2.5	190	470	1220	159	2	141	19

SHAKES & DESSERTS—continued

	Serving Weight (g)	kCal	kCals from fat	Fat – Total (g)	Saturated Fat (g)	Trans Fat (g)	Cholesterol (mg)	Sodium (mg)	Potassium (mg)	Total CHO (g)	Dietary Fiber (g)	Sugars (g)	Protein (g)
Chocolate Overload Cake	93	300	60	7	1.5	0	40	350	260	57	2	34	4
Egg Nog Shake – 16oz cup (seasonal only)	414	870	400	44	31	2	135	280	750	103	0	78	13
Egg Nog Shake – 24oz cup (seasonal only)	576	1210	510	57	39	3	190	390	1040	152	1	110	18
OREO® Cookie Ice Cream Shake – 16oz cup	404	910	440	49	32	2	135	420	750	102	1	80	14
OREO® Cookie Ice Cream Shake – 24oz cup	556	1290	600	67	42	2.5	190	650	1030	148	2	115	20
Strawberry Ice Cream Shake – 16oz cup	417	880	400	44	31	2	135	290	750	105	0	88	13
Strawberry Ice Cream Shake – 24oz cup	582	1220	510	57	39	2.5	190	390	1030	155	1	131	18
Vanilla Ice Cream Shake – 16oz cup	379	790	400	44	31	2	135	280	750	83	0	70	13
Vanilla Ice Cream Shake – 24oz cup	506	1050	510	57	39	2.5	190	380	1030	112	1	94	18

Salads

	Serving Weight (g)	kCal	kCals from fat	Fat – Total (g)	Saturated Fat (g)	Trans Fat (g)	Cholesterol (mg)	Sodium (mg)	Potassium (mg)	Total CHO (g)	Dietary Fiber (g)	Sugars (g)	Protein (g)
Asian Chicken Salad (with Grilled Chicken)*	365	160	15	1.5	0	0	65	380	870	18	5	11	22
Asian Chicken Salad (with Crispy Chicken)*	394	330	120	13	3	3	40	650	830	34	7	11	21
Chicken Club Salad (with Grilled Chicken)*	373	320	140	16	6	0	105	780	830	11	4	5	34
Chicken Club Salad (with Crispy Chicken)*	402	480	250	27	9	3	80	1060	800	28	6	5	33

*Nutritional data does not include dressing or condiments.

Side Salad*	Serving Weight (g)	kCal	kCals from fat	Fat – Total (g)	Saturated Fat (g)	Trans Fat (g)	Cholesterol (mg)	Sodium (mg)	Potassium (mg)	Total CHO (g)	Dietary Fiber (g)	Sugars (g)	Protein (g)
Side Salad*	123	50	25	3	1.5	0	10	60	260	5	2	2	3
Southwest Chicken Salad (with Grilled Chicken)*	430	320	110	12	6	0	90	760	950	27	7	5	31
Southwest Chicken Salad (with Crispy Chicken)*	459	480	210	23	8	3	70	1040	920	44	9	5	30

Snacks & Extras	Serving Weight (g)	kCal	kCals from fat	Fat – Total (g)	Saturated Fat (g)	Trans Fat (g)	Cholesterol (mg)	Sodium (mg)	Potassium (mg)	Total CHO (g)	Dietary Fiber (g)	Sugars (g)	Protein (g)
Bacon Cheddar Potato Wedges	257	720	430	48	15	12	45	1360	950	52	4	2	21
Beef Monster Taco®	112	240	130	15	5	2	20	390	220	20	3	4	8
Egg Roll (1)	57	130	60	6	2	1	5	310	140	15	2	1	5
Egg Rolls (2)	170	400	170	19	6	3	15	920	430	44	6	4	14
Fruit Cup	198	90	5	0	0	0	0	20	400	22	2	18	1
Mozzarella Cheese Sticks (3)	71	240	110	12	5	2	25	420	60	21	1	1	11
Mozzarella Cheese Sticks (6)	138	483	244	27	11	4	46	1018	210	39	2	1	20
Natural Cut Fries – small	124	340	160	17	4	5	0	620	860	41	5	1	5
Natural Cut Fries – medium	166	450	210	23	5	7	0	830	1150	54	6	1	6
Natural Cut Fries – large	236	640	300	33	8	10	0	1180	1630	77	9	1	9
Onion Rings (8)	119	500	270	30	6	10	0	420	140	51	3	3	6
Regular Beef Taco	76	160	70	8	3	1	15	270	190	15	2	4	5
Sampler Trio	236	750	350	39	14	7	85	1760	440	65	5	4	35
Spicy Chicken Bites (7)	93	290	130	14	3	3	45	660	270	21	3	1	18
Spicy Chicken Bites (16)	213	650	290	33	7	7	100	1500	630	49	6	1	41
Seasoned Curly Fries – small	84	270	140	15	3	5	0	590	390	30	3	1	4
Seasoned Curly Fries – medium	125	400	200	23	5	7	0	890	580	45	5	1	6
Seasoned Curly Fries – large	170	550	280	31	6	10	0	1200	790	60	6	1	8
Stuffed Jalapenos (3)	72	230	110	13	6	2	20	690	105	22	2	2	7
Stuffed Jalapenos (7)	168	530	270	30	13	4.5	45	1600	240	51	4	5	15

McDonald's

Sandwiches

	Serving Size	kcal	kCals from Fat	Total Fat (g)	% Daily Value**	Saturated Fat (g)	% Daily Value**	Trans Fat (g)	Cholesterol (mg)	% Daily Value**	Sodium (mg)	% Daily Value**	CHO (g)	% Daily Value**	Dietary Fiber (g)	% Daily Value**	Sugars (g)	Protein (g)	Vitamin A % DV	Vitamin C % DV	Calcium % DV	Iron %DV
Hamburger	3.5 oz (100 g)	250	80	9	13	3.5	16	0.5	25	9	520	22	31	10	2	6	6	12	0	2	10	15
Cheeseburger	4 oz (114 g)	300	110	12	19	6	28	0.5	40	13	750	31	33	11	2	7	6	15	6	2	20	15
Double Cheeseburger	5.8 oz (165 g)	440	210	23	35	11	54	1.5	80	26	1150	48	34	11	2	8	7	25	10	2	25	20
Quarter Pounder®+	6 oz (169 g)	410	170	19	29	7	37	1	65	22	730	30	37	12	3	10	8	24	2	4	15	20
Quarter Pounder® with Cheese+	7 oz (198 g)	510	230	26	40	12	61	1.5	90	30	1190	50	40	13	3	12	9	29	10	4	30	25
Double Quarter Pounder® with Cheese++	9.8 oz (279 g)	740	380	42	65	19	96	2.5	155	52	1380	57	40	13	3	12	9	48	10	4	30	35
Big Mac®	7.5 oz (214 g)	540	260	29	45	10	51	1.5	75	25	1040	43	45	15	3	13	9	25	6	2	25	25
Big N' Tasty®	7.2 oz (206 g)	460	220	24	37	8	42	1.5	70	23	720	30	37	12	3	12	8	24	6	8	15	25
Big N' Tasty® with Cheese	7.7 oz (220 g)	510	250	28	43	11	54	1.5	85	28	960	40	38	13	3	12	8	27	10	8	20	25
Filet-O-Fish®	5.1 oz (143 g)	380	160	18	28	4	20	1	35	12	660	28	38	13	2	8	5	15	2	0	15	10
McChicken®	5.2 oz (147 g)	360	150	16	25	3.5	18	1	40	14	790	33	40	13	1	5	5	14	0	2	10	15
Premium Grilled Chicken Classic Sandwich	7.9 oz (226 g)	420	90	10	15	2	11	0	70	23	1190	50	51	17	3	13	11	32	4	10	8	20
Premium Crispy Chicken Classic Sandwich	8.1 oz (229 g)	500	150	17	26	3.5	16	1.5	50	16	1330	55	61	20	3	13	10	27	4	10	8	20
Premium Grilled Chicken Club Sandwich	9.1 oz (260 g)	570	190	21	32	7	35	0	100	34	1720	72	52	17	4	14	12	44	8	10	20	20
Premium Crispy Chicken Club Sandwich	9.3 oz (263 g)	660	250	28	43	8	41	1.5	80	27	1860	77	63	21	4	14	11	39	8	10	20	20

Item	Serving Size	kcal	kCals from Fat	Total Fat (g)	% Daily Value**	Saturated Fat (g)	% Daily Value**	Trans Fat (g)	Cholesterol (mg)	% Daily Value**	Sodium (mg)	% Daily Value**	CHO (g)	% Daily Value**	Dietary Fiber (g)	% Daily Value**	Sugars (g)	Protein (g)	Vitamin A % DV	Vitamin C % DV	Calcium % DV	Iron %DV
Premium Grilled Chicken Ranch BLT Sandwich	8.6 oz (246 g)	520	140	16	24	4	21	0	90	30	1760	73	53	18	3	14	13	40	4	10	10	20
Premium Crispy Chicken Ranch BLT Sandwich	8.8 oz (249 g)	600	200	23	35	5	27	1.5	70	23	1900	79	64	21	3	14	12	35	4	10	8	20
Ranch Snack Wrap™ with Crispy Chicken	4.1 oz (115 g)	330	140	16	25	4.5	24	1	30	10	780	32	32	11	2	6	2	14	2	2	10	10
Ranch Snack Wrap™ with Grilled Chicken	4.3 oz (122 g)	270	90	10	15	4	19	0	45	15	830	34	26	9	1	4	2	18	2	2	10	10
Honey Mustard Snack Wrap™ with Crispy Chicken	4.1 oz (117 g)	320	130	15	22	4.5	22	1	30	10	750	31	34	11	1	6	4	14	2	2	10	10
Honey Mustard Snack Wrap™ with Grilled Chicken	4.4 oz (124 g)	260	80	9	13	3.5	18	0	45	15	800	33	27	9	1	4	4	18	2	2	10	10
Chipotle BBQ Snack Wrap™ with Crispy Chicken	4.2 oz (118 g)	320	130	14	22	4.5	22	1	25	9	780	32	35	12	2	6	4	14	4	2	10	10
Chipotle BBQ Snack Wrap™ with Grilled Chicken	4.4 oz (125 g)	260	80	8	13	3.5	18	0	45	14	820	34	28	9	1	5	5	18	4	2	10	10

French Fries

Item	Serving Size	kcal	kCals from Fat	Total Fat (g)	% Daily Value**	Saturated Fat (g)	% Daily Value**	Trans Fat (g)	Cholesterol (mg)	% Daily Value**	Sodium (mg)	% Daily Value**	CHO (g)	% Daily Value**	Dietary Fiber (g)	% Daily Value**	Sugars (g)	Protein (g)	Vitamin A % DV	Vitamin C % DV	Calcium % DV	Iron %DV
Small French Fries	2.6 oz (74 g)	250	120	13	20	2.5	13	3.5	0	0	140	6	30	10	3	12	0	2	0	6	2	4
Medium French Fries	4 oz (114 g)	380	180	20	31	4	20	5	0	0	220	9	47	16	5	19	0	4	0	10	2	6
Large French Fries	6 oz (170 g)	570	270	30	47	6	30	8	0	0	330	14	70	23	7	28	0	6	0	15	2	10
Ketchup Packet	1 pkg (10 g)	15	0	0	0	0	0	0	0	0	110	5	3	1	0	0	2	0	2	2	0	0
Salt Packet	1 pkg (0.7 g)	0	0	0	0	0	0	0	0	0	270	11	0	0	0	0	0	0	0	0	0	0

Chicken McNuggets®/ Chicken Selects® Premium Breast Strips/ Sauces	Serving Size	kCal	kCals from Fat	Total Fat (g)	% Daily Value**	Saturated Fat (g)	% Daily Value**	Trans Fat (g)	Cholesterol (mg)	% Daily Value**	Sodium (mg)	% Daily Value**	CHO (g)	% Daily Value**	Dietary Fiber (g)	% Daily Value**	Sugars (g)	Protein (g)	Vitamin A % DV	Vitamin C % DV	Calcium % DV	Iron % DV
Chicken McNuggets® (4 piece)	2.3 oz (64 g)	170	90	10	15	2	11	1	25	8	450	19	10	3	0	0	0	10	2	2	0	2
Chicken McNuggets® (6 piece)	3.4 oz (96 g)	250	130	15	22	3	16	1.5	35	12	670	28	15	5	0	0	0	15	2	2	2	4
Chicken McNuggets® (10 piece)	5.6 oz (160 g)	420	220	24	37	5	27	2.5	60	21	1120	47	26	9	0	0	0	25	4	2	2	6
Barbeque sauce	1 pkg (28 g)	50	0	0	0	0	0	0	0	0	260	11	12	4	0	0	10	0	2	0	0	0
Honey	1 pkg (14 g)	50	0	0	0	0	0	0	0	0	0	0	12	4	0	0	11	0	0	0	0	0
Hot Mustard Sauce	1 pkg (28 g)	60	20	2.5	4	0	0	0	5	1	250	10	9	3	2	8	6	1	0	0	0	2
Sweet 'N Sour Sauce	1 pkg (28 g)	50	0	0	0	0	0	0	0	0	150	6	12	4	0	0	10	0	2	0	0	0
Chicken Selects® Premium Breast Strips (3 pc)	4.7 oz (133 g)	380	180	20	30	3.5	19	2.5	55	18	930	39	28	9	0	0	0	23	0	4	2	4
Chicken Selects® Premium Breast Strips (5 pc)	7.8 oz (221 g)	630	300	33	51	6	31	4.5	90	30	1550	65	46	15	0	0	0	39	0	6	4	8
Spicy Buffalo Sauce	1.5 oz (43 g)	70	60	7	11	1	5	0	0	0	960	40	1	0	0	0	0	0	6	2	0	2
Creamy Ranch Sauce	1.5 oz (43 g)	200	200	22	33	3.5	17	0	10	3	320	13	2	1	0	0	1	0	0	0	2	0
Tangy Honey Mustard Sauce	1.5 oz (43 g)	70	20	2.5	4	0	0	0	5	2	170	7	13	4	0	0	9	1	0	0	0	0
Southwestern Chipotle Barbeque Sauce	1.5 oz (43 g)	70	0	0	0	0	0	0	0	0	260	11	18	6	1	3	13	0	4	0	2	4

Salads

Salads	Serving Size	kCal	kCals from Fat	Total Fat (g)	% Daily Value**	Saturated Fat (g)	% Daily Value**	Trans Fat (g)	Cholesterol (mg)	% Daily Value**	Sodium (mg)	% Daily Value**	CHO (g)	% Daily Value**	Dietary Fiber (g)	% Daily Value**	Sugars (g)	Protein (g)	Vitamin A % DV	Vitamin C % DV	Calcium % DV	Iron %DV
Southwest Salad with Grilled Chicken	12.3 oz (350 g)	320	90	9	15	3	14	0	70	24	970	40	30	10	7	27	11	30	130	50	15	15
Southwest Salad with Crispy Chicken	12.4 oz (352 g)	400	150	16	25	4	20	1.5	50	17	1110	46	41	14	7	27	10	25	130	50	15	15
Southwest Salad (without chicken)	8.1 oz (230 g)	140	40	4.5	7	2	9	0	10	3	150	6	20	7	6	24	5	6	130	45	15	10
Asian Salad with Grilled Chicken	12.7 oz (362 g)	300	90	10	15	1	6	0	65	21	890	37	23	8	5	21	12	32	130	90	15	15
Asian Salad with Crispy Chicken	12.9 oz (365 g)	380	150	17	26	2.5	12	1.5	45	15	1030	43	33	11	5	21	12	27	130	80	15	15
Asian Salad (without chicken)	8.6 oz (243 g)	150	70	7	11	0.5	3	0	0	0	35	1	15	5	5	21	9	8	130	70	15	15
Bacon Ranch Salad with Grilled Chicken	11.2 oz (321 g)	260	90	9	15	4	21	0	90	30	1010	42	12	4	3	13	5	33	130	50	15	10
Bacon Ranch Salad with Crispy Chicken	11.4 oz (323 g)	350	150	16	25	5	27	1.5	70	23	1150	48	23	8	3	13	4	28	130	50	15	10
Bacon Ranch Salad (without chicken)	7.8 oz (223 g)	140	70	7	11	3.5	18	0	25	9	300	12	10	3	3	13	4	9	130	50	15	8
Caesar Salad with Grilled Chicken	10.9 oz (311 g)	220	60	6	10	3	15	0	75	25	890	37	12	4	3	13	5	30	130	50	20	10
Caesar Salad with Crispy Chicken	11 oz (313 g)	300	120	13	20	4	21	1.5	55	18	1020	43	22	7	3	13	4	25	130	50	20	10
Caesar Salad (without chicken)	7.5 oz (213 g)	90	35	4	6	2.5	12	0	10	4	180	7	9	3	3	13	4	7	130	50	20	8
Side Salad	3.1 oz (87 g)	20	0	0	0	0	0	0	0	0	10	0	4	1	1	6	2	1	45	25	2	4
Butter Garlic Croutons	0.5 oz (14 g)	60	15	1.5	3	0	0	0	0	0	140	6	10	3	1	2	0	2	0	0	2	4
Snack Size Fruit & Walnut Salad	1 pkg (163 g)	210	70	8	13	1.5	7	0	5	2	60	2	31	10	2	9	25	4	0	170	8	2

Salad Dressings

	Serving Size	kcal	kCals from Fat	Total Fat (g)	% Daily Value**	Saturated Fat (g)	% Daily Value**	Trans Fat (g)	Cholesterol (mg)	% Daily Value**	Sodium (mg)	% Daily Value**	CHO (g)	% Daily Value**	Dietary Fiber (g)	% Daily Value**	Sugars (g)	Protein (g)	Vitamin A % DV	Vitamin C % DV	Calcium % DV	Iron %DV
Newman's Own® Creamy Southwest Dressing	1.5 fl oz (44 ml)	100	50	6	9	1	5	0	20	7	340	14	11	4	0	0	3	1	0	0	2	2
Newman's Own® Creamy Caesar Dressing	2 fl oz (59 ml)	190	170	18	28	3.5	17	0	20	7	500	21	4	1	0	0	2	2	0	0	6	0
Newman's Own® Low Fat Balsamic Vinaigrette	1.5 fl oz (44 ml)	40	25	3	4	0	0	0	0	0	730	30	4	1	0	0	3	0	0	4	0	0
Newman's Own® Low Fat Family Recipe Italian Dressing	1.5 fl oz (44 ml)	60	20	2.5	4	0	0	0	0	0	730	30	8	3	0	0	1	1	0	0	0	0
Newman's Own® Low Fat Sesame Ginger Dressing	1.5 fl oz (44 ml)	90	20	2.5	4	0	0	0	0	0	740	31	15	5	0	0	10	1	0	0	0	0
Newman's Own® Ranch Dressing	2 fl oz (59 ml)	170	130	15	23	2.5	12	0	20	6	530	22	9	3	0	0	4	1	0	0	4	0

Breakfast

	Serving Size	kcal	kCals from Fat	Total Fat (g)	% Daily Value**	Saturated Fat (g)	% Daily Value**	Trans Fat (g)	Cholesterol (mg)	% Daily Value**	Sodium (mg)	% Daily Value**	CHO (g)	% Daily Value**	Dietary Fiber (g)	% Daily Value**	Sugars (g)	Protein (g)	Vitamin A % DV	Vitamin C % DV	Calcium % DV	Iron %DV
Egg McMuffin®	4.8 oz (139 g)	300	110	12	19	5	24	0	260	87	820	34	30	10	2	8	3	18	10	0	30	20
Sausage McMuffin®	3.9 oz (114 g)	370	200	22	34	8	42	0	45	15	850	35	29	10	2	8	2	14	6	2	25	15
Sausage McMuffin® with Egg	5.7 oz (164 g)	450	250	27	42	10	51	0	285	95	920	38	30	10	2	8	2	21	10	2	30	20
English Muffin	2 oz (57 g)	140	15	1.5	2	0	0	0	0	0	260	11	27	9	2	7	2	5	0	0	15	10

Item	Serving																				
Bacon, Egg & Cheese Biscuit (Regular Size Biscuit)	5.1 oz (144 g)	450	230	25	39	11	53	0	245	82	1360	57	36	12	2	7	3	18	10	0	15	15
Bacon, Egg & Cheese Biscuit (Large Size Biscuit)	5.7 oz (162 g)	520	270	30	46	13	67	0	245	82	1520	63	43	14	3	12	4	19	15	0	15	20
Biscuit with Egg (Regular Size Biscuit)	5.6 oz (159 g)	500	290	32	50	12	60	0	250	83	1130	47	35	12	2	6	2	17	6	0	10	20
Sausage Biscuit with Egg (Large Size Biscuit)	6.2 oz (177 g)	570	330	37	57	15	74	0	250	83	1280	53	42	14	3	11	3	18	10	0	10	20
Sausage Biscuit (Large Size Biscuit)	4 oz (113 g)	410	240	27	41	10	51	0	30	10	1040	43	33	11	2	6	2	11	0	0	6	15
Biscuit (Regular Size)	4.6 oz (131 g)	480	280	31	48	13	65	0	30	10	1190	50	39	13	3	11	3	11	4	0	8	15
Biscuit (Large Size)	2.5 oz (72 g)	250	100	11	17	5	24	0	0	0	700	29	32	11	2	6	2	4	0	0	6	10
Bacon, Egg & Cheese McGriddles®	3.2 oz (90 g)	320	140	16	25	8	38	0	0	0	850	36	39	13	3	11	3	5	4	0	6	15
Sausage, Egg & Cheese McGriddles®	6.1 oz (173 g)	460	190	21	33	9	43	0	245	82	1360	56	48	16	2	8	16	19	10	0	20	15
Sausage McGriddles®	7.1 oz (202 g)	560	290	32	49	12	62	0	265	88	1360	56	48	16	2	8	15	20	10	0	20	15
Big Breakfast® (Regular Size Biscuit)	5 oz (141 g)	420	200	22	34	8	40	0	35	11	1030	43	44	15	2	8	15	11	0	0	8	10
Big Breakfast® (Large Size Biscuit)	9.2 oz (262 g)	720	410	46	71	16	78	2.5	555	185	1500	63	49	16	3	13	3	27	15	20	15	25
Deluxe Breakfast (Reg. Size Biscuit) w/o Syrup & Margarine	9.9 oz (280 g)	790	460	51	78	18	92	2.5	555	185	1660	69	55	18	4	18	3	28	15	2	15	30

Breakfast—continued

	Serving Size	kCal	kCals from Fat	Total Fat (g)	% Daily Value**	Saturated Fat (g)	% Daily Value**	Trans Fat (g)	Cholesterol (mg)	% Daily Value**	Sodium (mg)	% Daily Value**	CHO (g)	% Daily Value**	Dietary Fiber (g)	% Daily Value**	Sugars (g)	Protein (g)	Vitamin A % DV	Vitamin C % DV	Calcium % DV	Iron % DV
Deluxe Breakfast (Large Size Biscuit) w/o Syrup & Margarine	14.6 oz (413 g)	1070	490	55	84	18	88	2.5	575	192	2090	87	109	36	6	23	17	36	15	2	25	40
Sausage Burrito	15.2 oz (431 g)	1140	530	59	91	20	101	2.5	575	192	2250	94	115	38	7	28	17	36	15	2	30	40
Hotcakes and Sausage (2 pats margarine & syrup)	3.9 oz (111 g)	300	140	16	25	7	33	0.5	130	43	830	35	26	9	1	4	2	12	10	2	15	15
Hotcakes (2 pats margarine & syrup)	9.3 oz (264 g)	780	300	33	51	9	46	4	50	17	1020	42	106	35	3	10	48	15	2	0	15	15
Sausage Patty	7.9 oz (223 g)	610	160	18	27	4	19	4	20	7	680	28	105	35	3	10	47	9	2	0	15	15
Scrambled Eggs (2)	1.4 oz (41 g)	170	140	15	23	5	27	0	520	174	340	14	1	0	0	0	0	15	15	0	2	2
Hash Browns	3.3 oz (96 g)	170	100	11	17	4	19	0	30	10	180	7	1	0	0	0	0	1	0	0	6	10
Grape Jam	1.9 oz (53 g)	140	70	8	13	1.5	8	2	0	0	290	12	15	5	2	7	0	0	0	2	0	2
Strawberry Preserves	0.5 oz (14 g)	35	0	0	0	0	0	0	0	0	0	0	9	3	0	0	9	0	0	2	0	0

Desserts/Shakes

	Serving Size	kCal	kCals from Fat	Total Fat (g)	% Daily Value**	Saturated Fat (g)	% Daily Value**	Trans Fat (g)	Cholesterol (mg)	% Daily Value**	Sodium (mg)	% Daily Value**	CHO (g)	% Daily Value**	Dietary Fiber (g)	% Daily Value**	Sugars (g)	Protein (g)	Vitamin A % DV	Vitamin C % DV	Calcium % DV	Iron % DV
Fruit 'n Yogurt Parfait»	5.3 oz (149 g)	160	20	2	3	1	5	0	5	2	85	4	31	10	1	3	21	4	0	15	15	4
Fruit 'n Yogurt Parfait (without granola)»	5 oz (142 g)	130	15	2	3	1	5	0	5	2	55	2	25	8	0	0	19	4	0	15	10	2
Apple Dippers	1 pkg (68 g)	35	0	0	0	0	0	0	0	0	0	0	8	3	0	0	6	0	0	310	4	0

Low Fat Caramel Dip	0.8 oz (21 g)	70	5	0.5	1	0	0	0	5	1	35	2	15	5	0	0	9	0	0	0	2	0
Vanilla Reduced Fat Ice Cream Cone	3.2 oz (90 g)	150	35	3.5	6	2	11	0	15	5	60	2	24	8	0	0	0	4	6	0	10	2
Kiddie Cone	1 oz (29 g)	45	10	1	2	0.5	4	0	5	2	20	1	8	3	0	0	6	1	2	0	4	0
Strawberry Sundae	6.3 oz (178 g)	280	60	6	10	4	20	0	25	8	95	4	49	16	1	6	45	6	10	4	20	0
Hot Caramel Sundae	6.4 oz (182 g)	340	70	8	12	5	25	0	30	10	160	7	60	20	1	6	44	7	10	0	25	0
Hot Fudge Sundae	6.3 oz (179 g)	330	90	10	15	7	35	0	25	8	180	8	54	18	2	8	48	8	10	0	25	6
Peanuts (for Sundaes)	0.3 oz (7 g)	45	30	3.5	5	0.5	3	0	0	0	0	0	2	1	1	2	0	2	0	0	0	0
Swamp Sludge McFlurry® (12 fl oz cup)	10 oz (283 g)	510	150	16	25	9	47	1	50	16	180	8	80	27	1	3	69	12	20	0	40	6
Swamp Sludge McFlurry® (16 fl oz cup)	13.5 oz (383 g)	710	200	23	35	13	65	1.5	65	22	250	11	110	37	1	5	95	16	25	0	50	8
McFlurry® with M&M'S® Candies (12 fl oz cup)	12.3 oz (348 g)	620	180	20	30	12	59	1	55	19	190	8	96	32	1	3	85	14	20	0	45	6
McFlurry® with OREO® Cookies (12 fl oz cup)	11.9 oz (337 g)	560	150	16	25	9	43	2	50	17	250	10	88	29	0	0	71	14	20	0	45	10
Minty Mudd Bath Triple Thick® Shake (12 fl oz cup)	266 g	430	90	10	15	6	30	0.5	40	13	150	6	75	25	0	0	63	10	15	0	30	4
Minty Mudd Bath Triple Thick® Shake (16 fl oz cup)	355 g	570	120	13	21	8	40	1	50	17	210	9	101	34	0	0	84	13	20	0	45	4
Minty Mudd Bath Triple Thick® Shake (21 fl oz cup)	472 g	760	160	18	27	11	54	1	70	23	270	11	134	45	0	0	112	17	30	0	60	6
Minty Mudd Bath Triple Thick® Shake (32 fl oz cup)	710 g	1150	240	27	41	16	81	2	100	34	410	17	201	67	0	0	169	26	40	0	90	8
Chocolate Triple Thick® Shake (12 fl oz cup)	333 ml	440	90	10	16	6	31	0.5	40	13	190	8	76	25	1	3	63	10	15	0	35	8
Chocolate Triple Thick® Shake (16 fl oz cup)	444 ml	580	120	14	21	8	41	1	50	17	250	11	102	34	1	4	84	13	20	0	45	10

Desserts/Shakes—continued	Serving Size	kCal	kCals from Fat	Total Fat (g)	% Daily Value**	Saturated Fat (g)	% Daily Value**	Trans Fat (g)	Cholesterol (mg)	% Daily Value**	Sodium (mg)	% Daily Value**	CHO (g)	% Daily Value**	Dietary Fiber (g)	% Daily Value**	Sugars (g)	Protein (g)	Vitamin A % DV	Vitamin C % DV	Calcium % DV	Iron % DV
Chocolate Triple Thick® Shake (21 fl oz cup)	583 ml	770	160	18	28	11	55	1	70	23	330	14	134	45	1	5	111	18	30	0	60	15
Chocolate Triple Thick® Shake (32 fl oz cup)	888 ml	1160	240	27	42	16	82	2	100	34	510	21	203	68	2	7	168	27	40	0	90	20
Strawberry Triple Thick® Shake (12 fl oz cup)	333 ml	420	90	10	15	6	30	0.5	40	13	130	5	73	24	0	0	63	10	15	2	30	2
Strawberry Triple Thick® Shake (16 fl oz cup)	444 ml	560	120	13	20	8	40	1	50	17	170	7	97	32	0	0	84	13	20	2	45	2
Strawberry Triple Thick® Shake (21 fl oz cup)	583 ml	740	160	18	27	11	53	1	70	23	230	10	128	43	0	0	111	17	30	2	60	2
Strawberry Triple Thick® Shake (32 fl oz cup)	888 ml	1110	240	26	41	16	80	2	100	34	350	15	194	65	0	0	168	25	40	4	90	4
Vanilla Triple Thick® Shake (12 fl oz cup)	333 ml	420	90	10	15	6	30	0.5	40	13	140	6	72	24	0	0	54	9	15	0	30	2
Vanilla Triple Thick® Shake (16 fl oz cup)	444 ml	550	120	13	20	8	40	1	50	17	190	8	96	32	0	0	72	13	20	0	45	2
Vanilla Triple Thick® Shake (21 fl oz cup)	583 ml	740	160	18	27	11	53	1	70	23	250	10	128	43	0	0	96	17	30	0	60	2
Vanilla Triple Thick® Shake (32 fl oz cup)	888 ml	1110	240	26	41	16	80	2	100	34	370	16	193	64	0	0	145	25	40	0	90	2
Baked Apple Pie	2.7 oz (76 g)	270	110	12	19	3.5	16	5	0	0	190	8	36	12	4	17	14	3	2	10	2	8
Cinnamon Melts	4 oz (114 g)	460	170	19	30	9	43	0	15	5	370	15	66	22	3	11	32	6	4	0	6	15
McDonaldland® Chocolate Chip Cookies	2 oz (56 g)	270	100	11	17	6	32	0	35	12	170	7	39	13	1	5	19	3	4	0	2	10
McDonaldland® Cookies	2 oz (57 g)	250	70	8	12	2	9	2.5	0	0	270	11	42	14	1	4	14	4	0	0	0	10
Chocolate Chip Cookie	1 cookie (33 g)	160	70	7	12	2.5	12	1.5	10	3	90	4	22	7	1	3	15	2	4	0	2	8

Oatmeal Raisin Cookie	1 cookie (33 g)	150	50	6	9	1.5	7	1.5	10	3	135	6	22	7	1	3	13	2	4	0	2	4
Sugar Cookie	1 cookie (32 g)	150	60	6	10	1.5	7	2	5	2	110	5	21	7	0	0	11	2	6	0	2	4

* Contains less than 2% of the Daily Value of these nutrients
† Available at participating McDonald's
+ Based on the weight before cooking 4 oz. (113.4g)
++ Based on the weight before cooking 8 oz. (226.8g)
§ The values represent the sodium derived from ingredients plus water. Sodium content of the water is based on the value listed for municipal water in the USDA National Nutrient Database. The actual amount of sodium may be higher or lower depending upon the sodium content of the water where the beverage is dispensed.
» Made with low fat yogurt
** Percent Daily Values (DV) are based on a 2,000 calorie diet. Your daily values may be higher or lower depending on your calorie needs.

Sonic

Burgers

	Serving Weight (g)	kcal	kcals from Fat	Total Fat (g)	Saturated Fat (g)	Trans Fat (g)	Cholesterol (mg)	Sodium (mg)	CHO (g)	Dietary Fiber (g)	Sugars (g)	Protein (g)	Vitamin A % DV	Vitamin C % DV	Calcium % DV	Iron % DV
Sonic® Burger (w/ Mustard)	235	540	230	25	9	2	60	730	52	4	9	24	6%	10%	15%	30%
Sonic® Burger (w/ Ketchup)	235	540	230	25	9	2	60	730	54	4	10	24	6%	10%	15%	30%
Sonic® Cheeseburger (w/ Mayonnaise)	260	700	380	42	14	2	85	1020	55	4	10	27	8%	10%	15%	30%
Sonic® Cheeseburger (w/ Mustard)	253	600	280	31	12	2	75	1050	54	4	10	27	10%	10%	25%	30%
Sonic® Cheeseburger (w/ Ketchup)	260	610	280	31	12	2	75	1120	57	4	13	28	10%	10%	25%	30%
Sonic® Bacon Cheeseburger	273	770	420	47	16	2	100	1280	55	4	10	32	15%	15%	25%	30%
Super Sonic® Cheeseburger (w/ Mayonnaise)	337	970	570	63	24	3.5	165	1420	56	4	11	45	10%	10%	25%	30%
Super Sonic® Cheeseburger (w/ Mustard)	330	870	470	52	23	3.5	155	1440	55	4	11	45	15%	10%	40%	35%
Super Sonic® Cheeseburger (w/ Ketchup)	337	880	470	52	23	3.5	155	1520	59	4	14	45	15%	10%	40%	35%
Jr. Burger	117	320	140	16	5	1	35	610	29	2	7	15	20%	15%	40%	35%
Jr. Cheeseburger	135	380	190	21	9	1.5	55	930	30	2	8	18	4%	4%	10%	10%
Dixie Burger	249	640	330	37	11	2	70	790	53	4	9	24	8%	4%	20%	10%
Dixie cheeseburger	267	710	380	42	14	2	85	1110	55	4	10	27	6%	10%	15%	30%
Thousand Island Jr. Cheeseburger	137	440	250	28	10	1.5	60	700	29	2	6	17	10%	10%	25%	30%
California Cheeseburger	260	670	340	38	13	2	80	1050	56	4	11	27	10%	0%	20%	10%
Super Sonic® Jalapeno Cheeseburger	286	860	470	52	23	3.5	155	1310	53	3	10	45	15%	10%	25%	30%
Thousand Island Cheeseburger	260	660	330	37	13	2	85	1110	56	4	11	28	15%	2%	35%	35%
Jalapeno Cheeseburger	209	600	270	30	12	2	75	910	52	3	9	27	15%	10%	25%	30%
Jalapeno Burger	191	530	230	25	9	2	60	590	50	3	8	24	8%	2%	25%	25%
Green Chili Cheeseburger	281	610	280	31	12	2	75	1050	55	4	10	27	2%	2%	15%	25%
Chili Cheeseburger	220	640	310	34	14	2	85	970	54	4	9	30	10%	25%	25%	30%
Hickory Cheeseburger	230	620	270	30	12	2	75	1150	60	4	15	27	10%	6%	25%	30%
Jr. Double Cheeseburger	190	570	320	36	16	2.5	110	1290	32	2	8	30	15%	4%	30%	15%

Add Ons

	Serving Weight (g)	kCal	kCals from Fat	Total Fat (g)	Saturated Fat (g)	Trans Fat (g)	Cholesterol (mg)	Sodium (mg)	CHO (g)	Dietary Fiber (g)	Sugars (g)	Protein (g)	Vitamin A % DV	Vitamin C % DV	Calcium % DV	Iron % DV
Cheese	18	60	45	5	3	0	20	310	2	0	1	3	6%	0%	10%	0%
Bacon	13	70	50	5	2	0	15	260	0	0	0	4	0%	0%	0%	2%
Chili	33	50	35	3.5	1.5	0	10	160	2	1	1	3	6%	2%	2%	2%
Jalapeno	21	5	0	0	0	0	0	280	1	1	0	0	2%	0%	2%	2%
Green Chiles	28	5	0	0	0	0	0	5	1	0	0	0	0%	15%	0%	0%
Slaw	28	45	30	3	0.5	0	5	45	4	1	1	0	4%	80%	2%	0%
Grilled Onions	28	25	10	1.5	0	0	0	200	2	1	2	0	4%	0%	0%	2%

Kids' Meal

	Serving Weight (g)	kCal	kCals from Fat	Total Fat (g)	Saturated Fat (g)	Trans Fat (g)	Cholesterol (mg)	Sodium (mg)	CHO (g)	Dietary Fiber (g)	Sugars (g)	Protein (g)	Vitamin A % DV	Vitamin C % DV	Calcium % DV	Iron % DV
Jr. Burger	117	320	140	16	5	1	35	610	29	2	7	15	4%	4%	10%	10%
Jr. Cheeseburger	135	380	190	21	9	1.5	55	930	30	2	8	18	8%	4%	20%	10%
Corn Dog	73	250	130	15	4	1.5	15	80	23	2	8	5	0%	0%	15%	6%
Grilled Cheese	118	390	150	17	8	1.5	35	1010	45	2	7	14	15%	0%	30%	10%
Chicken Strips (2)	72	210	100	11	2	2	35	430	13	1	0	14	0%	0%	2%	4%

Toaster® Sandwiches

	Serving Weight (g)	kCal	kCals from Fat	Total Fat (g)	Saturated Fat (g)	Trans Fat (g)	Cholesterol (mg)	Sodium (mg)	CHO (g)	Dietary Fiber (g)	Sugars (g)	Protein (g)	Vitamin A % DV	Vitamin C % DV	Calcium % DV	Iron % DV
Chicken Club Toaster® Sandwich	265	690	310	35	10	3	80	1900	64	4	11	32	15%	6%	25%	15%
Bacon Cheeseburger Toaster® Sandwich	251	690	330	37	14	3	90	1410	58	3	13	31	15%	10%	30%	20%

Fresh Tastes® Salads

	Serving Weight (g)	kCal	kCals from Fat	Total Fat (g)	Saturated Fat (g)	Trans Fat (g)	Cholesterol (mg)	Sodium (mg)	CHO (g)	Dietary Fiber (g)	Sugars (g)	Protein (g)	Vitamin A % DV	Vitamin C % DV	Calcium % DV	Iron % DV
Grilled Chicken Salad	351	310	130	14	6	1	95	1050	19	4	8	28	110%	40%	25%	10%
Jumbo Popcorn Chicken® Salad	354	490	250	28	9	4	60	1440	39	5	8	22	110%	40%	30%	10%
Santa Fe Chicken Salad	399	370	140	15	6	1	95	1140	29	6	8	30	120%	50%	25%	10%

Hidden Valley® Ranch Dressings

	Serving Weight (g)	kCal	kCals from Fat	Total Fat (g)	Saturated Fat (g)	Trans Fat (g)	Cholesterol (mg)	Sodium (mg)	CHO (g)	Dietary Fiber (g)	Sugars (g)	Protein (g)	Vitamin A % DV	Vitamin C % DV	Calcium % DV	Iron % DV
Original Ranch Dressing	57	260	250	28	4.5	0	20	490	0	0	0	0	0%	0%	0%	0%
Original Light Ranch Dressing	57	120	60	7	1	0	15	740	14	0	5	1	0%	0%	2%	0%
Honey Mustard	57	240	190	21	3	0	15	300	14	0	12	1	0%	0%	0%	0%
Fat Free Golden Italian	57	50	0	0	0	0	0	600	13	0	4	0	0%	0%	0%	0%
Southwest Ranch	57	120	60	7	1	0	15	770	15	0	5	1	4%	0%	0%	0%
Thousand Island	57	250	230	25	4	0	30	590	9	0	7	1	15%	4%	0%	0%

Wraps

	Serving Weight (g)	kcal	kCals from Fat	Total Fat (g)	Saturated Fat (g)	Trans Fat (g)	Cholesterol (mg)	Sodium (mg)	CHO (g)	Dietary Fiber (g)	Sugars (g)	Protein (g)	Vitamin A % DV	Vitamin C % DV	Calcium % DV	Iron % DV
Grilled Chicken Wrap	247	380	100	11	2.5	1	75	1300	44	4	3	27	8%	8%	25%	15%
Chicken Strip Wrap	234	480	180	20	4	3	40	1170	56	5	3	20	8%	8%	25%	15%
FRITOS® Chili Cheese Wrap	239	670	340	38	12	1.5	50	1260	66	6	3	22	25%	4%	40%	20%

Chicken

	Serving Weight (g)	kcal	kCals from Fat	Total Fat (g)	Saturated Fat (g)	Trans Fat (g)	Cholesterol (mg)	Sodium (mg)	CHO (g)	Dietary Fiber (g)	Sugars (g)	Protein (g)	Vitamin A % DV	Vitamin C % DV	Calcium % DV	Iron % DV
Chicken Strip Dinner (4)	382	920	390	43	8	8	70	1730	97	9	8	36	2%	15%	15%	20%
Grilled Chicken On Ciabatta with Mayonnaise	213	410	160	18	3	0.5	80	980	34	2	5	29	6%	6%	10%	15%
Breaded Chicken On Ciabatta	215	540	260	29	5	2.5	55	1190	47	4	5	24	8%	6%	10%	15%
Jumbo Popcorn Chicken® - Snack	113	370	190	21	4	4	40	1270	27	2	0	19	0%	0%	4%	6%
Jumbo Popcorn Chicken® - Large	170	560	290	32	6	6	65	1910	41	3	0	28	0%	0%	6%	8%
Ranch Sauce	28	150	140	16	2.5	0	10	210	1	0	1	0	0%	0%	0%	0%
Honey Mustard Sauce	28	90	70	7	1	0	10	190	7	0	5	0	0%	0%	0%	0%
BBQ Sauce	28	45	0	0	0	0	0	390	11	0	7	0	2%	0%	0%	2%

Coneys

	Serving Weight (g)	kcal	kCals from Fat	Total Fat (g)	Saturated Fat (g)	Trans Fat (g)	Cholesterol (mg)	Sodium (mg)	CHO (g)	Dietary Fiber (g)	Sugars (g)	Protein (g)	Vitamin A % DV	Vitamin C % DV	Calcium % DV	Iron % DV
Extra-Long Chili Cheese Coney	237	600	290	33	11	1	75	1700	54	4	7	24	10%	2%	15%	25%
Corn Dog	73	250	130	15	4	1.5	15	80	23	2	8	5	0%	0%	15%	6%
Extra-Long Slaw Dog	280	670	340	38	12	1	80	1770	60	4	8	24	15%	120%	20%	25%

Other Items

	Serving Weight (g)	kcal	kCals from Fat	Total Fat (g)	Saturated Fat (g)	Trans Fat (g)	Cholesterol (mg)	Sodium (mg)	CHO (g)	Dietary Fiber (g)	Sugars (g)	Protein (g)	Vitamin A % DV	Vitamin C % DV	Calcium % DV	Iron % DV
FRITOS® Chili Pie	275	940	570	64	18	1	65	1540	72	6	3	25	30%	4%	35%	10%
Fish Sandwich	245	640	280	31	5	3	35	1180	69	5	10	22	2%	2%	15%	25%
Breaded Pork Fritter Sandwich	274	720	330	36	7	3.5	45	1010	71	5	12	27	6%	6%	15%	30%
Burrito	120	370	180	20	7	1	15	520	37	3	13	11	4%	0%	4%	15%
Burrito Deluxe	144	400	200	22	8	1.5	25	640	36	3	13	13	10%	2%	6%	20%
Tacos	118	310	160	18	6	2	25	370	30	4	1	12	10%	0%	15%	8%

Sides

	Serving Weight (g)	kcal	kCals from Fat	Total Fat (g)	Saturated Fat (g)	Trans Fat (g)	Cholesterol (mg)	Sodium (mg)	CHO (g)	Dietary Fiber (g)	Sugars (g)	Protein (g)	Vitamin A % DV	Vitamin C % DV	Calcium % DV	Iron % DV
Onion Rings – Regular	156	500	250	28	5	6	0	210	55	4	13	6	0%	0%	40%	8%
Onion Rings - Large	227	720	370	41	7	8	0	300	79	5	18	9	0%	0%	60%	10%
Tater Tots – Regular	84	220	120	14	2.5	3	0	600	23	3	0	2	0%	2%	0%	4%
Tater Tots – Large	126	330	180	20	3.5	4	0	890	35	4	0	3	0%	4%	2%	6%
Tater Tots - SONIC Size	168	440	240	27	4.5	6	0	1190	46	5	0	3	0%	6%	2%	8%
French Fries – Regular	75	210	90	10	2	2	0	260	28	4	0	3	0%	15%	2%	4%
French Fries – Large	98	280	120	13	2.5	3	0	340	37	5	1	4	0%	15%	2%	6%
French Fries - SONIC Size	134	380	160	18	3.5	4	0	470	50	7	1	5	0%	20%	2%	8%
French Fries w/cheese – Regular	93	280	140	15	5	2.5	20	570	29	4	1	6	6%	15%	10%	4%
French Fries w/cheese – Large	125	380	190	21	7	3	25	810	39	5	2	8	8%	15%	15%	6%
French Fries w/cheese - SONIC Size	170	510	250	28	10	4	35	1090	53	7	3	11	10%	20%	20%	8%
French Fries w/chili & cheese – Regular	122	300	160	18	6	2.5	25	530	31	5	1	9	10%	15%	15%	8%
French Fries w/chili & cheese – Large	186	440	240	27	10	3.5	40	820	43	6	2	14	15%	20%	20%	10%

	Serving Weight (g)	kcal	Kcals from Fat	Total Fat (g)	Saturated Fat (g)	Trans Fat (g)	Cholesterol (mg)	Sodium (mg)	CHO (g)	Dietary Fiber (g)	Sugars (g)	Protein (g)	Vitamin A % DV	Vitamin C % DV	Calcium % DV	Iron % DV
French Fries w/chili & cheese - SONIC Size	262	620	330	37	13	4.5	55	1160	58	9	3	20	25%	25%	25%	15%
Tater Tots w/cheese – Regular	102	290	170	19	6	3	20	910	25	3	1	5	6%	2%	10%	4%
Tater Tots w/cheese – Large	153	430	250	28	8	4.5	25	1360	37	4	1	7	8%	4%	15%	6%
Tater Tots w/cheese - SONIC Size	204	570	340	38	11	6	35	1820	49	5	2	9	10%	6%	20%	8%
Tater Tots w/chili & cheese – Regular	131	310	190	21	7	3	25	860	26	3	1	8	10%	4%	10%	6%
Tater Tots w/chili & cheese – Large	193	440	250	28	7	4.5	20	1220	40	5	2	8	10%	6%	4%	10%
Tater Tots w/chili & cheese - SONIC Size	296	680	420	47	15	6	55	1880	55	7	2	18	25%	8%	25%	15%
Mozzarella Sticks	135	410	190	21	9	2.5	40	1040	35	2	0	19	10%	0%	35%	4%
Ched 'R' Bites	108	360	190	21	9	2	40	910	28	2	0	17	10%	0%	40%	0%
Ched 'R' Peppers	112	290	150	17	6	2.5	20	1040	28	2	1	8	8%	0%	15%	4%
Sonic Blast®																
Oreo® Sonic Blast® - Regular (14 oz)	390	660	250	28	18	1	60	220	94	1	84	8	15%	0%	30%	10%
Oreo® Sonic Blast® - Large (20 oz)	559	960	360	40	25	1	85	310	139	2	124	12	20%	0%	45%	15%
M&M's® Sonic Blast® - Regular (14 oz)	390	660	250	28	18	1	60	220	95	1	84	8	15%	0%	30%	10%
M&M's® Sonic Blast® - Large (20 oz)	559	960	360	40	25	1	85	310	139	2	124	12	20%	0%	45%	15%
Reese's Peanut Butter Cups® Sonic Blast® - Regular (14 oz)	387	620	200	22	14	0.5	65	270	96	1	79	10	15%	0%	30%	8%
Reese's Peanut Butter Cups® Sonic Blast® - Large (20 oz)	555	900	270	30	19	1	90	400	142	2	115	15	20%	0%	40%	10%
Butterfinger® Sonic Blast® - Regular (14 oz)	389	670	280	31	19	1	60	250	89	1	77	9	10%	0%	25%	8%
Butterfinger® Sonic Blast® - Large (20 oz)	557	980	400	45	26	1.5	85	360	131	1	112	13	15%	0%	35%	10%

Shakes

	Serving Weight (g)	kCal	kCals from Fat	Total Fat (g)	Saturated Fat (g)	Trans Fat (g)	Cholesterol (mg)	Sodium (mg)	CHO (g)	Dietary Fiber (g)	Sugars (g)	Protein (g)	Vitamin A % DV	Vitamin C % DV	Calcium % DV	Iron % DV
Vanilla Shake - Regular (14 oz)	417	540	180	20	12	1	75	230	82	0	72	8	15%	0%	30%	8%
Vanilla Shake - Large (20 oz)	603	780	260	29	18	1	105	330	118	0	104	11	20%	0%	45%	10%
Chocolate Shake - Regular (14 oz)	433	610	170	19	12	0.5	70	300	101	0	84	7	15%	0%	30%	8%
Chocolate Shake - Large (20 oz)	637	920	240	27	16	1	100	470	156	0	129	11	20%	0%	40%	10%
Strawberry Shake - Regular (14 oz)	430	580	170	19	12	0.5	70	220	94	1	79	8	15%	15%	30%	8%
Strawberry Shake - Large (20 oz)	631	860	240	27	16	1	100	320	143	1	118	11	20%	25%	40%	15%
Banana Shake - Regular (14 oz)	436	550	170	19	12	0.5	70	220	87	1	73	8	15%	6%	30%	8%
Banana Shake - Large (20 oz)	637	790	240	27	17	1	100	310	127	2	106	11	20%	10%	40%	10%
Pineapple Shake - Regular (14 oz)	430	570	170	19	12	0.5	70	230	92	0	76	7	15%	80%	30%	8%
Pineapple Shake - Large (20 oz)	631	840	240	27	16	1	100	330	138	0	113	10	20%	160%	40%	10%
Peanut Butter Shake-Regular (14 oz)	426	710	330	37	15	0.5	70	330	87	0	73	11	15%	0%	30%	8%
Peanut Butter Shake-Large-20 oz)	623	1120	570	63	22	1	100	540	128	0	107	18	20%	0%	40%	10%
Peanut Butter Fudge Shake-Reg (14 oz)	430	680	280	31	15	0.5	70	300	92	1	77	9	15%	0%	30%	8%
Peanut Butter Fudge Shake-Large (20 oz)	610	990	430	47	22	1	100	450	128	1	108	14	20%	0%	40%	10%
Hot Fudge Shake-Regular (14 oz)	431	640	220	24	16	0.5	70	270	97	1	81	7	15%	0%	30%	10%
Hot Fudge Shake-Large (20 oz)	633	980	330	37	25	1	100	420	148	2	123	10	20%	0%	40%	15%

Malts

	Serving Weight (g)	kCal	kCals from Fat	Total Fat (g)	Saturated Fat (g)	Trans Fat (g)	Cholesterol (mg)	Sodium (mg)	CHO (g)	Dietary Fiber (g)	Sugars (g)	Protein (g)	Vitamin A % DV	Vitamin C % DV	Calcium % DV	Iron % DV
Vanilla Malt - Regular (14 oz)	420	550	190	21	13	1	75	240	84	0	73	8	15%	0%	30%	8%
Vanilla Malt - Large (20 oz)	609	810	270	30	19	1	110	350	122	0	107	12	20%	0%	45%	10%

	Serving Weight (g)	kCal	kCals from Fat	Total Fat (g)	Saturated Fat (g)	Trans Fat (g)	Cholesterol (mg)	Sodium (mg)	CHO (g)	Dietary Fiber (g)	Sugars (g)	Protein (g)	Vitamin A % DV	Vitamin C % DV	Calcium % DV	Iron % DV
Chocolate Malt - Regular (14 oz)	436	630	180	20	12	0.5	70	310	102	0	86	8	15%	0%	30%	436
Chocolate Malt - Large (20 oz)	643	950	260	28	17	1	100	490	160	0	132	11	20%	0%	40%	643
Strawberry Malt - Regular (14 oz)	433	590	180	20	12	0.5	70	230	96	1	80	8	15%	15%	30%	433
Strawberry Malt - Large (20 oz)	637	890	260	28	17	1	100	340	147	1	121	12	20%	25%	45%	637
Banana Malt - Regular (14 oz)	439	560	180	20	12	0.5	70	230	89	1	75	8	15%	6%	30%	439
Banana Malt - Large (20 oz)	643	820	260	29	17	1	100	330	131	2	109	12	20%	10%	45%	643
Pineapple Malt - Regular (14 oz)	433	590	180	20	12	0.5	70	240	93	0	78	8	15%	80%	30%	433
Pineapple Malt - Large (20 oz)	637	870	260	28	17	1	100	350	142	0	116	11	20%	160%	40%	637

CreamSlush® Treat

	Serving Weight (g)	kCal	kCals from Fat	Total Fat (g)	Saturated Fat (g)	Trans Fat (g)	Cholesterol (mg)	Sodium (mg)	CHO (g)	Dietary Fiber (g)	Sugars (g)	Protein (g)	Vitamin A % DV	Vitamin C % DV	Calcium % DV	Iron % DV
Strawberry CreamSlush® Treat - Regular (14 oz)	441	450	100	12	7	0	45	150	84	1	72	5	8%	15%	20%	441
Strawberry CreamSlush® Treat - Large (20 oz)	578	620	130	15	9	0.5	55	200	118	1	99	7	10%	25%	25%	578
Orange CreamSlush® Treat - Regular (14 oz)	437	430	110	13	8	0	45	160	77	0	70	5	8%	0%	20%	437
Orange CreamSlush® Treat - Large (20 oz)	569	580	150	17	10	0.5	60	210	104	0	94	6	10%	0%	25%	569
Cherry CreamSlush® Treat - Regular (14 oz)	437	440	110	13	8	0	45	160	77	0	71	5	8%	0%	20%	437
Cherry CreamSlush® Treat - Large (20 oz)	569	590	150	17	10	0.5	60	210	105	0	96	6	10%	0%	25%	569
Grape CreamSlush® Treat - Regular (14 oz)	437	430	110	13	8	0	45	160	76	0	70	5	8%	0%	20%	437
Grape CreamSlush® Treat - Large (20 oz)	569	580	150	17	10	0.5	60	220	103	0	94	7	10%	0%	25%	569
Watermelon CreamSlush® Treat - Regular (14 oz)	437	440	110	13	8	0	45	160	77	0	70	5	8%	0%	20%	437
Watermelon CreamSlush® Treat - Large (20 oz)	570	590	150	17	10	0.5	60	210	105	0	94	7	10%	0%	25%	570
Blue Coconut CreamSlush® Treat - Regular (14 oz)	437	430	110	13	8	0	45	160	76	0	69	5	8%	0%	20%	437
Blue Coconut CreamSlush® Treat - Large (20 oz)	569	580	150	17	10	0.5	60	210	102	0	92	7	10%	0%	25%	569
Lemon CreamSlush® Treat - Regular (14 oz)	446	430	110	13	8	0	45	160	77	0	69	5	8%	8%	20%	446

CreamSlush® Treat—continued

	Serving Weight (g)	kCal	kCals from Fat	Total Fat (g)	Saturated Fat (g)	Trans Fat (g)	Cholesterol (mg)	Sodium (mg)	CHO (g)	Dietary Fiber (g)	Sugars (g)	Protein (g)	Vitamin A % DV	Vitamin C % DV	Calcium % DV	Iron % DV
Lemon CreamSlush® Treat - Large (20 oz)	587	590	150	17	10	0.5	60	210	104	0	92	7	10%	15%	25%	587
Lemon-Berry CreamSlush® Treat - Regular (14 oz)	450	460	100	12	7	0	45	150	85	1	73	5	8%	20%	20%	450
Lemon-Berry CreamSlush® Treat - Large (20 oz)	596	630	130	15	9	0.5	55	200	119	1	99	7	10%	40%	25%	596
Lime CreamSlush® Treat - Regular (14 oz)	444	430	110	13	8	0	45	160	77	0	69	5	8%	4%	20%	444
Lime CreamSlush® Treat - Large (20 oz)	583	580	150	17	10	0.5	60	210	104	0	92	7	10%	8%	25%	583

Cream Pie Shakes

	Serving Weight (g)	kCal	kCals from Fat	Total Fat (g)	Saturated Fat (g)	Trans Fat (g)	Cholesterol (mg)	Sodium (mg)	CHO (g)	Dietary Fiber (g)	Sugars (g)	Protein (g)	Vitamin A % DV	Vitamin C % DV	Calcium % DV	Iron % DV
Banana Cream Pie Shake – Regular (14 oz)	477	690	210	23	15	1	65	230	113	1	96	8	15%	6%	30%	8%
Banana Cream Pie Shake - Large (20 oz)	698	1000	280	31	19	1.5	90	300	171	3	146	11	20%	10%	40%	10%
Coconut Cream Pie Shake - Regular (14 oz)	458	680	220	24	15	1	70	240	108	1	94	8	15%	0%	30%	8%
Coconut Cream Pie Shake - Large (20 oz)	665	990	290	32	20	1.5	100	330	162	1	144	11	20%	0%	40%	10%
Chocolate Cream Pie Shake - Regular (14 oz)	475	750	210	23	15	1	65	310	127	1	107	8	10%	0%	30%	8%
Chocolate Cream Pie Shake - Large (20 oz)	698	1130	270	30	19	1.5	90	470	200	1	169	11	15%	0%	40%	10%
Strawberry Cream Pie Shake - Regular (14 oz)	472	720	210	23	15	1	65	240	120	1	101	8	10%	15%	30%	8%
Strawberry Cream Pie Shake - Large (20 oz)	692	1070	270	30	19	1.5	90	330	187	2	158	11	15%	25%	40%	15%

Floats/Blended Floats

	Serving Weight (g)	kCal	kCals from Fat	Total Fat (g)	Saturated Fat (g)	Trans Fat (g)	Cholesterol (mg)	Sodium (mg)	CHO (g)	Dietary Fiber (g)	Sugars (g)	Protein (g)	Vitamin A % DV	Vitamin C % DV	Calcium % DV	Iron % DV
Coca-Cola® Float/Blended Float - Regular (14 oz)	355	290	70	8	5	0	30	95	54	0	50	3	6%	0%	10%	4%
Coca-Cola® Float/Blended Float - Large (20 oz)	501	430	110	12	7	0	45	140	77	0	71	5	8%	0%	20%	4%
Diet Coke® Float/Blended Float - Regular (14 oz)	348	220	70	8	5	0	30	100	33	0	29	3	6%	0%	10%	4%
Diet Coke® Float/Blended Float - Large (20 oz)	492	330	110	12	7	0	45	150	50	0	44	5	8%	0%	20%	4%
Dr. Pepper® Float/Blended Float - Regular (14 oz)	407	310	70	8	5	0	30	120	58	0	54	3	6%	0%	10%	4%
Dr. Pepper® Float/Blended Float - Large (20 oz)	502	420	110	12	7	0	45	170	76	0	70	5	8%	0%	20%	4%
Diet Dr. Pepper® Float/Blended Float - Regular (14 oz)	348	220	70	8	5	0	30	130	33	0	29	3	6%	0%	10%	4%
Diet Dr. Pepper® Float/Blended Float - Large (20 oz)	492	330	110	12	7	0	45	190	50	0	44	5	8%	0%	20%	4%
Barq's® Root Beer Float/Blended Float - Regular (14 oz)	356	300	70	8	5	0	30	110	56	0	52	3	6%	0%	10%	4%
Barq's® Root Beer Float/Blended Float - Large (20 oz)	503	440	110	12	7	0	45	160	80	0	74	5	8%	0%	20%	4%

Desserts

	Serving Weight (g)	kCals	kCals from Fat	Total Fat (g)	Saturated Fat (g)	Trans Fat (g)	Cholesterol (mg)	Sodium (mg)	CHO (g)	Dietary Fiber (g)	Sugars (g)	Protein (g)	Vitamin A % DV	Vitamin C % DV	Calcium % DV	Iron % DV
Junior Banana Split	139	200	40	4.5	3.5	0	10	60	38	1	27	2	6%	60%	15%	4%
Hot Fudge Cake Sundae	280	530	200	23	14	0	50	310	75	2	58	5	2%	30%	4%	2%
Banana Fudge	293	480	160	18	13	0	35	170	72	2	57	4	6%	0%	15%	30%

Single Topping Sundaes

	Serving Weight (g)	kcal	kCals from Fat	Total Fat (g)	Saturated Fat (g)	Trans Fat (g)	Cholesterol (mg)	Sodium (mg)	CHO (g)	Dietary Fiber (g)	Sugars (g)	Protein (g)	Vitamin A % DV	Vitamin C % DV	Calcium % DV	Iron % DV
Hot Fudge	253	440	160	18	13	0	35	170	63	1	52	4	6%	0%	15%	6%
Peanut Butter	248	510	280	31	12	0	35	230	53	0	44	8	6%	0%	15%	4%
Peanut Butter Fudge	250	470	220	25	13	0	35	200	58	1	48	6	6%	0%	15%	4%
Strawberry	252	380	120	13	9	0	35	120	61	1	49	4	6%	15%	15%	4%
Chocolate	255	410	120	13	9	0	35	190	67	0	55	4	6%	0%	15%	4%
Pineapple	252	370	120	13	9	0	35	125	58	0	47	4	6%	80%	15%	4%
Nuts Add-on	3.5	20	15	1.5	0	0	0	0	1	0	0	1	0%	0%	0%	0%

Cones and Dishes

	Serving Weight (g)	kcal	kCals from Fat	Total Fat (g)	Saturated Fat (g)	Trans Fat (g)	Cholesterol (mg)	Sodium (mg)	CHO (g)	Dietary Fiber (g)	Sugars (g)	Protein (g)	Vitamin A % DV	Vitamin C % DV	Calcium % DV	Iron % DV
Vanilla Cone	133	180	60	6	4	0	25	80	30	0	22	2	4%	0%	10%	2%
Vanilla Dish	184	240	80	9	5	0	35	100	36	0	32	3	6%	0%	15%	4%

Real Fruit Slushes

	Serving Weight (g)	kcal	kCals from Fat	Total Fat (g)	Saturated Fat (g)	Trans Fat (g)	Cholesterol (mg)	Sodium (mg)	CHO (g)	Dietary Fiber (g)	Sugars (g)	Protein (g)	Vitamin A % DV	Vitamin C % DV	Calcium % DV	Iron % DV
Lemon Real Fruit Slush - Small (14 oz)	399	200	0	0	0	0	0	30	53	0	50	0	0%	8%	0%	0%
Lemon Real Fruit Slush - Large (32 oz)	921	460	0	0	0	0	0	70	124	0	117	0	0%	20%	0%	2%
Lemon-Berry Real Fruit Slush - Small (14 oz)	401	210	0	0	0	0	0	30	55	0	52	0	0%	15%	0%	0%
Lemon-Berry Real Fruit Slush - Large (32 oz)	925	500	0	0	0	0	0	75	132	1	121	1	0%	40%	0%	2%
Lime Real Fruit Slush - Small (14 oz)	397	200	0	0	0	0	0	30	52	0	50	0	0%	4%	0%	0%

	Serving Weight (g)	kCal	kCals from Fat	Total Fat (g)	Saturated Fat (g)	Trans Fat (g)	Cholesterol (mg)	Sodium (mg)	CHO (g)	Dietary Fiber (g)	Sugars (g)	Protein (g)	Vitamin A % DV	Vitamin C % DV	Calcium % DV	Iron % DV
Lime Real Fruit Slush - Large (32 oz)	915	460	0	0	0	0	0	70	123	0	117	0	0%	10%	0%	2%
Strawberry Real Fruit Slush - Small (14 oz)	392	210	0	0	0	0	0	30	55	0	52	0	0%	6%	0%	0%
Strawberry Real Fruit Slush - Large (32 oz)	898	490	0	0	0	0	0	75	129	1	120	1	0%	20%	0%	2%

Slushes

	Serving Weight (g)	kCal	kCals from Fat	Total Fat (g)	Saturated Fat (g)	Trans Fat (g)	Cholesterol (mg)	Sodium (mg)	CHO (g)	Dietary Fiber (g)	Sugars (g)	Protein (g)	Vitamin A % DV	Vitamin C % DV	Calcium % DV	Iron % DV
Cherry Slush – Small (14 oz)	391	200	0	0	0	0	0	30	53	0	53	0	0%	0%	0%	0%
Cherry Slush – Large (32 oz)	895	470	0	0	0	0	0	70	124	0	124	0	0%	0%	0%	0%
Grape Slush – Small (14 oz)	391	190	0	0	0	0	0	35	52	0	52	0	0%	0%	0%	0%
Grape Slush – Large (32 oz)	895	460	0	0	0	0	0	80	121	0	121	0	0%	0%	0%	0%
Orange Slush – Small (14 oz)	390	200	0	0	0	0	0	30	52	0	51	0	0%	0%	0%	0%
Orange Slush – Large (32 oz)	894	460	0	0	0	0	0	75	122	0	120	0	0%	0%	0%	0%
Blue Coconut Slush – Small (14 oz)	390	190	0	0	0	0	0	30	52	0	51	0	0%	0%	0%	0%
Blue Coconut Slush – Large (32 oz)	894	450	0	0	0	0	0	70	121	0	118	0	0%	0%	0%	2%
Watermelon Slush – Small (14 oz)	391	200	0	0	0	0	0	30	53	0	51	0	0%	0%	0%	0%
Watermelon Slush – Large (32 oz)	895	470	0	0	0	0	0	75	124	0	120	0	0%	0%	0%	0%
Green Apple Slush – Small (14 oz)	391	200	0	0	0	0	0	30	54	0	53	0	0%	0%	0%	0%
Green Apple Slush – Large (32 oz)	897	490	0	0	0	0	0	75	129	0	124	0	0%	0%	0%	0%
Bubble Gum Slush – Small (14 oz)	391	190	0	0	0	0	0	35	52	0	51	0	0%	0%	0%	0%
Bubble Gum Slush – Large (32 oz)	895	460	0	0	0	0	0	85	121	1	120	0	0%	0%	0%	0%

Breakfast Foods

	Serving Weight (g)	kCal	kCals from Fat	Total Fat (g)	Saturated Fat (g)	Trans Fat (g)	Cholesterol (mg)	Sodium (mg)	CHO (g)	Dietary Fiber (g)	Sugars (g)	Protein (g)	Vitamin A % DV	Vitamin C % DV	Calcium % DV	Iron % DV
Breakfast Bistro - Bacon, Egg & Cheese	156	470	250	27	9	1	320	1370	35	2	6	21	15%	0%	20%	20%
Breakfast Bistro - Ham, Egg & Cheese	175	430	190	21	7	1	325	1640	35	2	6	25	15%	0%	20%	20%
Breakfast Bistro - Sausage, Egg & Cheese	183	560	330	37	12	1.5	340	1320	35	2	6	22	15%	0%	20%	20%
BREAKFAST TOASTER® - Sausage, Egg & Cheese	202	630	350	39	13	1.5	340	1380	46	2	7	23	15%	0%	25%	20%
BREAKFAST TOASTER® - Bacon, Egg & Cheese	175	540	270	30	10	1.5	325	1440	46	2	7	22	15%	0%	25%	15%
BREAKFAST TOASTER® - Ham, Egg & Cheese	194	500	210	23	7	1.5	325	1700	46	2	7	26	15%	0%	25%	15%
Breakfast Burritos - Sausage, Egg & Cheese	167	470	270	30	11	1.5	325	1040	38	3	2	19	15%	0%	40%	20%
Breakfast Burritos - Bacon, Egg & Cheese	157	450	240	27	10	1.5	320	1140	38	3	2	20	15%	0%	40%	15%
Breakfast Burritos - Ham, Egg & Cheese	183	440	210	23	8	1.5	330	1530	37	3	2	25	15%	0%	40%	20%
Super Sonic® Breakfast Burrito	216	550	310	35	11	2.5	325	1240	47	4	2	19	20%	4%	40%	25%
French Toast Sticks (4)	136	500	230	26	5	4.5	25	580	59	2	12	8	0%	0%	10%	15%
Syrup	28	80	0	0	0	0	0	0	21	0	19	0	0%	0%	0%	0%

Fruit Smoothies

	Serving Weight (g)	kCal	kCals from Fat	Total Fat (g)	Saturated Fat (g)	Trans Fat (g)	Cholesterol (mg)	Sodium (mg)	CHO (g)	Dietary Fiber (g)	Sugars (g)	Protein (g)	Vitamin A % DV	Vitamin C % DV	Calcium % DV	Iron % DV
Strawberry Fruit Smoothie – Regular (14 oz)	435	460	0	0	0	0	0	180	113	8	91	1	160%	240%	150%	8%
Strawberry-Banana Fruit Smoothie – Regular (14 oz)	415	440	0	0	0	0	0	160	108	3	76	1	150%	160%	150%	10%
Tropical Fruit Smoothie – Regular (14 oz)	420	500	0	0	0	0	0	170	124	4	98	1	150%	270%	140%	10%

http://www.sonicdrivein.com/pdfs/menu/SonicNutritionGuide.pdf

Taco Bell
"Fresco" Style* Nutrition Guide

Our most popular "Fresco" Style Items Under 10 Grams of Fat	Serving Size (g)	kcal	Kcals from Fat	Total Fat (g)	% Daily Value**	Saturated Fat (g)	% Daily Value**	Trans Fat (g)	Cholesterol (mg)	% Daily Value**	Sodium (mg)	% Daily Value**	CHO	% Daily Value**	Dietary Fiber (g)	% Daily Value**	Sugars (g)	Protein (g)	Vitamin A % DV	Vitamin C % DV	Calcium % DV	Iron % DV
Crunchy Taco	92	150	70	8	12	2.5	13	0	20	7	370	15	13	4	3	12	1	7	6	4	4	6
Crunchy TACO SUPREME®	106	150	70	8	12	2.5	13	0	20	7	370	15	14	5	3	12	2	7	6	8	4	6
Soft Taco – Beef	113	180	70	7	11	3	15	0	20	7	650	27	21	7	3	12	2	8	6	4	8	10
Soft Taco Supreme® – Beef	128	190	70	7	11	3	15	0	20	7	650	27	22	7	3	12	3	9	6	8	8	10
Ranchero Chicken Soft Taco	135	170	35	4	6	1.5	8	0	25	8	730	30	21	7	3	12	3	12	8	8	8	10
Grilled Steak Soft Taco	128	160	40	4.5	7	1.5	8	0	20	7	550	23	20	7	2	8	3	10	4	10	8	10
Bean Burrito	213	320	60	7	11	2.5	13	0.5	0	0	1200	50	54	18	9	36	4	12	10	10	15	25
7-Layer Burrito	248	380	80	8	12	2.5	13	0.5	0	0	1190	50	62	21	9	36	4	13	6	10	15	25
Chili Cheese Burrito	149	270	70	8	12	3	15	0	15	5	930	39	39	13	4	16	3	10	6	4	15	20
½ lb.† Cheesy Bean & Rice Burrito	198	330	70	7	11	2	10	0	0	0	1080	45	55	18	6	24	4	10	8	6	15	20
Enchirito® – Beef	206	230	80	8	12	3.5	18	0.5	20	7	1300	54	34	11	7	28	3	12	20	15	10	15
MexiMelt®	120	190	70	7	11	3	15	0	20	7	710	30	22	7	3	12	3	8	8	6	8	10
Steak Grilled Taquitos	135	260	60	7	11	2.5	13	0	20	7	830	35	37	12	3	12	3	13	4	4	10	20
Mexican Rice	138	120	25	3	5	0.5	3	0	0	0	760	32	23	8	2	8	1	3	15	10	2	8
Pintos 'n Cheese	135	100	20	2	3	0.5	3	0.5	0	0	640	27	19	6	7	28	1	6	10	10	4	8

Nutrition Guide–Original Items (Note: Any item with cheese and/or sauce can be made "Fresco" Style)

	Serving Size (g)	kCal	kCals from Fat	Total Fat (g)	% Daily Value**	Saturated Fat (g)	% Daily Value**	Trans Fat (g)	Cholesterol (mg)	% Daily Value**	Sodium (mg)	% Daily Value**	CHO	% Daily Value**	Dietary Fiber (g)	% Daily Value**	Sugars (g)	Protein (g)	Vitamin A %DV	Vitamin C %DV	Calcium %DV	Iron %DV
TACOS																						
Crunchy Taco	78	170	90	10	15	3.5	18	0	25	8	350	15	13	4	3	12	1	8	4	2	8	6
Crunchy TACO SUPREME®	113	210	120	13	20	6	30	0	40	13	370	15	15	5	3	12	2	9	10	6	10	6
DOUBLE DECKER® Taco Supreme®	191	370	150	17	26	7	35	1	40	13	820	34	40	13	7	28	4	14	10	6	15	20
Soft Taco – Beef	99	200	80	9	14	4	20	0	25	8	630	26	21	7	3	12	2	10	4	2	10	10
Soft Taco Supreme® – Beef	135	250	120	13	20	6	30	0.5	40	13	650	27	23	8	3	12	3	11	10	6	15	15
Ranchero Chicken Soft Taco	135	270	130	14	22	4	20	0	35	12	820	34	21	7	2	8	3	14	6	6	15	10
Grilled Steak Soft Taco	128	270	150	16	25	4.5	23	0	35	12	660	28	20	7	2	8	3	12	4	6	10	15
GORDITAS																						
Gordita Supreme® – Beef	153	310	140	16	25	6	30	0.5	40	13	620	26	29	10	3	12	6	14	8	6	15	15
Gordita Supreme® – Chicken	153	290	110	12	18	5	25	0	45	15	650	27	28	9	2	8	6	17	8	8	15	10
Gordita Supreme® – Steak	153	290	120	13	20	5	25	0	40	13	530	22	28	9	2	8	6	15	6	6	10	15
Gordita Baja® – Beef	153	340	170	19	29	5	25	0	35	12	780	33	29	10	4	16	6	13	8	4	10	15
Gordita Baja® – Chicken	153	320	140	16	25	3.5	18	0	40	13	800	33	28	9	3	12	6	17	8	6	10	10
Gordita Baja® – Steak	153	320	150	17	26	4	20	0	35	12	690	29	27	9	3	12	5	15	6	4	10	15
Gordita Nacho Cheese – Beef	153	300	130	14	22	4	20	1.5	25	8	770	32	31	10	3	12	6	12	4	6	10	15
Gordita Nacho Cheese – Chicken	153	280	100	11	17	2.5	13	1	25	8	800	33	29	10	2	8	6	16	4	8	10	10
Gordita Nacho Cheese – Steak	153	270	100	12	18	3	13	1	20	7	680	28	29	10	2	8	6	14	2	6	8	15
CHALUPAS																						
Chalupa Supreme – Beef	153	380	210	23	35	7	35	0.5	40	13	620	26	30	10	3	12	4	14	8	6	15	15
Chalupa Supreme – Chicken	153	360	180	20	31	5	25	0	45	15	650	27	29	10	2	8	4	17	8	8	15	10
Chalupa Supreme – Steak	153	360	180	21	32	6	30	0	40	13	530	22	28	9	2	8	4	15	6	6	10	15
Chalupa Baja – Beef	153	410	240	27	42	6	30	0	35	12	780	33	30	10	4	16	4	13	8	4	10	15

Item																						
Chalupa Baja – Chicken	153	390	210	23	35	4	20	0	40	13	800	33	29	10	3	12	4	17	8	6	10	10
Chalupa Baja –Steak	153	390	220	24	37	4.5	23	0	35	12	690	29	28	9	3	12	3	15	6	4	10	15
Chalupa Nacho Cheese – Beef	153	370	190	22	34	4.5	23	1.5	20	7	770	32	32	11	3	12	4	12	4	6	10	15
Chalupa Nacho Cheese – Chicken	153	350	160	18	28	3	15	1	25	8	790	33	30	10	2	8	4	16	4	8	10	10
Chalupa Nacho Cheese – Steak	153	340	170	19	29	3.5	18	1.5	20	7	680	28	30	10	2	8	4	14	2	6	8	15
BURRITOS																						
Bean Burrito	198	340	80	9	14	3.5	18	0.5	5	2	1190	50	54	18	8	32	4	13	10	8	20	25
7-Layer Burrito	283	490	170	18	28	7	35	1	25	8	1350	56	65	22	9	36	5	17	10	25	25	30
Burrito Supreme® – Beef	248	410	150	17	26	8	40	1	40	13	1340	56	51	17	7	28	5	17	15	10	20	25
Burrito Supreme® – Chicken	248	390	120	13	20	6	30	0.5	45	15	1360	57	49	16	6	24	5	20	15	15	20	25
Burrito Supreme® – Steak	248	380	130	14	22	7	35	0.5	40	13	1250	52	49	16	6	24	5	18	15	15	20	25
Fiesta Burrito – Beef	184	370	120	13	20	5	25	0	25	8	1200	50	49	16	4	16	4	14	8	4	20	25
Fiesta Burrito – Chicken	184	350	90	10	15	3.5	18	0	30	10	1220	51	47	16	3	12	4	18	8	4	20	20
Fiesta Burrito – Steak	184	340	100	11	17	4	20	0	25	8	1110	46	47	16	3	12	3	15	6	4	20	20
Grilled Stuft Burrito – Beef	325	680	270	30	46	10	50	1	55	18	2120	88	76	25	9	36	6	27	15	4	30	40
Grilled Stuft Burrito – Chicken	325	640	210	23	35	7	35	0.5	65	22	2160	90	73	24	7	28	6	34	10	6	30	35
Grilled Stuft Burrito – Steak	325	630	220	25	38	8	40	1	55	18	1930	80	72	24	7	28	5	30	10	8	30	40
BIG BELL VALUE MENU®																						
Grande Soft Taco	206	430	180	20	31	8	40	1.5	45	15	1440	60	43	14	5	20	5	19	8	2	20	25
DOUBLE DECKER® Taco	156	320	120	13	20	5	25	0.5	25	8	810	34	38	13	6	24	2	14	6	2	15	15
Spicy Chicken Soft Taco	113	170	50	6	9	2	10	0	25	8	580	24	20	7	2	8	2	10	8	4	10	10
Spicy Chicken Burrito	191	400	150	17	26	4	20	0	30	10	1190	50	48	16	3	12	4	14	10	4	15	20
½ lb.† Beef Combo Burrito	241	430	160	18	28	8	40	1	45	15	1630	68	51	17	8	32	4	21	15	6	20	30
½ lb.† Beef & Potato Burrito	252	520	210	23	35	7	35	1	30	10	1720	72	66	22	6	24	4	15	15	6	15	25
½ lb.† Cheesy Bean & Rice Burrito	227	470	180	20	31	6	30	1.5	15	5	1400	58	58	19	6	24	5	13	8	4	20	25
Cheesy Fiesta Potatoes	138	290	150	17	26	4	20	1.5	15	5	830	35	30	10	3	12	2	4	6	6	6	6
Caramel Apple Empanada	85	290	120	14	22	2.5	13	1.5	5	2	300	13	37	12	1	4	13	3	2	15	4	6

SPECIALTIES

	Serving Size (g)	kcal	kCals from Fat	Total Fat (g)	% Daily Value**	Saturated Fat (g)	% Daily Value**	Trans Fat (g)	Cholesterol (mg)	% Daily Value**	Sodium (mg)	% Daily Value**	CHO	% Daily Value**	Dietary Fiber (g)	% Daily Value**	Sugars (g)	Protein (g)	Vitamin A % DV	Vitamin C % DV	Calcium % DV	Iron % DV
Crunchwrap Supreme®	254	560	220	24	37	8	40	1.5	35	12	1430	60	68	23	5	20	7	17	8	8	25	30
Spicy Chicken CRUNCHWRAP SUPREME®	254	540	200	23	35	7	35	1.5	40	13	1360	57	67	22	4	16	7	19	10	8	30	30
Mexican Pizza	216	530	270	30	46	8	40	1	40	13	1000	42	46	15	7	28	3	20	10	8	35	20
Enchirito® – Beef	213	340	150	17	26	9	45	1	50	17	1420	59	34	11	7	28	3	18	25	10	30	20
Enchirito® – Chicken	213	320	120	13	20	7	35	0.5	50	17	1450	60	33	11	6	24	3	22	25	15	30	15
Enchirito® – Steak	213	310	130	14	22	7	35	1	45	15	1330	55	33	11	6	24	3	20	25	15	30	15
MexiMelt®	128	280	130	14	22	7	35	0.5	40	13	860	36	22	7	3	12	2	15	10	4	25	15
Fiesta Taco Salad	548	840	400	45	69	11	55	1.5	65	22	1780	74	80	27	15	60	10	30	25	20	45	40
Fiesta Taco Salad without Shell	479	470	220	24	37	10	50	1.5	65	22	1510	63	41	14	13	52	9	23	25	20	30	25
Chicken Fiesta Taco Salad	548	800	340	38	58	8	40	1	75	25	1830	76	77	26	13	52	10	37	25	25	40	35
Chicken Fiesta Taco Salad without Shell	479	430	160	18	28	6	30	1	75	25	1560	65	38	13	11	44	9	30	25	25	30	20
Express Taco Salad	479	610	290	32	49	10	50	1.5	65	22	1420	59	56	19	14	56	8	25	20	20	30	25
Steak Grilled Taquitos with Guacamole	170	380	150	17	26	6	30	0.5	35	12	1040	43	41	14	4	16	4	17	4	30	20	20
Steak Grilled Taquitos with Salsa	170	320	100	11	17	5	25	0	35	12	1030	43	39	13	3	12	5	16	10	6	25	20
Steak Grilled Taquitos with Sour Cream	170	390	170	19	29	10	50	0.5	60	20	900	38	39	13	2	8	5	17	10	2	30	20
Chicken Quesadilla	184	520	250	28	43	12	60	0.5	75	25	1420	59	59	13	3	12	4	28	10	2	45	20
Steak Quesadilla	184	520	260	28	43	13	65	1	70	23	1300	54	54	13	3	12	4	26	10	0	45	20
Zesty Chicken BORDER BOWL®	418	640	310	35	54	6	30	1	30	10	1800	75	75	20	10	40	4	22	15	15	15	25
Zesty Chicken BORDER BOWL® without Dressing	376	440	130	15	23	2.5	13	0.5	30	10	1540	64	64	19	10	40	3	21	15	15	15	20
Southwest Steak BORDER BOWL®	443	600	220	24	37	6	30	1	55	18	2120	88	88	23	9	36	3	28	20	15	20	35

NACHOS AND SIDES

Item																						
Nachos	99	330	180	21	32	3.5	18	2	5	2	530	22	32	11	2	8	3	4	0	0	8	4
Nachos Supreme	195	450	230	26	40	7	35	1.5	35	12	800	33	41	14	7	28	3	12	8	8	10	10
Nachos BellGrande®	308	770	390	44	68	9	45	3	35	12	1280	53	77	26	12	48	5	19	8	8	20	20
Pintos 'n Cheese	128	150	50	6	9	3	15	0.5	15	5	670	28	19	6	7	28	1	9	10	6	15	8
Mexican Rice	131	170	60	7	11	3	15	0	15	5	790	33	23	8	1	4	1	6	15	15	10	8
Cinnamon Twists	35	170	60	7	11	0	0	0	0	0	200	8	26	9	1	4	12	1	0	0	0	2

REGIONAL MENU ITEMS

Item																						
Cheese Quesadilla	142	470	240	26	40	12	60	0.5	50	17	1100	46	39	13	2	8	4	19	10	2	45	20
Chili Cheese Burrito	156	370	140	16	25	8	40	0.5	40	13	1060	44	40	13	3	12	3	16	10	0	30	20
Tostada	170	230	90	10	15	3.5	18	0.5	15	5	730	30	27	9	7	28	2	11	10	8	20	10

**Percent daily values are based on a 2,000 calorie diet.
* "Fresco" Style fat reduction varies per menu item and not all menu items will meet a 25% reduction in fat.
† ½ lb. claim based on average weight. Individual product weights necessarily vary.
http://www.yum.com/nutrition/documents/tb_nutrition.pdf

Wendy's

Garden Sensations® Salads Flavor-Packed Entrée Salads* Prepared Fresh Daily	kCal	Total Fat (g)	Saturated Fat (g)	Trams Fat (g)	Cholesterol (mg)	Sodium (mg)	Total CHO (g)	Dietary Fiber (g)	Sugars (g)	Protein (g)
Mandarin Chicken® Salad	170	2.5	0.5	0	60	520	16	3	12	21
Crispy Noodles	70	2.5	0	0	0	190	10	0	0	1
Roasted Almonds	130	11	1	0	0	70	4	2	1	5
Oriental Sesame Dressing	170	9	1.5	0	0	430	19	0	17	1
Chicken Caesar Salad	180	6	2.5	0	70	660	8	3	3	25
Homestyle Garlic Croutons	70	2.5	0	0	0	125	9	0	0	2
Caesar Dressing	120	13	2.5	0	20	220	1	0	0	1
Chicken BLT Salad	330	18	9	0	105	1050	11	4	5	33
Homestyle Garlic Croutons	70	2.5	0	0	0	125	9	0	0	2
Honey Mustard Dressing	250	23	3.5	0	20	330	9	0	9	1
Southwest Taco Salad	430	22	12	1	80	1090	30	8	9	30
Reduced Fat Acidified Sour Cream	50	4	2.5	0	10	30	2	0	1	1
Seasoned Tortilla Strips	110	5	1	0	0	160	13	1	0	2
Ancho Chipotle Ranch Dressing	90	8	1.5	0	10	270	3	0	2	1
Additional Salad Dressings										
Fat Free French	70	0	0	0	0	190	17	0	14	0
Reduced Fat Creamy Ranch**	90	7	1.5	0	10	400	6	1	3	1
Low Fat Honey Mustard**	100	2.5	0	0	0	300	19	0	14	0
Italian Vinaigrette	130	11	1.5	0	0	360	8	0	7	0
Creamy Ranch	200	20	3.5	0	15	400	4	0	2	1
Blue Cheese**	260	27	4.5	0	35	480	2	0	1	2
Thousand Island**	230	22	3.5	0	20	400	7	0	5	1

Toppings and Salad Dressings listed separately.
**Not available in all locations.*

Side Selections Numerous Options for a Balanced Meal	kCal	Total Fat (g)	Saturated Fat (g)	Trams Fat (g)	Cholesterol (mg)	Sodium (mg)	Total CHO (g)	Dietary Fiber (g)	Sugars (g)	Protein (g)
Side Salad	35	0	0	0	0	25	8	2	4	1
Caesar Side Salad	80	4.5	2	0	10	240	6	2	1	6
Mandarin Orange Cup	80	0	0	0	0	15	19	1	17	1
Low Fat Strawberry Flavored Yogurt	140	1.5	1	0	5	90	27	0	24	6
Granola Topping	110	4.5	0.5	0	0	0	15	1	6	2
Plain Baked Potato (avg. wgt. 10oz.)	270	0	0	0	0	25	61	7	3	7
Sour Cream & Chives Baked Potato	320	4	2.5	0	10	55	63	7	4	9
Buttery Best Spread	50	6	1	0	0	90	0	0	0	0
Small Chili	220	6	2.5	0	35	780	23	5	6	17
Large Chili	330	9	3.5	0.5	55	1170	35	8	9	25
Hot Chili Seasoning	5	0	0	0	0	270	2	0	1	0
Saltine Crackers	25	0.5	0	0	0	95	4	0	0	0
Cheddar Cheese, Shredded	70	6	3.5	0	15	110	1	0	0	4
Kid's Meal French Fries*	210	10	1.5	0	0	210	26	3	0	3
Small French Fries*	330	16	2.5	0.5	0	340	42	4	0	4
Medium French Fries*	420	20	3	1	0	430	53	5	0	6
Large French Fries*	520	24	3.5	1	0	550	69	7	0	7

*Recommended portion sizes. French fries are individually portioned at every restaurant. Variations will exist from restaurant to restaurant.

Beverages and Frosty™ Refreshments for Everyone's Thirst	kCal	Total Fat (g)	Saturated Fat (g)	Trams Fat (g)	Cholesterol (mg)	Sodium (mg)	Total CHO (g)	Dietary Fiber (g)	Sugars (g)	Protein (g)
Milk, 2% Reduced Fat Milk	120	4.5	3	0	20	125	12	0	11	7
Milk, 1% Low Fat Chocolate	170	2.5	1.5	0	15	200	28	0	26	8
Diet Coke®, Small Cup	0	0	0	0	0	15+	0	0	0	0
Sprite®, Small Cup	130	0	0	0	0	30+	34	0	34	0
Coca-Cola®, Small Cup	140	0	0	0	0	0+	37	0	37	0
Dasani® Water	0	0	0	0	0	0	0	0	0	0
Chocolate Frosty Junior	160	4	2.5	0	15	75	28	0	21	4
Chocolate Frosty Small	330	8	5	0	35	150	56	0	42	8
Chocolate Frosty Medium	430	11	7	0	45	200	74	0	55	10
Vanilla Frosty Junior	150	4	2.5	0	20	90	26	0	21	4
Vanilla Frosty Small	310	8	5	0	35	180	52	0	43	8
Vanilla Frosty Medium	410	10	6	0.5	45	240	68	0	57	11
Vanilla Frosty Float with Coca-Cola*	410	8	5	0	35	190+	78	0	69	8
Chocolate Frosty Fix 'N Mix	170	4	2.5	0	20	80	29	0	22	4
Vanilla Frosty Fix 'N Mix	160	4	2.5	0	20	95	27	0	22	4
Oreo® Cookie Crumbles*	100	4	1.5	0	0	115	15	1	9	1
Butterfinger® Candy Crumbles*	130	5	2.5	0	0	65	20	1	13	2
M&M® Candy Crumbles*	140	6	3.5	0	5	15	20	1	18	1

*Coca-Cola®, Diet Coke®, Sprite® and Dasani® are trademarks of The Coca-Cola Company.
Baked! Lays® is a trademark of Frito Lay®.
OREO® is a trademark of Kraft Foods Holdings, Inc.
NESTLÉ® and BUTTERFINGER® are registered trademarks of Société Des Produits Nestlé S.A., Vevey, Switzerland.
M&M's® is a registered trademark of Mars, Incorporated.

Sandwiches

Made when you order it using each sandwich's standard toppings

	kCal	Total Fat (g)	Saturated Fat (g)	Trams Fat (g)	Cholesterol (mg)	Sodium (mg)	Total CHO (g)	Dietary Fiber (g)	Sugars (g)	Protein (g)
Jr. Hamburger	230	8	3	0	25	500	26	1	5	13
Jr. Cheeseburger	270	11	5	0.5	35	710	26	1	6	15
Jr. Cheeseburger Deluxe	300	14	5	0.5	40	760	28	2	7	15
Jr. Bacon Cheeseburger	310	16	6	0.5	45	690	26	1	5	17
Hamburger, Kids' Meal	220	8	3	0	25	500	25	1	5	13
Cheeseburger, Kids' Meal	260	11	5	0.5	35	710	26	1	5	15
Ham & Cheese Sandwich, Kids' Meal	200	5	2.5	0	30	810	25	1	4	13
Turkey & Cheese Sandwich, Kids' Meal	210	6	2.5	0	25	830	27	1	4	12
Single w/Everything	430	20	7	1	65	900	37	2	9	25
Double w/Everything and Cheese	700	40	16	2.5	140	1500	38	2	9	48
Triple w/Everything and Cheese	980	59	25	3.5	215	2090	38	2	9	70
Baconator™	830	51	22	2.5	170	1920	35	1	8	57
Ultimate Chicken Grill Sandwich	320	7	1.5	0	70	950	36	2	8	28
Spicy Chicken Fillet Sandwich	440	16	2.5	0	60	1320	46	3	6	28
Homestyle Chicken Fillet Sandwich	430	16	2.5	0	45	1140	48	2	6	25
Chicken Club Sandwich	540	25	7	0.5	75	1410	49	2	7	33
Crispy Chicken Sandwich	320	14	2.5	0	30	660	34	1	4	15
Black Forest Ham & Swiss Frescata®	460	19	6	0	60	1470	50	4	8	27
Roasted Turkey & Swiss Frescata	470	20	6	0	60	1520	51	4	4	25
Frescata Club	440	17	3.5	0	50	1600	49	4	5	23

Crispy Chicken Nuggets Crispy All-White Meat for Full Flavor Dipping	kCal	Total Fat (g)	Saturated Fat (g)	Trams Fat (g)	Cholesterol (mg)	Sodium (mg)	Total CHO (g)	Dietary Fiber (g)	Sugars (g)	Protein (g)
4 Piece Kids' Meal Chicken Nuggets	190	12	2	0	30	420	10	0	0	10
5 Piece Chicken Nuggets	230	15	3	0	35	520	12	0	0	12
10 Piece Chicken Nuggets	460	30	6	0	70	1040	24	0	0	24
Barbecue Nugget Sauce	45	0	0	0	0	170	10	0	8	1
Sweet & Sour Nugget Sauce	50	0	0	0	0	120	13	0	11	0
Honey Mustard Nugget Sauce	130	12	2	0	10	220	6	0	5	0
Heartland Ranch Dipping Sauce	160	17	2.5	0	15	220	1	0	1	0

http://www.wendys.com/food/pdf/us/nutrition.pdf

APPENDIX B

Energy Expenditure in Household, Occupational, Recreational, and Sports Activities[a,b]

HOW TO USE APPENDIX B

Refer to the column that comes closest to your present body mass. Multiply the number in this column by the number of minutes you spend in an activity. Suppose that an individual weighing 80.0 kg (176 lb) spends 45 minutes working out with free weights. To determine the energy cost of participation, multiply the caloric value per minute (6.8 kCal) by 45 to obtain the 45-minute gross expenditure of 306 kCal. If the same individual does aerobic dance for 60 minutes, the gross (value includes resting energy expenditure) energy expended would be calculated as 7.8 kCal × 60 minutes, or 468 kCal.

[a] All values for energy expenditure expressed in kilocalories per minute.

[b] Copyright © 1999, 2004 by Frank I. Katch, Victor L. Katch, and William D. McArdle, and Fitness Technologies, Inc., 5043 Via Lara Lane, Santa Barbara, CA, 93111. No part of this appendix may be reproduced in any manner without written permission from the copyright holders.

YOUR BODY WEIGHT

Activity	kg / lb	47 / 104	50 / 110	53 / 117	56 / 123	59 / 130	62 / 137	65 / 143	68 / 150
Archery		3.1	3.3	3.4	3.6	3.8	4.0	4.2	4.4
Backpacking									
without load		5.7	6.1	6.4	6.8	7.1	7.5	7.9	8.2
with 11 pound load		6.1	6.5	6.8	7.2	7.6	8.0	8.4	8.8
with 22 pound load		6.6	7.0	7.4	7.8	8.3	8.7	9.1	9.5
with 44 pound load		7.0	7.4	7.8	8.2	8.7	9.1	9.6	10.0
Badminton									
leisure		4.6	4.9	5.1	5.4	5.7	6.0	6.3	6.6
tournament		7.0	7.3	7.7	8.1	8.6	9.0	9.4	9.9
Baking, general (F)		1.6	1.8	1.9	2.0	2.1	2.2	2.3	2.4
Baseball									
fielder		2.8	3.0	3.2	3.4	3.6	3.8	4.0	4.1
pitcher		4.2	4.5	4.8	5.0	5.3	5.6	5.9	6.2
Basketball									
competition		7.1	7.4	7.9	8.3	8.7	9.2	9.6	10.1
practice		6.5	6.9	7.3	7.7	8.1	8.6	9.0	9.4
Baton twirling		6.3	6.8	7.3	7.6	8.1	8.5	8.9	9.3
Billiards ("pool")		2.0	2.1	2.2	2.4	2.5	2.6	2.7	2.9
Bookbinding		1.8	1.9	2.0	2.1	2.2	2.4	2.5	2.6
Bowling		4.4	4.8	5.2	5.4	5.7	6.0	6.3	6.6
Boxing									
in ring, match		10.4	11.1	11.8	12.4	13.1	13.8	14.4	15.1
sparring, practice		6.5	6.9	7.3	7.7	8.1	8.6	9.0	9.4
Calisthenics, warm-ups		3.4	3.7	4.0	4.2	4.4	4.7	4.9	5.1
Canoeing									
leisure (2.5 mph)		2.1	2.2	2.3	2.5	2.6	2.7	2.9	3.0
racing ("fast")		4.8	5.2	5.5	5.8	6.1	6.4	6.7	7.0
Car washing		3.3	3.5	3.7	3.9	4.1	4.3	4.5	4.8
Card playing		1.2	1.3	1.3	1.4	1.5	1.6	1.6	1.7
Carpentry, general		2.4	2.6	2.8	2.9	3.1	3.2	3.4	3.5
Carpet sweeping (F)		2.2	2.3	2.4	2.5	2.7	2.8	2.9	3.1
Carpet sweeping (M)		2.3	2.4	2.5	2.7	2.8	3.0	3.1	3.3
Circuit resistance training									
Free weights		4.0	4.3	4.5	4.8	5.0	5.3	5.5	5.8
Hydra-Fitness		6.2	6.6	7.0	7.4	7.8	8.2	8.6	9.0
Nautilus		4.3	4.6	4.9	5.2	5.5	5.8	6.0	6.3
Universal		5.3	5.8	6.2	6.5	6.9	7.2	7.5	7.9
Cleaning (F)		2.9	3.1	3.3	3.5	3.7	3.8	4.0	4.2
Cleaning (M)		2.7	2.9	3.1	3.2	3.4	3.6	3.8	3.9
Coal mining									
drilling coal, rock		4.4	4.7	5.0	5.3	5.5	5.8	6.1	6.4
erecting supports		4.1	4.4	4.7	4.9	5.2	5.5	5.7	6.0
shoveling coal		5.1	5.4	5.7	6.0	6.4	6.7	7.0	7.3
Cooking (F)		2.1	2.3	2.4	2.5	2.7	2.8	2.9	3.1
Cooking (M)		2.3	2.4	2.5	2.7	2.8	3.0	3.1	3.3
Cricket									
batting		3.9	4.2	4.4	4.6	4.9	5.1	5.4	5.6
bowling		4.2	4.5	4.8	5.0	5.3	5.6	5.9	6.1
fielding		3.7	3.9	4.1	4.3	4.8	4.8	5.0	5.3

Note: Symbols (M) and (F) denote experiments for males and females, respectively.

| 71 | 74 | 77 | 80 | 83 | 86 | 89 | 92 | 95 | 98 |
157	163	170	176	183	190	196	203	209	216
4.6	4.8	5.0	5.2	5.4	5.6	5.8	6.0	6.2	6.4
8.6	9.0	9.3	9.7	10.0	10.4	10.8	11.1	11.5	11.9
9.2	9.5	9.9	10.3	10.7	11.1	11.5	11.9	12.3	12.6
9.9	10.4	10.8	11.2	11.6	12.0	12.5	12.9	13.3	13.7
10.4	10.9	11.3	11.8	12.2	12.6	13.1	13.5	14.0	14.4
6.9	7.2	7.5	7.8	8.1	8.3	8.6	8.9	9.2	9.5
10.4	10.8	11.2	11.6	12.1	12.5	12.9	13.4	13.8	14.3
2.5	2.6	2.7	2.8	2.9	3.0	3.1	3.2	3.3	3.4
4.3	4.5	4.7	4.9	5.1	5.2	5.4	5.6	5.8	6.0
6.4	6.7	7.0	7.2	7.5	7.8	8.0	8.3	8.6	8.9
10.5	10.9	11.4	11.8	12.3	12.7	13.1	13.6	14.0	14.5
9.8	10.2	10.6	11.0	11.5	11.9	12.3	12.7	13.1	13.5
9.5	9.7	9.9	10.1	10.4	10.6	10.8	11.0	11.2	11.4
3.0	3.1	3.2	3.4	3.5	3.6	3.7	3.9	4.0	4.1
2.7	2.8	2.9	3.0	3.2	3.3	3.4	3.5	3.6	3.7
6.9	7.2	7.5	7.7	8.1	8.4	8.6	8.9	9.2	9.5
15.8	16.4	17.1	17.8	18.4	19.1	19.8	20.4	21.1	21.8
9.8	10.2	10.6	11.0	11.5	11.9	12.3	12.7	13.1	13.5
5.3	5.5	5.8	6.0	6.2	6.5	6.7	6.9	7.1	7.3
3.1	3.3	3.4	3.5	3.7	3.8	3.9	4.0	4.2	4.3
7.3	7.6	7.9	8.2	8.5	8.9	9.2	9.5	9.8	10.1
5.0	5.2	5.5	5.7	5.7	5.9	6.1	6.3	6.5	6.9
1.8	1.9	1.9	2.0	2.1	2.2	2.2	2.3	2.4	2.5
3.7	3.8	4.0	4.2	4.3	4.5	4.6	4.8	4.9	5.1
3.2	3.3	3.5	3.6	3.7	3.9	4.0	4.1	4.3	4.4
3.4	3.6	3.7	3.8	4.0	4.1	4.3	4.4	4.6	4.7
6.1	6.3	6.6	6.8	7.1	7.4	7.6	7.9	8.1	8.4
9.4	9.7	10.2	10.5	10.9	11.4	11.7	12.1	12.5	12.9
6.6	6.8	7.1	7.4	7.7	8.0	8.2	8.5	8.8	9.1
8.3	8.6	8.9	9.3	9.6	10.0	10.3	10.7	11.0	11.4
4.4	4.6	4.8	5.0	5.1	5.3	5.5	5.7	5.9	6.1
4.1	4.3	4.5	4.6	4.8	5.0	5.2	5.3	5.5	5.7
6.7	7.0	7.2	7.5	7.8	8.1	8.4	8.6	8.9	9.2
6.2	6.5	6.8	7.0	7.3	7.6	7.8	8.1	8.4	8.6
7.7	8.0	8.3	8.6	9.0	9.3	9.6	9.9	10.3	10.6
3.2	3.3	3.5	3.6	3.7	3.9	4.0	4.1	4.3	4.4
3.4	3.6	3.7	3.8	4.0	4.1	4.3	4.4	4.6	4.7
5.9	6.1	6.4	6.6	6.9	7.1	7.4	7.6	7.9	8.1
6.4	6.7	6.9	7.2	7.5	7.7	8.0	8.3	8.6	8.8
5.6	5.9	6.2	6.5	6.8	7.1	7.4	7.7	8.0	8.3

YOUR BODY WEIGHT—*continued*

Activity	kg	47	50	53	56	59	62	65	68
	lb	104	110	117	123	130	137	143	150
Croquet		2.8	3.0	3.1	3.3	3.5	3.7	3.8	4.0
Cycling									
leisure, 5.5 mph		3.0	3.2	3.4	3.6	3.8	4.0	4.2	4.4
leisure, 9.4 mph		4.8	5.0	5.3	5.6	5.9	6.2	6.5	6.8
racing, fast		8.0	8.5	9.0	9.5	10.0	10.5	11.0	11.5
Dancing									
aerobic, easy		4.3	4.8	5.2	5.6	5.9	6.2	6.4	6.7
aerobic, medium		4.8	5.2	5.5	5.8	6.1	6.4	6.7	7.0
aerobic, intense		6.3	6.7	7.1	7.5	7.9	8.3	8.7	9.2
ballroom		2.4	2.6	2.7	2.9	3.0	3.2	3.3	3.5
choreographed		5.0	5.2	5.5	5.8	6.1	6.4	6.7	7.0
"twist," "lambada"		8.0	8.4	8.9	9.4	9.9	10.4	10.9	11.4
modern		3.4	3.6	3.8	4.0	4.3	4.5	4.7	4.9
Digging trenches		6.8	7.3	7.7	8.1	8.6	9.0	9.4	9.9
Drawing (standing)		1.7	1.8	1.9	2.0	2.1	2.2	2.3	2.4
Eating (sitting)		1.1	1.2	1.2	1.3	1.4	1.4	1.5	1.6
Electrical work		2.7	2.9	3.1	3.2	3.4	3.6	3.8	3.9
Farming									
barn cleaning		6.3	6.8	7.2	7.6	8.0	8.4	8.8	9.2
driving harvester		1.9	2.0	2.1	2.2	2.4	2.5	2.6	2.7
driving tractor		1.8	1.9	2.0	2.1	2.2	2.3	2.4	2.5
feeding cattle		4.2	4.3	4.5	4.8	5.0	5.3	5.5	5.8
feeding animals		3.1	3.3	3.4	3.6	3.8	4.0	4.2	4.4
forking straw bales		6.7	6.9	7.3	7.7	8.1	8.6	9.0	9.4
milking by hand		2.5	2.7	2.9	3.0	3.2	3.3	3.5	3.7
milking by machine		1.1	1.2	1.2	1.3	1.4	1.4	1.5	1.6
shoveling grain		4.2	4.3	4.5	4.8	5.0	5.3	5.5	5.8
Fencing									
competition		7.2	7.6	8.1	8.5	9.0	9.4	9.9	10.8
practice		3.6	3.9	4.2	4.4	4.6	4.9	5.1	5.3
Field hockey		6.5	6.7	7.1	7.5	7.9	8.3	8.7	9.1
Fishing		3.0	3.1	3.3	3.5	3.7	3.8	4.0	4.2
Food shopping (F)		3.0	3.1	3.3	3.5	3.7	3.8	4.0	4.2
Football, competition		6.2	6.6	7.0	7.4	7.8	8.2	8.6	9.0
Forestry									
ax chopping, fast		14.0	14.9	15.7	16.6	17.5	18.4	19.3	20.2
ax chopping, slow		4.0	4.3	4.5	4.8	5.0	5.3	5.5	5.8
barking trees		5.8	6.2	6.5	6.9	7.3	7.6	8.0	8.4
carrying logs		8.7	9.3	9.9	10.4	11.0	11.5	12.1	12.6
felling trees		6.2	6.6	7.0	7.4	7.8	8.2	8.6	9.0
hoeing		4.2	4.6	4.8	5.1	5.4	5.6	5.9	6.2
planting by hand		5.1	5.5	5.8	6.1	6.4	6.8	7.1	7.4
sawing by hand		5.7	6.1	6.5	6.8	7.2	7.6	7.9	8.3
sawing, power		3.5	3.8	4.0	4.2	4.4	4.7	4.9	5.1
stacking firewood		4.2	4.4	4.7	4.9	5.2	5.5	5.7	6.0
trimming trees		6.1	6.5	6.8	7.2	7.6	8.0	8.4	8.8
weeding		3.4	3.6	3.8	4.0	4.2	4.5	4.7	4.9
Frisbee		4.7	5.0	5.3	5.5	5.9	6.2	6.4	6.8
Furriery		3.9	4.2	4.4	4.6	4.9	5.1	5.4	5.6

71 157	74 163	77 170	80 176	83 183	86 190	89 196	92 203	95 209	98 216
4.2	4.4	4.5	4.7	4.9	5.1	5.3	5.4	5.6	5.8
4.5	4.7	4.9	5.1	5.3	5.5	5.7	5.9	6.1	6.3
7.1	7.4	7.7	8.0	8.3	8.6	8.9	9.2	9.5	9.8
12.0	12.5	13.0	13.5	14.0	14.5	15.0	15.5	16.1	16.6
6.9	7.2	7.5	7.8	8.1	8.4	8.8	9.1	9.4	9.7
7.3	7.6	7.9	8.2	8.5	8.9	9.2	9.5	9.8	10.1
9.6	10.0	10.4	10.8	11.2	11.6	12.0	12.4	12.8	13.2
3.6	3.8	3.9	4.1	4.2	4.4	4.5	4.7	4.8	5.0
7.3	7.6	7.9	8.2	8.5	8.9	9.2	9.5	9.8	10.1
11.9	12.4	12.9	13.4	13.9	14.4	15.0	15.5	16.0	16.5
5.1	5.3	5.6	5.8	6.0	6.2	6.4	6.7	6.9	7.1
10.3	10.7	11.2	11.6	12.0	12.5	12.9	13.3	13.8	14.2
2.6	2.7	2.8	2.9	3.0	3.1	3.2	3.3	3.4	3.5
1.6	1.7	1.8	1.8	1.9	2.0	2.0	2.1	2.2	2.3
4.1	4.3	4.5	4.6	4.8	5.0	5.2	5.3	5.5	5.7
9.6	10.0	10.4	10.8	11.2	11.6	12.0	12.4	12.8	13.2
2.8	3.0	3.1	3.2	3.3	3.4	3.6	3.7	3.8	3.9
2.6	2.7	2.8	3.0	3.1	3.2	3.3	3.4	3.5	3.6
6.0	6.3	6.5	6.8	7.1	7.3	7.6	7.8	8.1	8.3
4.6	4.8	5.0	5.2	5.4	5.6	5.8	6.0	6.2	6.4
9.8	10.2	10.6	11.0	11.5	11.9	12.3	12.7	13.1	13.5
3.8	4.0	4.2	4.3	4.5	4.6	4.8	5.0	5.1	5.3
1.6	1.7	1.8	1.8	1.9	2.0	2.0	2.1	2.2	2.3
6.0	6.3	6.5	6.8	7.1	7.3	7.6	7.8	8.1	8.3
11.2	11.7	12.1	12.6	13.1	13.5	14.0	14.4	14.9	15.5
5.6	5.8	6.1	6.3	6.5	6.8	7.0	7.2	7.4	7.7
9.5	9.9	10.3	10.7	11.1	11.5	11.9	12.3	12.7	13.1
4.4	4.6	4.8	5.0	5.1	5.3	5.5	5.7	5.9	6.1
4.4	4.6	4.8	5.0	5.1	5.3	5.5	5.7	5.9	6.1
9.4	9.8	10.2	10.6	11.0	11.4	11.7	12.1	12.5	12.9
21.1	22.0	22.9	23.8	24.7	25.5	26.4	27.3	28.2	29.1
6.0	6.3	6.5	6.8	7.1	7.3	7.6	7.8	8.1	8.3
8.7	9.1	9.5	9.8	10.2	10.6	10.9	11.3	11.7	12.1
13.2	13.8	14.3	14.9	15.4	16.0	16.6	17.1	17.7	18.2
9.4	9.8	10.2	10.6	11.0	11.4	11.7	12.1	12.5	12.9
6.5	6.7	7.0	7.3	7.6	7.8	8.1	8.4	8.6	8.9
7.7	8.1	8.4	8.7	9.0	9.4	9.7	10.0	10.4	10.7
8.7	9.0	9.4	9.8	10.1	10.5	10.9	11.2	11.6	12.0
5.3	5.6	5.8	6.0	6.2	6.5	6.7	6.9	7.1	7.4
6.2	6.5	6.8	7.0	7.3	7.6	7.8	8.1	8.4	8.6
9.2	9.5	9.9	10.3	10.7	11.1	11.5	11.9	12.3	12.6
5.1	5.3	5.5	5.8	6.0	6.2	6.4	6.6	6.8	7.1
7.1	7.4	7.7	8.0	8.2	8.5	8.8	9.1	9.4	9.7
5.9	6.1	6.4	6.6	6.9	7.1	7.4	7.6	7.9	8.1

YOUR BODY WEIGHT—*continued*

Activity	kg lb	47 104	50 110	53 117	56 123	59 130	62 137	65 143	68 150
Gardening									
digging		5.9	6.3	6.7	7.1	7.4	7.8	8.2	8.6
hedging		3.3	3.9	4.1	4.3	4.5	4.8	5.0	5.2
mowing		5.3	5.6	5.9	6.3	6.6	6.9	7.3	7.6
raking		2.5	2.7	2.9	3.0	3.2	3.3	3.5	3.7
Golf		4.0	4.3	4.5	4.8	5.0	5.3	5.5	5.8
Gymnastics		3.0	3.3	3.5	3.7	3.9	4.1	4.3	4.5
Handball		6.9	7.2	7.7	8.1	8.5	9.0	9.4	9.8
orse-grooming		6.0	6.4	6.8	7.2	7.6	7.9	8.3	8.7
Horseback riding									
galloping		6.4	6.9	7.3	7.7	8.1	8.5	8.9	9.3
trotting		5.2	5.5	5.8	6.2	6.5	6.8	7.2	7.5
walking		1.9	2.1	2.2	2.3	2.4	2.5	2.7	2.8
Horseshoes		3.3	3.4	3.5	3.7	3.9	4.1	4.3	4.5
Housework									
mopping floors		2.8	3.1	3.3	3.5	3.7	3.8	4.0	4.2
dusting		3.0	3.3	3.4	3.6	3.8	4.0	4.2	4.4
laundry		3.1	3.4	3.5	3.7	3.9	4.1	4.3	4.5
washing windows		3.2	3.5	3.6	3.8	4.0	4.2	4.4	4.6
vacuuming		3.0	3.3	3.4	3.6	3.8	4.0	4.2	4.4
Hunting		4.1	4.4	4.7	4.9	5.2	5.5	5.7	6.0
Ice hockey		7.4	7.7	8.2	8.6	9.1	9.6	10.0	10.5
Ironing clothes		1.6	1.7	1.7	1.8	1.9	2.0	2.1	2.2
Judo		9.2	9.8	10.3	10.9	11.5	12.1	12.7	13.3
Jumping rope									
70 per min		7.6	8.1	8.6	9.1	9.6	10.0	10.5	11.0
80 per min		7.7	8.2	8.7	9.2	9.7	10.2	10.7	11.2
125 per min		8.3	8.9	9.4	9.9	10.4	11.0	11.5	12.0
145 per min		9.3	9.9	10.4	11.0	11.6	12.2	12.8	13.4
Karate		9.5	9.8	10.3	10.9	11.5	12.1	12.7	13.3
Kendo		9.3	9.7	10.2	10.8	11.4	12.0	12.6	13.2
Knitting, sewing		1.1	1.1	1.2	1.2	1.3	1.4	1.4	1.5
Lacrosse		7.0	7.4	7.9	8.3	8.7	9.2	9.6	10.1
Locksmith		2.8	2.9	3.0	3.2	3.4	3.5	3.7	3.9
Lying at ease		1.0	1.1	1.2	1.2	1.3	1.4	1.4	1.5
Machine-tooling									
machining		2.3	2.4	2.5	2.7	2.8	3.0	3.1	3.3
operating lathe		2.5	2.6	2.8	2.9	3.1	3.2	3.4	3.5
operating punch press		4.2	4.4	4.7	4.9	5.2	5.5	5.7	6.0
tapping and drilling		3.2	3.3	3.4	3.6	3.8	4.0	4.2	4.4
welding		2.4	2.6	2.8	2.9	3.1	3.2	3.4	3.5
working sheet metal		2.3	2.4	2.5	2.7	2.8	3.0	3.1	3.3
Marching, rapid		6.7	7.1	7.5	8.0	8.4	8.8	9.2	9.7
Mountain climbing		7.4	7.9	8.4	8.9	9.4	9.9	10.3	10.8
Motorcycle riding		6.5	6.9	7.3	7.7	8.1	8.5	8.9	9.3

| 71 | 74 | 77 | 80 | 83 | 86 | 89 | 92 | 95 | 98 |
157	*163*	*170*	*176*	*183*	*190*	*196*	*203*	*209*	*216*
8.9	9.3	9.7	10.1	10.5	10.8	11.2	11.6	12.0	12.3
5.5	5.7	5.9	6.2	6.4	6.6	6.9	7.1	7.3	7.5
8.0	8.3	8.6	9.0	9.3	9.6	10.0	10.3	10.6	11.0
3.8	4.0	4.2	4.3	4.5	4.6	4.8	5.0	5.1	5.3
6.0	6.3	6.5	6.8	7.1	7.3	7.6	7.8	8.1	8.3
4.7	4.9	5.1	5.3	5.5	5.7	5.9	6.1	6.3	6.5
10.3	10.7	11.2	11.5	12.0	12.5	12.9	13.3	13.7	14.2
9.1	9.5	9.9	10.2	10.6	11.0	11.4	11.8	12.2	12.5
9.7	10.1	10.6	11.0	11.4	11.8	12.2	12.6	13.0	13.4
7.8	8.1	8.5	8.8	9.1	9.5	9.8	10.1	10.5	10.8
2.9	3.0	3.2	3.3	3.4	3.5	3.6	3.8	3.9	4.0
4.7	4.9	5.1	5.3	5.5	5.7	5.9	6.1	6.3	6.5
4.4	4.6	4.8	5.0	5.2	5.4	5.6	5.8	6.0	6.2
4.6	4.7	4.9	5.1	5.3	5.5	5.7	5.9	6.1	6.3
4.7	4.9	5.1	5.3	5.5	5.7	5.9	6.1	6.3	6.5
4.8	5.0	5.2	5.4	5.6	5.8	6.0	6.2	6.4	6.6
4.6	4.8	5.0	5.2	5.4	5.6	5.8	6.0	6.2	6.4
6.2	6.5	6.7	7.0	7.2	7.5	7.8	8.0	8.2	8.5
11.0	11.5	12.0	12.5	13.1	13.6	14.1	14.6	15.1	15.7
2.3	2.4	2.5	2.6	2.7	2.8	2.9	3.0	3.1	3.2
13.8	14.4	15.0	15.6	16.2	16.8	17.4	17.9	18.5	19.1
11.5	12.0	12.5	13.0	13.4	13.9	14.4	14.9	15.4	15.9
11.6	12.1	12.6	13.1	13.6	14.1	14.6	14.6	15.6	16.1
12.6	13.1	13.6	14.2	14.7	15.2	15.8	16.3	16.8	17.3
14.0	14.6	15.2	15.8	16.4	16.9	17.5	18.1	18.7	19.3
13.8	14.4	15.0	15.6	16.2	16.8	17.4	17.9	18.5	19.1
13.7	14.3	14.9	15.5	16.1	16.7	17.3	17.8	18.4	19.0
1.6	1.6	1.7	1.8	1.8	1.9	2.0	2.0	2.1	2.2
10.4	10.7	11.0	11.2	11.5	11.8	12.1	12.4	12.7	13.0
4.0	4.2	4.4	4.6	4.7	4.9	5.1	5.2	5.4	5.6
1.6	1.6	1.7	1.8	1.8	1.9	2.0	2.0	2.1	2.2
3.4	3.6	3.7	3.8	4.0	4.1	4.3	4.4	4.6	4.7
3.7	3.8	4.0	4.2	4.3	4.5	4.6	4.8	4.9	5.1
6.2	6.5	6.8	7.0	7.3	7.6	7.8	8.1	8.4	8.6
4.6	4.8	5.0	5.2	5.4	5.6	5.8	6.0	6.2	6.4
3.7	3.8	4.0	4.2	4.3	4.5	4.6	4.8	4.9	5.1
3.4	3.6	3.7	3.8	4.0	4.1	4.3	4.4	4.6	4.7
10.1	10.5	10.9	11.4	11.8	12.2	12.6	13.1	13.5	13.9
11.3	11.7	12.2	12.7	13.2	13.7	14.1	14.6	15.0	15.6
9.7	10.1	10.5	10.9	11.3	11.7	12.1	12.5	12.9	13.3

YOUR BODY WEIGHT—*continued*

Activity	kg	47	50	53	56	59	62	65	68
	lb	104	110	117	123	130	137	143	150
Music playing									
accordion (sitting)		1.5	1.6	1.7	1.8	1.9	2.0	2.1	2.2
cello (sitting)		2.0	2.1	2.2	2.3	2.4	2.5	2.7	2.8
conducting		1.9	2.0	2.1	2.2	2.3	2.4	2.5	2.7
drums (sitting)		3.1	3.3	3.5	3.7	3.9	4.1	4.3	4.5
flute (sitting)		1.7	1.8	1.9	2.0	2.1	2.2	2.3	2.4
horn (sitting)		1.4	1.5	1.5	1.6	1.7	1.8	1.9	2.0
organ (sitting)		2.6	2.7	2.8	3.0	3.1	3.3	3.4	3.6
piano (sitting)		1.9	2.0	2.1	2.2	2.4	2.5	2.6	2.7
trumpet (standing)		1.5	1.6	1.6	1.7	1.8	1.9	2.0	2.1
violin (sitting)		2.2	2.3	2.4	2.5	2.7	2.8	2.9	3.1
woodwind (sitting)		1.5	1.6	1.7	1.8	1.9	2.0	2.1	2.2
Paddleball		8.5	8.9	9.4	10.0	10.5	11.0	11.6	12.1
Paddle tennis		8.4	8.6	9.1	9.6	10.1	10.7	11.1	11.7
Painting									
inside projects		1.6	1.7	1.8	1.9	2.0	2.1	2.2	2.3
outside projects		3.7	3.9	4.1	4.3	4.5	4.8	5.0	5.2
scraping		3.1	3.2	3.3	3.5	3.7	3.9	4.1	4.3
Planting seedings		3.3	3.5	3.7	3.9	4.1	4.3	4.6	4.8
Plastering		3.7	3.9	4.1	4.4	4.6	4.8	5.1	5.3
Printing press work		1.7	1.8	1.9	2.0	2.1	2.2	2.3	2.4
Racquetball		8.4	8.9	9.4	10.0	10.5	11.0	11.6	12.1
Roller skating, leisure		5.3	5.8	6.2	6.5	6.9	7.3	7.3	8.0
Rope jumping									
110 rpm		6.7	7.1	7.5	7.9	8.4	8.8	9.2	9.7
120 rpm		6.4	6.8	7.3	7.7	8.1	8.5	8.9	9.3
130 rpm		6.0	6.4	6.8	7.1	7.5	7.7	8.3	8.7
Rowing									
machine, moderate		5.7	6.0	6.3	6.7	7.0	7.4	7.7	8.1
machine, race pace		8.6	8.9	9.4	10.0	10.5	11.0	11.6	12.1
skull, leisure		4.7	5.0	5.3	5.5	5.9	6.2	6.4	6.8
skull, race pace		8.7	8.9	9.4	10.0	10.5	11.0	11.6	12.1
Running, cross-country		7.8	8.2	8.6	9.1	9.6	10.1	10.6	11.1
Running, on flat surface									
11 min, 30 s per mile		6.3	6.8	7.2	7.6	8.0	8.4	8.8	9.2
9 min per mile		9.1	9.7	10.2	10.8	11.4	12.0	12.5	13.1
8 min per mile		9.8	10.8	11.3	11.9	12.5	13.1	13.6	14.2
7 min per mile		10.7	12.2	12.7	13.3	13.9	14.5	15.0	15.6
6 min per mile		11.8	13.9	14.4	15.0	15.6	16.2	16.7	17.3
5 min, 30 s per mile		13.6	14.5	15.3	16.2	17.1	17.9	18.8	19.7
Sailing, leisure		2.1	2.2	2.3	2.5	2.6	2.7	2.9	3.0
Scrubbing floors		5.1	5.5	5.8	6.1	6.4	6.8	7.1	7.4
Scuba diving		10.9	11.2	11.5	11.8	12.1	12.4	12.7	13.0
Shoe repair, general		2.2	2.3	2.4	2.5	2.7	2.8	2.9	3.1
Sitting quietly		1.0	1.1	1.1	1.2	1.2	1.3	1.4	1.4
Skateboarding		5.6	5.8	6.2	6.5	6.9	7.2	7.5	7.9
Skiing, hard snow									
level, moderate speed		5.6	6.0	6.3	6.7	7.0	7.4	7.7	8.1
level, walking speed		6.7	7.2	7.6	8.0	8.4	8.9	9.3	9.7
uphill, "fast" speed		12.9	13.7	14.5	15.3	16.2	17.0	17.8	18.6

71 157	74 163	77 170	80 176	83 183	86 190	89 196	92 203	95 209	98 216
2.3	2.4	2.5	2.6	2.7	2.8	2.8	2.9	3.0	3.1
2.9	3.0	3.2	3.3	3.4	3.5	3.6	3.8	3.9	4.0
2.8	2.9	3.0	3.1	3.2	3.4	3.5	3.6	3.7	3.8
4.7	4.9	5.1	5.3	5.5	5.7	5.9	6.1	6.3	6.6
2.5	2.6	2.7	2.8	2.9	3.0	3.1	3.2	3.3	3.4
2.1	2.1	2.2	2.3	2.4	2.5	2.6	2.7	2.8	2.8
3.8	3.9	4.1	4.2	4.4	4.6	4.7	4.9	5.0	5.2
2.8	3.0	3.1	3.2	3.3	3.4	3.6	3.7	3.8	3.9
2.2	2.3	2.4	2.5	2.6	2.7	2.8	2.9	2.9	3.0
3.2	3.3	3.5	3.6	3.7	3.9	4.0	4.1	4.3	4.4
2.3	2.4	2.5	2.6	2.7	2.8	2.8	2.9	3.0	3.1
12.6	13.2	13.7	14.2	14.8	15.3	15.8	16.4	16.9	17.4
12.2	12.7	13.2	13.7	14.2	14.2	15.2	15.8	16.3	16.8
2.4	2.5	2.6	2.7	2.8	2.9	3.0	3.1	3.2	3.3
5.5	5.7	5.9	6.2	6.4	6.6	6.9	7.1	7.3	7.5
4.5	4.7	4.9	5.0	5.2	5.4	5.6	5.8	6.0	6.2
5.0	5.2	5.4	5.6	5.8	6.0	6.2	6.4	6.7	6.9
5.5	5.8	6.0	6.2	6.5	6.7	6.9	7.2	7.4	7.6
2.5	2.6	2.7	2.8	2.9	3.0	3.1	3.2	3.3	3.4
12.6	13.2	13.7	14.2	14.8	15.3	15.8	16.4	16.9	17.4
8.3	8.6	9.0	9.3	9.7	10.1	10.4	10.8	11.1	11.4
10.1	10.5	10.5	11.3	11.8	12.2	12.6	13.1	13.5	13.9
9.8	10.1	10.6	10.9	11.4	11.8	12.2	12.6	13.0	13.4
9.1	9.4	9.8	10.2	10.6	11.0	11.3	11.7	12.1	12.5
8.5	8.9	9.3	9.7	10.1	10.6	11.1	11.6	12.1	12.6
12.6	13.2	13.7	14.2	14.8	15.3	15.8	16.4	16.9	17.4
7.2	7.6	8.0	8.4	8.8	9.2	9.6	10.0	10.4	10.8
12.6	13.2	13.7	14.2	14.8	15.3	15.8	16.4	16.9	17.4
11.6	12.1	12.6	13.0	13.5	14.0	14.5	15.0	15.5	16.0
9.6	10.0	10.5	10.9	11.3	11.7	12.1	12.5	12.9	13.3
13.7	14.3	14.9	15.4	16.0	16.6	17.2	17.8	18.3	18.9
14.8	15.4	16.0	16.5	17.1	17.7	18.3	18.9	19.4	20.0
16.2	16.8	17.4	17.9	18.5	19.1	19.7	20.3	20.8	21.4
17.9	18.5	19.1	19.6	20.2	20.8	21.4	22.0	22.5	23.1
20.5	21.4	22.3	23.1	24.0	24.9	25.7	26.6	27.5	28.3
3.1	3.3	3.4	3.5	3.7	3.8	3.9	4.1	4.2	4.3
7.7	8.1	8.4	8.7	9.0	9.4	9.7	10.0	10.4	10.7
13.3	13.6	13.9	14.2	14.5	14.8	15.1	15.4	15.7	16.0
3.2	3.3	3.5	3.6	3.7	3.9	4.0	4.1	4.3	4.4
1.5	1.6	1.6	1.7	1.7	1.8	1.9	1.9	2.0	2.1
8.3	8.6	8.9	9.3	9.6	10.0	10.3	10.7	11.0	11.4
8.4	8.8	9.2	9.5	9.9	10.2	10.6	10.9	11.3	11.7
10.2	10.6	11.0	11.4	11.9	12.3	12.7	13.2	13.6	14.0
19.5	20.3	21.1	21.9	22.7	23.6	24.4	25.2	26.0	26.9

YOUR BODY WEIGHT—*continued*

Activity	kg lb	47 104	50 110	53 117	56 123	59 130	62 137	65 143	68 150
Skiing, soft snow									
leisure (F)		4.6	4.9	5.2	5.5	5.8	6.1	6.4	6.7
leisure (M)		5.2	5.6	5.9	6.2	6.5	6.9	7.2	7.5
Skindiving									
considerable motion		13.0	13.8	14.6	15.5	16.3	17.1	17.9	18.8
moderate motion		9.7	10.3	10.9	11.5	12.2	12.8	13.4	14.0
Snorkeling		4.3	4.6	4.9	5.2	5.5	5.8	6.0	6.3
Snowshoeing, soft snow		7.8	8.3	8.8	9.3	9.8	10.3	10.8	11.3
Snowmobiling		3.4	3.7	4.0	4.2	4.4	4.7	4.9	5.1
Soccer		6.5	6.8	7.3	7.7	8.1	8.5	8.9	9.3
Softball		3.3	3.5	3.7	3.9	4.1	4.3	4.5	4.7
Squash		10.0	10.6	11.2	11.9	12.5	13.1	13.8	14.4
Standing quietly (M)		1.3	1.4	1.4	1.5	1.6	1.7	1.8	1.8
Steel mill, working in									
fettling		4.3	4.5	4.7	5.0	5.3	5.5	5.8	6.1
forging		4.7	5.0	5.3	5.6	5.9	6.2	6.5	6.8
hand rolling		6.4	6.9	7.3	7.7	8.1	8.5	8.9	9.3
merchant mill rolling		6.8	7.3	7.7	8.1	8.6	9.0	9.4	9.9
removing slag		8.4	8.9	9.4	10.0	10.5	11.0	11.6	12.1
tending furnace		5.9	6.3	6.7	7.1	7.4	7.8	8.2	8.6
tipping molds		4.3	4.6	4.9	5.2	5.4	5.7	6.0	6.3
Surfing		3.9	4.1	4.3	4.5	4.8	5.0	5.3	5.5
Stock clerking		2.5	2.7	2.9	3.0	3.2	3.3	3.5	3.7
Swimming, fitness swims									
back stroke		7.9	8.5	9.0	9.5	10.0	10.5	11.0	11.5
breast stroke		7.6	8.1	8.6	9.1	9.6	10.0	10.5	11.0
butterfly			8.6	9.1	9.6	10.1	10.7	11.1	11.7
crawl, fast		7.3	7.8	8.3	8.7	9.2	9.7	10.1	10.6
crawl, slow		6.0	6.4	6.8	7.2	7.6	7.9	8.3	8.7
side stroke		5.7	6.1	6.5	6.8	7.2	7.6	7.9	8.3
treading, fast		8.0	8.5	9.0	9.5	10.0	10.5	11.1	11.6
treading, normal		2.9	3.1	3.3	3.5	3.7	3.8	4.0	4.2
Table tennis (ping pong)		3.2	3.4	3.6	3.8	4.0	4.2	4.4	4.6
Tailoring									
cutting		2.0	2.1	2.2	2.3	2.4	2.5	2.7	2.8
hand-sewing		1.5	1.6	1.7	1.8	1.9	2.0	2.1	2.2
machine-sewing		2.2	2.3	2.4	2.5	2.7	2.8	2.9	3.1
pressing		2.9	3.1	3.3	3.5	3.7	3.8	4.0	4.2
Tennis									
competition		6.9	7.3	7.8	8.2	8.7	9.1	9.5	9.9
recreational		5.1	5.5	5.8	6.1	6.4	6.8	7.1	7.4
Typing									
electric (computer)		1.3	1.4	1.4	1.5	1.6	1.7	1.8	1.8
manual		1.5	1.6	1.6	1.7	1.8	1.9	2.0	2.1
Volleyball									
competition		5.9	7.3	7.8	8.2	8.7	9.1	9.5	10.0
recreational		2.4	2.5	2.7	2.8	3.0	3.1	3.3	3.4

| 71 | 74 | 77 | 80 | 83 | 86 | 89 | 92 | 95 | 98 |
157	163	170	176	183	190	196	203	209	216
7.0	7.3	7.5	7.8	8.1	8.4	8.7	9.0	9.3	9.6
7.9	8.2	8.5	8.9	9.2	9.5	9.9	10.2	10.5	10.9
19.6	20.4	21.3	22.1	22.9	23.7	24.6	25.4	26.2	27.0
14.6	15.2	15.9	16.5	17.1	17.7	18.3	19.0	19.6	20.2
6.6	6.8	7.1	7.4	7.7	8.0	8.2	8.5	8.8	9.1
11.8	12.3	12.8	13.3	13.8	14.3	14.8	15.3	15.8	16.3
5.3	5.5	5.8	6.0	6.2	6.5	6.7	6.9	7.1	7.3
9.8	10.1	10.6	10.9	11.4	11.8	12.2	12.6	13.0	13.4
4.9	5.1	5.3	5.5	5.7	5.9	6.1	6.3	6.5	6.7
15.1	15.7	16.3	17.0	17.6	18.2	18.9	19.5	20.1	20.8
1.9	2.0	2.1	2.2	2.2	2.3	2.4	2.5	2.6	2.6
6.3	6.6	6.9	7.1	7.4	7.7	7.9	8.2	8.5	8.7
7.1	7.4	7.7	8.0	8.3	8.6	8.9	9.2	9.5	9.8
9.7	10.1	10.6	11.0	11.4	11.8	12.2	12.6	13.0	13.4
10.3	10.7	11.2	11.6	12.0	12.5	12.9	13.3	13.8	14.2
12.6	13.2	13.7	14.2	14.8	15.3	15.8	16.4	16.9	17.4
8.9	9.3	9.7	10.1	10.5	10.8	11.2	11.6	12.0	12.3
6.5	6.8	7.1	7.4	7.6	7.9	8.2	8.5	8.7	9.0
5.7	6.0	6.3	6.5	6.8	7.0	7.2	7.4	7.6	7.9
3.8	4.0	4.2	4.3	4.5	4.6	4.8	5.0	5.1	5.3
12.0	12.5	13.0	13.5	14.0	14.5	15.0	15.5	16.1	16.6
11.5	12.0	12.5	13.0	13.4	13.9	14.4	14.9	15.4	15.9
12.2	12.7	13.2	13.7	14.2	14.2	15.2	15.8	16.3	16.8
11.1	11.5	12.0	12.5	12.9	13.4	13.9	14.4	14.8	15.3
9.1	9.5	9.9	10.2	10.6	11.0	11.4	11.8	12.2	12.5
8.7	9.0	9.4	9.8	10.1	10.5	10.9	11.2	11.6	12.0
12.1	12.6	13.1	13.6	14.1	14.6	15.1	15.6	16.2	16.7
4.4	4.6	4.8	5.0	5.1	5.3	5.5	5.7	5.9	6.1
4.8	5.0	5.2	5.4	5.6	5.8	6.1	6.3	6.5	6.7
2.9	3.0	3.2	3.3	3.4	3.5	3.6	3.8	3.9	4.0
2.3	2.4	2.5	2.6	2.7	2.8	2.8	2.9	3.0	3.1
3.2	3.3	3.5	3.6	3.7	3.9	4.0	4.1	4.3	4.4
4.4	4.6	4.8	5.0	5.1	5.3	5.5	5.7	5.9	6.1
10.2	10.6	11.1	11.5	11.9	12.4	12.8	13.2	13.7	14.1
7.7	8.1	8.4	8.7	9.0	9.4	9.7	10.0	10.4	10.7
1.9	2.0	2.1	2.2	2.2	2.3	2.4	2.5	2.6	2.6
2.2	2.3	2.4	2.5	2.6	2.7	2.8	2.9	2.9	3.0
3.6	3.7	3.9	4.0	4.2	4.3	4.5	4.6	4.8	4.9
10.5	10.9	11.4	11.8	12.3	12.7	13.1	13.6	14.0	14.5

YOUR BODY WEIGHT—*continued*

Activity	kg lb	47 104	50 110	53 117	56 123	59 130	62 137	65 143	68 150
Walking, leisure outdoors									
asphalt road		3.8	4.0	4.2	4.5	4.7	5.0	5.2	5.4
fields and hillsides		3.9	4.1	4.3	4.6	4.8	5.1	5.3	5.6
grass track		3.8	4.1	4.3	4.5	4.8	5.0	5.3	5.5
plowed field		3.6	3.9	4.1	4.3	4.5	4.8	5.0	5.2
Walking, treadmill level									
2.0 mph		2.4	2.6	2.8	3.0	3.1	3.3	3.4	3.6
2.5 mph		3.0	3.2	3.4	3.6	3.8	4.0	4.2	4.4
3.0 mph		3.6	3.8	4.0	4.2	4.4	4.6	4.8	5.0
3.5 mph		4.0	4.3	4.6	4.8	5.1	5.3	5.6	6.1
4.0 mph		4.6	4.9	5.2	5.4	5.7	6.0	6.3	6.6
Wallpapering		2.3	2.4	2.5	2.7	2.8	3.0	3.1	3.3
Water polo, recreation		7.0	7.4	7.7	8.1	8.5	8.9	9.3	9.7
Water polo, competition		9.4	9.9	10.4	11.0	11.5	12.0	12.5	13.1
Water-skiing		5.6	6.0	6.4	6.7	7.1	7.5	7.8	8.2
Watch repairing		1.2	1.3	1.3	1.4	1.5	1.6	1.6	1.7
Whitewater rafting, recreational		4.1	4.4	4.6	4.9	5.2	5.4	5.7	6.0
Window cleaning		2.9	3.0	3.1	3.3	3.5	3.7	3.8	4.0
Wind surfing		3.3	3.5	3.7	3.9	4.1	4.3	4.6	4.8
Wrestling, competition		9.1	9.7	10.3	10.8	11.4	12.0	12.6	13.2
Writing (sitting)		1.4	1.5	1.5	1.6	1.7	1.8	1.9	2.0
Yoga		2.9	3.1	3.3	3.5	3.7	3.8	4.0	4.2

| 71 | 74 | 77 | 80 | 83 | 86 | 89 | 92 | 95 | 98 |
157	163	170	176	183	190	196	203	209	216
5.7	5.9	6.2	6.4	6.6	6.9	7.1	7.4	7.6	7.8
5.8	6.1	6.3	6.6	6.8	7.1	7.3	7.5	7.8	8.0
5.8	6.0	6.2	6.5	6.7	7.0	7.2	7.5	7.7	7.9
5.5	5.7	5.9	6.2	6.4	6.6	6.9	7.1	7.3	7.5
3.7	3.9	4.1	4.2	4.4	4.5	4.7	4.9	5.0	5.2
4.5	4.7	4.9	5.1	5.3	5.5	5.7	5.9	6.1	6.3
5.3	5.5	5.7	5.9	6.2	6.5	6.7	6.9	7.1	7.3
6.1	6.4	6.6	6.9	7.1	7.4	7.7	7.9	8.2	8.4
6.9	7.2	7.5	7.8	8.1	8.4	8.7	8.9	9.2	9.5
3.4	3.6	3.7	3.8	4.0	4.1	4.3	4.4	4.6	4.7
10.1	10.5	10.9	11.3	11.7	12.1	12.5	12.9	13.3	13.7
13.6	14.1	14.7	15.2	15.7	16.3	16.8	17.3	17.9	18.4
8.7	9.1	9.4	9.8	10.1	10.5	10.9	11.2	11.6	12.0
1.8	1.9	1.9	2.0	2.1	2.2	2.2	2.3	2.4	2.5
6.2	6.5	6.7	7.0	7.3	7.5	7.8	8.1	8.3	8.6
4.2	4.4	4.5	4.7	4.9	5.1	5.3	5.4	5.6	5.8
5.0	5.2	5.4	5.6	5.8	6.0	6.2	6.4	6.7	6.9
13.8	14.3	14.9	15.5	16.1	16.7	17.2	17.8	18.4	19.0
2.1	2.1	2.2	2.3	2.4	2.5	2.6	2.7	2.8	2.8
4.4	4.6	4.8	5.0	5.1	5.3	5.5	5.7	5.9	6.1

APPENDIX C Assessment of Energy and Nutrient Intake: Three-Day Dietary Survey

The three-day dietary survey represents a relatively simple yet accurate method to determine the nutritional quality and total calories of food consumed daily. The key to successfully accomplish these goals requires a daily log of food intake for three days that represent your normal eating pattern (including at least one weekend).

Experiments have shown that calculations of caloric intake made from records of daily food consumption are usually within 10% of the number of calories actually consumed. For example, suppose a bomb calorimeter determined that your daily food intake equaled 2130 kCal. If you kept a three-day dietary history and estimated your calorie intake, the daily value would likely be within 10% of the actual value (1920 and 2350 kCal).

Use four items to measure food: (1) plastic ruler, (2) standard measuring cup, (3) measuring spoons, and (4) balance or weighing scale. Use Appendix A or consult one of several sources that list the nutritional content of foods including: Pennington JAT, Douglass JP. Bowes & Church's food values of portions commonly used. 18th ed. Baltimore: Lippincott Williams & Wilkins, 2005. You may also wish to consult the following URL: http://nat.crgq.com/mainnat.html.

Measure or weight each of the food items in your diet. This represents the only reliable way to obtain an accurate estimate of the size of a food portion. Be sure to do the following:

- List specific types, brands, and method of preparation.

Example	*List as:*
Milk	8 fl oz, 2% milk
1/2 chicken breast	3 oz breast, baked, without skin
Margarine	1 tsp. Fleishmann's Light Margarine

- Use these guidelines to estimate cooked portion sizes for these food categories:

Meat and Fish
Measure the portion of meat or fish by thickness, length, and width, or record weight on the scale.

Vegetables, Potatoes, Rice, Cereals, Salads
Measure the portion in a measuring cup or record weight on the scale.

Cream or Sugar Added to Coffee or Tea
Measure with measuring spoons before adding to the drink, or record weight on the scale.

Fluids and Bottled Drinks
Check the labels for volume or empty the container into the measuring cup. If you weigh the fluid, be sure to subtract the weight of the cup or glass. Sugar-free soft drinks usually have kCal values listed on their labels.

Cookies, Cakes, Pies
Measure the diameter and thickness with a ruler, or weigh on the scale. Evaluate frosting or sauces separately.

Fruits
Cut them in half before eating and measure the diameters, or weight them on the scale. For fruits that must be peeled or have rinds or cores, be sure to subtract the weight of the non-edible portion from the total weight of the food. Do this for items such as oranges, apples, and bananas.

Jam, Salad Dressing, Catsup, Mayonnaise
Measure the condiment with the measuring spoon or weigh the portion on the scale.

Record all the foods you consume using the blank 3-day food logs on the pages of this appendix. We encourage you to keep the sheets with you and record the pertinent information about the foods as you consume them.

DIRECTIONS FOR COMPUTING YOUR THREE-DAY DIETARY SURVEY

Step 1 Prepare a table (similar to Table C.1) indicating the intake of food items during a day. Include the amount (g or oz); caloric value; and carbohydrate, lipid, and protein content; the minerals Ca and Fe; and vitamins C, B_1 (thiamine), and B_2 (riboflavin); fiber; and cholesterol.

Step 2 List each food you consume for breakfast, lunch, dinner, between-meal eating, and snacks. Include food items that are used in preparing the meal (e.g., butter, oils, margarine, bread crumbs, egg coating, etc.).

Step 3 Weigh, measure or approximate the size of each portion of food that you eat. Record these values on your daily record chart (e.g., 3 oz of salad oil, 1/8 piece of 8″ diameter apple pie, etc.).

Step 4 Record your daily calorie and nutrient intake on a chart similar to Table C.1, which was recorded for a 21-year-old college student. Record the daily totals for the caloric and nutrient headings on the "Daily and Average Daily Summary Chart" (Table C.2). When you've completed your three-day survey, compute the three-day total by adding up the values for days 1, 2, and 3; then divide by 3 to determine the daily average of each nutrient category.

Step 5   Using each of the average daily nutrient values, calculate the percentage of the RDA consumed for that particular nutrient and graph your results as shown in Figure C.1 An example for calculating the percentage of the RDA is shown in Table C.3, along with the specific RDA values for men and women.

Step 6   Be as accurate and honest as possible. Do not include unusual or atypical days in your dietary survey (e.g., days that you are sick, special occasions such as birthdays, or eating out at restaurants unless that is normal for you).

Step 7   Remember that the protein RDA equals 0.8 g protein per kilogram of body mass (1 kg = 2.2 lb).

Step 8   Compute the percentage of your total calories supplied from carbohydrate, lipid, and protein.

> For example, if total average daily caloric intake is 2450 kCal/day, and 1600 kCal are from carbohydrates, the daily percentage of total calories from carbohydrates equals: 1600/2450 × 100 = 65%

Step 9   While there is no specific RDA for lipid or carbohydrate, a prudent recommendation is that lipid should not exceed more than 30% of your total caloric intake; for active men and women, carbohydrates should be approximately 60% of the total calories ingested.

> For example, if 50% of your average daily calories comes from lipid, you are taking in 167% of the recommended value ("RDA") for this nutrient: [50% divided by 30% (recommended percentage) × 100 = 167%]

Step 10   As was the case for lipid and carbohydrate, no RDA exists for average daily caloric intake. Any recommendation for energy intake must consider body fat level and current daily energy expenditure. However, average values for daily caloric intake have been published for the typical young adult and equal about 2100 kCal for young women and 3000 kCal for young men. Thus, for graphing purposes in Figure C.1, you can evaluate your average daily caloric intake against the "average" values for your sex and age.

> For example, if you are a 20-year-old female and you consume an average of 2400 kCal daily, your energy intake would equal 114% of the average ("RDA") for your age and sex. [2400 kCal divided by 2100 kCal (average)× 100 = 114%]. This does not mean that you need to go on a diet and reduce food intake to bring you in line with the average U.S. value. To the contrary, your higher-than-average caloric intake may be required to power your active lifestyle that contributes to maintaining a desirable body mass and body composition.

If you eat a food item not listed in Appendix A, try to make an intelligent guess as to its composition and amount consumed. It is better to overestimate the amount of food consumed than to underestimate or to make no estimation at all. If you go to a restaurant for dinner, or to a friend's house where it may be inappropriate to measure the food, then omit this day from the counting procedure and resume record keeping the following day.

Record-keeping for 3 days is extremely important so an accurate appraisal can be made of the average daily energy and nutrient intake. **Be sure to record everything you eat.** If you are not completely honest, you are wasting your time. Most people find it easier to keep accurate records if they record food items while preparing a meal or immediately afterwards when eating snack items.

TABLE C.1   Sample One-Day Caloric and Nutrient Intake for a 21-year-old College Student

Food Item	Amount	kCal	Protein (g)	CHO (g)	Lipid (g)	Ca (mg)	Fe (mg)	Fiber (g)	Cholesterol (mg)	Thiam[a] (mg)	Ribofl[a] (mg)
Breakfast											
Eggs, hard boiled	2 (2 oz ea)	160	14.1	1.4	11.2	55.2	1.9	0.0	452	0.06	0.53
Orange juice	8 oz	104	0.9	86.4	0.5	72.4	0.8	0.9	0.0	0.20	0.06
Corn flakes	1 cup/1 oz	110	2.3	24.4	0.5	1.0	1.8	0.6	0.0	0.37	0.42
Skim milk	8 oz	80	7.8	10.6	0.6	279.2	0.1	0.0	3.7	0.08	0.32
Snack											
None											
Lunch											
Tuna fish (oil pack)	2 oz	112	16.5	0.0	68.0	7.8	0.8	0.0	10.0	0.02	0.06
White bread (toast)	2 pieces	168	5.3	31.4	2.5	81.2	1.8	1.3	0.0	0.24	0.21
Mayonnaise	1 oz	203	0.3	0.8	22.6	5.7	0.2	0.0	16.8	0.01	0.01
Skim milk	8 oz	80	7.8	10.6	0.6	279.2	0.1	0.0	3.7	0.08	0.32
Plums	4 (2 oz ea)	128	1.8	29.5	1.4	10.3	0.2	4.4	0.0	0.10	0.22
Snack											
Chocolate milkshake	8 oz	288	7.7	46.4	8.4	256	0.7	0.3	29.6	0.13	0.55
Dinner											
Sirloin steak, lean	8 oz	456	64.8	0.0	20.2	18.6	5.8	0.0	173.6	0.21	0.47
French fries, veg. oil	6 oz	540	6.8	67.2	28.1	34.2	1.3	3.4	0.0	0.30	0.05
Cole slaw	4 oz	80	1.4	14.1	3.0	51.2	0.7	2.3	9.2	0.08	0.07
Italian bread	2 oz	156	5.1	32.0	1.0	9.4	1.5	0.9	0.0	0.23	0.13
Light beer	8 oz	96	0.6	8.8	0.0	11.2	0.1	0.5	0.0	0.02	0.06
Snack											
Yogurt, whole milk	6 oz	102	5.9	7.9	5.5	205.8	0.1	0.0	22.1	0.05	0.24
Daily Total		**2863**	**149.1**	**371.5**	**174.1**	**1378.4**	**17.2**	**14.6**	**720.7**	**2.18**	**3.72**

[a]*Thiam, thiamin; Ribofl, riboflavin.*

TABLE C.2   Daily and Average Summary Chart of the Intake of Calories and Specific Food Nutrients

Day	kCal	Protein[a] (g)	Lipid[a] (g)	CHO[a] (g)	Ca (mg)	Fe (mg)	Thiamine (mg)	Riboflavin (mg)	Fiber (g)	Cholesterol (mg)
#1										
#2										
#3										
Three-day total										
Average Daily Value[b]										

[a]Use the following caloric transformations to convert your average daily grams of carbohydrate (CHO), lipid, and protein to average daily calories:

1 g CHO = 4 kCal

1 g Lipid = 9 kCal

1 g Protein = 4 kCal

[b]Use the Average Daily Value to determine the percentage of the RDA for your graph. See Table 1 for sample calculations. Figure C.1 shows a bar graph for the nutrient values as a percentage of the average or recommended value for each item.

TABLE C.3   RDA Values for Selected Nutrients Including Sample Computations for Deriving the Percent of RDA from Your Dietary Survey. Values Listed in Table C.1 are 100% Values for Graphing your Dietary Survey

					Men				
Age	kCal[a]	Protein (g/kg)	Ca (mg)	Fe (mg)	Thiamine (mg)	Riboflavin (mg)	Fiber[a] (g)	Cholesterol[a] (mg)
19–22	3000	0.8	1200	10	1.5	1.7	30	300
23–50	2700	0.8	800	10	1.5	1.7	30	300

					Women				
Age	kCal[a]	Protein (g/kg)	Ca (mg)	Fe (mg)	Thiamine (mg)	Riboflavin (mg)	Fiber[a] (g)	Cholesterol[a] (mg)
19–22	2100	0.8	1200	15	1.1	1.3	30	300
23–50	2000	0.8	800	15	1.1	1.3	30	300

Source: Recommended Dietary Allowances, Revised 1989, Washington, DC: Food and Nutrition Board, National Academy of Sciences-National Research Council, 1989.

[a]No RDA exists for daily caloric intake or for the intake of fiber or cholesterol. Values for caloric intake represent an average for adult Americans, while fiber and cholesterol values are recommended as being prudent for maintaining good health.

How to determine the percentage of the RDA from your dietary survey

Example #1: Percentage of RDA for protein for a 70-kg
person
    Daily protein intake = 68 g
    RDA = (70 kg × 0.8 g/kg) = 56 g
    % of RDA = 56/68 × 100 = 121%

Example #2: Percentage of RDA for iron (female)
    Daily iron intake = 7.5 mg
    RDA = 15 mg
    % of RDA = 7.5/15 × 100 = 50%

Figure C.1
Example of a bar graph to illustrate the food and nutrient intake expressed as a
percentage of recommended values.

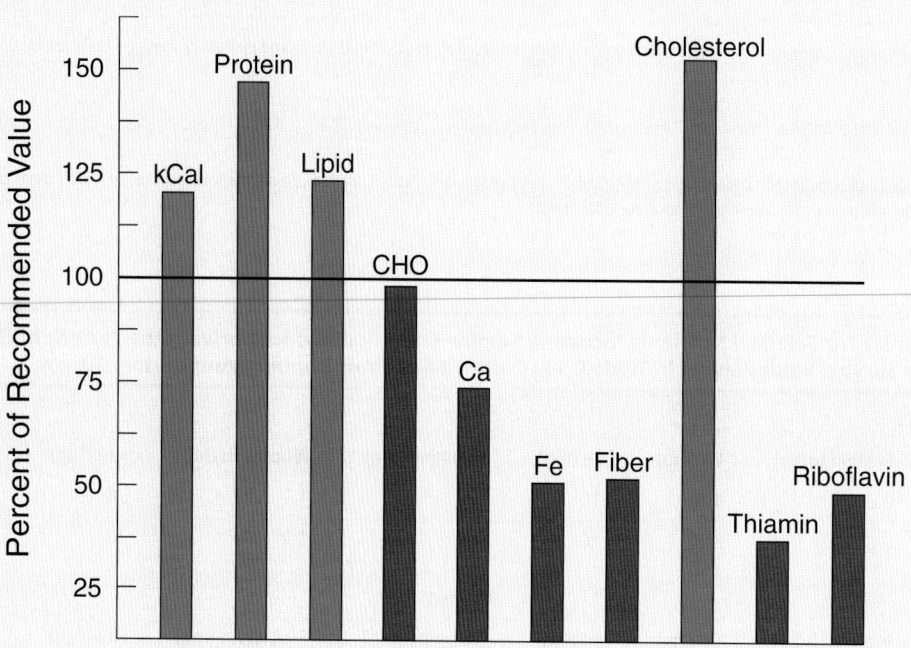

100% Value Represents

kCal:	3000 kCal for men age 19—22
	2700 kCal for men age 23—50
	2100 kCal for women age 19—22
	2000 kCal for women age 23—50
Lipid:	30% of total calories
CHO:	60% of total calories
Fiber:	30 g
Cholesterol:	300 mg

Sample Food Record

Time	Place	Amount	Description (including preparation)	Comments/Questions
8 AM	Home	3/4 cup	Kellogg's Corn Flakes	Breakfast
		1/2 cup	Skim milk	
		1 large	Orange	
		8 fl. oz.	Coffee, black	
		2 tsp	White sugar	
11:30 AM	Away	1/2 cup	Tuna, water packed	Lunch
		2 Tbls	Mayonnaise, light	
		2 slices	White bread	
		1 cup	Campbell's tomato soup	
		4 rounds	Melba toast (crackers)	
		1 oz.	Potato chips, Lay's	
		1 piece	Apple pie	
3:00 PM	Away	1 large	Apple, red delicious	Snack
6:00 PM	Home	4 oz.	Chicken breast, baked, no skin	Dinner
		1 medium	Baked potato, flesh and skin	
		3 tsp	Light margarine	
		1 cup	Broccoli, steamed, plain	
		1 cup	Salad lettuce, romaine	
		3 whole	Cherry tomatoes	
		5 slices	Cucumber	1/4 inch each
		2 Tbls	Ranch dressing, regular	
		2 cups	Water	
8:30 PM	Home	3 cups	Popcorn, air popped, plain	Snack
		12 oz. can	Orange soda, regular	
		1	Donut, chocolate	Dunkin Donuts
10:00 PM		2 cups	Ice cream, chocolate	Rich but good
10:45 PM		4 oz.	Chocolate bar, regular	Hershey's
11:10 PM		1 large	Apple, Macintosh	
11:30 PM		6 oz.	Apple cider	Hot
11:35 PM		1 small	Cookie, chocolate chip	

3-Day Food Record				Day 1
Time	**Place**	**Amount**	**Description** (including preparation)	**Comments/Questions**

3-Day Food Record				Day 2
Time	**Place**	**Amount**	**Description** **(including preparation)**	**Comments/Questions**

3-Day Food Record				Day 3
Time	Place	Amount	Description (including preparation)	Comments/Questions

APPENDIX D   Body Composition Assessment[a]

This appendix contains the age- and sex-specific equations to predict body fat percentage based on three girth measurements. There are four charts, one each for young and older men and women. In our experience, it is important to calibrate the tape measure prior to its use. Use a meter stick as the standard and check the markings on the cloth tape at 10-cm increments. A cloth tape is preferred over a metal one because little skin compression occurs when applying a cloth tape to the skin's surface at a relatively constant tension.

To use the charts, measure the three girths at the sites indicated in Figure 13.11, which shows the anatomic landmarks. The specific equation to predict percentage body fat with its corresponding constant is presented at the bottom of each of the four charts (Charts 2 to 5).

CHART 1
BODY SITES MEASURED BY THE CIRCUMFERENCE METHOD

Age (years)	Sex	Site Measured		
		A	B	C
18–26	M	Right upper arm	Abdomen	Right forearm
	F	Abdomen	Right thigh	Right forearm
27–50	M	Buttocks	Abdomen	Right forearm
	F	Abdomen	Right thigh	Right calf

CHART 2
CONVERSION CONSTANTS TO PREDICT PERCENTAGE BODY FAT FOR YOUNG MEN

Upper Arm			Abdomen			Forearm		
in	cm	Constant A	in	cm	Constant B	in	cm	Constant C
7.00	17.78	25.91	21.00	53.34	27.56	7.00	17.78	38.01
7.25	18.41	26.83	21.25	53.97	27.88	7.25	18.41	39.37
7.50	19.05	27.76	21.50	54.61	28.21	7.50	19.05	40.72
7.75	19.68	28.68	21.75	55.24	28.54	7.75	19.68	42.08
8.00	20.32	29.61	22.00	55.88	28.87	8.00	20.32	43.44
8.25	20.95	30.53	22.25	56.51	29.20	8.25	20.95	44.80
8.50	21.59	31.46	22.50	57.15	29.52	8.50	21.59	46.15
8.75	22.22	32.38	22.75	57.78	29.85	8.75	22.22	47.51
9.00	22.86	33.31	23.00	58.42	30.18	9.00	22.86	48.87
9.25	23.49	34.24	23.25	59.05	30.51	9.25	23.49	50.23
9.50	24.13	35.16	23.50	59.69	30.84	9.50	24.13	51.58
9.75	24.76	36.09	23.75	60.32	31.16	9.75	24.76	52.94
10.00	25.40	37.01	24.00	60.96	31.49	10.00	25.40	54.30
10.25	26.03	37.94	24.25	61.59	31.82	10.25	26.03	55.65
10.50	26.67	38.86	24.50	62.23	32.15	10.50	26.67	57.01

CHART 2—*continued*

Upper Arm			Abdomen			Forearm		
in	*cm*	*Constant A*	*in*	*cm*	*Constant B*	*in*	*cm*	*Constant C*
10.75	27.30	39.79	24.75	62.86	32.48	10.75	27.30	58.37
11.00	27.94	40.71	25.00	63.50	32.80	11.00	27.94	59.73
11.25	28.57	41.64	25.25	64.13	33.13	11.25	28.57	61.08
11.50	29.21	42.56	25.50	64.77	33.46	11.50	29.21	62.44
11.75	29.84	43.49	25.75	65.40	33.79	11.75	29.84	63.80
12.00	30.48	44.41	26.00	66.04	34.12	12.00	30.48	65.16
12.25	31.11	45.34	26.25	66.67	34.44	12.25	31.11	66.51
12.50	31.75	46.26	26.50	67.31	34.77	12.50	31.75	67.87
12.75	32.38	47.19	26.75	67.94	35.10	12.75	32.38	69.23
13.00	33.02	48.11	27.00	68.58	35.43	13.00	33.02	70.59
13.25	33.65	49.04	27.25	69.21	35.76	13.25	33.65	71.94
13.50	34.29	49.96	27.50	69.85	36.09	13.50	34.29	73.30
13.75	34.92	50.89	27.75	70.48	36.41	13.75	34.92	74.66
14.00	35.56	51.82	28.00	71.12	36.74	14.00	35.56	76.02
14.25	36.19	52.74	28.25	71.75	37.07	14.25	36.19	77.37
14.50	36.83	53.67	28.50	72.39	37.40	14.50	36.83	78.73
14.75	37.46	54.59	28.75	73.02	37.73	14.75	37.46	80.09
15.00	38.10	55.52	29.00	73.66	38.05	15.00	38.10	81.45
15.25	38.73	56.44	29.25	74.29	38.38	15.25	38.73	82.80
15.50	39.37	57.37	29.50	74.93	38.71	15.50	39.37	84.16
15.75	40.00	58.29	29.75	75.56	39.04	15.75	40.00	85.52
16.00	40.64	59.22	30.00	76.20	39.37	16.00	40.64	86.88
16.25	41.27	60.14	30.25	76.83	39.69	16.25	41.27	88.23
16.50	41.91	61.07	30.50	77.47	40.02	16.50	41.91	89.59
16.75	42.54	61.99	30.75	78.10	40.35	16.75	42.54	90.95
17.00	43.18	62.92	31.00	78.74	40.68	17.00	43.18	92.31
17.25	43.81	63.84	31.25	79.37	41.01	17.25	43.81	93.66
17.50	44.45	64.77	31.50	80.01	41.33	17.50	44.45	95.02
17.75	45.08	65.69	31.75	80.64	41.66	17.75	45.08	96.38
18.00	45.72	66.62	32.00	81.28	41.99	18.00	45.72	97.74
18.25	46.35	67.54	32.25	81.91	42.32	18.25	46.35	99.09
18.50	46.99	68.47	32.50	82.55	42.65	18.50	46.99	100.45
18.75	47.62	69.40	32.75	83.18	42.97	18.75	47.62	101.81
19.00	48.26	70.32	33.00	83.82	43.30	19.00	48.26	103.17
19.25	48.89	71.25	33.25	84.45	43.63	19.25	48.89	104.52
19.50	49.53	72.17	33.50	85.09	43.96	19.50	49.53	105.88
19.75	50.16	73.10	33.75	85.72	44.29	19.75	50.16	107.24
20.00	50.80	74.02	34.00	86.36	44.61	20.00	50.80	108.60
20.25	51.43	74.95	34.25	86.99	44.94	20.25	51.43	109.95
20.50	52.07	75.87	34.50	87.63	45.27	20.50	52.07	111.31
20.75	52.70	76.80	34.75	88.26	45.60	20.75	52.70	112.67
21.00	53.34	77.72	35.00	88.90	45.93	21.00	53.34	114.02
21.25	53.97	78.65	35.25	89.53	46.25	21.25	53.97	115.38
21.50	54.61	79.57	35.50	90.17	46.58	21.50	54.61	116.74
21.75	55.24	80.50	35.75	90.80	46.91	21.75	55.24	118.10
22.00	55.88	81.42	36.00	91.44	47.24	22.00	55.88	119.45
			36.25	92.07	47.57			
			36.50	92.71	47.89			
			36.75	93.34	48.22			
			37.00	93.98	48.55			
			37.25	94.61	48.88			
			37.50	95.25	49.21			
			37.75	95.88	49.54			

CHART 2—*continued*

Upper Arm			Abdomen			Forearm		
in	*cm*	*Constant A*	*in*	*cm*	*Constant B*	*in*	*cm*	*Constant C*
			38.00	96.52	49.86			
			38.25	97.15	50.19			
			38.50	97.79	50.52			
			38.75	98.42	50.85			
			39.00	99.06	51.18			
			39.25	99.69	51.50			
			39.50	100.33	51.83			
			39.75	100.96	52.16			
			40.00	101.60	52.49			
			40.25	102.23	52.82			
			40.50	102.87	53.14			
			40.75	103.50	53.47			
			41.00	104.14	53.80			
			41.25	104.77	54.13			
			41.50	105.41	54.46			
			41.75	106.04	54.78			
			42.00	106.68	55.11			

Note: Percent Fat = Constant A + Constant B − Constant C − 10.2

CHART 3
CONVERSION CONSTANTS TO PREDICT PERCENTAGE BODY FAT FOR OLDER MEN

Buttocks			Abdomen			Forearm		
in	*cm*	*Constant A*	*in*	*cm*	*Constant B*	*in*	*cm*	*Constant C*
28.00	71.12	29.34	25.50	64.77	22.84	7.00	17.78	21.01
28.25	71.75	29.60	25.75	65.40	23.06	7.25	18.41	21.76
28.50	72.39	29.87	26.00	66.04	23.29	7.50	19.05	22.52
28.75	73.02	30.13	26.25	66.67	23.51	7.75	19.68	23.26
29.00	73.66	30.39	26.50	67.31	23.73	8.00	20.32	24.02
29.25	74.29	30.65	26.75	67.94	23.96	8.25	20.95	24.76
29.50	74.93	30.92	27.00	68.58	24.18	8.50	21.59	25.52
29.75	75.56	31.18	27.25	69.21	24.40	8.75	22.22	26.26
30.00	76.20	31.44	27.50	69.85	24.63	9.00	22.86	27.02
30.25	76.83	31.70	27.75	70.48	24.85	9.25	23.49	27.76
30.50	77.47	31.96	28.00	71.12	25.08	9.50	24.13	28.52
30.75	78.10	32.22	28.25	71.75	25.29	9.75	24.76	29.26
31.00	78.74	32.49	28.50	72.39	25.52	10.00	25.40	30.02
31.25	79.37	32.75	28.75	73.02	25.75	10.25	26.03	30.76
31.50	80.01	33.01	29.00	73.66	25.97	10.50	26.67	31.52
31.75	80.64	33.27	29.25	74.29	26.19	10.75	27.30	32.27
32.00	81.28	33.54	29.50	74.93	26.42	11.00	27.94	33.02
32.25	81.91	33.80	29.75	75.56	26.64	11.25	28.57	33.77
32.50	82.55	34.06	30.00	76.20	26.87	11.50	29.21	34.52
32.75	83.18	34.32	30.25	76.83	27.09	11.75	29.84	35.27
33.00	83.82	34.58	30.50	77.47	27.32	12.00	30.48	36.02
33.25	84.45	34.84	30.75	78.10	27.54	12.25	31.11	36.77
33.50	85.09	35.11	31.00	78.74	27.76	12.50	31.75	37.53

CHART 3 — *continued*

Buttocks			Abdomen			Forearm		
in	*cm*	*Constant A*	*in*	*cm*	*Constant B*	*in*	*cm*	*Constant C*
33.75	85.72	35.37	31.25	79.37	27.98	12.75	32.38	38.27
34.00	86.36	35.63	31.50	80.01	28.21	13.00	33.02	39.03
34.25	86.99	35.89	31.75	80.64	28.43	13.25	33.65	39.77
34.50	87.63	36.16	32.00	81.28	28.66	13.50	34.29	40.53
34.75	88.26	36.42	32.25	81.91	28.88	13.75	34.92	41.27
35.00	88.90	36.68	32.50	82.55	29.11	14.00	35.56	42.03
35.25	89.53	36.94	32.75	83.18	29.33	14.25	36.19	42.77
35.50	90.17	37.20	33.00	83.82	29.55	14.50	36.83	43.53
35.75	90.80	37.46	33.25	84.45	29.78	14.75	37.46	44.27
36.00	91.44	37.73	33.50	85.09	30.00	15.00	38.10	45.03
36.25	92.07	37.99	33.75	85.72	30.22	15.25	38.73	45.77
36.50	92.71	38.25	34.00	86.36	30.45	15.50	39.37	46.53
36.75	93.34	38.51	34.25	86.99	30.67	15.75	40.00	47.28
37.00	93.98	38.78	34.50	87.63	30.89	16.00	40.64	48.03
37.25	94.61	39.04	34.75	88.26	31.12	16.25	41.27	48.78
37.50	95.25	39.30	35.00	88.90	31.35	16.50	41.91	49.53
37.75	95.88	39.56	35.25	89.53	31.57	16.75	42.54	50.28
38.00	96.52	39.82	35.50	90.17	31.79	17.00	43.18	51.03
38.25	97.15	40.08	35.75	90.80	32.02	17.25	43.81	51.78
38.50	97.79	40.35	36.00	91.44	32.24	17.50	44.45	52.54
38.75	98.42	40.61	36.25	92.07	32.46	17.75	45.08	53.28
39.00	99.06	40.87	36.50	92.71	32.69	18.00	45.72	54.04
39.25	99.69	41.13	36.75	93.34	32.91	18.25	46.35	54.78
39.50	100.33	41.39	37.00	93.98	33.14			
39.75	100.96	41.66	37.25	94.61	33.36			
40.00	101.60	41.92	37.50	95.25	33.58			
40.25	102.23	42.18	37.75	95.88	33.81			
40.50	102.87	42.44	38.00	96.52	34.03			
40.75	103.50	42.70	38.25	97.15	34.26			
41.00	104.14	42.97	38.50	97.79	34.48			
41.25	104.77	43.23	38.75	98.42	34.70			
41.50	105.41	43.49	39.00	99.06	34.93			
41.75	106.04	43.75	39.25	99.69	35.15			
42.00	106.68	44.02	39.50	100.33	35.38			
42.25	107.31	44.28	39.75	100.96	35.59			
42.50	107.95	44.54	40.00	101.60	35.82			
42.75	108.58	44.80	40.25	102.23	36.05			
43.00	109.22	45.06	40.50	102.87	36.27			
43.25	109.85	45.32	40.75	103.50	36.49			
43.50	110.49	45.59	41.00	104.14	36.72			
43.75	111.12	45.85	41.25	104.77	36.94			
44.00	111.76	46.12	41.50	105.41	37.17			
44.25	112.39	46.37	41.75	106.04	37.39			
44.50	113.03	46.64	42.00	106.68	37.62			
44.75	113.66	46.89	42.25	107.31	37.87			
45.00	114.30	47.16	42.50	107.95	38.06			
45.25	114.93	47.42	42.75	108.58	38.28			
45.50	115.57	47.68	43.00	109.22	38.51			
45.75	116.20	47.94	43.25	109.85	38.73			
46.00	116.84	48.21	43.50	110.49	38.96			
46.25	117.47	48.47	43.75	111.12	39.18			
46.50	118.11	48.73	44.00	111.76	39.41			
46.75	118.74	48.99	44.25	112.39	39.63			

CHART 3— *continued*

Buttocks			Abdomen			Forearm		
in	*cm*	*Constant A*	*in*	*cm*	*Constant B*	*in*	*cm*	*Constant C*
47.00	119.38	49.26	44.50	113.03	39.85			
47.25	120.01	49.52	44.75	113.66	40.08			
47.50	120.65	49.78	45.00	114.30	40.30			
47.75	121.28	50.04						
48.00	121.92	50.30						
48.25	122.55	50.56						
48.50	123.19	50.83						
48.75	123.82	51.09						
49.00	124.46	51.35						

Note: Percent Fat = Constant A + Constant B − Constant C − 15.0

CHART 4
CONVERSION CONSTANTS TO PREDICT PERCENTAGE BODY FAT FOR YOUNG WOMEN

Abdomen			Thigh			Forearm		
in	*cm*	*Constant A*	*in*	*cm*	*Constant B*	*in*	*cm*	*Constant C*
20.00	50.80	26.74	14.00	35.56	29.13	6.00	15.24	25.86
20.25	51.43	27.07	14.25	36.19	29.65	6.25	15.87	26.94
20.50	52.07	27.41	14.50	36.83	30.17	6.50	16.51	28.02
20.75	52.70	27.74	14.75	37.46	30.69	6.75	17.14	29.10
21.00	53.34	28.07	15.00	38.10	31.21	7.00	17.78	30.17
21.25	53.97	28.41	15.25	38.73	31.73	7.25	18.41	31.25
21.50	54.61	28.74	15.50	39.37	32.25	7.50	19.05	32.33
21.75	55.24	29.08	15.75	40.00	32.77	7.75	19.68	33.41
22.00	55.88	29.41	16.00	40.64	33.29	8.00	20.32	34.48
22.25	56.51	29.74	16.25	41.27	33.81	8.25	20.95	35.56
22.50	57.15	30.08	16.50	41.91	34.33	8.50	21.59	36.64
22.75	57.78	30.41	16.75	42.54	34.85	8.75	22.22	37.72
23.00	58.42	30.75	17.00	43.18	35.37	9.00	22.86	38.79
23.25	59.05	31.08	17.25	43.81	35.89	9.25	23.49	39.87
23.50	59.69	31.42	17.50	44.45	36.41	9.50	24.13	40.95
23.75	60.32	31.75	17.75	45.08	36.93	9.75	24.76	42.03
24.00	60.96	32.08	18.00	45.72	37.45	10.00	25.40	43.10
24.25	61.59	32.42	18.25	46.35	37.97	10.25	26.03	44.18
24.50	62.23	32.75	18.50	46.99	38.49	10.50	26.67	45.26
24.75	62.86	33.09	18.75	47.62	39.01	10.75	27.30	46.34
25.00	63.50	33.42	19.00	48.26	39.53	11.00	27.94	47.41
25.25	64.13	33.76	19.25	48.89	40.05	11.25	28.57	48.49
25.50	64.77	34.09	19.50	49.53	40.57	11.50	29.21	49.57
25.75	65.40	34.42	19.75	50.16	41.09	11.75	29.84	50.65
26.00	66.04	34.76	20.00	50.80	41.61	12.00	30.48	51.73
26.25	66.67	35.09	20.25	51.43	42.13	12.25	31.11	52.80
26.50	67.31	35.43	20.50	52.07	42.65	12.50	31.75	53.88
26.75	67.94	35.76	20.75	52.70	43.17	12.75	32.38	54.96
27.00	68.58	36.10	21.00	53.34	43.69	13.00	33.02	56.04
27.25	69.21	36.43	21.25	53.97	44.21	13.25	33.65	57.11
27.50	69.85	36.76	21.50	54.61	44.73	13.50	34.29	58.19

CHART 4— *continued*

Abdomen			Thigh			Forearm		
in	*cm*	*Constant A*	*in*	*cm*	*Constant B*	*in*	*cm*	*Constant C*
27.75	70.48	37.10	21.75	55.24	45.25	13.75	34.92	59.27
28.00	71.12	37.43	22.00	55.88	45.77	14.00	35.56	60.35
28.25	71.75	37.77	22.25	56.51	46.29	14.25	36.19	61.42
28.50	72.39	38.10	22.50	57.15	46.81	14.50	36.83	62.50
28.75	73.02	38.43	22.75	57.78	47.33	14.75	37.46	63.58
29.00	73.66	38.77	23.00	58.42	47.85	15.00	38.10	64.66
29.25	74.29	39.10	23.25	59.05	48.37	15.25	38.73	65.73
29.50	74.93	39.44	23.50	59.69	48.89	15.50	39.37	66.81
29.75	75.56	39.77	23.75	60.32	49.41	15.75	40.00	67.89
30.00	76.20	40.11	24.00	60.96	49.93	16.00	40.64	68.97
30.25	76.83	40.44	24.25	61.59	50.45	16.25	41.27	70.04
30.50	77.47	40.77	24.50	62.23	50.97	16.50	41.91	71.12
30.75	78.10	41.11	24.75	62.86	51.49	16.75	42.54	72.20
31.00	78.74	41.44	25.00	63.50	52.01	17.00	43.18	73.28
31.25	79.37	41.78	25.25	64.13	52.53	17.25	43.81	74.36
31.50	80.01	42.11	25.50	64.77	53.05	17.50	44.45	75.43
31.75	80.64	42.45	25.75	65.40	53.57	17.75	45.08	76.51
32.00	81.28	42.78	26.00	66.04	54.09	18.00	45.72	77.59
32.25	81.91	43.11	26.25	66.67	54.61	18.25	46.35	78.67
32.50	82.55	43.45	26.50	67.31	55.13	18.50	46.99	79.74
32.75	83.18	43.78	26.75	67.94	55.65	18.75	47.62	80.82
33.00	83.82	44.12	27.00	68.58	56.17	19.00	48.26	81.90
33.25	84.45	44.45	27.25	69.21	56.69	19.25	48.89	82.98
33.50	85.09	44.78	27.50	69.85	57.21	19.50	49.53	84.05
33.75	85.72	45.12	27.75	70.48	57.73	19.75	50.16	85.13
34.00	86.36	45.45	28.00	71.12	58.26	20.00	50.80	86.21
34.25	86.99	45.79	28.25	71.75	58.78			
34.50	87.63	46.12	28.50	72.39	59.30			
34.75	88.26	46.46	38.75	73.02	59.82			
35.00	88.90	46.79	29.00	73.66	60.34			
35.25	89.53	47.12	29.25	74.29	60.86			
35.50	90.17	47.46	29.50	74.93	61.38			
35.75	90.80	47.79	29.75	75.56	61.90			
36.00	91.44	48.13	30.00	76.20	62.42			
36.25	92.07	48.46	30.25	76.83	62.94			
36.50	92.71	48.80	30.50	77.47	63.46			
36.75	93.34	49.13	30.75	78.10	63.98			
37.00	93.98	49.46	31.00	78.74	64.50			
37.25	94.61	49.80	31.25	79.37	65.02			
37.50	95.25	50.13	31.50	80.01	65.54			
37.75	95.88	50.47	31.75	80.64	66.06			
38.00	96.52	50.80	32.00	81.28	66.58			
38.25	97.15	51.13	32.25	81.91	67.10			
38.50	97.79	51.47	32.50	82.55	67.62			
38.75	98.42	51.80	32.75	83.18	68.14			
39.00	99.06	52.14	33.00	83.82	68.66			
39.25	99.69	52.47	33.25	84.45	69.18			
39.50	100.33	52.81	33.50	85.09	69.70			
39.75	100.96	53.14	33.75	85.72	70.22			
40.00	101.60	53.47	34.00	86.36	70.74			

Note: Percent Fat = Constant A + Constant B − Constant C − 19.6

CHART 5
CONVERSION CONSTANTS TO PREDICT PERCENTAGE BODY FAT FOR OLDER WOMEN

Abdomen			Thigh			Forearm		
in	cm	Constant A	in	cm	Constant B	in	cm	Constant C
25.00	63.50	29.69	14.00	35.56	17.31	10.00	25.40	14.46
25.25	64.13	29.98	14.25	36.19	17.62	10.25	26.03	14.82
25.50	64.77	30.28	14.50	36.83	17.93	10.50	26.67	15.18
25.75	65.40	30.58	14.75	37.46	18.24	10.75	27.30	15.54
26.00	66.04	30.87	15.00	38.10	18.55	11.00	27.94	15.91
26.25	66.67	31.17	15.25	38.73	18.86	11.25	28.57	16.27
26.50	67.31	31.47	15.50	39.37	19.17	11.50	29.21	16.63
26.75	67.94	31.76	15.75	40.00	19.47	11.75	29.84	16.99
27.00	68.58	32.06	16.00	40.64	19.78	12.00	30.48	17.35
27.25	69.21	32.36	16.25	41.27	20.09	12.25	31.11	17.71
27.50	69.85	32.65	16.50	41.91	20.40	12.50	31.75	18.08
27.75	70.48	32.95	16.75	42.54	20.71	12.75	32.38	18.44
28.00	71.12	33.25	17.00	43.18	21.02	13.00	33.02	18.80
28.25	71.75	33.55	17.25	43.81	21.33	13.25	33.65	19.16
28.50	72.39	33.84	17.50	44.45	21.64	13.50	34.29	19.52
28.75	73.02	34.14	17.75	45.08	21.95	13.75	34.92	19.88
29.00	73.66	34.44	18.00	45.72	22.26	14.00	35.56	20.24
29.25	74.29	34.73	18.25	46.35	22.57	14.25	36.19	20.61
29.50	74.93	35.03	18.50	46.99	22.87	14.50	36.83	20.97
29.75	75.56	35.33	18.75	47.62	23.18	14.75	37.46	21.33
30.00	76.20	35.62	19.00	38.26	23.49	15.00	38.10	21.69
30.25	76.83	35.92	19.25	48.89	23.80	15.25	38.73	22.05
30.50	77.47	36.22	19.50	49.53	24.11	15.50	39.37	22.41
30.75	78.10	36.51	19.75	50.16	24.42	15.75	40.00	22.77
31.00	78.74	36.81	20.00	50.80	24.73	16.00	40.64	23.14
31.25	79.37	37.11	20.25	51.43	25.04	16.25	41.27	23.50
31.50	80.01	37.40	20.50	52.07	25.35	16.50	41.91	23.86
31.75	80.64	37.70	20.75	52.70	25.66	16.75	42.54	24.22
32.00	81.28	38.00	21.00	53.34	25.97	17.00	43.18	24.58
32.25	81.91	38.30	21.25	53.97	26.28	17.25	43.81	24.94
32.50	82.55	38.59	21.50	54.61	26.58	17.50	44.45	25.31
32.75	83.18	38.89	21.75	55.24	26.89	17.75	45.08	25.67
33.00	83.82	39.19	22.00	55.88	27.20	18.00	45.72	26.03
33.25	84.45	39.48	22.25	56.51	27.51	18.25	46.35	26.39
33.50	85.09	39.78	22.50	57.15	27.82	18.50	46.99	26.75
33.75	85.72	40.08	22.75	57.78	28.13	18.75	47.62	27.11
34.00	86.36	40.37	23.00	58.42	28.44	19.00	48.26	27.47
34.25	86.99	40.67	23.25	59.05	28.75	19.25	48.89	27.84
34.50	87.63	40.97	23.50	59.69	29.06	19.50	49.53	28.20
34.75	88.26	41.26	23.75	60.32	29.37	19.75	50.16	28.56
35.00	88.90	41.56	24.00	60.96	29.68	20.00	50.80	28.92
35.25	89.53	41.86	24.25	61.59	29.98	20.25	51.43	29.28
35.50	90.17	42.15	24.50	62.23	30.29	20.50	52.07	29.64
35.75	90.80	42.45	24.75	62.86	30.60	20.75	52.70	30.00
36.00	91.44	42.75	25.00	63.50	30.91	21.00	53.34	30.37
36.25	92.07	43.05	25.25	64.13	31.22	21.25	53.97	30.73
36.50	92.71	43.34	25.50	64.77	31.53	21.50	54.61	31.09
36.75	93.35	43.64	25.75	65.40	31.84	21.75	55.24	31.45
37.00	93.98	43.94	26.00	66.04	32.15	22.00	55.88	31.81
37.25	94.62	44.23	26.25	66.67	32.46	22.25	56.51	32.17
37.50	95.25	44.53	26.50	67.31	32.77	22.50	57.15	32.54

CHART 5—*continued*

Abdomen			Thigh			Forearm		
in	*cm*	*Constant A*	*in*	*cm*	*Constant B*	*in*	*cm*	*Constant C*
37.75	95.89	44.83	26.75	67.94	33.08	22.75	57.78	32.90
38.00	96.52	45.12	27.00	68.58	33.38	23.00	58.42	33.26
38.25	97.16	45.42	27.25	69.21	33.69	23.25	59.05	33.62
38.50	97.79	45.72	27.50	69.85	34.00	23.50	59.69	33.98
38.75	98.43	46.01	27.75	70.48	34.31	23.75	60.32	34.34
39.00	99.06	46.31	28.00	71.12	34.62	24.00	60.96	34.70
39.25	99.70	46.61	28.25	71.75	34.93	24.25	61.59	35.07
39.50	100.33	46.90	28.50	72.39	35.24	24.50	62.23	35.43
39.75	100.97	47.20	28.75	73.02	35.55	24.75	62.86	35.79
40.00	101.60	47.50	29.00	73.66	35.86	25.00	63.50	36.15
40.25	101.24	47.79	29.25	74.29	36.17			
40.50	102.87	48.09	29.50	74.93	36.48			
40.75	103.51	48.39	29.75	75.56	36.79			
41.00	104.14	48.69	30.00	76.20	37.09			
41.25	104.78	48.98	30.25	76.83	37.40			
41.50	105.41	49.28	30.50	77.47	37.71			
41.75	106.05	49.58	30.75	78.10	38.02			
42.00	106.68	49.87	31.00	78.74	38.33			
42.25	107.32	50.17	31.25	79.37	38.64			
42.50	107.95	50.47	31.50	80.01	38.95			
42.75	108.59	50.76	31.75	80.64	39.26			
43.00	109.22	51.06	32.00	81.28	39.57			
43.25	109.86	51.36	32.25	81.91	39.88			
43.50	110.49	51.65	32.50	82.55	40.19			
43.75	111.13	51.95	32.75	83.18	40.49			
44.00	111.76	52.25	33.00	83.82	40.80			
44.25	112.40	52.54	33.25	84.45	41.11			
44.50	113.03	52.84	33.50	85.09	41.42			
44.75	113.67	53.14	33.75	85.72	41.73			
45.00	114.30	53.44	34.00	86.36	42.04			

Note: **Percentage Fat = Constant A + Constant B – Constant C – 18.4**

Body Composition Characteristics of Athletes in Different Sports[a,b]

Sport	Sex	N	Age (y)	Stature (cm)	Mass (kg)	Body Fat (%)	Reference Number
Ballet							
	F	34	21.9 ±4.3	168.0 ±6.8	54.4 ±6.0	16.9 ±4.7	3
Baseball and softball							
Baseball	M		27.4	183.1	88.0	12.6	39
Softball	F	14	22.6 ±4.1	167.1 ±6.1	59.6 ±5.8	19.1 ±5.0	41
Basketball	F	49	19.3 ±1.4	176.5 ±8.8	±6.8 ±6.7	19.2 ±4.6	34
	M	10	20.9 ±1.3	194.3 ±10.2	87.5 ±7.2	10.5 ±3.8	27
Biathlon	F	9	25.1 ±5.3	165.9 ±7.1	59.0 ±7.1	15.0 ±2.2	2
Bicycling	M	11	22.2 ±3.6	176.4 ±7.1	±8.5 ±6.4	10.5 ±2.4	40
Field events							
Decathlon	M	3	22.5 ±2.2	186.3 ±1.4	84.1 ±9.2	8.4 ±5.1	40
Pentathlon	F	9	21.5 ±3.1	175.4 ±3.0	±5.4 ±5.7	11.0 ±3.3	15
Throwing	F	9	18.8 ±3.0	173.9 ±6.9	80.8 ±21.1	27.0 ±8.4	38
Discus	M	7	28.3 ±5.0	186.1 ±2.6	104.7 ±13.2	16.4 ±4.3	6
Shot	M	5	27.0 ±3.9	188.2 ±3.6	112.5 ±7.3	16.5 ±4.3	6
Jumping	F	13	17.4 ±0.9	173.6 ±8.0	57.1 ±6.0	12.9 ±2.5	33
	M	16	17.6 ±0.8	181.7 ±6.1	±9.2 ±7.2	8.5 ±2.1	33
Hammer, elite	M	10	24.8 ±3.2	187.3 ±3.1	104.2 ±9.1	15.1 ±4.2	20
Shotput, elite	M	10	23.5 ±4.2	187.0 ±4.0	112.3 ±6.2	14.8 ±3.4	20
Discus, elite	M	10	23.5 ±4.5	191.7 ±4.7	108.2 ±6.9	13.2 ±4.6	20
Javelin, elite	M	10	21.9 ±3.7	186.0 ±5.1	90.6 ±6.1	8.5 ±3.2	20
Field hockey	F	13	19.8 ±1.4	159.8 ±5.5	58.1 ±6.6	21.3 ±7.2	31
Football							
Defensive backs, Pro	M	26	24.5 ±3.2	182.5 ±4.5	84.8 ±5.2	9.6 ±4.2	37
College	M	15		178.3	77.3	11.5	18
College	M	12		179.9	83.1	8.8	
College	M	15		183.0	83.7	9.6	

continued

Sport	Sex	N	Age (y)	Stature (cm)	Mass (kg)	Body Fat (%)	Reference Number
Football, *continued*							
Pro, current	M	26		182.5	84.8	9.6	
Pro, older	M	25		183.0	91.2	10.7	
Offensive backs and	M	40	24.7	183.8	90.7	9.4	37
wide receivers, Pro			±3.0	±4.1	±8.4	±4.0	
College	M	15		179.7	79.8	12.4	36
College	M	29		181.8	84.1	9.5	18
College	M	18		185.6	86.1	9.9	
Pro, current	M	40		183.8	90.7	9.4	
Pro, older	M	25		183.0	91.7	10.0	
Line backers, Pro	M	28	24.2	188.6	102.2	14.0	37
			±2.4	±2.9	±6.3	±4.6	
College	M	7		180.1	87.2	13.4	36
College	M	17		186.1	97.1	13.1	18
College	M	17		185.6	98.8	13.2	
Pro, current	M	28		188.6	102.2	14.0	
Offensive line, Pro	M	38	24.7	193.0	112.6	15.6	37
			±3.2	±3.5	±6.8	±3.8	
College	M	13		186.0	99.2	19.1	36
College	M	23		187.5	107.6	19.5	18
College	M	25		191.1	106.5	15.3	
Pro, current	M	38		193.0	112.6	15.6	
Defensive line, Pro	M	32	25.7	192.4	117.1	18.2	37
			±3.4	±6.5	±10.3	±5.4	
College	M	15		186.6	97.8	18.5	36
College	M	8		188.8	114.3	19.5	18
College	M	13		191.1	109.3	14.7	
Pro, current	M	32		192.4	117.1	18.2	
Pro, older	M	25		185.7	97.1	14.0	
Quarterbacks, Pro	M	16	24.1	185.0	90.1	14.4	37
			±2.7	±5.4	±11.3	±6.5	
Total Team							
College	M	65		182.5	88.0	15.0	36
College	M	91		184.9	97.3	13.9	18
College	M	88		186.6	96.6	11.4	
Pro, current	M	164		188.1	101.5	13.4	
Pro, older	M	25		183.1	91.2	10.4	
Dallas-Jets	M	107		188.2	100.4	12.6	
Gymnastics							
	F	44	19.4	160.6	53.7	15.3	30
			±1.1	±4.4	±5.9	±4.0	
	F	97	15.7	162.4	54.0	8.2	5
			±1.1	±5.6	±6.5		
	M	19		168.7	±5.8	±.5	32
				±6.7	±4.3	±2.4	
Lacrosse	F	17	24.4	166.3	±0.6	19.3	41
			±4.5	±7.5	±7.3	±5.7	
	M	26	26.7	177.6	74.0	12.3	40
			±4.2	±5.5	±8.6	±4.3	
Orienteering	M	7	25.9	176.2	±4.7	10.7	40
			±8.5	±6.8	±5.0	±2.9	
Racket sports							
Badminton	F	6	23.0	167.7	±1.5	21.0	41
			±5.3	±2.5	±2.6	±2.1	
	M	7	24.5	180.0	71.2	12.8	40
			±3.6	±5.2	±5.6	±3.1	

Sport	Sex	N	Age (y)	Stature (cm)	Mass (kg)	Body Fat (%)	Reference Number
Racket sports, *continued*							
Tennis	F	7	21.3	164.7	59.6	22.4	31
			±0.9	±4.2	±4.6	±2.0	
	M	9		179.1	73.8	11.3	32
				±4.5	±7.3	±5.2	
Squash	M	9	22.6	177.5	71.9	11.2	40
			±6.8	±4.1	±8.3	±3.7	
Rowers	M	18	20.6	185.8	86.3	12.2	13
			±1.9	±2.2	±6.4	±4.1	
Skating							
Ice hockey	M	27	24.9	182.9	85.6	9.2	1
			±3.6	±6.1	±7.1	±4.6	
Speed skating	F	9	19.7	165.0	±1.2	16.5	23
			±3.0	±6.0	±6.9	±4.1	
	M	6	22.2	178.0	73.3	7.4	23
			±4.1	±7.1	±7.1	±2.5	
Skiing							
(Nordic)	F	5	23.5	164.5	56.9	16.1	29
			±4.7	±3.3	±1.1	±1.6	
Alpine	F	6	19.6	165.0	±3.6	16.6	35
	F	5	20.2	164.7	±0.1	18.5	12
	M	8	19.8	173.0	72.6	±.5	35
	M	5	21.2	175.5	73.0	7.2	12
	M	11	22.8	179.0	71.8	7.2	29
			±1.9	±5.0	±5.4	±1.9	
Soccer	F	11	22.1	164.9	±1.2	22.0	41
			±4.1	±5.6	±8.6	±6.8	
	M	19		176.8	72.4	9.5	32
				±6.6	±8.9	±4.9	
Swimming	F	9	13.5	164.5	53.3	17.2	19
			±0.9	±7.4	±5.3	±3.6	
	F	13	16.4	168.8	57.9	15.6	
			±0.9	±7.1	±5.5	±4.0	
	F	19	19.2	169.6	56.0	16.1	
			±0.8	±4.7	±3.1	±3.7	
	M	27		178.3	71.0	8.8	32
				±6.4	±5.9	±3.2	
Channel swimmers	M	11	38.2	173.8	87.5	22.4	24
			±10.2	±7.4	±10.4	±7.5	
Track events							
Distance runners	F	15	27	161.0	47.2	14.3	8
				±4.0	±4.6	±3.3	
	M	20		177.0	±3.1	4.7	22
				±6.0	±4.8	±3.1	
Masters and competitors	M	11	40–49	180.7	±3.1	4.7	21
		5	50–59	174.2	±7.2	10.9	
		6	±0–69	175.4	±7.1	11.3	
		3	70.8	175.6	±6.7	13.6	
Sprinters and hurdlers	F	8	15.8	166.5	54.0	10.9	38
			±2.7	±9.3	±8.4	±3.6	
	M	5	28.4	179.9	±6.8	8.3	40
			±0.1	±0.7	±0.9	±5.2	
Walkers	F	4	24.9	163.4	51.7	18.1	41
			±6.3	±3.9	±4.8	±4.4	

continued

Sport	Sex	N	Age (y)	Stature (cm)	Mass (kg)	Body Fat (%)	Reference Number
Track events, *continued*							
Walkers	M	3	20.3	178.4	±6.1	7.3	40
			±2.0	±2.1	±1.8	±1.3	
Triathlon	F	16	24.2	162.1	55.2	16.5	16
			±4.3	±6.3	±4.6	±1.4	
	M	14	36.0	176.4	73.3	12.5	17
			±9.9	±8.6	±8.6	±5.9	
	M	8	29.6	180.0	73.9	7.9	26
			±2.6	±2.4	±2.1	±0.5	
Volleyball	F	14	21.6	178.3	70.5	17.9	25
			±0.8	±4.2	±5.5	±3.6	
	M	11	20.9	185.3	78.3	9.8	40
			±3.7	±10.2	±12.0	±2.9	
Weight lifting and body building							
Power lift	F	10	25.2	164.6	±8.6	21.5	10
			±6.0	±3.7	±3.6	±1.3	
	M	13	24.8	173.5	80.8	9.1	11
			±1.6	±2.8	±3.2	±1.2	
Body builders	F	10	30.4	165.2	56.5	13.5	10
			±8.2	±5.6	±0.9	±1.5	
	F	10	27.0	160.8	53.8	13.2	7
	M	16	28.0	175.1	86.2	12.5	4
			±1.8	±1.7	±3.1	±3.4	
	M	18	27.8	177.1	82.4	9.3	11
			±1.8	±1.1	±1.0	±0.8	
	M	14	31.6	170.8	83.8	10.9	14
			±6.7	±5.6	±9.2	±2.4	
Wrestling[c]							
Adult	M	37	19.6	174.6	74.8	8.8	28
			±1.34	±7.0	±12.2	±4.1	
Adolescent	M	409	16.2	171.0	±3.2	11.0	9
			±1.0	±7.1	±10.0	±4.0	
Sumo (seki-tori)	M	37	21.1	178.9	115.9	26.1	14
			±3.6	±5.2	±27.4	±6.4	

[a]Values reported as means ± SD.

[b]Modified from Sinning, W.E.: Body composition in athletes. In Human Body Composition. Roche AF, et al, eds. Human Kinetics, Champaign, IL, 1996.

[c]Note: consult our web page (http://www.lww.com/mkk) for the recent NCAA policy about minimal wrestling weight certification.

References

1. Agre JC, et al. Professional ice hockey players: Physiologic, anthropometric, and musculoskeletal characteristics. *Arch Phys Med Rehab* 1988;69:188.

2. Bacharach DW, et al. Relationship of blood urea nitrogen to training intensity of elite female biathlon skiers. *J Strength Cond Res* 1996;10:105.

3. Calabrese LH, et al. Menstrual abnormalities, nutrition patterns, and body composition in female classical ballet dancers. *Phys Sportsmed* 1983;11:86.

4. Cordain L, et al. Variability of body composition assessment in men exhibiting extreme muscular hypertrophy. *J Strength Cond Res* 1995;9:85.

5. Eckerson JM, et al. Validity of bioelectrical impedence equations for estimating fat-free weight in high school female gymnasts. *Med Sci Exerc Sports* 1997;29:962.

6. Fahey TD, et al. Body composition and $\dot{V}O_{2max}$ of exceptional weight trained athletes. *J Appl Physiol* 1975;39:559.

7. Freedson PF, et al. Physique, body composition, and psychological characteristics of competitive female body builders. *Phys Sportsmed* 1983;11:85.

8. Graves JE, et al. Body composition of elite female distance runners. *Int J Sports Med* 1987;8:96.

9. Housh TJ, et al. Validity of anthropometric estimations of body composition in high school wrestlers. *Res Q Exerc Sport* 1989;60:239.

10. Johnson GO, et al. A physiological profile comparison of female body builders and power lifters. *J Sports Med Phys Fitness* 1990;30:361.

11. Katch VL, et al. Muscular development and lean body weight in body builders and weight lifters. *Med Sci Sports* 1980;12:340.

12. Katch FI. Body composition of elite male and female alpine skiers. Unpublished data. University of Massachusetts, 1998.

13. Katch FI. Physiological characteristics of lightweight and heavyweight male collegiate rowers. Unpublished data. University of Massachusetts, 1999.

14. Kondo M, et al. Upper limit of fat-free mass in humans: a study on Japanese Sumo wrestlers. *Am J Human Biol* 1994;6:613.

15. Krahenbuhl GS, et al. Characteristics of national and world class female pentathletes. *Med Sci Sports*, 1979;11:20.

16. Leake CN, and Carter, J.E. Comparison of body composition and somatotype of trained female triathletes. *J Sports Sci* 1991;9:125.

17. Lofton M, et al. Peak physiological function and performance of recreational triathletes. *J Sports Med Phys Fitness* 1988;28:33.

18. McArdle WD, et al. *Exercise Physiology.* 4th edition. Baltimore: Williams & Wilkins, 1996:590.

19. Meleski BW, et al. Size, physique and body composition of competitive female swimmers 11 through 20 years of age. *Human Biol* 1982;54:609.

20. Morrow JR, et al. Anthropometric strength, and performance characteristics of American world class throwers. *J Sports Med Phys Fitness* 1982;22:73.

21. Pollock ML, et al. Physiological characteristics of champion American track athletes 40 to 75 years of age. *J Gerontol* 1974;29:645.

22. Pollock ML, et al. Body composition of elite class distance runners. *Ann New York Acad Sci* 1977;301:361.

23. Pollock ML, et al. Comparison of male and female speedskating candidates. In: DM Landers (ed). *Sports and Elite Performance.* Champaign, IL: Human Kinetics, 143–152.

24. Pugh LG, et al. A physiological study of channel swimming. *Clin Sci* 1955;19:257.

25. Puhl J, et al. Physical and physiological characteristics of elite volleyball players. *Res Q Exerc Sport* 1982;53:257.

26. Rowbottom DG, et al. Training adaptation and biological changes among well-trained male triathletes. *Med Sci Sports Exerc* 1997;29:1233.

27. Siders WA, et al. Effects of participation in a collegiate sport season on body composition. *J Sports Med Phys Fitness* 1991;31:571.

28. Sinning WE. Body composition assessment of college wrestlers. *Med Sci Sports* 1974;6:139.

29. Sinning WE, et al. Body composition and somatotype of male and female Nordic skiers. *Res Q* 1977;48:741.

30. Sinning WE. Anthropometric estimation of body density, fat, and lean body weight in women gymnasts. *Med Sci Sports* 1978;10:243.

31. Sinning WE, and Wilson JR. Validity of "generalized" equations for body composition analysis in women athletes. *Res Q Exerc Sports* 1984;55:153.

32. Sinning WE, et al. Validity of generalized equations for body composition analysis in male athletes. *Med Sci Sports Exerc* 1985;17:124.

33. Thorland WG, et al. Body composition and somatotype characteristics of junior olympic athletes. *Med Sci Sports Exerc* 1981;13:332.

34. Walsh FK, et al. Estimation of body composition of female intercollegiate basketball players. *Phys Sportsmed* 1984;12:74.

35. White A, and Johnson S. Physiological comparison of international, national, and regional alpine skiers. *Int J Sports Med* 1991;12:374.

36. Wickkiser JD, and Kelly JM. The body composition of a college football team. *Med Sci Sports* 1975;7:199.

37. Wilmore JH, et al. Football pro's strengths and CV weaknesses charted. *Phys Sportsmed* 1976;4:45.

38. Wilmore JH, et al. Body physique and composition of the female distance runner. *Ann New York Acad Sci* 1977;301:764.

39. Wilmore JH. Body composition in sport and exercise: Directions for future research. *Med Sci Sports Exerc* 1983;15:21.

40. Withers RT, et al. Relative body fat and anthropometric prediction of body density of male athletes. *Eur J Appl Physiol* 1987;56:191.

41. Withers RT, et al. Relative body fat and anthropometric prediction of body density of female athletes. *Eur J Appl Physiol* 1987;56:169.

APPENDIX F   Three-Day Physical Activity Log

A three-day log of physical activities provides a relatively simple yet accurate way to assess average daily energy expenditure.

Step 1 Review Table 1 which provides an example of a daily physical activity log for one of your textbook authors. Note that the list includes mostly typical activities of daily living.

Step 2 Record your daily physical activities on each of the log entry forms for three typical days. Be specific for the beginning and ending times of activity; round off to the nearest minute.

Step 3 Consolidate the information from the three log entry forms (Step 2) to the Master Log in Table 2. If you devote more than 120 minutes to one of the recreational and sports activities, check the 120 minute box. For typical household activities, list activities by minutes and hours.

Step 4 Determine your basal metabolic rate (BMR) in kCal·h^{-1} as follows:

Men
BMR (kCal·h^{-1}) = 38 kCal·m^2·h^{-1} × surface area^a (m^2)

Women
BMR (kCal·h^{-1}) = 38 kCal·m^2·h^{-1} × surface area^a (m^2)

Example of BMR Calculations
Data: Male
Age, 40y
Stature, 182 cm (72 in)
Body mass, 86.4 kg (190 lb)
Body surface area^a = 2.08 m^2
kCal·m^2·h^{-1} = 38.0

Calculations
a. kCal·h^{-1} = 38.0 × 2.08 = 79.0
b. kCal·min^{-1} = 79.0 ÷ 60 = 1.3

Step 5 Determine energy expenditure (kCal·min^{-1}) for each of the activities in the Master Log (Table 2). Use Appendix B to determine caloric expenditure per minute. The values represent gross values plus resting. If an activity is not included, list one most similar to yours. The bottom of the Daily Log form includes a box to record daily total kCal.

Step 6 Multiply energy expenditure for each activity by the number of minutes of participation.

Step 7 Sum the total energy expenditure for each activity, including the value for sleep, to arrive at your TOTAL daily energy expenditure.

Step 8 Repeat Steps 5–7 for Days 2 and 3. Calculate average daily calorie by summing the total calories expended for three days and divide by 3.

Total energy expenditure (kCal) = Day 1 kCal + Day 2 kCal + Day 3 kCal

= ___ kCal + ___ kCal + ___ kCal

Average daily energy expenditure = Total kCal ÷ 3

= _____ kCal ÷ 3

---

^{a}Compute body surface area (BSA, m^2) as: Body mass, kg$^{0.425}$ × stature, cm$^{0.725}$ × 0.007184
Example: Body Mass=162 lb (73.5 kg); stature = 5′9″ (175.3 cm)
    BSA, m^2 = 73.5$^{0.425}$ × 175.3$^{0.725}$ × 0.007184
        = 6.210 × 42.332 × 0.007184
        = 1.89

TABLE F.1 **Example of Daily Physical Activity Log. [Column 5 Lists Activities Similar to those in Column 1.]**

Activity	Begin Time	End Time	Total Minutes	Similar Activity[a]	kcal · min^{-1}	Total kCal
Wake, bathroom use	6:45AM	6:53AM	8	Standing quietly	2.3	18.4
Go back to bed	6:53	7:30	38	BMR	1.3	48.1
Eat breakfast	7:30	7:50	10	Eating, sitting	2.0	40.0
Use bathroom	7:50	8:00	10	Standing quietly	2.3	23.0
Dress	8:00	8:06	6	Standing quietly	2.3	13.8
Drive to school	8:06	8:17	11	Sitting quietly	2.0	22.0
Walk to office	8:17	8:25	8	Walking, normal pace	6.9	55.8
Work in office, pick up mail	8:25	10:00	95	Writing, sitting	2.5	237.5
Up/down stairs	10:00	10:10	10	11 min 30 s pace	11.7	117.0
Work in office	10:10	12:10PM	120	Writing, sitting	2.5	300.0
Go to locker	12:10PM	12:12	2	Walking, normal pace	6.9	13.8
Get dressed	12:12	12:16	4	Standing quietly	2.3	9.2
Walk to track	12:16	12:20	4	Walk, normal pace	6.9	27.6
Wait for friend	12:20	12:30	10	Standing quietly	2.3	23.0
Run to park, back	12:30	2:00	90	8-min mile pace	17.2	1553.0
Walk to locker	2:00	2:04	4	Walk, normal pace	6.9	27.6
Shower, dress	2:04	2:20	16	Quiet standing	2.3	36.8
Walk to office	2:20	2:24	4	Walk, normal pace	6.9	27.6
Meeting/lunch	2:24	3:00	36	Eating, sitting	2.0	72.0
Work in office	3:00	5:05	125	Writing, sitting	2.5	312.5
Walk to library	5:05	5:12	7	Walk, normal pace	6.9	48.3
Work in library	5:12	6:05	53	Writing, sitting	2.5	132.5
Walk to dean	6:05	6:10	5	Walk, normal pace	6.9	34.5
Meeting, dean	6:10	6:35	25	Writing, sitting	2.5	62.5
Walk to office	6:35	6:43	8	Walk, normal pace	6.9	55.2
Walk to car	6:43	6:51	8	Walk, normal pace	6.9	55.2
Drive home	6:51	7:03	12	Sitting quietly	1.8	21.6
Change clothes	7:03	7:07	4	Standing quietly	2.3	9.2
Wash-up	7:07	7:11	4	Standing quietly	2.3	9.2
Cook dinner	7:11	8:00	49	Cooking	4.1	200.9
Watch TV	8:00	8:30	30	Sitting quietly	1.8	54.0
Eat dinner	8:30	9:00	30	Eating, sitting	2.0	60.0
Mail letter	9:00	9:05	5	Walk, normal pace	6.9	34.5
Listen to stereo	9:05	9:30	25	Sitting quietly	1.8	45.0
Watch TV	9:30	10:30	60	Sitting quietly	1.8	108.0
Wash-up	10:30	10:38	8	Standing quietly	2.3	18.4
Read in bed	10:38	11:15	37	Lying at ease	1.9	70.3

DAILY TOTAL = 4583

[a]When you cannot match a specific activity with a table value in Appendix B, select a similar activity and base the kCal value on that activity.

DAY 2. **Physical Activity Log**						
Activity	Begin Time	End Time	Total Minutes	Similar Activity[a]	kCal · min⁻¹	Total kCal

DAILY TOTAL =

DAY 3.   Physical Activity Log

Activity	Begin Time	End Time	Total Minutes	Similar Activity[a]	kCal · min^{-1}	Total kCal

DAILY TOTAL =

TABLE F.2	Master Log of Physical Activity

Activity	Day 1	2	3	Minutes 0–10	10–20	20–30	30–40	40–50	50–60	60–70	70–80	80–90	90–100	100–110	110–120	kCal
Aerobics	☐	☐	☐	☐	☐	☐	☐	☐	☐	☐	☐	☐	☐	☐	☐	___
Basketball	☐	☐	☐	☐	☐	☐	☐	☐	☐	☐	☐	☐	☐	☐	☐	___
Fitness Center	☐	☐	☐	☐	☐	☐	☐	☐	☐	☐	☐	☐	☐	☐	☐	___
Rowing Machine	☐	☐	☐	☐	☐	☐	☐	☐	☐	☐	☐	☐	☐	☐	☐	___
Stair Master	☐	☐	☐	☐	☐	☐	☐	☐	☐	☐	☐	☐	☐	☐	☐	___
Stationary Bike	☐	☐	☐	☐	☐	☐	☐	☐	☐	☐	☐	☐	☐	☐	☐	___
Treadmill	☐	☐	☐	☐	☐	☐	☐	☐	☐	☐	☐	☐	☐	☐	☐	___
Weight Lifting	☐	☐	☐	☐	☐	☐	☐	☐	☐	☐	☐	☐	☐	☐	☐	___
_____	☐	☐	☐	☐	☐	☐	☐	☐	☐	☐	☐	☐	☐	☐	☐	___
_____	☐	☐	☐	☐	☐	☐	☐	☐	☐	☐	☐	☐	☐	☐	☐	___
_____	☐	☐	☐	☐	☐	☐	☐	☐	☐	☐	☐	☐	☐	☐	☐	___
_____	☐	☐	☐	☐	☐	☐	☐	☐	☐	☐	☐	☐	☐	☐	☐	___
Cycling	☐	☐	☐	☐	☐	☐	☐	☐	☐	☐	☐	☐	☐	☐	☐	___
Field Hockey	☐	☐	☐	☐	☐	☐	☐	☐	☐	☐	☐	☐	☐	☐	☐	___
Hiking	☐	☐	☐	☐	☐	☐	☐	☐	☐	☐	☐	☐	☐	☐	☐	___
Jogging/Running	☐	☐	☐	☐	☐	☐	☐	☐	☐	☐	☐	☐	☐	☐	☐	___
Soccer	☐	☐	☐	☐	☐	☐	☐	☐	☐	☐	☐	☐	☐	☐	☐	___
Softball	☐	☐	☐	☐	☐	☐	☐	☐	☐	☐	☐	☐	☐	☐	☐	___
Swimming	☐	☐	☐	☐	☐	☐	☐	☐	☐	☐	☐	☐	☐	☐	☐	___
Racket Sports	☐	☐	☐	☐	☐	☐	☐	☐	☐	☐	☐	☐	☐	☐	☐	___
Martial Arts	☐	☐	☐	☐	☐	☐	☐	☐	☐	☐	☐	☐	☐	☐	☐	___
_____	☐	☐	☐	☐	☐	☐	☐	☐	☐	☐	☐	☐	☐	☐	☐	___
_____	☐	☐	☐	☐	☐	☐	☐	☐	☐	☐	☐	☐	☐	☐	☐	___
_____	☐	☐	☐	☐	☐	☐	☐	☐	☐	☐	☐	☐	☐	☐	☐	___
_____	☐	☐	☐	☐	☐	☐	☐	☐	☐	☐	☐	☐	☐	☐	☐	___
				☐	☐	☐	☐	☐	☐	☐	☐	☐	☐	☐	☐	

Activity	Day 1	2	3	Minutes 0–10	10–20	20–30	30–40	40–50	50–60	Hours 1	2	3	4	5	6	7	8	kCal
Sleep	☐	☐	☐	☐	☐	☐	☐	☐	☐	☐	☐	☐	☐	☐	☐	☐	☐	___
Walking	☐	☐	☐	☐	☐	☐	☐	☐	☐	☐	☐	☐	☐	☐	☐	☐	☐	___
Resting	☐	☐	☐	☐	☐	☐	☐	☐	☐	☐	☐	☐	☐	☐	☐	☐	☐	___
Personal Hygiene	☐	☐	☐	☐	☐	☐	☐	☐	☐	☐	☐	☐	☐	☐	☐	☐	☐	___
Watch TV	☐	☐	☐	☐	☐	☐	☐	☐	☐	☐	☐	☐	☐	☐	☐	☐	☐	___
Attend Class	☐	☐	☐	☐	☐	☐	☐	☐	☐	☐	☐	☐	☐	☐	☐	☐	☐	
Homework	☐	☐	☐	☐	☐	☐	☐	☐	☐	☐	☐	☐	☐	☐	☐	☐	☐	
Computer	☐	☐	☐	☐	☐	☐	☐	☐	☐	☐	☐	☐	☐	☐	☐	☐	☐	
Eating	☐	☐	☐	☐	☐	☐	☐	☐	☐	☐	☐	☐	☐	☐	☐	☐	☐	
_____	☐	☐	☐	☐	☐	☐	☐	☐	☐	☐	☐	☐	☐	☐	☐	☐	☐	___
_____	☐	☐	☐	☐	☐	☐	☐	☐	☐	☐	☐	☐	☐	☐	☐	☐	☐	___
_____	☐	☐	☐	☐	☐	☐	☐	☐	☐	☐	☐	☐	☐	☐	☐	☐	☐	___
_____	☐	☐	☐	☐	☐	☐	☐	☐	☐	☐	☐	☐	☐	☐	☐	☐	☐	___
_____	☐	☐	☐	☐	☐	☐	☐	☐	☐	☐	☐	☐	☐	☐	☐	☐	☐	___

Index

Page numbers in *italics* indicate figures. Page numbers ending in "t" indicate tables.

A

Abdomen, percentage fat, 636–642
Absolute oxygen consumption, 183
Absorption of food nutrients
    acid-base concentration, 98–101
    biology and chemistry, 91–101
    carbohydrate digestion and, 106–108
    condensation, *92*, 92–93
    dietary intake
        analyzing, 116
        assessing, 116
    digestive process, 106–112
    enzymes, 93–95, *94*
    gastrointestinal tract, 102–106
    glucose, *239*
    hydrolysis, 91–92, *92*
    intestinal fluid, *243*
    iron, 75
    lipid digestion and, 108–110, *109*
    minerals, 111, 111, *112*
    protein digestion and, 110
    vitamins, 110–111
    water, 111–112
    water-soluble vitamins, 110, 111
Acclimatization to heat, 305–306
    physiologic adjustments during, 306t
Acesulfame-K, 6t
Acid, 98–99
Acid-base concentration, 98–101
Acidosis, 15–16, 99
Acquired immunity, 217
Acromegaly, 330
ACSM. *See* American College of Sports
    Medicine (ACSM)
Activation energy, 93
Active site, 94
Active transport processes, 97–98
Activity log, three-day physical, 648–652
Acute gastroenteritis, 115
Addiction to exercise, 503–504
Adenosine diphosphate (ADP), 130
Adenosine monophosphate (AMP), 73
Adenosine 3′, 5′-cyclic monophosphate, 143
Adenosine triphosphate (ATP), 73, *138*
    body energy supply and, 130–131
    from energy transfer, *145*
    formation of, *131*
    phosphate bond energy and, *133*
    total energy for, 156t
Adequate intake (AI), 51
ADH. *See* Antidiuretic hormone (ADH)
Adipocytes, 143, 145
Adolescents, central body fat distribution, 419
ADP. *See* Adenosine diphosphate (ADP)
Adults
    annual food intake, 451
    hyperlipidemia in, 26–27
    obesity in, 457

Advertising, food, 258–259, 263
Aerobic, 125, 163
    anaerobic *vs.*, 138
Aerobic Center Longitudinal Study, 206
Aerobic glycolysis, 140
Aerobic training, fat-burning adaptations with,
    163
Age, of male athletes, 427t
Aging
    creatine supplementation and, 374
    energy output and, 461, *462*
    rehydration and, 301
AHA. *See* American Heart Association
    (AHA)
AI. *See* Adequate intake (AI)
Alanine
    amino acid, structure of, *34*
    glucose cycle, 40, *41*
Alanine-glucose cycle, 40, *40*
Albuterol, 329–330
Alcohol
    benefit of, 347
    CAGE questionnaire to screen abuse of,
        346
    effect on athletic performance,
        343–344
    fluid replacement and, 344–347
    guidelines for use of, 346
    intake of, 346
    metabolism and use, 345–346
    use among athletes, 343
Alcoholic beverages, nutritive values for,
    552–553
Aldosterone, 78, 220, 295
Alkalosis, 99
Alternative sweeteners, 6t
AMA. *See* American Medical Association
    (AMA)
Ambient temperature, 419–421
    heat loss at, 294
Amenorrhea, exercise-related, 72
American Academy of Eating Disorders, 404
American Cancer Society, 28, *397*
American College of Sports Medicine (ACSM),
    196, 324, 327, 347, 479
    WB-GT recommendations, 307
American Diabetes Association, 7, 258
American diet, 6
American Dietetic Association, 196
American football players, 433–434, 438
American ginseng, 319t
American Heart Association (AHA)
    dietary guidelines, 201
    recommendations, 201–202
    recommendations and classifications for
        cholesterol and HDL-LDL and
        triacylglycerol, 29t
American Medical Association (AMA), 479
American Psychiatric Association, 492

Americans
    eating habits of, 271, 273
    portion size distortion, 274–275
    supersizing of food, 275–276
Amino acid alanine, chemical structure of, *34*
Amino acid homocysteine, *57*
Amino acids, 33, *63*
    essential, 33
    fate after nitrogen removal, 38–39
    nonessential, 33
    simple, 210
Amino acid supplements, 365–368
AMP. *See* Adenosine monophosphate (AMP)
Amphetamines, 335–336
    athletic performance and use of, 336
    dangers of, 336
Amylopectin, 6
Amylose, 6
Anabolic, defined, 93
Anabolic-androgenic steroids, 327, *328*
Anabolic phase, 176
Anabolic steroids, 323–328
    American College of Sports Medicine
        stand on, 327
    side effects and medical risks of, 328t
Anabolism, 38, *63*
Anaerobic, 125
    vs. aerobic, 138
Anaerobic energy metabolism, *156*
Anaerobic glycolysis, 140
Anaerobic macronutrient, 139–141
Anaerobic sources, 155–156
Anal (two sphincters), 104t
Androstenedione, 334–335, *335*
Anemia
    functional, 77
    iron deficiency, 74
    sports, 76
Animal polysaccharides, 10–11
    glycogen dynamics, 10–11
Animal protein, 471t
Anorexia athletica, 502, 502t
Anorexia nervosa, 492–493, 507–509
    body compositions, 509t
    common signs and symptoms of, 510t
    DSM-IV clinical criteria for, 508t
    physical and medical consequences of,
        509
    physical consequences of, 508
Anthropometric equations, 479t
Anthropometric measurements, 430t
Anticortisol compounds, 349–350
Antidepressants, for treating eating disorders,
    517
Antidiuretic hormone (ADH), 295
Antioxidants, 214–215, 261
    and disease protection, 53–56
Anxiolytic effect, 343
Arby's, nutritive values for, 555–559